T0294952

The **Psyche** in **Chinese Medicine**

Commissioning Editor: ***Mary Law/Karen Morley***
Development Editors: ***Kerry McGechie/Veronika Watkins***
Project Manager: ***Emma Riley***
Designer: ***Charles Gray***
Illustration Manager: ***Merlyn Harvey***

The **Psyche** in Chinese Medicine

Treatment of Emotional and Mental Disharmonies with Acupuncture and Chinese Herbs

Giovanni Maciocia CAc (Nanjing)

Acupuncturist and Medical Herbalist, UK;
Visiting Associate Professor at the Nanjing University of Traditional Chinese Medicine, Nanjing, People's Republic of China

Foreword by
Peter Deadman

Illustrators:
Michael Courtney, Richard Morris and Jonathan Haste

CHURCHILL LIVINGSTONE

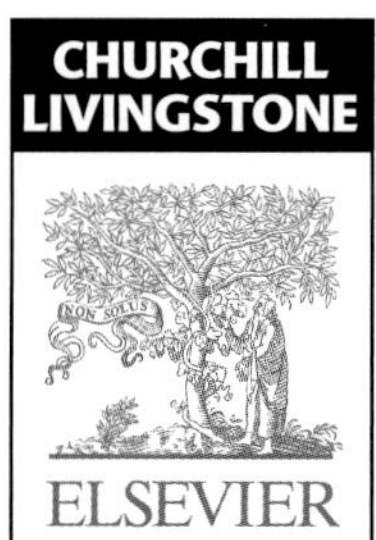

Edinburgh • London • New York • Oxford • Philadelphia • St Louis • Sydney • Toronto • 2009

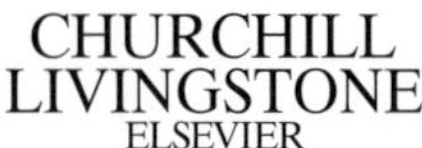

ISBN: 978-0-7020-2988-2

British Library Cataloguing in Publication Data
A catalogue record for this book is available from the British Library

Library of Congress Cataloging in Publication Data
A catalog record for this book is available from the Library of Congress

Notice

Knowledge and best practice in this field are constantly changing. As new research and experience broaden our knowledge, changes in practice, treatment and drug therapy may become necessary or appropriate. Readers are advised to check the most current information provided (i) on procedures featured or (ii) by the manufacturer of each product to be administered, to verify the recommended dose or formula, the method and duration of administration, and contraindications. It is the responsibility of the practitioner, relying on their own experience and knowledge of the patient, to make diagnoses, to determine dosages and the best treatment for each individual patient, and to take all appropriate safety precautions. To the fullest extent of the law, neither the Publisher nor the Author assumes any liability for any injury and/or damage to persons or property arising out of or related to any use of the material contained in this book.

The Publisher

Printed in India

Last digit is the print number: 19 18 17 16 15

CONTENTS

Foreword *xiii*
Preface *xv*
Acknowledgements *xxi*
Note on the translation of Chinese medical terms *xxiii*

CHAPTER 1

THE PSYCHE IN CHINESE MEDICINE *1*

THE SPIRIT AND SOUL IN WESTERN PHILOSOPHY ***1***
The spirit ***1***
The soul ***3***

THE SPIRIT, SOUL AND MIND IN CHINESE MEDICINE ***3***
Terminology ***3***
The Spirit (*Shen*) in Chinese medicine ***4***
The concept of "body" in China ***6***
The Soul in Chinese medicine ***6***
The Mind (*Shen*) in Chinese medicine ***8***
Meaning of the word *shen* in Chinese medicine ***9***
Mental illness in ancient Chinese medicine ***10***

CHAPTER 2

THE NATURE OF THE MIND (*SHEN*) IN CHINESE MEDICINE *15*

THE NATURE OF THE MIND (*SHEN*) IN CHINESE MEDICINE ***15***
Terminology ***15***
Chinese characters for *Shen* ***16***
Nature of the Mind and of the "Three Treasures" ***16***
Functions of the Mind ***18***
The Mind and the senses ***20***
Coordinating and integrating function of the Mind ***21***

"MIND" VERSUS "SPIRIT" AS A TRANSLATION OF *SHEN* ***22***

CLINICAL APPLICATION ***23***

CHAPTER 3

THE ETHEREAL SOUL (*HUN*) *25*

SLEEP AND DREAMING ***29***

THE MOVEMENT OF THE ETHEREAL SOUL AND MENTAL ACTIVITIES ***31***

BALANCE OF EMOTIONS ***32***

EYES AND SIGHT ***34***

COURAGE ***34***

PLANNING ***35***

RELATIONSHIP WITH THE MIND ***36***
Relationship between the Ethereal Soul and the Mind ***36***
Mild "manic" behavior in clinical practice ***38***
Examples of the nature of the Ethereal Soul ***38***
The Ethereal Soul and modern diseases ***40***
The Ethereal Soul and Buddhist psychology ***40***
The Ethereal Soul and Jungian psychology ***41***
The movement of the Ethereal Soul and expansion/contraction ***42***
Clinical patterns of pathologies of the Ethereal Soul ***43***

CLINICAL APPLICATION ***44***
Acupuncture ***44***
Herbal therapy ***45***

CHAPTER 4

THE CORPOREAL SOUL (*PO*) *47*

THE CORPOREAL SOUL AND THE ESSENCE (*JING*) ***48***

INFANCY ***51***

SENSES ***51***

PHYSIOLOGICAL ACTIVITY ***52***

EMOTIONS ***53***

BREATHING ***54***

THE CORPOREAL SOUL AND INDIVIDUAL LIFE ***54***

THE CORPOREAL SOUL AND THE *GUI* ***54***

THE CORPOREAL SOUL AND THE ANUS ***55***

RELATIONSHIP BETWEEN CORPOREAL SOUL AND ETHEREAL SOUL ***55***

CLINICAL APPLICATION ***60***
Contraction of the Corporeal Soul ***60***
Expansion of the Corporeal Soul ***60***

CHAPTER 5
THE INTELLECT (*YI*) *63*

MEMORY ***63***

GENERATION OF IDEAS ***64***

STUDYING AND CONCENTRATING ***64***

FOCUSING ***65***

RELATIONSHIP WITH THE MIND (*SHEN*) ***65***

CLINICAL APPLICATION ***65***

CHAPTER 6
THE WILL-POWER (*ZHI*) *67*

ZHI AS MEMORY ***67***

ZHI AS WILL-POWER ***68***

CLINICAL APPLICATION ***69***

CHAPTER 7
THE *GUI* 71

GUI AS SPIRIT, GHOST ***71***

GUI AS MOVEMENT OF THE ETHEREAL SOUL AND CORPOREAL SOUL ***75***

GUI AS A CENTRIPETAL, SEPARATING, FRAGMENTING FORCE ***76***

GUI IN RELATION TO THE CORPOREAL SOUL ***77***

GUI AS A SYMBOL OF CONTRACTION, COUNTERPOLE OF *SHEN* (EXPANSION) ***79***

GUI AS DARK FORCE OF THE PSYCHE AND ITS CONNECTION WITH THE JUNGIAN SHADOW ***83***

ACUPUNCTURE POINTS WITH "*GUI*" IN THEIR NAMES ***84***

CHAPTER 8
THE 12 INTERNAL ORGANS AND THE PSYCHE *87*

HEART ***90***

LUNGS ***93***

LIVER ***94***

SPLEEN ***96***

KIDNEYS ***97***

PERICARDIUM ***100***

SMALL INTESTINE ***102***

LARGE INTESTINE ***104***

GALL-BLADDER ***104***

STOMACH ***107***

BLADDER ***110***

TRIPLE BURNER ***110***

CHAPTER 9
THE EMOTIONS *115*

THE EMOTIONS ***122***
Anger ***122***
Joy ***126***
Worry ***127***
Pensiveness ***129***
Sadness and grief ***131***
Fear ***133***
Shock ***134***
Love ***135***
Craving ***136***
Guilt ***138***
Shame ***140***

THE PATHOLOGY OF QI AND MINISTER FIRE IN EMOTIONAL PROBLEMS ***143***
The effect of emotions on the body's Qi ***143***
The pathology of the Minister Fire in emotional problems ***148***

THE TRIUNE BRAIN AND CHINESE MEDICINE ***155***
The triune brain, the Mind, Ethereal Soul and Corporeal Soul ***157***

CHAPTER 10
ETIOLOGY OF MENTAL-EMOTIONAL PROBLEMS *161*

CONSTITUTION ***162***
Wood type ***162***
Fire type ***163***
Earth type ***164***
Metal type ***164***
Water type ***165***

DIET ***166***
Excessive consumption of hot-energy foods ***166***
Excessive consumption of Damp-producing foods ***166***
Excessive consumption of cold-energy foods ***167***
Irregular eating habits ***167***
Insufficient eating ***167***

OVERWORK ***167***

EXCESSIVE SEXUAL ACTIVITY ***167***

DRUGS ***167***
Cannabis ***168***
Cocaine ***168***

Ecstasy *169*

PREVENTION OF MENTAL-EMOTIONAL PROBLEMS *169*

CHAPTER 11

DIAGNOSIS OF MENTAL-EMOTIONAL PROBLEMS *171*

COMPLEXION *171*

EYES *173*

PULSE *174*
The pulse and the emotions *174*
The Heart pulse *175*
General pulse qualities and the emotions *176*

TONGUE *177*
Red tip *177*
Heart crack *178*
Sides of the tongue *179*
Body shape *179*
Combined Stomach and Heart crack *180*

CHAPTER 12

PATTERNS IN MENTAL-EMOTIONAL PROBLEMS AND THEIR TREATMENT WITH HERBAL MEDICINE AND ACUPUNCTURE *183*

THE EFFECT OF MENTAL-EMOTIONAL PROBLEMS ON QI, BLOOD, YIN AND PATHOGENIC FACTORS *183*
Effects on Qi *184*
Effects on Blood *185*
Effects on Yin *188*
Pathogenic factors in mental-emotional problems *190*

MIND OBSTRUCTED, UNSETTLED, WEAKENED *196*
Mind Obstructed *196*
Mind Unsettled *196*
Mind Weakened *197*
Herbal treatment methods for Mind Obstructed, Unsettled or Weakened *198*
Treatment principles *199*

MIND OBSTRUCTED *200*
Qi stagnation *200*
Blood stasis *205*
Phlegm misting the Mind *208*

MIND UNSETTLED *212*
Blood deficiency *212*
Yin deficiency *213*
Yin deficiency with Empty Heat *217*
Qi stagnation *221*
Blood stasis *221*
Fire *221*
Phlegm-Fire *226*

MIND WEAKENED *228*
Qi and Blood deficiency *228*
Yang deficiency *232*
Blood deficiency *234*
Yin deficiency *234*

CHAPTER 13

ACUPUNCTURE IN THE TREATMENT OF MENTAL-EMOTIONAL PROBLEMS *243*

LUNG CHANNEL *245*
LU-3 Tianfu *245*
LU-7 Lieque *246*
LU-10 Yuji *246*

LARGE INTESTINE CHANNEL *247*
L.I.-4 Hegu *247*
L.I.-5 Yangxi *247*
L.I.-7 Wenliu *247*

STOMACH CHANNEL *248*
ST-25 Tianshu *248*
ST-40 Fenglong *249*
ST-41 Jiexi *249*
ST-42 Chongyang *249*
ST-45 Lidui *249*

SPLEEN CHANNEL *250*
SP-1 Yinbai *250*
SP-3 Taibai *250*
SP-4 Gongsun *251*
SP-5 Shangqiu *251*
SP-6 Sanyinjiao *251*

HEART CHANNEL *252*
HE-3 Shaohai *252*
HE-4 Lingdao *252*
HE-5 Tongli *252*
HE-7 Shenmen *253*
HE-8 Shaofu *253*
HE-9 Shaochong *253*

SMALL INTESTINE CHANNEL *254*
S.I.-5 Yanggu *254*
S.I.-7 Zhizheng *255*
S.I.-16 Tianchuang *255*

BLADDER CHANNEL *255*
BL-10 Tianzhu *255*
BL-13 Feishu *256*
BL-15 Xinshu *256*
BL-23 Shenshu *257*
BL-42 Pohu *257*
BL-44 Shentang *258*
BL-47 Hunmen *258*
BL-49 Yishe *259*
BL-52 Zhishi *259*
BL-62 Shenmai *259*

KIDNEY CHANNEL *260*
KI-1 Yongquan *260*
KI-3 Taixi *261*
KI-4 Dazhong *261*
KI-6 Zhaohai *261*
KI-9 Zhubin *261*
KI-16 Huangshu *262*

PERICARDIUM CHANNEL *263*
P-3 Quze *264*
P-4 Ximen *264*
P-5 Jianshi *264*
P-6 Neiguan *264*
P-7 Daling *266*
P-8 Laogong *267*

TRIPLE BURNER CHANNEL *268*
T.B.-3 Zhongzhu *268*
T.B.-10 Tianjing *268*

GALL-BLADDER CHANNEL *268*
G.B.-9 Tianchong *268*
G.B.-12 Wangu *268*
G.B.-13 Benshen *268*
G.B.-15 Linqi *270*
G.B.-17 Zhengying *270*
G.B.-18 Chengling *270*
G.B.-19 Naokong *270*
G.B.-40 Qiuxu *270*
G.B.-44 Zuqiaoyin *270*

LIVER CHANNEL *271*
LIV-2 Xingjian *271*
LIV-3 Taichong *271*

DIRECTING VESSEL (*REN MAI*) *272*
Ren-4 Guanyuan *272*
Ren-8 Shenque *272*
Ren-12 Zhongwan *273*
Ren-14 Juque *273*
Ren-15 Jiuwei *275*

GOVERNING VESSEL (*DU MAI*) *276*
Du-4 Mingmen *276*
Du-10 Lingtai *277*
Du-11 Shendao *277*
Du-12 Shenzhu *277*
Du-14 Dazhui *278*
Du-16 Fengfu *278*
Du-17 Naohu *278*
Du-18 Qiangjian *278*
Du-19 Houding *278*
Du-20 Baihui *278*
Du-24 Shenting *278*

EXTRA POINTS *280*
Hunshe *280*
Yintang *280*

POINTS FOR MENTAL PROBLEMS FROM NANJING AFFILIATED HOSPITAL *281*

EXAMPLES OF POINT COMBINATIONS FOR MENTAL-EMOTIONAL PROBLEMS *281*

CHAPTER 14

EMOTIONS AND CONCEPT OF SELF IN WESTERN PHILOSOPHY *283*

ANCIENT THEORIES ON EMOTIONS *285*
Pythagoras *285*
Heraclitus *285*
Socrates *286*
Plato *286*
Aristotle *286*
Stoics *287*
Middle Ages and Christianity *288*
St Augustine *288*
Thomas Aquinas *288*
Descartes *290*
Thomas Willis *290*
Spinoza *291*
Hume *291*
Kant *291*

EARLY MODERN THEORIES ABOUT EMOTIONS *291*

THE JAMES–LANGE THEORY OF EMOTIONS *292*

MODERN THEORIES ABOUT EMOTIONS *294*
Sartre *295*
Solomon's theory of emotions *295*
Bockover's theory of emotions *297*
Damasio's theory of emotions *297*

FREUD, JUNG AND BOWLBY *299*
Freud *299*
Jung *300*
Bowlby *302*

MODERN NEUROPHYSIOLOGICAL VIEW ON EMOTIONS *303*
Neurophysiology of emotions *303*
The triune brain *306*

SUMMARY *309*

CHAPTER 15

THE INFLUENCE OF CONFUCIANISM ON THE CHINESE VIEW OF THE MIND AND SPIRIT *313*

CONFUCIANISM *315*
Confucius *315*
Tian (Heaven) *316*
Confucian ethics *317*
Confucian ethics, society and state *320*

NEO-CONFUCIANISM *323*
Human nature (*Xing*) *325*
Li (Principle) *326*

THE CONCEPT OF SELF IN WESTERN AND CHINESE PHILOSOPHY *327*

EMOTIONS IN NEO-CONFUCIANISM *332*

INFLUENCE OF NEO-CONFUCIANISM ON CHINESE MEDICINE *336*

CONCLUSIONS *339*

CHAPTER 16
DEPRESSION *341*

DEFINITION AND WESTERN MEDICINE'S VIEW ***342***
Major depressive syndrome ***343***

PATHOLOGY OF DEPRESSION IN CHINESE MEDICINE ***344***
Yu as stagnation ***344***
Yu as mental depression ***345***
Depression and the relationship between the Mind (*Shen*) and the Ethereal Soul (*Hun*) ***345***
The Will-Power (*Zhi*) of the Kidneys in Depression ***346***
Distinction between Depression in *Yu* Syndrome and in *Dian* Syndrome ***346***
Lilium Syndrome (*Bai He Bing*) ***347***
Agitation (*Zang Zao*) ***348***
Plum-Stone Syndrome (*Mei He Qi*) ***349***
Palpitations and Anxiety (*Xin Ji Zheng Chong*) ***350***
Liver-Qi deficiency ***351***
"Neurasthenia" and Depression ***353***
Elements of pathology of Depression ***353***

ETIOLOGY ***354***
Emotional stress ***354***
Constitutional traits ***355***
Irregular diet ***356***
Overwork ***356***

PATHOLOGY ***356***

IDENTIFICATION OF PATTERNS AND TREATMENT ***357***
Liver-Qi stagnation ***358***
Heart- and Lung-Qi stagnation ***361***
Stagnant Liver-Qi turning into Heat ***362***
Phlegm-Heat harassing the Mind ***364***
Blood stasis obstructing the Mind ***365***
Qi stagnation with Phlegm ***367***
Diaphragm Heat ***369***
Worry injuring the Mind ***370***
Heart and Spleen deficiency ***372***
Heart-Yang deficiency ***373***
Kidney- and Heart-Yin deficiency, Empty Heat blazing ***375***
Kidney-Yang deficiency ***376***

ACUPUNCTURE POINTS FOR DEPRESSION ***378***

HERBS FOR DEPRESSION ***386***

MODERN CHINESE LITERATURE ***389***

CLINICAL TRIALS ***392***

CASE HISTORIES ***399***

PATIENTS' STATISTICS ***407***

WESTERN DRUG TREATMENT ***407***
Introduction and pharmacology ***408***
Clinical use ***410***
Types of antidepressants ***410***
Combination of Chinese and Western medicine ***415***

CHAPTER 17
ANXIETY *417*

ANXIETY IN WESTERN MEDICINE ***417***

ANXIETY IN CHINESE MEDICINE ***418***
Chinese disease entities corresponding to anxiety ***419***
Rebellious Qi of the Penetrating Vessel (*Chong Mai*) ***419***
Palpitations in Chinese diagnosis ***422***
Difference between Mind Unsettled and Mind Obstructed in anxiety ***422***

ETIOLOGY ***422***
Emotional stress ***422***
Constitution ***423***
Irregular diet ***423***
Loss of blood ***423***
Overwork ***423***

PATHOLOGY AND TREATMENT PRINCIPLES ***423***
Heart ***424***
Lungs ***425***
Kidneys ***426***
Spleen ***427***
Liver ***427***

ACUPUNCTURE TREATMENT OF ANXIETY ***427***
Distal points according to channel ***427***
Head points ***428***

IDENTIFICATION OF PATTERNS AND TREATMENT ***430***
Heart and Gall-Bladder deficiency ***430***
Heart-Blood deficiency ***431***
Kidney- and Heart-Yin deficiency with Empty Heat ***432***
Heart-Yang deficiency ***433***
Lung- and Heart-Qi deficiency ***434***
Lung- and Heart-Qi stagnation ***435***
Lung- and Heart-Yin deficiency ***435***
Heart-Blood stasis ***436***
Phlegm-Heat harassing the Heart ***437***

MODERN CHINESE LITERATURE ***438***

CLINICAL TRIALS ***439***

CASE HISTORIES ***443***

CHAPTER 18
INSOMNIA *447*

ETIOLOGY ***450***
Emotional stress ***450***
Overwork ***450***
"Gall-Bladder timid" ***450***
Irregular diet ***450***
Childbirth ***451***
Residual Heat ***451***
Excessive sexual activity ***451***

PATHOLOGY ***451***

DIAGNOSIS ***454***

Sleep **454**
Dreams **454**
Sleeping positions **455**
Snoring **455**

IDENTIFICATION OF PATTERNS AND TREATMENT **456**
Liver-Fire blazing **456**
Heart-Fire blazing **457**
Phlegm-Heat harassing the Mind **459**
Heart-Qi stagnation **460**
Heart-Blood stasis **461**
Residual Heat in the diaphragm **462**
Retention of Food **464**
Liver-Qi stagnation **465**
Heart- and Spleen-Blood deficiency **466**
Heart-Yin deficiency **468**
Heart and Kidneys not harmonized **468**
Heart and Gall-Bladder deficiency **470**
Liver-Yin deficiency **471**
Liver- and Kidney-Yin deficiency **473**

MODERN CHINESE LITERATURE **475**

CLINICAL TRIALS **478**

PATIENTS' STATISTICS **484**

APPENDIX 1 EXCESSIVE DREAMING **484**

IDENTIFICATION OF PATTERNS AND TREATMENT **486**
Phlegm-Heat **486**
Liver-Fire **486**
Deficiency of Qi of Heart and Gall-Bladder **487**
Heart- and Lung-Qi deficiency **487**
Deficiency of Heart and Spleen **488**
Heart and Kidneys not harmonized **489**

APPENDIX 2 SOMNOLENCE **489**

IDENTIFICATION OF PATTERNS AND TREATMENT **489**
Dampness obstructing the Brain **489**
Phlegm misting the Brain **490**
Spleen deficiency **491**
Kidney-Yang deficiency (Deficiency of Sea of Marrow) **492**

APPENDIX 3 POOR MEMORY **493**

ETIOLOGY **493**
Worry and pensiveness **493**
Overwork and excessive sexual activity **493**
Childbirth **493**
Sadness **493**
"Recreational" drugs **493**

IDENTIFICATION OF PATTERNS AND TREATMENT **494**
Spleen deficiency **494**
Kidney-Essence deficiency **494**
Heart deficiency **495**

CHAPTER 19

BIPOLAR DISORDER (MANIC-DEPRESSION) 497

BIPOLAR DISORDER IN WESTERN MEDICINE **498**
Symptoms of bipolar disorder **498**
Diagnosis of bipolar disorder **500**
Course of bipolar disorder **501**
Treatment of bipolar disorder **501**
History **502**

BIPOLAR DISORDER IN CHINESE MEDICINE **503**
Historical development of *Dian Kuang* in Chinese medicine **503**
Correspondences and differences between bipolar disorder and *Dian Kuang* **504**
Pathology of *Dian Kuang* **506**

ETIOLOGY OF *DIAN KUANG* **508**
Emotional stress **508**
Diet **508**
Constitution **508**

PATHOLOGY AND TREATMENT PRINCIPLES OF *DIAN KUANG* **509**
Pathology of *Dian Kuang* **509**
Treatment principles for *Dian Kuang* **511**
How to adapt the patterns and treatment of *Dian Kuang* to the treatment of bipolar disorder **513**

ACUPUNCTURE TREATMENT **514**
Points that open the Mind's orifices **514**
Sun Si Miao's 13 ghost points **515**
The Pericardium channel in Manic-Depression **515**

IDENTIFICATION OF PATTERNS AND TREATMENT **516**
Dian **516**
Qi stagnation and Phlegm **516**
Heart and Spleen deficiency with Phlegm **518**
Qi deficiency with Phlegm **519**
Phlegm obstructing the Heart orifices **520**
Kuang **521**
Phlegm-Fire harassing upwards **521**
Fire in Bright Yang **524**
Gall Bladder- and Liver-Fire **524**
Fire injuring Yin with Phlegm **525**
Qi stagnation, Blood stasis, Phlegm **526**
Yin deficiency with Empty Heat **527**

MODERN CHINESE LITERATURE **528**

CLINICAL TRIALS **532**

CHAPTER 20

NIGHT TERRORS 535

ETIOLOGY **536**
Emotional stress **536**
Overwork **536**
Irregular diet **536**
Loss of blood during childbirth **536**

PATHOLOGY ***536***

IDENTIFICATION OF PATTERNS AND TREATMENT ***537***
Liver- and Heart-Fire ***537***
Phlegm-Heat harassing the Ethereal Soul and the Mind ***537***
Liver- and Heart-Blood Deficiency ***538***
Liver- and Heart-Yin Deficiency ***539***
Shock displacing the Mind ***540***

CHAPTER 21
ATTENTION DEFICIT DISORDER (ADD) AND ATTENTION DEFICIT HYPERACTIVITY DISORDER (ADHD) ***543***

ATTENTION DEFICIT DISORDER (ADD) AND ATTENTION DEFICIT HYPERACTIVITY DISORDER (ADHD) ***544***

ATTENTION DEFICIT DISORDER IN WESTERN MEDICINE ***544***

SYMPTOMS ***544***
Hyperactivity–impulsiveness ***544***
Inattention ***545***

POSSIBLE CAUSES OF ADHD AND ADD ***545***
Environmental agents ***545***
Brain injury ***545***
Food additives and sugar ***545***
Genetics ***545***

TREATMENT OF ADHD AND ADD ***546***

ATTENTION DEFICIT HYPERACTIVITY DISORDER IN ADULTS ***547***
Diagnosis ***547***
Treatment ***547***

ATTENTION DEFICIT DISORDER IN CHINESE MEDICINE ***548***

PATHOLOGY ***548***
The Mind (*Shen*) ***548***
The Ethereal Soul (*Hun*) ***548***
The Intellect (*Yi*) ***548***
Organ pathology ***549***
Phlegm ***549***

ETIOLOGY ***550***
Heredity ***550***
Diet ***550***
Emotional stress ***550***
Pregnancy and labor ***551***

ACUPUNCTURE TREATMENT ***551***
Heart ***551***
Spleen ***551***
Liver ***552***
Governing Vessel ***552***
Other points ***553***
The experience of teachers from the Nanjing University of Traditional Chinese Medicine ***554***

IDENTIFICATION OF PATTERNS AND TREATMENT ***555***
Deficiency of Heart- and Spleen-Blood ***555***
Heart- and Kidney-Yin deficiency ***556***
Kidney- and Liver-Yin deficiency with Liver-Yang rising ***556***
Heart- and Spleen-Qi deficiency ***557***
Liver- and Heart-Fire ***557***
Heart and Spleen deficiency with Phlegm ***558***

WESTERN MEDICINE CLINICAL TRIALS ***559***

CHINESE MEDICINE CLINICAL TRIALS ***561***

CHAPTER 22
EPILOGUE: THE ROLE OF CHINESE MEDICINE IN DISORDERS OF THE PSYCHE ***565***

APPENDIX 1 HERBAL PRESCRIPTIONS ***571***

APPENDIX 2 SUGGESTED SUBSTITUTIONS OF CHINESE HERBS ***597***

APPENDIX 3 THE CLASSICS OF CHINESE MEDICINE ***599***

APPENDIX 4 TERMINOLOGY OF TREATMENT PRINCIPLES ***605***

ENGLISH–PINYIN GLOSSARY OF CHINESE TERMS ***607***

PINYIN–ENGLISH GLOSSARY OF CHINESE TERMS ***615***

CHRONOLOGY OF CHINESE DYNASTIES ***623***

COMPARATIVE TIMELINE OF WESTERN AND CHINESE PHILOSOPHERS AND DOCTORS ***625***

BIBLIOGRAPHY ***627***

INDEX ***633***

FOREWORD

For many Westerners encountering Chinese medicine, one of the great attractions is that it appears to address the whole person, seamlessly integrating body, mind and spirit within its understanding of human health and disease. This is considered to be in stark contrast to a Western view which, for various reasons, has tended to separate the material from the emotional and spiritual, especially since the 17th century. Even as far back as the 4th century BCE, Plato was complaining, "The greatest mistake in the treatment of diseases is that there are physicians for the body and physicians for the soul, although the two cannot be separated."

So strong has been the attraction of this integrated Chinese perspective that it has been the primary factor motivating many individuals to study and practice Chinese medicine. And even more, it has led to schools of thought within the new Western traditions of Chinese medicine which consider addressing the emotional and even spiritual dimensions of a patient to be a pre-requisite of healing, perhaps in the process according more obviously physical concerns a lesser significance.

There may indeed be some historical basis for this emphasis. Certainly in the teachings of "yang sheng fa", the art of nourishing life, we find that training and regulating the mind and emotions is the starting point of health-promoting behavior.

This is spelled out in the Yellow Emperor's Inner Classic: "If one is calm, peaceful, empty, without desire, then true Qi follows. If essence and spirit are protected inside, from where can illness come? If will is at rest and there are few desires, the heart is in peace and there is no fear." (Huang Di Nei Jing Su Wen, chapter 1), and even earlier in the Nei Ye (Inward Training), 4th century BCE, "Those who keep their minds unimpaired within, Externally keep their bodies unimpaired...."

This is reflected, also, in the Yellow Emperor's Inner Classic theory of the heart as Emperor of the body. The heart houses the Shen and if the heart is strong and in harmony, then the other organs of the body – performing their different "official" roles – will naturally follow, in the same way that a wise Emperor was thought to ensure the well-being of the Empire.

Understanding the historical discussion of the Shen and its relationship to health and well-being is not, however, straightforward. As Giovanni Maciocia emphasizes throughout this book, when attempting to absorb the teachings and medical practices of a culture so distant in both geography and time, the first requisite is to understand what is actually being said when terms such as mind, will and spirit are used. Without this understanding, we risk imposing our own cultural and personal prejudices on what we read, study and teach.

What is meant, however, by classical discussions of the *Shen*, is only one of the many important questions this vital subject demands that we consider. To what degree can treatment, administered by another, help resolve our emotional or spiritual distress; to what degree do we consider that the content of the emotional landscape is the true measure of an individual; how should we try to manage (and teach our patients to manage) emotions; to what degree should we fully embrace and inhabit them and to what degree should we try to train and restrain them? These are all questions that relate both to our own personal development and to our ideas about our role as practitioners.

If we look at some of the traditional Chinese teachings on regulating the mind and emotions, we find the following advice from the great Daoist 7th century doctor Sun Si Miao:

"To live long, people should take care not to worry too much, not to get too angry, not to get too sad, not to get too frightened, not to do too much, talk too much or laugh too much. One should not have too many desires nor face numerous upsetting conditions. All these are harmful to health."

How can we reconcile this seemingly arid denial of the emotions with our own belief in the health-giving richness of exploring, freeing and expressing these emotions?

In the culture we find ourselves in, reconciling these two perspectives can be a challenge – both in our work with patients and in our own lives. It may be that – as so often – it is the harmonization of these seeming opposites that offers a solution. Quietening the mind and dwelling in the present allows us to connect with what is universal and withdraw from the peripheral, debilitating noise of what is emotionally unnecessary. At the same time, cultivating this deeper awareness allows us to feel and explore the truer currents of our emotional life. Perhaps in that way we can hold a vision of emotional health that is neither repressive nor self-indulgent.

In this essential work, Giovanni Maciocia has addressed all these important questions, whether in his detailed exploration of classical Chinese and classical and modern Western perspectives, his thorough exposition of the most common and distressing manifestations of emotional disorder, and his personal reflections on his own extensive clinical experience. This book will add significantly to the body of work that, through unremitting authorship over decades, Giovanni Maciocia has been compiling on the theory and practice of this human treasure, Chinese medicine.

Peter Deadman, 2009

PREFACE

The seeds for the writing of this book were planted 35 years ago when I first started practicing acupuncture. I can say that not a day went by in my practice that I did not question the nature of *Shen* and its meaning in the context of modern Western patients. After practicing for only a few weeks, it became obvious to me that very many patients presented with emotional suffering which was either at the root of their medical problem or a contributory factor to it.

I also started noticing straight away that acupuncture had a profound influence on the emotional and mental state of my patients, alleviating depression and anxiety even when the patient may have come simply to have a shoulder-joint problem fixed. I came to experience for myself the "unity of body and mind" that my teachers talked about.

In the past 10 years or so, I have been totally absorbed in the study of the *Shen* in Chinese medicine seen in its historical, social and philosophical contexts and, as a result, my research developed along four strands:

1. The study of Confucian philosophy
2. A research into the influence of Confucian philosophy on Chinese medicine and particularly on its view of the *Shen* and emotions
3. A research on the emotions in Western philosophy
4. An analysis of the differences between the concept of Self in the West and in China.

I have been absorbed by the above studies because I have come to realize that Confucianism had a much bigger influence on Chinese medicine than we think. In my opinion, we tend to overemphasize the influence of Daoism on Chinese medicine and overlook that of Confucianism. One simple reason why the influence of Daoism on Chinese medicine is overemphasized is probably because whenever we read the word "*Dao*" in Chinese texts, we assume it reflects the Daoist philosophy. However, the Confucians also constantly refer to the *Dao*. This is discussed in Chapter 15.

In particular, I believe that the concept of Self in Chinese medicine and its view of emotions is Confucian. These ideas are discussed in Chapters 14 and 15 which the reader is urged to read (although they can be read quite separately from the other chapters and not necessarily in the order in which they appear). I do realize that these two chapters do not make "light reading" but I do urge the reader to read them carefully as the ideas expounded therein permeate the whole book.

When adapting Chinese medicine to Western patients in the emotional and mental field, we should be aware of such differences in the concept of Self and in the view of emotions between the West and China.

The Self as an individual, autonomous, inward-looking self, center of our emotional life simply does not exist as a concept in Confucianism: under the Confucian influence, the Chinese self is socially determined. As Fingarette says:[1]

I must emphasize that my point is not that Confucius words are intended to exclude reference to the inner psyche. He could have done this if he had such a basic metaphor in mind, had seen its plausibility, but on reflection, had decided to reject it. But this is not what I am arguing here. My thesis is that the entire notion never entered his head. The metaphor of an inner psychic life, in all its ramifications so familiar to us, simply is not present in the Analects, not even as a rejected possibility. Hence when I say that in the above passages using Yu *(the opposite of* Ren *indicating anxiety, worry, unhappiness) there is no reference to the inner, subjective states. I do not mean that these passages clearly and explicitly exclude such elaboration, but that they make no use of it and do not require it for intelligibility or validity.*

The Self as an individual, autonomous, inward-looking self, center of our emotional life, is the result of a 2500-year evolution of thought in Western philosophy, starting from ancient Greece down to Freud and Jung: the journey from "soul" to "self" in Western civilization was a long one, and one that did not take place in China.

The Chinese (Confucian) view of the Self as socially constructed is evident from the character for *ren*, the Confucian quality that is sometimes erroneously translated as "compassion" or "benevolence"; this character shows a "person" and the number "two" (see Figures 15.2, 15.4 and 15.5 in Chapter 15). Ames says:[2]

This etymological analysis underscores the Confucian assumption that one cannot become a person by oneself – we are, from our inchoate beginnings, irreducibly social. Fingarette has stated the matter concisely: 'For Confucius, unless there are at least two human beings, there can be no human being'.

Ames therefore clearly thinks that *ren* is not a psychological disposition of an individual self, a concept which simply does not exist in Confucian philosophy. Fingarette states very clearly:[3]

Ren *seems to emphasize the individual, the subjective: it seems in short a psychological notion. The problem of interpreting* ren *thus becomes particularly acute if one thinks, as I do, that it is of the essence of the Analects that the thought expressed in it is not based on psychological notions. And, indeed, one of the chief results of the present analysis of* ren *will be to reveal how Confucius could handle in a non-psychological way basic issues which we in the West naturally cast in psychological terms.*

The implication of the above passages is profound: it means that the concept of an individual self as an autonomous psychological center of consciousness and whose emotional life is influenced by the complex of past experiences of such an individual, autonomous self, simply did not exist in Confucian philosophy and, by extension, in Chinese medicine. The Chinese self is a social construct and the result of family and social relationships.

This means that the modern Western view of an individual psychological self whose emotional life is affected deeply by our childhood experiences is absent in Chinese medicine. For example, Chinese medicine considers that anger makes Qi rise and the correct treatment therefore consists of making Qi descend but it does not delve into the person's psyche to probe whether the anger may be due to a projection that has its roots in sibling relationships (for example) or whether it may be due to a thwarted manifestation of guilt.

To give another example, I find that anger is often a manifestation of a shadow projection. When we see in others traits that make us angry, it often (although not always) indicates that we are projecting our shadow onto the other person and that their traits that make us angry are traits of our own shadow. Chinese medicine had no such psychological insights precisely because such insights require a concept of an inner-life, autonomous, individual self that Chinese culture does not have.

That might also explain the omission of many emotions from the list usually presented in Chinese medicine. For example, there is no envy, pride or guilt. One explanation of this omission is that these three emotions require a concept of self (we are proud of our self, we feel guilty about our self) that is different in Chinese medicine and culture.

I have personally a deep interest in Jungian psychology and always try to see emotional suffering of a patient in the light of their projections, complexes, relationship with their *animus/anima* and shadow projection. Such a view gives me a perspective of a patient's psyche and emotions that I believe Chinese medicine simply does not have. Chinese medicine correctly identifies the emotion involved in a patient's suffering but I have never seen in a Chinese book (modern or ancient) any mention that such an emotion may be due to that person's mother being cold and undemonstrative in her affection (for example).

I believe that real healing from emotional suffering can take place only when the self is analyzed deeply with a conscious (and extremely difficult) effort of the patient. Of course, that is not to say that every patient should undergo psychotherapy as psychological problems occur with different depths and not all require deep psychotherapy. Moreover, Chinese medicine *always* has a positive role to play in alleviating emotional suffering. It creates a space where healing can take place, whether the patient delves into his/her psyche or not.

Chinese medicine alleviates emotional suffering in many different ways and I personally feel we should not adhere rigidly to a scheme. If the patient is willing to delve deeply into his/her psyche in order to really get to the root of their suffering, then Chinese medicine provides a wonderful complement to this work. I believe it can also greatly shorten the course of therapy necessary.

An interesting passage by Xu Chun Fu (1570) discusses the combination of herbal treatment by a doctor with incantations by a shaman. He said that a pre-existing weakness in the person's Qi made an attack by an evil spirit possible and he advocated combining herbal therapy with incantation in a very interesting passage:[4]

If these two methods of treatment are combined [herbal therapy and incantation], inner and outer are forged into a whole producing a prompt cure of the illness. Anyone who engages an exorcist and avoids the application of drugs will be unable to eliminate his illness, for a principle is lacking that could bring about a cure. He who takes only drugs and does not call upon an exorcist to drive out existing doubts, will be cured, but relief will be achieved slowly. Consequently the inner and outer must be treated together; only in this way is rapid success possible.

The classification of "inner" and "outer" methods of treatment (herbal drugs and exorcisms, respectively) is interesting and his advocating a combination of these two methods is significant: it is tempting to substitute "psychotherapist" for "exorcist" and infer that Xu Chun Fu advocated combining a physical therapy such as herbal medicine with psychotherapy. It is also interesting to note the difference in outcome when each therapy is used: if one goes only to an exorcist he or she "*will be unable to eliminate the illness*", whereas if one goes to a herbalist, he or she "*will be cured*" (albeit more slowly).

If the patient is not prepared to undergo psychotherapy, Chinese medicine helps greatly by alleviating emotional suffering. It also creates a space where Qi is flowing, the Mind (*Shen*) and Ethereal Soul (*Hun*) are more coordinated in their activities, the Corporeal Soul (*Po*) is animating the body better and the Will-Power (*Zhi*) is strong.

I also noticed another phenomenon when treating patients with mental-emotional problems. The treatment seems to make people more aware and more receptive to emotional work spontaneously. The treatment modulates the relationship between the Mind and the Ethereal Soul, relieving depression and anxiety; however, beyond the mere relief of emotional suffering, the treatment seems to nourish the Mind and regulate the Ethereal Soul so that the individual is more open and receptive. For example, I have noticed several times that, after a series of treatments, a patient may take up an art form that they have neglected for years, for example playing an instrument or painting.

The very way Chinese medicine sees emotions as forces that disrupt the proper direction of movement of Qi ("anger makes Qi rise, fear makes Qi descend, etc.") reflects, in my opinion, the absence of an individual, psychological self in Confucian philosophy. In other words, anger makes Qi rise, independently from a self: it is an objective force that disrupts the movement of Qi and the cognitive part of the Mind plays no role in it. The rising of Qi from anger generates a picture of disharmony that is at once physical (headaches, dizziness) and emotional (irritability, outbursts of anger) and it does not really even require the concept of an individual self as the center of consciousness.

In my opinion, the way in which Chinese medicine sees emotions is Confucian: they are bodily and psychic forces that cloud reason and obscure our human nature. As we know from Western views on emotions, these are far more than that: to some, they are an essential way in which our psyche works and what gives meaning to our life, from both an existential and a purely neurological point of view. As discussed in Chapter 14, the development of the higher cortex also depends partly on the limbic system.

One particular feature of the book is the space dedicated to the relationship between the Mind (*Shen*) and Ethereal Soul (*Hun*). Over the years of dealing with mental-emotional problems, I have come to attach great importance to the role of the Ethereal Soul and its relationship with the Mind. For example, I think that every case of depression is characterized by a deficient movement of the Ethereal Soul (and "manic behavior" by an excessive movement of the Ethereal Soul).

More and more I see the relationship between the Mind and Ethereal Soul as a mirror of that between the cortex and the limbic system (although the Mind cannot be reduced simply to the cortex or the Ethereal Soul to the limbic system). In particular, the prefrontal cortex seems to be the arena of the interplay between the Mind and the Ethereal Soul.

The prefrontal cortex (located just behind the forehead) is responsible for the executive functions, which include mediating conflicting thoughts, making choices between right and wrong or good and bad, predicting future events, and governing social control – such as suppressing emotional or sexual urges. The basic activity of this brain region is considered to be orchestration of thoughts and actions in accordance with internal goals.

These functions depend very much on the relationship between the Mind and the Ethereal Soul and, especially, on the normal control and integration exercised by the Mind towards the Ethereal Soul.

In my opinion, a disturbance of the relationship between Mind and Ethereal Soul is implicated in modern diseases such as autism (in which the movement of the Ethereal Soul is insufficient) or attention deficit hyperactivity disorder (in which the movement of the Ethereal Soul is excessive and the Mind's control and integration of the Ethereal Soul is insufficient).

After researching extensively on the emotions in Western philosophy and modern neurophysiology, and on the influence of Neo-Confucianism on Chinese medicine, I have come to the (perhaps controversial) conclusion that the "emotions" we talk about in the West are simply not the emotions of Chinese medicine.

As discussed in Chapter 14, emotions are, on the one hand, what gives meaning to our life from an existential, spiritual point of view; on the other hand, in a modern neurophysiological sense, they are an essential part to the functioning of the cortex and our cognitive faculties. Emotions assist reasoning.[5] This is a far cry from the Chinese view of emotions as factors that "cloud" the Mind and obscure our human nature: Sartre and Nietzsche for a start would say that emotions *are* our human nature.

It could be argued that it is emotions, not reason, that distinguishes us as human beings. Far from being factors that make us lose our human nature (as the Neo-Confucianists say), emotions *are* our human nature. For better or for worse, emotions make us "human". We can be driven not only by hatred but also by deep love, empathy and compassion which define us as human beings.

I have come to the conclusion that the "emotions" as considered in Chinese medicine are merely *pathologies of Qi*: anger *is* the arousal of Qi with its psychological and (most of all) physical manifestations. They are pathologies of Qi that are disengaged from the self because the Confucian self is not the individualized, inward-looking, autonomous self of Western culture.

Another momentous consequence of the different views of the self in China and the West is that Chinese medicine totally lacks a view of the self as a psychological center formed from birth, through our childhood experiences and adult life with all its unconscious material, projections, complexes and defences.

That is *not* to say that Chinese medicine cannot play a major role in the interpretation and treatment of deep disturbances of the self: indeed it can. But this work will require the painstaking effort, research and clinical enquiry of *generations* of Chinese medicine practitioners. I also believe that, due to the different concepts of the self in China and in the West, most of this work will have to be carried out by Western practitioners. But for this process to happen, we need to be conscious of the Confucian influence on Chinese medicine, take what applies to us and discard what does not, and abandon an unrealistic view of Chinese medicine.

By "unrealistic" view of Chinese medicine, I mean three things. First, a somewhat nebulous view of Qi as the basis of all pathology and treatment. Every mental-emotional disharmony can be diagnosed and treated as a disharmony of Qi: that does not mean that all will be cured.

Second, in the process of adapting Chinese medicine to the West, to Western patients and to our Western concept of self, we need to stay true to the roots of Chinese medicine and avoid attributing powers to Chinese medicine that (in my opinion) it cannot have.

Third, having said that we need to stay true to the roots of Chinese medicine, it is equally important that we see through the influence of Confucianism on Chinese medicine and therefore discard some of the views that do not apply to Westerners and a Western concept of self. I feel this is very important: if we persist in having a "romantic" view of Chinese medicine and take as gold nuggets everything we read in the classics without seeing its Confucian veneer, we will never accomplish the task of truly adapting Chinese medicine to the Western world.

Such work is already being done by many of our colleagues and, although ideas often diverge, together we can develop a Chinese medicine that is truly integrated in the West and that addresses the emotional, mental and spiritual issues of Westerners.

As in my previous books, contrary to all other English-language authors, I continue to translate *Shen* (of the Heart) as "Mind" rather than "Spirit", reserving the term "Spirit" for the complex of the five, i.e. Mind, Ethereal Soul, Corporeal Soul, Intellect and Will-Power. The reasons for this are explained in Chapters 1 and 2. Please note that I am not saying that the word "*shen*" cannot mean "spirit": of course it does. What I am saying is that, based on the functions of the *Shen* of the Heart, "Mind" is a better translation of it and call "Spirit" the total of the five. The problem is not merely semantic: if we call the *Shen* of the Heart "Spirit" we overlook the role of the Ethereal Soul, Corporeal Soul and Will-Power in mental, emotional and spiritual problems.

To see this from a Jungian perspective, we can say that the *Shen* of the Heart is the ego while the total of the five (and especially Mind and Ethereal Soul together) is the Self.

Interestingly, in mental illness the *Shen* of the Heart is obstructed but what is obstructed is the Mind, not the Spirit. We can seen this clearly in the lives of very many great artists whose *Shen* of the Heart was obstructed but whose spirit soared to produce masterpieces of universal, spiritual value.

In this book, I deliberately restrict the conditions treated to the few that account for the overwhelming majority of mental-emotional problems we see, i.e. depression, anxiety and insomnia. To these, I added a few others and notably bipolar disorder and attention deficit hyperactivity disorder.

As I have done in my last book, the second edition of the *Practice of Chinese Medicine*, I report both Western and Chinese clinical trials to give the reader a general idea of the clinical use of acupuncture and herbs. In each chapter, the section on "Modern Chinese Literature" reports a few clinical trials conducted in China. Most of these trials are conducted to a standard that would not be acceptable: however, they are reported to show the treatment principle adopted by modern Chinese doctors.

Both Western and Chinese clinical trials suffer from flaws. Chinese trials often suffer from poor design to a standard that would not be accepted in the West. On the other hand, many of the Western clinical trials, although well designed, suffer from other flaws, often to do with the choice of treatment (points or formulae). An example of a Western trial suffering from poor design from the point of view of Chinese medicine could be that of a trial on the use of Chinese herbal medicine in the treatment of bipolar disorder (see Chapter 19). One such trial selected the formula Xiao Yao San *Free and Easy Wanderer Powder*, a very strange choice indeed for the treatment of bipolar disorder.

Another example of poor design is that of a clinical trial on depression after stroke using only five points (P-6 Neiguan, Du-26 Renzhong, Du-20 Baihui, Yintang, and SP-6 Sanyinjiao) and the same ones in every patient. Moreover, the points were used on the "affected" side: this is a strange choice as, if the points were chosen to treat the depression rather than the paralysis resulting from stroke, it is not clear why they would be used only on the affected side (see Chapter 16).

As in my previous books, I report Chinese herbal formulae as they were formulated in China. This means that many formulae will contain animal or mineral products. As legislation in herbal medicine differs from country to country, the reader is urged to familiarize him or herself with the laws of their country. Some substances used are illegal for reasons to do with protection of endangered species (animal or vegetable) and some to do with animal cruelty. Again, I present the formulae as they were in Chinese books so that the reader can make intelligent substitutions of unacceptable ingredients. For this reason, Appendix 2 lists suggested substitutions for mineral and animal substances.

Appendix 4 explains some of the treatment principles listed in the book when these are not self-evident; for example, the difference between "rooting the Ethereal Soul" and "settling the Ethereal Soul".

Finally, the reader is urged to read the "Epilogue" that concludes the book. In it, I describe the issues I wrestled with over many years when treating patients suffering from emotional turmoil and I propose my own ideas about the integration of Chinese medicine into a Western practice.

My study of emotions in Western philosophy and in modern neurophysiology has led me to realize that emotions are far more than just the causes of disease envisaged by Chinese medicine. Far from obscuring our human nature, as the Neo-Confucianists tell us, they define our human nature and give meaning to our life. Together we need to develop a Chinese medicine that is based on a Western (rather than Confucian) concept of self and a view of the emotions that sees them not only as causes of disease but also as psychic factors that define us as human beings.

Giovanni Maciocia
Santa Barbara, April 2008

END NOTES

1. Fingarette H 1972 Confucius – The Secular as Sacred. Waveland Press, Prospect Heights, Illinois, p. 45.
2. Ames RT, Rosemont H 1999 The Analects of Confucius – A Philosophical Translation. Ballantine Books, New York, p. 48.
3. Confucius – The Secular as Sacred, p. 37.
4. Unschuld P 1985 Medicine in China – A History of Ideas. University of California Press, Berkeley, p. 200.
5. Damasio A 1994 Descartes' Error – Emotion, Reason and the Human Brain. Penguin Books, London, p. xii.

ACKNOWLEDGEMENTS

My first trip to China where I attended my first acupuncture course at the Nanjing University of Traditional Chinese Medicine in 1980 was an important milestone in my professional development. My first teacher there was the late Dr Su Xin Ming who played an important role in the development of my acupuncture skills. I am indebted to him for the patient way in which he communicated his skills to me.

I am grateful to Dr Zhou Zhong Ying of the Nanjing University of Chinese Medicine for teaching me his knowledge and skills in diagnosis and herbal medicine. I am indebted to many other teachers and clinical teachers from the Nanjing University of Traditional Chinese Medicine.

I am indebted to Fi Lyburn for her exceptional attention to detail in checking the manuscript for consistency and generally helping with editing. Backed by his considerable teaching and clinical experience, Peter Valaskatgis helped greatly with his constant feedback and his extremely valuable suggestions which enhanced the book.

I am grateful to Suzanne Turner for her help with research and editing. Dr J.D. Van Buren was my very first teacher 35 years ago: from him I learned the importance of diagnosis and especially of pulse diagnosis. I owe him a debt of gratitude for being my first source of inspiration in Chinese medicine.

Finally, I would like to thank Karen Morley, Kerry McGechie and Mary Law of Elsevier for their professionalism and support.

Giovanni Maciocia
Santa Barbara, 2009

NOTE ON THE TRANSLATION OF CHINESE MEDICAL TERMS

The terminology used in this book generally follows that used in the second edition of *Foundations of Chinese Medicine, Obstetrics and Gynaecology in Chinese Medicine, Diagnosis in Chinese Medicine* and the second edition of the *Practice of Chinese Medicine*. As in those books, I have opted for translating all Chinese medical terms with the exception of Yin, Yang, Qi and *cun* (unit of measurement).

I have also continued using initial capitals for the terms which are specific to Chinese medicine. For example, "Blood" indicates one of the vital substances of Chinese medicine, whereas "blood" denotes the liquid flowing in the blood vessels (e.g. "In Blood deficiency the menstrual blood may be pale."). I use initial capitals also for all pulse qualities and for pathological colors and shapes of the tongue body.

This system has served readers of my previous books well. As most teachers (including myself) use Chinese terms when lecturing (e.g. *Yuan Qi* rather than Original Qi), I have given each term in Pinyin whenever it is introduced for the first time. One change I have introduced in this book (as in the second editions of *Foundations of Chinese Medicine* and *Practice of Chinese Medicine*) is to use the Pinyin terms more often throughout the text and at least once in each chapter when the Chinese term is first introduced. I have done this to reduce the frequency with which the reader may need to consult the glossary.

I made the choice of translating all Chinese terms (with the exceptions indicated above) mostly for reasons of style: I believe that a well-written English text reads better than one peppered with Chinese terms in Pinyin. Leaving Chinese terms in Pinyin is probably the easiest option but this is not ideal because a single Pinyin word can often have more than one meaning; for example, *jing* can mean "channels", "periods", "Essence" or "shock", while *shen* can mean "Kidneys", "Mind" or "Spirit".

I am conscious of the fact that there is no such thing as a "right" translation of a Chinese medicine term and my terminology is not proposed in this spirit; in fact, Chinese medicine terms are essentially impossible to translate. The greatest difficulty in translating Chinese terms is probably that a term has many facets and different meanings in different contexts: thus it would be impossible for one translation to be "right" in every situation and every context. For example, the term *Jue* (厥) has many different meanings; a translation can illustrate only one aspect of a multifaceted term. In fact, *Jue* can mean a state of collapse with unconsciousness; coldness of hands and feet; or a critical situation of retention of urine. In other contexts it has other meanings, for example *Jue qi* (厥气), a condition of chaotic Qi; *Jue Xin Tong* (厥心痛), a condition of violent chest pain with cold hands; and *Jue Yin Zheng* (厥阴证), the Terminal Yin pattern within the Six Stage identification of patterns characterized by Heat above and Cold below.

Many sinologists concur that Chinese philosophical terms are essentially impossible to translate and that, the moment we translate them, we distort them with a worldview that is not Chinese. Ames is particularly clear about the intrinsic distortion of Chinese concepts when they are translated. He gives examples of Chinese terms that are distorted when translated, such as *Tian* 天 ("Heaven"), *You-Wu* 有无 ("Being" and "Non-Being"), *Dao* 道 ("Way"), *Xing* 性 ("human nature"), *Ren* 仁 ("benevolence"), *Li* 理 ("Principle"), *Qi* 气 ("primal substance"), etc.[1]

Ames is particularly forceful in rejecting a single, one-to-one translation of a Chinese term into a Western one in the introduction of his book *Focusing the Familiar* (a translation of the Confucian text *Zhong Yong*).[2] Ames says:[3]

> *Our Western languages are substance-oriented and are therefore most relevant to the descriptions of a world*

defined by discreteness, objectivity and permanence. Such languages are ill disposed to describe and interpret a world, such as that of the Chinese, that is primarily characterized by continuity, process and becoming.

Ames then gives some examples of what he considers to be serious mistranslations of Chinese philosophical terms. The important thing is that these are not "mistranslations" because the terms are "wrong" but because of the intrinsic difference between Chinese and Western thinking and therefore the inherent inability of Western terms to convey Chinese philosophical ideas. Ames says:[4]

For example, You 有*and* Wu 無*have often been uncritically rendered as "Being" and "Non-being". Influential translators, until quite recently, have rendered* wu xing 五行 *as "Five Elements".* Xing 性 *is still most often translated as "nature". All these translations promote the fixed and univocal characterizations of objects or essences emergent from a language rooted in a substantialist perspective* [our Western languages].

Ames stresses that the use of a "substances language" (i.e. a Western language) to translate Chinese insights into a world of process and change has led to seriously inappropriate interpretations of the Chinese sensibility. Ames asserts that it is the very difference between Chinese and Western philosophy that makes translation of Chinese terms virtually impossible. He says:[5]

In the classical traditions of the West, being takes precedence over becoming and thus becoming is ultimately unreal. Whatever becomes is realized by achieving its end – that is, coming into being. In the Chinese world, becoming takes precedence over being. "Being" is interpreted as a transitory state marked by further transition.

Ames then says:[6]

The Chinese world is a phenomenal world of continuity, becoming and change. In such a world there is no final discreteness. Things cannot be understood as objects. Without this notion of objectivity, there can only be the flux of passing circumstances in which things dissolve into the flux and flow. A processive language precludes the assumption that objects serve as references of linguistic expressions. The precise referential language of denotation and description is to be replaced by a language of "deference" in which meanings both allude to and defer to one another in a shifting field of significance. A referential language [Western language] *characterizes an event, object, or state of affairs through an act of naming meant to indicate a particular thing. On the other hand, the language of deference* [Chinese] *does not employ proper names simply as indicators of particular individuals or things, but invokes hints, suggestions, or allusions to indicate foci in a field of meanings.*

As an example of this intrinsic impossibility of translating a Chinese philosophical term into a Western language, Ames then cites Steve Owen's reluctance in translating *shi* 诗 as "poem". Owen says:[7]

If we translate "shi" *as "poem", it is merely for the sake of convenience.* "Shi" *is not a "poem":* "shi" *is not a thing made in the same way one makes a bed, a painting or a shoe. A* "shi" *can be worked on, polished and crafted; but that has nothing to do with what a* "shi" *fundamentally "is" ...* "Shi" *is not the "object" of its writer: it is the writer, the outside of an inside.*

Ames gives various translations of *Li* (a Confucian concept) as an example of how a multiplicity of terms may apply to a single Chinese term and how none of them is "wrong". He says that *Li* has been variously translated as "ritual", "rites", "customs", "etiquette", "propriety", "morals", "rules of proper behavior" and "worship". Ames says:[8]

Properly contextualized, each of these English terms can render Li on occasion. In classical Chinese, however, the character carries all of these meanings on every occasion of its use.

This confirms clearly how, by the very translation, we limit a Chinese term that is rich with multiple meanings to a single meaning in Chinese.

Ames says that in classical Chinese philosophical texts, allusive and connotatively rich language is more highly prized than clarity, precision and argumentative rigor. This rather dramatic contrast between Chinese and Western languages with respect to the issue of clarity presents the translator of Chinese philosophical texts with a peculiar burden.

For the Chinese, the opposite of clarity is not confusion, but something like *vagueness*. Vague ideas are really determinable in the sense that a *variety* of meanings are associated with them. Each Chinese term constitutes a field of meanings which may be focused by any of a number of its meanings. Ames says that in the translation of Chinese texts we must avoid what Whitehead called the "Fallacy of the Perfect Dictionary". By this, he means the assumption that there exists a complete semantic repository of terms of which we may adequately characterize the variety and depth of our experience and that, ideally, one may seek a one-to-one correspondence between word and meaning.

With this "fallacy" in mind, Ames and Hall say:[9]

We challenge the wisdom and accuracy of proposing "one-to-one" equivalencies in translating terms from one language to another. We introduce the notion of "linguistic clustering" as an alternative strategy to "literal translation" that allows us to put the semantic value of a term first by parsing [describe grammatically] *its range of meaning according to context, with the assumption that a range of meaning with a different configuration of emphasis is present on each appearance of the term.*

These ideas could not be more apt to illustrate the problems in translating Chinese medicine terms. Of course we must strive for precision and consistency but to think that there is a one-to-one, "right" correspondence between a Chinese medicine idea and a Western term is a misunderstanding of the very essence of Chinese medicine.

For example, to say that the only "right" translation of *Chong Mai* is "Thoroughfare Vessel" makes us fall into the trap of what Whitehead calls the "Fallacy of the Perfect Dictionary". Of course, *Chong Mai can* be translated as "Thoroughfare Vessel", but that is only one of its meanings and it is absolutely *impossible* for a single Western term to convey the richness of ideas behind the word *Chong Mai* (which I translate as "Penetrating Vessel"): to think that we can reduce a rich Chinese medicine idea to a single, one-to-one term in a Western language reveals, in my opinion, a misunderstanding of the very essence of Chinese medicine.

Ames makes this point very forcefully. He says:[10]

The Fallacy of the Perfect Dictionary is largely a consequence of our analytical bias towards univocity. We would suggest that this bias does not serve us well when approaching Chinese texts. Not only is there the continued possibility of novel experiences requiring appeal to novel terminologies, but also there is seldom, if ever, a simple, one-to-one translation of Chinese terms into Western languages. The allusiveness of the classical Chinese language is hardly conducive to univocal translations. We would contend that, in translating Chinese texts into Western languages, it is most unproductive to seek a single equivalent for a Chinese character. In fact, rather than trying to avoid ambiguity by a dogged use of formally stipulated terms, the translator might have to concede that characters often require a cluster of words to do justice to their range of meanings – all of which are suggested in any given rendering of the character. In fact, any attempt to employ univocal translations of Chinese terms justified by appeal to the criteria of clarity or univocity often reduces philosophical insight to nonsense and poetry to doggerel. Such an approach to translation serves only to numb Western readers to the provocative significance harboured within the richly vague and allusive language of the Chinese texts.

As an example of the multiplicity of meanings of a Chinese term and therefore of the fact that it is perfectly legitimate to translate a single Chinese idea into more than one term according to different contexts, Ames says that he translates the term *zhong* ("center" or "central") in the title of the Confucian text sometimes as "focus", sometimes as "focusing" and other times as "equilibrium". Other times, he even translates it as "center" or "impartiality". He says strongly:[11]

The Chinese language is not logocentric. Words do not name essences. Rather, they indicate always-transitory processes and events. It is important therefore to stress the gerundative character of the language. The language of process is vague, allusive and suggestive.

Rosemont makes the same point with regard to the translation of *Li* (rituals). He says *Li* could be translated as "customs", "mores", "propriety", "etiquette", "rites", "rituals", "rules of proper behavior", and "worship". He says:[12]

If we can agree that, appropriately contextualized, each of these English terms can translate Li on occasion, we should conclude that the Chinese graph must have all of these meanings on every occasion of its use, and that selecting only one of them can lead only to the result that something is lost in translation.

According to Ames, in the field of philosophy, two terms particularly stand out as being influenced by a

Western thinking when translated, i.e. *Tian* ("Heaven") and *Ren* ("benevolence"). Ames says:[13]

When we translate Tian *as "Heaven", like it or not, we invoke in the Western reader a notion of transcendent creator Deity, along with the language of soul, sin and afterlife ... When we translate* Ren *as "benevolence", we psychologize and make altruistic a term which originally had a radically different range of sociological connotations. Being altruistic, for example, implies being selfless in the service of others. But this "self-sacrifice" implicitly entails a notion of "self" which exists independently of others and that can be surrendered – a notion of self which we believe is alien to the world of the Analects* [of Confucius]*: indeed, such a reading* [of the term "ren"] *transforms what is fundamentally a strategy for self-realization into one of self-abnegation.*

With regard to Chinese medicine, the term *Xue* 血 ("Blood") is a good example of the above-mentioned problem reported by Ames. When we translate the word *Xue* as "Blood" we immediately alter its essential character and give it a Western medical connotation; in fact, in Chinese medicine, *Xue* is itself actually a form of Qi and one that is closely bound with Nutritive Qi (*Ying Qi*). Indeed, the term *mai* 脉 appearing in the *Yellow Emperor's Classic of Internal Medicine* is often ambiguous as it sometimes clearly refers to the acupuncture channels and other times to the blood vessels.

After highlighting the problems in translating Chinese terms, Ames confirms that a single Chinese term may have different meaning in different contexts. For example, the term *shen* 神 in some cases means "human spirituality", in others it means "divinity".[14] As he considers only the philosophical meanings of the word *shen*, we could actually add many others in the context of Chinese medicine, for example "mind", "spirit" and "lustre" (in the context of diagnosis).

Graham says:[15]

Every Western sinologist knows that there is no exact equivalent in his own language for such a word as ren 仁 *or* de 德, *and that as long as he thinks of it as synonymous with "benevolence" or "virtue" he will impose Western preconceptions on the thought he is studying.*

Ames then surveys the options that are presented to a translator and seems to favor simply transliterating the Chinese terms and leave them untranslated. He says:[16]

To some, this approach may appear to be simply the laziest way out of a difficult problem. But "ritual" has a narrowly circumscribed set of meanings in English, and Li an importantly different and less circumscribed set. Just as no Indological scholar would look for English equivalent for "karma", "dharma" and so on, perhaps it is time to do the same for classical Chinese, the homonymity of the language notwithstanding.

Hall confirms that a single Chinese term may have a plurality of meanings. He says:[17]

The Chinese have traditionally affirmed as the ground of their intellectual and institutional harmony the recognition of the co-presence of a plurality of significances with which any given term might easily resonate.

Finally, another sinologist, Yung Sik Kim, discusses the difficulty presented by the plurality of meanings of a single Chinese term. He says:[18]

I have adopted the policy of sticking to one English translation for a particular Chinese word whenever possible ... Of course, exceptions cannot be avoided altogether. I have had to resort to different translations for such characters as "xin" 心 *which means both "heart" and "mind";* "tian" 天, *both "heaven" and "sky".*

In another passage, Yung Sik Kim affirms that transliteration of a Chinese term with a plurality of meanings is the only alternative:[19]

The term "li" 理 is difficult to define. It is difficult even to translate because there is no single word in Western languages that covers all facets of what "li" meant to the traditional Chinese mind. The existence of many translations for the term, which often leaves transliteration as the only viable option, bespeaks the difficulty.

Although a diversity of translation of Chinese terms may present its problems, these are easily overcome if an author explains the translation in a glossary and, most importantly, explains the meaning of a given Chinese term in its context (in our case, Chinese medicine).

In my books, I have chosen to translate all Chinese medicine terms rather than using Pinyin purely for reasons of style as a sentence written half in English and half in Pinyin is often awkward. Moreover, if we use Pinyin terms in writing, it could be argued that we should be consistent and use Pinyin terms for *all* Chinese medicine terms and this would not make for very clear reading. Consider the following sentence: "*To treat* Pi-Yang Xu *we adopt the* zhi fa *of* bu pi *and* wen Yang" ("*To treat Spleen-Yang deficiency we adopt the treatment principle of tonifying the Spleen and warming Yang*").

Moreover, the problem arises only in the written form as, in my experience, most lecturers in colleges throughout the Western world normally prefer using Pinyin terms rather than their counterparts in English (or any other Western languages). Thus, a lecturer will refer to Kidney-*Jing* rather than Kidney-Essence. Indeed, when I myself lecture, I generally use the Pinyin terms rather than their English translation. Again, most lecturers use a pragmatic approach, translating some terms into English (such as "treatment principle" instead of *zhi fa*) and leaving others in Pinyin such as *Yuan Qi* or *Chong Mai*.

When I lecture I always try to give the participants an idea of the meaning of a particular Chinese character and its significance and application in Chinese medicine. Indeed, the use of Pinyin when lecturing renders Chinese medicine truly international as I can lecture in the Czech Republic and mention *Jing*, *Yang Qiao Mai*, *Wei Qi*, etc., knowing that I will be understood by everyone. A diversity of translation of Chinese terms may even have a positive aspect as each author may highlight a particular facet of a Chinese term so that diversity actually enriches our understanding of Chinese medicine. If someone translates *Zong Qi* 宗气 as "Initial Qi", for example, we learn something about that author's view and understanding of *Zong Qi*; the translation cannot be branded as "wrong" (I translate this term as "Gathering Qi"). Another example: if someone translates *yang qiao mai* as "Yang Motility Vessel", the translation captures one aspect of this vessel's nature; again, this could not be defined as wrong (I translate the name of this vessel as "Yang Stepping Vessel").

Trying to impose a standard, "right" translation of Chinese medicine terms may lead to suppression of healthy debate; I therefore hope that readers will continue to benefit from the diversity of translation of Chinese medical terms and draw inspiration from the rich heritage of Chinese medicine that it represents.

I firmly believe that the future lies not in trying to establish a rigid, embalmed, fossilized, "right" terminology based on single, one-to-one translations of Chinese ideas. Indeed, I believe this is a potentially dangerous trend as it would, in my opinion, lead students and practitioners away from the richness of Chinese language and richness of meanings of Chinese medicine ideas. The adoption of a standardized, "approved" terminology of Chinese medical terms may indeed, in time, divorce students and practitioners from the essence of Chinese medicine. If an "official", standardized translation of Chinese terms took hold, then students would be less inclined to study the Chinese terms to explore their meaning.

Ames and Hall make the same point:[20]

> *Such translations have been "legitimized" by their gradual insinuation into the standard Chinese-English dictionaries and glossaries. By encouraging the uncritical assumption in those who consult these reference works that this formula of translations provides the student with a "literal" rendering of the terms, these lexicons have become complicit in an entrenched cultural equivocation that we strive to avoid.*

They then further make the point that using a one-to-one translation of Chinese terms ignores the cultural background from which they came:[21]

> *Our argument is that it is in fact these formulaic usages that are radical interpretations. To our mind, to consciously or unconsciously transplant a text from its own historical and intellectual soil and replant it in one that has a decidedly different philosophical landscape is to take liberties with the text and is radical in the sense it tampers with its very roots.*

As I said above, an "official", standardized translation of Chinese terms may make students and practitioners less inclined to study the Chinese terms to explore their meaning with their own interpretation. Ames and Hall say:[22]

> *Our goal is not to replace one inadequate formula with another. Our translations are intended as no more than suggestive "placeholders" that refer readers back to this glossary to negotiate their own meaning, and, we hope, to appropriate the Chinese terms for themselves.*

Moreover, imposing an "approved" terminology in English betrays an Anglocentric worldview: to be consistent, we should then have an "approved" terminology in every major language of the world. It seems to me much better to try to understand the spirit and the essence of Chinese medicine by studying its characters and their *clinical* significance and using Pinyin transliteration whenever appropriate.

Trying to fossilize Chinese medicine terms into an imposed terminology goes against the very essence of the Chinese language which, as Ames says, is not logocentric and in which words do not name essences: rather, they indicate always-transitory processes and events. The language of process is vague, allusive and suggestive.

Because Chinese language is a language of *process*, the question arises also whether practicing Chinese medicine actually helps the understanding of Chinese medical terminology: in my opinion, in many cases it does. For example, I feel that clinical experience helps us to understand the nature of the *Chong Mai* (Penetrating Vessel) and therefore helps us to understand the term *chong* in a "knowing practice" way (as Farquhar defines it)[23] rather than a theoretical way.

Of course, a translator of Chinese books should strive for precision and consistency, but we must accept that there is a rich multiplicity of meanings for any given idea of Chinese medicine. The *Chong Mai* is a good example of this multiplicity as the term *chong* could be translated as "thoroughfare", "strategic cross-roads", "to penetrate", "to rush", "to rush upwards", "to charge", "activity", "movement" and "free passage". Which of these translations is "correct"? They are all correct as they all convey an idea of the nature and function of the *Chong Mai*.

I therefore think that the future of teaching Chinese medicine lies not in trying to impose the straightjacket of a rigid terminology of the rich ideas of Chinese medicine, but in teaching students more and more Chinese characters explaining the richness of meanings associated with them in the context of Chinese medicine. I myself would not like my own terminology to be "adopted" as the "correct" or "official" one: I would rather see colleges teaching more and more Chinese to their students by illustrating the rich meanings of Chinese medicine terms. As mentioned above, my main motive for translating all terms is purely for reasons of style in an English-language textbook; when I lecture I generally use Pinyin terms but, most of all, I show the students the Chinese characters and try to convey their meaning in the context of Chinese medicine.

Finally, I would like to explain my continued translation of *Wu Xing* as "Five Elements". The term "Five Elements" has been used by most Western practitioners of Chinese medicine for a long time (also in French and other European languages). Some authors consider this to be a misunderstanding of the meaning of the Chinese term *Wu Xing*, perpetuated over the years. *Wu* means "five" and *Xing* means "movement", "process", "to go", "conduct" or "behavior". Most authors therefore think that the word *Xing* cannot indicate "element" as a basic constituent of Nature, as was supposedly intended in ancient Greek philosophy.

This is, in my opinion, only partly true as the elements, as they were conceived by various Greek philosophers over the centuries, were not always considered "basic constituents" of Nature or "passive motionless fundamental substances".[24] Some Greek philosophers conceived the elements as dynamic qualities of Nature, in a way similar to Chinese philosophy.

For example, Aristotle gave a definite dynamic interpretation to the four elements and called them "primary form" (*prota somata*). He said:[25]

Earth and Fire are opposites also due to the opposition of the respective qualities with which they are revealed to our senses: Fire is hot, Earth is cold. Besides the fundamental opposition of hot and cold, there is another one, i.e. that of dry and wet: hence the four possible combinations of hot-dry [Fire], *hot-wet* [Air], *cold-dry* [Earth] *and cold-wet* [Water] ... *the elements can mix with each other and can even transform into one another ... thus Earth, which is cold and dry, can generate Water if wetness replaces dryness.*

To Aristotle, therefore, the four elements became the four basic qualities of natural phenomena, classified as combinations of four qualities: hot, cold, dry and wet. As is apparent from the above statement, the Aristotelian elements could even transform into one another and generate each other.

This interpretation is very similar to the Chinese one, in which the elements are *qualities* of Nature. Furthermore, it is interesting to note the similarity with the Chinese theory of Yin-Yang: the four Aristotelian elements derive from the interaction of the basic Yin-Yang qualities of cold-hot and dry-wet.

Thus, it is not entirely true to say that the Greek elements were conceived only as the basic constituents of matter, the "building blocks" of Nature, which would make the use of the word "element" wrong to indicate *xing*. Furthermore, the word "elements" does not necessarily imply that: it does so only in its modern chemical interpretation.

In conclusion, for the above reasons I have kept the word "element" as a translation of the Chinese word *xing*. According to Wang, the term "Five Elements" could be translated in a number of ways, for example "agents", "entities", "goings", "conduct", "doings", "forces", "activities" and "stages of change".[26]

Recently, the term "Five Phases" is gaining acceptance, but some sinologists disagree with this translation and propose returning to "Five Elements". Friedrich and Lackner, for example, suggest restoring the term "elements".[27] Graham uses the term "Five Processes".[28] I would probably agree that "processes" is the best translation of *Wu Xing*. In fact, the book *Shang Shu* written during the Western Zhou dynasty (1000–771 BC) said:[29]

The Five Elements are Water, Fire, Wood, Metal and Earth. Water moistens downwards; Fire flares upwards; Wood can be bent and straightened; Metal can be moulded and can harden; Earth allows sowing, growing and reaping.

Some sinologists (e.g. Needham and Fung Yu Lan) still use the term "element". Fung Yu Lan suggests that a possible translation of *wu xing* could be "Five Activities" or "Five Agents".[30] Although the term "five phases" has gained some acceptance as a translation of *wu xing*, I find this term restrictive as it clearly refers to only one aspect of the Five Elements, i.e. phases of a (seasonal) cycle.

A glossary with Pinyin terms, Chinese characters and English translation appears at the end of the book. I have included both a Pinyin–English and an English–Pinyin glossary.

END NOTES

1. Ames RT, Rosemont H 1999 The Analects of Confucius – A Philosophical Translation. Ballantine Books, New York, p. 311.
2. Ames RT, Hall DL 2001 Focusing the Familiar – A Translation and Philosophical Interpretation of the *Zhong Yong*. University of Hawai'i Press, Honolulu, pp. 6–16.
3. Ibid., p. 6.
4. Ibid., p. 6.
5. Ibid., p. 10.
6. Ibid., p. 10.
7. Ibid., p. 13.
8. Ibid., p. 69.
9. Ames RT, Hall DL 2003 Daodejing – Making This Life Significant: A Philosophical Translation. Ballantine Books, New York, p. 56.
10. Ibid., p. 16.
11. Ibid., p. 16.
12. Bockover M (ed) 1991 Rules, Ritual and Responsibility – Essays Dedicated to Herbert Fingarette. Open Court, La Salle, Illinois, p. 98.
13. The Analects of Confucius, p. 312.
14. Ibid., p. 313.
15. Hall DL, Ames RT 1998 Thinking from the Han – Self, Truth and Transcendence in Chinese and Western Culture. State University of New York Press, New York, p. 238.
16. The Analects of Confucius, p. 314.
17. Thinking from the Han, p. 4.
18. Kim Yung Sik 2000 The Natural Philosophy of Chu Hsi. American Philosophical Society, Philadelphia, p. 11.
19. Ibid., p. 19.
20. Daodejing – Making This Life Significant, p. 55.
21. Ibid., pp. 55–56.
22. Ibid., p. 56.
23. Farquhar J 1994 Knowing Practice – The Clinical Encounter of Chinese Medicine. Westview Press, Boulder, Colorado.
24. Needham J 1977 Science and Civilization in China, vol. 2. Cambridge University Press, Cambridge, p. 244.
25. Lamanna EP 1967 Storia della Filosofia [History of Philosophy], vol. 1. Le Monnier, Florence, pp. 220–221.
26. Wang Ai He 1999 Cosmology and Political Culture in Early China. Cambridge University Press, Cambridge, p. 3.
27. Friedrich M, Lackner M. Once again: the concept of Wu Xing. Early China 9–10: 218–219.
28. Graham AC 1986 Yin-Yang and the Nature of Correlative Thinking. Institute of East Asian Philosophies, Singapore, pp. 42–66 and 70–92.
29. Shang Shu (*c*.659 BC), cited in 1980 Shi Yong Zhong Yi Xue 实用中医学 [Practical Chinese Medicine]. Beijing Publishing House, Beijing, p. 32. The book *Shang Shu* is placed by some in the early Zhou dynasty (hence *c*.1000 BC), but the prevalent opinion is that it was written sometime between 659 BC and 627 BC.
30. Fung Yu Lan 1966 A Short History of Chinese Philosophy. Free Press, New York, p. 131.

A GUIDE TO MACIOCIA'S BOOKS

FOUNDATIONS OF CHINESE MEDICINE

PRACTICE OF CHINESE MEDICINE

DIAGNOSIS IN CHINESE MEDICINE

THE CHANNELS OF ACUPUNCTURE

OBSTETRICS AND GYNECOLOGY IN CHINESE MEDICINE

THE PSYCHE IN CHINESE MEDICINE

FOUNDATIONS OF CHINESE MEDICINE

First published in 1989 (with a second edition in 2005), this was and remains the first textbook that discusses the basic theories of Chinese medicine in detail. The knowledge derived from the book constitutes the necessary basis for the training in the theory of Chinese medicine. This applies to both acupuncturists and herbalists.

PRACTICE OF CHINESE MEDICINE

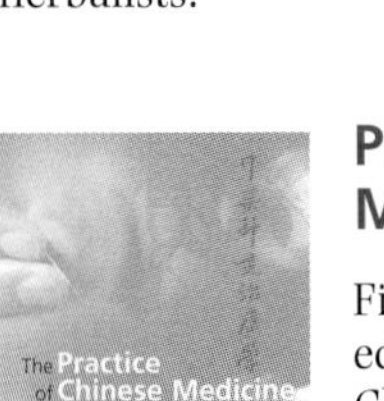

First published in 1994 (with a second edition in 2008), the Practice of Chinese Medicine is the logical companion to the *Foundations of Chinese Medicine*, illustrating the application of the principles of Chinese Medicine to the treatment of diseases. It is a clinical manual that helps practitioners diagnose the patterns of disease, the etiology of diseases and that discusses the treatment of each disease with both acupuncture and herbal medicine in great detail.

The book contains more that 150 case histories with detailed explanation of the diagnostic process and analysis of treatment. An 8-page color plate section with tongue slides is added to clarify diagnoses.

DIAGNOSIS IN CHINESE MEDICINE

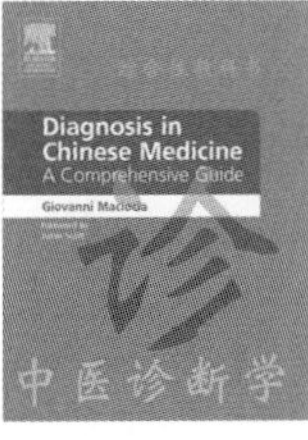

Published in 2004, this book still remains the most voluminous, extensive and detailed text on Chinese medicine diagnosis. Comprising of over 1,000 pages, this book is an essential desk companion in every Chinese medicine practitioner's clinic.

THE CHANNELS OF ACUPUNCTURE

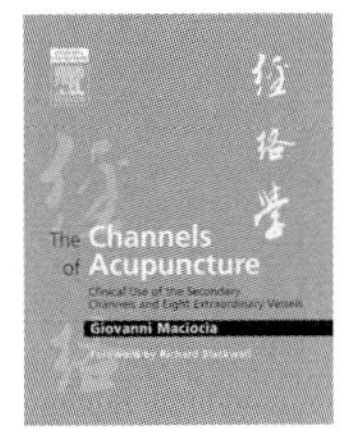

Published in 2006, this book complements all the other texts in so far as it is entirely dedicated to acupuncture, the channels and acupuncture treatments. This books deals with the physiology, diagnosis, pathology and treatment of the acupuncture channels in great depth and detail.

OBSTETRICS AND GYNECOLOGY IN CHINESE MEDICINE

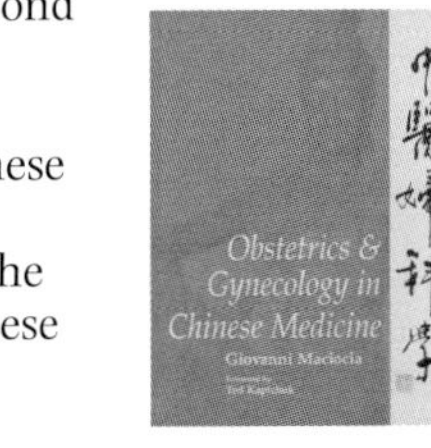

The scope of this textbook is the same as that of the Practice of Chinese Medicine, i.e. to illustrate the application of the theory of Chinese Medicine to the treatment of diseases, in this case, gynaecological diseases.

THE PSYCHE IN CHINESE MEDICINE

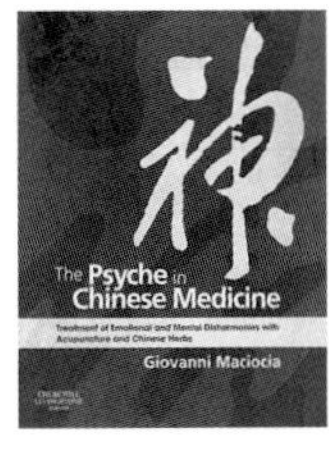

This is one of very few books dedicated entirely to the treatment of mental-emotional problems. The book first describes the functions and nature of the five 'spirits' (*Shen, Hun, Po, Yi* and *Zhi*) in a depth and detail not seen previously in the English language. The nature and functions of the five spirits are creatively explained in light of modern conditions such as autism, ADD and bipolar disorder.

The book then discusses the treatment of the most common psychiatric conditions seen in a Western clinic, i.e. depression, anxiety and bipolar disorder. For each condition, the author discusses the etiology, pathology and treatment both with acupuncture and herbal medicine.

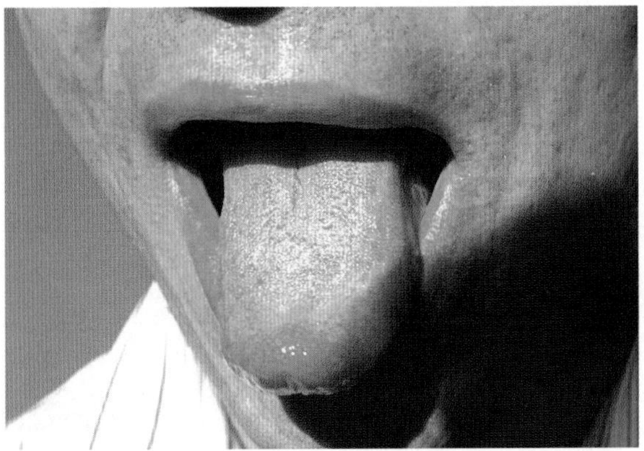

Plate 11.1 Red tip of the tongue, indicating mental-emotional stress, page 177.

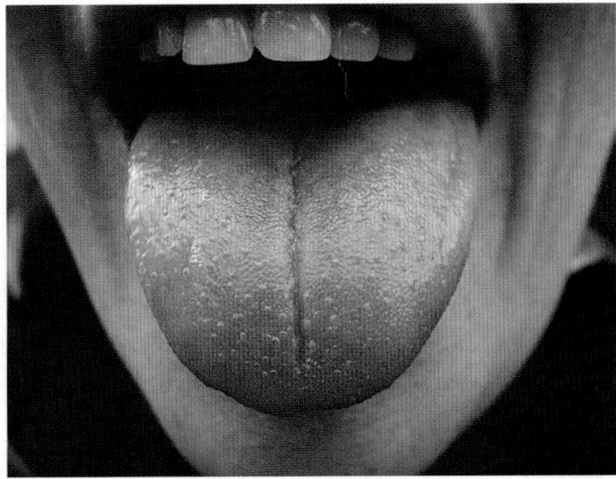

Plate 11.2 Heart crack, page 178.

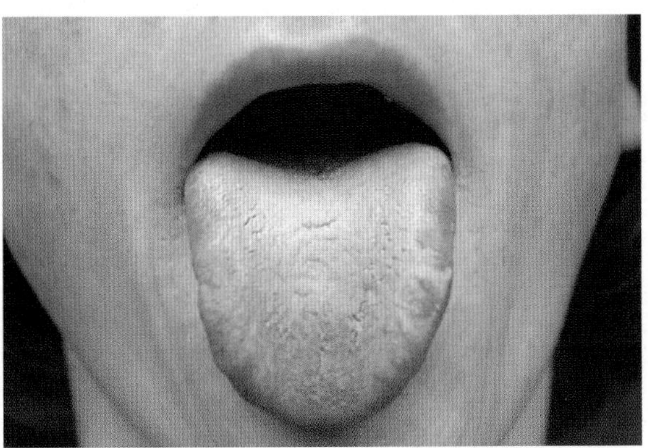

Plate 11.3 Red sides of the tongue related to Liver-Heat, page 179.

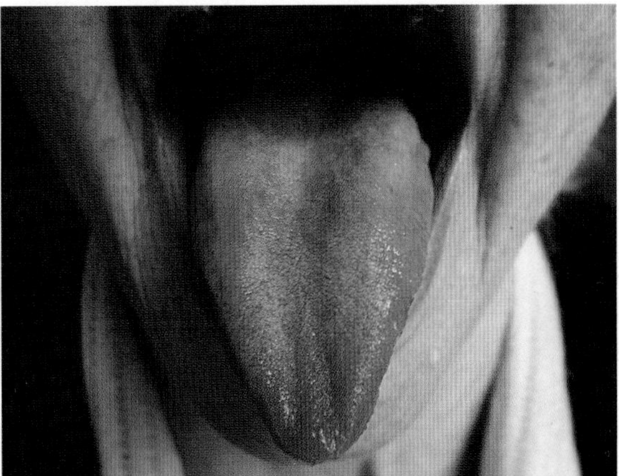

Plate 11.4 Red sides and tip related to Liver- and Heart-Heat, page 179.

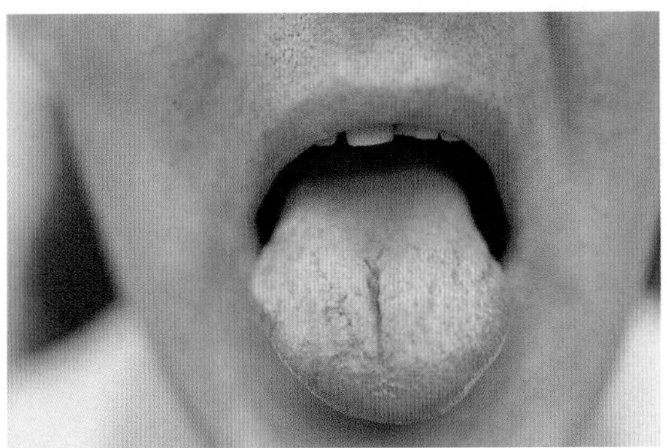

Plate 11.5 Abnormal swelling of front third of tongue, indicating chest/breast pathology, page 179.

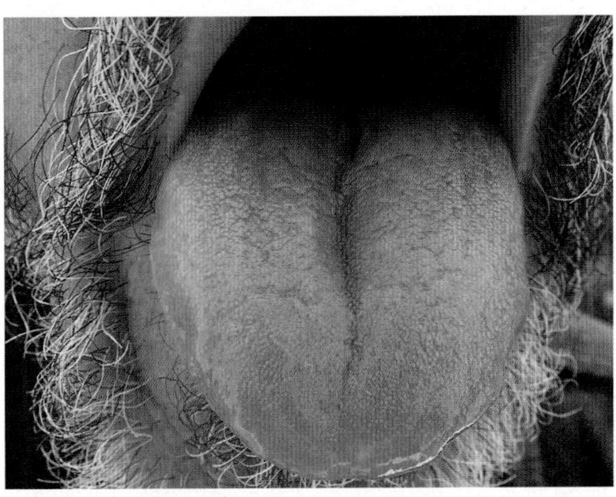

Plate 11.6 Combined Stomach–Heart crack, page 180.

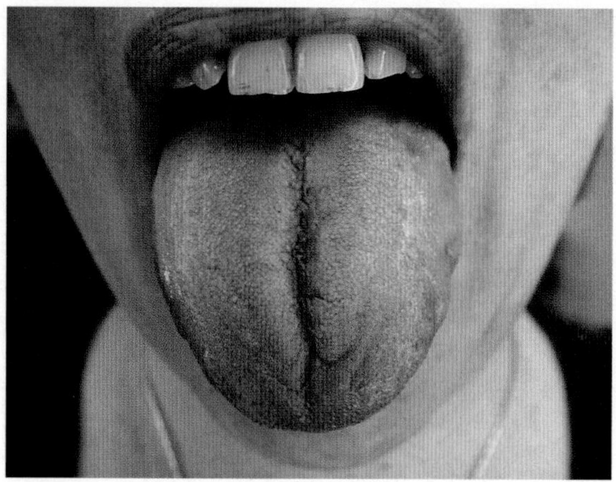

Plate 11.7 Combined Stomach–Heart crack with rough-sticky-yellow coating in crack, page 180.

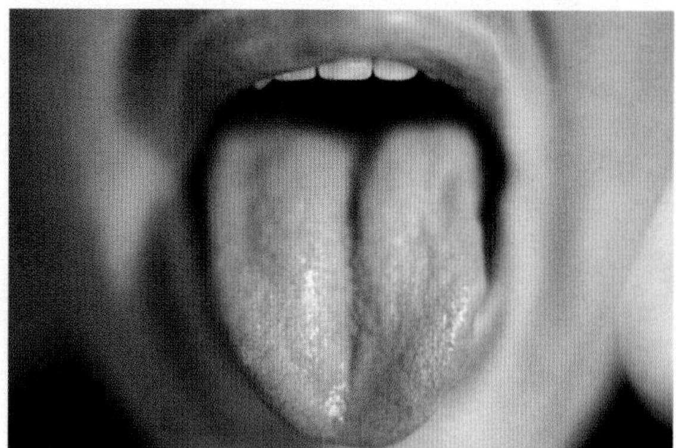

Plate 12.1 Stomach–Heart crack, page 198.

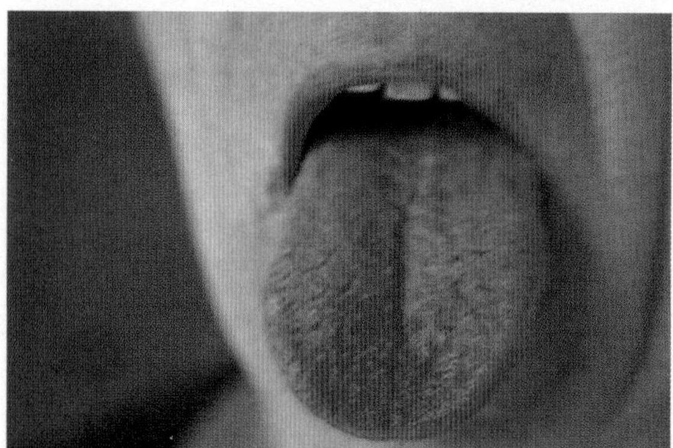

Plate 12.2 Red tongue without coating and with Heart crack, page 210.

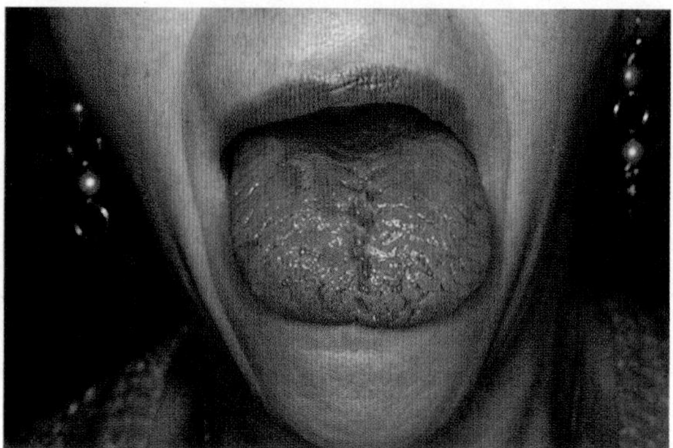

Plate 12.3 Slightly Red, Swollen on the sides, cracked and with a rootless coating, Heart crack in the middle, page 218.

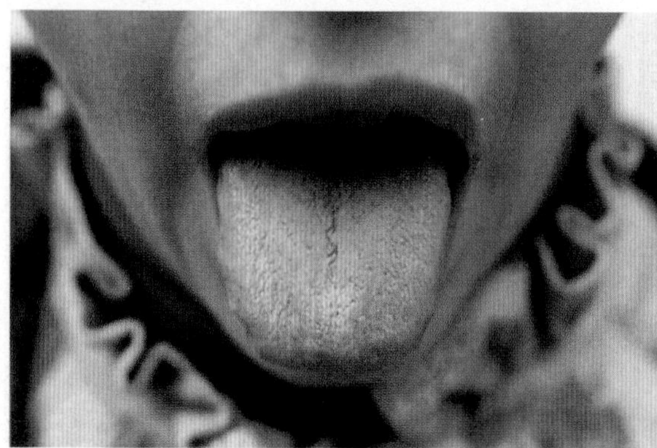

Plate 12.4 Red, redder on the sides, with a yellow coating, page 225.

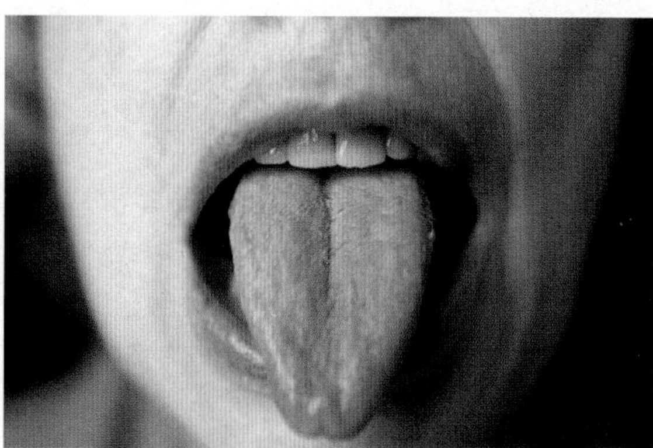

Plate 12.5 Reddish-Purple, Stiff, Swollen, with a Stomach crack in the center, thick-sticky-yellow coating, page 227.

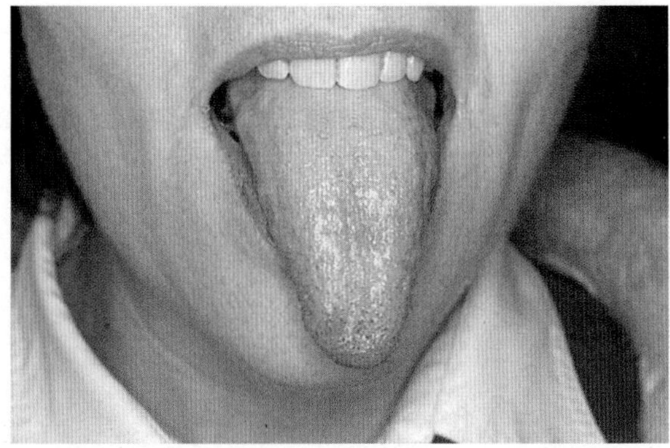

Plate 12.6 Slightly Pale with a Red tip with red points, page 233.

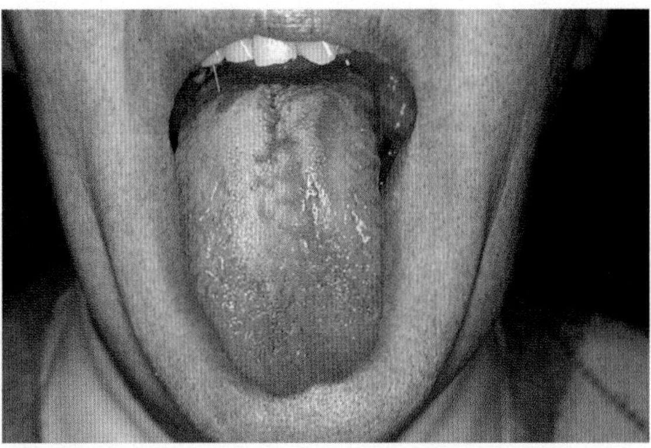

Plate 12.7 Red, with a Heart crack and without enough coating, page 236.

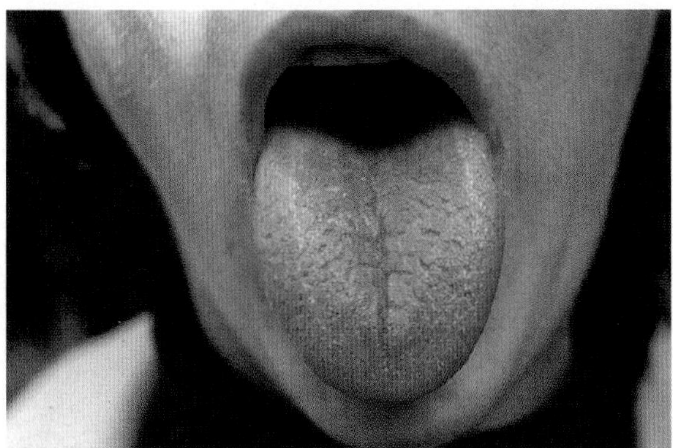

Plate 12.8 Red, with a Heart crack, almost entirely without coating, page 238.

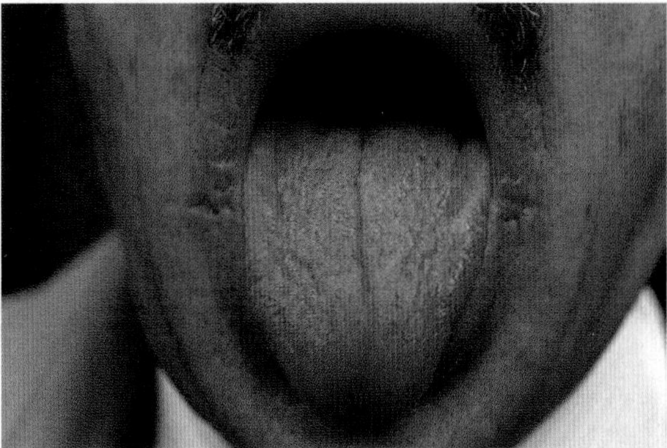

Plate 18.1 Tongue of a 61-year-old man with insomnia, page 472.

五神

CHAPTER 1

THE PSYCHE IN CHINESE MEDICINE

THE SPIRIT AND SOUL IN WESTERN PHILOSOPHY *1*
The spirit *1*
The soul *3*
THE SPIRIT, SOUL AND MIND IN CHINESE MEDICINE *3*
Terminology *3*
The Spirit (*Shen*) in Chinese medicine *4*
The concept of "body" in China *6*
The Soul in Chinese medicine *6*
The Mind (*Shen*) in Chinese medicine *8*
Meaning of the word *shen* in Chinese medicine *9*
Mental illness in ancient Chinese medicine *10*

THE PSYCHE IN CHINESE MEDICINE

A discussion of the treatment of mental and emotional problems is not possible without first exploring the concept of the mind and spirit in Chinese medicine. It is only by understanding this concept of the mind and spirit in Chinese culture that we can truly grasp how to treat psychological and emotional problems with acupuncture and Chinese herbs. We must be careful not to interpret the Chinese concepts of "mind" and "spirit" in terms of Western (and often Christian) concepts of "mind" and "spirit".

However, in order to grasp the differences between Western and Chinese views of the psyche, soul and spirit, I will first investigate the Western concepts. A longer discussion of Western concepts of self, soul, mind and emotions is in Chapter 14.

The discussion of the spirit and soul in this chapter will be conducted according to the following topics.

- The spirit and soul in Western philosophy
- The spirit, soul and Mind in Chinese medicine

THE SPIRIT AND SOUL IN WESTERN PHILOSOPHY

The spirit

The Oxford English Dictionary definition of "spirit" highlights an important feature of this concept in Western philosophy and illustrates its difference from Chinese philosophy. The dictionary's opening definition of "spirit" is: "*The animating or vital principle in man (and animals); that which gives life to the physical organism, in contrast to its purely material elements; the breath of life.*"[1]

The definition of "spirit" as "*that which gives life to the physical organism, in contrast to its purely material elements*" illustrates the duality between body and spirit that has been typical of most of Western philosophy, a duality that is absent from Chinese medicine. However, as we shall see, the difference between Western and Chinese philosophy is not that simple, for some Western philosophers also conceived the "spirit" as a refined form of matter (as the Chinese do). And vice versa, some Chinese philosophers (notably some Neo-Confucian philosophers) conceived of a metaphysical reality distinct from the physical one.

!

The Oxford English Dictionary definition of "spirit" is: "The animating or vital principle in man (and animals); that which gives life to the physical organism, in contrast to its purely material elements; the breath of life."

The word "spirit" means "breath" and comes from *spiritus*, the Latin rendering of the Greek *pneuma* (πνευμα), which also means "breath" or "air". "Spirit" has the same meaning as the Latin word *anima* (later used by Jung in a different sense) which derives from the Greek *anemos* (ανεμος), meaning "breath" or "wind"; this is related to the Sanskrit *atman* which also means "breath". Therefore, it is clear from its etymology that "spirit" is something subtle, ethereal in nature, like air.

Interestingly, the Greek Stoics conceived "spirit" as a refined form of matter, in the form of a subtle fire, of which the individual souls (or spirits) were particles. The concept of "vital spirit" animating the body became elaborated by ancient Greek doctors such as Erasistratus who distinguished between a psychic spirit (*pneuma zotikon*, πνευμα ζωτικον) residing in the heart and flowing in the blood vessels, and a physical spirit (*pneuma physicon*, πνευμα ψυχικον) residing in the brain and flowing in the nerves. The placing of the psychic spirit in the heart is interesting as it coincides with the Chinese view. Erasistratus's view that there are two spirits, one psychic and one physical, is also interesting as he was a practitioner of what we might today call psychosomatic medicine.

Furthermore, Erasistratus's view of two spirits, one psychic and one physical, resembles the Chinese view of the Mind (*Shen*) and Corporeal Soul (*Po*).

> **!**
>
> The ancient Greek doctor Erasistratus distinguished between a psychic spirit (*pneuma zotikon*, πνευμα ζωτικον) residing in the heart and flowing in the blood vessels, and a physical spirit (*pneuma physicon*, πνευμα ψυχικον) residing in the brain and flowing in the nerves.

With the Christian religion, the duality between a subtle, non-material "spirit" and a material body became firmly established. In the Christian religion, the "spirit" is the soul of a human being and is contrasted with the body; at death, the soul survives the body. From the advent of Christianity, the spirit is counterposed to the body. Interestingly, St Paul thought that the "body" should not be seen as the material body but as the "carnal spirit" (πνευμα σαρκικον). This is interesting as it resonates with the Chinese concept of a "corporeal soul" (*Po*).

The opposition and separation between spirit and body are reaffirmed in the philosophy of Descartes (1596–1650) and his rationalism. Descartes also mentions "animal spirits" as St Paul did. In the *Passions of the Soul*, Descartes defines these emotions as follows: "*Perceptions or sensations or excitations of the soul which are referred to it in particular and which are caused, maintained, and strengthened by some movement of the spirits.*"[2] The "spirits" mentioned here are the "animal spirits" central to Descartes's account of physiology. Descartes explains that the animal spirits are produced by the blood and are responsible for stimulating the body's movement. By affecting the muscles, for example, the animal spirits "*move the body in all the different ways in which it can be moved*". This description sounds very similar to that of the Corporeal Soul.

Henry More (1614–1687) was one of the main English exponents of the idealist, Neo-Platonic school. More's dualistic theology of body and soul was heavily indebted to Neo-Platonic thought. More is notable as a rationalist theologian who tried to use the details of the mechanical philosophy, as developed by René Descartes, to establish the existence of immaterial substance, or spirit, and, therefore, God.

John Locke (1632–1704) attributes to the spirit the same reality as that of the body. He says:[3]

> *Positing a substance in which reside thought, knowing, doubting and the power of movement, we obtain a notion of the spirit that is no less real than that of the body; the former is the substratum of the ideas we receive from the external world, the latter of the ideas from ourselves.*

George Berkeley (1685–1753) was an exponent of the Idealism school of philosophy according to which an object exists first as an idea. Ideas are the main reality. He equated spirit with mind and soul and believed that ideas exist in someone's mind and spirit. He said: "*It is evident that there is no other reality than the spirit who is the one that perceives.*"[4]

Immanuel Kant (1724–1804) considered that the spirit is the life-giving principle of the soul, the productive power of reason, the originality of thought. He also discussed the spirit in the context of art; in his opinion, "spirit" is also the unfathomable quality of beautiful art.

G.W.F. Hegel (1770–1831) considered the whole in all its complexity as the Absolute. The Absolute is spiritual.[5] Hegel's philosophical system is the culmination of the Idealism school of philosophy according to which ideas precede material objects. Hegel considered Spirit to be the one immutably homogeneous entity.[6]

The soul

The soul, according to many religious and philosophical traditions, is a self-aware *ethereal substance* unique to a particular living being. The soul differs from the spirit in so far as the latter may or may not be eternal, while the former is usually considered to survive the body after death.

The concept of the soul has strong links with notions of an afterlife, but each religion has its own views as to what happens to the soul after death. The English word "soul" derives from the Old English *sawol*. "Sawol" has possible etymological links with an old German word *se(u)la*, which means "belonging to the sea". The association between "soul" and the "sea" is interesting because it is a theme that recurs in many religions and in fairytales. In the Jungian interpretation of dreams, the sea is often a symbol for the unconscious.

In Greek, the soul is called *psyche* (φυχη); in modern languages and psychology, the term "psyche" is now different from "soul". The Oxford English Dictionary defines "psyche" as "the conscious and unconscious mind and emotions, especially as influencing and affecting the whole person". In Latin, it is called *anima*, which derives from the Greek *anemos* (ανεμος), meaning "breath" or "wind".

In pre-Socratic ancient Greece, the word "soul" indicated something that distinguishes the living from the dead and the animate from the inanimate; when we die, the soul leaves the body and goes into an "underworld". In later times, a wide variety of activities and responses, cognitive as well as emotional, were attributed to the soul and this was also thought to be the source of such virtues as courage, temperance and justice. In other words, some of the activities of the "soul" were activities of what we would call the "mind" (e.g. cognition).

However, the soul was obviously more than just the mind as some Greek philosophers attributed a soul also to animals and plants; this presents interesting parallels with Chinese thinking which describes three Ethereal Souls (plants have one, animals two and human beings all three).

Plato considered the soul as the essence of a person's being. He regarded this essence as an incorporeal, eternal occupant of our being and held that, after death, it is reborn in another body. Plato thinks that body and soul differ in kind, the former being perceptible and perishable, the latter being intelligible and exempt from destruction. The Platonic soul comprises three parts: the *logos* (mind, nous), the *thymos* (emotions) and the *pathos* (carnal). We could say that it was with Plato that the great Western divide between soul and body, spirit and body, mind and body started.

The soul, as Plato conceives it, is therefore characterized by cognitive and intellectual features; it is something that reasons; something that regulates and controls the body and its desires and affections, "especially if it is a wise soul". However, the soul is not simply the "mind" as we conceive it. It is broader than that, in that Plato retains the traditional idea of soul as distinguishing the animate from the inanimate.

Aristotle, following Plato, defined the soul as the core essence of a being, but argued against its having a separate existence. He did not consider the soul as some kind of separate, ghostly occupant of the body. As the soul, in Aristotle's view, is an *activity* of the body, it cannot be immortal. According to Aristotle's theory, a soul is a particular kind of nature, a principle that accounts for change and rest in the particular case of living bodies, i.e. plants, non-human animals and human beings. The relation between soul and body, in Aristotle's view, is also an instance of the more general relation between form and matter; thus an ensouled, living body is a particular kind of in-formed matter.

Both Epicurus and the Stoics thought that the soul is corporeal. The Stoics argued that the soul is a body because only bodies affect one another, and soul and body do affect one another, for instance in cases of bodily damage and emotion.

Epicurus held that the soul is a particularly fine kind of body, diffused all the way through the perceptible (flesh-and-blood) body of the animate organism. Epicurus thinks that the soul is dispersed at death along with its constituent atoms, losing the powers that it has while it is contained by the body of the organism that it ensouls. These views are remarkably similar to the Chinese views of the Corporeal Soul.

THE SPIRIT, SOUL AND MIND IN CHINESE MEDICINE

Terminology

Throughout this book, I shall use the word "spirit" generally in a Chinese sense to denote the complex of the spiritual aspects of the Yin organs, i.e. the Mind (*Shen*) of the Heart, the Ethereal Soul (*Hun*) of the Liver, the Corporeal Soul (*Po*) of the Lungs, the Intellect (*Yi*) of the Spleen and the Will-Power (*Zhi*) of the Kidneys.

I shall call "Mind", the *Shen* that resides in the Heart. Most authors translate *Shen* as "spirit" in English; I believe the term "spirit" describes more accurately the complex of *Shen, Hun, Po, Yi* and *Zhi*. The implication of this is not merely semantic as, if we translate the *Shen* of the Heart as "spirit", we ignore the influence of the Ethereal Soul and Corporeal Soul on the spirit. This question is discussed also in Chapter 2.

I shall use the term "soul" mostly in relation to the Ethereal Soul (*Hun*). Although I regard "psyche" as a synonym of the word "spirit", I employ it in a more general sense to include all the mental, spiritual and emotional phenomena of a human being.

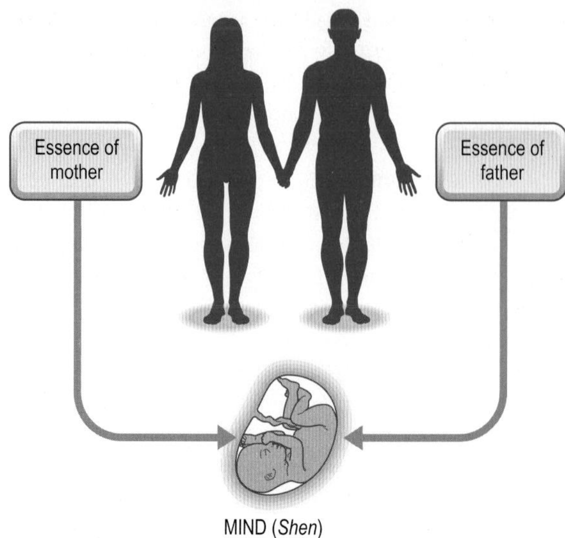

Figure 1.1 Union of Essences to form Mind.

The Spirit (*Shen*) in Chinese medicine

The "spirit" as defined above in the context of Chinese medicine includes all mental phenomena (thinking, reason, including that of the Ethereal Soul), emotional phenomena and bodily phenomena. The term is used without any reference to a particular religion and no inference is made on the spirit's destiny after death.

As any practitioner of Chinese medicine knows, the unity of spirit and body is a distinctive and central feature of Chinese medicine. The spirit is not something that "animates" a body. Instead, spirit and body are nothing but two different states of condensation and aggregation of Qi. Both spirit and body are manifestations of Qi, the spirit being the most rarefied form. Indeed, the presence of a Corporeal Soul (*Po*) in the Chinese view of the spirit confirms this; the Corporeal Soul is a "physical" soul responsible for all physiological processes.

For example, the commentary to Chapter 23 of the *Simple Questions*, which is based on passages from the *Spiritual Axis*, clearly expresses the unity of spirit and body when it says: "*The Mind [Shen] is a transformation of Essence and Qi; both Essences* [i.e. the Prenatal and Postnatal Essences] *contribute to forming the Mind.*"[7] See Figure 1.1.

Xi Kang, a Daoist philosopher (AD 223–262), said: "*Therefore the gentleman knows that the body depends on the spirit to stand, but the spirit requires the body to exist.*"[8] Thus, there is no question of a spirit being "trapped" in a body, as in Western philosophy; instead, the spirit itself is material, being simply an especially refined product of the same constituent of the body, i.e. Qi. The spirit and the body are nothing but two manifestations of aggregation of Qi; when Qi disperses, it is spirit; when it condenses, it is matter.

The same Daoist philosopher said:[9]

Although the spirit is a subtle thing, it certainly is still something that is transformed by Yin and Yang. With transformation it is born, and with another transformation it is dead. As it is brought together it begins, and as it disperses again it ends. The very fine and the very coarse are composed of the same Qi and, first and last, abide together.

Yang Quan, a Daoist philosopher of the third century AD, said:[10]

People contain Qi and so live. When their essence is exhausted, they die. It is like being drained dry or being extinguished. It may be compared to fire. When the fuel is exhausted and the fire is extinguished, there is no light. Therefore, in the remains of a fire that has been extinguished, there is no residual flame. After a man dies there is no residual spirit.

Yang Quan also wrote that "a stone is a lump of Qi" and so is a human being, as is the spirit.[11]

For thinkers of the Han dynasty, in other words, the spirit itself was merely an especially rarefied version of the same Qi that composed the body. Fan Chen, a later

Daoist thinker (AD 450–515) said that body and spirit are actually different facets of the same thing. Body is a word for its material substance and spirit is a word for its function, "like the sharpness of a knife". There is no question of one knife's sharpness surviving the destruction of its blade.[12]

Many of the ideas about the spirit and body being two manifestations of a state of rarefaction and condensation of Qi, respectively, derive from the Neo-Confucianist philosopher Zhang Zai (1020–1077). He discussed the condensation and dispersal of Qi at length, the former giving rise to matter and the latter to "spirit" (or non-material states of existence).

For Zhang Zai, Qi includes matter and the forces that govern interactions between matter, Yin and Yang. In its dispersed, rarefied state, Qi is invisible and insubstantial, but when it condenses it becomes a solid or liquid and takes on new properties. All material things are composed of condensed Qi; rocks, trees, human beings. Such ideas that we take for granted in Chinese medicine actually derived mostly from Zhang Zai.

Zhang believed that Qi is never created or destroyed; the same Qi goes through a continuous process of condensation and dispersion. He compared it to water; water in liquid form or frozen into ice is still the same water. Similarly, condensed Qi which forms things or dispersed Qi is still the same substance. Condensation is the Yin force of Qi and dispersion is the *yang* force.

Zhang Zai says:[13]

When Qi consolidates itself it has shape and becomes visible to our eyes. When Qi does not consolidate itself and has no shape, it will not be visible to the eye. After its consolidation it manifests itself in the external world. When it dissolves, can one say that it becomes nothingness?

The last sentence of this statement is dictated by Zhang's concern to rebut the Buddhist theory of Emptiness, as is also the following statement:[14]

The fact that Qi consolidates or disperses itself into the Void is just like ice consolidating or dissolving itself into water. If one knows that the Void consists of Qi one will find that there is no such thing as Emptiness.

What looks like creation and destruction is just the never-ending movements of Qi. These processes of condensation and dispersion have no outside cause; they are just part of the nature of Qi. Zhang wholly naturalized the workings of Qi and rejected any idea of an anthropomorphic Heaven that controlled things. While many Chinese thinkers talked of the workings of ghosts and spirits, he reinterpreted these terms to mean the extending and receding of Qi from and back to the Great Void. It is all a naturally occurring process.

To sum up, Western thinking is broadly dominated by "dualism", i.e. a fundamentally indeterminate, unconditioned power is posited as determining the essential meaning and order of the world. Ames says:[15]

It is a dualism because of the radical separation between the transcendent and non-dependent creative source, and the determinate and dependent object of its creation. The creative source does not require reference to its creature for explanation. This dualism, in many various forms, has been a prevailing force in the development of Western cosmogonies; supernatural/natural, reality/appearance, being/becoming, self/others, subject/object, mind/matter, form/matter, animate/inanimate and so forth.

Ames counterposes the Western dualism to the "polarism" of Chinese philosophy, i.e. a symbiosis and the unity of two (opposite) organismic processes, both of which require the other as a necessary condition for being what each is. Western dualism of mind/matter and spirit/body is replaced by the Chinese polarism in which two opposites are manifestations of the same process and depend on each other for their existence.

The main distinguishing feature of polarism is that each pole can be explained only by reference to the other; left requires right, up requires down, Yin requires Yang, spirit requires body, mind requires matter, self requires other.

Ames continues:[16]

The separateness implicit in dualistic explanations of relationships conduces to an essentialistic interpretation of the world, a world of 'things' characterized by discreteness, finality, closedness, determinateness, independence, a world in which one thing is related to the other extrinsically. By contrast, a polar explanation of relationships gives rise to an organismic interpretation of the world, a world of 'processes' characterized by interconnectedness, interdependence, openness, mutuality, indeterminateness, complementarity, correlativity, a world in which continuous processes are related to each other intrinsically.

The concept of "body" in China

Even the very concept of "body" is different in Western and Chinese philosophy. Interestingly, the etymology of the word "body" is from Old High German *botah* or *potah* which implies the idea of a "tub", "vat", "cask", i.e. a container. This is interesting as it highlights the Western dualism of spirit/body in which the body is a "container" (prison or temple, depending on the viewpoint) for the spirit which has an independent existence from it.

By contrast, in Chinese there are three terms for the body: *shen* 身, *xing* 形 and *ti* 体. Interestingly, the word *shen* (for "body") does not always simply indicate the body but instead often denotes one's entire psychosomatic person. Ames thinks it is not by chance that *shen* as "body" and *Shen* as "Mind" (of the Heart) are phonetically the same (although denoted by different characters). He thinks it suggestive that a person was seen as having correlative physical and spiritual aspects denoted by the above instances of *shen*.[17]

That the word *shen* refers to more than just a "body" is also highlighted by the fact that many Chinese expressions containing the word *shen* can be translated into English only by using words such as "person", "self" or "life". The following are some Chinese expressions containing the word *shen* with their English translations (first a literal one, then a contemporary one):[18]

- *an shen*: make one's body peaceful = "settle down in life"
- *chu shen*: put forth one's body = "start one's career"
- *shen fen*: one's body allocation = "personal status"
- *shen shi*: body's world = "one's lifetime experiences"
- *zhong shen*: to body's end = "to the end of one's life"
- *ben shen*: basic body = "oneself"
- *sui shen*: following the body = "on one's person".

The Soul in Chinese medicine

I use the word "soul" in relation to the Ethereal Soul and the Corporeal Soul and especially to the former. Indeed, most translations of the word "soul" in Chinese refer to the Ethereal Soul, e.g. *Hun*, *Hun-Po*, *Ling-Hun*, *Hun-Ling* or *Gui-Hun* (the last one indicating specifically the soul of a dead person).

As we have just seen, the Mind, and therefore the Heart, plays a pivotal and leading role in all mental activities. Yu Chang in *Principles of Medical Practice* (1658) says clearly: "*The Mind [Shen] of the Heart gathers and unites the Ethereal Soul [Hun] and the Corporeal Soul [Po] and it combines the Intellect [Yi] and the Will-Power [Zhi].*"[19] However, all other organs also take part in mental, emotional and spiritual activities, their roles very often overlapping with that of the Heart. In particular, the Yin organs are more directly responsible for mental activities. Each Yin organ "houses" a particular mental-spiritual aspect of a human being. These are:

- Mind (*Shen*) – Heart
- Ethereal Soul (*Hun*) – Liver
- Corporeal Soul (*Po*) – Lungs
- Intellect (*Yi*) – Spleen
- Will-Power (*Zhi*) – Kidneys.

The *Simple Questions* in Chapter 23 says: "*The Heart houses the Mind, the Lungs house the Corporeal Soul, the Liver houses the Ethereal Soul, the Spleen houses the Intellect and the Kidneys house the Will-Power.*"[20]

In Chapter 9 it says:[21]

The Heart is the root of life and the origin of the Mind ... the Lungs are the root of Qi and the dwelling of the Corporeal Soul ... the Kidneys are the root of sealed storage [Essence] and the dwelling of Will-Power ... the Liver is the root of harmonization and the residence of the Ethereal Soul.

The commentary to Chapter 23 of the *Simple Questions*, also based on passages from the *Spiritual Axis* (see Fig. 1.2) says:[22]

The Mind is a transformation of Essence and Qi; both Essences [i.e. the Prenatal and Postnatal Essences] contribute to forming the Mind. The Corporeal Soul is the assistant of the Essence and Qi; it is close to Essence but it moves in and out. The Ethereal Soul complements the Mind and Qi; it is close to the Mind but it comes and goes. The Intellect corresponds to memory; it is the memory which depends on the Heart. The Will-Power is like a purposeful and focused mind; the Kidneys store Essence ... and through the Will-Power they can fulfil our destiny.

These five aspects together form the "Spirit" which is also called *Shen* or sometimes the "Five *Shen*" in the old classics. The five Yin organs are the residences of *Shen*, i.e. the Spirit, and they are sometimes also called the "Five-*Shen* residences", as in Chapter 9 of the *Simple Questions*.[23]

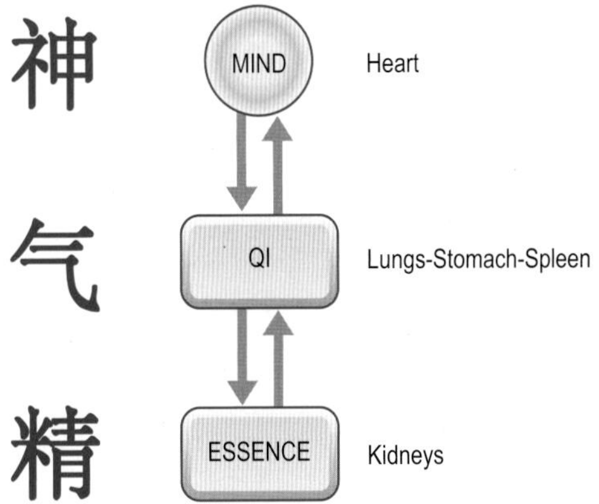

Figure 1.2 The Three Treasures (Essence, Qi, Mind).

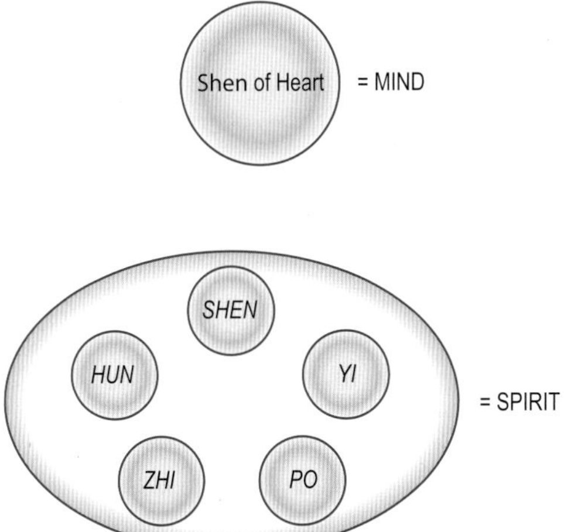

Figure 1.3 The two meanings of *Shen*.

As indicated above, I use the term "Mind" to indicate the *Shen* that resides in the Heart and is responsible for thinking, cognition, consciousness, self-identity, insight, emotions and memory, and the term "Spirit" to denote the *Shen* as the complex of all five mental-spiritual aspects of a human being, i.e. the Mind itself of the Heart, the Ethereal Soul (*Hun*) of the Liver, the Corporeal Soul (*Po*) of the Lungs, the Intellect (*Yi*) of the Spleen and the Will-Power (*Zhi*) of the Kidneys (Fig. 1.3).

The Mind and the Ethereal Soul are closely interrelated and are both Yang in nature; the Ethereal Soul is described as the "coming and going" of the Mind. The Corporeal Soul and the Essence (*Jing*) are closely interrelated. The Corporeal Soul is described as the "entering and exiting" of the Essence. The Intellect (*Yi*) resides in the Spleen and depends on Postnatal Qi (Fig. 1.4).

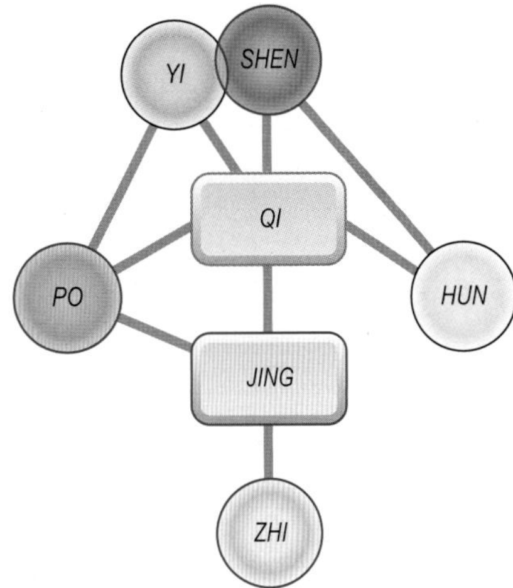

Figure 1.4 The landscape of the psyche in Chinese medicine.

The five Yin organs are the physiological basis of the Spirit. The indissoluble relationship between them is well known to any practitioner of Chinese medicine. The state of Qi and Blood of each organ can influence the Mind or Spirit and, conversely, alterations of the Mind or Spirit will affect one or more of the internal organs.

Of course, Western medicine recognizes the interrelationship between the mind and the body too, but its way of doing so differs from that of Chinese medicine. The Western view of the mind-body integration is essentially like a top-down pyramid from the mind to the body. In other words, emotional stimuli induce changes in the autonomic nervous system which will affect the viscera (Fig. 1.5).

By contrast, in Chinese medicine, there is a two-way interaction between the brain (or Mind of the Heart) and the viscera; emotional stimuli affecting the Mind may cause a disharmony of the viscera and, vice versa, a disharmony of the viscera may cause an emotional imbalance.

More importantly, Chinese medicine sees the body and the Mind (and the Spirit) as two poles of the same substance, i.e. Qi; the former is a very rarefied manifestation and the latter is a condensed version. Emotions also are at the same physical and psychic phenomena.

Interestingly, the James–Lange theory of emotions, developed at the beginning of the 20th century, presents some analogy with the Chinese view of body-mind.

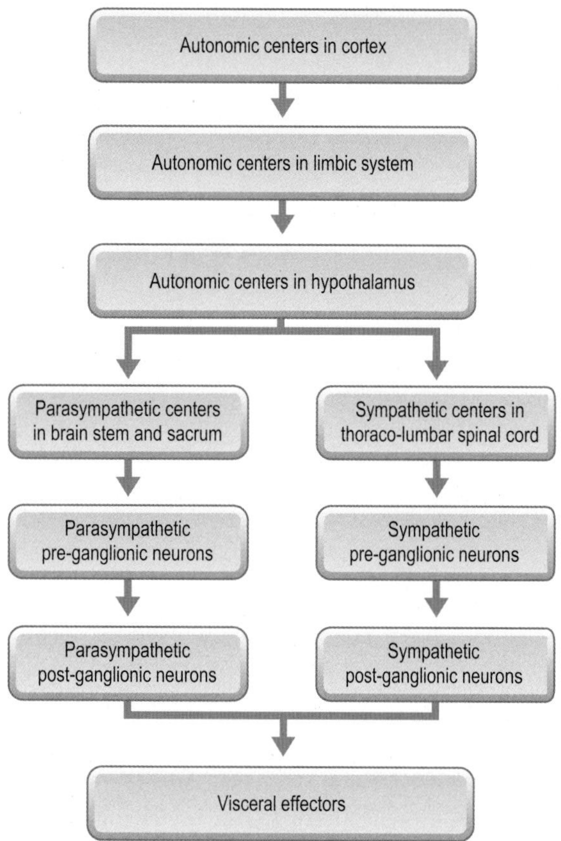

Figure 1.5 Influence of emotional stimuli on the viscera in Western physiology.

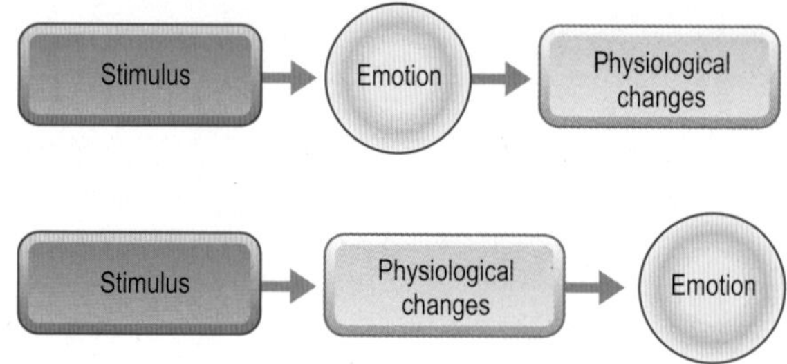

Figure 1.6 The James–Lange theory of emotions.

The James–Lange theory refers to a hypothesis on the origin and nature of emotions developed independently by two 19th-century researchers, William James and Carl Lange. The theory states that, in human beings, the autonomic nervous system creates physiological events such as muscular tension, a rise in heart rate, perspiration and dryness of the mouth as a response to experiences in the world.

Emotions are feelings that come about as a *result* of these physiological changes, rather than being their cause. James and Lange arrived at the theory independently. Lange specifically stated that vasomotor changes *are* emotions. This theory proposes that emotions happen *as a result* of these, rather than being the cause of them. Figure 1.6 illustrates the conventional view of emotions in the upper part and the James–Lange view in the lower part. The James–Lange theory of emotions is described more at length in Chapter 14.

The Mind (*Shen*) in Chinese medicine

The Mind (*Shen*) resides in the Heart and is responsible for consciousness, cognition, thinking and emotional life. A whole school of Neo-Confucian thought was dedicated to the Mind and this school became known as the "School of Mind" (*Xin Jia*), bearing in mind that all modern and ancient Chinese philosophers equate "Heart" (*Xin*) with Mind (*Shen*).

As explained below, the term *Shen* has many meanings but the two main ones in psychology are that it denotes both the *Shen* residing in the Heart, which I translate as "Mind", and the complex of Mind, Ethereal Soul (*Hun*), Corporeal Soul (*Po*), Intellect (*Yi*) and Will-Power (*Zhi*), which I translate as "Spirit".

Most sinologists translate the *Shen* of the Heart as "Mind". For example, Kim Yung Sik says: "*Zhu Xi did not concern himself with a description of the viscera. The only exception was the heart which he considered to be the site of the Mind.*"[24]

According to Zhang Zai and Zhu Xi, two Neo-Confucian philosophers of the Song dynasty, the Mind unites human nature (*xing*) and emotions (*qing*). The Mind is not the same as human nature but is the meeting of human nature and consciousness. Zhu Xi says: "*Human nature [xing] is the seat of consciousness; the Mind is that which has consciousness.*"[25] Thus, according to Zhu Xi, the Mind is endowed with consciousness and cognitive faculty.

Zhu Xi further clarifies the relationship between Mind, human nature and emotions:[26]

Human nature [xing] is the Principle [Li] of the Mind [xin]; emotions [qing] are the Mind in action. Human nature is passive, emotions are active and the Mind is both active and passive; the Mind is the most intellectual. The Mind is the controlling ruler.

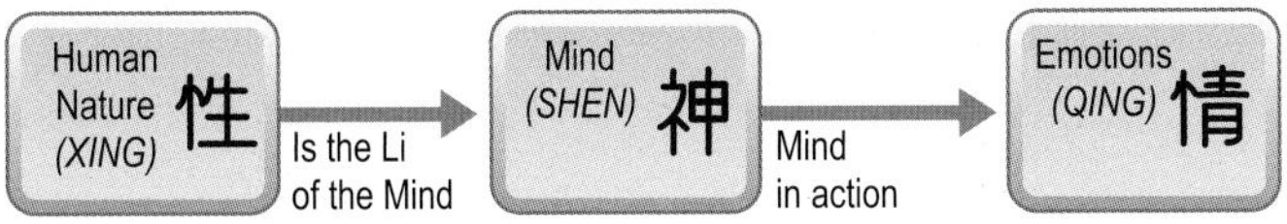

Human Nature (*XING*) 性 → Is the Li of the Mind → Mind (*SHEN*) 神 → Mind in action → Emotions (*QING*) 情

Figure 1.7 Relationship among Human Nature, Mind and emotions in the philosophy of Zhu Xi.

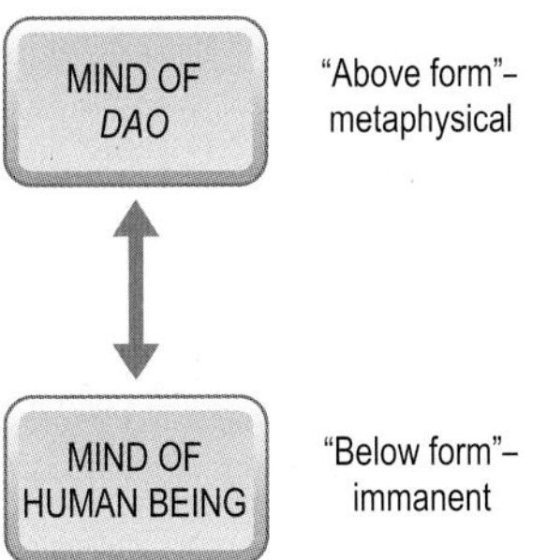

Figure 1.8 Relationship between Above-Form Mind and Below-Form Mind according to Zhu Xi.

The last sentence is interesting as it is clearly borrowed from Chinese medicine's view of the Heart as the monarch of the other 11 Internal Organs (Fig. 1.7).

Zhu Xi also described the Heart as the "organ that thinks"; he considered this to be the key function of the Mind. He believed that the thinking activity was continuous even during sleep (as in dreams). Wisdom and knowledge also come from the Mind. There are many passages in which Zhu Xi spoke of the Mind's role in perception.[27] Finally, he also said that the Mind rules humankind's nature, emotions and talent.[28]

> **!**
>
> Zhu Xi described the Heart as the "organ that thinks"; he considered this to be the key function of the Mind.

Zhu Xi also considered the Mind as the link between the metaphysical ("above form") and physical ("below form") worlds (Fig. 1.8). He said that the Mind, in its original state, is pure, transparent and has reality in itself; it belongs to the world of "above form" and is referred to as the Mind of the Dao. The other aspect of the Mind is the Mind of a human being or cognitive Mind which comes into contact with external things, responds to them and belongs to the realm of "below form".

The Confucian School of Mind even equated Mind with Principle (*Li*). Lu Xiang Shan (1139–1193) says:[29]

Mind and Principle are one in principle. Mind is one mind and Principle is one principle. Oneness pertains to them throughout, and even in their most subtle meaning, they contain no duality. This Mind and this Principle truly do not admit any dualism.

Meaning of the word *shen* in Chinese medicine

It is interesting to note that the word *shen* has multiple meanings in Chinese medicine, and that "Mind" or "Spirit" are only two of them. The following are further meanings (in addition to "Mind" or "Spirit") given to the word *shen* in the *Yellow Emperor's Classic of Internal Medicine*.

Unfathomable natural phenomena

The word *shen* is sometimes used to denote the changes and transformations of unfathomable natural phenomena. For example, Chapter 66 of the *Simple Questions* says: "*The beginning of things is called transformation; the development of things is called change; the unfathomable changes of Yin and Yang are called Shen.*"[30]

The physiological activities

The word *shen* is sometimes used to denote physiological activities. For example, Chapter 54 of the *Spiritual Axis* says: "*What is called Shen?* [*Shen* is the term used when] *Qi and Blood are harmonious; Nutritive and Defensive Qi circulate freely; the Five Yin Organs have been formed; the Mind resides in the Heart; the Ethereal and Corporeal Souls have been generated. Under these conditions a person is formed.*"[31] The same passage says earlier: "*When there is no Shen, there is death; when there is Shen, there is life.*"[32]

A condition of lustre in diagnosis

The word *shen* is frequently used in diagnosis to denote a condition of "lustre" or "flourishing". This is applied especially to the eyes and complexion but also to the tongue and pulse. For example, a complexion with *shen* has a lustrous appearance and looks flourishing even if it is pathological, e.g. a complexion may be pathologically red but this redness may be red with *shen* or red without *shen*. The presence of *shen* in diagnosis indicates a good prognosis.

Needling sensation

The word *shen* is sometimes used to denote the needling sensation. For example, Chapter 16 of the *Simple Questions* says: "*In Autumn needle the skin and the space between skin and muscles; stop when the needling sensation* [*shen*] *arrives.*"[33]

The doctor's skill

The word *shen* is sometimes used to denote the acupuncturist's skill. For example, Chapter 4 of the *Spiritual Axis* says: "*When pressing on a channel* [the doctor is capable of] *understanding the disease, this is called shen.*"[34]

A term for various vital substances

The word *shen* is often used to indicate various vital substances. For example, Chapter 26 of the *Simple Questions* says: "*The Qi of Blood is the shen of a person.*"[35] Chapter 32 of the *Spiritual Axis* says: "*Shen is the refined Qi of water and grains.*"[36]

Chapter 1 of the *Spiritual Axis* says: "*Shen is the Upright Qi* [*Zheng Qi*]."[37]

The spirit of a dead person

The word *shen* is sometimes used to denote the spirit or ghost of a dead person. For example, Chapter 25 of the *Simple Questions* says: "*The Dao has nothing to do with ghosts* [*gui-shen*]."[38] Incidentally, this passage is also interesting because it contains a critique of demonic medicine (i.e. the attributing of a disease's origin to an attack by evil spirits) and it upholds natural medicine. It says:[39]

If the treatment is given according to the laws of Heaven and Earth [i.e. natural laws] and it is modified with flexibility, a cure will follow the treatment like the shadow follows the body. The Dao has nothing to do with ghosts.

Mental illness in ancient Chinese medicine

The main categories of mental illness mentioned in the classics are as follows:

- *Bai He Bing* 百合病: Lilium Syndrome. This is mentioned in *Essential Prescriptions of the Golden Chest* (*Jin Gui Yao Lue Fang Lun*), Chapter 3-1[40]
- *Yu Zheng* 郁证 Depression
- *Mei He Qi* 梅核气: Plum-Stone Syndrome
- *Zang Zao* 脏燥: Agitation
- *Xin Ji Zheng Chong* 心悸怔忡: Palpitations and Anxiety
- *Dian Kuang* 癫狂: Manic-depression
- *Dian Xian* 癫痫: Epilepsy.

Lilium Syndrome (*Bai He Bing*)

The Lilium Syndrome (*Bai He Bing*) is described in the *Essential Prescriptions of the Golden Chest* (*Jin Gui Yao Lue*, c.AD 220), Chapter 3-1. This syndrome sounds remarkably like the description of a depressed patient. It says:[41]

The patient wants to eat, but is reluctant to swallow food and unwilling to speak. He or she wants to lie in bed but cannot lie quietly as he or she is restless. He or she wants to walk but is soon tired. Now and then he or she may enjoy eating but cannot tolerate the smell of food. He or she feels cold or hot but without fever or chills, bitter taste or dark urine [i.e. it is not external Wind or internal Heat]. No drugs are able to cure this syndrome. After taking the medicine the patient may vomit or have diarrhoea. The disease haunts the patient [hu huo; hu means "fox" and huo means "bewildered"] and, although he or she looks normal, he or she is suffering. The pulse is rapid.

Modern books describe the syndrome with the following symptoms: "as if in a trance" or "absent-minded" (*huang hu*), mental restlessness, bitter taste, dark urine, anxiety, depression, red tongue (which may be without coating), rapid pulse.

The treatment principle recommended by modern doctors is to moisten and nourish the Heart and Lungs, tonify Qi, nourish Yin, clear Heat (or Empty Heat), calm the Mind, strengthen the Will-Power (*Zhi*).

The formula recommended in the original text is Bai He Zhi Mu Tang *Lilium-Anemarrhena Decoction* composed of only Bai He *Bulbus Lilii* and Zhi Mu *Radix Anemarrhenae*.

SUMMARY

Lilium syndrome (*Bai He Bing*)

- The patient wants to eat, but is reluctant to swallow food.
- The patient is unwilling to speak.
- He or she wants to lie in bed but cannot lie quietly because of restlessness.
- He or she wants to walk but is soon tired.
- He or she cannot tolerate the smell of food.
- He or she feels cold or hot.
- Rapid pulse.

CLINICAL NOTE

Bai He (*Bulbus Lilii*) and Zhi Mu (*Radix Anemarrhenae*)

I use the combination of Bai He *Bulbus Lilii* and Zhi Mu *Radix Anemarrhenae* to treat Lilium Syndrome (*Bai He Bing*). In fact, I use these two herbs in any situation when a patient is depressed against a background of a Lung and Heart syndrome, but especially for Qi and Yin deficiency of these two organs or for Heart-Heat. The combination of these two herbs is particularly good to treat sadness and grief. In such cases, I frequently add these two herbs to whatever formula I am using.

Depression (*Yu Zheng*)

The Chinese term for depression is *Yu*. *Yu* has the double meaning of "depression" or "stagnation".

The *Simple Questions* in Chapter 71 talks about the five stagnations of Wood, Fire, Earth, Metal and Water. It says: "*When Wood stagnates it extends, when Fire stagnates it rises, when Earth stagnates it seizes, when Metal stagnates it discharges, when Water stagnates it pours.*"[42]

The *Essential Method of Dan Xi* (*Dan Xi Xin Fa*, 1347) talks about six stagnations of Qi, Blood, Dampness, Phlegm, Heat and Food. It says:[43]

When Qi and Blood are harmonized, no disease arises. If they stagnate diseases arise. Many diseases are due to stagnation. Stagnation makes things accumulate so that they would like to descend but cannot, they would like to transform but cannot ... thus the six stagnations come into being.

The *Complete Book of Jing Yue* (*Jing Yue Quan Shu*, 1624) gives it an emotional interpretation and talks about six stagnations of anger, pensiveness, worry, sadness, shock and fear. This confirms that all emotions can lead to stagnation of Qi. He said: "*In the six stagnations, stagnation is the cause of the disease. In emotional stagnation, the disease* [i.e. the emotion] *is the cause of the stagnation.*"[44]

Depression is discussed in Chapter 16. The formula for depression recommended by Zhu Dan Xi is Yue Ju Wan *Gardenia-Chuanxiong Pill*.

Plum-Stone Syndrome (*Mei He Qi*)

Plum-Stone Syndrome was first described in the chapter *Pulse, Syndromes and Treatment of Miscellaneous Gynecological Diseases* of the *Essential Prescriptions of the Golden Chest* (*Jin Gui Yao Lue*, c.AD 220). This text says: "*The patient has a suffocating feeling as if there was a piece of roast meat stuck in the throat. Use Ban Xia Hou Po Tang.*"[45]

It can be seen from the above statement that the symptom of Plum-Stone Syndrome was originally compared to the feeling of having a piece of meat (rather than a plum stone) stuck in the throat. The etiology of this syndrome is emotional and is due to depression.

Subsequent Chinese books attributed this syndrome to the combination of Qi stagnation and Phlegm obstructing the throat. This type of Phlegm is actually called Qi-Phlegm and it is the most non-substantial type of Phlegm.

Although modern books relate the Plum-Stone Syndrome to Liver-Qi stagnation, the original text related to the Qi stagnation of the Lungs and Stomach. The formula recommended by the original text is Ban Xia Hou Po Tang *Pinellia-Magnolia Decoction*.

Agitation (*Zang Zao*)

Zang Zao, literally meaning "visceral restlessness", was first mentioned in the chapter *Pulse, Syndromes and Treatment of Miscellaneous Gynecological Diseases* of the

Essential Prescriptions of the Golden Chest (*Jin Gui Yao Lue*, c.AD 220). This text says:[46]

The patient suffers from Agitation [Zang Zao], feels sad and tends to weep constantly as if she were haunted. She stretches frequently and yawns repeatedly. The decoction of Fu Xiao Mai, Zhi Gan Cao and Da Zao can calm the patient.

The formula for Agitation (*Zang Zao*) is Gan Mai Da Zao Tang *Glycyrrhiza-Triticum-Jujuba Decoction*. Agitation is discussed in Chapter 17.

Palpitations and Anxiety (*Xin Ji Zheng Chong*)

The condition called "Palpitations and Anxiety" corresponds to two separate Chinese disease entities, i.e. *Xin Ji* (which is more often called *Jing Ji* in modern Chinese medicine) and *Zheng Chong*. Both *Jing Ji* (or *Xin Ji*) and *Zheng Chong* involve a state of fear, worry and anxiety, the first with palpitations and the second with a throbbing sensation in the chest and below the umbilicus. *Jing Ji* is usually caused by external events such as a fright or shock and it comes and goes; it is more frequently of a Full nature.

Zheng Chong is not caused by external events and it is continuous; this condition is usually of an Empty nature and is more serious than the first. In chronic cases, *Jing Ji* may turn into *Zheng Chong*. In severe cases, *Zheng Chong* may correspond to panic attacks. Despite the fact that the name *Jing Ji* means "fear and palpitations", such states of fear and anxiety may occur without palpitations.

Palpitations and Anxiety are discussed in Chapter 17.

Manic-depression (*Dian Kuang*)

Bipolar disorder follows closely the symptoms of the ancient Chinese disease of *Dian Kuang* which may be translated as "dullness and raving" or "dullness and mania":

- *Dian* indicates a depressive state, indifference, being withdrawn, worry, quietness, unresponsiveness, incoherent speech, inappropriate laughter, taciturnity
- *Kuang* indicates agitation, shouting, scolding and hitting people, irritability, aggressive behavior, offensive speech, inappropriate laughter, singing, climbing high places, wild behavior, smashing objects, unusual physical strength, refusing sleep and food.

Dian Kuang is discussed in Chapter 19. As explained in this chapter, *Dian Kuang* does not necessarily correspond exactly to bipolar disorder.

Epilepsy (*Dian Xian*)

Epilepsy has been discussed in Chinese medicine since very early times and it is mentioned in the *Yellow Emperor's Classic of Internal Medicine*. In ancient times, epilepsy was wrongly included among mental illnesses.

END NOTES

1. Oxford English Dictionary CD-ROM, 2nd edn. Oxford University Press, Oxford.
2. Battaglia F et al 1957 Encyclopedia Filosofica. Casa Editrice Sansoni, Firenze, p. 895.
3. Ibid., p. 898.
4. Ibid., p. 898.
5. Russell B 2002 History of Western Philosophy. Routledge, London, p. 702.
6. Ibid., p. 707.
7. 1979 Huang Di Nei Jing Su Wen 黄帝内经素问 [The Yellow Emperor's Classic of Internal Medicine – Simple Questions]. People's Health Publishing House, Beijing, p. 153. First published c.100 BC.
8. Holcombe C 1994 In the Shadow of the Han. University of Hawaii, Honolulu, p. 100.
9. Ibid., p. 100.
10. Ibid., p. 100.
11. Ibid., p. 101.
12. Ibid., p. 101.
13. Chang C 1977 The Development of Neo-Confucian Thought. Greenwood Press Publishers, Westport, Connecticut, p. 172.
14. Ibid., pp. 172–173.
15. Kasulis TP, Ames RT, Dissanayke W 1993 Self as Body in Asian Theory and Practice. State University of New York Press, New York, p. 159.
16. Ibid., p. 160.
17. Ibid., p. 165.
18. Ibid., pp. 219–220.
19. Yu Chang 1658 Yi Men Fa Lu [Principles of Medical Practice], cited in Wang Ke Qin 1988 Zhong Yi Shen Zhu Xue Shuo 中医神主学说 [Theory of the Mind in Chinese Medicine]. Ancient Chinese Medical Texts Publishing House, Beijing, p. 39.
20. Simple Questions, p. 153.
21. Ibid., pp. 67–68.
22. Ibid., p. 153.
23. Ibid., p. 63.
24. Kim Yung Sik 2000 The Natural Philosophy of Chu Hsi. American Philosophical Society, Philadelphia, p. 211.
25. Huang Siu-chi 1999 Essentials of Neo-Confucianism. Greenwood Press, Westport, Connecticut, p. 137.
26. Ibid., p. 150.
27. The Natural Philosophy of Chu Hsi, p. 213.
28. Essentials of Neo-Confucianism, p. 214.
29. Ibid., p. 174.
30. Simple Questions, p. 361.

31. Tian Dai Hua 2005 Ling Shu Jing 灵枢经 [Spiritual Axis]. People's Health Publishing House, Beijing, p. 110. First published *c.*100 BC.
32. Ibid., p. 110.
33. Simple Questions, p. 92.
34. Spiritual Axis, p. 12.
35. Simple Questions, p. 168.
36. Spiritual Axis, p. 77.
37. Ibid., p. 3.
38. Simple Questions, p. 162.
39. Ibid., p. 162.
40. 1981 Jin Gui Yao Lue Fang Xin Jie 金匮要略方新解[A New Explanation of the Essential Prescriptions of the Golden Chest]. Zhejiang Scientific Publishing House, Zhejiang, pp. 24–26. The *Essential Prescriptions of the Golden Chest* was written by Zhang Zhong Jing and first published *c.*AD 220.
41. Ibid., p. 26.
42. Simple Questions, pp. 501–502.
43. Cited in Zhang Bo Yu 1986 Zhong Yi Nei Ke Xue 中医内科学 [Chinese Internal Medicine]. Shanghai Science Publishing House, Shanghai, p. 121.
44. Ibid., p. 121.
45. A New Explanation of the Essential Prescriptions of the Golden Chest, p. 185.
46. Ibid., p. 185.

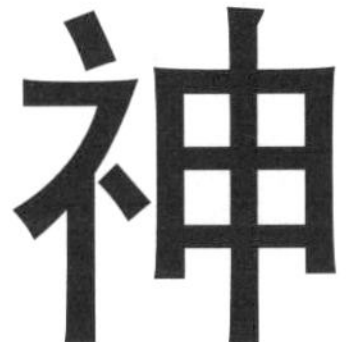

CHAPTER 2

THE NATURE OF THE MIND (*SHEN*) IN CHINESE MEDICINE

THE NATURE OF THE MIND (*SHEN*) IN CHINESE MEDICINE *15*

Terminology *15*

Chinese characters for *Shen* *16*

Nature of the Mind and of the "Three Treasures" *16*

Functions of the Mind *18*

The Mind and the senses *20*

Coordinating and integrating function of the Mind *21*

"MIND" VERSUS "SPIRIT" AS A TRANSLATION OF *SHEN* *22*

CLINICAL APPLICATION *23*

THE NATURE OF THE MIND (*SHEN*) IN CHINESE MEDICINE

This chapter will be discussed according to the following topics.

- The nature of the Mind (*Shen*) in Chinese medicine
- "Mind" versus "Spirit" as a translation of *Shen*
- Clinical application

THE NATURE OF THE MIND (*SHEN*) IN CHINESE MEDICINE

The Mind (*Shen*) is one of the vital substances of the body. It is the most subtle and non-material type of Qi.

Terminology

Most authors translate the word *Shen* as "spirit"; for reasons which will be clearer as the discussion progresses, I prefer to translate *Shen* of the Heart as "Mind" rather than as "Spirit". I translate as "Spirit" the complex of all five mental-spiritual aspects of a human being, i.e. the Ethereal Soul (*Hun*), the Corporeal Soul (*Po*), the Intellect (*Yi*), the Will-Power (*Zhi*) and the Mind (*Shen*) itself. In the ancient classics, these five are sometimes called the "Five *Shen*".

Strictly speaking, even the translation of *Shen* as "Mind" is not completely accurate because Mind is not the same as consciousness and the *Shen* could be more appropriately called "Consciousness". Damasio says:[1]

Consciousness and mind are not synonymous. In the strict sense, consciousness is the process whereby a mind is imbued with a reference we call self, and is said to know of its own existence and the existence of objects around it. In certain neurological conditions there is evidence that the mind process continues but consciousness is impaired.

Chapter 54 of the *Spiritual Axis* clearly shows how the term *Shen* can refer both to the Mind residing in the Heart or to the complex of the five mental-spiritual aspects:[2]

The mother provides the foundation, the father the fertilization. If there is no Shen there is death; if there is Shen, there is life. When Blood and Qi are harmonized, the Nutritive and Defensive Qi communicating, the five viscera are complete, the Mind [Shen] is housed in the Heart, the Ethereal and Corporeal Soul are complete, then a human being is formed.

In this passage, the first reference to *Shen* is to be interpreted as the "spirit" and the second as the "mind".

All sinologists who write about the Confucian and Neo-Confucian philosophers of the Song and Ming dynasty translate "School of *Xin*" as "School of Mind", i.e. they translate the word *Xin* (meaning Heart) as "Mind". Lau and Ames also translate *Xin* as "Mind", illustrating the close connection between the Heart and the "Mind" rather than "Spirit". They say:[3]

Xin, normally translated as 'heart-mind', precludes the assumption of distinctions between thinking and feeling, or idea and affect. Xin is perhaps most frequently translated simply as 'heart', but since it is the seat of thinking and judgement, the notion of Mind must be included in its characterization if the term is to be properly understood. Indeed the functional equivalent of what we often think of as 'purpose' or 'intention' is also to be included in the notion of Xin.

Rosemont says:[4]

The term Xin [heart] has often been translated as 'mind'. There is much justification for this, because a number of passages in the texts can only be rendered intelligible on the basis of the xin thinking.

The word *Shen* is used in the *Yellow Emperor's Classic of Internal Medicine* with many different meanings. The two main meanings which concern us are the following:

1. *Shen* indicates the activity of thinking, consciousness, self-identity, insight and memory, all of which depend on and "reside" in the Heart. I translate this as "Mind".
2. *Shen* indicates the complex of all five mental-spiritual aspects of a human being, i.e. the Mind itself of the Heart, the Ethereal Soul (*Hun*) of the Liver, the Corporeal Soul (*Po*) of the Lungs, the Intellect (*Yi*) of the Spleen and the Will-Power (*Zhi*) of the Kidneys. I translate this as "Spirit".

There is another meaning to the word *Shen* which is frequently mentioned in relation to diagnosis. In this context the word *shen* indicates an indefinable and subtle quality of "life", "flourishing" or "lustre" which can be observed in health. This quality can be observed in the complexion, the eyes, the tongue and the pulse, as will be explained in Chapter 11.

Chinese characters for *Shen*

The Chinese character for *Shen* 神 is composed of two parts. The left-hand part of the character, called *shi* 示, indicates "influx from heaven; auspicious or inauspicious signs by which the will of Heaven is known to mankind"; this character is itself composed of two horizontal lines at the top indicating what is above, high

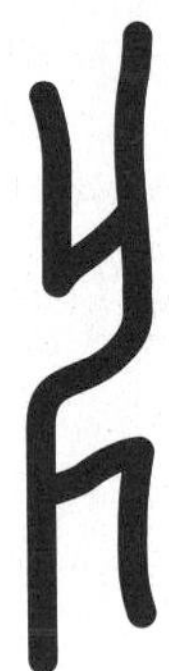

Figure 2.1 Ancient Chinese script for *shi*.

and therefore Heaven, and three vertical lines representing what is hanging from Heaven, i.e. the sun, the moon and the stars, the mutations of which reveal to people transcendent things.

The right-hand part of the character is the word *shen* 申 meaning "to state, to express, to explain, to stretch, to extend". As we shall see later, the quality of "extending" has an important psychological implication in the life of the Mind (*Shen*). This part of the character, called *shen*, is also phonetic, i.e. it gives the word its sound ("shen").

The ancient seal writing shows two hands stretching a rope and hence the idea of stretching, expansion (Fig. 2.1). The combination is probably phonetic but the idea of spirit may have some connection with an increased or extended spiritual revelation.

The combination of the radical *shi* with that of *shen* therefore indicates that the *Shen* of the Heart is a subtle form of Qi, something spiritual, an immaterial quality that "extends" towards others.

> **!**
>
> The Chinese character for *Shen* (Mind) conveys two ideas: "spiritual manifestation" and "to extend", "to stretch". It is therefore a pure and subtle Vital Substance that "extends" outwards towards others and mediates the relationship between the individual and other people.

Nature of the Mind and of the "Three Treasures"

What is then the Chinese view of the Mind? As explained above, the Mind, like other vital substances,

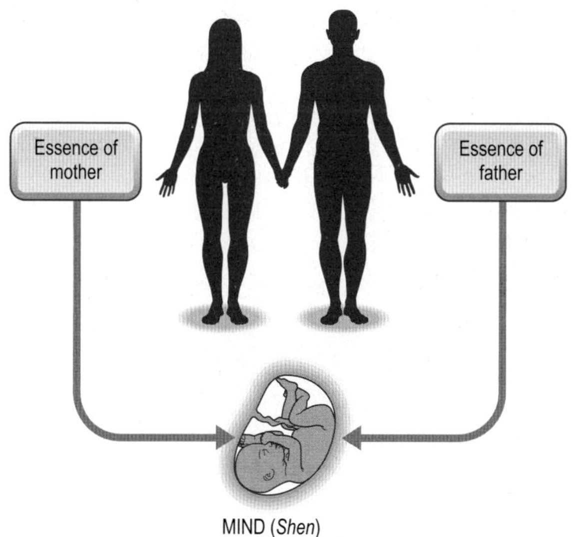

Figure 2.2 Union of Essences to form Mind.

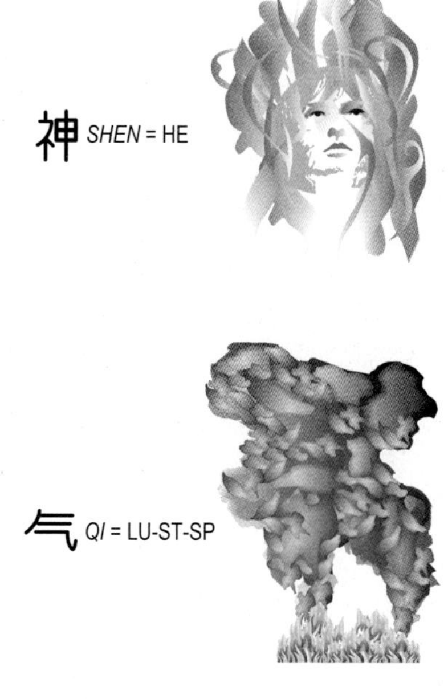

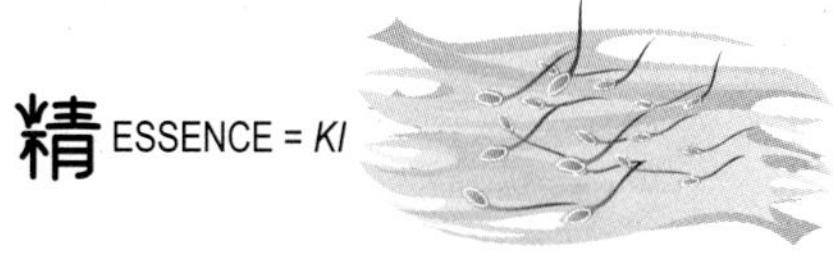

Figure 2.3 The Three Treasures (Essence, Qi, Mind).

is a form of Qi; in fact, the most subtle and non-material type of Qi. One of the most important characteristics of Chinese medicine is the close integration of body and Mind which is highlighted by the integration of the three Vital Substances of Essence (*Jing*), Qi and Mind (*Shen*), called the "Three Treasures".

The Essence is the origin and biological basis of the Mind. The *Spiritual Axis* says in Chapter 8: "*Life comes about through the Essence; when the two Essences* [of mother and father] *unite, they form the Mind.*"[5] Zhang Jie Bin says: "*The two Essences, one Yin, one Yang, unite to form life; the Essences of mother and father unite to form the Mind.*"[6] See Figure 2.2.

The Prenatal Essences of the mother and father combine to produce the Mind of a newly conceived being. After birth, its Prenatal Essence is stored in the Kidneys and it provides the biological foundation for the Mind. The life and Mind of a newborn baby, however, also depend on the nourishment from its own Postnatal Essence.

The *Spiritual Axis* in Chapter 30 says:[7]

> *When the Stomach and Intestines are coordinated, the five Yin organs are peaceful, Blood is harmonized and mental activity is stable. The Mind derives from the refined essence of water and food.*

Thus the Mind draws its biological basis and nourishment from the Prenatal Essence stored in the Kidneys and the Postnatal Essence produced by Lungs, Stomach and Spleen. Hence the Three Treasures (Fig. 2.3):

Mind (*Shen*) = HEART

Qi = Lungs-Stomach-Spleen

Essence (*Jing*) = Kidneys.

These Three Treasures represent three different states of condensation or aggregation of Qi, the Essence being the densest, Qi more rarefied, and the Mind the most subtle and non-material. The activity of the Mind relies on the Essence and Qi as its fundamental basis. Hence the Essence is said to be the "foundation of the body and the root of the Mind".

Thus, if Essence and Qi are strong and flourishing, the Mind will be happy, balanced and alert; if Essence and Qi are depleted, the Mind will suffer and may become unhappy, depressed, anxious or clouded. Zhang Jie Bin says: "*If the Essence is strong, Qi flourishes; if Qi flourishes, the Mind is whole.*"[8]

However, the state of the Mind in turn affects Qi and Essence. If the Mind is disturbed by emotional stress, becoming unhappy, depressed, anxious or unstable, it will definitely affect Qi and/or the Essence. Since all emotional stress upsets the normal functioning of Qi, in most cases it will affect Qi first. Emotional stress will tend to weaken the Essence, either when it is combined with overwork and/or excessive sexual activity, or when the Fire generated by long-term emotional tensions injures Yin and Essence.

The mutual interaction among Essence, Qi and Mind is a defining aspect of the Chinese view of the body and mind, in that bodily imbalances affect the Mind and mental-emotional stress of the Mind produces bodily pathology.

CLINICAL NOTE

The Three Treasures

The Essence (*Jing*), Qi and Mind (*Shen*) interact with and influence each other in both directions, i.e. from the Essence to Qi and the Mind, and from the Mind to Qi and the Essence.

Functions of the Mind

Of all the organs, the Mind is most closely related to the Heart, which is said to be its "residence". The *Simple Questions* in Chapter 8 says: "*The Heart is the Monarch and it governs the Mind ...*"[9] The *Spiritual Axis* in Chapter 71 says: "*The Heart is the Monarch of the five Yin organs and six Yang organs and it is the residence of the Mind.*"[10]

The "Mind" residing in the Heart or Heart-Mind is responsible for many different mental activities including:

- thinking
- memory
- consciousness
- insight
- emotional life
- cognition
- sleep
- intelligence
- wisdom
- ideas.

In addition to these, the Mind of the Heart is also responsible for hearing, sight, touch, taste and smell. Of course many of the above activities are also carried out by other organs and there is often an overlap between the functions of various organs. For example, although the Mind is mainly responsible for memory, the Spleen and Kidneys (and therefore Intellect and Will-Power) also play a role.

CLINICAL NOTE

In order to stimulate the thinking function that is associated with the Heart, I use the points HE-5 Tongli and BL-15 Xinshu.

Let us now briefly look at the above functions in more detail.

Thinking

Thinking depends on the Mind. If the Mind is strong, thinking will be clear. If the Mind is weak or disturbed, thinking will be slow and dull. The Chinese characters for "thought" (*yi*), "to think" (*xiang*) and "pensiveness" (*si*) all have the character for "heart" as their radical.

Memory

Memory has two different meanings. On the one hand it indicates the capacity of memorizing data when one is studying or working. On the other hand, it refers to the ability to remember past events. Both of these depend on the Mind and therefore on the Heart, although also on the Spleen and Kidneys.

Modern neuroscience distinguishes between *explicit* and *implicit* memory. Explicit memory is responsible for remembering past events and facts. In other words, remembering what we did 2 months ago depends on extrinsic memory, and so does remembering the location of acupuncture points when we study acupuncture. Explicit memory of past events depends on both the Heart (Mind) and Kidneys (Memory); explicit memory of facts depends primarily on the Spleen.

Implicit memory is the one that allows us to remember how to knit, ride a bike or play the piano even after years of not performing those acts. This means that the neural record describing how to knit or ride a bike must be stored differently from the event memory. While explicit memory serves itself up for conscious reflec-

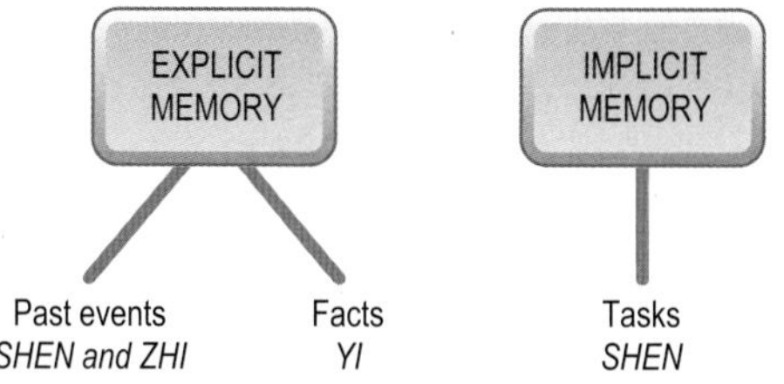

Figure 2.4 Explicit and implicit memory in Chinese medicine.

tion, implicit memory does not.[11] Implicit memory depends primarily on the Mind (*Shen*) and therefore the Heart (Fig. 2.4).

Consciousness

Consciousness indicates the totality of thoughts and perceptions as well as the state of being conscious. In the first sense, the Mind is responsible for the recognition of thoughts, perceptions and feelings. In the latter sense, when the Mind is clear, we are conscious; if the Mind is obfuscated or suddenly depleted, we lose consciousness.

In a broader sense, when the Mind is obstructed, consciousness is affected not in the sense that we lose consciousness but that we may have irrational thoughts. In extreme degrees, obstruction of the Mind exists in mental illness; however, obstruction of the Mind may also exist in milder degrees, manifesting, for example, with phobias, obsessive thoughts, or panic attacks with an irrational fear of death.

Insight

Insight indicates our capacity of self-knowledge, self-recognition and identity of self. I am not using the word "insight" here in the normal everyday sense of the word, which describes the power of perception, of seeing through a surface to what lies behind it. In psychiatry, "insight" is responsible for our identity of self as individuals. This is lost in serious mental illness such as schizophrenia. In psychiatry, insight also refers to the patient's awareness of being ill in a mental or emotional sphere. A person with insight appreciates that a personal experience (a symptom) is not normal, seeks help from a formal source that can identify an illness producing the experience, appreciates the need for a treatment plan for this illness and complies with an agreed treatment plan. Birchwood distinguishes three components to insight: awareness of illness, need for treatment, and attribution of symptoms.[12]

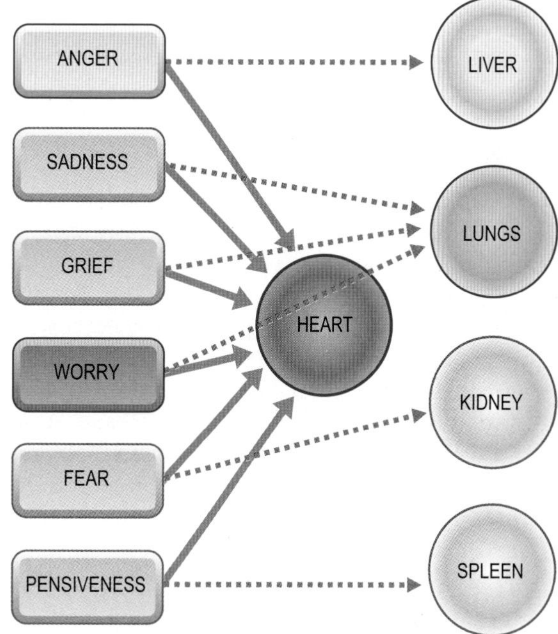

Figure 2.5 Affliction of the Heart by all emotions.

Emotional life

Emotional life refers to the perception and feeling of emotional stimuli. With regard to emotions, only the Mind (and therefore the Heart) can "feel" them. Of course, emotions definitely affect all the other organs too, but it is only the Mind that actually recognizes, feels and assesses them. For example, anger affects the Liver, but the Liver cannot feel it because it does not house the Mind. Only the Heart can feel it because it houses the Mind which is responsible for insight. When one feels sad, angry or worried, it is the Mind of the Heart that feels these emotions (Fig. 2.5).

It is for this reason that all emotions eventually affect the Heart (in addition to other specific organs), and it is in this sense that the Heart is the "emperor" of all the other organs. It is for this reason that a red tip of the tongue is such a common occurrence in practice: any emotion can lead to a red tip of the tongue because the tip reflects the condition of the Heart and all emotions affect the Heart.

CLINICAL NOTE

Only the Mind (and therefore the Heart) can "feel" the emotions. Each emotion affects one or more organs but it is only the Mind that actually recognizes, feels and assesses them.

It is for this reason that all emotions eventually affect the Heart (in addition to other specific organs), and it is in this sense that the Heart is the "emperor" of all the other organs.

Emotions usually tend to cause some Heat, and this is the reason why a red tip of the tongue is such a common sign as all emotions affect the Heart.

The best point to treat when the Heart is affected by emotional stress is HE-7 Shenmen.

Cognition

Cognition indicates the activity of the Mind in perceiving and conceiving, in reaction to stimuli.

Sleep

Sleep is dependent on the state of the Mind. If the Mind is calm and balanced, a person sleeps well. If the Mind is restless, the person sleeps badly. However, the Ethereal Soul of the Liver is also responsible for sleep.

Intelligence

Intelligence also depends on the Heart and the Mind. A strong Heart and Mind will make a person intelligent and bright. A weak Heart and Mind will render a person slow and dull. It should be remembered, however, that the Essence, and therefore heredity, plays a role in determining a person's intelligence. However, intelligence depends also on the Intellect of the Spleen.

Wisdom

Wisdom derives from a strong Heart and a healthy Mind. As the Mind is responsible for knowing and perceiving, it also gives us the sagacity to apply this knowledge critically and wisely.

Ideas

Ideas are another function of the Mind. The Heart and Mind are responsible for our ideas, our projects and the dreams which give our lives purpose. However, the Ethereal Soul plays a crucial role in this area in providing the Heart with ideas in the sense of life dreams. Moreover, the Intellect of the Spleen is also responsible for ideas but in a sense that differs from that of the Ethereal Soul: the Spleen is responsible more for specific ideas in one's field of work or study rather than "ideas" in the sense of life dreams.

Thus, if the Heart is strong and the Mind healthy, a person can think clearly, memory is good, the state of consciousness and the insight are sharp, the cognition is clear, sleep is sound, intelligence is bright, the emotional life is balanced, ideas flow easily and he or she acts wisely. If the Heart is affected and the Mind weak or disturbed, a person is unable to think clearly, memory is poor, the consciousness is clouded, insight is poor, cognition is hazy, sleep is restless, intelligence is lacking, the emotional life is unbalanced, ideas are muddled and he or she acts unwisely.

The Mind and the senses

The Mind of the Heart is also responsible for all senses in coordination with the relevant organs. For example, the Liver influences the eyes and sight, but sight also needs the input of the Mind. The following is an overview of how the Mind of the Heart controls the senses.

Eyesight

The eyes and sight are obviously related to the Liver, especially Liver-Blood, and the Ethereal Soul. The book *The Essence of Medical Classics on the Convergence of Chinese and Western Medicine* (1892) says: "*When the Ethereal Soul swims to the eyes they can see.*"[13] However, although the eyes rely on the nourishment from Liver-Blood, blood flows to the eyes through blood vessels which are under the control of the Heart. On the other hand, the Mind "gathers" the Ethereal Soul and, in this way, it has an influence on sight.

The *Simple Questions* says in Chapter 10: "*Blood vessels influence the eyes.*"[14] It should be noted here that when the *Simple Questions* or *Spiritual Axis* refers to one of the five tissues (skin, muscles, sinews, blood vessels and bones), sometime these are code words for the Internal Organs (Lungs, Spleen, Liver, Heart and Kidneys, respectively).

In fact, the *Simple Questions* also lists excessive use of the eyes as harmful to the blood vessels and Heart. It says in Chapter 23: "*Excessive use of the eyes injures Blood* [i.e. the Heart]."[15] Ren Ying Qiu in *Theories of Chinese Medicine Doctors* says: "*The Heart governs the Mind ... sight is a manifestation of the activity of the Mind.*"[16] Wang Ken Tang in *Standards of Diagnosis and Treatment* (1602) says: "*The eye is an orifice of the Liver ... but a function of the Heart.*"[17]

From the point of view of channels, both the Heart Main and the Heart Connecting (*Luo*) channels flow to the eye.

Hearing

Hearing depends on the Kidneys but the Heart also has an influence on it in so far as it brings Qi and Blood to the ears. The *Simple Questions* in Chapter 4 says: "*The color of the Southern direction is red; it is related to the Heart which opens into the ears.*"[18] Some types of tinnitus are due to Heart-Qi's being deficient and not reaching the ears.

Smell

The sense of smell is also dependent on the Heart and Mind besides the Lungs. The *Simple Questions* in Chapter 11 says: "*The five odours enter the nose and are stored by Lungs and Heart; if Lungs and Heart are diseased, the nose cannot smell.*"[19]

Taste

The sense of taste naturally depends on the Heart and Mind as the tongue is an offshoot of the Heart.

Touch

The sense of touch is also dependent on the Heart and Mind as this is responsible for the cognition and organization of external stimuli sensations. However, the Corporeal Soul plays an important role in the sense of touch.

To sum up, all sensations of sight, hearing, smell, taste and touch depend on the Mind in much the same way as they depend on the brain in Western medicine. Most of the above functions of the Mind are attributed to the brain in Western medicine. During the course of development of Chinese medicine too, there have been doctors who attributed mental functions to the brain rather than the Heart: in particular, Sun Si Miao of the Tang dynasty, Zhao You Qin of the Yuan dynasty, Li Shi Zhen of the Ming dynasty and especially Wang Qing Ren of the Qing dynasty.

Coordinating and integrating function of the Mind

Finally, the Mind of the Heart performs the very important function of *coordinating* and *integrating* the various parts of our mental-emotional life into an individual whole: this is probably its most important characteristic and function. It is really in this sense that the Heart is the "emperor" or "monarch" of the other organs. The Mind of the Heart needs to integrate, coordinate and somewhat control the psychic influence of the other four mental-spiritual aspects of the Organs, i.e. the Ethereal Soul, the Corporeal Soul, the Intellect and the Will-Power (Fig. 2.6).

As the Heart controls all mental activities of the Mind and is responsible for insight and cognition, which other organs do not have, this is another reason why it is the "emperor" of all the other organs. For this reason, the Heart is also called the "root of life" as in Chapter 9 of the *Simple Questions*: "*The Heart is the root of life and the origin of mental life.*"[20]

Therefore, the Mind (*Shen*) of the Heart is the Qi that performs the following functions. It:

- forms life from the union of the Essence of the parents (but life needs also the Corporeal and Ethereal Souls)
- allows the individual to be conscious of his or her self
- permits the cohesion of various parts of our psyche and emotions
- defines us as individuals
- feels and assesses the emotions
- is responsible for perceptions and senses

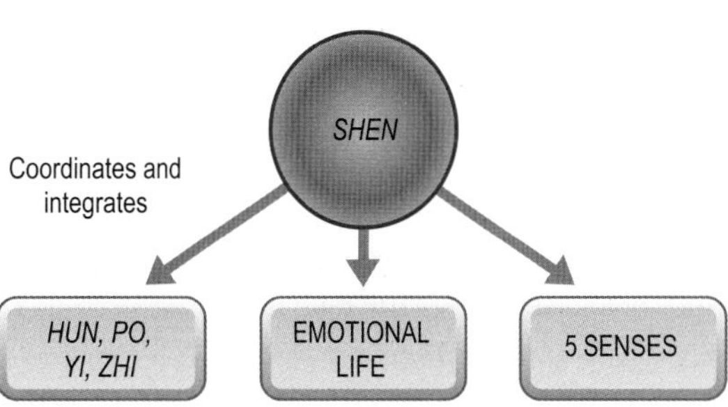

Figure 2.6 The coordinating and integrating function of the Mind (*Shen*).

- is responsible for thinking, memory, intelligence, wisdom, ideas
- determines consciousness
- allows insight and identity of self
- is responsible for cognition
- influences sleep
- governs the five senses (sight, hearing, smelling, taste, touch).

SUMMARY

The nature of the Mind (*Shen*) in Chinese medicine

- I translate the *Shen* of the Heart as "Mind" rather than Spirit.
- The Chinese character for *Shen* implies the idea of "extending, projecting outwards, expressing".
- The Mind is the most subtle and refined Vital Substance of the Three Treasures, i.e. Essence (*Jing*), Qi and Mind (*Shen*). The Essence, Qi and Mind interact with and influence each other.
- The Mind is responsible for thinking, memory, consciousness, insight, emotional life, cognition, sleep, intelligence, wisdom and ideation.
- The Mind is responsible for sight, hearing, smell, taste and touch.
- The Mind is responsible for self-consciousness and the integration of various parts of our psyche.

"MIND" VERSUS "SPIRIT" AS A TRANSLATION OF *SHEN*

The translation of *Shen* as "Mind" rather than "Spirit" has repercussions beyond pure semantics. As we have seen, the *Shen* functions of memory, thinking, emotions and consciousness are typically those of the Mind. "Spirit" has a much broader meaning than Mind and it includes metaphysical aspects.

The Oxford English Dictionary defines "spirit" as "the animating or vital principle in man (and animals); that which gives life to the physical organism, in contrast to its purely material elements; the breath of life". This very description, i.e. the spirit "giving life" to the physical organism, highlights the dichotomy between body and spirit that has pervaded Western philosophy for millennia.

Most authors assert that Chinese philosophy (and therefore medicine) is free from such dichotomy, i.e. that the body and spirit have always been seen as an indivisible whole. Needham makes this point very eloquently:[21]

Europe has the macrocosm-microcosm doctrine, yes, and to that extent, a primitive form of organic naturalism, together with its minor counterpart, the state-analogy, but both were subject to what I shall call the characteristic European schizophrenia or split-personality. Europeans could only think in terms either of Democritean mechanical materialism or of Platonic theological spiritualism. A deus always had to be found for a machina. Animas, entelechias, souls, archaei, dance processionally through the history of European thinking. When the living animal organism, as apprehended in beasts, other men, and the self, was projected onto the universe, the chief anxiety of Europeans, dominated by the idea of a personal God or gods, was to find the 'guiding principle'. Yet this was exactly the path that Chinese philosophy had not taken.

Needham further stresses the influence of Daoist thinking on Chinese medicine and attributes to it a belief in an "organism" that works spontaneously by itself following natural laws. He says:[22]

The classical statement of the organismic idea by Chuang Zi in the 4th century BC *has set the tone for later formulations, expressly avoiding the idea of any spiritual rector. The parts, in their organisational relations, whether of a living body or of the universe, were sufficient to account, by a kind of harmony of wills, for the observed phenomena.*

To illustrate this point, Needham quotes a passage from Chuang Zi:[23]

The hands and feet differ in their duties; the five viscera differ in their functions. They never associate with each other; yet the hundred parts [of the body] are held together with them in a common unity. Thus do they associate in non-association. They never force themselves to cooperate; and yet, both within and without, all complete one another. This is the way in which they cooperate in non-cooperation.

Needham concludes: "*The cooperation of the component parts of the organism is therefore not forced but absolutely spontaneous, even involuntary.*"[24]

Although Daoism exerted an influence on Chinese medicine, it did so more in the field of medical *qigong* and sexual hygiene and there is little evidence in ancient medical texts of a belief in a self-regulating and homoeostatic organism. Chinese medicine has been profoundly influenced by Confucian and Neo-Confucian philosophy; for example, the view of the internal organs as "officials" of a government is clearly of Confucian origin. Moreover, there is little if any adherence to a Daoist "non-action" in Chinese medicine: when symptoms occur, these are not considered to resolve spontaneously following a spontaneous harmony of the organism but they have to be actively treated with acupuncture or herbs: if there are hot symptoms, one must apply cold medicaments and vice versa; if there is a pathogenic factor it must be expelled (rather than relying on an innate *vis medicatrix* of the body as in naturopathic medicine).

As for the absence of a metaphysical current in Chinese philosophy, the Neo-Confucian theory of *Li* is certainly an expression of a metaphysical view of the world, i.e. of the existence of two separate realities, a physical and a metaphysical one. In fact, Neo-Confucians considered reality to be made of *Qi* in an imminent (i.e. physical) sense and *Li* in a transcendent (i.e. non-physical) sense. Qi forms matter (with "matter" intended in a broad sense to include subtle forms of it) while *Li* is the transcendent principle infused in reality.

Specifically in Chinese medicine, the concept of Ethereal Soul is certainly metaphysical. This is confirmed by the presence of the radical for *gui* in its character (*see Chapter 3*). *Gui* is the spirit of a dead person that goes on living after the death of the body and the Ethereal Soul pertains to this nature. This is also confirmed by the fact that the Ethereal Soul is not formed at conception (as are the Mind and the Corporeal Soul): it enters the body 3 days after birth and it is "imparted" by the father.

This is another reason why I prefer to call *Shen* the Mind and reserve the term "Spirit" for the total of the Five *Shen* (i.e. the Mind itself, the Ethereal Soul, the Corporeal Soul, the Intellect and the Will-Power). The problem is not only semantic; the important implication is that if we call the *Shen* of the Heart "spirit", we give undue importance to the Heart in the treatment of mental and spiritual problems to the detriment of the other four *Shen* and especially of the Ethereal Soul (*see Chapter 3*). Of course, translating the *Shen* of the Heart as "Mind" does not mean that it cannot be used for "spiritual" problems: as the Heart (and therefore the Mind) is the monarch and leader of all the other four *Shen*, it certainly treats emotional, mental and spiritual problems (Fig. 2.7).

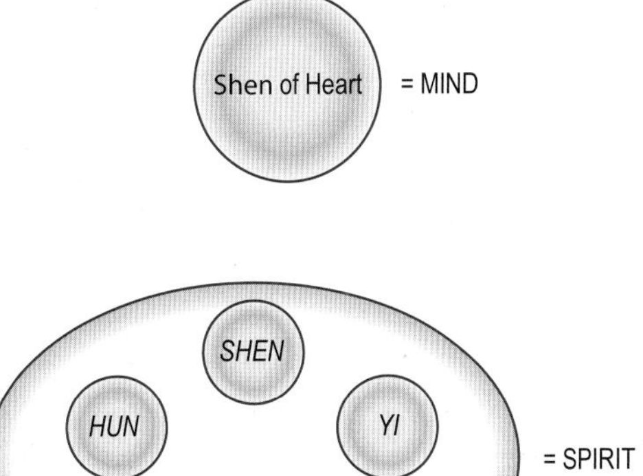

Figure 2.7 The two meanings of *Shen*.

CLINICAL APPLICATION

The clinical application of the Mind is extremely wide, with three broad areas.

1. As it encompasses the emotional life, it can be used when the person is affected by emotional stress (anger, sadness, etc.).
2. As the Mind controls memory, thinking and consciousness, it can be treated in problems of memory, cognition, thinking and consciousness; for example, it is used to treat poor memory or slow thinking in the elderly.
3. As the Mind of the Heart is the leader and coordinator of the other four *Shen*, it can be used to treat spiritual problems, e.g. when a person questions the meaning of life, is depressed, etc.

The points I use most frequently to treat the Mind are: HE-7 Shenmen, HE-5 Tongli, BL-15 Xinshu, Ren-15 Jiuwei and Du-24 Shenting.

HE-7 Shenmen

I use HE-7 Shenmen primarily to nourish Heart-Blood. I use it to treat emotional stress which may be caused by anger, sadness, grief, worry, fear or guilt. As it nourishes Heart-Blood, it also treats problems of the Mind such as poor memory and slow thinking. In a spiritual sense, I use HE-7 to nourish the Mind and to help the person find a sense of direction in life.

HE-5 Tongli

I use HE-5 Tongli primarily to tonify and move Heart-Qi. I see it as a more dynamic point than HE-7 Shenmen and use it to tonify Heart-Qi when the person is depressed. In terms of the Mind's function, as this point tonifies Qi, it can help to treat memory and thinking. In an emotional sense, I use it to treat sadness and grief.

BL-15 Xinshu

I use BL-15 Xinshu primarily to tonify Heart-Qi but also to nourish Heart-Blood. I use it to tonify the Mind's memory and thinking. In an emotional sense, I use it to lift the Mind when the person is sad; in a spiritual sense, I use it when the person is depressed.

BL-15 Xinshu is also used to clear Heart-Heat when the person is anxious and restless.

Ren-15 Jiuwei

I use Ren-15 Jiuwei to nourish the Heart more frequently than Ren-14 Juque which is the Front-Collecting point of the Heart. I use Ren-15 to nourish Heart-Blood and calm the Mind. In an emotional sense, I use this point to treat sadness, grief and worry especially; in a spiritual sense, I use this point for depression.

Du-24 Shenting

Du-24 Shenting stimulates memory and has a dual effect on the Mind as it can lift mood in depression and calm the Mind in anxiety and insomnia. As its name implies, it is the "courtyard" of the *Shen* (in this instance meaning both Mind and Spirit); it is a very important point to treat the Mind and Spirit and to harmonize the Mind with the Ethereal Soul.

END NOTES

1. Damasio A 2003 Looking for Spinoza – Joy, Sorrow and the Feeling Brain. Harcourt, San Diego, p. 184.
2. Tian Dai Hua 2005 Ling Shu Jing 灵枢经 [Spiritual Axis]. People's Health Publishing House, Beijing, p. 110. First published *c*.100 BC.
3. Lau DC, Ames RT 1998 Yuan Dao – Tracing Dao to its Source. Ballantine Books, New York, p. 45.
4. Bockover M (ed) 1991 Rules, Ritual and Responsibility – Essays Dedicated to Herbert Fingarette. Open Court, La Salle, Illinois, p. 100.
5. 1981 Ling Shu Jing 灵枢经 [Spiritual Axis]. People's Health Publishing House, Beijing, p. 23. First published *c*.100 BC.
6. 1982 Lei Jing 类经 [Classic of Categories]. People's Health Publishing House, Beijing, p. 49. The *Classic of Categories* was written by Zhang Jie Bin and first published in 1624.
7. 1981 Spiritual Axis, p. 71.
8. Classic of Categories, p. 63.
9. 1979 Huang Di Nei Jing Su Wen 黄帝内经素问 [The Yellow Emperor's Classic of Internal Medicine – Simple Questions]. People's Health Publishing House, Beijing, p. 58. First published *c*.100 BC.
10. Spiritual Axis, p. 128.
11. Lewis T, Amini F, Lannon R 2000 A General Theory of Love. Random House, New York, p. 107.
12. Birchwood M et al 1994 A self-report insight scale for psychosis, reliability, validity and sensitivity to change. Acta Psychiatrica Scandinavica 89: 62–67.
13. Tang Zong Hai 1892 Zhong Xi Hui Tong Yi Jing Jing Yi [The Essence of Medical Classics on the Convergence of Chinese and Western Medicine], cited in Wang Ke Qin 1988 Zhong Yi Shen Zhu Xue Shuo 中医神主学说) [Theory of the Mind in Chinese Medicine]. Ancient Chinese Medical Texts Publishing House, Beijing, p. 22.
14. Simple Questions, p. 72.
15. Ibid., p. 154.
16. Ren Ying Qiu 1985 Zhong Yi Ge Jia Xue Shuo [Theories of Chinese Medicine Doctors], cited in Wang Ke Qin, Theory of the Mind in Chinese Medicine, p. 22.
17. Wang Ken Tang 1602 Zheng Zhi Zhun Sheng [Standards of Diagnosis and Treatment], cited in Wang Ke Qin, Theory of the Mind in Chinese Medicine, p. 22.
18. Simple Questions, p. 26.
19. Ibid., p. 78.
20. Ibid., p. 67.
21. Needham J 1977 Science and Civilisation in China, Vol. 2. Cambridge University Press, Cambridge, p. 302.
22. Ibid.
23. Ibid.
24. Ibid.

魂

CHAPTER 3

THE ETHEREAL SOUL (*HUN*)

SLEEP AND DREAMING *29*

THE MOVEMENT OF THE ETHEREAL SOUL AND MENTAL ACTIVITIES *31*

BALANCE OF EMOTIONS *32*

EYES AND SIGHT *34*

COURAGE *34*

PLANNING *35*

RELATIONSHIP WITH THE MIND *36*

Relationship between the Ethereal Soul and the Mind *36*
Mild "manic" behavior in clinical practice *38*
Examples of the nature of the Ethereal Soul *38*
The Ethereal Soul and modern diseases *40*
The Ethereal Soul and Buddhist psychology *40*
The Ethereal Soul and Jungian psychology *41*
The movement of the Ethereal Soul and expansion/contraction *42*
Clinical patterns of pathologies of the Ethereal Soul *43*

CLINICAL APPLICATION *44*

Acupuncture *44*
Herbal therapy *45*

THE ETHEREAL SOUL (*HUN*)

The Ethereal Soul broadly corresponds to our Western concept of "soul". According to ancient Chinese beliefs it enters the body shortly after birth; to be precise, it does so 3 days after birth. It is imparted by the father. Ethereal in nature, after death it survives the body and flows back to "Heaven" (*Tian*); this is the ancient Chinese concept of "Heaven", i.e. a state of subtle and non-material energies and beings, which has therefore nothing to do with the Western and Christian concept of "Heaven". The Ethereal Soul can be described as "*that part of the Soul* [as opposed to the Corporeal Soul] *which at death leaves the body, carrying with it an appearance of physical form*".[1]

The Chinese character for Ethereal Soul is as follows:

魂

This is composed of the following parts:

云 = clouds

鬼 = spirit, ghost (*gui*)

The ancient form of this last radical is depicted in Figure 3.1. This form is itself composed of two parts (Fig. 3.2), meaning a swirling movement.

This ancient radical therefore depicts the bodiless head of a dead person flowing to Heaven in a swirling movement or wandering in the realm of spirits and ghosts. The cloud radical on the left is partly phonetic ("cloud" is pronounced *yun* which is similar to *hun*) but it also signifies that the Ethereal Soul is ethereal in nature and therefore Yang.

The combination of the two characters for "cloud" and "spirit" in the character for Ethereal Soul conveys the idea of its nature; it is like a "ghost" or the spirit of a dead person but it is Yang and ethereal in nature and essentially harmless, i.e. it is not one of the evil spirits (hence the presence of the "cloud" radical).

Bearing in mind that the character for Corporeal Soul (*Po*) is based on that for *gui* plus that for "white", quoting an ancient text, *Chinese Medicine Psychology* says:[2]

Spirit (gui) plus 'cloud' makes the character for Ethereal Soul; spirit plus 'white' makes the character for Corporeal Soul. Cloud is wind, wind pertains to Wood. White corresponds to Qi, Qi pertains to Metal. Wind is light and scatters so that the Corporeal Soul can follow the rising of the Ethereal Soul. Metal is heavy so that the Ethereal Soul can follow the descent of the Corporeal Soul.

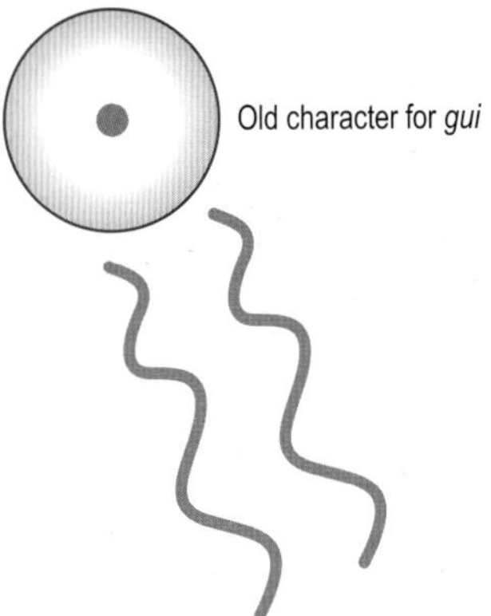

Figure 3.1 Old Chinese character for *gui*.

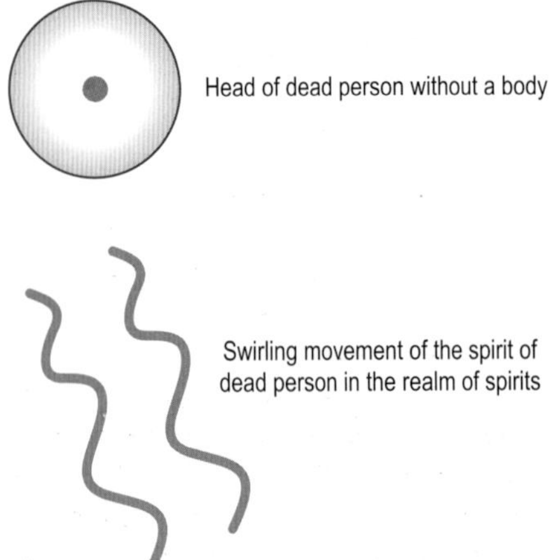

Figure 3.2 Component parts of old Chinese character for *gui*.

> **!**
>
> The Chinese character for Ethereal Soul (*Hun*) contains the radical for *gui*, i.e. "ghost, spirit, demon". This immediately conveys the idea that the Ethereal Soul is a "dark", subterranean part of our psyche with its own independent existence.

There are three types of Ethereal Soul: a vegetative one (called *Shuang Ling* or "Clear Spirit") common to plants, animals and human beings; an animal one (called *Tai Guang* or "Brilliant Light") common to animals and human beings; and a human one (called *You Jing* or "Dark Essence") which is present only in human beings (Fig. 3.3).

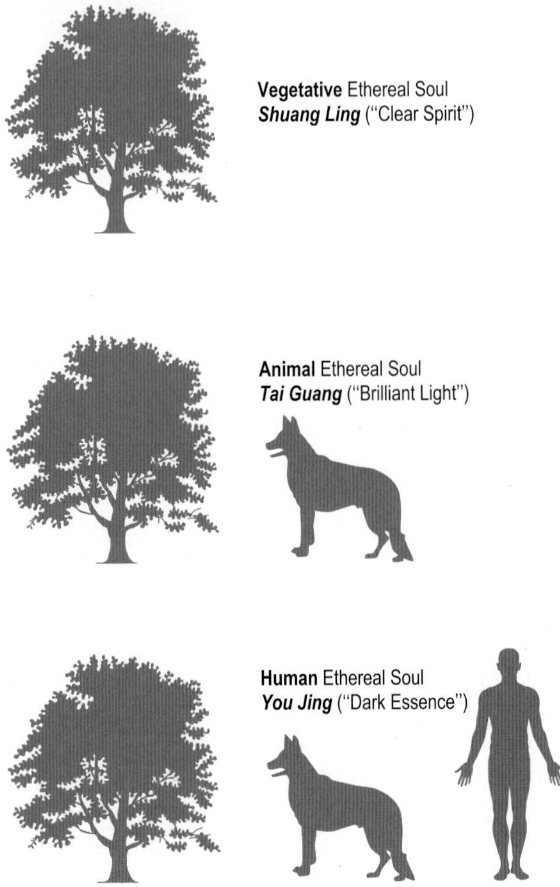

Figure 3.3 The three Ethereal Souls.

Zhang Jie Bin in the *Classic of Categories* says: "*The Mind and Ethereal Soul are Yang, the Ethereal Soul follows the Mind; if the Mind is unconscious the Ethereal Soul is swept away.*"[3] He also says: "*The Mind corresponds to Yang within Yang, the Ethereal Soul corresponds to Yin within Yang.*"[4] The *Spiritual Axis* in Chapter 8 says: "*The Ethereal Soul is the coming and going of the Mind.*"[5] See Figure 3.4.

The concept of the Ethereal Soul is closely linked to the ancient Chinese beliefs in spirits, ghosts and demons. According to these beliefs, spirits, ghosts and demons are spirit-like creatures that preserve a physical appearance after death and wander in the world of spirit. Some are good and some are evil.

The belief in a soul that survives the body after death is very ancient and pre-dates the times when the main theories of Chinese medicine developed, i.e. the Warring States period (475–221 BC) and the Han

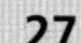

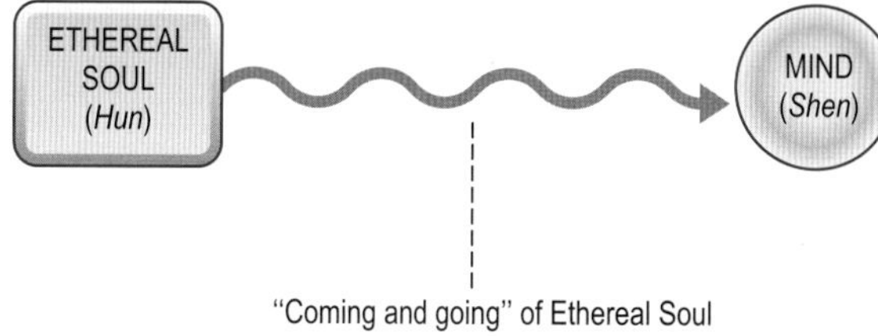

Figure 3.4 Relationship between Ethereal Soul and Mind.

dynasty (221–207 BC). The text *Record of Rites* (*Li Ji*) is a Warring States period text that recollects practices from the mid-Zhou dynasty times (11th century to 771 BC). This text refers to a soul that survives the body after death and calls it "spirit Ethereal Soul" (*Ling Hun* 灵魂). It says that flesh and bones die at death and return to Earth while the "spirit Ethereal Soul" survives the body and wanders off.[6]

In the times prior to the Warring States period, such spirits were considered to be the main cause of disease. Following the Warring States period, a belief in naturalistic causes of disease (such as weather or lifestyle) gradually came to the fore. The very first chapter of the *Simple Questions* (dating back to approximately 100 BC) is testimony to this change. In fact, the *Simple Questions* opens with the Yellow Emperor asking his chief physician Qi Bo why it is that in ancient times people lived a very long life and nowadays they die young. Qi Bo's answer is very significant; he does not say that people die young because they are attacked by evil spirits, but that they die young because of their lifestyle. Hence this text marks the transition from demonic medicine (in which illness is due to attack by evil spirits) to natural medicine (in which illness is due to inappropriate lifestyle).

However, the belief in spirits has never really disappeared in Chinese medicine and all the ancient doctors, including eminent ones like Sun Si Miao or Li Shi Zhen, believed in evil spirits as causes of disease and prescribed various incantations in addition to herbal treatment. The belief in evil spirits is present even in modern China after 60 years of Marxist ideology (*see Chapter 7, The gui*).[7]

What is the Ethereal Soul then and what does it do? An analysis of the Chinese character depicting the Ethereal Soul is essential to gain an understanding of and a feeling for what it is. The presence of the radical for *gui* within its character immediately tells us that the Ethereal Soul has a somewhat "dark" nature; in ancient Greek philosophy, we would say it has a "Dionysian" nature. It pertains to a "subterranean" world that is different from the world of the Mind.

The Ethereal Soul is the *gui*, i.e. the "dark", intuitive, non-rational side of human nature. Yang in character, it enters and exits through the nose and communicates with Heaven. The *gui* in the character *hun* for the "Ethereal Soul" has also another important meaning. The fact that the Ethereal Soul has the nature of *gui* means that its existence is *independent* from that of the Mind (*Shen*). The Ethereal Soul has its own life and "agenda" over which the Mind has no say; the interaction and integration of the Mind with the Ethereal Soul form the basis for our rich psychic life.

Unlike the Ethereal Soul, the other two mental-spiritual aspects of Intellect (*Yi* of the Spleen) and Will-Power (*Zhi* of the Kidneys) do not have an independent existence but could be said to be aspects of the Mind (*Shen*) of the Heart.

As we shall see below, the character for "Corporeal Soul" (*Po*) also contains the character for *gui*; like the Ethereal Soul, the Corporeal Soul also has its own independent existence although on a physical level. Thus, the Ethereal Soul and the Corporeal Soul have their own separate existence from the Mind, the former on a psychic level and the latter on a physical level.

Chapter 54 of the *Spiritual Axis* confirms this when it describes how a human being comes into existence; it clearly says that this happens when the body, Mind (*Shen*) and Ethereal and Corporeal Souls come into existence:[8]

The mother provides the foundation, the father the fertilization. If there is no Shen, there is death; if there is Shen, there is life. When Blood and Qi are harmonized, the Nutritive and Defensive Qi communicating, the five viscera are complete, the Mind is housed in the Heart, the Ethereal and Corporeal Soul are complete, then a human being is formed.

This passage confirms that the Ethereal and Corporeal Souls are independent of the Mind and they are necessary components of a human being.

The Chinese character for Ethereal Soul should be compared and contrasted with that for the Mind (*Shen*). The radical *gui* in the character for "Ethereal Soul" is a ghost, a spirit; it is "dark" and leads its own independent existence separate from that of the Mind. The character *shen*, by contrast, indicates the influx from Heaven, something pure, spiritual.

The Ethereal Soul can be described as the part of the soul (as opposed to the Corporeal Soul) that at death leaves the body, carrying with it an appearance of physical form. From this point of view therefore, the soul is regarded as having an independent existence just as was believed in the ancient Greek–Roman civilization and during the Middle Ages.

At death, the Ethereal Soul survives the body and returns to "Heaven", the Corporeal Soul dies with the body and returns to Earth, and the Mind is simply extinguished. It is interesting to note that, when describing the changes occurring at death, Chinese books say that it is the Ethereal Soul and not the Mind (*Shen*) that returns to "Heaven"; this would seem to confirm that the *Shen* has indeed the nature of Mind rather than of "Spirit".

Quoting an ancient text, *Chinese Medicine Psychology* says:[9]

> *At birth, the Ethereal Soul joins the Corporeal Soul and this restrains the former; at death, the Ethereal Soul floats away and returns to Heaven while the Corporeal Soul sinks back to Earth. Motion depends on the Ethereal Soul; absence of it is due to the Corporeal Soul. Yin controls storage and, for this reason, the Corporeal Soul* [being Yin in comparison to the Ethereal Soul], *controls memory. Yang controls motion and for this reason the Ethereal Soul can extend and come and go. These two* [souls] *are inseparable: when Essence (Jing) gathers, the Corporeal Soul comes into being; when Qi gathers, the Ethereal Soul comes into being.*

Figure 3.5 uses the image of a cigarette to convey the different destinies of the Ethereal Soul, the Corporeal Soul and the Mind at death; the cigarette itself is the Mind (*Shen*), the smoke is the Ethereal Soul, the ashes the Corporeal Soul, and the tobacco the Essence (*Jing*).

When the cigarette is extinguished, the Ethereal Soul survives and drifts away to "Heaven" in the form of smoke, and the Corporeal Soul dies with the body and returns to Earth in the form of ashes. The Mind (the cigarette itself) is extinguished and the Essence (in the form of tobacco) has been used up.

> **!**
>
> At death, the Ethereal Soul survives the body and returns to "Heaven", the Corporeal Soul dies with the body and returns to Earth, and the Mind is simply extinguished.

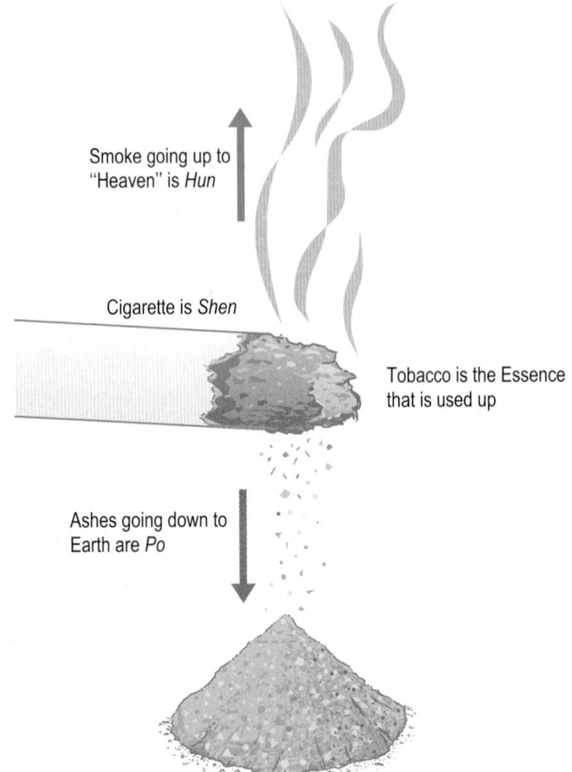

Figure 3.5 Comparison between Ethereal Soul, Mind, Corporeal Soul and Essence.

According to ancient Chinese beliefs, the Ethereal Soul was imparted by the father 3 days after birth during a naming ceremony, i.e. the baby was given a name and the father "imparted" the Ethereal Soul to him or her.

The fact that the Ethereal Soul is imparted by the father after birth should not be taken literally; it is significant in that it is symbolic of the social, relational nature of the Ethereal Soul (as opposed to the Corporeal Soul). The Ethereal Soul is responsible for relationships and our relating to other people in the family and society. The ceremony during which the father imparted the Ethereal Soul and the name to the baby 3 days after birth is therefore symbolic of the fact that, through this ceremony, the baby was assigned his or her place in the family and society. The Ethereal Soul corresponds to our individuality, but an individuality within the family and society.

When describing the Ethereal Soul, the theme of "movement", "swirling", "wandering" is ever present. As we have seen above, the old form of the Chinese radical within the word *Hun* depicts the swirling movement of the soul of a dead person in the realm of spirit. The Ethereal Soul provides "movement" to the psyche in many ways; movement of the soul out of the body as in dreaming, movement out of one's everyday life as in life dreams and ideas, movement towards others in human relationships, movement in terms of plans and projects.

CLINICAL NOTE

The Ethereal Soul provides movement to the psyche in many ways; movement of the soul out of the body as in dreaming, movement out of one's everyday life as in movement towards others in human relationships, movement in terms of plans, projects, ideas, life dreams, inspiration, creativity.

The best points to stimulate the movement of the Ethereal Soul are G.B.-40 Qiuxu together with BL-47 Hunmen.

To sum up, the Ethereal Soul is basically another level of consciousness, different from the Mind but closely related to it. It is a part of the psyche that is not rational like the Mind (*Shen*) but is responsible for intuition, inspiration, ideas, life dreams, relations with others, artistic inspiration; it is also responsible for the "movement" of our psyche towards the environment and other people in relationships.

CLINICAL NOTE

The Ethereal Soul is another level of consciousness, different from the Mind but closely related to it. It is a part of the psyche that, unlike the Mind (*Shen*), is not rational but is responsible for intuition, inspiration, ideas, life dreams, artistic inspiration; it is also responsible for the "movement" of our psyche towards the environment and other people in relationships. The point BL-47 Hunmen regulates the movement of the Ethereal Soul.

The Ethereal Soul is rooted in the Liver and in particular Liver-Yin (which includes Liver-Blood). If Liver-Blood and/or Liver-Yin are depleted, the Ethereal Soul is deprived of its residence and becomes rootless. This can result in insomnia or restless sleep with many dreams. The Ethereal Soul, deprived of its residence, wanders without aim.

At death, the Ethereal Soul survives and goes to "Heaven" while the Corporeal Soul dies and returns to Earth.

The discussion of the nature and functions of the Ethereal Soul in this chapter will be conducted according to the following topics.

- Sleep and dreaming
- The movement of the Ethereal Soul and mental activities
- Balance of emotions
- Eyes and sight
- Courage
- Planning
- Relationship with the Mind

SLEEP AND DREAMING

The Ethereal Soul influences sleep and dreaming. The length and quality of sleep are related to the state of the Ethereal Soul. If this is well rooted in the Liver (Liver-Blood or Liver-Yin), sleep is normal and sound and without too many dreams. If Liver-Yin or Liver-Blood is deficient, or if Heat agitates the Ethereal Soul, this is deprived of its residence and wanders off at night, causing a restless sleep with many tiring dreams (Fig. 3.6).

Sleep disturbances linked to excessive dreaming are particularly related to the Ethereal Soul. As it is in the nature of the Ethereal Soul to "wander", it does so at night, giving rise to dreams. Tang Zong Hai says: "*At night during sleep the Ethereal Soul returns to the Liver; if the Ethereal Soul is not peaceful there are a lot of dreams.*"[10]

The *Secret of the Golden Flower* in Chapter 2 says:[11]

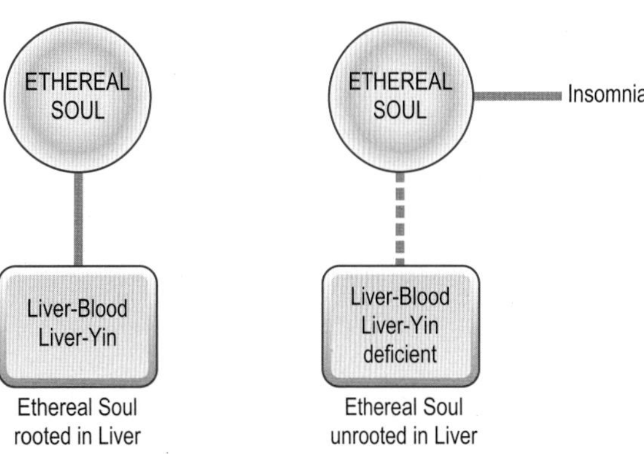

Figure 3.6 Ethereal Soul and sleep.

In the daytime the Ethereal Soul is in the eyes and at night in the Liver. When it is in the eyes we can see; when it is in the Liver we dream.

It also says:[12]

Dreams constitute the wandering of the Ethereal Soul in the Nine Heavens and Nine Earths. When one wakes up one feels obscure and confused [because] *one is constrained by the Corporeal Soul.*

Quoting an ancient text, *Chinese Medicine Psychology* says:[13]

The Ethereal Soul goes to the eyes and to the Liver at night. When in the eyes, it allows us to see; when in the Liver, it makes us dream. When we dream a lot, the Corporeal Soul is restricting the hun; when we wake up, the Ethereal Soul is victorious over the Corporeal Soul.

Hardly any Chinese book defines "excessive dreaming". In my experience, dreaming can be defined as excessive either when the sleeper has nightmares or when he or she has unpleasant or anxiety-causing dreams the whole night, waking up exhausted.

Dr Wang Ke Qin defines "normal" dreaming as that characterized by short, pleasant dreams, and not too many of them. "Excessive" dreaming is characterized by nightmares and too many dreams, and by ones that are very long.[14]

Some doctors classify dreams as "chaotic dreams" – dreams of fear, dreams of shock, strange dreams, "absurd dreams". They are considered pathological. These are due to the Mind's and the Ethereal Soul's being unsettled and to the "Ethereal Soul leaving the body".

The *Classic of Categories* by Zhang Jie Bin distinguishes six types of dream:[15]

1. Normal dreams not associated with any particular emotion
2. "Shock" dreams characterized by a feeling of fear
3. "Worry" dreams characterized by a feeling of worry about the events of the day
4. "Sleep" dreams in which, at the time of waking up, one is still dreaming
5. "Pleasure" dreams
6. "Fear" dreams characterized by fear and anxiety dreaming.

If excessive dreaming and insomnia are caused by an excessive wandering of the Ethereal Soul at night from its not being rooted in Liver-Blood and Liver-Yin, one should nourish Liver-Yin with sour and absorbing herbs such as Mu Li *Concha Ostreae*, Long Chi *Fossilia Dentis Mastodi*, Suan Zao Ren *Semen Ziziphi spinosae* or Bai Shao *Radix Paeoniae alba*. There is an interesting correlation between the astringent and absorbing quality of such herbs on a physical level and their use in calming the Mind and "absorbing" the Ethereal Soul to draw it back into the Liver.

CLINICAL NOTE

In order to nourish Liver-Blood and anchor the Ethereal Soul into the Liver, I use LIV-8 Ququan, Ren-4 Guanyuan and SP-6 Sanyinjiao (with reinforcing method).

If Liver-Yin is very depleted, the Ethereal Soul may sometimes even leave the body temporarily at night during or just before sleep. Those who suffer from severe deficiency of Yin may experience a floating sensation in the few moments just before falling asleep; this is said to be due to the "floating" of the Ethereal Soul not rooted in Yin.

We have just discussed Liver-Blood and/or Liver-Yin deficiency as a cause of the Ethereal Soul's not being rooted in the Liver and causing insomnia or excessive dreaming. This is an Empty cause. However, the Ethereal Soul may also fail to be rooted in the Liver when it is agitated by pathogenic factors such as Heat or Fire. This lack of rooting of the Ethereal Soul in the Liver is due to a Full cause (Fig. 3.7). Dreams caused by Full conditions are called the "12 Excesses" and dreams caused by Empty conditions are called the "15 Deficiencies" (*see Chapter 18, Insomnia*).

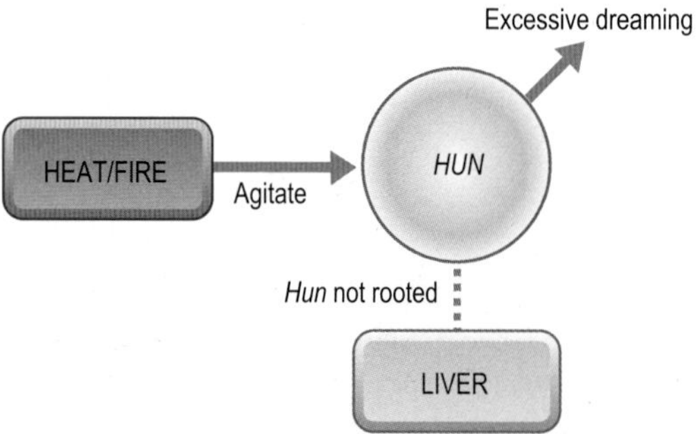

Figure 3.7 Causes of excessive dreaming from failure of rooting of the Ethereal Soul in the Liver.

Of course, the length and quality of sleep also depend on the state of Heart-Blood and there is an overlap between the influence of Heart-Blood and Liver-Blood on sleep.

Besides dreaming at night, the Ethereal Soul influences dreaming in a broad sense, i.e. the dreams, aims and projects of our life. When one has a life "dream", this is dependent on the activity of the Ethereal Soul. The Ethereal Soul is therefore also responsible for "dreaming" in a positive sense, i.e. having a sense of purpose in life and "dreams" in the sense of goals. As we shall see later, the lack of a sense of direction and purpose and the absence of life dreams and goals are important features of depression and are due to a lack of "movement" of the Ethereal Soul.

Thus, the Ethereal Soul influences dreaming at night and "life dreams" in our wakeful state. When the Ethereal Soul is in the eyes we have external visualization; when it is in the Liver we have internal visualization as in dreams or life dreams.

Finally, the Ethereal Soul is also responsible for daydreaming. Zhang Jie Bin says in the *Classic of Categories*: "*Absent-mindedness as if in a trance is due to the Ethereal Soul wandering outside its residence.*"[16] He also says: "*When one is in a trance like in a dream, it is due to the swimming of the Ethereal Soul at the borders* [of consciousness]."[17] Thus, if Liver-Blood or Liver-Yin is deficient, the Ethereal Soul wanders off in a daydream and the person has no clear sense of direction in life. Attention deficit disorder (ADD) may also be characterized by the movement of the Ethereal Soul in daydreaming.

The Ethereal Soul may even leave the body temporarily; some Chinese idiomatic expressions confirm this. For example, *fan hun* (literally "Hun returning") means "to come back to life", as after being in a trance during which the soul leaves the body. *Hun fei po san* (literally "hun flying, po scattered") means "to be scared out of one's wits" or also "to be struck dumb", for example by love.

SUMMARY

The Ethereal Soul, sleep and dreaming

- The Ethereal Soul is responsible for sound sleep and a normal amount of dreaming.
- When the Ethereal Soul flows to the eyes in daytime, we can see; when it flows to the eyes at night, we dream.
- If the Ethereal Soul is not rooted in Liver-Blood and Liver-Yin, or if it is agitated by Heat, it may wander too much and we have too many dreams or unpleasant dreams.
- The Ethereal Soul is responsible for life dreams.

THE MOVEMENT OF THE ETHEREAL SOUL AND MENTAL ACTIVITIES

The Ethereal Soul assists the Mind in its mental activities. The *Five-Channel Righteousness*, a text from the Tang dynasty, says: "*Knowledge is dependent on the sharpness of the Ethereal Soul.*"[18] The Ethereal Soul provides the Mind, which is responsible for rational thinking, with intuition and inspiration. It also gives the Mind "movement" in the sense that it allows the Mind the capacity of self-insight and introspection, as well as the ability to project outwards and relate to other people. This capacity for movement and outward projection is closely related to the Liver-Qi quality of quick and free movement.

The modern doctor Wang Ke Qin says: "*Hun implies movement.*"[19] Interestingly, he also says: "*The Ethereal Soul is a second layer of mental activity.*"[20] Chapter 9 of the *Simple Questions* says: "*Movement depends on the Mind and the Ethereal Soul; the Liver houses the Ethereal Soul, and it is the root for stopping extremes* [i.e. the regulating and balancing organ]."[21]

It will be remembered that the descriptions "movement", "coming and going" and "wandering" are often used in connection with the Ethereal Soul. For example, as mentioned above, the Ethereal Soul is the "*coming and going of the Mind*", or "*when the Ethereal Soul swims to the eyes, they can see*". It is interesting to compare this quality of the Ethereal Soul with the swirling movement of a spirit depicted in its old character on an ethereal level, and, on a physical level, with the smooth flow of Liver-Qi. Indeed, the smooth flow of Liver-Qi in all directions is the physical counterpart of the psychic movement of the Ethereal Soul towards the Mind.

The Ethereal Soul is always described as the "coming and going of the Mind (*Shen*)" (*sui Shen wang lai wei zhi Hun*) or, to put it differently, "what follows the Mind in its coming and going is the Ethereal Soul". On a psychic level, this means that the Ethereal Soul provides the Mind with "movement" in the sense of intuition, inspiration, movement towards others in relationships, creativity, dreaming (in the sense of life dreams), planning, imagination, projects, symbols and archetypes. The Ethereal Soul gives the Mind the necessary psychic tension of Wood. The Mind without the Ethereal Soul would be like a powerful computer without software.

Interestingly, some modern philosophers say the same. For example, Searle says:[22]

The way the system works is that the brain is a digital computer and what we call the 'mind' is a digital computer program or set of programs. The mind is to the brain as the software is to the hardware.

> **CLINICAL NOTE**
>
> On a psychic level, the Ethereal Soul provides the Mind with "movement" in the sense of intuition, inspiration, movement towards others in relationships, creativity, dreaming (in the sense of life dreams), planning, imagination, projects, symbols and archetypes. The Ethereal Soul gives the Mind the necessary psychic tension of Wood. In order to stimulate the movement of the Ethereal Soul I use BL-47 Hunmen and G.B.-40 Qiuxu.

An important aspect of the movement of the Ethereal Soul is the movement of the individual towards other people in relationships; this affects all types of relationships such as marriage, loving friendships, relationships within the family and at work. The Ethereal Soul is responsible for our capacity of relating to, interacting with and empathizing with other people.

> **CLINICAL NOTE**
>
> It could be said that autism is a pathology of the Ethereal Soul's function of projecting outwards towards others and responding emotionally to others.

The relationship between the Mind, responsible for rational thinking (but also for our emotional life), and the Ethereal Soul, responsible for intuition and inspiration, is somewhat similar to the relationship between Athena and Dionysus in Greek mythology. In fact, Athena is the goddess of reason and wisdom while Dionysus is the god of mystery religions, religious ecstasy, personal delivery from the daily world through spiritual intoxication, and initiation into secret rites. A delightful illustration on an ancient Greek vase depicts Athena sitting on a swing and Dionysus pushing it (Fig. 3.8). This illustrates the necessary coordination and integration of the rational side of the psyche (symbolized by Athena) with the "dark", inspirational and non-rational side (symbolized by Dionysus).

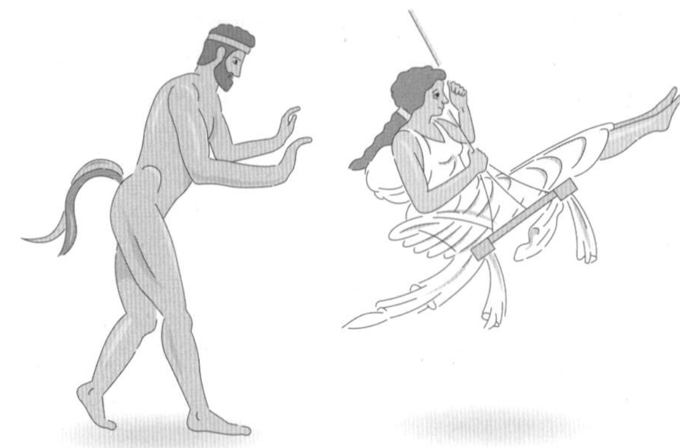

Figure 3.8 Comparison between the relationship between Ethereal Soul and Mind with that between Dionysus and Athena.

This Greek painting is a good illustration of the "movement" that the Ethereal Soul imparts to the Mind symbolized by the movement of the swing as Dionysus pushes it forward.

There are other connections between Dionysus and the Ethereal Soul. According to Trimble, Dionysus represents "*a force that is beyond human control but that we cannot shut out: the force that takes possession of our minds or places us outside ourselves, in 'ecstasy'.*"[23]

> **SUMMARY**
>
> **The movement of the Ethereal Soul and mental activities**
>
> - The Ethereal Soul contributes to the mental activities of the Mind (*Shen*) by providing it with ideas, intuition, images and creativity.
> - This activity of the Ethereal Soul depends on its "coming and going".

BALANCE OF EMOTIONS

The Ethereal Soul is responsible for maintaining a normal balance between excitation and restraint of the emotional life, under the leadership of the Heart and the Mind. Emotions are a normal part of our mental life; we all experience anger, sadness, worry or fear on occasions in the course of our life and these do not normally lead to disease. The Ethereal Soul, being responsible for the more intuitive and subconscious part of the Mind, plays a role in keeping an emotional balance and, most of all, prevents the emotions from becoming excessive and therefore turning into causes of disease.

This regulatory function of the Ethereal Soul is closely related to the balance between Liver-Blood (the Yin part of the Liver) and Liver-Qi (the Yang part of the Liver). Liver-Blood and Liver-Qi need to be harmonized and Liver-Blood must root Liver-Qi to prevent its becoming stagnant or rebelling upwards. On a mental-emotional level, Liver-Blood needs to root the Ethereal Soul, thus allowing a balanced and happy emotional life. This is one of the meanings, on a mental level, of the Liver's being a "regulating and harmonizing" organ (Fig. 3.9).

Chapter 9 of the *Simple Questions* says: "*The Liver houses the Ethereal Soul, and it is the root for stopping extremes* [i.e. the regulating and balancing organ]."[24] If Liver-Blood is deficient there will be fear and anxiety; if Liver-Yang is in excess there will be anger. The *Spiritual Axis* in Chapter 8 says: "*If the Liver is deficient there will be fear; if it is in excess there will be anger.*"[25] Tang Zong Hai in the *Discussion on Blood Patterns* says: "*If Liver-Blood is deficient, Fire agitates the Ethereal Soul resulting in nocturnal emissions with dreams.*"[26]

Tang Zong Hai clearly describes the balance between Liver-Blood and Liver-Qi when he says:[27]

The Ethereal Soul is the Yang of the Essence [Jing] and the spirit of Qi. The body's Qi is Yang and Blood is Yin. Yang cannot exist without Yin, Qi cannot exist without Blood. The Liver governs Blood and contains Yang; this is a function of the Ethereal Soul.

This statement is interesting because the last sentence clearly says that it is the Ethereal Soul that keeps the balance between Liver-Blood and Liver-Qi, i.e. between the Yin and the Yang aspects of the Liver. In an emotional sense, this means that the Ethereal Soul keeps the balance in the free flow of Liver-Qi.

The free flow of Liver-Qi is the physical counterpart of the "coming and going" of the Ethereal Soul; this "coming and going" should be regulated and balanced. If it is deficient (as in Liver-Qi stagnation), the person is depressed and out of touch with his or her emotions; if it is excessive (as in Liver-Yang rising or Liver-Fire), the person may be agitated, angry or too emotional, or may show a degree of mania (Figs 3.10 and 3.11).

Movement of Ethereal Soul

LIVER-QI

LIVER-BLOOD

Roots the Ethereal Soul

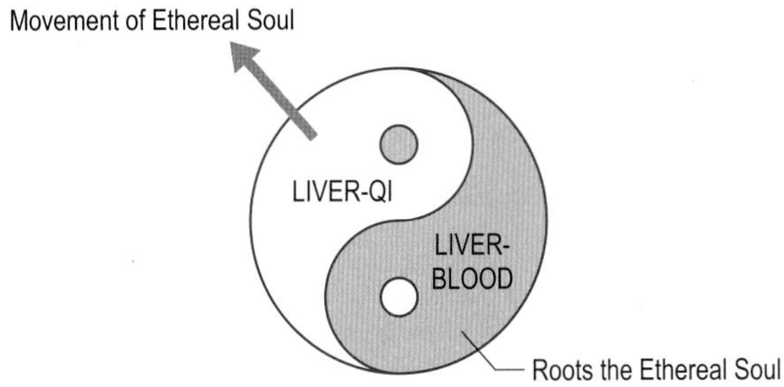

Figure 3.9 Relationship between Liver-Qi and Liver-Blood and the Ethereal Soul.

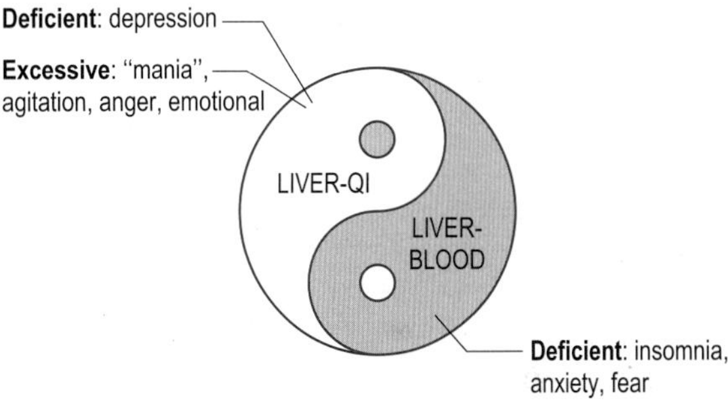

Figure 3.10 Pathological states of the relationship between Liver-Qi and Liver-Blood.

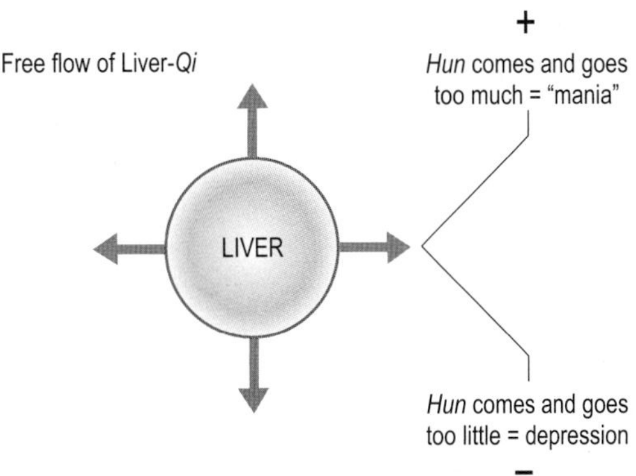

Figure 3.11 Pathology of excessive or deficient movement of Liver-Qi.

CLINICAL NOTE

The free flow of Liver-Qi is the physical counterpart of the "coming and going" of the Ethereal Soul; this "coming and going" should be regulated and balanced. If it is deficient (as in Liver-Qi stagnation), the person is depressed and not in touch with his or her emotions; if it is excessive (as in Liver-Yang rising or Liver-Fire), the person may be agitated, angry, too emotional or slightly manic. The best points to regulate and balance the coming and going of the Ethereal Soul are LIV-3 Taichong and BL-47 Hunmen.

These two opposing emotional states, characterized by a hyperactive Liver-Qi (with excessive "coming and going" of the Ethereal Soul) or a stagnant Liver-Qi (with insufficient "coming and going" of the Ethereal Soul), are described in the *Simple Questions* as "Fullness" and "Emptiness" of the Mind (*Shen*). Chapter 62 of the *Simple Questions* says:[28]

What are the symptoms of Fullness and Emptiness of the Mind [Shen]? When the Mind is in Excess, the person laughs uncontrollably; when the Mind is Deficient, the person is sad.

SUMMARY

The Ethereal Soul's balance of emotions

- The Ethereal Soul is responsible for maintaining a normal balance between excitation and restraint of the emotional life, under the leadership of the Heart and the Mind.
- On an emotional level, Liver-Blood needs to root the Ethereal Soul, thus allowing a balanced and happy emotional life.
- The free flow of Liver-Qi is the physical counterpart of the "coming and going" of the Ethereal Soul; this "coming and going" should be regulated and balanced. If it is deficient (as in Liver-Qi stagnation), the person is depressed and not in touch with his or her emotions; if it is excessive (as in Liver-Yang rising or Liver-Fire), the person may be agitated, angry, too emotional or slightly manic.

EYES AND SIGHT

The Ethereal Soul relates to the eyes and sight. Tang Zong Hai says: "*When the Ethereal Soul wanders to the eyes, they can see.*"[29] The *Secret of the Golden Flower* in Chapter 2 says:[30]

In the daytime the Ethereal Soul is in the eyes and at night in the Liver. When it is in the eyes we can see. When it is in the Liver we dream.

Apart from physical sight, the Ethereal Soul also gives us "vision" in life, i.e. the capacity to have life dreams, projects and creativity.

CLINICAL NOTE

The best points to influence the Ethereal Soul and sight are G.B.-37 Guangming, LIV-2 Xingjian and BL-18 Ganshu.

This connection with the eyes can easily be related to the rooting of the Ethereal Soul in Liver-Blood as this nourishes the eyes.

On a psychic level, the Ethereal Soul gives us "vision" and insight. At night, the Ethereal Soul makes us "see" when we dream. Thus, the Ethereal Soul is responsible for vision in three ways: physical sight, "seeing" at night in the form of dreams and "vision" in life (Fig. 3.12).

SUMMARY

The Ethereal Soul, eyes and sight

- The Ethereal Soul relates to the eyes and sight.
- In the daytime the Ethereal Soul is in the eyes and at night in the Liver. When it is in the eyes we can see; when it is in the Liver we dream.
- On a psychic level, the Ethereal Soul gives us "vision" and insight.

COURAGE

The Ethereal Soul is related to courage or to its lack, cowardice, and for this reason the Liver is sometimes called the "resolute organ". Tang Zong Hai says: "*When the Ethereal Soul is not strong, the person is timid.*"[31] The

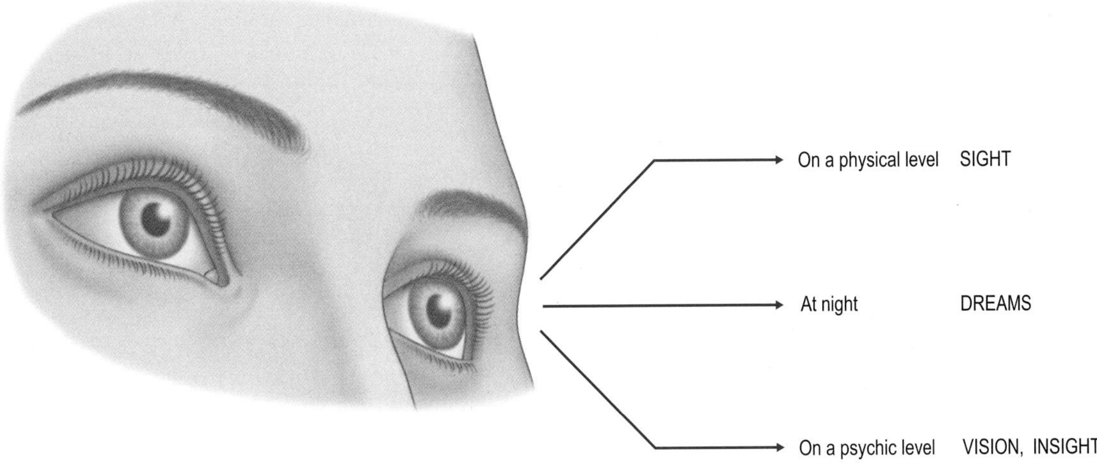

Figure 3.12 The three influences of the Ethereal Soul on "seeing".

"strength" of the Ethereal Soul in this connection derives mainly from Liver-Blood. If Liver-Blood is abundant, the person is fearless and is able to face up to life's difficulties without being easily discouraged.

Just as in disease Liver-Yang easily flares upwards causing anger, in health the same type of mental energy deriving from Liver-Blood can give a person courage and resoluteness. If Liver-Blood and Liver-Qi are deficient and the Ethereal Soul is dithering, the person lacks courage and resolve, cannot face up to difficulties or make decisions, and is easily discouraged. A vague feeling of fear at night before falling asleep is also due to a lack of rooting of the Ethereal Soul.

CLINICAL NOTE

In order to stimulate the "courage" of the Ethereal Soul I use the point G.B.-40 Qiuxu.

The quality of courage and resoluteness is also dependent on the strength of Gall-Bladder Qi.

SUMMARY

The Ethereal Soul and courage

- The Ethereal Soul is related to courage or to its lack, cowardice, and for this reason the Liver is sometimes called the "resolute organ".
- If Liver-Blood is abundant, the person is fearless and is able to face up to life's difficulties with an indomitable spirit; if Liver-Blood is deficient and the Ethereal Soul is dithering, the person lacks courage and resolve, cannot face up to difficulties or making decisions, and is easily discouraged.

PLANNING

The Ethereal Soul influences the capacity to plan one's life and give it a sense of direction. A lack of direction in life and a sense of spiritual confusion may be compared to the aimless wandering of the Ethereal Soul; such a loss of purpose and such inability to plan are due to the insufficient "coming and going" of the Ethereal Soul.

If the Liver is flourishing and the Ethereal Soul, while firmly rooted, is also capable of sufficient movement, we are helped to plan our life with vision, wisdom and creativity. If Liver-Blood and Liver-Qi are deficient, the Ethereal Soul does not "come and go" enough and we lack a sense of direction and vision in life.

This lack of a sense of direction and this absence of life dreams are a common spiritual problem and an important feature of depression.

SUMMARY

The Ethereal Soul and planning

- The Ethereal Soul influences our capacity for planning our life and giving it a sense of direction.
- If the Liver is flourishing the Ethereal Soul is firmly rooted and can help us to plan our life with vision, wisdom and creativity; if Liver-Blood and Liver-Qi are deficient, the Ethereal Soul does not "come and go" enough and we lack a sense of direction and vision in life.
- The lack of a sense of direction and the absence of life dreams are important features of depression.

RELATIONSHIP WITH THE MIND

This section will be divided into the following topics.

- Relationship between the Ethereal Soul and Mind
- Mild "manic" behavior in clinical practice
- Examples of the nature of the Ethereal Soul
- The Ethereal Soul and modern diseases
- The Ethereal Soul and Buddhist psychology
- The Ethereal Soul and Jungian psychology
- The movement of the Ethereal Soul and expansion/contraction
- Clinical patterns of pathologies of the Ethereal Soul

Relationship between the Ethereal Soul and the Mind

It is important to consider the relationship between the Mind (*Shen*) and the Ethereal Soul (*Hun*). Both Yang in nature, they are closely connected to each other and both partake in all the mental activities of a human being. We have already seen that the Ethereal Soul is described as the "coming and going" of the Mind. This means that, through the Ethereal Soul, the Mind can project outwards to the external world and to other people and can also turn inwards to receive the intuition, inspiration, dreams and images deriving from the unconscious.

As we have seen above, the modern doctor Wang Ke Qin describes the Ethereal Soul as "another layer of consciousness". This is a good description of the Ethereal Soul's nature; it is another part of our psyche that is independent of the Mind (*Shen*) but is an essential element of our psyche. In a psychoanalytic sense, "another layer of consciousness" could be interpreted as the unconscious, although one has to exercise caution when making direct parallels between ancient Chinese ideas and modern psychoanalysis.

Essential to this nature of the Ethereal Soul is, as described above, its *independent* existence from the Mind as evidenced by the presence of the radical for *gui* in its pictogram; it is the *gui* of our psyche. Here the term *gui* is not used in the sense of the "spirit" of a dead person or "ghost", but has a metaphorical meaning; it is the subterranean part of our psyche, the repository of ideas, inspiration, creativity, projects, life dreams, archetypes.

Thus, if Liver-Blood and Liver-Qi are abundant and the Ethereal Soul is firm, a healthy flow of inspiration, ideas, creativity and plans will stem from it to the Mind. On the other hand, because the Mind provides control and integration to the Ethereal Soul, it must exercise some form of "control" over the material flowing from the Ethereal Soul, and, most of all, must integrate it into the overall psyche.

The perfect relationship between the Mind and the Ethereal Soul is one in which the latter provides the former with "movement" manifesting as aims, intuition, creativity, ideas, life dreams, plans, etc., while the former exercises some control over the psychic influences coming from the latter and integrates them. Left to itself, it is in the nature of the Ethereal Soul to "move" and "wander"; the Ethereal Soul is always searching and always comes up with ideas, projects, aspirations, etc. However, the Mind can deal with only one at a time and must integrate these in the overall psyche. Figure 3.13 illustrates the concept that the Ethereal Soul is the source of several ideas, plans, projects, inspiration and life dreams which the Mind must deal with one at a time.

Zhang Jie Bin says in the *Classic of Categories*: "*The Shen of Qi is called Hun*"; "*The Mind and Ethereal Soul are Yang in nature. The Ethereal Soul follows the Mind, if the Mind is unconscious, the Ethereal Soul is swept away*"; and "*The Mind is Yang within Yang; the Ethereal Soul is Yin within Yang.*"[32]

Figure 3.13 illustrates the ideal relationship between the Mind and the Ethereal Soul in which the movement of the Ethereal Soul is normal and the control and integration of the Mind are also normal.

Being the source of ideas and life dreams for the Mind, the Ethereal Soul may be compared to a sea; its

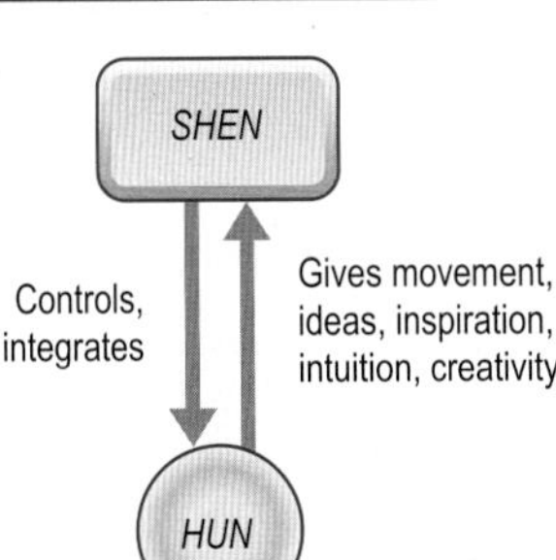

Figure 3.13 Normal relationship between Ethereal Soul and Mind.

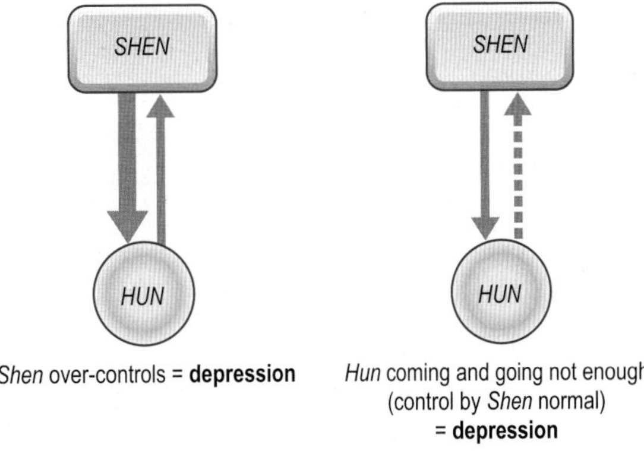

Figure 3.14 Deficient movement of the Ethereal Soul.

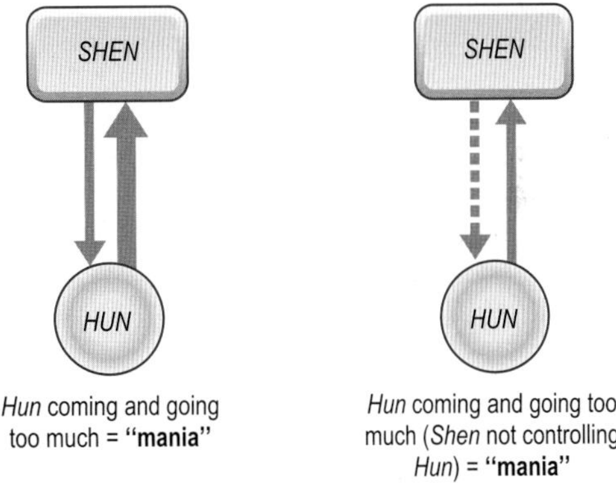

Figure 3.15 Excessive movement of the Ethereal Soul.

world is subterranean and undifferentiated, and it is also the world of *gui*. The Ethereal Soul is the *gui* of the Mind's mental-emotional-spiritual life.

The Mind can cope with only one idea at a time originating from the Ethereal Soul and it must therefore exercise some form of control over the material coming from this source. It must also integrate the material deriving from the Ethereal Soul in the general psychic life. If the Mind is strong and the Ethereal Soul properly "gathered", there will be harmony between the two and the person has calm vision, insight and wisdom.

If the Ethereal Soul does not "come and go" enough, it may lack movement and inspiration, and the person may be depressed, lacking aims and life dreams. The Ethereal Soul may be restrained in its movement either by itself or because the Mind is over-controlling it. This happens, for example, in people who are rigid in their views and repressed. Figure 3.14 illustrates the two situations when the "coming and going" of the Ethereal Soul is restrained either by itself (on the right-hand side) or because the Mind is over-controlling it (on the left-hand side).

Conversely, if the movement of the Ethereal Soul is excessive, there is a surge of ideas, plans, projects, inspiration, etc. flowing out of the Ethereal Soul and flooding the Mind, which cannot control and integrate it. This can be observed in some people who are always full of ideas, dreams and projects, none of which ever comes to fruition because of the chaotic state of the Mind which is unable to restrain the Ethereal Soul.

There are two possible factors leading to this situation. If the Mind is weak and fails in its restraint and control, the Ethereal Soul may be too restless and its "movement" excessive, only bringing confusion and chaos to the Mind, making the person restive, unsettled and, to some degree, manic. On the other hand, the movement of the Ethereal Soul may in itself be excessive (not because the Mind is failing to control it); the result is the same, i.e. an excessive amount of ideas, life dreams, plans and projects flowing out of the Ethereal Soul and making the person, to some degree, manic. Figure 3.15 illustrates the two situations when the "coming and going" of the Ethereal Soul is excessive either in itself (on the left-hand side) or because the Mind does not control it enough (on the right-hand side).

The Mind should integrate the Ethereal Soul so that images, symbols and dreams coming from it can be assimilated. For the conscious Mind this means bringing together two disparate ways of seeing the world; the conscious and rational one (of the Mind) and the entirely different one in which the Ethereal Soul holds sway. If not, the Mind may be flooded by the contents of the Ethereal Soul with a risk of obstruction of the Mind and, in serious cases, of psychosis. If, however, the Mind is weak, or if the Ethereal Soul "comes and goes" too much, the material breaking through from the Ethereal Soul cannot be integrated by the Mind.

> **!**
>
> The key words that describe the function of the Mind in relation to the Ethereal Soul are *control* and *integration*.

Mild "manic" behavior in clinical practice

As I have mentioned the terms "manic" and "mania" a few times in connection with the situation when the Ethereal Soul is not restrained by the Mind and its "coming and going" is excessive, I should define what I mean by this term.

In psychiatric terms, signs and symptoms of *mania* (or a *manic episode*) include:[33]

- increased energy, activity, and restlessness
- an excessively "high", overly good, euphoric mood
- extreme irritability
- racing thoughts and talking very fast, jumping from one idea to another
- distractibility, inability to concentrate well
- little sleep needed
- unrealistic beliefs in one's abilities and powers
- poor judgment
- spending sprees
- a style of behavior that differs from the usual and that proves lasting
- increased sexual drive
- abuse of drugs, particularly cocaine, alcohol or sleeping medications
- provocative, intrusive or aggressive behavior
- denial that anything is wrong.

Full-blown mania will be discussed in Chapter 19. The important thing to realize is that mania and manic behavior can occur in many degrees of severity, i.e. the border between "mental illness" and "normality" is not a clear-cut separation between the two but there is a broad area of behaviors that, while not normal, do not constitute "mental illness". In other words, in their milder forms, "mania" and "manic behavior" are relatively common. Whenever the "coming and going" of the Ethereal Soul is excessive, there is the possibility of "manic" behavior.

> **CLINICAL NOTE**
>
> Mania and manic behavior can occur in many degrees of severity, i.e. the border between "mental illness" and "normality" is not a clear-cut separation between the two but there is a broad area of behaviors that, while not normal, do not constitute "mental illness". In other words, in their milder forms, "mania" and "manic behavior", are relatively common. Whenever the "coming and going" of the Ethereal Soul is excessive, there is the possibility of "manic" behavior.

My own criteria for diagnosing mild "mania" (i.e. in normal people who are not mentally ill) are as follows:

- mental restlessness, agitation
- hyperactivity
- working and being active at night
- spending a lot
- having many projects simultaneously, none of which comes to fruition
- embarking on risky projects
- high sex drive and seeking multiple partners
- an almost messianic drive in one's chosen field
- mental confusion
- obsessive thoughts
- laughing a lot
- talking a lot and/or fast
- propensity to taking risks
- often artistic.

Examples of the nature of the Ethereal Soul

In order to give the reader a feel for the actions of the Ethereal Soul, I have listed six things (Fig. 3.16):

1. children
2. artistic inspiration
3. dreams
4. sleepwalking
5. guided daydreams
6. coma.

Children

Children are a good example of the activity of the Ethereal Soul. In small children, the Mind (*Shen*) is "immature" and it therefore does not control and restrain the

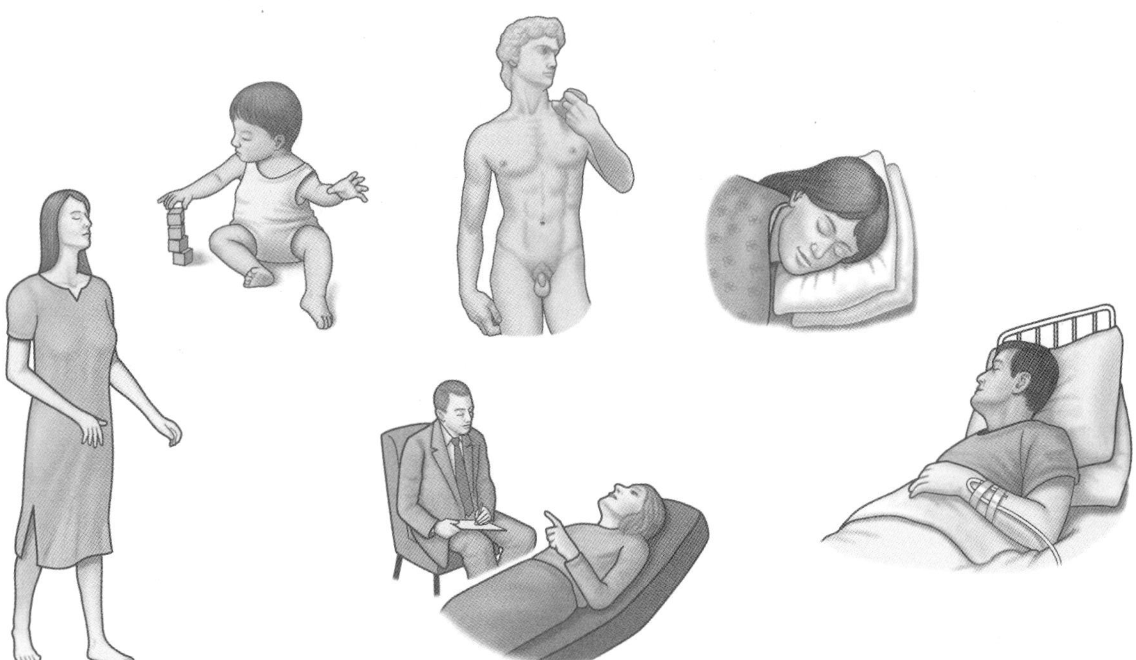

Figure 3.16 Six illustrations of the activity of the Ethereal Soul.

Ethereal Soul. In adults, this is a pathological situation which is illustrated on the right-hand side of Figure 3.15. In children, however, it is perfectly normal.

The result is that, from the age of about 2 to about 7, children live in the world of the Ethereal Soul, a world of wild imagination and fantasy where inanimate objects come to life. Behaviors that are normal in children would be considered mental illness in adults. After the age of about 7, the Mind (*Shen*) is more mature and it starts to control and restrain the Ethereal Soul.

Artistic inspiration

Artistic inspiration is another good example of the activity of the Ethereal Soul. In Western art, at least, artistic inspiration derives from the Ethereal Soul, not the Mind.[34] The Ethereal Soul is the source from which creativity and inspiration spring forth. The same psychic energy that, in pathological conditions, leads to manic behavior is also responsible for artistic inspiration. In fact, this is the result of the "coming and going" of the Ethereal Soul; it is the Ethereal Soul that is the source of images coming forth in an artist's mind and work. It is interesting to note that, among the artistic community, there is a disproportionate incidence of bipolar disorder compared to the general population.[35]

Dreams

Dreams derive from the wandering of the Ethereal Soul at night; when the Ethereal Soul goes to the eyes in daytime, we see; when it goes to the eyes at night, we dream. It is interesting that most dreaming takes place during the rapid eye movement (REM) periods of sleep. It could be argued that the REM is due to the Ethereal Soul's going to the eyes at night! It is also interesting to note that we suffer more from dream deprivation than from lack of sleep.

The "language" of dreams is also interesting. Dreams speak to us in a symbolic language precisely because they derive from the Ethereal Soul and not from the Mind.

Dream sleep is a good illustration of the respective roles of the Mind (*Shen* of the Heart) and of the Ethereal Soul (*Hun*). When we are asleep, the Mind is temporarily disabled (so to speak) but during dream there is some consciousness; this is provided by the movement of the Ethereal Soul at night.

From a Western perspective, Damasio says something similar. He says that wakefulness and consciousness generally go together but there are situations when that is not the case. During dream sleep, we have some consciousness but not wakefulness; that is because the Mind is asleep but the Ethereal Soul is moving, producing some form of consciousness. There are neurological conditions when the opposite happens, i.e. there is no consciousness but there is wakefulness. This happens, for example, during the episodes of petit mal epilepsy.[36]

Sleepwalking

In sleepwalking, the Mind is inactive but the Ethereal Soul is active; the Ethereal Soul wanders at night and leads to sleepwalking. Interestingly, the point BL-47 Hunmen (the Door of the *Hun*) was used to treat sleepwalking.

Guided daydreams

Guided daydreams are a technique used in psychotherapy whereby the therapist sets a certain scene for the client who is asked to imagine him or herself in that scene and to proceed as if in a dream. The aim of this exercise is to bypass the critical analysis of the Mind and bring forth psychological material from the Ethereal Soul as happens in dreams.

Jung described this technique:[37]

We learn to sit and simply observe a fragment of a dream without any attempt to guide, control or interfere with it. The aim is to allow the image to come to life of its own autonomous psychic energy [= Ethereal Soul], *our ego* [= Mind] *letting go of all expectations, presuppositions, or interpretations. After a certain period of practice and initial coaching by the therapist, this inner image will start to move in some way and our observing ego* [Mind] *learns to participate in the story very much like a dream.*

Coma

In coma, the Mind is completely devoid of residence and it therefore cannot function at all, and yet the person is not dead. This means that there are other mental aspects at play, and these are the Ethereal Soul and the Corporeal Soul. In fact, for death to occur, not only must the Mind die, but the Ethereal Soul must leave the body and the Corporeal Soul return to Earth.

The Ethereal Soul and modern diseases

The movement (or lack of movement) of the Ethereal Soul and its relationship with the Mind play a crucial role in many modern pathologies. For example, besides accounting for depression and manic behavior as described above, a dysfunction of the movement of the Ethereal Soul (either deficient or excessive) may explain autism and attention deficit hyperactivity disorder (ADHD).

In fact, autism could be seen as a pathology characterized by an insufficient movement of the Ethereal Soul causing the autistic person to find projection towards other people difficult; unlike depression (also characterized by a deficient movement of the Ethereal Soul), in autism the Mind (*Shen*) fails, too, in its integrative function. By contrast, in ADHD, there is an excessive movement of the Ethereal Soul and a deficient controlling function of the Mind.

The Ethereal Soul and Buddhist psychology

Drawing from Buddhist ideas, the Mind could be said to be the individual Mind, and the Ethereal Soul the link between the individual Mind and the Universal Mind. This can be represented with a diagram (Fig. 3.17).

The Universal Mind is the repository of images, archetypes, symbols and ideas belonging to the collective unconscious in Jungian psychology. These often manifest to our Mind as myths, symbols and dreams.

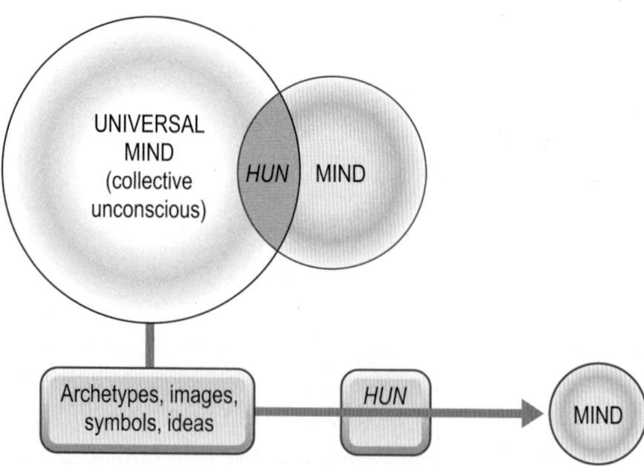

Figure 3.17 The relationship between Ethereal Soul and Mind from Buddhist and Jungian viewpoint.

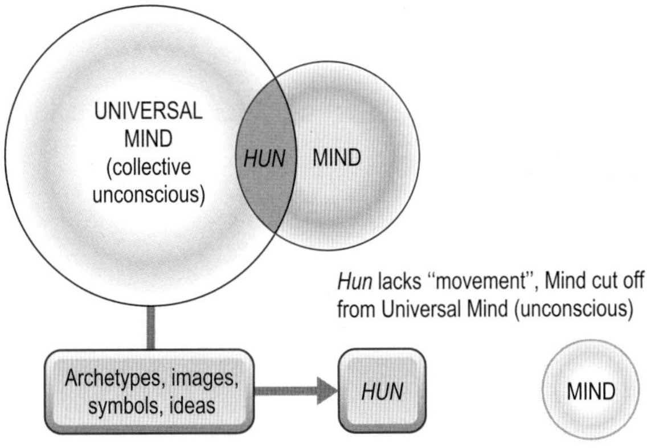

Figure 3.18 Deficient movement of the Ethereal Soul and its relation with Universal Unconscious.

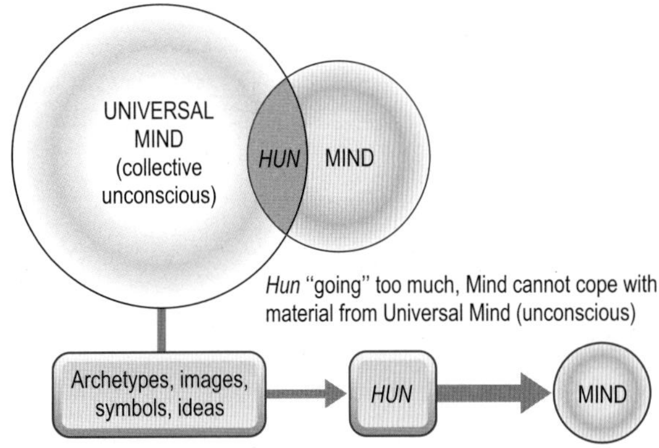

Figure 3.19 Excessive movement of the Ethereal Soul and its relation with Universal Unconscious.

They come into our consciousness (individual Mind) via the Ethereal Soul since this belongs to the world of image and ideas. Thus the Ethereal Soul is the vehicle through which images, ideas and symbols from the Universal Mind (or the collective unconscious) emerge into our individual Mind (consciousness).

This shows the vital importance of the Ethereal Soul for our mental and spiritual life. Without the Ethereal Soul, our mental and spiritual life would be quite sterile and deprived of images, ideas and dreams. If the Liver is strong and the Ethereal Soul firm and flowing harmoniously, ideas and images from the Universal Mind will flow freely and the mental and spiritual state will be happy, creative and fruitful. If the "coming and going" of the Ethereal Soul is insufficient, the individual Mind will be cut off from the Universal Mind and will be unhappy, confused, isolated, aimless, sterile and without dreams (Fig. 3.18).

On the other hand, if the Mind is clouded and cannot exercise its proper control over the Ethereal Soul, it cannot integrate material breaking through from the Ethereal Soul (Fig. 3.19). It is important for the Mind to assume an integrating position towards the Ethereal Soul so that images, symbols and dreams coming from it can be assimilated. If not, the Mind may be flooded by the contents of the Ethereal Soul with a risk of obstruction of the Mind and, in serious cases, of psychosis.

The Ethereal Soul and Jungian psychology

According to Jung, the unconscious is compensatory to consciousness. He said: "*The psyche is a self-regulating system that maintains itself in equilibrium. Every process*

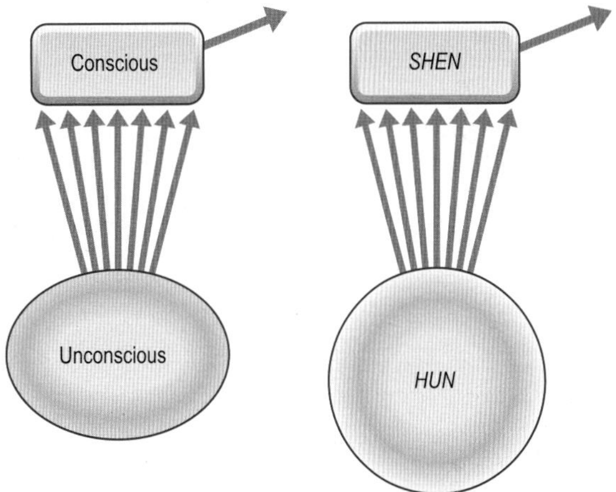

Figure 3.20 Comparison of the relationship between the Ethereal Soul and Mind with that between the unconscious and conscious.

that goes too far immediately and inevitably calls forth a compensatory activity."[38] This compensatory relationship between the unconscious and consciousness resembles the balancing relationship between the Ethereal Soul and the Mind.

The Mind discriminates and differentiates, whereas the Ethereal Soul is like an undifferentiated sea which flows around, under and above the Mind, eroding certain parts and depositing fresh material. The psyche as a whole, i.e. the sum total of Mind, Ethereal Soul, Corporeal Soul, Intellect and Will-Power, contains all possibilities, whereas the Mind can work with only one possibility at a time (Fig. 3.20). Figure 3.20 shows many arrows from the Ethereal Soul to the Mind (indicating the material in the form of ideas coming from

Figure 3.21 Total absorption of the Mind within the Ethereal Soul in mental illness.

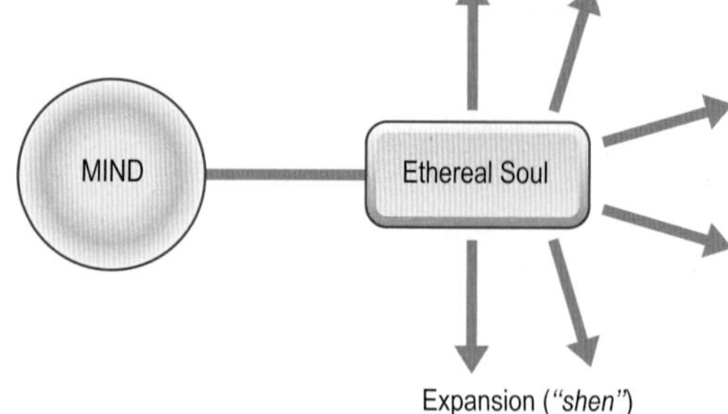

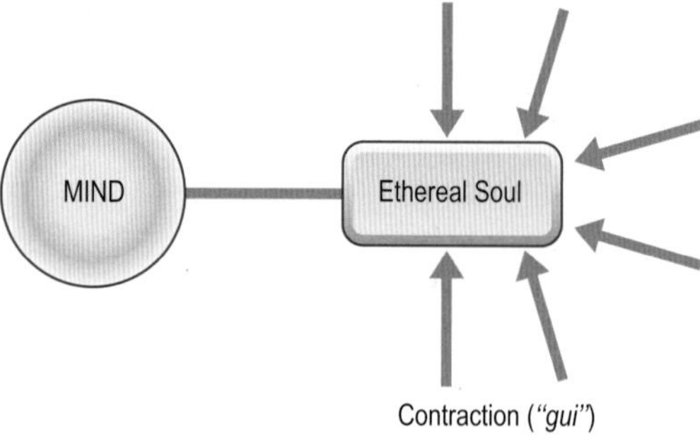

Figure 3.22 Expansion and contraction of the Ethereal Soul.

the Ethereal Soul) but only one arrow coming out of the Mind.

It is no wonder that in myths and fairytales the unconscious is often symbolized by the sea. The Ethereal Soul is an underwater world and a total immersion of the Mind in it means insanity (Fig. 3.21). In Figure 3.21, the Mind is totally enclosed by the Ethereal Soul; this image is used to depict mental illness.

In Christian mythology too, baptism uses water and the sea as a spiritual symbol, as does the parting of the waters by God. Like an ocean, it is the source of archetypes, symbols, ideas, images; the Mind draws from this sea through the intermediary of the Ethereal Soul. The material coming forth is controlled and, item by item, integrated by the Mind (hence the key words "control" and "integration" expressing the Mind's function in relation to the Ethereal Soul).

The movement of the Ethereal Soul and expansion/contraction

The relationship between the Mind and the Ethereal Soul is all about expansion (stimulation of the "coming and going" of the Ethereal Soul) and contraction (restraint of the "coming and going" of the Ethereal Soul) in our psychic life. *Shen* and *gui* can be interpreted as the two opposing states of expansion (*shen*) and contraction (*gui*) in our psychic life (Fig. 3.22).

Expansion and contraction in our psychic life are two normal, physiological states that alternate naturally. When we feel "up", we are in an extroverted mood, we feel like going out and we are active; that is, we are then in a state of expansion and the Ethereal Soul is "coming and going" normally. When we feel "down", we are in an introverted mood, we do not want to go out and we are passive; that is, we are then in a state of contraction and the Ethereal Soul's "coming and going" is restrained.[39]

The proper alternation of expansion (stimulation of the coming and going of the Ethereal Soul) and contraction (restraint of the coming and going of the Ethereal Soul) in our psychic life allows for it to be healthy and normal.

Chinese herbal medicine reflects this polarity of expansion and contraction in our psychic life as, within the category of herbs that calm the Mind, some are pungent and stimulate expansion (and therefore the coming and going of the Ethereal Soul), while others are sour and astringent and stimulate contraction (and therefore restrain the coming and going of the Ethereal Soul).

The two important herbs Yuan Zhi *Radix Polygalae* and Suan Zao Ren *Semen Ziziphi spinosae* are representative of this polarity of expansion and contraction. The actions of these two herbs are described below.

- Yuan Zhi *Radix Polygalae*: pungent, bitter, warm, dispersing and draining, resolves Phlegm, opens the Heart orifices = stimulates expansion, i.e. the coming and going of Ethereal Soul.
- Suan Zao Ren *Semen Ziziphi spinosae*: sour, sweet, astringent, promotes sleep, anchors the Ethereal Soul = stimulates contraction, i.e. restraint of the coming and going of the Ethereal Soul.

Clinical patterns of pathologies of the Ethereal Soul

In terms of patterns, what are those that arise from the Ethereal Soul's "coming and going", too much or too little? The coming and going of the Ethereal Soul may become excessive either from Full conditions of Heat or Fire or from Empty conditions with a deficiency of Liver-Blood and/or Liver-Yin.

In the case of Full conditions with Heat or Fire, these agitate the Ethereal Soul and stimulate its coming and going excessively; in the case of Empty conditions with deficiency of Liver-Blood and/or Liver-Yin, these fail to anchor the Ethereal Soul so that this becomes agitated and its coming and going becomes excessive. Although the end result is the same, the symptoms and signs of the Ethereal Soul's coming and going too much from Full conditions and coming and going too much from Empty conditions will be different. Excessive coming and going of the Ethereal Soul results in "manic behavior" as described above.

The coming and going of the Ethereal Soul may become deficient under three conditions: Liver-Qi stagnation, Liver-Blood and Liver-Qi deficiency, and deficiency of Yang of the Spleen and Kidneys may all impair its coming and going and result in depression. It is worth remembering that the Ethereal Soul, although residing in the Liver, is affected by many other organs. In particular, the movement of the Ethereal Soul relies on Yang Qi and therefore a deficiency of Spleen- and Kidney-Yang often impairs this movement, resulting in depression.

I should explain the pattern of Liver-Qi deficiency in more detail. Although we are often told that "Liver-Qi cannot be deficient", this is not quite true. Deficiency of Liver-Qi does exist and it manifests primarily in the psychic sphere with depression.

As we know, every organ's Qi should flow in a proper, correct direction, e.g. Stomach-Qi descends, Spleen-Qi ascends, etc. Liver-Qi should flow in all directions; this is the manifestation of the free flow of Liver-Qi. However, the normal, correct flow of Liver-Qi is also ascending; its ascending movement is coordinated with the descending of Lung-Qi.

Where does Liver-Qi ascend to? One important aspect of this movement is Liver-Qi's ascension towards the Heart and the Mind (*Shen*). The ascending of Liver-Qi towards the Mind is an important way in which the Ethereal Soul stimulates the "coming and going" of the Mind (Fig. 3.23). A deficiency of Liver-Qi always implies a failure of Liver-Qi to ascend to the Mind and therefore results in depression.

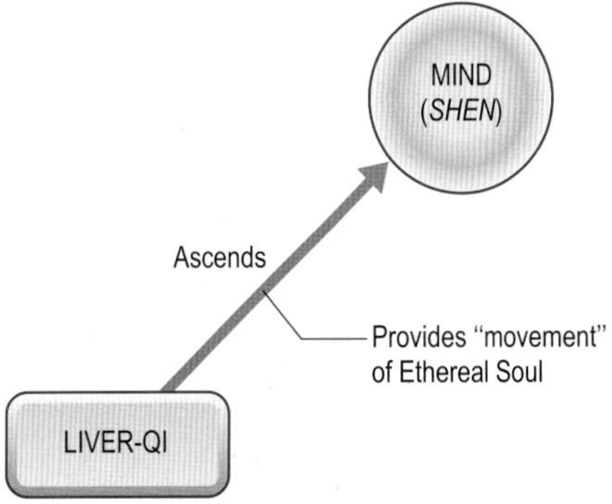

Figure 3.23 Ascending movement of Liver-Qi in relation to the Ethereal Soul.

What are the symptoms of Liver-Qi deficiency? First, they include all the symptoms of Liver-Blood deficiency (blurred vision, tingling of limbs, dry hair and skin); second, they include symptoms such as sighing, tiredness and depression.

The patterns manifesting in excessive or insufficient movement of the Ethereal Soul are listed below:

- Ethereal Soul coming and going too much ("manic" behavior)
  - Heat or Fire
  - Phlegm-Fire (in which case the Mind is also obstructed)
  - Liver-Blood and/or Liver-Yin deficiency
- Ethereal Soul coming and going too little (depression)
  - Liver-Qi stagnation
  - Liver-Blood and Liver-Qi deficiency
  - Spleen- and Kidney-Yang deficiency.

SUMMARY

Relationship between the Mind and the Ethereal Soul

- The Ethereal Soul is the "coming and going" of the Mind.
- Through the Ethereal Soul, the Mind can project outwards to the external world and to other people and can also turn inwards to receive the intuition, inspiration, dreams and images deriving from the unconscious.

- The Ethereal Soul provides the Mind with "movement" manifesting with aims, intuition, creativity, ideas, life dreams, plans, etc.; on the other hand, the Mind provides control and integration to the Ethereal Soul.
- If the Ethereal Soul does not "come and go" enough, it may lack movement and inspiration and the person may be depressed, aimless or without life dreams.
- If the Mind is weak and fails to restrain and control the Ethereal Soul, this may be too restless and its "movement" excessive, only bringing confusion and chaos to the Mind, and making the person scattered, unsettled and, to a slight degree, manic.
- The nature and activity of the Ethereal Soul may be observed in six areas, i.e. children's fantasy, artistic inspiration, dreams, sleepwalking, guided daydreams and coma.
- The patterns that arise from the Ethereal Soul's "coming and going" too much are Full conditions of Heat or Fire or Empty conditions with a deficiency of Liver-Blood and/or Liver-Yin; the patterns that arise from the Ethereal Soul's coming and going too little are Liver-Qi stagnation, Liver-Blood and Liver-Qi deficiency and deficiency of Yang of the Spleen and Kidneys.

SUMMARY

The Ethereal Soul

- The Ethereal Soul enters the body 3 days after birth; at death, it survives the body and returns to "Heaven".
- It resides in the Liver and is anchored in Liver-Blood and Liver-Yin.
- It is responsible for:
  - sleep and dreaming
  - mental activities in association with the Mind (*Shen*)
  - emotional balance
  - sight
  - courage
  - planning
  - giving the Mind "movement" in the sense of ideas, vision, plans, life dreams, intuition, creativity.

CLINICAL APPLICATION

The Ethereal Soul is of huge clinical significance; it is an essential component of our psyche and a crucial companion of the Mind (*Shen*). As discussed above, the Mind could not function without the input of the Ethereal Soul.

From a practical, clinical viewpoint, it is very important to realize that the Ethereal Soul's residing in the Liver does not mean that it is influenced only by the Liver; it may be influenced by any organ. For example, Heat of any organ (e.g. Heart, Lungs, Stomach, Kidneys), besides that of the Liver, can agitate the Ethereal Soul.

As we have seen, a deficient movement or an excessive movement are the two main pathological conditions of the Ethereal Soul. A deficient movement may lead to depression, while an excessive one may lead to behavior that is, to a slight degree, manic. Both conditions can be aggravated by the presence of Phlegm obstructing the Mind.

I will outline below the treatment of the main pathological conditions with acupuncture and herbs.

Acupuncture

Deficient movement of the Ethereal Soul (depression)

General points to stimulate movement of the Ethereal Soul

G.B.-40 Qiuxu, BL-47 Hunmen, P-6 Neiguan, Du-20 Baihui, Hunshe extra point (see Fig. 3.24). Reinforcing method.

Points according to pattern

Qi stagnation

- Liver-Qi stagnation: P-6 Neiguan, G.B.-40 Qiuxu, LIV-3 Taichong, BL-47 Hunmen, Du-20 Baihui, Hunshe. If there is Phlegm, add ST-40 Fenglong, Ren-9 Shuifen and SP-6 Sanyinjiao. Reducing or even method.
- Heart- and Lung-Qi stagnation: P-6 Neiguan, BL-47 Hunmen, Du-20 Baihui, Hunshe, LU-7 Lieque, Ren-17 Shanzhong. If there is Phlegm, add ST-40

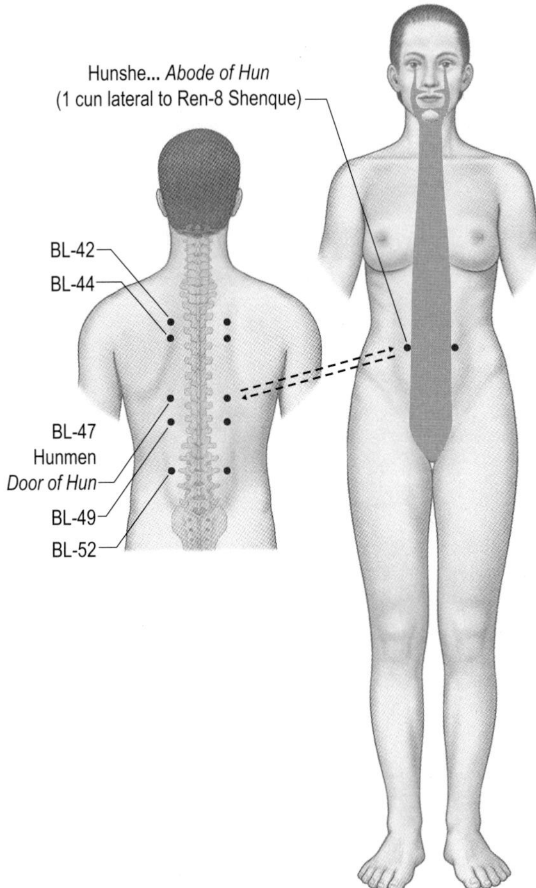

Figure 3.24 Location of extra point Hunshe.

Fenglong, Ren-9 Shuifen and SP-6 Sanyinjiao. Reducing or even method.

Liver-Blood and Liver-Qi deficiency

G.B.-40 Qiuxu, Du-20 Baihui, BL-47 Hunmen, Hunshe, LIV-8 Ququan, ST-36 Zusanli, SP-6 Sanyinjiao, Ren-4 Guanyuan. Reinforcing method.

Spleen- and Kidney-Yang deficiency

G.B.-40 Qiuxu, Du-20 Baihui, BL-47 Hunmen, Hunshe, Ren-12 Zhongwan, ST-36 Zusanli, KI-3 Taixi, BL-20 Pishu, BL-23 Shenshu, BL-52 Zhishi. Reinforcing method. Moxa is applicable.

Excessive movement of the Ethereal Soul (slightly manic behavior)

General points to restrain the movement of the Ethereal Soul

LIV-3 Taichong, BL-47 Hunmen, P-7 Daling, Hunshe. Reducing or even method.

Points according to pattern

Heat or Fire

- Liver-Fire: LIV-2 Xingjian, LIV-3 Taichong, P-7 Daling, BL-47 Hunmen, Hunshe. Reducing or even method.
- Heart-Fire: LIV-3 Taichong, BL-47 Hunmen, Hunshe, P-7 Daling, HE-8 Shaofu. Reducing or even method.

Phlegm-Fire

- Phlegm-Fire in the Liver: LIV-3 Taichong, BL-47 Hunmen, Hunshe, P-7 Daling, LIV-2 Xingjian, G.B.-13 Benshen, G.B.-17 Zhengying, G.B.-18 Chengling (plus general points to resolve Phlegm). Reducing or even method.
- Phlegm-Heat in the Lungs and Heart: BL-47 Hunmen, Hunshe, P-7 Daling, P-5 Jianshi, Ren-15 Jiuwei, G.B.-17 Zhengying, G.B.-18 Chengling (plus general points to resolve Phlegm). Reducing or even method.

Liver-Blood and/or Liver-Yin deficiency

LIV-3 Taichong, BL-47 Hunmen, Hunshe, P-7 Daling, HE-7 Shenmen, Ren-4 Guanyuan, LIV-8 Ququan, ST-36 Zusanli, SP-6 Sanyinjiao. Reinforcing method.

Herbal therapy

Deficient movement of the Ethereal Soul (depression)

Qi stagnation

- Liver-Qi stagnation: Yue Ju Wan *Gardenia-Chuanxiong Pill.*
- Heart- and Lung-Qi stagnation: Ban Xia Hou Po Tang *Pinellia-Magnolia Decoction.*

Liver-Blood and Liver-Qi deficiency

Empirical prescription by Dr Chen Jia Xu.[40]

Spleen- and Kidney-Yang deficiency

You Gui Wan *Restoring the Right* [Kidney] *Pill*.

Excessive movement of the Ethereal Soul (slightly manic behavior)

Heat or Fire

- Liver-Fire: Long Dan Xie Gan Tang *Gentiana Draining the Liver Decoction* plus Fu Shen *Sclerotium Poriae pararadicis*, Long Gu *Mastodi Ossis fossilia*, Mu Li *Concha Ostreae*, Ye Jiao Teng *Caulis Polygoni multiflori*.
- Heart-Fire: Dao Chi San *Eliminating Redness Powder* plus Lian Zi Xin *Plumula Nelumbinis* and Huang Qin *Radix Scutellariae*.

Phlegm-Fire

- Phlegm-Fire in Liver: Ling Jiao Gou Teng Tang *Cornu Saigae-Uncaria Decoction* plus Zhu Ru *Caulis Bambusae in Taeniam* and Gua Lou *Fructus Trichosanthis*.
- Phlegm-Fire in Heart: Wen Dan Tang *Warming the Gall-Bladder Decoction*.

Liver-Blood and/or Liver-Yin deficiency

Suan Zao Ren Tang *Ziziphus Decoction*.

END NOTES

1. Giles H 1912 Chinese-English Dictionary. Kelly & Walsh, Shanghai, p. 650.
2. Gu Yu Qi 2005 Zhong Yi Xin Li Xue 中医心理学[Chinese Medicine Psychology]. China Medicine Science and Technology Publishing House, Beijing, p. 35.
3. 1982 Lei Jing 类经 [Classic of Categories]. People's Health Publishing House, Beijing, p. 50. The *Classic of Categories* was written by Zhang Jie Bin (also called Zhang Jing Yue) and first published in 1624.
4. Ibid., p. 50.
5. 1981 Ling Shu Jing 灵枢经 [Spiritual Axis]. People's Health Publishing House, Beijing, p. 23. First published *c* 100 BC.
6. Chinese Medicine Psychology, p. 3.
7. Recently (April 2008) the General Secretary of the Communist Party of Tibet called the Dalai Lama an "evil spirit" (gui). For him to call the Dalai Lama that, it clearly shows that he believes in *gui*, which is strange after 60 years of Marxist education in China.
8. Tian Dai Hua 2005 Ling Shu Jing 灵枢经 [Spiritual Axis]. People's Health Publishing House, Beijing, p. 110. First published *c*.100 BC.
9. Chinese Medicine Psychology, p. 35.
10. 1979 Xue Zheng Lun 血证论 [Discussion on Blood Patterns]. People's Health Publishing House, Beijing, p. 29. The *Discussion on Blood Patterns* was written by Tang Zong Hai and first published in 1884.
11. Wilhelm R (translator) 1962 The Secret of the Golden Flower. Harcourt, Brace & World, New York, p. 26.
12. Ibid., p. 26.
13. Chinese Medicine Psychology, p. 35.
14. Wang Ke Qin 1988 Zhong Yi Shen Zhu Xue Shuo 中医神主学说 [Theory of the Mind in Chinese Medicine]. Ancient Chinese Medical Texts Publishing House, Beijing, pp. 94–95.
15. Classic of Categories, p. 48.
16. Classic of Categories, p. 50.
17. Cited in Wang Ke Qin 1988 Theory of the Mind in Chinese Medicine, p. 8.
18. Kong Ying Da Wu Jing Zheng Yi [Five-Channel Righteousness], cited in Theory of the Mind in Chinese Medicine, p. 37.
19. Theory of the Mind in Chinese Medicine, p. 36.
20. Ibid.
21. 1979 Huang Di Nei Jing Su Wen 黄帝内经素问[The Yellow Emperor's Classic of Internal Medicine – Simple Questions]. People's Health Publishing House, Beijing, p. 58. First published *c*.100 BC.
22. Searle JR 2004 Mind. Oxford University Press, Oxford.
23. Trimble MR 2007 The Soul in the Brain. Johns Hopkins University Press, Baltimore, p. 194.
24. Simple Questions, p. 68.
25. Spiritual Axis, p. 24.
26. Discussion on Blood Patterns, p. 29.
27. Cited in Theory of the Mind in Chinese Medicine, p. 37.
28. Simple Questions, p. 335.
29. The Essence of the Convergence between Chinese and Western Medicine, cited in Theory of the Mind in Chinese Medicine, p. 36.
30. The Secret of the Golden Flower, p. 26.
31. Cited in Theory of the Mind in Chinese Medicine, p. 36.
32. Ibid., p. 36.
33. National Institute of Mental Health website: www.nimh.nih.gov [Accessed 2008].
34. It is interesting to note that this statement probably applies to Western, not Chinese, art. Chinese art (painting, calligraphy, music and poetry) was traditionally carried out by the educated Confucian gentleman, not as an expression of his inner self, but as an artistic pursuit conducted according to rigid rules. It could therefore be said that this type of Chinese art derives from the Mind rather than the Ethereal Soul. I am using the word "gentleman" with reason as, according to Confucian philosophy, such activities were the domain of men, with women confined to cooking, sewing and looking after the household.
35. Redfield Jamison K 1993 Touched with Fire – Manic-Depressive Illness and the Artistic Temperament. Free Press, New York.
36. Damasio A 1999 The Feeling of What Happens – Body and Emotion in the Making of Consciousness. Harcourt, San Diego, pp. 89–90.
37. Jung CG 1961 Modern Man in Search of a Soul, Routledge & Kegan Paul, London.
38. Ibid.
39. Many pieces of classical music display such alternation of expansion and contraction, none more than Beethoven's. Many of Beethoven's works are characterized by musical phrases of intense, deep, romantic feeling ("expansion") to be followed quickly by phrases of turbulent and dark passion ("contraction"). The best example of such an alternation of feelings is Beethoven's Violin Sonata No. 5 ("Spring").
40. Chen Jia Xu 1994 Discussion on the syndrome of Liver-Qi deficiency. Journal of Chinese Medicine (*Zhong Yi Za Zhi*) 5: 264–267.

魄

CHAPTER 4

THE CORPOREAL SOUL (*PO*)

THE CORPOREAL SOUL AND THE ESSENCE (*JING*) *48*

INFANCY *51*

SENSES *51*

PHYSIOLOGICAL ACTIVITY *52*

EMOTIONS *53*

BREATHING *54*

THE CORPOREAL SOUL AND INDIVIDUAL LIFE *54*

THE CORPOREAL SOUL AND THE *GUI* *54*

THE CORPOREAL SOUL AND THE ANUS *55*

RELATIONSHIP BETWEEN CORPOREAL SOUL AND ETHEREAL SOUL *55*

CLINICAL APPLICATION *60*

Contraction of the Corporeal Soul *60*

Expansion of the Corporeal Soul *60*

THE CORPOREAL SOUL (*PO*)

The Corporeal Soul (*Po*) resides in the Lungs and is the physical counterpart of the Ethereal Soul. Its Chinese character is composed of two parts: one (on the right) is the radical *gui*, which means "spirit" or "ghost", the other (on the left) is the radical for *bai* (or *bo*), meaning "white".

The character for Corporeal Soul is *Po*:

魄

This is composed of the radical *gui* for "spirit" or "ghost":

鬼

and the character for "white":

白

The radical for "white" in the character for *Po* can have several interpretations. The *bai* (or *bo*) meaning "white" within the character is related not only to the light of the waxing moon, but is also phonetic, i.e. it gives the character the sound *po*. The association with the waxing moon (Yin) is in keeping with the association of the Corporeal Soul with Yin (as opposed to the Ethereal Soul that is Yang). The connection between the Corporeal Soul and the moon is also related to the fact that this physical soul comes into being on the third day after conception, analogous to the thin crescent on the third day of the rising moon.

Finally, the association with the color white somewhat tempers the radical for the dark *gui* and it conveys the idea that the Corporeal Soul, although related to *gui*, is a human, physical soul. See Figure 4.1.

Hence there is a connection between the Corporeal Soul and the embryonic lunar light (Yin) as opposed to the hot (Yang) sun light of the Ethereal Soul. In fact, in ancient times, the Corporeal Soul was also called "Moon-Po". As the waxing moon is in the West, one can therefore build the following correspondence:

WEST – WHITE – METAL – CORPOREAL SOUL – LUNGS.

The Corporeal Soul can be defined as "*that part of the Soul* [as opposed to the Ethereal Soul] *which is indissolubly attached to the body and goes down to Earth with it at death*".[1] It is closely linked to the body and could be described as the somatic expression of the Soul or, conversely, the organizational principle of the body. However, it is important not to interpret the Corporeal

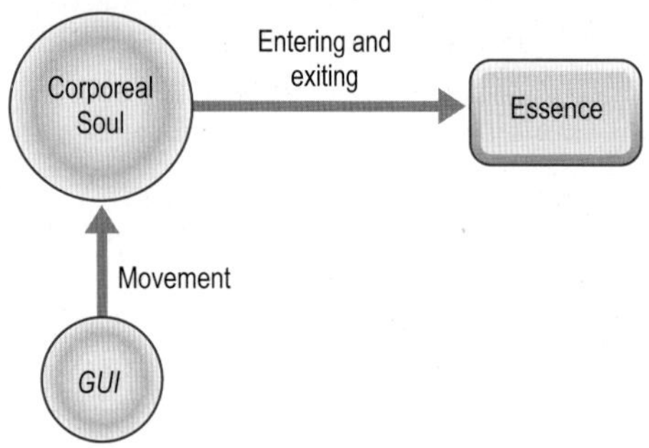

Figure 4.1 *Gui* within the Corporeal Soul.

Soul in terms of the Western duality between the inert, physical body and a "soul" that inhabits it and gives it life. From the point of view of Chinese medicine, the Corporeal Soul is the physiological activity of the body and this, itself, is the soul.

The Corporeal Soul could also be described as the organization of the organism and the coordinating force of all physiological processes. Zhang Jie Bin says:[2]

In the beginning of an individual's life the body is formed; the spirit of the body is the Corporeal Soul. When the Corporeal Soul is in the Interior there is [enough] *Yang Qi.*

The Corporeal Soul is active from conception and it shapes the body. In the traditional view, the Corporeal Soul entered the body 3 days after conception, analogous to the third day of the rising moon.

The great Neo-Confucian philosopher Zhu Xi said:[3]

As for the birth of a human being, the first change and transformation produce physical form. The numinous part of the physical form is named Corporeal Soul. After the Corporeal Soul has been produced, there spontaneously is Yang Qi inside Corporeal Soul. The Shen part of Qi is named Ethereal Soul.

At death, unlike the Ethereal Soul, the Corporeal Soul dies with the body but it is thought to adhere to the corpse for some time, especially the bones, before returning to Earth. This explains the importance of looking after the bones of the dead in ancient Chinese culture. Some years after death, relatives of the dead used to clean the bones of the skeleton carefully and place them in neat bundles.

There are seven types of Corporeal Soul: the five senses, the limbs and the Corporeal Soul as a whole. The link between the five senses and the Corporeal Soul will be explained shortly.

As we have seen for the Ethereal Soul, the ancient character for *gui* conveys the idea of movement, an expression of the swirling movement of the bodiless head of a dead person in the realm of spirits. The Ethereal Soul is responsible for movement in a psychic sense and the Corporeal Soul in a physical sense.

The movement related to the Corporeal Soul is a physical movement of this soul in all physiological processes of the body. Also, the Corporeal Soul gives the body the capacity of movement, agility, balance and coordination of movements.

The Ethereal Soul is described as the "coming and going" of the Mind while the Corporeal Soul is described as the "entering and exiting" of the Essence (see below).

As we shall see below, the Corporeal Soul is in relation with *gui*. Confucius said: "*Qi is the fullness of the Shen; the Corporeal Soul is the fullness of gui.*"[4] He Shang Gong said:[5]

The turbid and humid five flavours form bones, flesh, blood, vessels and the six passions ... this gui is called Corporeal Soul. This is Yin in character and enters and exits through the mouth and communicates with Earth.

The discussion of the Corporeal Soul will be conducted according to the following topics.

- The Corporeal Soul and the Essence (*Jing*)
- Infancy
- Senses
- Physiological activity
- Emotions
- Breathing
- The Corporeal Soul and individual life
- The Corporeal Soul and the *gui*
- The Corporeal Soul and the anus
- Relationship between Corporeal Soul and Ethereal Soul
- Clinical application

THE CORPOREAL SOUL AND ESSENCE (*JING*)

The Corporeal Soul is closely linked to the Essence (*Jing*) and is described in Chapter 8 of the *Spiritual Axis* as the "*exiting and entering of Essence*".[6] The Corporeal Soul derives from the mother and arises at conception (in theory, 3 days after conception) soon after the Prenatal Essence of a newly conceived being is formed. Thus the Corporeal Soul, closely linked to Essence, is the first to come into being after conception. Both Essence and Corporeal Soul represent the organizational principles of life which shape the body from conception (the Extraordinary Vessels are the channels through which this happens).

"Entering and exiting" implies an Interior and Exterior, i.e. a separation of the individual from the environment. It also implies a vertical movement as *ru* 入 (to enter) evokes "roots" and *chu* 出 (to exit) evokes "branches". Thus the centripetal, separating, materializing movement of the Corporeal Soul (see below) also depends on the vertical exiting and entering of the Essence (Fig. 4.2).

The Corporeal Soul could be described as the manifestation of the Essence in the sphere of sensations and feelings. Just as the Ethereal Soul provides psychic movement to the Mind ("*coming and going of the Mind*"), the Corporeal Soul provides physical movement to the Essence, i.e. it brings the Essence into play in all physiological processes of the body.

This is a very important function of the Corporeal Soul as without it, the Essence would be an inert, albeit precious, vital substance. The Corporeal Soul is the closest to the Essence and is the intermediary between it and the other vital substances of the body. In fact, Zhang Jie Bin in the *Classic of Categories* says: "*If the Essence is exhausted, the Corporeal Soul declines, Qi is scattered and the Ethereal Soul swims without a residence.*"[7]

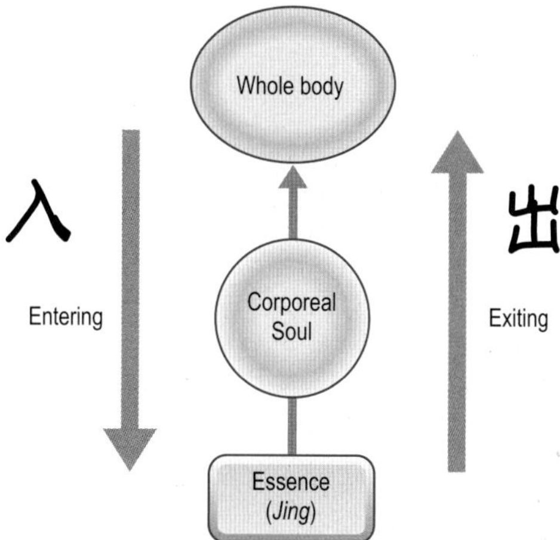

Figure 4.2 The entering and exiting of the Essence.

CLINICAL NOTE

Through the Corporeal Soul, the Essence (*Jing*) of the Kidneys plays a role in all physiological processes. This is further confirmation that the Essence, although a precious, partly inherited and constitutional Essence, does not simply "reside" in the Lower *Dan Tian*. Through the Corporeal Soul, it "enters and exits" in all parts of the body, playing a role in all physiological activities. The implication of this is that, when nourishing the Essence (through tonification of the Kidneys), it is better to also strengthen the Corporeal Soul (through tonification of the Lungs). This may be an explanation why the opening points of the Directing Vessel (*Ren Mai*), the best vessel to nourish the Essence, are one on the Lung and the other on the Kidney channel (LU-7 Lieque and KI-6 Zhaohai).

The relationship between Corporeal Soul and Essence also explains the eruption of atopic eczema and asthma in babies. From the Chinese point of view, eczema in babies is due to the surfacing of Toxic Heat from the uterus; it is therefore closely linked with the Prenatal Essence of the baby (Fig. 4.3). Since the Essence is related to the Corporeal Soul which manifests on the skin (with itching and pain), the Toxic Heat from the uterus erupts on the baby's skin in the form of eczema.

CLINICAL NOTE

As I interpret the pathology of atopic eczema as being due to a deficiency of the Lung and Kidney's Defensive-Qi systems, when using herbal medicine in children, I modify the classic formulae with the addition of Tu Si Zi *Semen Cuscutae* and Mai Men Dong *Radix Ophiopogonis* to tonify the Kidneys and the Lungs, respectively (and therefore the Essence and the Corporeal Soul).

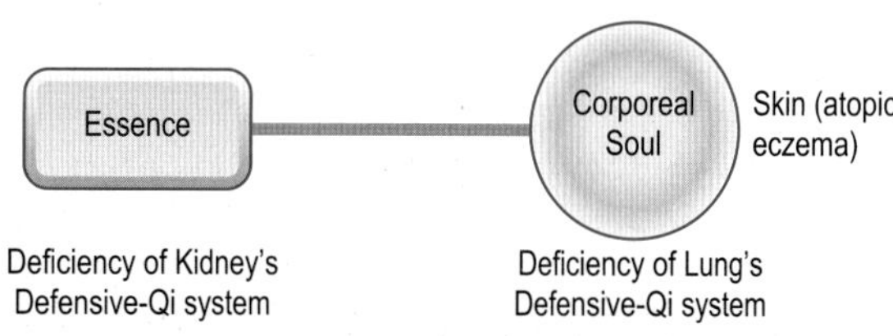

Figure 4.3 The Corporeal Soul and atopic eczema.

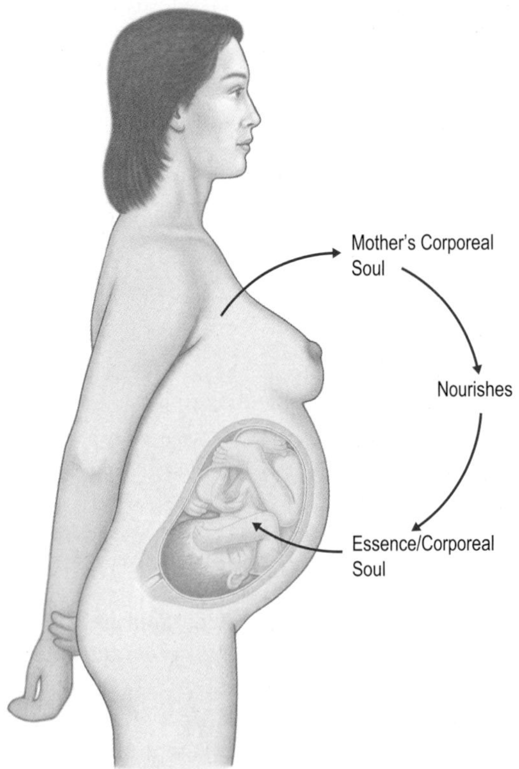

Figure 4.4 The Corporeal Soul during pregnancy.

Asthma can be explained in the same way as the deficient Essence of the baby fails to root its Corporeal Soul and therefore its Lungs.

During gestation, the fetus is "all Corporeal Soul and Essence" and is nourished by the Corporeal Soul of the mother (Fig. 4.4). This is of clinical importance, as we are inclined to think that it is the Kidneys of the mother that nourish the fetus; this is certainly so, but the Lungs and Corporeal Soul of the mother also play an important role in nourishing the fetus.

The connection between Corporeal Soul and fetal life is very ancient; Granet calls the Corporeal Soul the "soul of blood". The fetus depends on the mother's Corporeal Soul, Blood and Essence for its nourishment.

By giving rise to the human form during gestation, the Corporeal Soul has a centripetal, separating, materializing, aggregating movement. As it separates, it aggregates and materializes into a separate existence in the fetus. As this separation is expressed by the skin (which separates the being from the world), there is a further connection between the Corporeal Soul, the skin and the Lungs.

This separating power of the Corporeal Soul allies itself with the centripetal forces of *gui*, which are constantly fragmenting and which, eventually, become the germ of death. With regard to the fragmenting of the Corporeal Soul and of *gui*, there is a resonance between the word *gui* 鬼 and the word *kuai* 塊 (formed by the radical for *gui* with "earth" in front) which means "pieces". This confirms the fragmentation tendency of the *gui* (and therefore of the Corporeal Soul) in its centripetal movement.

Although contraction and fragmentation may seem to be contradictory, they are not and there are several examples of this process in the natural world. Gravity is an inward-directed, centripetal force (like that of the *gui*). When a star has burned all its nuclear fuel, the centripetal force of gravity causes it to collapse into a black hole.[8] Another example of the connection between contraction and fragmentation is the fragmentation of myofibrils in muscles as a result of contraction.[9]

The Corporeal Soul is therefore linked to a "thirst for existence", centripetal, materializing life force, aggregating into a separate existence and eventually ending in death.

SUMMARY

The Corporeal Soul and Essence (*Jing*)

- The Corporeal Soul is closely linked to the Essence (*Jing*) and is described in Chapter 8 of the *Spiritual Axis* as the *"exiting and entering of Essence"*.
- The Corporeal Soul derives from the mother and arises at conception (in theory, 3 days after conception) soon after the Prenatal Essence of a newly conceived being is formed.
- The Corporeal Soul provides physical movement to the Essence, i.e. it brings the Essence into play in all physiological processes of the body.
- During gestation, the fetus is "all Corporeal Soul and Essence" and is nourished by the Corporeal Soul of the mother.
- The Corporeal Soul has a centripetal, separating, materializing, aggregating movement. This separating power of the Corporeal Soul allies itself with the centripetal forces of *gui*, which are constantly fragmenting and which, eventually, become the germ of death.

INFANCY

Being the closest to the Essence, the Corporeal Soul is responsible for the first physiological processes after birth. Zhang Jie Bin says: "*In the beginning of life, ears, eyes and Heart perceive, hands and feet move and breathing starts; all this is due to the sharpness of the Corporeal Soul.*"[10]

It is said that in the first month of life especially, the baby is "all Corporeal Soul". As it resides in the Lungs, the Corporeal Soul is responsible for touch and skin sensations and it is nourished by the mother's Corporeal Soul through breast feeding and touching. This explains the importance of touching in a baby's life; it not only establishes a bonding between mother and baby but it also physically nourishes the Corporeal Soul and therefore the Lungs.

Sleep scientist McKenna found that a sleeping mother and an infant share far more than a mattress. Their physiological rhythms in slumber exhibit mutual concordances and synchronicities that McKenna thinks are life sustaining for the child. He says:[11]

The temporal unfolding of particular sleep stages and awake periods of the mother and infant become entwined. On a minute-to-minute basis, throughout the night, much sensory communication is occurring between them.

This is a clear confirmation of the connection between the mother's and the baby's Corporeal Souls.

CLINICAL NOTE

In the first month of life, the baby is "all Corporeal Soul", i.e. its life revolves around its Corporeal Soul (breast feeding, touch from the mother) and its Corporeal Soul is nourished by the mother's Corporeal Soul.

SUMMARY

Infancy

- Being the closest to the Essence, the Corporeal Soul is responsible for the first physiological processes after birth.
- In the first month of life especially, the baby is "all Corporeal Soul". As it resides in the Lungs, the Corporeal Soul is responsible for touch and skin sensations and it is nourished by the mother's Corporeal Soul through breast feeding and touching.

SENSES

Later in life, the Corporeal Soul gives us the capacity of sensation, feeling, hearing and sight. When the Corporeal Soul is flourishing, ears and eyes are keen and can register. The decline of hearing and sight in old people is due not only to a decline of Kidney-Essence but also to a weakening of the Corporeal Soul. We often attribute the decline of sensory acuity in the elderly to the decline of the Kidneys and of the Essence; this may certainly be so but the influence of the Corporeal Soul in this decline should not be underestimated.

Zhu Xi said:[12]

The Corporeal Soul is like water. Because of it, man's seeing can be bright, hearing can be acute and the Mind can be vigorous and can memorize well. When a man has this Corporeal Soul, then he has this Shen.

Zhang Jie Bin says: "*The Corporeal Soul can move and do things and* [when it is active] *pain and itching can be felt.*"[13] This shows that the Corporeal Soul is responsible for sensations and itching and is therefore closely related to the skin through which such sensations are experienced.

This explains the somatic expression on the skin of emotional tension which affects the Corporeal Soul and the connection between the Corporeal Soul, Lungs and skin (Fig. 4.5). The Corporeal Soul, being closely

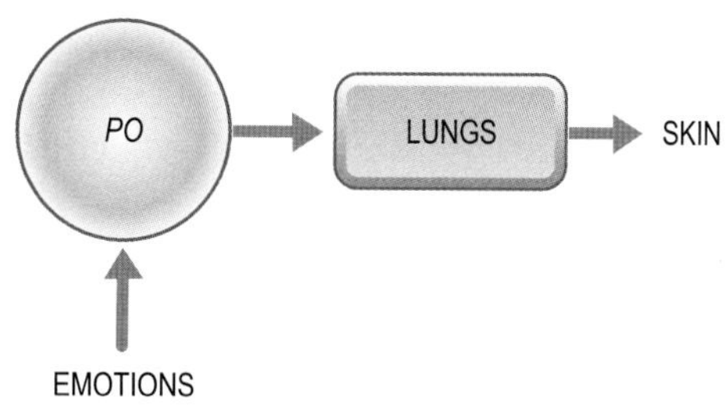

Figure 4.5 The Corporeal Soul, emotions and the skin.

related to the body, is the first to be affected when needles are inserted; the almost immediate feeling of relaxation following the insertion of needles is due to the unwinding of the Corporeal Soul. Through it, the Mind, Ethereal Soul, Intellect and Will-Power are all affected.

SUMMARY

Senses

- The Corporeal Soul gives us the capacity of sensation, feeling, hearing and sight.
- When the Corporeal Soul is flourishing, ears and eyes are keen and can register.
- The decline of hearing and sight in old people is due not only to a decline of Kidney-Essence but also to a weakening of the Corporeal Soul.

PHYSIOLOGICAL ACTIVITY

Some modern doctors consider the Corporeal Soul the "*basic regulatory activity of all physiological functions of the body*".[14] In this sense, it is the manifestation of the Lung's function of regulating all physiological activities.

Chapter 8 of the *Simple Questions* says: "*The Lungs are like a Prime Minister in charge of regulation.*"[15] This description of the Lungs' function in the *Simple Questions* should be seen in context. In fact, the sentence preceding the above concerning the function of the Heart says: "*The Heart is like the Emperor, in charge of the Spirit (Shen Ming).*"[16]

Thus, the Heart is compared to an Emperor and the Lungs to a Prime Minister assisting the Emperor.[17] This relationship is an expression of the close relationship between Qi and Blood. The Lungs govern Qi and the Heart governs Blood; Qi is the "commander of Blood" (it moves Blood) and Blood is the "mother of Qi". Qi and Blood assist and depend on each other, hence the comparison of the relationship between the Heart and Lungs to that between an Emperor and his Prime Minister.

After saying that the Lungs are like a Prime Minister, the *Simple Questions* says that the Lungs are in charge of "regulation". This means that, just as the Prime Minister regulates all administrative functions, the Lungs help to regulate all physiological activities in every organ and every part of the body, just as the Prime Minister's office controls and directs the administrative functions of all government departments.

The Lungs regulate all physiological activities in various ways:

- by governing Qi
- by controlling all channels and blood vessels
- by governing breathing.

As Qi is the basis for all physiological activities, the Lungs, by governing Qi, are naturally in charge of all physiological activities. This regulatory function is dependent also on the Lungs' action in moving Qi around the body.

Thus, the Corporeal Soul is the expression of the Lungs' regulatory function in all physiological processes; the Corporeal Soul is the physical soul that makes this regulation possible.

The Corporeal Soul's regulation of physiological processes has another very important aspect in relation to consciousness. From a Chinese perspective, consciousness is shared among the Mind (*Shen* of the Heart), Ethereal Soul and Corporeal Soul.

- The center of consciousness is, of course, the Mind; it corresponds to the activity not only of the cortex but also of the limbic system.
- The Ethereal Soul is responsible for our "consciousness" when we sleep (when the wakefulness of the Mind is not there) and its "movement" corresponds to the limbic system of Western neurophysiology.
- The Corporeal Soul corresponds to the reptilian brain (*see Chapters 1 and 14*) and is responsible for the "consciousness" that keeps our breathing going. For example, when a person is in a coma, the Mind is disabled but the Corporeal Soul is functioning and maintaining the brain centers responsible for breathing and heartbeat.

Damasio's definition of *core* and *extended consciousness* presents interesting similarities with Chinese medicine. He calls *core consciousness* the one that provides the organism with a sense of self about one moment (now) and about one place (here). The scope of core consciousness is here and now. This is similar to the function of the Corporeal Soul. He calls *extended consciousness* the one that provides "*the organism with an elaborate sense of self and places the person at a point in individual historical time, richly aware of the lived past and of the anticipated future.*"[18] This is a function of the Mind (*Shen* of the Heart) in Chinese medicine.

SUMMARY

Physiological activity

- Some modern doctors consider the Corporeal Soul the "basic regulatory activity of all physiological functions of the body".
- The Corporeal Soul is the expression of the Lung's regulatory function in all physiological processes; the Corporeal Soul is the physical soul that makes this regulation possible.
- The Corporeal Soul's regulation of physiological processes has another very important aspect in relation to consciousness; the Corporeal Soul corresponds to the reptilian brain (as described in Chapters 1 and 14) and is responsible for the "consciousness" that maintains our breathing.

EMOTIONS

As we have seen in Chapter 3, the Ethereal Soul is primarily responsible for our emotional life; its "movement" is responsible for our emotional balance and our dreams and aspirations.

However, the Corporeal Soul also plays a role in our emotional life. The relationship between the *cognitive* aspect of an emotion ("I have been offended and I am angry") and its *feeling* ("I feel angry") has been the subject of controversy for over 2000 years in Western philosophy. The general consensus is, however, that emotions do involve a feeling. Interestingly, some of these feelings may even be below the level of consciousness; of course, eventually, they all reach consciousness.

Interestingly, Damasio makes a distinction between *feeling* and *emotion*. He says that feelings are inwardly directed and private, while emotions are outwardly directed and public. Damasio maintains that there are feelings of which we are conscious and feelings of which we are not conscious. He says:[19]

An organism may represent in mental and neural patterns the state that we conscious creatures call a feeling without ever knowing that the feeling is taking place.

This is an interesting distinction and one that presents intriguing similarities with Chinese medicine. In fact, we could say that the feelings of which we are not conscious pertain to the Corporeal Soul (*Po*) while emotions involve the Mind (*Shen*) and Ethereal Soul (*Hun*). Damasio says: "*Emotions and core consciousness tend to go together in the literal sense by being present together or absent together.*"[20]

The above presents interesting connections with Chinese medicine as core consciousness (as described above) is akin to the Corporeal Soul and therefore the Corporeal Soul modulates all feelings at a deep, autonomic and automatic level. In other words, as explained in Chapter 2, the Mind (*Shen* of the Heart) is responsible for consciousness and it is the one that recognizes the emotions at a cognitive level and also "feels" them. For this reason, all emotions affect the Heart. However, not only all emotions but especially all feelings that have not yet come to consciousness affect the Corporeal Soul. For this reason, treatment of the Lungs (especially with LU-7 Lieque and LU-3 Tianfu) is very important in emotional problems to soothe the Corporeal Soul and, through that, the Mind. With herbal medicine, I use especially the herb Bai He *Bulbus Lilii* to achieve the same effect.

CLINICAL NOTE

I use the points LU-7 Lieque and LU-3 Tianfu and the herb Bai He to soothe the Corporeal Soul when it is affected by emotions and feelings.

More specifically, the Corporeal Soul is also related to weeping and crying. Just as the Corporeal Soul makes us feel pain on a physical level, it also makes us cry and weep when subject to grief and sadness.

Unexpressed grief in particular constricts the Corporeal Soul and gives rise to accumulation of Qi. Emotional stress (especially worry, pensiveness, grief and sadness) "constricts" the Corporeal Soul and causes Lung-Qi stagnation in the chest. Lung-Qi stagnation affects the breasts and may give rise to the formation of lumps.

Indeed, one could say that all emotions affect the Corporeal Soul because they all affect Qi and the Lung governs Qi.

CLINICAL NOTE

The fact that all emotions affect the Corporeal Soul explains the powerful emotional effect of the point LU-7 Lieque; it moves Qi and frees emotional constraint.

SUMMARY

Emotions

- The Corporeal Soul plays a role in our emotional life.
- Feelings we are not conscious of pertain to the Corporeal Soul (*Po*) while emotions involve the Mind (*Shen*) and Ethereal Soul (*Hun*).
- More specifically, the Corporeal Soul is also related to weeping and crying.
- Unexpressed grief constricts the Corporeal Soul and gives rise to accumulation of Qi.
- Emotional stress (especially worry, pensiveness, grief and sadness) "constricts" the Corporeal Soul and causes Lung-Qi stagnation in the chest.

BREATHING

Residing in the Lungs, the Corporeal Soul is closely linked to breathing. Breathing can be seen as the pulsating of the Corporeal Soul. Meditation makes use of the link between breathing and the Corporeal Soul. By concentrating on the breathing, someone who is meditating quietens the Corporeal Soul, the Mind becomes still and empty, and through this the Ethereal Soul becomes open and gets in touch with the Universal Mind.

Therefore, on a physical level, breathing is not only an expression of Lung-Qi, but also an expression of the pulsation of the Corporeal Soul.

THE CORPOREAL SOUL AND INDIVIDUAL LIFE

The Corporeal Soul is related to our life as individuals while the Ethereal Soul is responsible for our relations with other people and the world. From this point of view, there is an important difference between the Ethereal Soul and the Corporeal Soul.

As we have seen, the Ethereal Soul is imparted by the father 3 days after birth; this shows that it is a soul that is responsible for an outward movement toward others in relationships and it therefore lets us take our place in the family and society.

By contrast, the Corporeal Soul is a physical, individual soul that is formed soon after conception; it is the "blind" force of a soul whose only function is the regulation of physical activity and of the life force itself. However, that is not to say, of course, that the Corporeal Soul is not affected by our emotional life. Emotional stress certainly always affects the Corporeal Soul but the Corporeal Soul does not control our emotional life in the same way that the Mind and Ethereal Soul do.

THE CORPOREAL SOUL AND THE *GUI*

Beyond its nature of "spirit" or "ghost", *gui* can have a very interesting psychological interpretation. *Gui* is like a "dark" force of the psyche which gives the Ethereal and Corporeal Souls its imprint; in fact, as we have seen, the Chinese characters for these two souls contain the radical *gui*. Apart from other implications, this tells us that these two souls have their own existence independent from that of the Mind; they are "dark" forces of the psyche, one on a psychic level, the other on a physical level (Fig. 4.6).

The *gui* within the Ethereal Soul gives it movement on a psychic level (*coming and going* of the Mind) which, as we have seen, generates ideas, intuition, creativity; the *gui* within the Corporeal Soul gives it movement on a physical level (*entering and exiting* of the Essence) in all the body's physiological processes.

Thus, the *gui* within the Corporeal Soul is the "dark" force that animates it in carrying out its function of promoting all physiological processes and of bringing the Essence into play in all parts of the body. There is

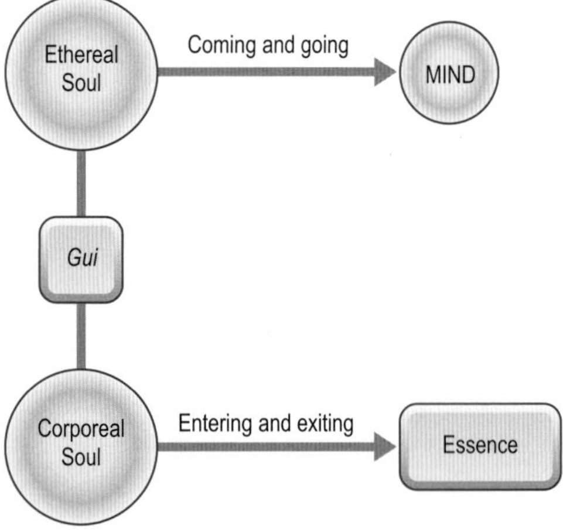

Figure 4.6 The *gui*, the Ethereal Soul and the Corporeal Soul.

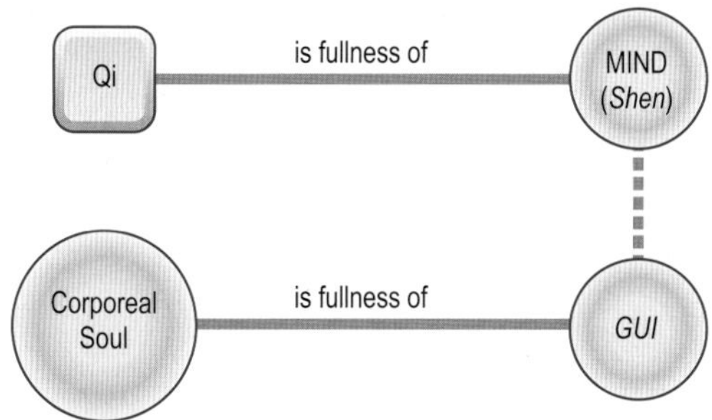

Figure 4.7 Qi, Mind, Corporeal Soul and *gui*.

a close connection between Corporeal Soul and *gui* intended in the sense of a contracting, centripetal, fragmenting, materializing force (Fig. 4.7).

As mentioned above, He Shang Gong says: "*The five turbid and humid flavours form bones, muscles, blood, vessels and the six passions ... these gui are called Corporeal Soul.*"[21] This statement illustrates the physical and "dark" nature of the Corporeal Soul which assimilates it to a *gui*; it is the soul of "bones, muscles and blood vessels". The statement also indicates the Corporeal Soul is related to all emotions ("the six passions").

SUMMARY

The Corporeal Soul and the *gui*

- *Gui* is like a "dark" force of the psyche which gives the Ethereal and Corporeal Souls its imprint.
- The *gui* within the Corporeal Soul gives it movement on a physical level (*entering and exiting* of the Essence) in all the body's physiological processes.
- The *gui* within the Corporeal Soul is the "dark" force that animates it in carrying out its function of promoting all physiological processes and of bringing the Essence into play in all parts of the body.
- There is a close connection between Corporeal Soul and *gui* intended in the sense of a contracting, centripetal, fragmenting, materializing force.

THE CORPOREAL SOUL AND THE ANUS

Because of the relationship between the Corporeal Soul and the Lungs and of that between these and the Large Intestine, the anus is sometimes called *po men*, the "door of the Po" as in Chapter 11 of the *Simple Questions*: "*The door of the Po* [anus] *is the messenger for the five viscera and it drains off water and food without storing them for too long.*"[22] In fact, the point BL-42 Pohu (the "Window of the Po") was indicated for incontinence of both urine and faeces from fright.

RELATIONSHIP BETWEEN CORPOREAL SOUL AND ETHEREAL SOUL

Since the Ethereal Soul and Corporeal Soul are two aspects of the soul, it is interesting to compare and contrast their various characteristics and functions (Table 4.1). Most of the characteristics indicated in Table 4.1 are derived from Zhang Jie Bin's *Classic of Categories*.[23]

As can be seen from Table 4.1, the Ethereal Soul is involved in problems occurring at night (although not exclusively), and the Corporeal Soul in problems occurring in daytime. The *Discussion of Blood Patterns* (1884) by Tang Zong Hai says:[24]

> *Restlessness at night with excessive dreaming is due to an unsettled Ethereal Soul; this is Yang and if at night it has no resting place the person is restless and dreams a lot. Restlessness in the daytime and a clouded Mind are due to an unsettled Corporeal Soul; this is Yin and if Yin is deficient in daytime, restlessness and mental confusion result.*

Table 4.2 lists the comparison of Ethereal Soul and Corporeal Soul by Zhu Xi.[25] This contains many interesting observations. The Ethereal Soul "moves and uses", "is able to move, use and take action", and is responsible for the "ability to think and plan". All these expressions confirm what was discussed in Chapter 3 regarding the Ethereal Soul being responsible for the "movement" of the Mind and for planning, ideas, projects and life dreams.

The Ethereal Soul pertains to the realm of Image and the Corporeal Soul to that of Form. This can be represented with a diagram (Fig. 4.8).

The Ethereal Soul is ethereal, is last to arrive (after birth) and first to go (after death); the Corporeal Soul is physical, it is the first to arrive (at conception) and the last to go after death (it lingers in the bones). According to Granet, the Ethereal Soul corresponds to the higher aspect of personality, to the personal name

Table 4.1 Comparison of Ethereal Soul and Corporeal Soul

ETHEREAL SOUL	CORPOREAL SOUL
Is the "coming and going of the Mind"	Is the "entering and exiting of the Essence"
Pertains to the Mind	Pertains to the body
Is the Qi of the Mind	Is the spirit of the body
Follows the changes of Qi	Follows the changes of the body
Is Yang and moves	Is Yin and is quiescent
Creates action with movement	Creates action without movement
Related to the Mind: when Qi gathers, the Ethereal Soul gathers	Related to the Essence: when this gathers, the Corporeal Soul gathers
At birth the Ethereal Soul joins with the Corporeal Soul	At birth the Corporeal Soul restrains the Ethereal Soul
At death it swims away and returns to Heaven	At death it dissolves and returns to Earth
Is bright and it lights the Corporeal Soul	Is dark and it roots the Ethereal Soul
Is like a fire: the more things you add, the more it burns	Is like a mirror: it shines, but holds only a reflection (of the Ethereal Soul)
Represents the movement of the Mind outwardly	Represents the movement of the Essence inwardly
Is rooted in Blood and Yin	Is connected to Qi and Yang
Disharmony causes problems with sleep at night	Disharmony causes problems in daytime
Disharmony causes lack of direction and inspiration, confusion	Disharmony causes lack of vigor and vitality
It is the link with the universal Mind	It is purely individual
Corresponds to full moon	Corresponds to new moon

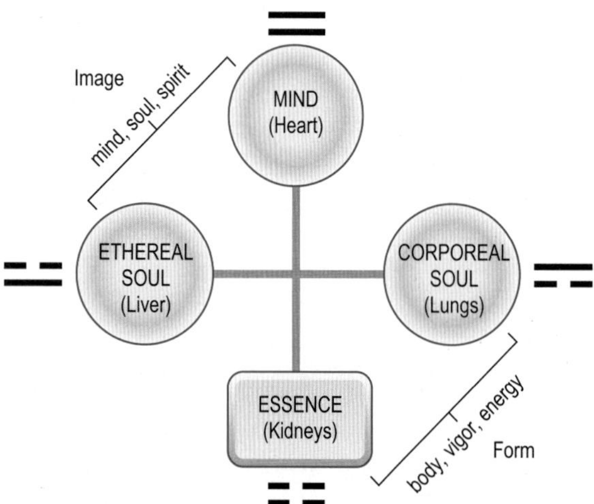

Figure 4.8 The realms of Image and Form and the Ethereal and Corporeal Souls.

through which each person takes his or her social and family place; the Ethereal Soul conferred one one's individuality but an individuality that finds its expression within family and society.

The *Huai Nan Zi* says: "*The Ethereal Soul derives from Heavenly Qi, the Corporeal Soul from Earthly Qi.*"[26] The *Wu Xing Da Yi* says: "*The Corporeal Soul is like the envelope, the Ethereal Soul is the source of Life's Qi.*"[27] These statements highlight the nature of the Corporeal Soul as the centripetal, materializing, separating force which produces Form and the body; hence it is like an "envelope" separating the body from the world. Consequently, the Corporeal Soul is constraining, contracting, centripetal; this constraining, separating and fragmenting movement eventually ends in death.

By contrast, the Ethereal Soul is expansive, it is constantly moving towards the world; hence it is expan-

Table 4.2 Comparison of Ethereal Soul and Corporeal Soul according to Zhu Xi

ETHEREAL SOUL	CORPOREAL SOUL
Yang	Yin
Shen of Yang	*Shen* of Yin
Shen	*Gui*
Qi	Essence
Shen of Qi	*Shen* of Essence
Qi	Blood
Qi	Body
Qi	Physical form
Shen	Essence
Movement	Rest
Warm	Cold
Sun	Moon
Fire	Water
Wood	Metal
3	7
Fire and sun (which have shadow outside)	Metal and Water (which have shadow inside)
Full moon	New moon
Moving and using	Storing and receiving
Able to move, use, take action	Unable to move, use and take action
Respiration of mouth and nose	Acuteness and brightness of ears and eyes
Perception and movement	Physical form and body
Speech and action	Essence and Blood
Spirit (*jing-shen*) and perception	The four limbs and the nine orifices and their essence and blood
Manifesting and using	Settling of Qi
Knowledge	Memory
Ability to think and account	Ability to memorize
Ability to think and plan	Ability to memorize and distinguish
Manifesting outward (like a lantern)	Ability to reflect (like mirror)

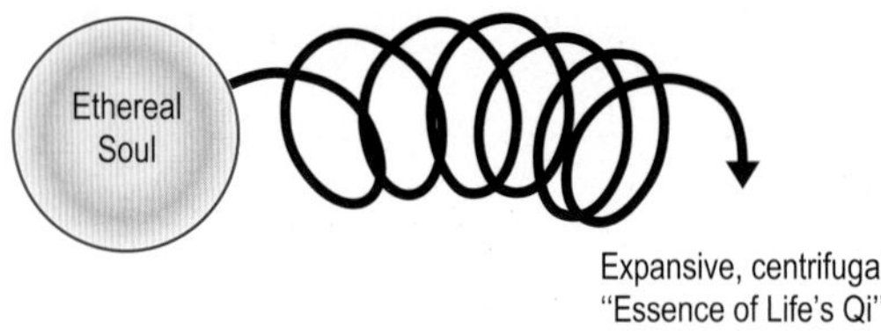

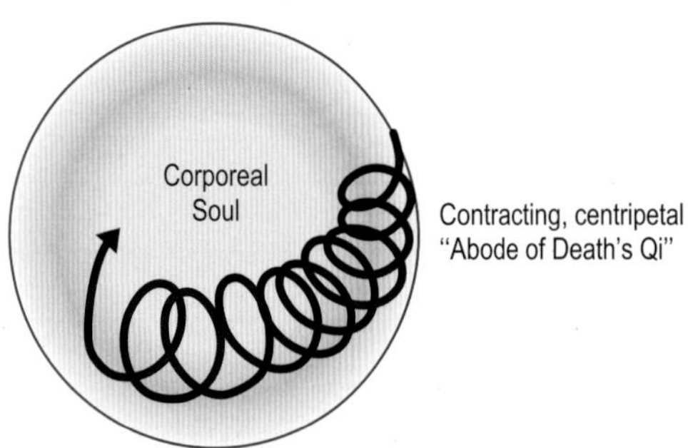

Figure 4.9 Expansive and contracting movements of Ethereal Soul and Corporeal Soul.

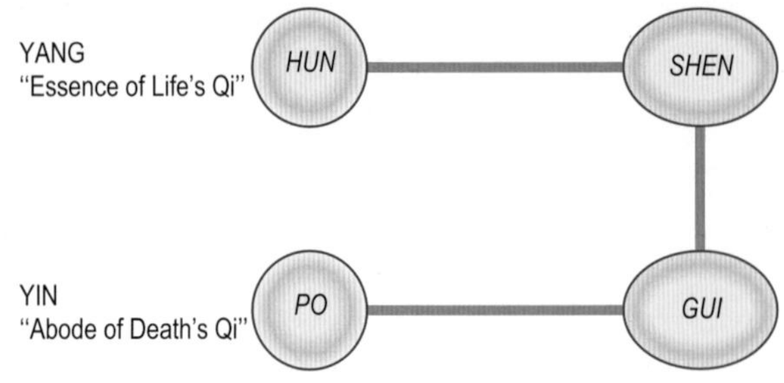

Figure 4.10 Ethereal Soul, Corporeal Soul, Mind and *gui*.

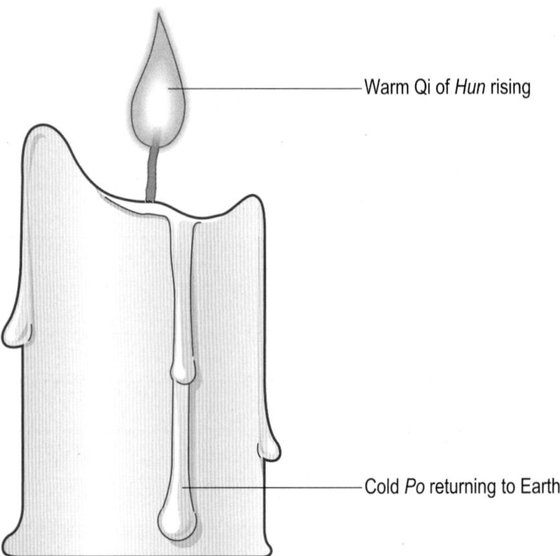

Figure 4.11 Ethereal Soul rising and Corporeal Soul falling at death.

sive, centrifugal. The Ethereal Soul is the source of Life's Qi, it is centrifugal, it has an outward movement and goes towards life. The Ethereal Soul is called the "Essence of Life's Qi" and the Corporeal Soul the "Abode of Death's Qi".

The connection of the Corporeal Soul with death is due to the fact that it is separating, constraining, fragmenting, contracting and it dies with the body (Fig. 4.9). The *Secret of the Golden Flower* says: "*The Corporeal Soul partakes of the nature of darkness. It is the energy of the heavy and turbid. The Ethereal Soul loves life; the Corporeal Soul seeks death.*"[28]

The *Wu Xing Da Yi* says:[29]

The Qi of the Ethereal Soul is the fullness [perfection] *of Shen; the Qi of the Corporeal Soul is the fullness* [perfection] *of Gui. Human life includes death. At death, one returns to Earth, that is called Gui.*

Zhu Xi said:[30]

Qi belongs to the Ethereal Soul and the body is governed by the Corporeal Soul. The Ethereal Soul is the spirit of Yang and the Corporeal Soul is the spirit of Yin. When a person is about to die the warm Qi leaves him or her and rises. This is called the Ethereal Soul rising. The lower part of the body gradually becomes cold. This is called the Corporeal Soul falling.

See Figures 4.10–4.14.

Zhu Xi also said:[31]

Qi is the flourishing of shen; Corporeal Soul is the flourishing of gui. Combining gui and shen is the supreme of teaching. All living things must die. Having died, they must return to Earth. This is called gui. Bones and flesh die and go down. The Yin becomes the Earth of the fields. Its Qi is emitted and displayed up high; it is bright and fuming up. This is the essence of the 100 things and the manifestation of Shen.

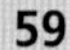

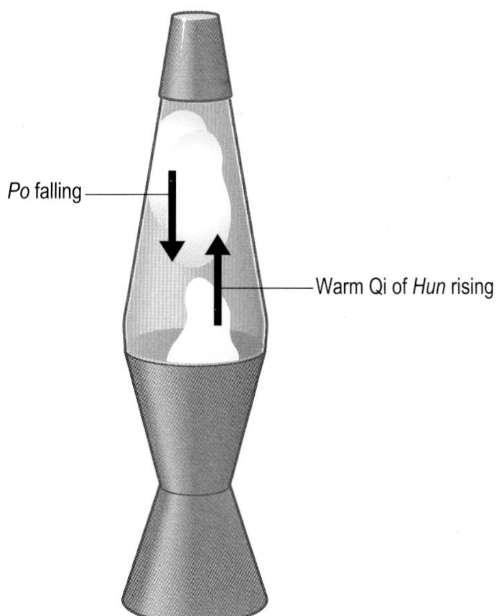

Figure 4.12 Rising of Ethereal Soul and falling of Corporeal Soul.

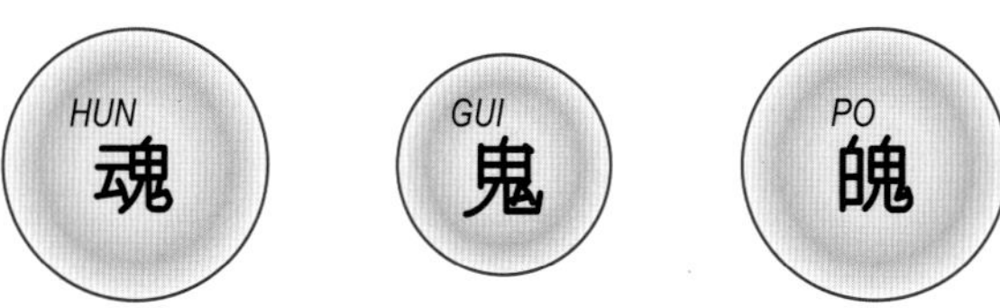

Figure 4.13 *Gui* in Ethereal Soul and Corporeal Soul.

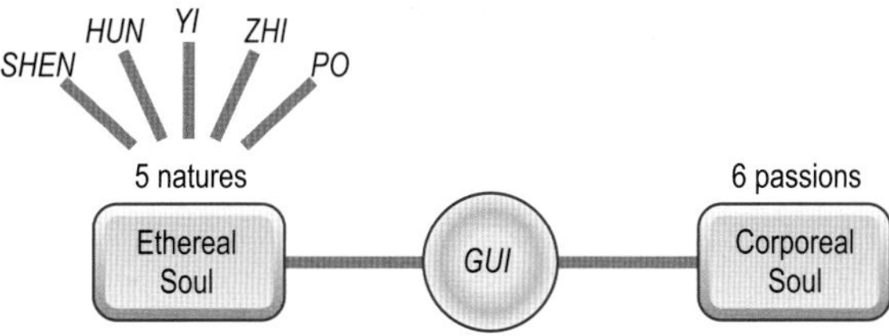

Figure 4.14 Ethereal Soul and Corporeal Soul as the *gui* of the 5 natures and 6 passions.

In another passage, Zhu Xi confirms that at death the Ethereal Soul goes to "Heaven" and the Corporeal Soul to Earth:[32]

When a man is alive, Ethereal Soul and Corporeal Soul meet each other. When he dies, they are separated and each is dispersed. The Hun, being Yang, is scattered upwards; the Po, being Yin, descends.

In another passage, Zhu Xi expands on the differences between Ethereal Soul and Corporeal Soul:[33]

In general, Ethereal Soul is hot and Corporeal Soul is cold; Ethereal Soul moves and Corporeal Soul is at rest. If it can be that Corporeal Soul is protected by Ethereal Soul, then the Ethereal Soul, for the sake of protecting, is also at rest. Because of Ethereal Soul, Corporeal Soul has life intent. Ethereal Soul, being hot, produces coolness; Corporeal Soul, being cold, produces warmth. Only when the two are not separated from each other, the Yang is not dry and Yin is not impeded, is their harmony achieved. Otherwise, the more the Ethereal Soul moves, the more at rest is Corporeal Soul; the hotter Ethereal Soul becomes, the colder the Corporeal Soul becomes. If the two are separated from each other, then their harmony is not achieved and the human being dies.

In ancient China, the dead were temporarily buried in the corner of the house where seeds were kept. This allowed the substance of the dead to penetrate the Earth in the house. The body of the dead decomposed in the corner where seeds were kept to symbolize the sprouting of new life from the seeds. In the same place was the marital bed, where new lives are conceived. As the Corporeal Soul returned to Earth after death, this allowed people to imagine that a new life sprouted from the Earth in the house and from the dead ancestors as if the baby had taken the substance of the ancestors.[34]

The bodiless *gui* were hovering around the marital bed waiting for a new incarnation. This continuity between dead and living allowed people to believe in an unbroken family lineage, in an eternal family substance like the Earth. A death did not diminish this family substance and a birth did not increase it. The family was formed of two parallel communities: the living (with their individualities in the Corporeal Soul) and the dead.

The Ethereal Soul's "coming and going" gives "horizontality" to life; the Corporeal Soul's "entering and exiting" gives "verticality" to life (Fig. 4.15).

"Horizontality" means that the Ethereal Soul is constantly exploring the bounds of consciousness into the world of ideas, creativity, art, exploration, dreams, etc. "Verticality" means that the Corporeal Soul is constantly materializing into the body in the spheres of physiological activities.

From what we have said about the Ethereal Soul and the Corporeal Soul, we can build the following sets of correspondences:

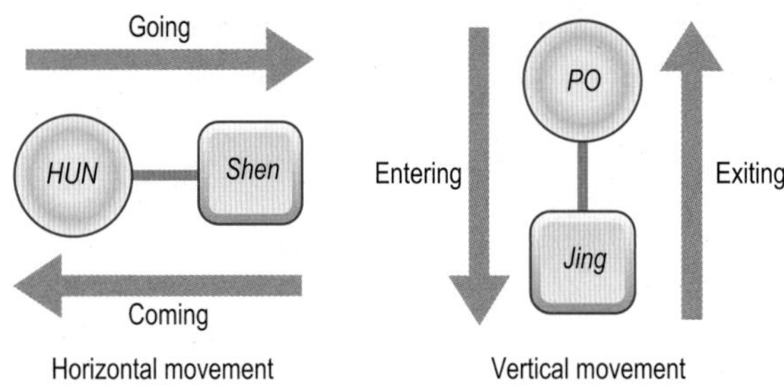

Figure 4.15 Verticality of Corporeal Soul and horizontality of Ethereal Soul.

ETHEREAL SOUL – YANG – MIND (*SHEN*) – CENTRIFUGAL – "ESSENCE OF LIFE'S QI"

CORPOREAL SOUL – YIN – *GUI* – CENTRIPETAL – "ABODE OF DEATH'S QI"

CLINICAL NOTE

Given the connection between the Corporeal Soul and death, it is interesting to note the association with death among the indications of three points related to the Lungs (and therefore Corporeal Soul).

- BL-13 Feishu: "suicidal"
- Du-12 Shenzhu: "desire to kill people"
- BL-42 Pohu: "three corpses flowing" (*see Chapter 13*).

CLINICAL APPLICATION

I shall discuss the clinical application of the Corporeal Soul under the separate headings of acupuncture and herbal therapy. For each of them, I will discuss the two pathological states of contraction and expansion of the Corporeal Soul. Bearing in mind that the Corporeal Soul influences the skin and the emotional life, a state of contraction involves skin problems such as redness, rashes, acne; emotionally, a state of contraction means that the patient suppresses his or her emotions and these cause stagnation of Qi of the Lungs and possibly depression.

A state of expansion of the Corporeal Soul with regard to the skin causes problems such as itching; with regard to the emotional life, a state of expansion causes anxiety and worry.

Contraction of the Corporeal Soul

Skin

Acupuncture

LU-7 Lieque, LU-5 Chize, LU-1 Zhongfu, L.I.-11 Quchi. Reducing or even method.

Herbal therapy

Sang Dan Xie Bai Tang Variation
Morus-Moutan Draining Whiteness Decoction Variation

Emotional life

Acupuncture

LU-7 Lieque, P-6 Neiguan, L.I.-4 Hegu. Reducing or even method.

Herbal therapy

Ban Xia Hou Po Tang
Pinellia-Magnolia Decoction

Expansion of the Corporeal Soul

Skin

Acupuncture

LU-5 Chize, BL-13 Feishu, Du-12 Shenzhu, T.B.-6 Zhigou. Reinforcing method.

Herbal therapy

Xiao Feng San from Imperial Grace Formulary
Eliminating Wind Powder from Imperial Grace Formulary

Emotional life

Acupuncture

BL-13 Feishu, Du-12 Zhenzhu, P-7 Daling, Du-19 Houding. Reinforcing method.

Herbal therapy

Bu Fei Tang Variation (*see Chapter 17, Anxiety, Lung- and Heart-Qi deficiency*)
Tonifying the Lungs Decoction Variation

SUMMARY

The Corporeal Soul

- It is a physical soul that resides in the Lungs.
- If is formed 3 days after conception.
- It is closely related to the Essence (*Jing*).
- It is the "entering and exiting" of Essence, bringing this into play in all physiological processes.
- During infancy, the baby's life revolves entirely around the Corporeal Soul.
- The Corporeal Soul is responsible for acuity of the sense organs.
- The Corporeal Soul is affected by all emotions, especially pensiveness, worry, grief and sadness.
- The Corporeal Soul is responsible for all physiological processes; it is the "soul" that animates all physiological activities.
- The Corporeal Soul is responsible for breathing.
- The Corporeal Soul is closely linked to *gui* as a centripetal, materializing, fragmenting force.
- The anus is related to the Corporeal Soul.

END NOTES

1. Giles H 1912 Chinese-English Dictionary. Kelly & Walsh, Shanghai, p. 1144.
2. 1982 Lei Jing 类经 [Classic of Categories]. People's Health Publishing House, Beijing, p. 63. The *Classic of Categories* was written by Zhang Jie Bin (also called Zhang Jing Yue) and first published in 1624.
3. Kim Yung Sik 2000 The Natural Philosophy of Chu Hsi. American Philosophical Society, Philadelphia, p. 224.
4. Eyssalet J-M 1990 Le Secret de la Maison des Ancêtres. Guy Trédaniel Editeur, Paris, p. 30.
5. Ibid., p. 31.
6. 1981 Ling Shu Jing 灵枢经 [Spiritual Axis]. People's Health Publishing House, Beijing, p. 23. First published *c.*100 BC.
7. Classic of Categories, p. 63.
8. Greene B 2000 The Elegant Universe. Vintage, London, p. 339.
9. Takahashi K, Hattori A, Yasu T 1970 Effect of contraction on the fragmentation of myofibrils. Journal of Biochemistry 67: 609–610. Another example of the effect of contraction on fragmentation is in muscles. The authors of this article found that the post-mortem fragmentation of myofibrils was caused by the post-mortem contraction of muscles and that the high degree of the fragmentation in isometric muscles was largely dependent on tension developed during the contraction.
10. Classic of Categories, p. 63.
11. Lewis T, Amini F, Lannon R 2000 A General Theory of Love. Random House, New York, p. 195.
12. Classic of Categories, p. 229.
13. Ibid., p. 63.
14. Zhao You Chen 1979 Liao Ning Journal of Chinese Medicine (*Liao Ning Zhong Yi* 了宁中医) 5: 24.
15. 1979 Huang Di Nei Jing Su Wen 黄帝内经素问 [The Yellow Emperor's Classic of Internal Medicine – Simple Questions]. People's Health Publishing House, Beijing, p. 58. First published *c.*100 BC.
16. Ibid., p. 58.
17. In order to understand the clinical significance of the Lungs being like a Prime Minister, we should see this statement in the context of the social and political situation of ancient China. In modern Western societies, the Prime Minister has primarily political responsibility and the administration of government is delegated to government departments (or the Civil Service in Britain). In ancient China, society was administered very tightly by a central, pyramidal bureaucracy with the Prime Minister at its apex; the Prime Minister, therefore, was the head of all government departments administering the country. It is in this context that the functions of the Lungs should be seen.
18. Damasio A 1999 The Feeling of What Happens – Body and Emotion in the Making of Consciousness. Harcourt, San Diego, p. 16.
19. Ibid., p. 136.
20. Ibid., p. 100.
21. Le Secret de la Maison des Ancêtres, p. 31.
22. Simple Questions, p. 77.
23. Classic of Categories, pp. 63–64.
24. Pei Zheng Xue 1979 Xue Zheng Lun Ping Shi 血证论评释 [A Commentary on the Discussion on Blood Patterns]. People's Health Publishing House, Beijing, p. 236. The *Discussion on Blood Patterns* was written by Tang Zong Hai and first published in 1884.
25. The Natural Philosophy of Chu Hsi, pp. 226–227.
26. Le Secret de la Maison des Ancêtres, p. 441.
27. Ibid., p. 441.
28. Wilhelm R (translator) 1962 The Secret of the Golden Flower. Harcourt, Brace & World, New York, p. 28.
29. Ibid., p. 453.
30. The Natural Philosophy of Chu Hsi, p. 224.
31. Ibid., p. 224.
32. Ibid., p. 225.
33. Ibid., p. 225.
34. Granet M 1973 La Religione dei Cinesi. Adelphi, Milano, p. 33.

意

CHAPTER 5

THE INTELLECT (*YI*)

MEMORY *63*

GENERATION OF IDEAS *64*

STUDYING AND CONCENTRATING *64*

FOCUSING *65*

RELATIONSHIP WITH THE MIND (*SHEN*) *65*

CLINICAL APPLICATION *65*

THE INTELLECT (*YI*)

The Chinese character for Intellect is *Yi* 意 which can mean "idea". I have chosen to translate this as "Intellect" as it is very close to the Mind (*Shen*) of the Heart. The Intellect (*Yi*) resides in the Spleen and is responsible for applied thinking, studying, memorizing, focusing, concentrating and generating ideas.

Specifically, the Intellect is responsible for the following aspects of mental activity:

- Memory
- Generation of ideas
- Studying and concentrating
- Focusing.

The Postnatal Qi and Blood are the physiological basis for the Intellect. Thus if the Spleen is strong, thinking will be clear, memory good and the capacity for concentrating, studying and generating ideas will also be good. If the Spleen is weak, the Intellect will be dull, thinking will be slow, memory poor and the capacity for studying, concentrating and focusing will all be weak.

However, it is important to remember that the state of the Intellect depends not only on the strength of the Spleen but also on the presence of pathogenic factors such as Dampness or Phlegm. Dampness and Phlegm in the head will interfere with the function of the Intellect and cause poor memory, a feeling of muzziness and difficulty in concentrating and focusing.

As we shall see later (Chapter 21), a weakness of the Intellect is an important feature of the pathology of attention deficit disorder.

The discussion of the function of the Intellect will be conducted according to the following topics.

- Memory
- Generation of ideas
- Studying and concentrating
- Focusing
- Relationship with the Mind (*Shen*)
- Clinical application

MEMORY

The Intellect is responsible for memory but specifically the memory that is needed when studying or researching in the course of one's study or work. Psychology distinguishes two types of memory, implicit and explicit. Graf and Birt describe these two types of memory: "*Implicit memory is revealed when performance on a task is facilitated in the absence of conscious recollection of previous experiences*", and "*Explicit memory is revealed by intentional recollection from a specific previous episode, whereas implicit memory is revealed when performance on a task is facilitated without deliberate recollection from a specific learning episode.*"[1]

For example, implicit memory is the one that allows one to cycle effortlessly even after years of not cycling. Explicit memory is the one that allows us to recall a telephone number we have memorized recently.

The Intellect (and therefore the Spleen) is particularly responsible for explicit memory, i.e. the capacity

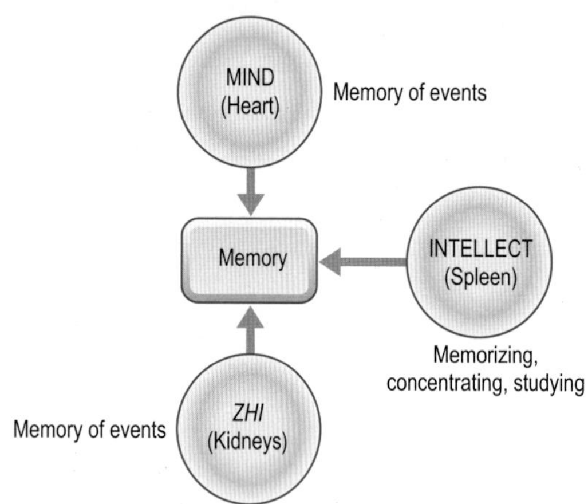

Figure 5.1 Relationship of Mind, Intellect and Will-Power with memory.

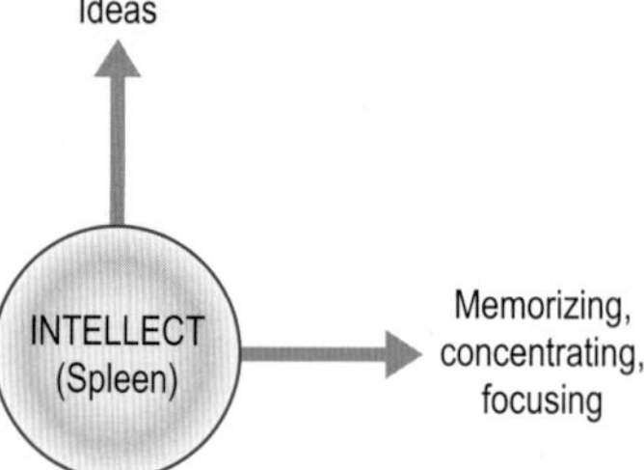

Figure 5.2 The Intellect as source of memorization and ideas.

of memorizing data in the course of one's study or work with a conscious effort; the Heart and the Spleen, and therefore the Mind and Intellect, together are responsible for the implicit memory.

In the sphere of memory, there is considerable overlap between the Intellect (*Yi* of Spleen), the Mind (*Shen* of Heart) and the Will-Power (*Zhi* of Kidneys). The main differentiating factor is that the Spleen is specifically responsible for memorizing data in the course of one's work or study (Fig. 5.1). For example, it is not uncommon for someone to have a brilliant memory in his or her field of study or research (a function of the Spleen), and yet be quite forgetful in daily life (a function of the Heart and Kidneys).

The Heart and Kidneys naturally contribute to this function, but they are also responsible for the memory of past events, whether recent or long past. In particular, the overlap between the Intellect and the Mind in thinking activity is very close, so much so that the *Spiritual Axis* says in Chapter 8: "*The Heart function of recollecting is called Intellect.*"[2] In turn, the memorizing function of the Intellect is so closely related to the Will-Power, or Memory (*Zhi* of the Kidneys) that the same chapter continues: "*The storing* [of data] *of the Intellect is called Will-Power* [*Zhi*]."[3] It should be noted here that I translate the mental aspect of the Kidneys' *Zhi* as Will-Power although it also has the meaning of "memory" or "mind". In the context of the passage just mentioned, *Zhi* is memory.

The Intellect of the Spleen and Will-Power (or Memory) of the Kidneys are closely connected; they are two aspects of memory, the former dependent on the Post-Heaven Qi, the latter on the Pre-Heaven Qi. As mentioned above, Chapter 8 of the *Spiritual Axis* seems to imply that the Will-Power (Memory) of the Kidneys is responsible for the long-term storage of memories. The same chapter also says "*Zhi is for the purpose of Yi except that* [its memories] *are not removed.*"[4]

GENERATION OF IDEAS

Another aspect of the Intellect of the Spleen is the generation of ideas (Fig. 5.2). As we have seen above, the Ethereal Soul also generates ideas, plans, projects, etc. The "ideas" generated by the Spleen differ from those deriving from the Ethereal Soul. The Ethereal Soul is responsible for "ideas" more in the sense of intuition, inspiration, life dreams and creativity; these are broad ideas also in the sense of vision.

The Intellect is responsible for "ideas" more in the sense of specific ideas in a given field. For example, the "idea" that allows us to carry out a repair job successfully derives from the Intellect of the Spleen; by contrast, the "idea" that gives us vision, a life dream and creativity derives from the Ethereal Soul of the Liver.

STUDYING AND CONCENTRATING

The Intellect is responsible for our capacity of studying and concentrating. Of course, such a function is carried out in conjunction with the Mind of the Heart. When the Intellect is clear, we can study hard and concentrate in a sustained way. When the Spleen is deficient and the Intellect weak, we find it difficult to study and concentrate.

From the point of view of thinking, studying and concentrating, the Intellect of Chinese medicine corresponds to the activity of the cerebral cortex in modern medicine. Interestingly, the two opposing views according to which the Mind resides in the Heart or in the Brain developed in parallel in Chinese medicine, even as early as the *Yellow Emperor's Classic of Internal Medicine* times.

Chapter 17 of the *Simple Questions* says: "*The head is the residence of Jing Ming.*"[5] The term *Jing Ming* can be interpreted in different ways but modern books generally interpret it as referring to *Jing* and *Shen*, i.e. the Essence and the Mind. Therefore, from this point of view, thinking and mental activity depend on the Brain. Sun Si Miao says: "*The head is the seat of the Shen.*"[6] Li Shi Zhen said: "*The Brain is the seat of the Original Shen.*"[7]

The Brain is a transformation of Marrow which in turn derives from the Kidney-Essence; therefore the Brain depends largely on the Pre-Heaven Essence of the Kidneys. However, the significance of the Spleen governing the Intellect is that the Brain depends also on the nourishment from the Post-Heaven Essence of the Stomach and Spleen.

Thus, the three organs of Heart, Spleen and Kidneys all influence the Brain through the Mind, Intellect and Will-Power (Memory). See Figure 5.3.

FOCUSING

Allied to the previous function of studying and concentrating is that of focusing. The Intellect of the Spleen allows us to focus on a study or job in hand with single-mindedness, clarity and concentration. The emotion pertaining to the Spleen (and therefore the Intellect) is pensiveness which, in extreme cases, includes that of obsessive thinking; this may derive from a Spleen deficiency or, vice versa, it may cause it.

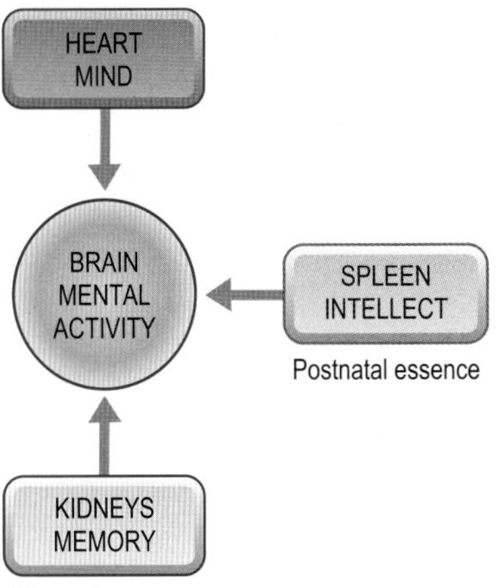

Figure 5.3 Relationship among Mind, Intellect and Will-Power in connection with the Brain.

It is interesting to note that obsessive thinking is nothing but the pathological counterpart of the ability to focus intensely.

RELATIONSHIP WITH THE MIND (*SHEN*)

The relationship between the Intellect of the Spleen and the Mind of the Heart is very close; one could say that the Intellect is but a sub-aspect of the Mind (*Shen*). As the Memory (*Zhi*) of the Kidneys is also closely related to the Mind of the Heart, we can see that the Ethereal Soul and Corporeal Soul stand out as being two independent aspects of our psyche with their own independent existence (the former on a psychic and the latter on a physical level).

Therefore, the Intellect is that part of the Mind that allows us to memorize data, study, concentrate and focus. There is a relationship of interdependence between the Intellect and the Mind. The Intellect depends on the directing and coordinating activity of the Mind, and the Mind, in turn, depends on the Intellect for memorizing, concentrating and focusing.

CLINICAL APPLICATION

In practice, the condition of the Intellect depends directly on the state of Stomach and Spleen; in other words, the Intellect relies on the nourishment deriving from the Postnatal Essence of the Stomach and Spleen.

The points that strengthen the Intellect are therefore: BL-20 Pishu, BL-21 Weishu, Du-20 Baihui, ST-36 Zusanli, SP-3 Taibai and BL-49 Yishe.

If there is Dampness obstructing the head and impairing the Intellect, the main points to use are: Ren-12 Zhongwan, Ren-9 Shuifen, LU-7 Lieque, L.I.-4 Hegu, SP-9 Yinlingquan, SP-6 Sanyinjiao, BL-22 Sanjiaoshu, Du-20 Baihui and ST-8 Touwei.

If there is Phlegm obstructing the head and impairing the Intellect, the main points to use are: Ren-12 Zhongwan, Ren-9 Shuifen, LU-7 Lieque, L.I.-4 Hegu, ST-40 Fenglong, SP-9 Yinlingquan, SP-6 Sanyinjiao, BL-22 Sanjiaoshu, Du-20 Baihui and ST-8 Touwei.

The herbal formulae to strengthen the Intellect will not be mentioned as any formula that tonifies the Stomach and Spleen will strengthen the Intellect.

SUMMARY

The Intellect (*Yi*)

The Intellect (*Yi*) resides in the Spleen and is responsible for applied thinking, studying, memorizing, focusing, concentrating and generating ideas.

Memory

The Intellect is responsible for memory but specifically the memory that is needed when studying or researching in the course of one's study or work. The Intellect (and therefore the Spleen) is particularly responsible for extrinsic memory, i.e. the capacity of memorizing data in the course of one's study or work with a conscious effort.

Generation of ideas

The Intellect of the Spleen is responsible for the generation of ideas in the sense of specific ideas in a given field.

Studying and concentrating

The Intellect is responsible for our capacity of studying and concentrating. When the Intellect is clear, we can study hard and concentrate in a sustained way. When the Spleen is deficient and the Intellect weak, we find it difficult to study and concentrate.

Focusing

The Intellect of the Spleen allows us to focus on a study or job in hand with single-mindedness, clarity and concentration.

*Relationship with the Mind (*Shen*)*

The relationship between the Intellect of the Spleen and the Mind of the Heart is very close; one could say that the Intellect is but a sub-aspect of the Mind (*Shen*). The Intellect is that part of the Mind that allows us to memorize data, study, concentrate and focus. There is a relationship of interdependence between the Intellect and the Mind. The Intellect depends on the directing and coordinating activity of the Mind and the Mind, in turn, depends on the Intellect for memorizing, concentrating and focusing.

Clinical application

The points that strengthen the Intellect are therefore: BL-20 Pishu, BL-21 Weishu, Du-20 Baihui, ST-36 Zusanli, SP-3 Taibai and BL-49 Yishe.

END NOTES

1. Graf P, Birt A 1996 Explicit and implicit memory retrieval: intentions and strategies. In: Reder L (ed) Implicit Memory and Metacognition. Lawrence Erlbaum Associates, Mahwah, NJ, p. 46.
2. 1981 Ling Shu Jing 灵枢经 [Spiritual Axis]. People's Health Publishing House, Beijing, p. 23. First published *c.*100 BC.
3. Ibid., p. 23.
4. Ibid., p. 23.
5. 1979 Huang Di Nei Jing Su Wen 黄帝内经素问 [The Yellow Emperor's Classic of Internal Medicine – Simple Questions]. People's Health Publishing House, Beijing, p. 100. First published *c.*100 BC.
6. Cited in Wang Ke Qin 1988 Zhong Yi Shen Zhu Xue Shuo 中医神主学说 [Theory of the Mind in Chinese Medicine]. Ancient Chinese Medical Texts Publishing House, Beijing, p. 9.
7. Ibid., p. 9.

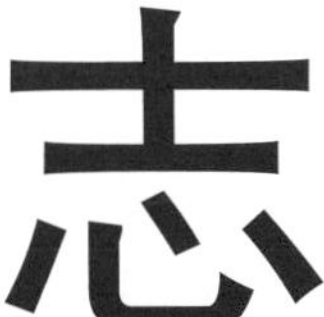

CHAPTER 6

THE WILL-POWER (*ZHI*)

ZHI AS MEMORY *67*

ZHI AS WILL-POWER *68*

CLINICAL APPLICATION *69*

THE WILL-POWER (*ZHI*)

The word *Zhi* 志 has at least three meanings:

1. it indicates "memory"
2. it means "will-power" (Fig. 6.1)
3. it is sometimes used to indicate the five emotions.

I translate "*Zhi*" of the Kidneys as Will-Power because it is its most important aspect in the mental-emotional field as we shall see when discussing Depression (Chapter 16). However, *Zhi* also means "memory", a translation which is also relevant to its nature and function; from this point of view, *Zhi* can be translated as "Memory".

The discussion of the *Zhi* of the Kidneys will be conducted according to the following topics.

- *Zhi* as Memory
- *Zhi* as Will-Power
- Clinical application

ZHI AS "MEMORY"

The Kidneys influence our capacity for memorizing and storing data. Some of the ancient doctors even said that the Intellect (of the Spleen) and the memory (of the Kidneys) are almost the same thing, except that the Intellect is responsible for memorizing in the course of studying and the memory of the Kidneys is responsible for the storing of data over the long term. Tang Zong Hai says: "*Memory* [*Zhi*] *indicates Intellect with a capacity for storing* [data]."[1]

Thus, in memory, three factors are involved: the Mind of the Heart, the Intellect of the Spleen and the Memory (*Zhi*) of the Kidneys. The Memory of the Kidneys is also a function of the Sea of Marrow which is formed by a transformation of Kidney-Essence. The decline in memory experienced by the elderly is often due to a decline of Kidney-Essence, a weakening of the Sea of Marrow and a decrease in Memory.

However, it is important to remember that the decline in memory experienced by the elderly is also frequently caused by Phlegm or Blood stasis obstructing the Brain.

CLINICAL NOTE

To strengthen the Memory (*Zhi*) of the Kidneys, use BL-23 Shenshu and BL-52 Zhishi. As Memory also depends on the Sea of Marrow and the Governing Vessel arises from between the Kidneys and enters the Brain, tonification of the Governing Vessel will also strengthen Memory. To strengthen the Governing Vessel, use S.I.-3 Houxi and BL-62 Shenmai in combination plus Du-16 Fengfu, Du-20 Baihui and BL-23 Shenshu.

Indeed, memory depends primarily on the *communication* between the Heart and Kidneys (Fig. 6.2). The Heart is above and houses the Mind (*Shen*) and the Kidneys are below and house the Essence (*Jing*) and memory (*Zhi*). One of the functions of the Mind of the Heart is memory and consciousness, and this faculty needs to descend towards the Kidneys. On the other hand, the Kidney-Essence and *Zhi* need to ascend towards the Heart and Brain. When this communication takes place, Essence can generate Qi and Qi, in turn, can generate the Mind and memory is good.

Thus, the Kidneys control memory in two ways: by its *Zhi* reaching the Heart and the Mind, and by its Essence reaching the Brain.

ZHI AS WILL-POWER

In the second and clinically more important sense, *Zhi* indicates will-power. The Kidneys house Will-Power which indicates drive, determination, single-mindedness in the pursuit of goals, enthusiasm and motivation. Zhang Jie Bin says in the *Classic of Categories*: "*When one thinks of something, decides on it and then acts on it, this is called Will-Power* [*Zhi*]."[2] The implication of this passage is that thinking of something (an "idea") derives from the Ethereal Soul or the Intellect depending on the kind of idea, making a decision depends on the Liver and Gall-Bladder (and the Ethereal Soul), and acting on it depends on the drive provided by the Will-Power (*Zhi*) of the Kidneys (Fig. 6.3).

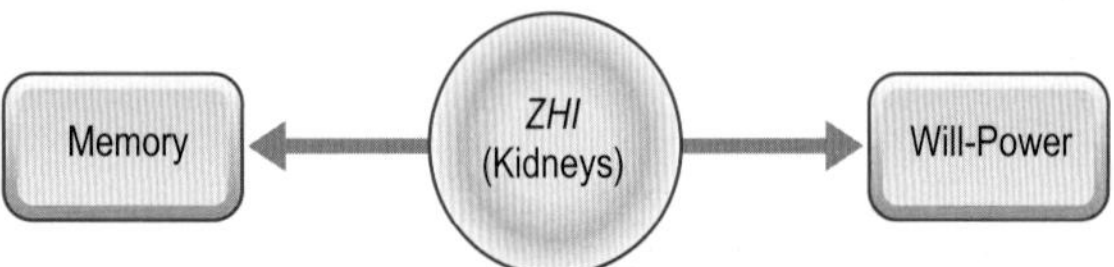

Figure 6.1 *Zhi* as "memory" and "will-power".

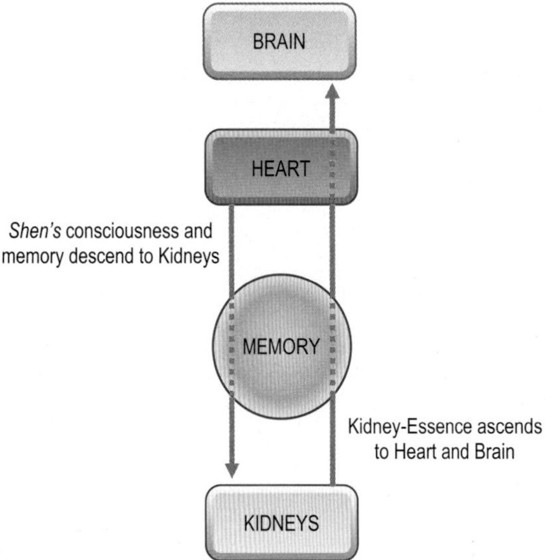

Figure 6.2 Communication between Heart and Kidneys in relation to memory.

Thus, if the Kidneys are strong, the Will-Power is strong and the person will have drive, enthusiasm, motivation and determination in the pursuit of goals. If the Kidneys are depleted and the Will-Power weakened, the person will lack drive and initiative, will be easily discouraged and swayed from his or her aims. A deficiency of the Kidneys and Will-Power is an important aspect of chronic depression.

> **CLINICAL NOTE**
>
> I always tonify the Kidneys in order to strengthen the Will-Power in depression, even in the absence of a specific Kidney pattern. To do so, I reinforce BL-23 Shenshu and BL-52 Zhishi.

The Will-Power (*Zhi*) must be coordinated with the Mind (*Shen*), just as on a physiological level, the Kidneys and Heart must communicate (Fig. 6.4). The Will-Power gives the Mind drive and determination in the pursuit of its goals, and the Mind directs and harnesses the Will-Power. If the Mind is clear in its aims and plans, and the Will-Power is strong, then the person will have the drive to pursue goals. Thus it is necessary for both Will-Power and Mind to be strong.

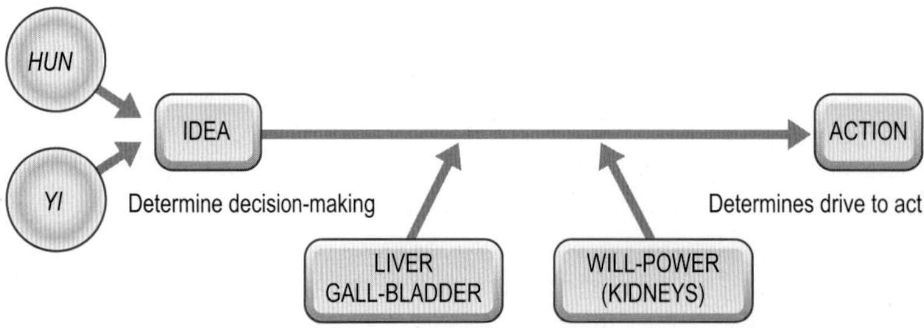

Figure 6.3 Respective roles of Liver, Gall-Bladder and Kidneys in transforming ideas into action.

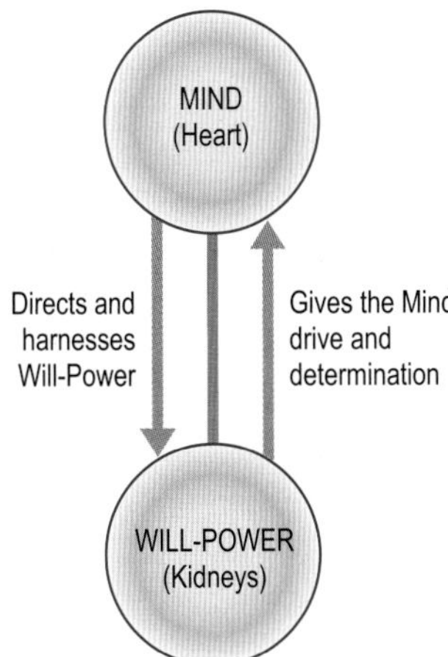

Figure 6.4 Relationship between Will-Power (*Zhi*) and Mind.

The Mind may be clear in its objectives, but if the Will-Power is weak, the person will have no drive to realize such objectives. Conversely, the Will-Power may be strong, but if the Mind is confused, the force of Will-Power will only become reckless and possibly destructive. Although not a pathology, a good example of this second situation may be seen in toddlers who have a strong Will-Power (the age at which they always say "*No!*") but an immature Mind (*Shen*). A similar situation in adults transforms the normal drive and determination of Will-Power (*Zhi*) into recklessness and excessive risk-taking.

CLINICAL APPLICATION

To strengthen the *Zhi* of the Kidneys (both in the sense of "Memory" and of "Will-Power"), I reinforce the following points:

- BL-23 Shenshu and BL-52 Zhishi.

As the Governing Vessel originates from the Kidneys and flows into the Brain, it is the vessel through which the Kidneys exert their influence on the Sea of Marrow and the Brain and therefore Memory and Will-Power. To strengthen this aspect of the Governing Vessel, I use the following points:

- S.I.-3 Houxi and BL-62 Shemai in combination plus Du-16 Fengfu, Du-20 Baihui and BL-23 Shenshu.

From the herbal point of view, any formula that tonifies the Kidneys (Yang or Yin) will strengthen both Will-Power and Memory. Please note that the names of some herbal formulae mentioned in this book contain the words "*ding Zhi*", i.e. "settle the *Zhi*". In this context, *Zhi* means neither Will-Power nor Memory but mostly "emotions" or "Mind".

SUMMARY

The Will-Power (*Zhi*)

- The word *Zhi* 志 has at least three meanings:
  1. it indicates "memory"
  2. it means "will-power "
  3. it is sometimes used to indicate the five emotions.
- In the sense of *Zhi* as memory, the Kidneys influence our capacity for memorizing and storing data.
- In the second sense of *Zhi* as will-power, the Kidneys house Will-Power which indicates drive, determination, enthusiasm, motivation, and single-mindedness in the pursuit of goals.
- A deficiency of the Kidneys and Will-Power is an important aspect of chronic depression.
- The Will-Power (*Zhi*) must be coordinated with the Mind (*Shen*). The Will-Power is the basis for the Mind and the Mind directs the Will-Power. If the Mind is clear in its aims and plans, and the Will-Power is strong, then the person will have the drive to pursue goals. Thus it is necessary for both Will-Power and Mind to be strong.

END NOTES

1. The Essence of Medical Classics on the Convergence of Chinese and Western Medicine, cited in Wang Ke Qin 1988 Zhong Yi Shen Zhu Xue Shuo 中医神主学说 [Theory of the Mind in Chinese Medicine]. Ancient Chinese Medical Texts Publishing House, Beijing. p. 38.
2. 1982 Lei Jing 类经 [Classic of Categories]. People's Health Publishing House, Beijing, p. 50. The *Classic of Categories* was written by Zhang Jie Bin (also called Zhang Jing Yue) and first published in 1624.

鬼

CHAPTER 7

THE *GUI*

GUI AS SPIRIT, GHOST *71*

GUI AS MOVEMENT OF THE ETHEREAL SOUL AND CORPOREAL SOUL *75*

GUI AS A CENTRIPETAL, SEPARATING, FRAGMENTING FORCE *76*

GUI IN RELATION TO THE CORPOREAL SOUL *77*

GUI AS A SYMBOL OF CONTRACTION, COUNTERPOLE OF *SHEN* (EXPANSION) *79*

GUI AS DARK FORCE OF THE PSYCHE AND ITS CONNECTION WITH THE JUNGIAN SHADOW *83*

ACUPUNCTURE POINTS WITH "*GUI*" IN THEIR NAMES *84*

THE *GUI*

Having discussed the nature and functions of the Mind (*Shen*), Ethereal Soul (*Hun*), Corporeal Soul (*Po*), Intellect (*Yi*) and Will-Power (*Zhi*), the overview of the Chinese view of the psyche would not be complete without a discussion of the nature and functions of *gui*. As discussed in Chapter 3, *gui* means "spirit" or "ghost" and it refers to the bodiless form of a deceased person after death (*see Figs 3.1 and 3.2*).

The concept of *gui* in Chinese philosophy and culture has important implications in Chinese medicine. *Gui* is an important complement to the Mind (*Shen*), Ethereal Soul (*Hun*), Corporeal Soul (*Po*), Intellect (*Yi*) and Will-Power (*Zhi*) in the Chinese view of the psyche.

As there are many different ways of looking at *gui* in Chinese medicine, the discussion of *gui* will be broken down into the following topics.

- *Gui* as spirit, ghost
- *Gui* as movement of the Ethereal Soul and Corporeal Soul
- *Gui* as a centripetal, separating, fragmenting force
- *Gui* in relation to the Corporeal Soul
- *Gui* as a symbol of contraction, counterpole of *Shen* (expansion)
- *Gui* as dark force of the psyche and its connection with the Jungian Shadow
- Acupuncture points with "*gui*" in their names

GUI AS SPIRIT, GHOST

As we have seen in Chapter 3, the old pictogram for *gui* depicts the bodiless head of a dead person in its swirling movement in the world of spirit. It therefore indicates the spirit of a dead person which survives after death. Initially, there was no evil connotation to this term, i.e. the spirits of dead people were neither benevolent nor malevolent. After the introduction of Buddhism into China, the word was used to indicate demons or *pretas*.

The belief in spirits of the dead is a cornerstone of Chinese culture, even today after nearly 60 years of Marxism–Leninism. The family is composed of two parts: the community of the living member and that of the dead members of the family. This provided the basis for the cult of ancestors which is so typical of Chinese society, even today.[1]

During the Shang dynasty (1751–1112 BC) and earlier, the influence of spirits dominated life and medicine. In medicine, the main cause of disease was attack by evil spirits and the treatment consisted of exorcism carried out by shamans to drive out evil spirits. The vocabulary of acupuncture is a testimony of this.

In fact, the very character for "medicine" during the Shang dynasty consisted of a quiver of arrows, the word "to take out" and the pictogram for "shaman" as follows:

医 "quiver of arrows"
殳 "to strike", "to kill", an ancient weapon made of bamboo
巫 "shaman".

It is interesting to note that, from the Warring States period (476–221 BC) onwards, the character for "medicine" changed by replacing the radical for "shaman" on the lower part of the character with that for "herbal wine"; this signified that treatment was no longer carried out by a shaman but by a herbalist.

!

Before the Warring States period (476–221 BC), the character for "medicine" contained the radical for "shaman"; after the Warring States period, it contained the radical for "herbal wine".

Later, the Zhou dynasty (1112–476 BC), and especially the Warring States period (476–221 BC), saw the beginning of humanism which reached its apex during the Han and, later on, during the Song-Yuan and Ming dynasties. During the Shang dynasty the influence of *gui* spirits on mankind had been almost total, for no important things could be done without first seeking their approval. During the Zhou dynasty, the *gui* were taken into account but they did not dominate life.

The *Book of Rites* says:

The people of Shang honour spiritual beings, serve them and put them ahead of ceremonies ... the people of Zhou honour ceremonies ... they serve the spiritual beings gui but keep them at a distance. They remain near to mankind and loyal to it.

Confucius also discouraged belief in ghosts and spirits or, at least, he maintained that they should not rule our life and that our life should be ruled by strict adherence to ethical rules. The Analects say:[2]

Fan Chi inquired about wisdom. The Master replied: 'To devote oneself to what is appropriate (Yi) for the people and to show respect for the ghosts and spirits while keeping them at a distance can be called wisdom'.

Demonic medicine, i.e. the belief that illnesses were due to negative influences from spirits whom we have displeased, and that treatment depended on exorcisms and incantations by a shaman to rid the body of such spirits, is indeed probably the origin of acupuncture. Exorcists and shamans used to run through the streets, gesturing and fending the air with spears and arrows to rid the inhabitants of evil spirits. It is quite conceivable that the step between fending the air with the spear and piercing the body to rid it of spirits is a very short one and this would have constituted the beginning of acupuncture.

Spirits and ghosts used to reside in holes or caves; the Chinese word for acupuncture point is *xue* which actually means "hole" or "cave". This is another possible link between demonic medicine and acupuncture, i.e. the acupuncture points were the "holes" where the spirits resided causing illness and requiring piercing of the skin to be driven out.

Some of the acupuncture terminology also supports the connection with demonic medicine. For example, the term *xie qi* 邪气 (nowadays translated as "pathogenic factor") literally means "evil Qi" and it evolved from the term *xie gui*, i.e. "evil spirit". With the transition from demonic to natural medicine that occurred during the Warring States period, diseases were not caused by "evil spirits" any longer but by "evil Qi".

Indeed, the very beginning of the first chapter of the *Simple Questions* confirms this. When the Yellow Emperor asks Qi Bo why in ancient times people lived to 100 years old while "nowadays" they grow old at 50, Qi Bo answers:[3]

The sages in ancient times knew the Dao, patterned themselves on Yin and Yang, cultivated health, they were moderate in eating and drinking, balanced work and rest and avoided overwork.

The above passage is very significant as, when asked why people fall ill, Qi Bo does not say it is because of evil spirits but because of their lifestyle; this marks the passage from demonic medicine to natural medicine and from the shaman to the doctor. However, it is important to remember that the belief in evil spirits did not disappear altogether but remained alive throughout the course of Chinese medicine in parallel with natural medicine.

In fact, even the greatest Chinese doctors believed in evil spirits and recommended various incantations and other methods to neutralize evil spirits. For example, Sun Si Miao (author of the *1000 Golden Ducats Prescriptions* of the Tang dynasty) prescribes the following treatment for an eye disease called "sparrow blindness":[4]

Let the person suffering from sparrow blindness behold a resting place of sparrows by the time of twilight. Then beat on something so that they rise in alarm. When the sparrows fly off, say the exorcism: 'Purple Lord, Purple Lord! I return blindness to you. You return clarity to me!' Do this every night three times; then the eyes will regain clarity. This has been tested and proven effective.

The term *Zhong Feng* 中风 (meaning Wind-Stroke) also suggests a demonic influence as *zhong* suggests an arrow hitting the target. Given the sudden collapse of a person suffering a stroke, it would have been easy to attribute that to being hit by the "arrow" of an evil spirit.

The term *Ji* 疾 for "illness" also bears testimony of the demonic thinking in medicine. This character is composed of the radicals for "bed" and "arrow"; its original meaning was that of a "person who is bedridden because of injury by third parties with an arrow". "Arrow" here is a symbol of being "hit" by an evil spirit.

In subsequent centuries, demonic medicine became to be integrated seamlessly with natural medicine and Chinese doctors, including very famous and eminent ones such as Sun Si Miao and Li Shi Zhen, were quite at ease integrating the practice of acupuncture and herbal medicine with that of exorcism and incantations.

There have been even examples of ancient doctors who gave quite a naturalistic (rather than supernatural) interpretation to *gui*. For example, some doctors maintained that, even when illness was caused by a demonic influence, this attack itself was made possible by a pre-existing organic imbalance; this represents an interesting and intriguing marriage of natural with demonic medicine.

In typical, Chinese, pragmatic fashion, some ancient doctors quite simply thought that if one has Yang deficiency he or she will be invaded by Cold; if one has deficiency of the Mind, he or she will be invaded by *gui*.

Xu Chun Fu (1570) said that a pre-existing weakness in a person's Qi made an attack by an evil spirit possible and, in a very interesting passage, he advocated combining herbal therapy with incantation:[5]

If these two methods of treatment are combined [herbal therapy and incantation], *inner and outer are forged into a whole, producing a prompt cure of the illness. Anyone who engages an exorcist and avoids the application of drugs will be unable to eliminate his illness, for a principle is lacking that could bring about a cure. He who takes only drugs and does not call upon an exorcist to drive out existing doubts, will be cured, but relief will be achieved slowly. Consequently the inner and outer must be treated together; only in this way is rapid success possible.*

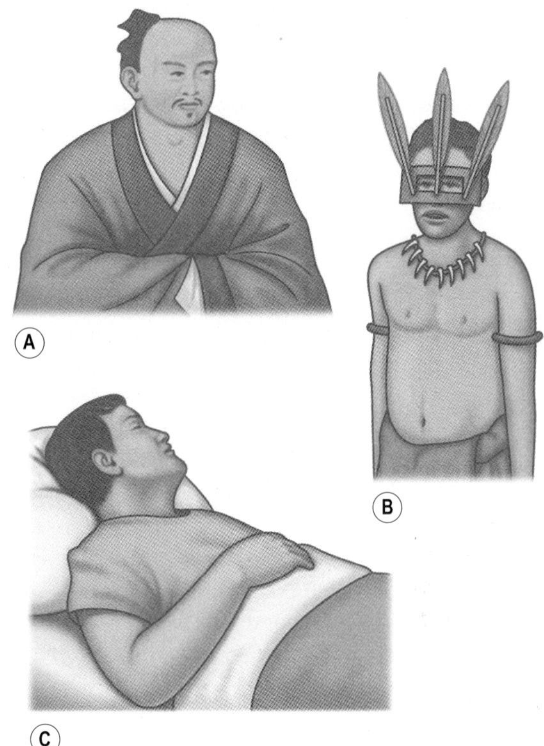

Figure 7.1 Combination of herbal therapy and incantations in ancient China.

See Figure 7.1.

The classification of "inner" and "outer" methods of treatment (herbal drugs and exorcisms respectively) is interesting and his advocating a combination of these two methods is significant; it is tempting to substitute "psychotherapist" for "exorcist" and infer that Xu Chun Fu advocated combining a physical therapy such as herbal medicine with psychotherapy.

!

Xu Chun Fu advocated combining herbal treatment with incantations.

It is also interesting to note the difference in outcome when each therapy is used; if one attends only an exorcist he or she "*will be unable to eliminate the illness*", whereas if one attends a herbalist, he or she "*will be cured*", albeit more slowly than he or she would have been had they hired the services of both a herbalist and an exorcist.

Zhang Jie Bin says something similar when he maintains that the invasion of spirits is made possible purely by the deficiency of the Mind (*Shen*). This is an interesting interpretation as it treats invasions of spirits as a natural phenomenon; just as external Cold invades the body when there is Yang deficiency, spirits invade the body when there is a "deficiency" of the Mind.

Zhang Jie Bin carried the integration of demonic with natural medicine a step further in the *Classic of Categories* (*Lei Jing*, 1624). He says that demons do exist but they are creations of the human mind due to an inner imbalance of Qi and Blood. He even correlated the color in which the demon appears to the patient with a Five-Element imbalance, e.g. if the Earth element is weak, the patient will see green demons (because green is the color of Wood which overacts on Earth).

> **!**
>
> Zhang Jie Bin (1624) carried the integration of demonic with natural medicine a step further. He says that demons do exist but they are creations of the human mind due to an inner imbalance of Qi and Blood. He even correlated the color in which the demon appears to the patient with a Five-Element imbalance, e.g. if the Earth element is weak, the patient will see green demons (because green is the color of Wood which overacts on Earth).

Zhang Jie Bin says in Chapter 43 of the *Classic of Categories* (*Lei Jing*, 1624) entitled "The needling method in case of external invasion of *gui* due to the loss of *Shen* from normal location of the 12 organs":[6]

Huang Di asks: 'When the body is weak Shen escapes and loses its normal location, it allows the external invasion of gui leading to early death. How can we keep the body intact? I would like to know the needling methods for such a condition to keep the body intact and keep the Shen intact.' When Shen is intact, evil spirits cannot invade the body. The combination of weak body and invasion of evil spirits may cause early death.

Dr Zhang says that when the coordination of the *Shen* of the 12 organs is lost, to prevent invasions of external factors (*xie*), one should needle the Source (*Yuan*) point of the relevant channel. Insert the needle, retain for three breaths, then insert another *fen* deeper and retain for one breath; withdraw needle slowly. The following are the point combinations given by Dr Zhang for invasion of evil spirits.

- If the Liver is deficient, the Ethereal Soul has no residence and it escapes, it "swims" away and the body is invaded by white *gui*. First use the Source (*Yuan*) point of the Gall-Bladder G.B.-40 Qiuxu and then the Back-Transporting point of the Liver BL-18 Ganshu at the same time as saying an incantation.
- If the Heart is deficient, the Emperor and Minister Fire do not perform normal functions, and the body is invaded by black *gui*. Use the Source (*Yuan*) point of the Triple Burner T.B.-4 Yangchi and the Back-Transporting point of the Heart BL-15 Xinshu at the same time as saying an incantation.
- If the Spleen is deficient, the body is invaded by green *gui*. Use the Source point of the Stomach ST-42 Chongyang and the Back-Transporting point of the Spleen BL-20 Pishu at the same time as saying an incantation.
- If the Lungs are deficient, the body is invaded by red *gui*. Use the Source point of the Large Intestine L.I.-4 Hegu and the Back-Transporting point of the Lungs, BL-13 Feishu at the same time as saying an incantation.
- If the Kidneys are deficient, the body is invaded by yellow *gui*. Use the Source point of the Bladder BL-64 Jinggu and the Back-Transporting point of the Kidneys, BL-23 Shenshu at the same time as saying an incantation.

As can be observed, the pattern of points used is that, when a Yin organ is deficient (e.g. Liver), Dr Zhang uses the Source (*Yuan*) point of its associated Yang organ (i.e. the Gall-Bladder, G.B.-40 Qiuxu) and the Back-Transporting point of the involved Yin Organ (i.e. the Liver, BL-18 Ganshu) (see Fig. 7.2).

The only exception is the Heart channel for which Dr Zhang uses not S.I.-4 Wangu (as would be logical) but T.B.-4 Yangchi instead, i.e. not the Source point of the associated Small Intestine channel but that of the Triple Burner.

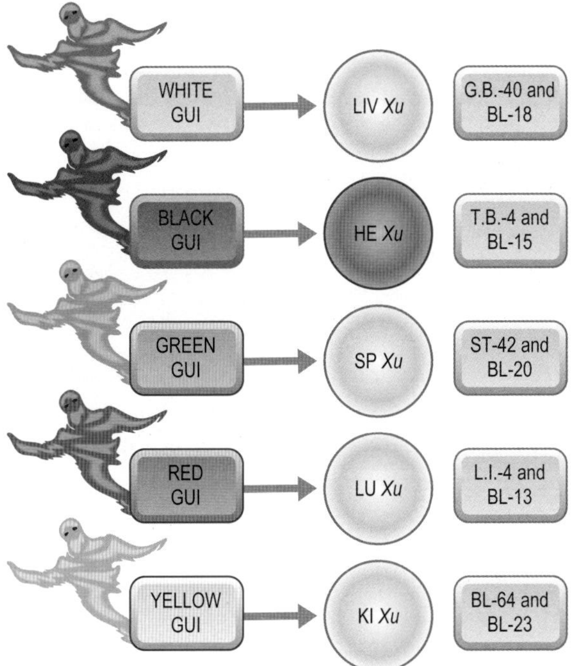

Figure 7.2 Acupuncture for demonic invasion according to Zhang Jie Bin.

- During the Shang dynasty (1751–1112 BC) and earlier, the influence of spirits dominated life and medicine. In medicine, the main cause of disease was attack by evil spirits and the treatment consisted of exorcism carried out by shamans to drive out evil spirits.
- Later, the Zhou dynasty (1112–476 BC), and especially the Warring States period (476–221 BC) saw the beginning of humanism and natural medicine.
- Demonic medicine, i.e. the belief that illnesses were due to negative influences from spirits whom we have displeased and that treatment depended on exorcisms and incantations by a shaman to rid the body of such spirits, dominated until the Warring States period.
- In subsequent centuries, demonic medicine became integrated seamlessly with natural medicine and Chinese doctors, including very famous and eminent ones such as Sun Si Miao and Li Shi Zhen, were quite at ease integrating the practice of acupuncture and herbal medicine with that of exorcism and incantations.
- Zhang Jie Bin maintained that the invasion of spirits is made possible purely by the deficiency of the Mind (*Shen*). He says that demons do exist but they are creations of the human mind due to an inner imbalance of Qi and Blood.

It is important to note that some of the ancient doctors dissented from the view that diseases may be caused by evil spirits. For example, Wang Tao has this to say about eye diseases:[7]

If someone suffers from an eye disease and does not go and see a brilliant physician but rather runs into some Daoist nun or Buddhist old woman, that person will be cheated with some false talk to the effect that he or she has offended a spirit or ghost, and either they restrain the demon inside by having some metal ring around, or they repeatedly fumigate with garlic, or they apply needle or cauterize with irons heated in fire. All this means that they do not know the source of the illness, and that the treatment is contrary to what is required. To stay with Yin and Yang is beneficial; the slightest aberration results in harm.

SUMMARY

Gui as spirit, ghost

- The old pictogram for *gui* depicts the bodiless head of a dead person in its swirling movement in the world of spirit. It therefore indicates the spirit of a dead person which survives after death.

GUI AS MOVEMENT OF THE ETHEREAL SOUL AND CORPOREAL SOUL

As we have seen above, the Chinese characters for both Ethereal Soul and Corporeal Soul contain the radical for *gui*, i.e. "spirit" or "ghost". An important significance of this is that, in relation to the Mind (*Shen*), the Ethereal Soul and Corporeal Soul have an independent existence just like that of a *gui* wandering in the realm of spirits (Fig. 7.3).

What is the significance of the Ethereal Soul and Corporeal Soul having an "independent existence"? It means that they are a part of the psyche that is beyond our consciousness expressed by the Mind (*Shen*): the Ethereal Soul on a psychic level and the Corporeal Soul on a physical level. From this point of view, these two souls are quite different from the other two

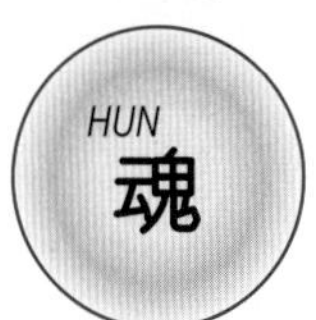

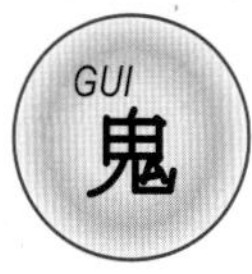

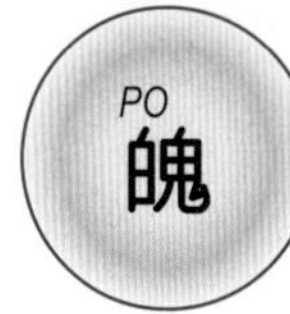

Figure 7.3 Chinese characters for *Hun*, *Gui* and *Po*.

mental-spiritual aspects of Intellect (*Yi*) and Will-Power (*Zhi*) which are really part of the Mind (*Shen*).

This means, especially in the case of the Ethereal Soul, that this soul is like a *gui* that has its own aims and that it cannot be controlled by the Mind.

It is important to see *gui*, Ethereal Soul and Corporeal Soul as a continuum of psychic forces; as the Chinese characters clearly show, Ethereal Soul and Corporeal Soul pertain to the world of *gui*; as is clear from the Chinese characters for "*Hun*" and "*Po*", *gui* is an integral part of the Ethereal and Corporeal Souls.

The significance of *gui* in the life of the Ethereal Soul and Corporeal Soul is "movement": the *gui* wanders and moves in the world of spirits after death. This movement extends to the Ethereal Soul and Corporeal Soul, the former on a psychic, the latter on a physical level. As we have seen in Chapter 3, the Ethereal Soul is described as the "coming and going" of the Mind. It provides "movement" to the Mind in the sense of ideas, plans, projects, life dreams, vision, intuition and creativity. This movement is absolutely essential to our psyche.

The Corporeal Soul, on the other hand, provides movement on a physical level and is described as the "entering and exiting of Essence". The Corporeal Soul's movement is essential to bring the Essence into play in all physiological processes.

A quote confirms the independent existence of *gui* and its influence on our psyche:

If you do something outrageous the wandering gui *has lost the address to his home. If you do something totally mad, the wandering* gui *has gone abroad.*

SUMMARY

Gui as movement of the Ethereal Soul and Corporeal Soul

- The Chinese characters of both Ethereal Soul and Corporeal Soul contain the radical for *gui*, i.e. "spirit" or "ghost".
- In relation to the Mind (*Shen*), the Ethereal Soul and Corporeal Soul have an independent existence just like that of a *gui* wandering in the realm of spirits.
- The Ethereal Soul and Corporeal Soul are a part of the psyche that is beyond our consciousness expressed by the Mind (*Shen*): the Ethereal Soul on a psychic level and the Corporeal Soul on a physical level.
- *Gui*, Ethereal Soul and Corporeal Soul are a continuum of psychic forces.

GUI AS A CENTRIPETAL, SEPARATING, FRAGMENTING FORCE

The phonetic similarity between the word *gui* meaning "spirit" and *gui* 归 meaning "to return" is not casual. The ghost – *gui* – is a dead person who *returns* as a ghost. "Returning" also implies that the spirit of the dead person returns to where it came from. The *Book of Lieh-Tzu* (a Daoist classic) says:[8]

What belongs to Heaven is pure and disperses; what belongs to Earth is dense and sticks together. When spirit departs from the body, each returns to its true state. That is why ghosts are called 'gui'; 'gui' means 'one who has gone home', they have gone back to their true home.

"Returning" also has the meaning of "to converge, to come together", indicating the centripetal, contracting movement of a *gui*, which is discussed below.

The Wu Xing Da Yi says: "*Gui are those that return. Ancient people called dead persons 'those who return'.*"[9] Wang Chong (AD 27–100) said:

When a person dies, his spirit ascends to Heaven and his flesh and bones return to Earth. To be an earthly gui *means to return ... to be a heavenly* shen *means to expand. When the expansion reaches its limit, it ends and begins again. A person is born of* gui *and at death returns to them. Yin and Yang are called* gui-shen. *After people die, they are also called* gui-shen.

See Figure 7.4.

The coming into being of a separate existence, of a living body, itself requires the *gui*'s centripetal, separating and "returning" movement; the *gui* look for the fragmentation into "pieces" of separate existence. The

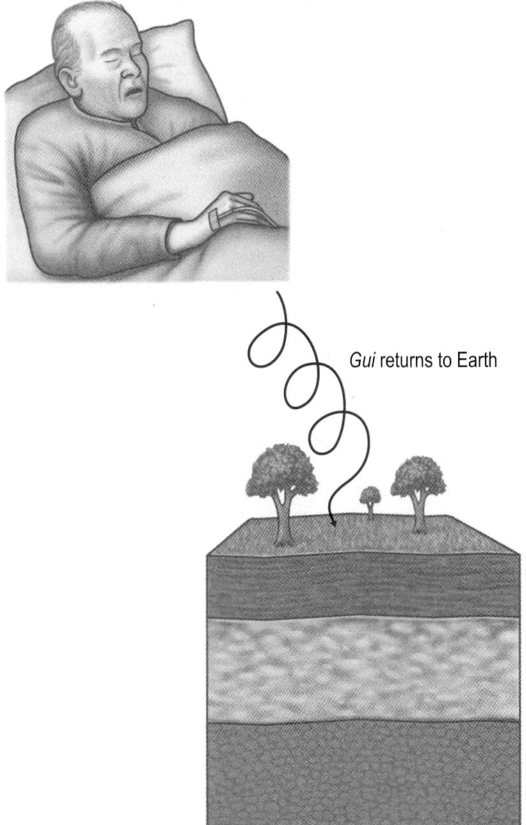

Figure 7.4 *Gui* as "that who returns".

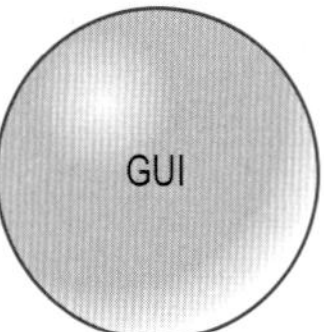

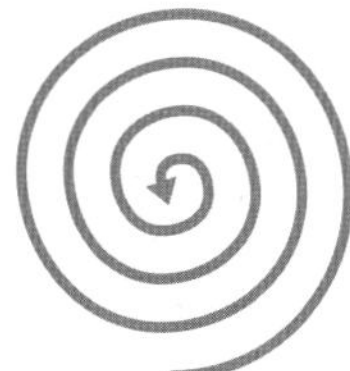

Figure 7.5 *Gui* as contracting, fragmenting force.

phonetic connection between *gui* 鬼 (ghosts) and *kuai* 塊 (pieces) is not coincidental. Thus, the *gui* represents a centripetal, materializing, separating and fragmenting force (Fig. 7.5).

Thus, from this point of view, *gui* is a metaphor for a contracting, centripetal force on both a physical and a psychic level. On a physical level, *gui* as a centripetal, contracting force is allied with the Corporeal Soul (see below). This contracting, centripetal force is manifested in the Yin phase of any physiological process. For example, inhalation is Yin and therefore *gui*, bending of a joint is Yin and therefore *gui*, falling asleep is Yin and therefore *gui*, etc.

The process of contraction eventually leads to fragmentation and, in the individual, death. As explained in Chapter 4, although contraction and fragmentation may seem to be contradictory, they are not and there are several examples of this process in the natural world. For this reason, thoughts of death are often due to an imbalance in the Lung organ which houses the Corporeal Soul.

On a psychic level, *gui* corresponds to movement of the Ethereal Soul which is essential to our psychic life. From this point of view, this movement is expansive, centrifugal; this is essential for our relationships with other people.

SUMMARY

Gui as a centripetal, separating, fragmenting force

- The phonetic similarity between the word *gui* meaning "spirit" and *gui* meaning "to return" indicates that the ghost – *gui* – is a dead person who *returns* as a ghost.
- "Returning" also has the meaning of "to converge, to come together", indicating the centripetal, contracting movement of a *gui*.
- The coming into being of a separate existence, of a living body, itself requires the *gui*'s centripetal, separating and "returning" movement; the *gui* look for the fragmentation into "pieces" of separate existence.
- There is a phonetic connection between *gui* (ghosts) and *kuai* (pieces).

GUI IN RELATION TO THE CORPOREAL SOUL

The centripetal, materializing, separating and fragmenting force of *gui* can be observed particularly in the

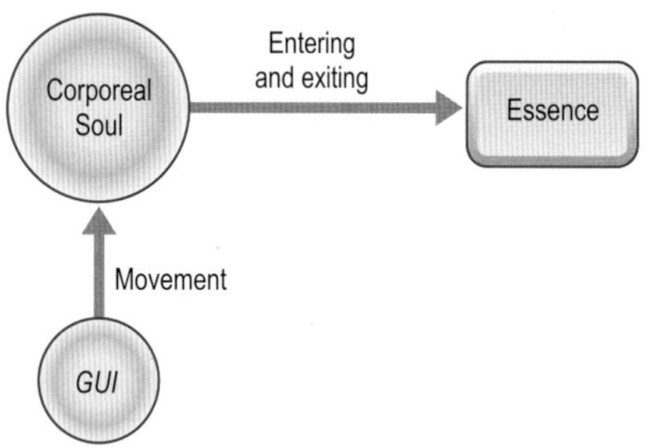

Figure 7.6 The *gui* and the movement of the Corporeal Soul.

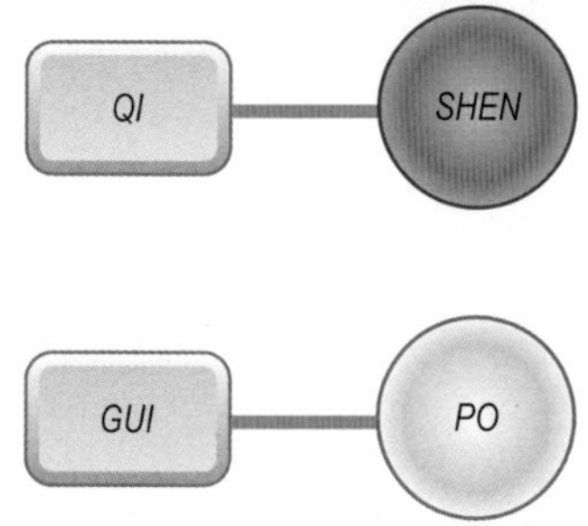

Figure 7.7 Relationship between Qi and Shen and between *gui* and Corporeal Soul.

activity of the Corporeal Soul. Indeed, Granet says that in life, this soul is called *Po*, while in death, it is called *gui*.[10] By contrast, the other soul is called *Hun* in life and *Shen* after death.

The *gui* within the Corporeal Soul gives it movement on a physical level (*entering and exiting* of the Essence) in all the body's physiological processes. As movement is intrinsic in the nature of the *gui*, this is the force that animates the movement of the Corporeal Soul in all physiological processes and in all parts of the body (Fig. 7.6).

Thus, the *gui* within the Corporeal Soul is the "dark" force that animates it in carrying out its function of promoting all physiological processes and of bringing the Essence into play in all parts of the body. Confucius said that "*Qi is the fullness* [perfection] *of Shen; Corporeal Soul is the fullness* [perfection] *of gui*" (Fig. 7.7). This means that the nature of the Mind (*Shen*) is Qi, while the nature of Corporeal Soul is *gui*. Thus, there is a close connection between Corporeal Soul and *gui* intended in the sense of a contracting, centripetal, fragmenting, materializing force; it is a force that the Corporeal Soul needs to carry out its functions and its movement.

The same centripetal, separating, materializing, contracting and fragmenting power of *gui* is active in the Corporeal Soul; the Corporeal Soul needs that type of contracting movement to carry out its functions. This is in opposition to the Ethereal Soul which requires an expansive movement.

He Shang Gong says: "*The five turbid and humid flavours form bones, muscles, blood, vessels and the six passions ... these* gui *are called Corporeal Soul.*"[11] In this statement, *gui* is considered to be the Qi of the physical form, such as bones, muscles, blood and, interestingly, the six "passions", i.e. emotions.

Thus *gui* is like a dark force of the body that is closely bound to the Corporeal Soul. To put it differently, one could say that the Ethereal Soul is the *gui* of the five natures, while the Corporeal Soul is the *gui* of the six passions (Fig. 7.8). The "five natures" here should be seen in the context of the Confucian concept of "human nature" (*xing*). According to Confucian philosophy, human nature is our true essential human nature (defined by propriety, adherence to rites, ethics, etc.), while the emotions (or "passions") cloud our human nature. This is discussed at length in Chapter 15.

In order to understand this statement, one must understand the Confucian view of human nature and emotions. According to Neo-Confucian philosophers of the Song and Ming dynasties, human nature (*xing* 性) is essentially pure and good; for some, it is a manifestation of *principle* (*Li* 理). Emotions tend to cloud true human nature. One can think of a clear pond; the purity and clarity of the water reflects the pure human nature. If we stir up the muddy bottom of the pond, the water becomes murky. The stirring up of mud is equivalent to the stirring up of emotions which cloud true human nature; when we are completely overtaken by emotions, then these *become* our human nature, i.e. we lose our human nature entirely.

Thus, the above passage needs to be seen in this context. The "five natures" of the five Yin organs are part of the Confucian "human nature" and the Ethereal Soul is the *gui*, i.e. the animating spirit of these five natures. The Corporeal Soul, by contrast, is the *gui*, i.e. the animating spirit of the passions (emotions) which cloud true human nature.

To put it differently, we could say that the five natures of the five Yin organs are like the "Ethereal Soul's aspects of each of the five mental-spiritual aspects of the organs" (see Fig. 7.8). In other words, each of the

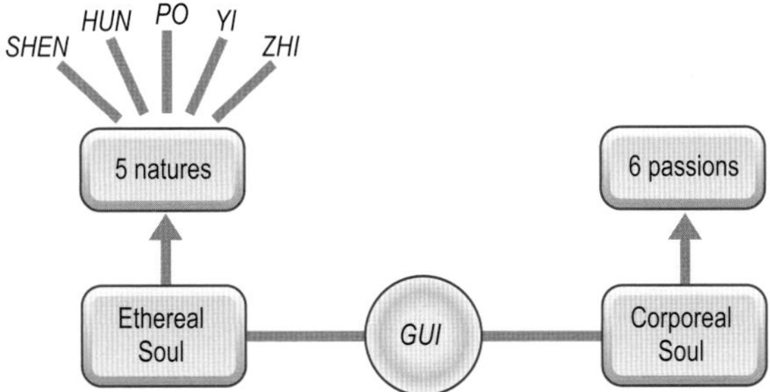

Figure 7.8 Role of *gui* in the 5 natures and 6 passions.

mental-spiritual aspects of each of the five Yin organs partakes of our human nature through the Ethereal Soul.

SUMMARY

Gui in relation to the Corporeal Soul

- The *gui* within the Corporeal Soul gives it movement on a physical level (*entering and exiting* of the Essence) in all the body's physiological processes.
- The *gui* within the Corporeal Soul is the "dark" force that animates it in carrying out its function of promoting all physiological processes and of bringing the Essence into play in all parts of the body.
- The same centripetal, separating, materializing, contracting and fragmenting power of *gui* is active in the Corporeal Soul; the Corporeal Soul needs that type of contracting movement to carry out its functions.

GUI AS A SYMBOL OF CONTRACTION, COUNTERPOLE OF *SHEN* (EXPANSION)

The dark powers of *gui* are complementary to *Shen* and they constantly oppose it at every turn to regain their freedom of action. The *gui* strive towards contraction, materialization and fragmentation; the *shen* strives towards expansion and wholeness (Fig. 7.9). However, this tension, this opposition, is relative and is a source of dynamism. On a psychic level, it generates opposition, desires and conflicts, but it is also the motive force of transformation and metamorphosis of the Spirit.

Wang Chong said;

Qi produces a person just as water becomes ice. As water freezes into ice, so Qi coagulates to form a person. When ice melts, it becomes water. When a person dies, he becomes a gui *spirit again. He is called* gui *just as melted ice changes its name to water. As people see that its name has changed, they say it has consciousness, can assume physical form, and can hurt people. But they have no basis for saying so.*

See Figure 7.10.

Wang Chong was a Confucian philosopher with a sceptical streak. In this passage, he considers the changes occurring at death in a naturalistic way, comparing them to the changes from water to ice and back. He compares the formation of human form to the freezing of water into ice and death to the melting of ice back into water. So death is nothing but a change in condensation of Qi. Wang Chong says that when people live, they are called *shen* and when they die, *gui*. According to Wang Chong this transformation is nothing but a natural change and *gui* is nothing other than a change in human Qi; therefore, they cannot assume physical form and hurt people. He therefore used this argument to contradict those who considered *gui* to be real and harmful to human beings.

Zhu Xi (1113–1200) said:[12]

Is expansion shen *and contraction* gui*? The teacher drew a circle on the desk with his hand and pointed to its center and said: Principle [Li] is like a circle. Within it there is differentiation like this. All cases of material force [Qi] which is coming forth belong to Yang and are* shen. *All cases of material force which is returning to its origin belong to Yin and are* gui. *In the day, forenoon is* shen, *afternoon is* gui. *In the month, from the 3rd day onward is* shen; *after the 16th day it is* gui. *The sun is* shen *and the moon is* gui. *Plants growing are* shen, *plants decaying are* gui. *A person from childhood to maturity is* shen, *while a person in his declining years and old age is* gui. *In breathing, breath going out is* shen, *breath coming in is* gui.

Table 7.1 summarizes Zhu Xi's view of *Shen* and *gui*. See also Figures 7.11 and 7.12.

Zhu Xi said: "*To arrive is called* shen *on account of its expansion; to turn back is called* gui *on account of its returning.*"[13] Zhu Xi also said:[14]

Qi is the flourishing of shen; *Po is the flourishing of* gui. *Combining* gui *and* shen *is the supreme of teaching. All*

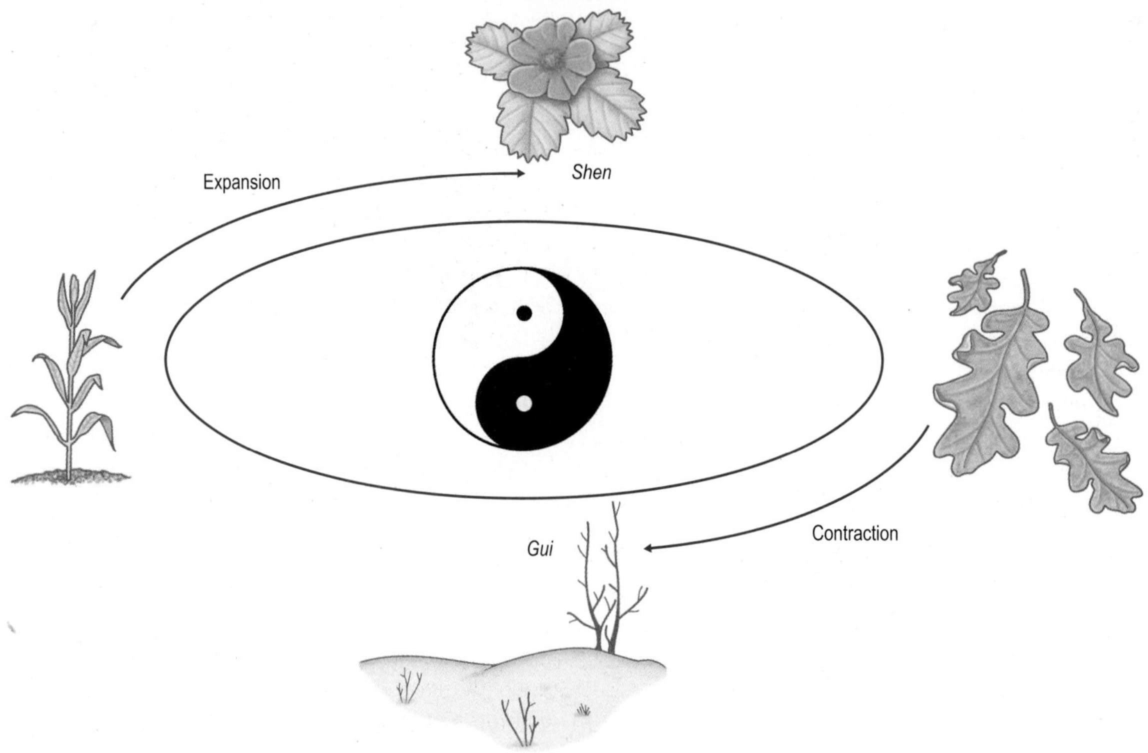

Figure 7.9 *Shen* and *gui* as expansion and contraction.

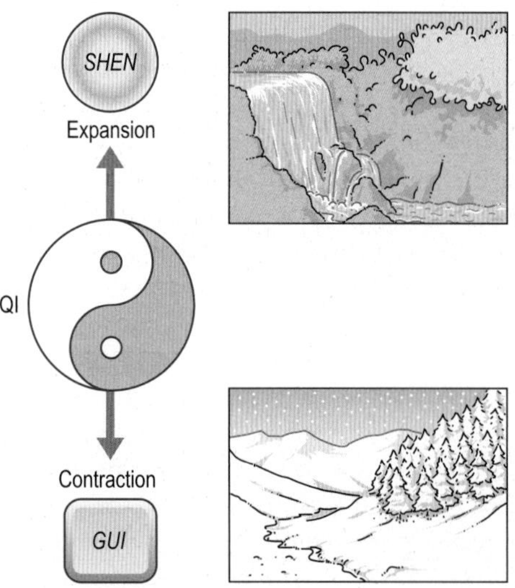

Figure 7.10 *Shen* and *gui* as expansion and contraction of Qi according to Wang Chong.

living things must die. Having died, they must return to Earth. This is called gui. *Bones and flesh die and go down. The Yin becomes the Earth of the fields. Its Qi is emitted and displayed up high; it is bright and fuming up. This is the essence of the 100 things and the manifestation of* shen.

These passages clearly show the important view according to which *gui* is synonymous with a centripetal, contractive movement and *shen* with a centrifugal, expansive movement in every human sphere. It is important to stress that, in this context, *shen* does not mean "Mind" or "Spirit" but is simply the symbol of an expansive movement. The opposition (and interaction) between *shen* and *gui* has important implications in psychology.

The Ethereal Soul and Corporeal Soul are the manifestations of *shen* and *gui* in the human body. Zhu Xi said:[15]

Table 7.1 *Shen* and *gui* as poles of Yang and Yin in Zhu Xi

SHEN	*GUI*
Expansion	Contraction
Qi coming forth	Qi returning to origin
Before noon	After noon
From 3rd day of month	From 16th day of month
Sun	Moon
Growing plants	Decaying plants
From childhood to adulthood	From adulthood to death
Breathing out	Breathing in
Yang	Yin
Arriving	Turning back
Bright	Dark
Manifest	Hidden
Alive	Dead
Movement	Rest
Dispersing	Aggregating
Day	Night
Youth	Old age
Spring and summer	Autumn and winter
Music	Rituals
Ethereal Soul	Corporeal Soul
Qi	Corporeal Soul
Qi	Essence
Speech	Silence

Before man dies, shen *is in control; after death* gui *is in control. Corporeal Soul is a speck of essence and Qi. When Qi meets, there is* shen. *The Ethereal Soul is that which is manifest and coming out, like the coming in and out of Qi in respiration. The Corporeal Soul is like water. Because of it, man's seeing can be bright, hearing can be acute and the Mind can be vigorous and can memorize well. When a man has this Corporeal Soul, then he has this* shen.

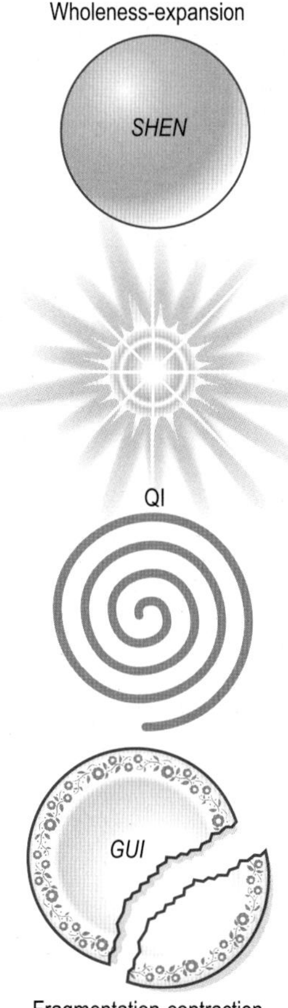

Figure 7.11 *Shen* and *gui* as expansion and contraction of Qi according to Zhu Xi.

Gui is often presented as the counterpole of *shen*. *Shen* pertains to Heaven and is the Heavenly spirit; *gui* pertains to Earth and is the Earthly spirit. In other words, they are the two polarities of utmost Yang and utmost Yin in the world of spirit and in our psyche.

This polarity was always considered relative in Chinese thinking. It basically signifies the tension, conflicts and contradictions between the subtle, dark, centripetal, contracting psychic forces of *gui* and the subtle, bright, centrifugal, expansive psychic forces of *shen*.

This polarity is made up of the two poles of Yin and Yang in the human psyche and their interplay animates our psyche. Hence *gui* is an integral part of the human psyche; it represents the centripetal, desire force seeking to separate itself and which must be nourished (like one feeds hungry pretas). In essence, *gui* can be seen as the Shadow within our psyche (see below).

Zhang Cai said:

SHEN

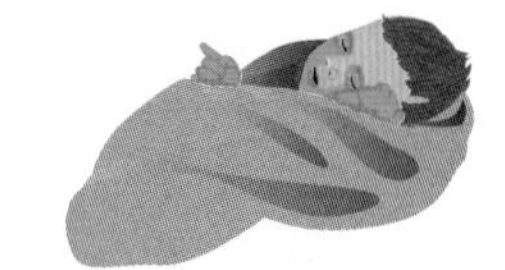

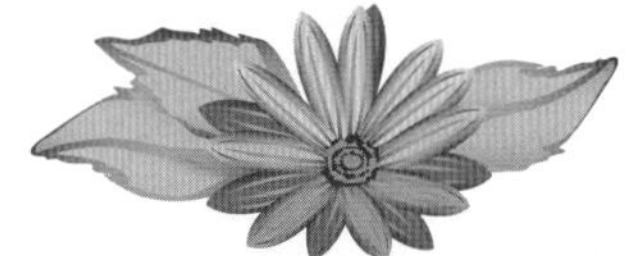

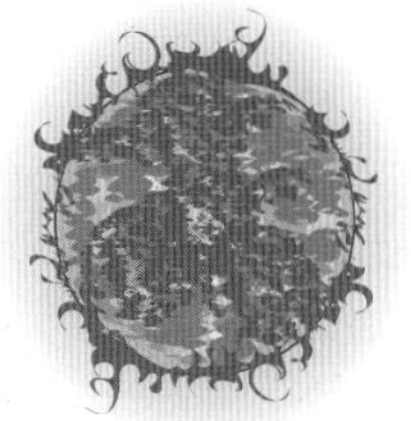

GUI

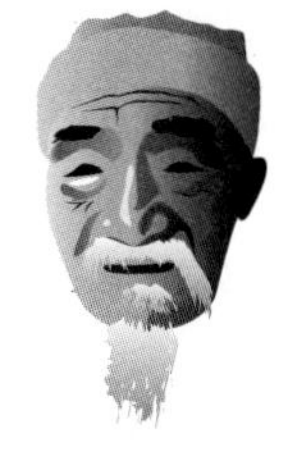

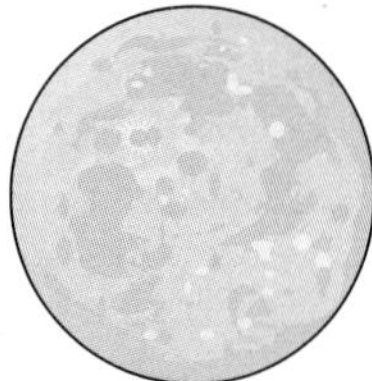

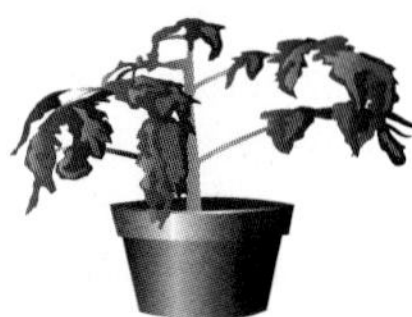

Figure 7.12 Examples of *Shen* and *gui* as expansion and contraction of Qi according to Zhu Xi.

Gui *and* shen *are the spontaneous activity of Yin and Yang ... the reality of* gui *and* shen *does not go beyond these two fundamental elements ... if Yin and Yang do not exist, the One cannot be revealed. Reality and unreality, motion and rest, integration and disintegration are two different substances. In the final analysis, however, they are one.*

He also said:

When a thing first comes into existence, material force [Qi] comes gradually into it to enrich its vitality. As it reaches its maturity, Qi gradually reverts to where it came from, wanders off and disperses. Its coming means shen *because it is expanding; its reversion means* gui *because it is returning.*

To sum up, in the psychic sphere *gui* and *shen* symbolize two opposing but complementary states of contraction and expansion. When we are "down", do not feel like going out, introvert or sad, we are in a state of *gui*; when we are up, feel like going out, extrovert or happy, we are in a state of *shen*. Table 7.2 summarizes my view of the polarity of *shen* and *gui* in our psychic life. Please note that Table 7.2 does not indicate two different personalities but the alternation of two emotional states in the *same* person at different times.

The psychic balance between *gui* and *shen* depends on the opposing activities of the Ethereal Soul and Corporeal Soul: one expansive, the other contracting. The two herbs Yuan Zhi *Radix Polygalae* and Suan Zao Ren *Semen Ziziphi spinosae* are representative of these two opposing expanding (*shen*) and contracting (*gui*) psychic movements. The former herb is pungent and stimulates the coming and going of the Ethereal Soul

Table 7.2 The polarity of *Shen* and *gui* in our psychic life

SHEN	*GUI*
Feeling up	Feeling down
Extrovert	Introvert
Wanting to go out	Wanting to stay in
Happy	Sad
Talking a lot	Wanting to be silent
Seeking company	Wanting to be alone
Heightened sexual desire	Lacking sexual desire
Ebullient	Melancholic

while the latter is sour and restrains the coming and going of the Ethereal Soul.

Thus we can build the following correspondences:

- *Shen* = heavenly, bright, ethereal, expanding, going, centrifugal, wholeness, life
- *Gui* = earthly, dark, corporeal, contracting, returning, centripetal, fragmenting, death (Fig. 7.13).

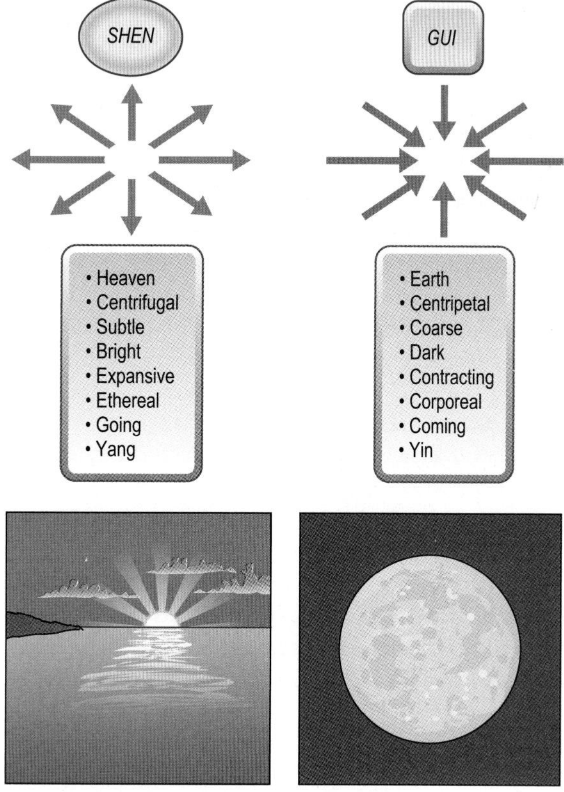

Figure 7.13 Polarity of *Shen* and *gui*.

SUMMARY

Gui as a symbol of contraction, counterpole of *shen* (expansion)

- The *gui* strives towards fragmentation, materialization and contraction; the *shen* strives towards expansion and wholeness.
- *Gui* is synonymous with a centripetal, contractive movement and *shen* with a centrifugal, expansive movement in every human sphere.
- This polarity is made up of the two poles of Yin and Yang in the human psyche and their interplay animates our psyche.
- In the psychic sphere *gui* and *shen* symbolize two opposing but complementary states of contraction and expansion.

GUI AS A DARK FORCE OF THE PSYCHE AND ITS CONNECTION WITH THE JUNGIAN SHADOW

Although I believe we should always be very careful in making direct correlations between Chinese medicine concepts and Western medicine, we could postulate that, from a psychological point of view, *gui* resembles the Jungian Shadow.

Traditionally, ghosts needed food offerings daily to be appeased; this is symbolic of the need to come to terms with and integrate the Shadow, the dark side of the psyche.

The Shadow is a psychological term introduced by Carl G. Jung. The shadow is an unconscious complex that is defined as the repressed and suppressed aspects of the conscious self. The Shadow often represents everything that the conscious person does not wish to acknowledge within themselves. For instance, someone who identifies as being kind has a shadow that is harsh or unkind.

The Shadow is made of dark, rejected aspects of our being which we do not want to see or admit to. There is also light, positive undeveloped potential in the Shadow but we are not concerned with that here.

Everyone has a Shadow and Jung considered an awareness and coming to terms with our Shadow an essential starting point in therapy. We all have a Shadow and a confrontation with the Shadow is essential for self-awareness. Jung thought that therapy cannot even start without an awareness of one's Shadow. We cannot learn about ourselves if we do not learn about our Shadow; if we do not, we will tend to be in denial of it and "project" onto others like a mirror. We see traits that we do not like in others but that is in reality a mirror of our own Shadow (although not always).

When the Shadow is acknowledged, we then realize that it is not a destructive force but a natural part of our psyche; in a certain sense, the Shadow is also power and originality.

In this sense, the Chinese concept of *gui* could be interpreted as a metaphor for the Shadow; it is the dark aspect that is part of the Ethereal Soul and Corporeal Soul, but an essential part of our being in providing "movement" to these two souls, the former on a psychic level, the latter on a physical one.

When seen as a "dark", contracting psychic force, the *gui* needs to be integrated into the psyche to prevent dis-association, splitting of contents of the psyche. Neurosis, psychosis, mania, etc. consist of dis-association of dark contents of the psyche. When this happens, the *gui* are perceived as external agents, evil spirits possessing the psyche, while they are actually a product of the psyche itself.

As Jung says: "*If tendencies towards dis-association were not inherent in the human psyche, parts would have never split off: in other words, neither spirits nor gods would ever have come to exist.*"[16] Thus we should learn to recognize the psychic forces symbolized by *gui* and not wait until (as Jung says) our moods "*make clear to us in the most painful way that we (i.e. the Mind) are not the only master of our house*".[17]

SUMMARY

Gui as a dark force of the psyche and its connection with the Jungian Shadow

- *Gui* needs to be integrated in the psyche to prevent dis-association, splitting of contents of the psyche.
- *Gui* is the equivalent of the Shadow in Jungian psychology.

ACUPUNCTURE POINTS WITH "*GUI*" IN THEIR NAMES

All acupuncture points have more than one name and the names we commonly use are only one of the possible names for each acupuncture point.

Many alternative names of points contain the word "*gui*"; generally speaking, all the points with the word "*gui*" in their names have a strong mental-emotional effect, particularly in opening the Mind's orifices when these are obstructed.

The following is a list of alternative names for common points with the word "*gui*" in their names.

GUI XIE L.I.-10 Shousanli and ST-36 Zusanli	"Evil spirit"
GUI CHEN L.I.-11 Quchi	"Spirit Minister"
GUI CHUANG ST-6 Jiache and LU-10 Yuji	"Spirit bed"
GUI XIN LU-9 Taiyuan and P-7 Daling	"Spirit heart"
GUI TANG LU-5 Chize and Du-23 Shangxing	"Spirit hall"
GUI XIN LU-11 Shaoshang	"Spirit believe"
GUI XIN L.I.-1 Shangyang	"Spirit letter"
GUI YAN SP-1 Dadu	"Spirit eye"
GUI LUO BL-62 Shenmai and P-5 Jianshi	"Spirit channel"
GUI KU P-8 Laogong	"Spirit cave"
GUI XUE Du-16 Fengfu	"Spirit hole", "Spirit cave"
GUI SHI Du-26 Renzhong and Ren-24 Chengjiang	"Spirit market", "Spirit city"
GUI MEN Du-22 Xinhui	"Spirit door"
GUI CANG Ren-1 Huiyin	"Hidden spirit"

Sun Si Miao's 13 Ghost points

Sun Si Miao's 13 Ghost points are almost the same as in the above list. The Ghost points were formulated by Sun Si Miao in his *1000 Golden Ducats Prescriptions* (*Qian Jin Yao Fang*, AD 652).[18] These points were used for severe mental illness such as manic-depression or psychosis.

Sun Si Miao's instructions were to needle the points in the order indicated, the left side in men and the right side in women, and then withdraw the needles in reverse order. Use one point at a time in succession. The point Ren-1 is not needled but direct moxa is applied to it.

Sun Si Miao's 13 Ghost points are listed in Table 7.3.

SUMMARY

The *gui*

- *Gui* as spirit, ghost.
- *Gui* as movement of Ethereal Soul and Corporeal Soul.
- *Gui* as a centripetal, separating, fragmenting force.
- *Gui* in relation to the Corporeal Soul.
- *Gui* as a symbol of contraction, counterpole of *Shen* (expansion).
- *Gui* as dark force of the psyche and its connection with the Jungian Shadow.

Table 7.3 Sun Si Miao's 13 Ghost points

POINT	NAME	ALTERNATIVE NAME	TRANSLATION	CHINESE
Du-26	Renzhong	Gui Gong	G. Palace	鬼宫
LU-11	Shaoshang	Gui Xin	G. True (Believe)	鬼信
SP-1	Yinbai	Gui Yan	G. Eye	鬼眼
P-7	Daling	Gui Xin	G. Heart	鬼心
BL-62	Shenmai	Gui Lu	G. Road	鬼路
Du-16	Fengfu	Gui Zhen	G. Pillow	鬼枕
ST-6	Jiache	Gui Chuang	G. Bed	鬼床
Ren-24	Chengjiang	Gui Shi	G. Market	鬼市
P-8	Laogong	Gui Ku	G. Cave	鬼窟
Du-23	Shangxing	Gui Tang	G. Hall	鬼堂
Ren-1	Huiyin	Gui Cang	G. Hidden	鬼藏
L.I.-11	Quchi	Gui Chen	G. Minister	鬼臣
Extra	Hai Quan	Gui Feng	G. Seal	鬼封

END NOTES

1. Granet M 1973 La Religione dei Cinesi. Adelphi, Milano, p. 34.
2. Ames RT, Rosemont H 1999 The Analects of Confucius – A Philosophical Translation. Ballantine Books, New York, p. 108.
3. 1979 Huang Ti Nei Jing Su Wen [黄帝内经素问] [The Yellow Emperor's Classic of Internal Medicine – Simple Questions]. People's Health Publishing House, Beijing, pp. 1–2. First published *c.*100 BC.
4. Cited in Kovacs J, Unschuld P 1998 Essential Subtleties on the Silver Sea – The Yin Hai Jing Wei: a Chinese Classic of Ophthalmology. University of California Press, Berkeley, p. 36.
5. Unschuld P 1985 Medicine in China – A History of Ideas. University of California Press, Berkeley, p. 220.
6. Ibid., p. 1018.
7. Cited in Essential Subtleties on the Silver Sea, p. 42.
8. Graham AC 1999 The Book of Lieh-Tzu – A Classic of Tao. Columbia University Press, New York, p. 23.
9. Eyssalet J-M 1990 Le Secret de la Maison des Ancêtres. Guy Trédaniel Editeur, Paris, p. 23.
10. La Religione dei Cinesi, p. 78.
11. Le Secret de la Maison des Ancêtres, p. 30.
12. Kim Yung Sik 2000 The Natural Philosophy of Chu Hsi. American Philosophical Society, Philadelphia, p. 101
13. Ibid., p. 101.
14. Ibid., p. 224.
15. Ibid., p. 229.
16. Wilhelm R (translator) 1962 The Secret of the Golden Flower. Harcourt, Brace & World, New York, p. 111.
17. Ibid., p. 113.
18. 1982 Qian Jin Yao Fang [千金要方] [Thousand Golden Ducats Prescriptions]. People's Health Publishing House, Beijing, p. 327. The *Thousand Golden Ducats* was written by Sun Si Miao in AD 652.

五神与脏腑的联系

CHAPTER 8

THE 12 INTERNAL ORGANS AND THE PSYCHE

HEART *90*

LUNGS *93*

LIVER *94*

SPLEEN *96*

KIDNEYS *97*

PERICARDIUM *100*

SMALL INTESTINE *102*

LARGE INTESTINE *104*

GALL-BLADDER *104*

STOMACH *107*

BLADDER *110*

TRIPLE BURNER *110*

THE 12 INTERNAL ORGANS AND THE PSYCHE

The nature and functions of the Mind (*Shen*), Ethereal Soul (*Hun*), Corporeal Soul (*Po*), Intellect (*Yi*) and Will-Power (*Zhi*) were discussed in Chapters 2, 3, 4, 5 and 6 respectively. These aspects of the psyche are connected to the relevant internal organ, i.e. Heart, Liver, Lungs, Spleen and Kidneys. We must now turn our attention to describing the influence of all 12 Internal Organs on the psyche by drawing primarily on the *Yellow Emperor's Classic of Internal Medicine* as a source.

Chapter 8 of the *Simple Questions* contains the core of the theory of the Internal Organs seen as the "officials" of a government. It states:[1]

The Heart is the official functioning as the Monarch: the Spirit originates from it. The Lungs are the official functioning as Minister: they are in charge of government. The Liver is the official functioning as general: planning originates from it. The Gall-Bladder is the official functioning as Minister of Justice: decision-making originates from it. The Pericardium is the official functioning as envoy: joy and happiness originate from it. The Spleen and Stomach are the official functioning as granary: the five flavours originate from them. The Large Intestine is the official functioning as Minister of Transport: change and transformation originate from it. The Small Intestine is the official in charge of reception: transformation originates from it. The Kidneys are the official in charge of power: skill originates from them. The Triple Burner is the official responsible for dredging of channels: regulation of water passages originates from it. The Bladder is the official functioning as a regional capital: fluids storage originates from it and they [fluids] *are excreted through transformation by Qi.*

The same passage continues with a typically Confucian view of the Internal Organs as the government of a State that is governed according to the Confucian principles of ethics:[2]

These 12 organs should not lose balance. If the Monarch is wise, the subordinates will be peaceful. Abidance by the rules of nourishment of life (yang sheng) will avoid any suffering all through life. Using this [rule], *the country will be prosperous. If the Monarch is not wise, all the 12 organs will be in danger and unable to function well, inevitably resulting in severe damage to the body. Using such a way to nourishing life (yang sheng) disasters will ensue. Using such a way to govern a country, it will be in great danger. Be on guard and heighten vigilance!*

This passage presents a typical Confucian view of the body: the body is like a country; the Internal Organs are like the officials in charge of government; the Heart is like the Monarch. According to Confucian political ethics, if the ruler behaved ethically, there was harmony in the country; vice versa, if the ruler behaved unethically, there would be chaos. In the above analogy between the body and a country, "nourishing life" according to the principles of Chinese medicine ensures health; not following them ensures danger. Similarly, in a country, good government ensures harmony and bad government, chaos.

"Nourishing life" (*yang sheng*) here refers to a lifestyle that fosters the preservation and cultivation of our Qi and Essence through a balanced diet, exercise, breathing exercises and sexual restraint.

Chapter 23 of the *Simple Questions* identifies the mental-spiritual aspects of the five Yin organs clearly:[3]

The housing of the Five Yin Organs is as follows: the Heart houses the Mind [Shen], the Lungs house the Corporeal Soul [Po], the Liver houses the Ethereal Soul [Hun], the Spleen houses the Intellect [Yi], the Kidneys house the Will-Power [Zhi].

A passage in Chapter 9 of the *Simple Questions* adds some more information to the functions of the Internal Organs. It describes the function of each organ, the place it manifests (e.g. Heart on the complexion) and the tissue it influences. In the following translation of this passage, I will omit these last two aspects to concentrate on the functions of the organs which are again compared to officials of a government.

Chapter 9 of the *Simple Questions* says:[4]

The Heart is the root of life and it houses the Mind. The Lungs are the root of Qi and they house the Corporeal Soul. The Kidneys are the root of sealed closure and storage; they house the Essence (Jing). The Liver is the root of stopping extremes (balancing and regulating) and they house the Ethereal Soul. The Spleen, Stomach, Large Intestine, Small Intestine, Triple Burner and Bladder are the root of granary and they house the Nutritive Qi (Ying Qi). These organs are called containers because they store food, transform waste and manage transformation and excretion of the flavours. All the 11 organs mentioned above depend on the decisions of the Gall-Bladder.

This passage is interesting for two reasons. First, it incongruously classifies the Spleen as a Yang (*Fu*) organ; secondly, it introduces the idea of the Gall-Bladder as a quite important organ on whose "decisions" all the other organs depend. This is an idea that does not recur frequently but that is used clinically by some doctors.

CLINICAL NOTE

G.B.-40 Qiuxu can be used to "motivate" all the other organs and to boost the effect of any treatment.

The clinical significance of this last statement is twofold. First, the Gall-Bladder is responsible for our capacity to take decisions; secondly, the Gall-Bladder's decision-making power can be used to "motivate" all the other organs. Interestingly, there are some modern Chinese doctors who use G.B.-40 Qiuxu with nearly every treatment to boost the effectiveness of the treatment.

Chapter 47 of the *Simple Questions* reinforces the idea that the Gall-Bladder is responsible for decision-taking in our life and also that the other organs depend on its decisions:[5]

What is the name and cause of the disease marked by bitter taste in the mouth? It is called Gall-Bladder Heat. The Liver is like a military general and its decisions depend on the Gall-Bladder, and the throat is like an envoy. The patient with such a problem frequently deliberates but never makes a decision, thus weakening the Gall-Bladder and driving its Qi to flow upwards into the mouth. This is why there is bitter taste.

It is interesting to note that the Heart is not always considered the Monarch in some passages of the *Yellow Emperor's Classic of Internal Medicine*. For example, in Chapter 44 of the *Simple Questions*, the Lungs are considered to be the most important organ and the leader of the other organs: "*The Lungs is the chief of the organs, and the lid of the Heart.*"[6]

In fact, the importance of the Lungs in the field of mental-emotional problems cannot be overstated for various reasons. First, the Lungs govern Qi and are in charge of "government": in practice, this means that the Lungs control the movement of Qi in every part of the body and every organ. We usually emphasize (and, in my opinion, overemphasize) the role of the Liver in the free flow of Qi, but the Lungs perform a similar role.

It follows that, especially in mental-emotional problems, there is stagnation of Lung-Qi. This is usually due to sadness, grief, worry or guilt and it manifests on a physical level primarily in the chest and throat with a feeling of tightness of the chest and/or throat, sighing, and a slight feeling of shortness of breath. From an emotional point of view, Lung-Qi stagnation manifests with sadness, worry, a tendency to crying and a tendency to self-criticism.

The other reason for the importance of the Lungs is that it is affected by emotions which play a huge role in Western patients, i.e. sadness and grief from loss, worry and guilt. Therefore it would not be inconceivable to consider the Lungs as the "monarch", especially in the mental-emotional field.

CLINICAL NOTE

Due to the importance of the Lungs in emotional problems, LU-7 Lieque is a major point for sadness and grief from loss, worry and grief. It acts on the throat and chest and has a "centripetal" movement in moving Qi and promoting the expression of emotions.

In Chapter 79 of the *Simple Questions*, Qi Bo implies that the Liver is the most important organ, although the Yellow Emperor himself disagrees:[7]

The Yellow Emperor asked Lei Gong which Organ is the most important one. Lei Gong answered that Spring corresponds to Jia and Yi (Heavenly Stems), to the green colour and to the Liver. He therefore thinks that the Liver is the most important organ. The Yellow Emperor said that according to the classics Shang Jing and Xia Jing, the Liver is the most unimportant organ.

Before discussing the mental-emotional sphere of each organ, I would like to describe my approach to the treatment of such problems with acupuncture and herbal medicine.

Over the years, I have come to think that, although treating according to patterns is essential, simply treating the Mind, Ethereal Soul, Corporeal Soul, Intellect and Will-Power can produce deep psychological changes.

In other words, although I always diagnose the patterns, I also diagnose in the general terms of the pathology of the Mind (*Shen*), Ethereal Soul (*Hun*), Corporeal Soul (*Po*), Intellect (*Yi*) or Will-Power (*Zhi*). I find that when these five *Shens* are "nourished" in a broad sense, it brings about deep mental-emotional changes, irrespective of the patterns. This applies especially to acupuncture. I tend to use acupuncture to "nourish" the five *Shens* while I tend to use herbal medicine to treat the patterns.

For example, irrespective of the patterns involved, I see depression as a manifestation of an insufficient movement of the Ethereal Soul, which, itself, may be due to an excessive control of the Mind over it. If the movement of the Ethereal Soul is deficient by itself, then I treat the Liver and Gall-Bladder; if the movement of the Ethereal Soul is insufficient due to over-control by the Mind, then I treat the Liver, Gall-Bladder and Heart.

If the person is slightly manic, it is due to an excessive movement of the Ethereal Soul, irrespective of the pattern, and I therefore treat the Liver. In autism, there is also an insufficient movement of the Ethereal Soul and a wounding of the Mind; I therefore treat Liver and Heart. Conversely, in attention deficit hyperactivity disorder (ADHD), there is an excessive movement of the Ethereal Soul, a lack of control of the Mind and a deficiency of the Intellect; I therefore treat the Liver, Heart and Spleen.

Case history

A case history of a young woman with attention deficit disorder (ADD) is a good illustration of this principle, i.e. of seeing a pathology in the light of the Mind, Ethereal Soul, Corporeal Soul, Intellect and Will-Power.

This very pleasant 23-year-old woman suffered from ADD. She found it very difficult to organize herself and to do anything on time; she also found it very difficult to concentrate and read. Every act of organization that comes naturally to most people required a huge effort on her part.

Although her main problem was ADD, she also occasionally became hyperactive, talked fast and had to exercise vigorously to discharge this hyperactive energy. Another feature of her problem was that she was extremely sensitive to music and lights. Some types of music drove her crazy (in her own words) and, if it was played in a restaurant, she had to leave. Similarly, she was very sensitive to naked lights and could not sit at a table with a naked bulb overhead.

There was nothing wrong with her mental capacity and intelligence. She was bright, very intuitive and emotionally very attuned and wise. Another feature, however, was a certain lack of motivation and determination in the pursuit of her goals.

Finally, she was prone to day-dreaming but she seldom dreamed at night.

Diagnosis We can see clearly in this case history an involvement of all the five *Shens*, i.e. the Mind, Ethereal Soul, Corporeal Soul, Intellect and Will-Power. I will list below the relevant manifestations according to each.

- *Mind*: lack of concentration, lack of control of the Mind over the Ethereal Soul. HE-7 Shenmen, Ren-15 Jiuwei and Du-24 Shenting.
- *Ethereal Soul*: day-dreaming, hyperactivity. The excessive movement of the Ethereal Soul on the one hand caused the hyperactive episodes and, on the other, it also interfered with normal cognition by the Mind. Interestingly, she probably did not dream at night because the Ethereal Soul was overactive in the daytime, giving rise to day-dreaming. LIV-3 Taichong.
- *Corporeal Soul*: hypersensitivity to music and lights. BL-13 Feishu and BL-42 Pohu.
- *Intellect*: difficulty in concentrating and studying. BL-20 Pishu and BL-49 Yishe.
- *Will-Power*: lack of motivation. BL-23 Shenshu and BL-52 Zhishi.

I shall now discuss the mental-emotional sphere of influence of each organ, in the following order.

- Heart
- Lungs
- Liver
- Spleen
- Kidneys
- Pericardium
- Small Intestine
- Large Intestine
- Gall-Bladder
- Stomach
- Bladder
- Triple Burner

HEART

The role of the Heart and Mind has been discussed at length in Chapter 2. As mentioned above, Chapter 8 of the *Simple Questions* says of the Heart: "*The Heart is the official functioning as the Monarch: the Spirit originates from it.*"[8] It is really in this sense that the Heart is the Monarch, i.e. it is the most important organ because it is the only one that houses the Mind which has a directing, integrating and coordinating function on our psychic life.

Indeed, in every other way, it would be difficult to argue that the Heart is the most important of the Internal Organs. From the point of view of physiology, it would be easy to argue that the Stomach and Spleen are the most important organs as they are the origin of Postnatal Qi. Indeed, Li Dong Yuan (1180–1251) made precisely this point.

On the other hand, it would be perfectly legitimate to argue that the Kidneys are the most important organ because they house the Prenatal Essence and because they are the source of the physiological Water and Fire of the whole body.

Thus, the Heart occupies an absolutely central role in the psychic sphere because it houses the Mind that is responsible for the very consciousness, our sense of identity, thinking, perceiving and for our emotional life. Moreover, the Heart (through the Mind) plays a most important coordinating and integrating role towards the Ethereal Soul, Corporeal Soul, Intellect and Memory.

Finally, the Heart occupies a central role in our psychic life because it is affected by all emotions; in fact, while each emotion affects a specific organ more (e.g. sadness affects the Lungs), the Heart is affected by all emotions because it houses the Mind which feels the emotions. When we feel sad, sadness affects the Lungs but it is the Heart that "feels" the sadness because only the Mind (*Shen*) feels the emotions (*see Fig. 2.5*).

For these reasons, treatment of the Heart is essential in all mental and emotional disorders. Apart from specific patterns, treatment of the Heart with acupuncture "nourishes" the Heart, the Mind (*Shen* of the Heart) and the Spirit. We should bear in mind that herbal medicine and acupuncture are modalities that act in different ways. Although acupuncture can, of course, be tailored to treat patterns (HE-8 Shaofu clears Heart-Heat while HE-7 Shenmen nourishes Heart-Blood), its effect is more general than that of herbal medicine.

Therefore, any Heart point, apart from its specific effect, also "nourishes" the Heart, Mind and Spirit. I am using "nourish" here in a general sense rather than in the specific sense of a Chinese medicine treatment method. Thus, for example, HE-8 Shaofu clears Heart-Heat and HE-7 nourishes Heart-Blood, but they both "nourish" the Mind and Spirit.

CLINICAL NOTE

The best point to influence the mental-emotional aspect of the Heart is HE-7 Shenmen.

As the Heart is the monarch that is affected by all emotions and that coordinates and integrates the actions of the other four *shens* (*Hun, Po, Yi* and *Zhi*), I treat the Heart channel in nearly every case of mental-emotional suffering. I have noticed in practice that treating the Heart "nourishes" the Mind and Spirit (in the sense described above) and has the effect of "softening" a person's Mind, making it more receptive and open to change.

My two favorite points for nourishing the Mind and Spirit are HE-7 Shenmen with Ren-15 Jiuwei. These two points nourish the Heart, Mind and Spirit, calm the Mind and relax the chest.

With regard to the Mind's coordinating and integrating function, this is particularly important in relation to the Ethereal Soul. The Mind and Ethereal Soul together are responsible for thinking, judgment, our emotional life, our evaluation of goals and the balance between the ideas, creating movement of the Ethereal Soul and the control of the Mind. Treatment of the Heart and Liver will automatically help the balance between the Mind and the Ethereal Soul. The two best points to achieve this are HE-7 Shenmen with LIV-3 Taichong, together with Du-24 Shenting and G.B.-13 Benshen.

I find the point Du-24 excellent in nourishing the Mind and Spirit and to help both depression and anxiety. This point is discussed at length in Chapter 13. I combine Du-24 with G.B.-13 Benshen when I want to coordinate and balance the control of the Mind with the movement of the Ethereal Soul.

The location of these two points at the top of the forehead presents interesting parallels with Western anatomy and neurology. The prefrontal cortex is behind these two points and, as we know, this structure is responsible for the executive functions, which include mediating conflicting thoughts, making choices between right and wrong or good and bad, predicting future events, and governing social control – such as suppressing emotional or sexual urges. The basic activity of this brain region is considered to be orchestration of thoughts and actions in accordance with internal goals. The mediating role of the prefrontal cortex is very similar to the balance between Mind and Ethereal Soul and the control of the Ethereal Soul by the Mind.

CLINICAL NOTE

HE-7 Shenmen and Ren-15 Jiuwei together nourish the Heart, Mind and Spirit, calm the Mind and relax the chest.

In my experience, treatment of the Heart is particularly important in men. Of course, the functions of the Mind (*Shen* of the Heart) are the same in men and women. There are, however, some subtle differences. Although the following is a broad generalization (which therefore suffers from many exceptions), men tend to function through the thinking and cognitive part of the Mind (*Shen*), of their Intellect (*Yi* of the Spleen) and of their Will-Power (*Zhi* of the Kidneys), whereas women tend to function more through the Ethereal Soul (*Hun* of the Liver). I may go so far as to say that while the Ethereal Soul is unconscious in men, it is conscious in women. Moreover, it could be said that the controlling function of the Mind over the Ethereal Soul is stronger in men than it is in women.

I think that explains why women are so much better at communicating than men. As in men the controlling function of the Mind is somewhat stronger than in women, many men find communicating hard and, in a clinical setting, they find expressing their emotions and sometimes even their physical symptoms difficult. Some psychotherapists say that it takes the average man 9 months to reach the point in psychotherapy where women *start*.

For this reason, I treat the Heart very frequently in men, and certainly more than in women. I treat the Heart very frequently in men to nourish the Mind, reduce the control of the Mind over the Ethereal Soul and promote the connection between the Mind and the Will-Power. To nourish the Mind in men, I use HE-7 Shenmen, Du-24 Shenting and Ren-15 Jiuwei.

Indeed, I find that the use of the Heart channel helps men in many other ways, for example in lower backache. If a man suffers from chronic lower backache occurring against a background of a Kidney deficiency and a disturbance of the Mind, I would use the following point combination:

- S.I.-3 on the left with BL-62 on the right (to open the Governing Vessel)
- HE-7 Shenmen on the right and KI-4 Dazhong on the left.

Claremont de Castillejo describes a masculine and a feminine aspect of the psyche that present interesting connections with that of Chinese medicine. Please note that the "masculine" and "feminine" qualities of the psyche apply equally to men and women, i.e. a woman could display "masculine" qualities of the psyche and a man "feminine" ones. However, every individual has both qualities although in different proportions.

Claremont de Castillejo calls the masculine aspect of the psyche "focused consciousness" and the feminine one "diffuse awareness". She describes "focused consciousness" thus:[9]

Focussed consciousness has emerged over thousands of years from the unconscious and it still is emerging. All our education is an attempt to produce and sharpen it in order to give us power to look at things and analyze them into their component parts, in order to give us the ability to formulate ideas and the capacity to change, invent, create. It is this focussed consciousness which we are all using in the everyday world all the time. Without it, there would have been no culture and no scientific discoveries.

We can see from this description that what Claremont calls "focused consciousness" corresponds to the Intellect (*Yi* of the Spleen) and to the thinking and cognitive part of the Mind (*Shen* of the Heart). Although obviously present in both men and women, men tend to function more from this standpoint than from the feminine one described below.

Claremont de Castillejo describes the feminine aspect of the psyche, "diffuse awareness", thus:[10]

It is, however, not the only kind of consciousness. Most children are born with, and many women retain, a diffuse awareness of the wholeness of nature, where everything is linked with everything else and they feel themselves to be part of a whole. It is from this layer of the psyche which is not yet broken into parts that comes the wise utterances of children. Here lies the wisdom of artists and the words of prophets.

From this description, we can draw some parallels with Chinese medicine and say that "diffuse awareness" corresponds to the Ethereal Soul. Although obviously both men and women have it, women tend to work more from its standpoint. Claremont's reference to children and artists is interesting as they both live in the world of the Ethereal Soul.

For this reason also, I tend to treat the Heart and the Mind in men very frequently to stimulate the "diffuse awareness" described above and to reduce the control of the Mind, thus stimulating the movement of the Ethereal Soul.

Finally, the nourishing effect on the Mind of Heart points has another repercussion. "Calming the Mind" (by treating the Heart channel) also has a pronounced analgesic action on any type of pain. This is an added reason for using HE-7 in the combination described above for chronic backache. In very many cases, a chronic pain is often the physical manifestation of an unspoken emotional pain; especially in these cases, the use of HE-7 is essential.

SUMMARY

The Heart

- The Heart is the Monarch, i.e. it is the most important organ because it is the only one that houses the Mind which has a directing, integrating and coordinating function on our psychic life.
- The Heart occupies a central role in the psychic sphere because it houses the Mind that is responsible for the very consciousness, our sense of identity, thinking, perceiving and for our emotional life.
- The Heart (through the Mind) plays a most important coordinating and integrating role towards the Ethereal Soul, Corporeal Soul, Intellect and Memory.
- The Heart occupies a central role in our psychic life because it is affected by all emotions since it houses the Mind which feels the emotions.
- Treatment of the Heart is essential in all mental and emotional disorders.
- "Calming the Mind" with HE-7 has a pain-killing effect on chronic pain, especially that deriving from emotional suffering.

Summary of Heart points

- HE-7 Shenmen: nourish Heart-Blood, calm the Mind, nourish the Mind, regulate the control of the Ethereal Soul by the Mind.
- HE-5 Tongli: tonify the Heart and the Mind, move Qi, depression.
- HE-8 Shaofu: drain Heart-Fire, calm the Mind.

Summary of Heart point combinations

- HE-7 Shenmen, Du-24 Shenting, Ren-15 Jiuwei: nourish the Mind, calm the Mind, tonify the Mind and the Heart, open the chest, regulate the control of the Ethereal Soul by the Mind.
- HE-7 Shenmen, LIV-3 Taichong, Du-24 Shenting and G.B.-13 Benshen: calm the Mind and the Spirit, restrain the movement of the Ethereal Soul.

LUNGS

According to Chapter 8 of the *Simple Questions*, "*The Lungs are the official functioning as Minister: they are in charge of government.*"[11] As they are the "Prime Minister", they are the second in command after the Heart. Being in charge of "government" is a reflection of their governing of Qi, i.e., through Qi, they are responsible for all physiological processes.

The Lung function of being in charge of "government" (*Zhi*) is significant in the mental-emotional sphere. We tend to think of the Liver influencing the circulation of Qi in all parts of the body; this is certainly true. But the Lungs also perform a similar function in all parts of the body; this is the meaning of their "governing of Qi".

In the mental-emotional sphere, the Lung's movement of Qi is particularly affected by sadness, grief, worry and guilt; these cause either a deficiency or a stagnation of Lung-Qi, or both. A stagnation of Lung-Qi manifests in the chest and throat and its physical manifestations include a slight shortness of breath, a feeling of tightness of the chest and/or throat and sighing. The Lung pulse feels relatively Tight. The emotional manifestations of Lung-Qi stagnation are sadness, worry, depression, a tendency to weeping and a tendency to self-criticism.

I use the point LU-7 Lieque for Lung-Qi stagnation. I see this point as having a "centripetal", moving effect; it encourages the expression of repressed emotions.

Treatment of the Lungs in mental-emotional problems is of paramount importance, given that sadness and grief deriving from loss are such pervasive emotions in Western patients. Interestingly, our modern world and lifestyle are based very much on development of the thinking part of the Mind and of the Intellect (*Yi*) and yet, our limbic systems remain as vulnerable as centuries ago. It is in the nature of higher mammals to seek nurturing and every loss resonates with the loss of nurturing. It can be loss of a spouse from death, divorce, separation, loss of a child from death or separation, loss of a job, loss of a friendship.

Loss is the major cause of sadness and grief affecting the Lungs. The Lungs are a "delicate" organ in that they are the first to be invaded by external pathogenic factors. However, they are "delicate" also from a psychological point of view and they are easily wounded by loss. To treat sadness and grief affecting the Lungs, again I use LU-7 Lieque but also LU-9 Taiyuan and BL-13 Feishu.

The Lungs house the Corporeal Soul and this also reflects them being responsible for all physiological processes; in fact, these depend on Qi but also on the movement and activity of the Corporeal Soul in all parts of the body.

From an emotional perspective, governing Qi in all physiological processes and housing the Corporeal Soul means that the Lungs are involved in all emotions, and not just those that pertain to the Lungs (such as sadness, grief and worry). Thus, all emotions affect the Lungs and the Corporeal Soul, hence the importance of LU-7 Lieque in the treatment of emotional problems.

The nature and functions of the Corporeal Soul were discussed in detail in Chapter 4.

CLINICAL NOTE

The best points to influence the mental aspect of the Lungs are LU-7 Lieque, BL-13 Feishu and BL-42 Pohu.

SUMMARY

The Lungs

- According to Chapter 8 of the Simple Questions, *"The Lungs are the official functioning as Minister: they are in charge of government."*

- As they are the "Prime Minister", they are the second in command after the Heart. Being in charge of "government" is a reflection of their governing of Qi, i.e. through Qi, they are responsible for all physiological processes.
- The Lungs house the Corporeal Soul and this also reflects them being responsible for all physiological processes.
- The Lungs are affected by sadness, grief, worry and guilt which tend to cause Lung-Qi stagnation, for which I use LU-7.
- Sadness and grief from loss are pervasive emotions in Western patients and they deeply affect the Lungs. I use LU-7, LU-9 and BL-13.
- From an emotional perspective, governing Qi in all physiological processes and housing the Corporeal Soul means that the Lungs are involved in all emotions.

Summary of Lung points

- LU-7 Lieque: stagnation of Lung-Qi from sadness, grief, worry or guilt, encourage the expression of repressed emotions, centripetal movement.
- LU-9 Taiyuan: deficiency of Lung-Qi from sadness and grief.
- LU-3 Tianfu: soothe the Corporeal Soul, calm the Mind, open the Mind's orifices, sadness, weeping.

Summary of Lung point combinations

- LU-7 Lieque, LU-9 Taiyuan and BL-13 Feishu: deficiency of Lung-Qi from sadness and grief, weeping, depression.
- LU-7 Lieque, BL-13 Feishu and BL-42 Pohu: depression or anxiety, sadness, grief, worry, guilt, soothe the Corporeal Soul, calm the Mind, nourish the Mind.

LIVER

Chapter 8 of the *Simple Questions* says: "*The Liver is the official functioning as general: planning originates from it.*"[12] This means that the Liver is responsible for deliberating and planning one's life; this is a function of the Ethereal Soul which is housed by the Liver.

The planning function of the Liver should not be confused with the decision-taking of the Gall-Bladder. When we act on something, there are usually two stages. In the first stage, we deliberate, we think about it and we plan a course of action; this depends on the Liver. In the second stage, we need the courage to act and take a decision on what has been planned; this depends on the Gall-Bladder.

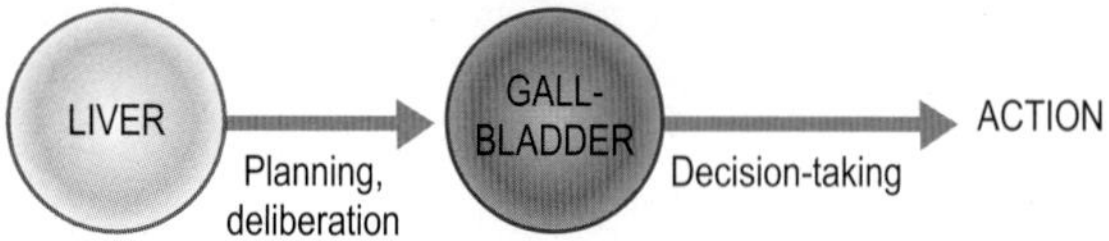

Figure 8.1 Planning of the Liver and decision-taking of the Gall-Bladder.

The planning of the Liver might be right, but if the Gall-Bladder is weak, we lack the courage to take a decision. We can observe this situation in our patients frequently and especially in the field of relationships and work. For example, a person may know that a certain relationship or job should be relinquished, but if the Gall-Bladder is weak, he or she will lack the courage to act on the planning and to take a decision (Fig. 8.1).

The reverse situation may also arise. The Gall-Bladder may be strong and the person takes decisions easily; however, if the Liver's planning function is compromised, that person may take reckless decisions every time.

CLINICAL NOTE

The best points to influence the mental aspect of the Liver are LIV-3 Taichong and BL-47 Hunmen.

The Liver plays a very important role in our emotional life because it houses the Ethereal Soul. As described in Chapter 3, the Ethereal Soul is responsible for our emotional life, our projection towards others in relationships, our plans, life dreams, inspiration and creativity. It is in the nature of the Ethereal Soul to always want to "move" and its movement is responsible for the above qualities; when this movement is normal, the person can project towards others, has life dreams, plans, inspiration and creativity.

The free flow of Liver-Qi is an expression of the psychic movement of the Ethereal Soul. The movement of the Ethereal Soul may be insufficient when Liver-Qi is deficient or stagnant. Please note that Liver-Qi *can* be deficient and its manifestations are the same as those of Liver-Blood deficiency plus mental depression. This is discussed in Chapter 3.

The movement of the Ethereal Soul may also be excessive, in which case the person will display a slightly manic behavior as described in Chapter 3.

The best point to stimulate the movement of the Ethereal Soul in depression is G.B.-40 Qiuxu, while LIV-3 Taichong, together with BL-47 Hunmen, can be used to restrain the movement of the Ethereal Soul.

Please note that although the Ethereal Soul resides in the Liver, it is affected by other organs too. For example, a deficiency of Yang of the Spleen and Kidneys may induce an insufficient movement of the Ethereal Soul, while Heart-Fire may cause it to move excessively.

As is of course well known, the Liver is affected by anger. I personally feel that anger is overemphasized both in China and in the West as a cause of disease. This is discussed at length in Chapter 9. The pulse is useful to identify anger as the emotional cause of disease; if it is anger, the pulse is Wiry; if the pulse is not at all Wiry, then anger is not the emotional cause of the disease.

Case history

A 32-year-old woman had been suffering from a slight asthma and allergic rhinitis. However, her main affliction was a slight depression, confusion about her direction in life, recurrent relationship problems and a tendency to cry. She was seeing a psychotherapist as she had been subject to some sexual harassment by her stepfather during her teenage years. Her psychotherapist had told her that she had repressed anger (related to the sexual harassment) and that she "should get it out".

She was very pale, and, apart from a tendency to crying, her voice had a weepy tone and was quite weak. Her tongue was Pale and her pulse was Choppy and Weak in general but the weakest was the right *cun* position, i.e. the Lung position.

I am presenting this case here as an example of overemphasis on anger as an emotional cause of disease, not only by the Chinese, but often also by Western psychotherapists. Every sign contradicted anger as a cause of disease: the voice, the weeping, the paleness and, most of all, the pulse being so Weak, especially on the Lung position.

Therefore, from my point of view, she was suffering from sadness and grief affecting the Lungs. Her psychotherapist had based her diagnosis on the pre-conceived idea that she would be angry at being sexually harassed. But every individual reacts in different ways to certain life events. After sexual harassment, a woman (or man) may be angry, another sad, some may even feel guilty; therefore we cannot work from pre-conceived ideas about anger.

Most of all, from the Chinese diagnosis point of view, I would say: "If the pulse is not Wiry, it is not anger."

We should not forget that the Liver is affected by other emotions too. In women, the Liver may be affected by sadness which leads to Liver-Blood deficiency. The Liver is also affected by worry which leads to Liver-Yang rising.

SUMMARY

The Liver

- The Liver is responsible for deliberating and planning one's life; this is a function of the Ethereal Soul which is housed by the Liver.
- The planning function of the Liver should not be confused with the decision-taking of the Gall-Bladder.
- The Liver plays a very important role in our emotional life because it houses the Ethereal Soul which is responsible for our emotional life, our projection towards others in relationships, our plans, life dreams, inspiration and creativity.
- The free flow of Liver-Qi is an expression of the psychic movement of the Ethereal Soul.
- The movement of the Ethereal Soul may be insufficient when Liver-Qi is deficient or stagnant.
- The movement of the Ethereal Soul may also be excessive in which case the person will display a slightly manic behavior.

Summary of Liver points

- G.B.-40 Qiuxu: stimulate the physiological rising of Liver-Qi, depression, indecision.
- LIV-3 Taichong: restrain the movement of the Ethereal Soul.

Summary of Liver point combinations

- LIV-3 Taichong and BL-47 Hunmen: regulate the movement of Ethereal Soul (especially restrain), depression, manic behavior, irritability, anger, repressed anger.
- LIV-3 Taichong, L.I.-4 Hegu, Du-24 Shenting, G.B.-13 Benshen: restrain the movement of the Ethereal Soul, calm the Spirit.

SPLEEN

As mentioned above, Chapter 8 of the *Simple Questions* says: "*The Spleen and Stomach are the official functioning as granary: the five flavours originate from them.*"[13] I will discuss the Spleen and Stomach separately.

The main aspect of the Spleen's function in the psyche is its housing of the Intellect (*Yi*); this is responsible for memory, focusing, concentration, mental application, studying and ideas. This function was discussed in detail in Chapter 5.

From the perspective of emotions, the Spleen is affected by pensiveness and worry. In severe cases, it may generate obsessive thinking.

> **CLINICAL NOTE**
> The best points to influence the mental aspect of the Spleen are SP-3 Taibai and BL-49 Yishe.

The Spleen belongs to Earth which is in the center, if we place the Five Elements in the shape of a cross with Fire at the top, Water at the bottom, Wood on the left and Metal on the right (Fig. 8.2). The central position of the Earth and of the Spleen is significant in a mental-emotional context.

A deficiency of the Spleen makes a person without a "center" in a psychological sense. This causes the person to be depressed and lack confidence. I see this situation frequently in young people who have just left their parents' home (which often happens too early in life). Young people suffering from a Spleen deficiency also tend to walk lifting their heels as if they were walking on the balls of the feet.

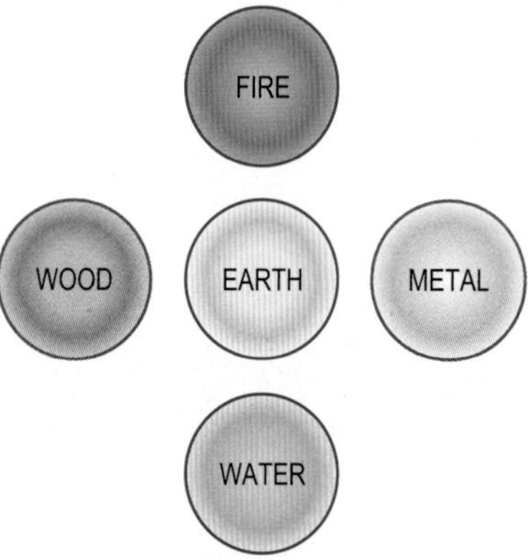

Figure 8.2 The Five Elements with Earth at the center.

The Spleen belongs to Earth which, among the Five Elements, is the granary. Spleen-Qi is the origin of Qi and Blood and, from a mental-emotional perspective, the Spleen is involved in issues of nourishment. This is nourishment on both a physical and psychic level. On a physical level, the Spleen is very much affected by our diet, both what we eat and how we eat.

From a mental-emotional perspective, the Spleen is responsible for "nourishment" and nurturing, and the Spleen is frequently affected by lack of nurturing from the parents. To tonify the Spleen when it is affected by nurturing (or the lack of it), I use the points Ren-12 Zhongwan, ST-36 Zusanli and BL-20 Pishu.

> **CLINICAL NOTE**
> To tonify the Spleen when it is affected by nurturing (or the lack of it), I use the points Ren-12 Zhongwan, ST-36 Zusanli and BL-20 Pishu.

Conversely, the Spleen may also be affected by excessive and suffocating nurturing from one or both of the parents. Such "nurturing" is actually not true nurturing as it is narcissistic.

SUMMARY

The Spleen

- "*The Spleen and Stomach are the official functioning as granary: the five flavours originate from them.*"
- The main aspect of the Spleen's function in the psyche is its housing of the Intellect (*Yi*); this is responsible for memory, focusing, concentration, mental application, studying and ideas.
- The Spleen is affected by pensiveness and worry. In severe cases, it may generate obsessive thinking.
- A deficiency of the Spleen makes a person without a "center" in a psychological sense. This causes the person to be depressed and lack confidence.
- Spleen-Qi is the origin of Qi and Blood and, from a mental-emotional perspective, the Spleen is involved in issues of nourishment, on both a physical and psychic level.

- On a physical level, the Spleen is very much affected by our diet, both what we eat and how we eat.
- From a mental-emotional perspective, the Spleen is responsible for "nourishment" and nurturing and the Spleen is frequently affected by lack of nurturing from the parents.
- The Spleen may also be affected by excessive and suffocating nurturing from one or both of the parents.

Summary of Spleen points

- SP-3 Taibai: tonify the Spleen, strengthen the Intellect (*Yi*).
- Ren-12 Zhongwan: tonify the Spleen, strengthen the Intellect.
- BL-20 Pishu: tonify the Spleen, strengthen the Intellect.
- BL-49 Yishe: pensiveness, obsessive thoughts.

Summary of Spleen point combinations

- Ren-12 Zhongwan, ST-36 Zusanli, BL-20 Pishu: tonify the Spleen, nourish the Intellect, treat nurturing issues.

KIDNEYS

As mentioned above, Chapter 23 of the *Simple Questions* says: *"The Kidneys house the Will-Power [Zhi]."*[14] *Zhi* may be translated as "Memory" or as "Will-Power". In the context of mental-emotional problems, the translation of *Zhi* as "will-power" is more clinically relevant.

The Will-Power of the Kidneys refers to drive, determination, enthusiasm, persistence, single-mindedness in the pursuit of one's objectives, and will-power. As will be noticed, the lack of these attributes is often a feature of depression.

CLINICAL NOTE

The best points to influence the mental aspect of the Kidneys and its Will-Power are KI-4 Dazhong, BL-23 Shenshu and BL-52 Zhishi.

Chapter 8 of the *Simple Questions* says: *"The Kidneys are the official in charge of power: skill originates from them."*[15] It is interesting that the *Simple Questions* mentions "power" in connection with the Kidneys. This has two meanings. From a physical point of view, "power" refers to the fact that the Kidneys are the root of Prenatal Qi and house the Essence; this determines our innate energy, strength or "power". In fact, the symptoms of fullness of the Sea of Marrow (originating from the Kidneys) are "full of vigour, great physical strength"). The Sea of Marrow is mentioned in Chapter 33 of the *Spiritual Axis*.[16]

From a mental point of view, "power" refers to the drive and steadfastness stemming from the Kidneys. This corresponds to *Zhi*, i.e. Will-Power. This was discussed in detail in Chapter 6.

The symptoms of fullness and emptiness of the Sea of Marrow have mental-emotional significance. The symptoms of fullness of the Sea of Marrow ("full of vigour, great physical strength") indicate a constitutional condition of strength of the individual; this is not only physical vigor but it also involves mental "vigour" which means that the person will be able to stand up to emotional stress, keeping the integrity of his or her *Shen*. Contrary to what we might think, many elderly people actually have a constitutional strength of the Sea of Marrow which makes their *Shen* strong and grounded.

The physical symptoms of deficiency of the Sea of Marrow are dizziness, tinnitus, weak legs, blurred vision and a desire to lie down. On a mental-emotional level, a person with a constitutional deficiency of the Sea of Marrow will be more prone to emotional stress; his or her *Shen* is more vulnerable and the person lacks mental strength and resilience. Under these conditions, the person is easily prone to depression when subject to emotional stress.

The points given by Chapter 33 of the *Spiritual Axis* for the Sea of Marrow are Du-20 Baihui (described by the *Spiritual Axis* as the "upper" point) and Du-16 (described as the "lower" point). I particularly use Du-20 to strengthen the Sea of Marrow, nourish the *Shen* and strengthen the Kidney's Will-Power (*Zhi*). For these reasons, Du-20 is a very important point for depression.

CLINICAL NOTE

The best point to influence the mental aspect of the Kidneys and strengthen the Sea of Marrow is Du-20 Baihui.

The Kidneys have a deep influence on the mental-emotional state through the Minister Fire. The Minister

Fire is the Fire aspect of the Kidneys. The Kidneys are a unique organ in that they are the origin of the physiological Water and Fire of the whole body. The Minister Fire can be assimilated with the Gate of Life (*Ming Men*).

The first discussion of the Gate of Life (*Ming Men*) can be found in the *Classic of Difficulties*, especially in Chapters 36 and 39. Chapter 36 says:[17]

The Kidneys are not really two, as the left Kidney is a Kidney proper and the right Kidney is the Ming Men. The Ming Men is the residence of the Shen and is related to the Yuan Qi: in men it stores Essence, in women it is connected to the uterus. That is why there is only one Kidney.

Chapter 39 says:[18]

Why does the classic say that there are 5 Yang and 6 Yin organs? The reason is that the Yin organs count as 6 since there are two Kidneys. The left Kidney is the Kidney proper, the right Kidney is the Ming Men ... the reason that there are 6 Yang organs is that each of the 5 Yin organs has a corresponding Yang organ, plus an extra one being the Triple Burner.

See Figure 8.3.

These two passages clearly show that according to the *Classic of Difficulties* the *Ming Men* corresponds to the right Kidney, and is therefore functionally inseparable from the Kidneys. The *Pulse Classic* (*Mai Jing*), written by Wang Shu He in the Han dynasty, confirms this in assigning the Kidney and *Ming Men* to the right-Rear (proximal) position on the pulse. Chen Wu Ze of the Song dynasty wrote: "*The ancients considered the left Kidney as Kidney proper, related to the Bladder, and the right Kidney as the* Ming Men *related to the Triple Burner*" (Fig. 8.4). However, for several centuries, up to the Ming dynasty, medical writers seldom discussed the *Ming Men* as something separate from the Kidney, and simply referred to it as "Kidney-Qi".

With the beginning of the Ming dynasty, the concept of *Ming Men* was greatly developed, and ideas on it differed from those expounded in the Nan Jing. During the Ming dynasty, Chinese physicians no longer considered the *Ming Men* as part of the right Kidney, but as occupying the place between the two Kidneys.

Zhang Jie Bin (1563–1640) said:

There are two Kidneys ... the Ming Men is in between them ... The Ming Men is the organ of Water and Fire, it is the residence of Yin and Yang, the Sea of Essence and it determines life and death.

Li Shi Zhen also said that the *Ming Men* is in between the two Kidneys (Fig. 8.5).

Zhao Xian He discussed the *Ming Men* in greatest depth in his book *Medicine Treasure* (*Yi Gui*) published in 1687. Most of this book deals with physiological and pathological aspects of the *Ming Men*. Zhao Xian He

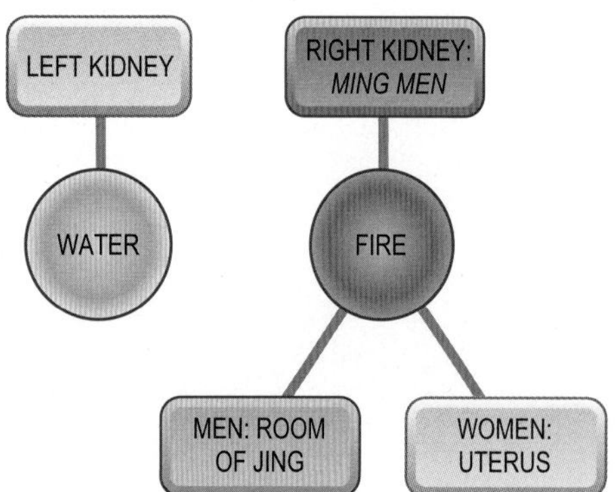

Figure 8.3 The *Ming Men* in the Nan Jing.

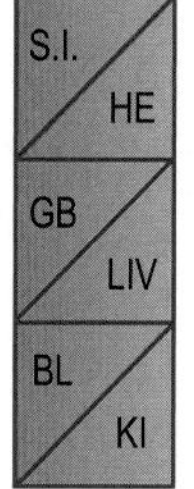

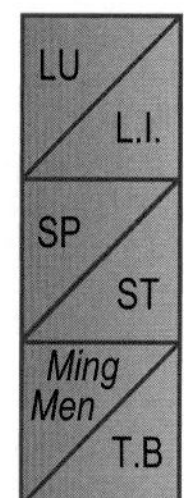

Figure 8.4 Assignment of Minister Fire to right-Rear position of the pulse.

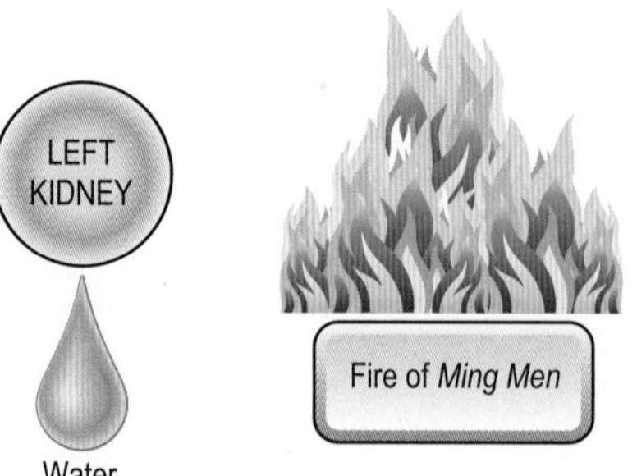

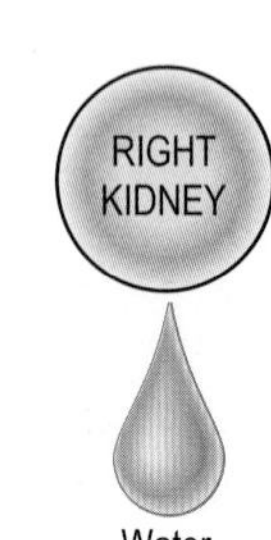

Figure 8.5 The Minister Fire in between the Kidneys.

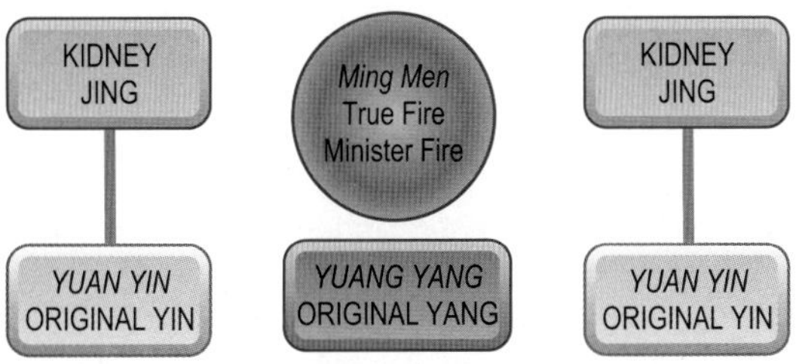

Figure 8.6 The Minister Fire as the Yang aspect of Essence.

also regarded the *Ming Men* as being between the two Kidneys. He wrote that the *Ming Men* is the motive force of all functional activities of the body, being the physiological Fire which is essential to life.

This Fire is also called "True Fire" or "Minister Fire" (in quite a different sense from that attributed to the Pericardium). The importance of the Fire nature of the *Ming Men* is that it provides heat for all our bodily functions and for the Kidney-Essence itself. The Kidneys are unlike any other organ in so far as they are the origin of Water and Fire of the body, the Primary Yin and Primary Yang. The *Ming Men* is the embodiment of the Fire within the Kidneys and the Minister Fire is a special type of Fire in that, not only does it not extinguish Water, but it can actually produce Water (Fig. 8.6).

In this respect the *Ming Men* theory is at variance with the Five-Element theory according to which the Minister Fire is the Triple Burner and Pericardium. However, there are ways in which the Pericardium is connected to the Minister Fire (see below).

In the context of mental-emotional problems, the Minister Fire is frequently and easily "stirred" by emotional stress with the creation of Heat and an upward movement of Qi which goes up to disturb the Heart and Pericardium. In emotional stress, Heat is frequently the result of Qi stagnation; however, it may also arise independently, without a preceding Qi stagnation (Fig. 8.7).

When Heat is formed under the influence of emotional stress, the Minister Fire becomes pathological; it is "stirred" out of its residence in the Lower Burner and flows upwards to the Heart and Pericardium. The physiological Minister Fire should be "concealed" in the Lower *Dan Tian* and it should not be seen. When there is Heat, the Minister Fire is seen.

To subdue the rising Minister Fire in emotional problems, one must use Heart and Pericardium points such as HE-8 Shaofu and P-7 Daling. The use of Pericardium

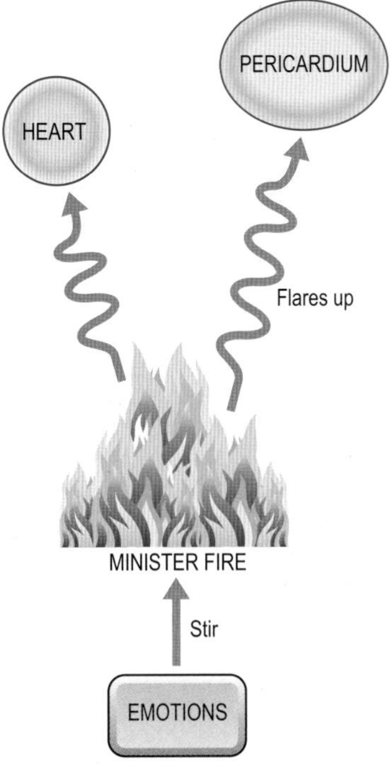

Figure 8.7 Minister Fire stirred by emotional stress.

points is particularly important because the pathological Minister Fire from emotional stress goes up to the Triple Burner and Pericardium (the "Minister Fire" channels).

CLINICAL NOTE

To subdue the pathological Minister Fire rising upwards from emotional stress, use points from the Triple Burner and Pericardium channels, e.g. T.B.-5 Waiguan, P-7 Daling or P-8 Laogong.

In addition, tonifying the physiological Minister Fire with points such as Ren-4 Guanyuan will also help to bring the Minister Fire back into its place of "concealment" and therefore to calm the Mind. By bringing the pathological Minister Fire back down into its place of concealment, Ren-4 Guanyuan calms the Mind.

CLINICAL NOTE

Ren-4 Guanyuan calms the Mind.

SUMMARY

Kidneys

- The Kidneys house the Will-Power (*Zhi*).
- The Will-Power of the Kidneys refers to drive, determination, enthusiasm, persistence, single-mindedness in the pursuit of one's objectives, and will-power.
- Chapter 8 of the *Simple Questions* says: *"The Kidneys are the official in charge of power: skill originates from them."*
- From a physical point of view, "power" refers to the fact that the Kidneys are the root of Prenatal Qi and house the Essence; this determines our innate energy, strength or "power".
- From a mental point of view, "power" refers to the drive and steadfastness stemming from the Kidneys. This corresponds to *Zhi*, i.e. Will-Power.
- The symptoms of fullness of the Sea of Marrow ("full of vigor, great physical strength") indicate a constitutional condition of strength of the individual; this is not only physical vigor but it also involves mental "vigor", which means that the person will be able to stand up to emotional stress, keeping the integrity of his or her *Shen*.
- In deficiency of the Sea of Marrow on a mental-emotional level, a person with a constitutional deficiency of the Sea of Marrow will be more prone to emotional stress; his or her *Shen* is more vulnerable and the person lacks mental strength and resilience.
- I particularly use Du-20 to strengthen the Sea of Marrow, nourish the *Shen* and strengthen the Kidney's Will-Power (*Zhi*).
- The Kidneys have a deep influence on the mental-emotional state through the Minister Fire.
- From the Ming dynasty onwards, the *Ming Men* was considered to be in between the Kidneys.
- In the context of mental-emotional problems, the Minister Fire is frequently and easily "stirred" by emotional stress with the creation of Heat and an upward movement of Qi which goes up to disturb the Heart and Pericardium.
- To subdue the rising Minister Fire in emotional problems, one must use Heart and Pericardium points such as HE-8 Shaofu and P-7 Daling.
- Tonifying the physiological Minister Fire with points such as Ren-4 Guanyuan will also help to bring the Minister Fire back into its place of "concealment" and therefore to calm the Mind.

Summary of Kidney points

- KI-4 Dazhong: tonify the Kidneys, move Qi, strengthen the communication between Heart and Kidneys, fear, anxiety.
- BL-52 Zhishi: strengthen Will-Power (*Zhi*), depression.
- KI-3 Taixi: strengthen Will-Power, depression.
- Du-20 Baihui: nourish the Sea of Marrow, depression.

Summary of Kidney point combinations

- BL-23 Shenshu and BL-52 Zhishi: strengthen Will-Power.

PERICARDIUM

Chapter 8 of the *Simple Questions* says: "*The Pericardium is the official functioning as envoy: joy and happiness originate from it.*"[19] Like the Heart, the Pericardium houses the Mind and it therefore influences our mental-emotional state deeply.

The Pericardium's function on the mental-emotional plane could be seen as the psychic equivalent of its physical function of moving Qi and Blood in the chest; just as it does that on a physical level, on a mental-emotional level, the Pericardium is responsible for "movement" towards others, i.e. in relationships.

Moreover, the "moving" nature of the Pericardium is also enhanced by its relationship with the Triple Burner as a channel (within the "Minister Fire" channels). As the Triple Burner is responsible for the free flow of Qi (together with the Liver), the Pericardium's relationship with the Triple Burner partly accounts for its action in moving Qi and Blood and its mental-emotional function of "movement" towards others.

Given that the Pericardium is related to the Liver within the Terminal-Yin channels, this "movement" is also related to the "movement" of the Ethereal Soul from the ego towards others in social relationships and familial interactions. For this reason, on a mental-emotional level, the Pericardium is particularly responsible for a healthy interaction with other people in social, love and family relationships. This is probably the meaning of the *Simple Questions* statement that "*joy and happiness derive from the Pericardium*" (Fig. 8.8).

The description of the Pericardium as an "envoy" is probably related to its role in relationships with others: the role of the envoy or ambassador is to relay messages from one state to another (Fig. 8.9).

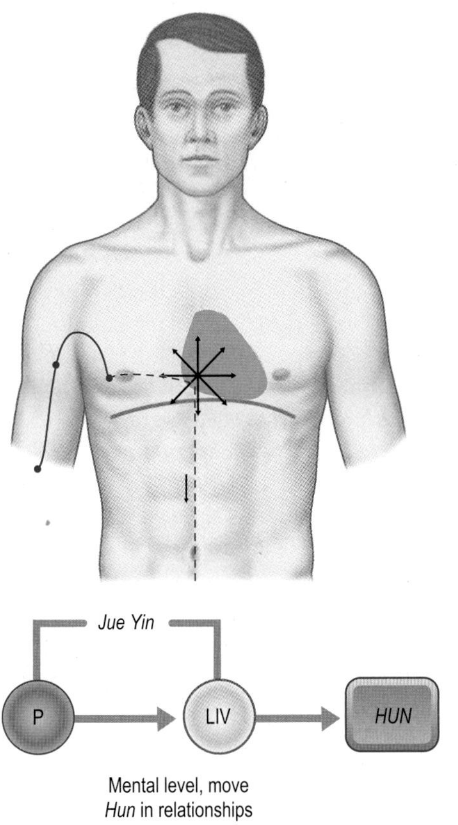

Figure 8.8 Relationship between Pericardium and Liver.

The Pericardium houses the Mind (with the Heart) and its pathology includes the following:

- Blood deficiency of the Pericardium will cause depression and slight anxiety.
- Blood Heat of the Pericardium will cause anxiety, insomnia and agitation.
- Phlegm in the Pericardium will cause mental confusion and, in severe cases, mental illness.
- The Pericardium affects emotional problems from relationship difficulties.

The Pericardium, together with the Triple Burner, pertains to the "Minister Fire". Although many doctors, such as Zhu Zhen Heng (1281–1358), identified "Ministerial Fire" with the Fire of the *Ming Men* (and therefore the Kidneys), others, such as Zhang Jie Bin (1563–1640), identified the "Ministerial Fire" with such internal organs as the Kidney, Liver, Triple Burner, Gall-Bladder and Pericardium. In fact, the Minister Fire is said to go upwards to the Liver, Gall-Bladder and Pericardium (in so doing it is compared to the "Fire Dragon flying to the top of a high mountain") and downwards to the Kidneys (in so doing it is compared to the "Fire Dragon immersing in the deep sea") (*see Figs 9.41 and 9.42*).

The mental-emotional aspect of the Pericardium is discussed further in Chapter 9.

> **CLINICAL NOTE**
>
> The best points to influence the mental aspect of the Pericardium are P-6 Neiguan to stimulate the movement of the Ethereal Soul or P-7 Daling to restrain it.

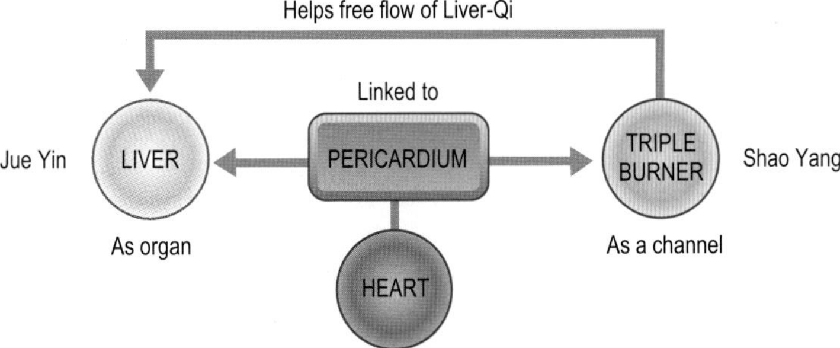

Figure 8.9 Pericardium relationships with Heart, Liver and Triple Burner.

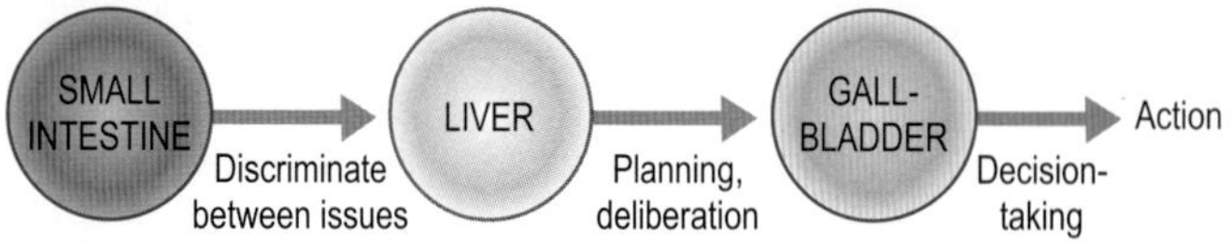

SMALL INTESTINE → Discriminate between issues → LIVER → Planning, deliberation → GALL-BLADDER → Decision-taking → Action

Figure 8.10 Small Intestine's function of discriminating between issues.

SUMMARY

Pericardium

- Like the Heart, the Pericardium houses the Mind and it therefore influences our mental-emotional state deeply.
- The Pericardium is responsible for "movement" towards others, i.e. in relationships.
- The Pericardium's relationship with the Triple Burner partly accounts for its action in moving Qi and Blood and its mental-emotional function of "movement" towards others.
- Given the relationship of the Pericardium with the Liver (within Terminal-Yin channels), and therefore the Ethereal Soul, it influences the movement of the ego towards others in social relationships and familial interactions.

Summary of Pericardium points

- P-6 Neiguan: stimulate the movement of the Ethereal Soul, depression, centripetal effect.
- P-7 Daling: restrain the movement of the Ethereal Soul, calm the Spirit, open the Mind's orifices, manic behavior.

Summary of Pericardium point combinations

- P-6 Neiguan and LIV-3 Taichong: stimulate the movement of the Ethereal Soul, move Qi, repressed anger, depression.
- P-6 Neiguan and ST-40 Fenglong: stimulate the movement of the Ethereal Soul, open the chest, calm the Mind, worry, nurturing issues.

SMALL INTESTINE

As mentioned above, Chapter 8 of the *Simple Questions* says: "*The Small Intestine is the official in charge of reception: transformation originates from it.*" This quotation refers to the Small Intestine's digestive function, i.e. that of receiving food from the Stomach and transforming it into a clear and a turbid part.

The Small Intestine also plays a role in separating a pure from a turbid part of fluids. It is this last function that has a psychic equivalent; just as this organ separates a clear from a turbid part of body fluids, so it helps us separate the "clear" from the "turbid" at a psychic level. This means that it helps us to discriminate between issues to determine what course of action we should take.

This function of the Small Intestine is different from the planning function of the Liver and it is coordinated with it. Before the planning of the Liver, it is necessary to have the Small Intestine's separation of "clear" from "turbid", i.e. discriminate between issues and determine what is "clear", i.e. usable, and what is "turbid", i.e. to be discarded (Fig. 8.10).

The Small Intestine allows us to make the first discrimination between issues in distinguishing what is appropriate in any given situation and what is not. Thereafter, it is the Liver's function of planning that takes over in deciding what is more appropriate to our particular circumstances.

An interesting aspect of the Small Intestine from the mental-emotional point of view is its coupling with the Heart, which seems rather tenuous. The relationships between the Large Intestine and Lungs, Stomach and Spleen, Bladder and Kidneys, and Gall-Bladder and Liver are much clearer and easier to explain.

There may, however, be a modern explanation of the relationship between the Small Intestine and the Heart and that is in the so-called "second brain". Dr Michael Gershon proposed the theory of a "second brain" located in the gut. Over one half of our nerve cells are located in the gut. The gut also contains neurons and neurotransmitters just like those found in the brain.

According to Dr Gershon, like the brain, the "gut brain" is also able to learn, remember and produce emotion-based feelings. The two brains communicate back and forth via the vagus nerve extending down from the base of the brain all the way into the abdomen. Through the vagus nerve, the two brains directly influence each other.

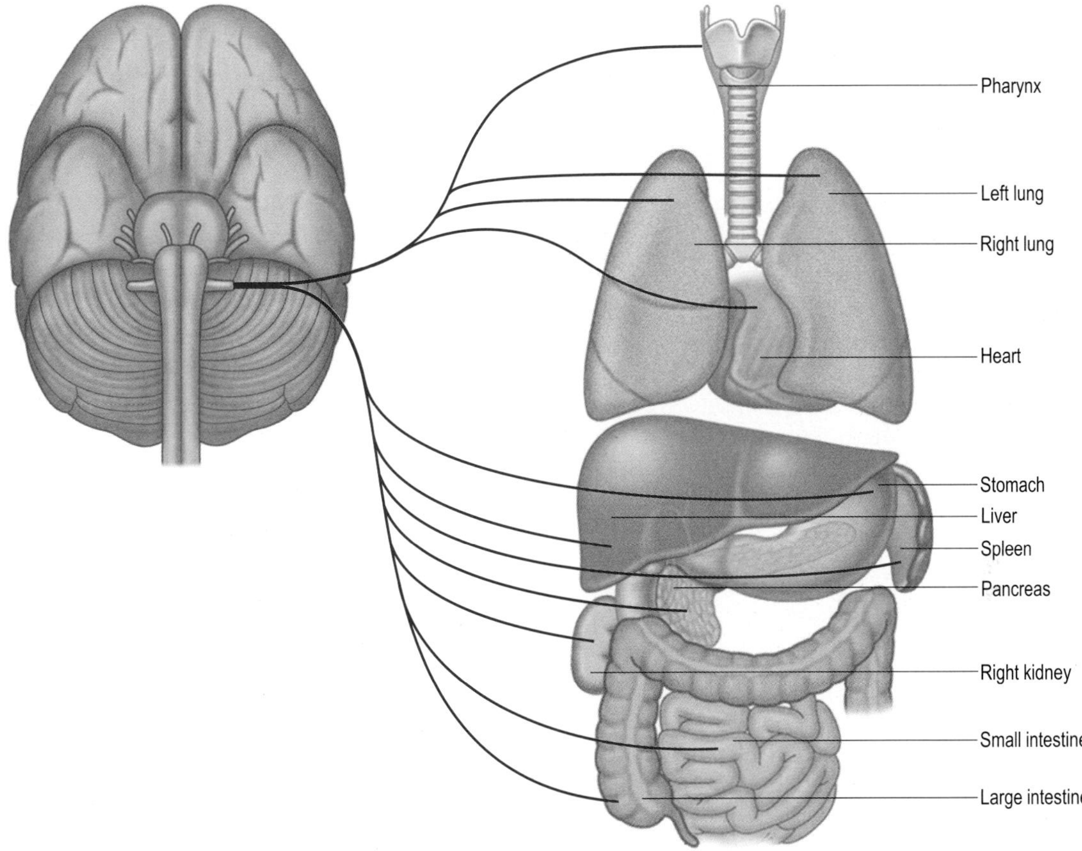

Figure 8.11 The vagus nerve.

During early fetal development, both the "gut" (esophagus, stomach, small intestine and colon) and the brain start to develop from the same clump of embryonic tissue. When that piece of tissue is divided, one piece grows into the central nervous system (brain and cranial nerves); the other section becomes the enteric nervous system (what Dr Gershon calls the "gut brain"). During later stages of fetal development, these two "brains" become connected via the vagus nerve. The vagus nerve creates a direct connection between the brain and the gut (Fig. 8.11).

The "gut brain", known as the enteric nervous system (ENS), is embedded in the sheaths of tissue lining the esophagus, stomach, small intestine and colon. One hundred million neurotransmitters line the length of the gut, approximately the same number as those found in the brain.

The modern connection between the brain and the gut might explain the strong mental-emotional effect of points such as S.I.-7 Zhizheng and L.I.-6 Pianli. In fact, among the indications of S.I.-7 are "*dullness-mania [Dian-Kuang], fear, fright, sadness, anxiety, agitation [Zang Zao]*". According to Deadman, the *Golden Mirror of Medicine* recommends S.I.-7 for depression and stagnation from all emotions.[20] The *Great Compendium of Acupuncture* also lists "sadness, grief, shock and worry" among the indications for S.I.-7.[21] Among the indications for S.I.-5 is "*dullness-mania*".[22] Among the indications of L.I.-6 Pianli is "manic behavior".

CLINICAL NOTE

The best points to influence the mental aspect of the Small Intestine are S.I.-5 Yanggu and S.I.-7 Zhizheng.

SUMMARY

Small Intestine

- The Small Intestine is the official in charge of reception and transformation.
- The Small Intestine also plays a role in separating a pure from a turbid part of fluids.
- It also helps us separate the "clear" from the "turbid" at a psychic level. This means that it helps us to discriminate between issues to determine what course of action we should take.
- This function of the Small Intestine is different from the planning function of the Liver and it is coordinated with it. Before the planning of the Liver, it is necessary to have the Small Intestine's separation of "clear" from "turbid", i.e. discriminate between issues and determine what is "clear", i.e. usable, and what is "turbid", i.e. to be discarded.

Summary of Small Intestine points

- S.I.-5 Yanggu: calm the Mind, stimulate the Small Intestine's function of discriminating between issues.
- S.I.-7 Zhizheng: calm the Spirit, open the Mind's orifices, manic behavior.

LARGE INTESTINE

Chapter 8 of the *Simple Questions* says: "*The Large Intestine is the official functioning as Minister of Transport: change and transformation originate from it.*"[23] This statement refers to the Large Intestine's function of transporting the dregs of food after separation by the Small Intestine for excretion.

On a psychic level, the Large Intestine's function of transporting dregs influences our capacity to let go. Chinese books do not discuss the mental-emotional aspects of the Yang organs with the same depth as for the Yin organs. Especially for the Large Intestine, information on its mental-emotional aspects is rather scanty in Chinese books.

I personally see the mental-emotional sphere of the Large Intestine as being influenced by that of the Lungs. The Lungs govern Qi and control its circulation in all organs; from an emotional perspective, they are therefore influenced by every emotion. However, they are particularly affected by sadness, grief, worry and guilt.

The Large Intestine is the Yang part of Metal and it therefore partakes of this mental-emotional aspect of the Lungs. In addition, being Yang, I see the influence of the Large Intestine in the mental-emotional sphere as being responsible for movement and expression of the emotions. For this reason, I use some Large Intestine points to stimulate the expression of the above emotions and, in this context, there is an interesting correlation with the Large Intestine's function of controlling evacuation.

The Large Intestine points I use most to stimulate emotional movement and the release of emotions are L.I.-4 Hegu and L.I.-6 Pianli. Among the indications of L.I.-6 Pianli is manic behavior.

CLINICAL NOTE

The best points to influence the mental aspect of the Large Intestine are L.I.-4 Hegu and L.I.-6 Pianli.

SUMMARY

Large Intestine

- The Large Intestine transports the dregs of food for excretion after separation by the Small Intestine.
- On a psychic level, the Large Intestine influences our capacity to let go.
- In addition, the mental-emotional sphere of the Large Intestine is influenced by that of the Lungs as both organs pertain to Metal, and the Large Intestine is therefore responsible for the movement and expression of the emotions.

Summary of Large Intestine points

- L.I.-4 Hegu: calm the Spirit, centripetal movement, stimulate the expression of emotions, regulate the movement of the Ethereal Soul.
- L.I-6 Pianli: restrain the movement of the Ethereal Soul, manic behavior.

GALL-BLADDER

Chapter 8 of the *Simple Questions* says: "*The Gall-Bladder is the official functioning as Minister of Justice: decision-making originates from it.*"[24] This statement clearly implies that the Gall-Bladder is responsible for our capacity of taking decisions; this stage comes after the

Liver's planning (see Fig. 8.1). This capacity of taking decisions (which may often be difficult ones) is also dependent on the Gall-Bladder's courage.

Chapter 9 of the *Simple Questions* says: *"All the 11 organs mentioned above depend on the decisions of the Gall-Bladder."*[25] This interesting statement implies that all other organs need the "motivation" provided by the Gall-Bladder. Chapter 47 of the *Simple Questions* reinforces the idea that the Gall-Bladder is responsible for decision-taking in our life and also that the other organs depend on its decisions:[26]

> *The Liver is like a military general and its decisions depend on the Gall-Bladder, and the throat is like an envoy. The patient with such a problem (bitter taste) frequently deliberates but never makes a decision.*

The Gall-Bladder is responsible for decisiveness, for the capacity of taking decisions.

Besides controlling decision-making, the Gall-Bladder is also said to give an individual courage and initiative. For this reason, in Chinese, there are several expressions such as "big gall-bladder" meaning "courageous" and "small gall-bladder" meaning "timid or fearful".

This is an important function of the Gall-Bladder on a psychological level. It controls the spirit of initiative and the courage to take decisions and make changes. Although the Kidneys control the "drive", will-power, enthusiasm and vitality, the Gall-Bladder gives us the capacity to turn this drive and vitality into positive and decisive action (Fig. 8.12). Thus a deficient Gall-Bladder will cause indecision, timidity and the affected person will be easily discouraged at the slightest adversity.

CLINICAL NOTE

G.B.-40 Qiuxu can be used to strengthen a person's capacity to take decisions.

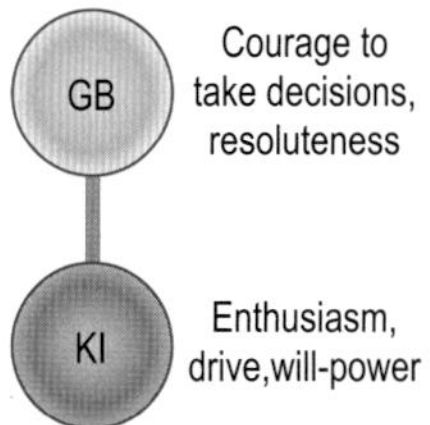

Figure 8.12 Relationship between Gall-Bladder and Kidneys.

The Gall-Bladder provides the courage for the Mind (*Shen*), governed by the Heart, to carry out decisions. This reflects the Mother–Child relationship existing between Gall-Bladder and Heart according to the Five Elements. In cases of weak Mind from Heart deficiency, it is often necessary to tonify the Gall-Bladder to support the Heart (Fig. 8.13). As a further confirmation of the relationship between the Gall-Bladder and the Heart, the Gall-Bladder Divergent channel flows through the heart.

On the other hand, the Mind provides the clarity and, most of all, the integration and control necessary to somehow "moderate" the decisiveness of the Gall-Bladder; without the control and integration of the Mind, the decisiveness of the Gall-Bladder may turn into recklessness (Fig. 8.14).

The Gall-Bladder influences mental-emotional life in yet another way. As described above, Gall-Bladder-Qi helps the ascending of Liver-Qi (relationship between Liver and Lungs). On a physical level, Gall-Bladder-Qi helps the ascending and free flow of Liver-Qi in relation to the Stomach and Spleen.

The ascending of Gall-Bladder-Qi has a psychological implication in that it stimulates the ascending and free

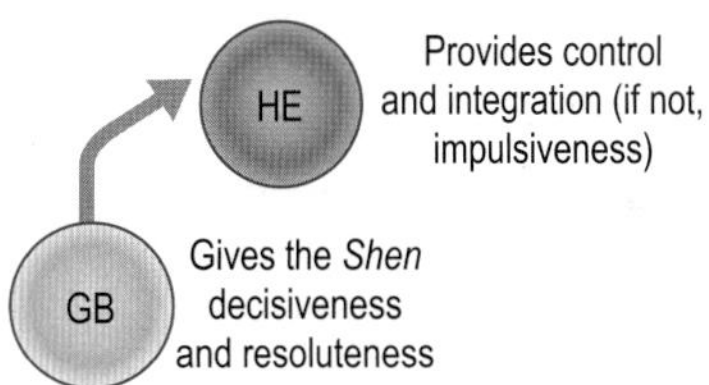

Figure 8.13 Relationship between Gall-Bladder and Heart.

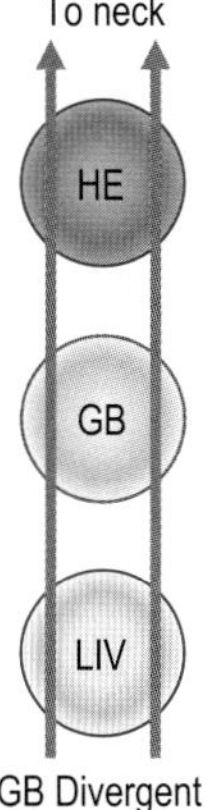

Figure 8.14 Relationship between Gall-Bladder and Heart and the Gall-Bladder Divergent channel.

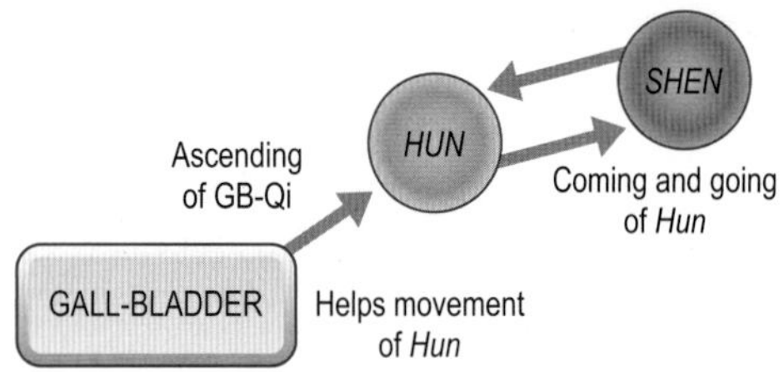

Figure 8.15 The Gall-Bladder and the ascending of Liver-Qi.

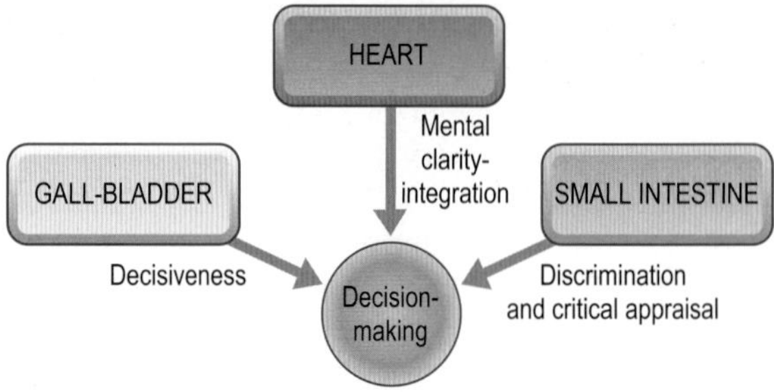

Figure 8.16 Relationship between Heart, Gall-Bladder and Small Intestine in planning.

flow of Liver-Qi on a mental level. As we have seen, the Ethereal Soul which is housed in the Liver gives "movement" to the Mind (*Shen*) of the Heart, providing it with inspiration, planning, ideas, initiative, life dreams and creativity. This "movement" of the Ethereal Soul depends on the ascending of Liver-Qi which, in turn, relies on Gall-Bladder-Qi. If this "movement" of the Ethereal Soul is lacking, the person will tend to be depressed; in this case, Liver-Qi is not ascending enough and Gall-Bladder-Qi is weak. If this movement is excessive, the person may be slightly manic (Fig. 8.15).

To stimulate the movement of the Ethereal Soul from the Gall-Bladder, I use G.B.-40.

CLINICAL NOTE

To stimulate the movement of the Ethereal Soul from the Gall-Bladder, I use G.B.-40.

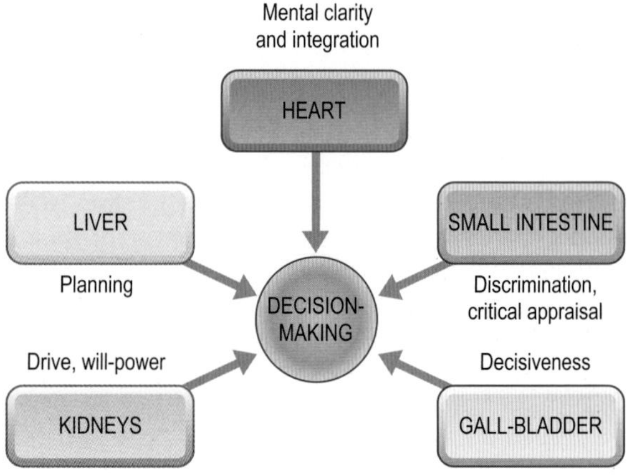

Figure 8.17 Role of organs in decision-making.

As for the mental-emotional-spiritual aspect of the Mind (Heart), Ethereal Soul (Liver), Will-Power (Kidneys), Gall-Bladder and Small Intestine, we can build a picture of how these organs are involved and coordinated in decision-making (Fig. 8.16):

- The capacity to plan our life, to have "dreams" and plans that is conferred by the Ethereal Soul (*Hun*) of the Liver
- The drive and will-power to want to make something of our lives that is conferred by the Will-Power (*Zhi*) of the Kidneys
- The capacity to discriminate between issues, to analyze issues with clarity, to distinguish what is relevant and what is not, that is conferred to us by the Small Intestine
- The capacity to take a decision with resoluteness once all issues have been analyzed, the courage to act that is conferred by the Gall-Bladder
- The integration and direction provided by the Mind (*Shen*) of the Heart (Fig. 8.17).

Gall-Bladder points have interesting psychological actions. Firstly, all Gall-Bladder points stimulate the Yang of the Liver. On a mental level the rising of Liver-Qi has two aspects:

- The coming and going of the Ethereal Soul
- Courage, decisiveness, resoluteness.

The Gall-Bladder stimulates the rising of clear Yang to the head and it does so in relation to all the other channels. Due to the connection between the Gall-Bladder and the rising of Liver-Qi, the rising of clear Yang Qi to all the channels depends on the Gall-Bladder. Obstruction in *any* of the other channels is reflected in the Gall-Bladder and, conversely, obstruction in any channel can be treated through the Gall-Bladder channel. In the 1930s to 1950s, a famous practitioner in Shanghai added the point G.B.-40 to every point prescription to increase the therapeutic effect.

!

Obstruction in any channel can be treated through the Gall-Bladder channel.

G.B.-40 is the main point to stimulate Liver-Qi on a mental level, stimulate the coming and going of the Ethereal Soul, stimulate courage, decisiveness, resoluteness. It is an important point for depression.

CLINICAL NOTE

G.B.-40 is the main point to stimulate Liver-Qi on a mental level, stimulate the coming and going of the Ethereal Soul, stimulate courage, decisiveness, resoluteness. It is an important point for depression.

Thus, it is important to distinguish the two ways in which the Gall-Bladder controls decision-making. On a personal level, it influences our capacity to take decisions and a person with a disharmony in the Gall-Bladder may be indecisive.

On the other hand, from the point of view of organs' physiology, all the organs depend on the "decision-making" or "motivation" of the Gall-Bladder.

CLINICAL NOTE

G.B.-40 Qiuxu can be used as an addition to any treatment to strengthen its effectiveness.

SUMMARY

Gall-Bladder

- The Gall-Bladder is the official functioning as Minister of Justice: decision-making originates from it.
- The Gall-Bladder is responsible for our capacity to take decisions.
- Chapter 9 of the *Simple Questions* says: *"All the 11 organs mentioned above depend on the decisions of the Gall-Bladder."* The Gall-Bladder is responsible for decisiveness, for the capacity to take decisions.
- The Gall-Bladder also gives an individual courage and initiative.
- On a psychological level the Gall-Bladder controls the spirit of initiative and the courage to take decisions and make changes.
- The Gall-Bladder provides the courage for the Mind (*Shen*), governed by the Heart, to carry out decisions. On the other hand, the Mind provides the clarity and most of all, the integration and control necessary to somehow "moderate" the decisiveness of the Gall-Bladder.
- Gall-Bladder-Qi helps the ascending of Liver-Qi and it stimulates the ascending and free flow of Liver-Qi on a mental level. The "movement" of the Ethereal Soul depends on the ascending of Liver-Qi which, in turn, relies on Gall-Bladder-Qi.
- To stimulate the movement of the Ethereal Soul from the Gall-Bladder, I use G.B.-40.
- All Gall-Bladder points stimulate the Yang of the Liver. On a mental level the rising of Liver-Qi affects the coming and going of the Ethereal Soul and courage, decisiveness and resoluteness.
- The Gall-Bladder stimulates the rising of clear Yang to the head and it does so in relation to all the other channels. Obstruction in *any* of the other channels is reflected in the Gall-Bladder and, conversely, obstruction in any channel can be treated through the Gall-Bladder channel.

Summary of Gall-Bladder points

- G.B.-40 Qiuxu: stimulate the physiological ascending of Liver-Qi, stimulate the movement of the Ethereal Soul, depression, indecision.

STOMACH

Chapter 8 of the *Simple Questions* states: "*The Spleen and Stomach are the official functioning as granary: the five flavours originate from them.*"[27] Chapter 9 of the *Simple Questions* says:[28]

The Spleen, Stomach, Large Intestine, Small Intestine, Triple Burner and Bladder are the root of granary and they house the Nutritive Qi (Ying Qi). These organs are called containers because they store food, transform waste and manage transformation and excretion of the flavours.

Thus, the first statement assimilates Stomach and Spleen together as the "granary" of the body; the second statement assimilates all Yang organs together as being responsible for digestion, transformation and excretion.

With regard to nutrition, what distinguishes the Stomach from the other Yang organs and from the Spleen? Firstly, with regard to the other Yang organs, the Stomach plays the most important role in nutrition because it is the first stage of that process. Food and drink enter the Stomach first where they are subjected to the first transformation leading to the production of Qi and Blood. Secondly, the Stomach is the Root of Post-Heaven Qi; this confirms its importance compared to that of other Yang organs.

When compared to the Spleen, the Stomach could be seen more as the container, the source of food and drink leading to the production of Qi and Blood; the Spleen can be seen more like the agent that transports and transforms the food and drink from the Stomach to produce Qi and Blood. Thus, it is almost as if the Yin–Yang qualities of these two organs were reversed: the Stomach is the container, the origin of nutrition (a Yin function) while the Spleen is the transformer (a Yang function). Indeed, in pathology, a deficiency of Stomach-Yin is very common, as is a deficiency of Spleen-Yang.

This is by far the Stomach's most important aspect: it is responsible for nutrition and for making Qi and Blood (together with the Spleen). It is the source of nutrition and of Nutritive Qi (*Ying Qi*). Indeed, the Stomach's function in relation to nutrition is so important that a popular Chinese saying states: "If there is Stomach-Qi, there is life; if there is no Stomach-Qi, there is death."

Therefore, a deficiency of the Stomach (whether it is of Yin or Yang) always involves a deficiency in nutrition which affects the whole organism. On a physical level this manifests primarily with tiredness and weak limbs. Apart from digestive symptoms, tiredness is a major symptom of Stomach deficiency (of course that is not to say that many other organs cause tiredness too).

A deficiency of the Stomach also has important psychological implications; the tiredness deriving from a Stomach deficiency may be frequently associated with a mild depression.

The psychic equivalent of the Stomach's digestive and nutritive function has to do with emotional nurturing. The Stomach pertains to Earth which provides nourishment. Just as the Stomach and the Earth Element provide nourishment on a physical level, they provide nourishment on a psychic level.

Therefore, on a psychic level, the Stomach influences our capacity to nurture and be nurtured. Emotional problems deriving from emotional nurturing issues (such as those between a mother and daughter for example) are common causes of Stomach disharmonies. Vice versa, when a person suffers from such emotional problems, it will help to tonify the Stomach.

The Stomach is affected particularly by pensiveness, sadness, grief, worry, fear and shame.

Case history

A 32-year-old woman had been suffering from digestive complaints for a long time. She often experienced fullness and distension after eating. The main problem, however, was a pronounced tiredness, a slight depression and a constant preoccupation with food. She paid great attention to her diet but very many foods seemed to influence her digestion. She felt very tired after eating and was losing weight.

Her voice had a slight weepy sound, she was pale and looked haunted. Her eyes lacked *shen*. Her tongue was unremarkable: it was only slightly Pale and had a sticky coating. Her pulse was Weak in general and Choppy, and it lacked a wave.

Diagnosis Strictly from the patterns point of view, there is a deficiency of the Spleen and Stomach with a slight deficiency of Spleen-Yang and of Stomach-Yin; this is not a contradiction and it is not uncommon.

However, the lack of *shen* of the eyes, the weepy sound of her voice, her somewhat obsessive preoccupation with food and the lack of wave of the pulse all indicate a disturbance of the *Shen* (Mind and Spirit). It was only through talking to her over many sessions that a picture began to emerge.

Her mother was a very cold and unaffectionate person; she seldom held or hugged her children and her love had a clear narcissistic quality. This had affected my patient deeply and the lack of emotional nourishment had affected the Stomach and Spleen (particularly the Stomach).

Case history

A 35-year-old woman suffered from tiredness, dizziness and lower backache. At first appearance, she appeared as a very pleasant and stable young woman. She was very pale and suffered the cold a lot. Her tongue was Pale; her pulse was Weak and especially so on the Stomach/ Spleen position. Besides being Weak, this position was also Fine.

Diagnosis At first, the diagnosis seemed "easy": deficiency of Stomach and Spleen, general deficiency of Qi and Blood and a slight Kidney-Yang deficiency. I gave her two remedies to take: *Precious Sea* (a variation of Ba Zhen Tang *Eight Precious Decoction*) to tonify Qi and Blood and *Strengthen the Root* (a variation of You Gui Wan *Restoring the Right* [Kidney] *Pill*) to tonify Kidney-Yang.

I also treated her with acupuncture even though she was very sensitive to needling and disliked the idea. Although she disliked needling, she still insisted in wanting to have acupuncture as she did feel better after each treatment. As she was so sensitive, I used only two points in total: these were usually ST-36 Zusanli, sometimes with SP-6 Sanyinjiao and sometimes with KI-3 Taixi.

As I was using only two points (and also two needles as I used them unilaterally to reduce the amount of needling), I noticed an interesting and strange reaction to ST-36 every time. As soon as I inserted the needle in ST-36, she became very emotional and started crying. This reaction puzzled me as I do not usually get it from using this point.

This led me to ask her more questions about her past history. I did ask her about her past history the first time but she told there was nothing remarkable to report. However, when I probed her more about her reaction to ST-36 being needled, she said that when she was a teenager, she suffered from an eating disorder with both anorexia and bulimia.

She was quite reluctant to talk about this and I respected her wish but I did manage to extract some information about her relationship with her mother. Her mother was a very controlling and domineering character while her father was a rather weak character. Thus, she had the "wrong" archetypal parents from the beginning, the female one being too strong and controlling and the male one being weak. This affected the nurturing of the Earth and led to the Stomach deficiency.

It was therefore for this reason that she became so emotional every time the Stomach was tonified; tonifying the Earth brought home all the painful memories of the lack of psychic nourishments from her parents. Interestingly, this reaction did not stop ST-36 from working and from helping her in the long run.

CLINICAL NOTE

The best points to influence the mental aspect of the Stomach are ST-36 Zusanli and ST-40 Fenglong.

SUMMARY

Stomach

- Chapter 8 of the *Simple Questions* states: *"The Spleen and Stomach are the official functioning as granary: the five flavours originate from them."*
- The Stomach is responsible for nutrition and for making Qi and Blood (together with the Spleen). It is the source of nutrition and of Nutritive Qi (*Ying Qi*).
- A deficiency of the Stomach (whether it is of Yin or Yang) always involves a deficiency in nutrition which affects the whole organism, manifesting with tiredness and weak limbs.
- The psychic equivalent of the Stomach's digestive and nutritive function has to do with emotional nourishment. Just as the Stomach and the Earth Element provide nourishment on a physical level, they provide nourishment on a psychic level.
- On a psychic level, the Stomach influences our capacity to nurture and be nurtured.
- The Stomach is affected particularly by pensiveness, sadness, grief, worry, fear and shame.

Summary of Stomach points

- ST-36 Zusanli: tonify Stomach and Spleen, strengthen the Mind and the Intellect, depression from deficiency.
- ST-40 Fenglong: subdue rebellious Stomach-Qi, resolve Phlegm, open the Mind's orifices, calm

the Spirit, open the chest, worry, sadness, grief, guilt, nurturing issues.

Summary of Stomach point combinations

- ST-40 Fenglong and P-6 Neiguan: stimulate the movement of the Ethereal Soul, open the chest, calm the Mind, worry, nurturing issues.
- ST-36 Zusanli and SP-6 Sanyinjiao: tonify Stomach and Spleen, nourish Blood, strengthen the Mind (*Shen* of the Heart), depression, nurturing issues.

BLADDER

Chapter 8 of the *Simple Questions* says: "*The Bladder is the official functioning as a regional capital: fluids storage originates from it and they* [fluids] *are excreted through transformation by Qi.*"[29]

The Bladder pertains to the Water Element and is responsible for the excretion of impure fluids. It is interesting to compare the Kidneys and Bladder's function in relation to the Water Element as they both pertain to this Element.

The Kidneys pertain to the Water Element but in the sense of them being the origin of Water, i.e. the Original Yin of the body; this is therefore a precious type of "Water" because the Kidney-Essence is part of it.

By contrast, the Bladder pertains to Water in the sense that it is responsible for the excretion of impure fluids; indeed it is the last stage of fluid transformation and therefore the fluids it excretes are the most "impure" ones. Thus the "Water" of the Kidneys is different from the "Water" of the Bladder.

On a psychic level, this means that the Bladder is affected by the incapacity of "excreting the impure" and therefore by "dark" emotions such as guilt, resentment and jealousy.

CLINICAL NOTE

The best point to influence the mental aspect of the Bladder is BL-60 Kunlun.

SUMMARY

Bladder

- Chapter 8 of the *Simple Questions* says: "*The Bladder is the official functioning as a regional capital: fluids storage originates from it and they* [fluids] *are excreted through transformation by Qi.*"
- The Bladder pertains to Water in the sense that it is responsible for the excretion of impure fluids; indeed it is the last stage of fluid transformation and therefore the fluids it excretes are the most "impure" ones.
- On a psychic level, the Bladder is affected by the incapacity of "excreting the impure" and therefore by "dark" emotions such as guilt, resentment and jealousy.
- The best point to influence the mental aspect of the Bladder is BL-60 Kunlun.

Summary of Bladder points

- BL-60 Kunlun: calm the Spirit, guilt, shame.

TRIPLE BURNER

Chapter 8 of the *Simple Questions* says: "*The Triple Burner is the official responsible for dredging of channels: regulation of water passages originates from it.*"[30]

The Triple Burner belongs to the Lesser Yang channels which are the "hinge" between the Greater Yang (opening onto the Exterior) and Bright Yang channels (opening onto the Interior). On a psychological level, being the "hinge" means that these channels are "mediators" in the sense that they can affect a person's capacity to relate to other people and the external world. The use of Triple Burner points is therefore important in emotional problems deriving from relationships (Fig. 8.18).

The Triple Burner and Pericardium channels also affect the mental-emotional state because the Minister Fire rises towards these two channels; therefore, when the Minister Fire is aroused by emotional problems and it rises towards the Pericardium and Triple Burner channels, points on these channels can be used to clear Heat and calm the Mind (Fig. 8.19). The main points are T.B.-5 Waiguan, P-7 Daling and P-8 Laogong.

Finally, the Pericardium and Triple Burner channels are symmetrical in so far as the former is the opening point of the Yin Linking Vessel (*Yin Wei Mai*) and the latter of the Yang Linking Vessel (*Yang Wei Mai*); this is another reason why these two channels connect the three Yin and three Yang respectively (Fig. 8.20).

The mental-emotional aspect of the Triple Burner is determined by its dual nature as pertaining to the character of both Fire and Wood. The Triple Burner pertains to Fire as it is not only exteriorly and interiorly related to the Pericardium but also because it is the emissary of the Original Qi (*Yuan Qi*) and of the Fire of the Gate of Life (*Ming Men*) (Fig. 8.21). It partakes of the character of Wood as it is connected to the Gall-Bladder within the Lesser Yang channels. These two aspects are not unrelated since, as we have seen, the Minister Fire between the Kidneys ascends to connect with the Triple Burner, the Gall-Bladder and the Pericardium (Fig. 8.22).

TAI YANG
Opens onto the Exterior
SHAO YANG
'Hinge'
YANG MING
Opens onto the Interior

Figure 8.18 Triple Burner as the hinge of the Yang channels.

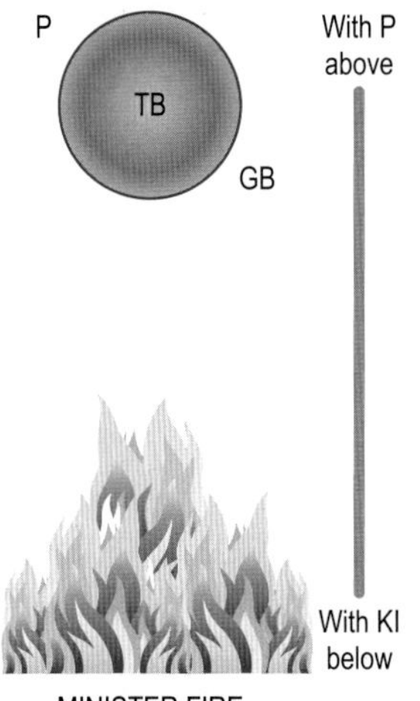

Figure 8.19 Minister Fire rising to Triple Burner and Pericardium.

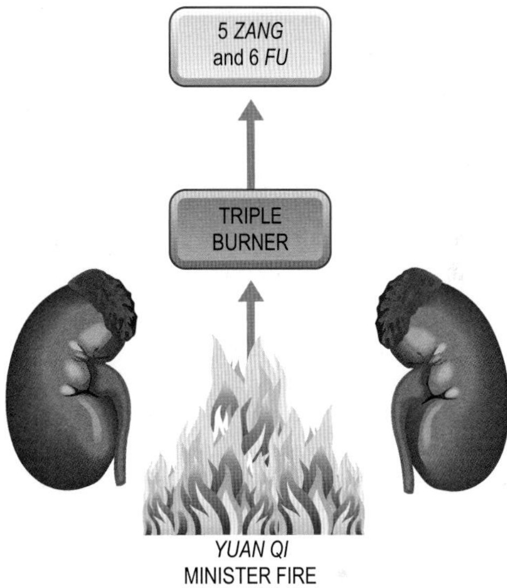

Figure 8.21 The Triple Burner as "emissary" of the Original Qi and Minister Fire.

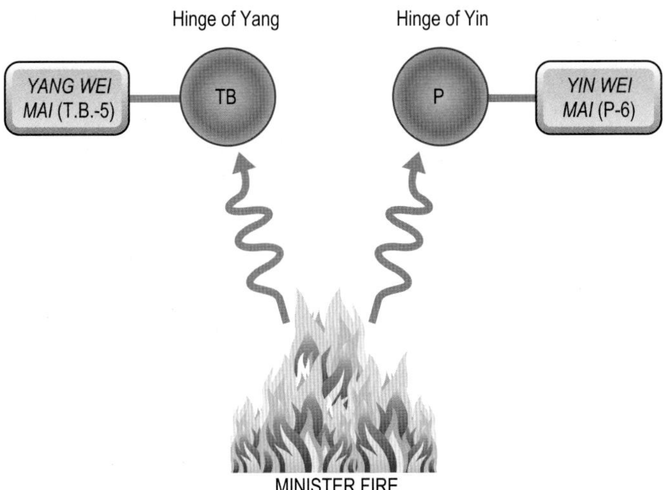

Figure 8.20 Triple Burner and Pericardium and Yang and Yin Linking Vessels.

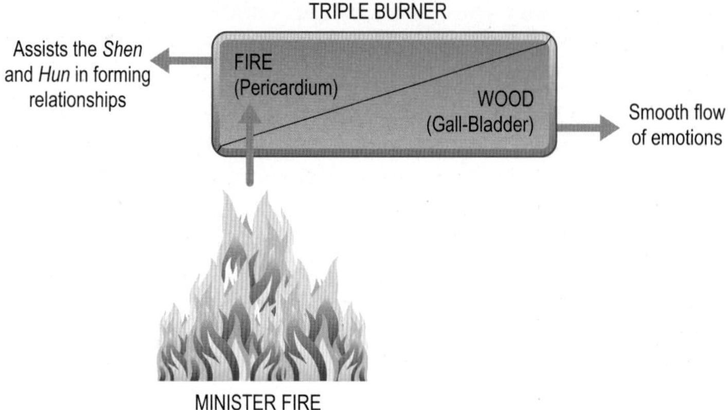

Figure 8.22 Dual nature of Triple Burner as pertaining to Wood and to Minister Fire.

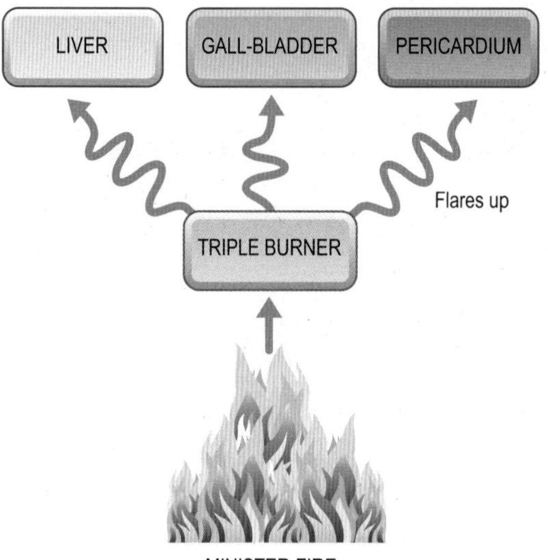

Figure 8.23 Connection of Triple Burner with Pericardium, Gall-Bladder and Minister Fire.

In so far as it shares the character of Wood, the Triple Burner has a similar mental-emotional influence as the Liver, i.e. it also promotes the "free flow" of emotions in a smooth way so that emotions are freely expressed and not repressed. Just as, on a physical level, the Triple Burner controls the movement of Qi in all organs and structures, on a mental-emotional level, it controls the smooth flow of Qi between the Mind and the Ethereal Soul so that emotions do not turn into "moods" which happens when Qi stagnates (Fig. 8.23).

CLINICAL NOTE

The best points to influence the mental aspect of the Triple Burner are T.B.-5 Waiguan and T.B.-3 Zhongzhu.

SUMMARY

Triple Burner

- Chapter 8 of the *Simple Questions* says: *"The Triple Burner is the official responsible for dredging of channels: regulation of water passages originates from it."*
- The Triple Burner belongs to the Lesser Yang channels which are the "hinge" between the Greater Yang (opening onto the Exterior) and Bright Yang channels (opening onto the Interior).
- On a psychological level, being the "hinge" means that these channels are "mediators" in the sense that they can affect a person's capacity to relate to other people and the external world.
- The Triple Burner and Pericardium channels also affect the mental-emotional state because the Minister Fire rises towards these two channels; therefore when the Minister Fire is aroused by emotional problems and it rises towards the Pericardium and Triple Burner channels, points of these channels can be used to clear Heat and calm the Mind. The main points are T.B.-5 Waiguan, P-7 Daling and P-8 Laogong.

- The mental-emotional aspect of the Triple Burner is determined by its dual nature as pertaining to the character of both Fire and Wood.
- In so far as it shares the character of Wood, the Triple Burner has a similar mental-emotional influence as the Liver, i.e. it also promotes the "free flow" of emotions in a smooth way so that emotions are freely expressed and not repressed.
- The best points to influence the mental aspect of the Triple Burner are T.B.-5 Waiguan and T.B.-3 Zhongzhu.

Summary of Triple Burner points

- T.B.-5 Waiguan: stimulate the movement of the Ethereal Soul, relationship problems, depression, Qi stagnation.
- T.B.-3 Zhongzhu: stimulate the movement of the Ethereal Soul, depression.

Summary of Triple Burner point combinations

- T.B.-5 Waiguan and P-7 Daling: calm the Spirit, restrain the movement of the Ethereal Soul, anxiety, relationship problems. Manic behaviors.
- T.B.-5 Waiguan and P-6 Neiguan: stimulate the movement of the Ethereal Soul, depression, relationship problems.

END NOTES

1. 1979 Huang Di Nei Jing Su Wen 黄帝内经素问[The Yellow Emperor's Classic of Internal Medicine – Simple Questions]. People's Health Publishing House, Beijing. pp. 58–59. First published *c.*100 BC.
2. Ibid., p. 59.
3. Ibid., p. 153.
4. Ibid., pp. 68–69.
5. Ibid., p. 262.
6. Ibid., p. 247.
7. Ibid., p. 561.
8. Ibid., p. 58.
9. Claremont de Castillejo I 1997 Knowing Woman – A Feminine Psychology. Shambhala, Boston, p. 15.
10. Ibid., p. 15.
11. Simple Questions, p. 58.
12. Ibid., p. 58.
13. Ibid., p. 58.
14. Ibid., p. 153.
15. Ibid., p. 58.
16. 1981 Ling Shu Jing 灵枢经 [Spiritual Axis]. People's Health Publishing House, Beijing. p. 77. First published *c.*100 BC.
17. Qin Yue Ren 2004 Nan Jing Jiao Shi 难经校释[Classic of Difficulties]. Scientific and Technical Documents Publishing House, Beijing, p. 22. First published *c.*AD 100.
18. Ibid, p. 23.
19. Simple Questions, p. 59.
20. Deadman P, Al-Khafaji M 2007 A Manual of Acupuncture. Journal of Chinese Medicine Publications, Hove, England, p. 238.
21. 1980 Zhen Jiu Da Cheng 针灸大成 [The Great Compendium of Acupuncture]. People's Health Publishing House, Beijing, p. 222. The *Great Compendium of Acupuncture* was written by Yang Ji Zhou and first published in 1601.
22. Ibid., p. 222.
23. Simple Questions, p. 59.
24. Ibid., p. 59.
25. Ibid., pp. 68–69.
26. Ibid., p. 262.
27. Ibid., pp. 58–59.
28. Ibid., pp. 68–69.
29. Ibid., p. 59.
30. Ibid., p. 59.

情志

CHAPTER 9

THE EMOTIONS

THE EMOTIONS 122

Anger 122

Joy 126

Worry 127

Pensiveness 129

Sadness and grief 131

Fear 133

Shock 134

Love 135

Craving 136

Guilt 138

Shame 140

THE PATHOLOGY OF QI AND MINISTER FIRE IN EMOTIONAL PROBLEMS 143

The effect of emotions on the body's Qi 143

The pathology of the Minister Fire in emotional problems 148

THE TRIUNE BRAIN AND CHINESE MEDICINE 155

The triune brain, the Mind, Ethereal Soul and Corporeal Soul 157

THE EMOTIONS

Le coeur a ses raisons que la Raison ne connait point (“The heart has its reasons which Reason does not know”)
Pascal, Pensees

In this chapter, I shall discuss the emotions as etiological factors in the origin of mental-emotional problems. I shall discuss the etiology of mental-emotional problems in two separate chapters. The present chapter discusses the emotions as causes of disease in Chinese medicine; these are obviously the main etiological factors in mental-emotional disharmonies. Chapter 10 will discuss other contributory factors such as diet and overwork; these are usually only contributory factors which aggravate the effect of the emotional causes of disease.

Please note that Chapter 14 discusses the emotions in Western philosophy (not necessarily as causes of disease) and Chapter 15 the influence of Confucianism on the way Chinese medicine sees the emotions. The reader is urged to read these two important chapters although these can be read not necessarily in the order in which they appear.

The Chinese term for what we translate as “emotion” is *qing* 情; this is composed of the radical for “heart” on the left and another component on the right (*qing* 青) that is partly phonetic and partly conveying the idea of “growing plants”. This is because the pictogram indicates the green color of growing plants; it is made up of the radical for life (*sheng* 生) and that for *dan* 丹, i.e. cinnabar.

The word “emotion” itself is not, in my opinion, a good term to indicate the Chinese view of the “emotional” causes of disease. The word “emotion” derives from Latin and it refers to “*e-movere*”, i.e. to “move out”; it is used to indicate any feeling of the mind “moving outwards” or “being moved” as distinct from the cognitive or volitional states of consciousness.

In this sense, the term “emotion” may refer to any feeling such as fear, joy, hope, surprise, desire, aversion, pleasure, pain, etc.; it is therefore not entirely suitable as a term denoting the emotions as intended in Chinese medicine. In fact, emotions are considered in Chinese medicine as causes of disease and some of the emotions just mentioned (e.g. surprise) are not causes of disease.

It is interesting to note that the word used to indicate a suffering of the mind (as they are in Chinese medicine) originally was “passion” rather than “emotion”. The word “passion” derives from the Latin verb “*patire*” which means "to suffer" and it would therefore be a better translation of the Chinese word "*qing*" in the context of emotions as causes of disease.

The word "emotion" replaced "passion" in the time between Descartes and Rousseau, i.e. between 1650 and 1750 (as the former used the word "passion" and the latter the word "emotion").

Thus, the word "passion" would convey the idea of mental suffering better than "emotion" also because it implies the idea of something that is "suffered", something that we are subject to. Indeed, feelings such as sadness, fear and anger become causes of disease when they take over our mind, when we no longer possess them but they "possess" us. In fact, the Chinese expression most Chinese books use to describe the "stimulation" or "excitation" produced by the emotions is *ci ji* 刺激 where "*ji*" contains the radical for "water" and means to "swash, surge" as a wave does, i.e. it denotes the surge of emotions like a wave that carries us away.

Damasio defines six basic emotions (or universal emotions). These are: happiness, sadness, fear, anger, surprise and disgust.[1] As we can see from this list, it obviously includes emotions that are not causes of disease (e.g. surprise or disgust). Hence the term "passion" might seem more appropriate. Chinese medicine considers only the emotions that become causes of disease.

We know that emotions played an important evolutionary role in our development and, besides becoming causes of disease under certain circumstances, they can also perform positive roles. For example, sadness can strengthen social bonds; anger allows us to mobilize and sustain energy at high levels; shame ensures social order and stability; fear motivates escape from dangerous situations, etc.[2]

Interestingly, Damasio makes a distinction between *feeling* and *emotion*. He says that feelings are inwardly directed and private, while emotions are outwardly directed and public. Damasio maintains that there are feelings we are conscious of and feelings that we are not. He says:[3]

> *An organism may represent in mental and neural patterns the state that we conscious creatures call a feeling without ever knowing that the feeling is taking place.*

This is an interesting distinction and one that presents intriguing similarities with Chinese medicine. In fact, we could say that the feelings we are not conscious of are the Corporeal Soul (*Po*) while emotions involve the Mind (*Shen*) and Ethereal Soul (*Hun*).

Emotions are mental stimuli which influence our affective life. Under normal circumstances, they are not a cause of disease. Hardly any human being can avoid being angry, sad, aggrieved, worried or afraid at some time in his or her life. For example, the death of a relative provokes a very natural feeling of grief.

Emotions become causes of disease only when they are either long-lasting or very intense. It is only when we are in a particular emotional state for a long time (months or years) that they become a cause of disease; for example, if a particular family or work situation makes us angry and frustrated in an ongoing way, this will affect the Liver and cause an internal disharmony. In a few cases, emotions can become a cause of disease in a very short time if they are intense enough; shock is the best example of such a situation.

CLINICAL NOTE

Emotions become causes of disease only when they are either long-lasting or very intense.

In Chinese medicine, emotions (intended as causes of disease) are mental stimuli which impair the circulation of Qi and disturb the Mind (*Shen*), Ethereal Soul (*Hun*) and Corporeal Soul (*Po*) and, through these, they alter the balance of the Internal Organs and the harmony of Qi and Blood. Thus, emotional stress is an internal cause of disease which injures the Internal Organs directly and is obviously the main cause of mental-emotional disharmonies. For this reason, Chinese medicine usually refers to emotional stress as "internal" cause of disease and climate as "external" cause of disease. On the other hand, and this is a very important feature of Chinese medicine, the state of the Internal Organs affects our emotional state.

The mutual interaction between the emotions and the Internal Organs and the unity of body and Mind is one of the most important and distinctive aspects of Chinese medicine. Emotional stress causes an imbalance in the Internal Organs and a disharmony of these (from causes other than emotional stress), in turn, will cause an emotional imbalance. For example, a prolonged state of anger will affect the Liver and, conversely, a Liver disharmony (perhaps from diet and overwork) will cause an emotional imbalance and cause the person to become irritable (Fig. 9.1).

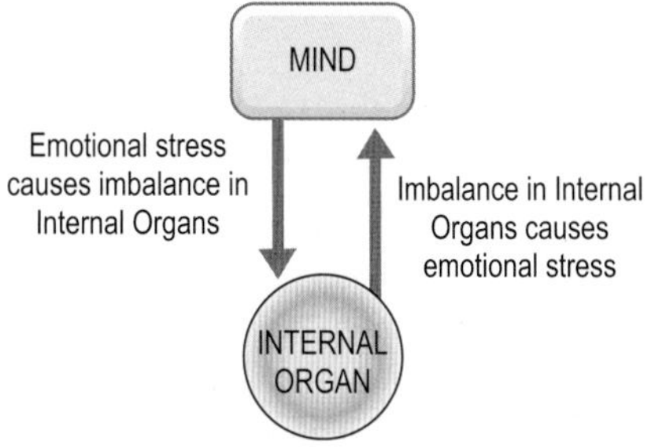

Figure 9.1 Mutual interaction between emotions and Internal Organs.

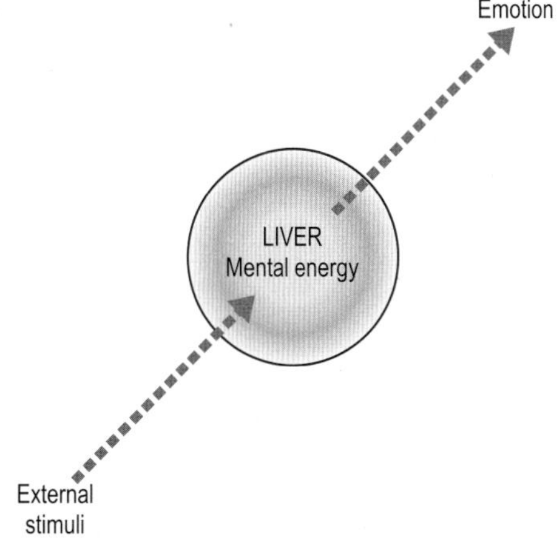

Figure 9.2 Conversion of organ's mental energy into "emotion".

For example, if Liver-Blood is deficient (perhaps from dietary factors) and causes Liver-Yang to rise, this may cause a person to become irritable all the time. Conversely, if a person is constantly angry about a certain situation or with a particular person, this may cause Liver-Yang to rise.

The *Spiritual Axis* in Chapter 8 clearly illustrates the reciprocal relationship between the emotions and the Internal Organs. It says:[4]

Worry, timidity, and pensiveness injure the Mind [Shen]; excess joy scatters the Mind which is therefore deprived of its residence. Sadness and grief block Qi and cause stagnation.

It also says:[5]

The Heart's fear, anxiety and pensiveness injure the Mind (Shen) ... the Spleen's worry injures the Intellect (Yi) ... the Liver's sadness and shock injure the Ethereal Soul (Hun) ... the Lung's excessive joy injures the Corporeal Soul (Po) ... the Kidney's anger injures the Will-Power (Zhi).

On the other hand, further on it says:[6]

If Liver-Qi is deficient there is fear, if it is in excess there is anger ... if Heart-Qi is deficient there is sadness, if it is in excess there is manic behaviour.

These passages clearly show that, on the one hand, emotional stress injures the Internal Organs and, on the other hand, disharmony of the Internal Organs causes emotional imbalance.

Each emotion stems from a psychic field which pertains to the relevant Yin organ. This, in fact, explains why a certain emotion affects a specific organ; that particular organ already produces a certain psychic energy with specific characteristics which, when subject to emotional stimuli, responds to or "resonates" with a particular emotion; for example, an external stimulus resonates with the Liver's psychic energy, giving rise to anger (Fig. 9.2). Thus the Internal Organs already have a psychic energy which turns into a negative emotion only when triggered by certain external circumstances.

For example, why does anger affect the Liver? If one considers the Liver's characteristics of free-going, easy and quick movement, with a tendency for its Qi to rise, its correspondence to Spring when the powerful Yang energy bursts outwards and upwards and its correspondence to Wood with its expansive movement, it is easy to understand that the Liver would be affected by anger. This emotion, with its quick outbursts, the rising of blood to the head that one feels when very angry, the destructive, expansive quality of rage, mimics, on an affective level, the characteristics of the Liver and Wood outlined above.

The emotions taken into consideration in Chinese medicine have varied over the years. Therefore, we should not be too rigid in adhering to the five emotions according to the Five Elements nor to the "seven emotions" as traditionally listed in Chinese books. As we shall see below, the emotions considered in Chinese medicine have varied over the centuries; moreover, as we shall see below, there are many emotions that have never been considered in Chinese medicine and yet are pervasive in Western people.

One of the oldest mention of emotions is from Confucius's *Book of Rites* (*Li Ji*) dating back to *c.*500 BC. In this book, Confucius lists seven emotions: joy, anger, grief, fear, love, hatred and desire.[7] According to *Chinese Medicine Psychology*, the Daoist Lao Zi lists seven emotions that differ from those listed by Confucius: these are joy, anger, worry, sadness, love, hatred and desire.[8] Other texts mention six emotions: love, hatred, desire, anger, grief and joy.[9]

From a Five-Element perspective, Chapter 5 of the *Simple Questions* considered five emotions, each one affecting a specific Yin organ:[10]

- anger affects the Liver
- joy affects the Heart
- pensiveness affects the Spleen
- worry affects the Lungs
- fear affects the Kidneys.[i]

SUMMARY

The emotions and the Five Elements
WOOD – ANGER – LIVER
FIRE – JOY – HEART
EARTH – PENSIVENESS – SPLEEN
METAL – WORRY – LUNGS
FEAR – WATER – KIDNEYS

However, the above five emotions are not by any means the only emotions discussed in the *Yellow Emperor's Classic*. In other passages sadness and shock are added, giving seven emotions as follows:

- anger affecting the Liver
- joy affecting the Heart
- worry affecting the Lungs and Spleen
- pensiveness affecting the Spleen
- sadness affecting the Lungs and Heart
- fear affecting the Kidneys
- shock affecting the Kidneys and Heart.

Chen Wu Ze (1174) lists the seven emotions that are usually discussed in modern books, i.e. joy, anger, worry, pensiveness, sadness, fear and shock.

Zhang Jie Bin mentions eight emotions in his *Classic of Categories*.[11] These are:

- joy
- anger
- pensiveness
- worry
- fright (*kong* 恐)
- shock
- sadness
- fear (*wei* 畏).

Although each emotion affects a particular Yin organ selectively, the relationship between a given emotion and a particular organ should not be interpreted too rigidly. Each emotion can and does affect more than one organ and often in a pattern that does not follow that of the Five Elements. This will be explained more in detail below.

Many passages from the *Spiritual Axis* and *Simple Questions* confirm that the relationship between an emotion and an organ (e.g. anger – Liver) should not be interpreted too restrictively because each emotion can affect several organs. For example, with regard to excess joy, Chapter 8 of the *Spiritual Axis* says: "*Excess joy of the Lungs injures the Corporeal Soul and this may cause manic behavior.*"[12]

With regard to anger, Chapter 23 of the *Simple Questions* says: "*When the Gall Bladder is diseased there is anger.*"[13] Chapter 62 of the *Simple Questions* says: "*When Blood rushes upwards and Qi downwards, the Heart is harassed and may cause anger.*"[14] Chapter 8 of the *Spiritual Axis* says: "*Anger affecting the Kidneys injures the Will-Power* [Zhi]."[15]

With regard to pensiveness, Chapter 39 of the *Simple Questions* says: "*Pensiveness makes the Heart* [Qi] *accumulate causing the Mind to stagnate: the Upright Qi settles and does not move and therefore Qi stagnates.*"[16]

With regard to worry, Chapter 23 of the *Simple Questions* says: "*When Qi rushes upwards it affects the Liver causing worry.*"[17] Chapter 8 of the *Spiritual Axis* says: "*Worry of the Spleen injures the Intellect.*"[18]

With regard to fear, Chapter 4 of the *Spiritual Axis* says: "*Worry and fear injure the Heart.*"[19] Chapter 62 of the *Simple Questions* says: "*When Blood* [of the Liver] *is deficient, there is fear.*"[20] Chapter 19 of the *Simple Questions* says: "*Fear makes Spleen-Qi stagnate.*"[21] Chapter 23 of the *Simple Questions* says: "*When Stomach-Qi rebels upwards there is vomiting and fear.*"[22]

Zhang Jie Bin summarizes the effect of each emotion on groups of organs in Chapter 216 of his book *Classic of Categories* (*Lei Jing*, 1624):[23]

The five emotions interact with each other in causing disease; for example, excess joy affects the Heart but it may also affect the Lungs and injure the Corporeal Soul. Excess joy derives from the Heart but moves to the Lungs. Anger affects the Liver but also the Gall Bladder;

Liver and Gall Bladder are interiorly–exteriorly related and when Liver-Qi is excessive it affects the Gall Bladder. [When there is anger] *Blood rushes upwards and Qi downwards and this harasses the Heart. Sometimes anger affects the Kidneys and it injures the Will-Power. Hence anger can affect the Liver, Gall Bladder, Heart and Kidneys. Pensiveness pertains to the Spleen but it also affects the Heart. The Heart is the Mother of the Spleen; when the Qi of the Mother does not move freely it affects the Child and therefore both Spleen and Heart are affected by pensiveness. Worry pertains to the Lungs but it also affects the Heart. Worry makes Qi rise and can affect the Liver; the Liver becomes overactive and it invades the Spleen. The Spleen is then affected by worry and this injures the Intellect* [Yi]. *Hence worry affects the Lungs, Heart, Liver and Spleen.*

To summarize what Zhang Jie Bin says in the above passage, each emotion affects groups of organs as follows:

- *Excess joy*: Heart and Lungs
- *Anger*: Liver, Gall-Bladder, Heart and Kidneys
- *Pensiveness*: Spleen and Heart
- *Worry*: Lungs, Heart, Liver and Spleen
- *Fear*: Kidneys, Heart, Liver, Spleen and Stomach.

Besides this, all emotions by definition affect the Heart because the Heart is the organ that houses the Mind (*Shen*) and it is the Mind that feels the emotions. When we feel angry, although anger will affect the Liver, it is the Mind of the Heart that feels the anger and knows we are angry. Therefore, by definition all emotions affect the Heart and that is why a red tip of the tongue (Heart area) is such a common clinical finding; it indicates emotional stress deriving from any of the emotions, not only those pertaining to the Heart.

Zhang Jie Bin explains how all emotions affect the Heart in his *Classic of Categories* (*Lei Jing*, 1624):[24]

The Heart is the ruler of the five Yin and six Yang organs, it gathers the Ethereal and Corporeal Souls and it includes the Intellect [Yi] *and Will-Power* [Zhi]. *Worry affects the Heart and then the Lungs; pensiveness affects the Heart and then the Spleen; anger affects the Heart and then the Liver; fear affects the Heart and then the Kidneys.*

Fei Bo Xiong (1800–1879) put it very clearly when he said:[25]

The seven emotions injure the five Yin organs selectively, but they all affect the Heart. Joy injures the Heart ... Anger injures the Liver, the Liver cannot recognize anger but the Heart can, hence it affects both Liver and Heart. Worry injures the Lungs, the Lungs cannot recognize it but the Heart can, hence it affects both Lungs and Heart. Pensiveness injures the Spleen, the Spleen cannot recognize it but the Heart can, hence it affects both Spleen and Heart.

Yu Chang in *Principles of Medical Practice* (1658) says:[26]

Worry agitates the Heart and has repercussions on the Lungs; pensiveness agitates the Heart and has repercussions on the Spleen; anger agitates the Heart and has repercussions on the Liver; fear agitates the Heart and has repercussions on the Kidneys. Therefore all the five emotions [including joy] *affect the Heart.*

Chapter 28 of the *Spiritual Axis* also says that all emotions affect the Heart: "*The Heart is the Master of the five Yin and six Yang organs ... sadness, shock and worry agitate the Heart; when the Heart is agitated the five Yin and six Yang organs are shaken.*"[27] Chinese writing clearly bears out the idea that all emotions affect the Heart since the characters for all seven emotions are based on the "heart" radical. This is probably the most important aspect of the Heart functions and the main reason for it being compared to a "monarch".

Chapter 8 of the *Spiritual Axis* deals with the mental effect of the emotions in quite some detail. It says:[28]

The method of needling should first of all be rooted in the Mind (Shen). Blood, blood vessels, Nutritive Qi (Ying Qi), Qi, and the spirit (Jingshen) are stored in the five Yin Organs. When they are out of harmony due to the emotions, the Essence (Jing) is lost, the Ethereal Soul (Hun) and Corporeal Soul (Po) are scattered, the Will-Power (Zhi) and Intellect (Yi) are chaotic and the person lacks wisdom and reflection: why is that? Heaven bestows us Virtue (De), Earth bestows us Qi. When Virtue flows and Qi pulsates, there is life. When the two Essences [of mother and father] *unite, the Mind comes into being. What follows the Mind in its coming and going is the Ethereal Soul, what follows the Essence in its entering and exiting is the Corporeal Soul. The Heart directs mental activities; it houses memory that is called Intellect (Yi); The storing* [of data] *of the Intellect is called Memory (Zhi); Memory generates pensiveness; pensiveness (si 思) generates reflection (lu 虑). Thus the wise nourish life (yang sheng) by following the four seasons, adapting to cold and heat, moderating joy and anger, regulating Yin and Yang and thus will enjoy long life.*

Fear, pensiveness and worry injure the Mind and Spirit. When the Spirit is injured, fear may run wild. When sadness agitates inside, it injures life. Joy scatters the Spirit out of its residence. Worry obstructs Qi so that it stagnates. Anger causes loss of self-control. Fear sweeps the Spirit away. Fright and pensiveness of the Heart injure the Spirit. Worry of the Spleen injures the Intellect. Sadness of the Liver injures the Ethereal Soul which may cause manic behaviour and mental confusion; there is contraction of the sinews, the hypochondrium cannot be raised, the hair withers. The joy of the Lungs injures the Corporeal Soul, when the Corporeal Soul is injured there is manic behaviour and the Yin cannot reside, the skin becomes like heated leather, the hair withers. Anger of the Kidneys injures the Will-Power, when the Will-Power is injured it affects the memory and one does not remember what they said, there is lower backache and inability to bend or extend the back, the hair withers. Fear injures the Essence, this injures the bones. Thus, the five Yin Organs which store the Essence should not be injured; if they are, Yin deficiency results and from this, Qi deficiency.

Therefore when needling one should observe the patient in order to know the condition of the Essence, Mind, Ethereal Soul, Corporeal Soul, and whether they have been preserved or not.

The Liver stores Blood and Blood houses the Ethereal Soul: when Liver-Qi is deficient there is fear; when full, anger. The Spleen stores nourishment and this houses the Intellect: when Spleen-Qi is deficient the four limbs are weak and there is an imbalance in the five Yin Organs; when full, there is abdominal distension and menstrual and urinary problems. The Heart stores the blood vessels and these house the Mind: when Heart-Qi is deficient, there is sadness; when full, incessant laughter. The Lungs store Qi and this houses the Corporeal Soul: when Lung-Qi is deficient, there is nasal obstruction; when full, breathlessness and a feeling of tightness of the chest. The Kidneys store the Essence and this houses Will-Power: when Kidney-Qi is deficient there is collapse; when full, distension and the five Yin Organs are not at peace.

See Figure 9.3.

An interesting aspect of the above passage from the *Spiritual Axis* are the sentences: "*Heaven bestows us Virtue (De), Earth bestows us Qi. When Virtue flows and Qi pulsates, there is life.*" These two sentences show very clearly the Confucian influence on Chinese medicine, i.e. the idea that "Heaven bestows Virtue"; the term "Virtue" is a translation of the Chinese term *De* 德, a typical Confucian term indicating the qualities of the

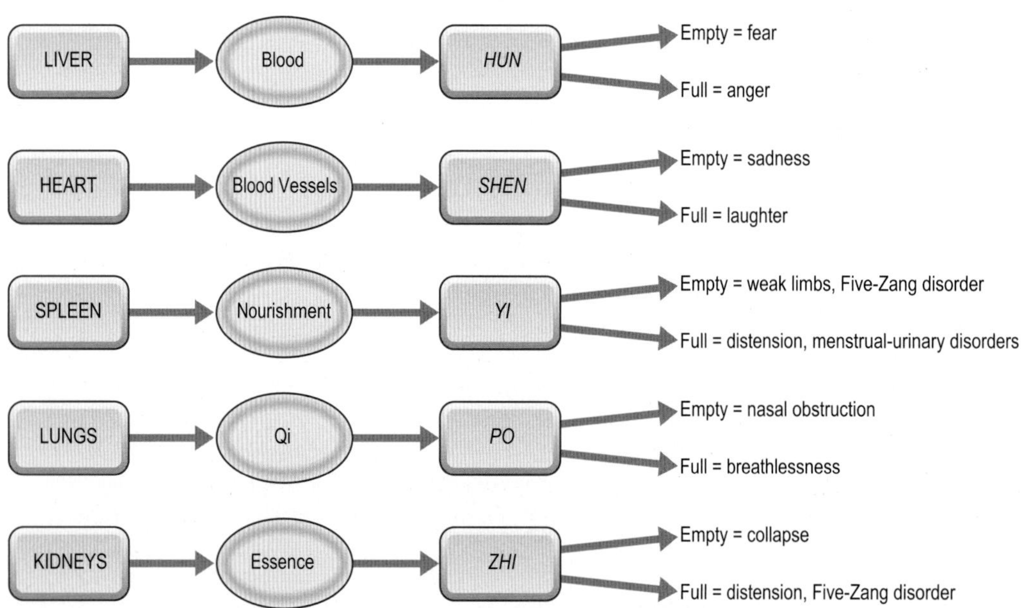

Figure 9.3 Effect of Internal Organs' disharmony on emotional state according to Chapter 8 of the *Spiritual Axis*.

Confucian sage; the translation as "virtue" is inevitably inadequate. This is discussed more fully below.

Chapter 5 of the *Simple Questions* says:[29]

> *Anger injures the Liver, sadness counteracts anger ... joy injures the Heart, fear counteracts joy ... pensiveness injures the Spleen, anger counteracts pensiveness ... worry injures the Lungs, joy counteracts worry ... fear injures the Kidneys, pensiveness counteracts fear.*

An interesting feature of this passage is that each emotion is said to counteract another along the Controlling Sequence of the Five Elements (Fig. 9.4). For example, fear pertains to the Kidneys and Water, Water controls Fire (Heart), the emotion related to the Heart is joy, hence fear counteracts joy. This thinking presents some interesting ideas which are certainly true in practice, e.g. that "anger counteracts pensiveness".

Thus, according to this scheme, emotions counteract each other as follows (Fig. 9.4):

- anger counteracts pensiveness
- joy counteracts sadness
- pensiveness counteracts fear
- sadness counteracts anger
- fear counteracts joy.

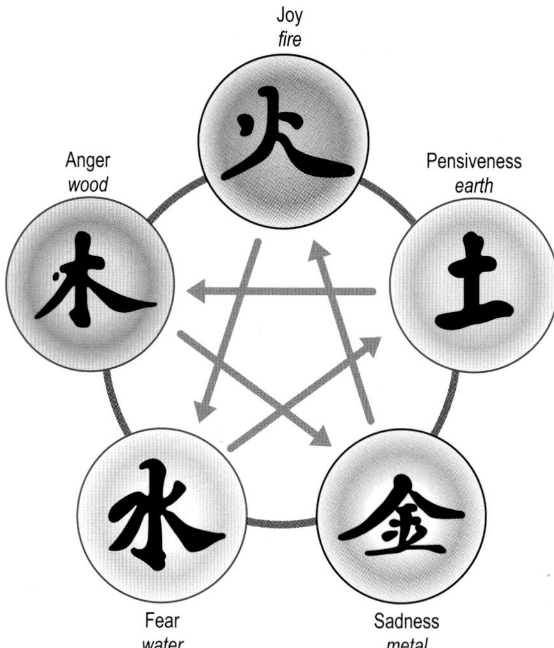

Figure 9.4 Emotions counteracting each other along the Controlling Sequence of the Five Elements.

Besides the above emotions, I shall also discuss some emotions that are not usually mentioned in modern Chinese books but were mentioned in the ancient ones. Moreover, I am also going to discuss some emotions that are never mentioned in Chinese books, modern or ancient. Indeed, the list of emotions that are *not* discussed in Chinese books is very long and the following are some examples:

- pride
- shame
- guilt
- envy
- contempt
- angst
- despair
- hopelessness
- frustration
- hatred
- rejection (being rejected)
- indignation
- humiliation
- regret
- remorse
- self-contempt
- self-hatred
- self-love (narcissism)
- spite
- vanity.

Some of the above emotions could be assimilated with one of the traditional Chinese emotions, e.g. frustration and indignation could be assimilated with "anger".

Besides the usual seven emotions, some Chinese doctors considered other emotions such as grief, love, hatred and desire. Grief would naturally be akin to sadness. "Love" here means not normal love, such as that of a mother towards her child or that between two lovers, but rather the condition when love becomes an obsession or when it is misdirected, as when a person loves someone who persistently hurts them.

Hatred is a common negative emotion which would be akin to anger. "Desire" means excessive craving. The inclusion of this as a cause of disease reflects the Daoist, Confucianist and Buddhist influence on Chinese medicine as all three major Chinese religions/philosophies considered excessive desire as the root of many emotional problems.

Indeed, according to Buddhist thought, desire is the ultimate cause of disease, i.e. clinging to external objects or other people and to life itself. Indeed, from a Buddhist perspective, it is the very "craving" for the warmth of a womb by a soul in the Bardo state (the state in between death and life) that brings our existence into being.

This excessive craving, which is one aspect of the emotion of "joy" in Chinese medicine, causes the Minister Fire to blaze upwards and harass the Mind. Craving as an emotional cause of disease will be discussed in greater detail below.

Finally, two emotions that are common in Western patients but not mentioned in Chinese books are guilt and shame, which will be discussed below.

Thus, the list of emotions could be expanded as follows and these are the emotions I will discuss:

- anger (including frustration and resentment) affecting the Liver
- joy affecting the Heart
- worry affecting the Lungs and Spleen
- pensiveness affecting the Spleen
- sadness and grief affecting the Lungs and Heart
- fear affecting the Kidneys
- shock affecting the Kidneys and Heart
- love affecting the Heart
- craving affecting the Heart
- guilt affecting the Kidneys and Heart
- shame affecting the Heart and Spleen.

I shall first discuss the effects of emotions on Qi in general and then discuss each emotion individually. The discussion of the emotions will be carried out according to the following topics:

- The emotions
- The pathology of Qi and Minister Fire in emotional problems
- The triune brain and Chinese medicine

THE EMOTIONS

As mentioned above, the emotions discussed are:

- anger
- joy
- worry
- pensiveness
- sadness and grief
- fear
- shock
- love
- craving
- guilt
- shame.

Anger

The term "anger", perhaps more than any other emotion, should be interpreted broadly to include several other allied emotional states, such as resentment, repressed anger, feeling aggrieved, frustration, irritation, rage, indignation, animosity or bitterness.

If they persist for a long time, any of these emotional states can affect the Liver, causing stagnation of Liver-Qi, stasis of Liver-Blood, rising of Liver-Yang or blazing of Liver-Fire. Anger (intended in the broad sense outlined above) usually makes Qi rise and many of the symptoms and signs will manifest in the head and neck, such as headaches, tinnitus, dizziness, red blotches on the front part of the neck, a red face, thirst, a bitter taste and a Red tongue with red sides (Fig. 9.5).

Chapter 8 of the *Spiritual Axis* says: "*Anger causes loss of self-control.*"[30] The *Simple Questions* in Chapter 39 says: "*Anger makes Qi rise and causes vomiting of blood and diarrhoea.*"[31] It causes vomiting of blood because it

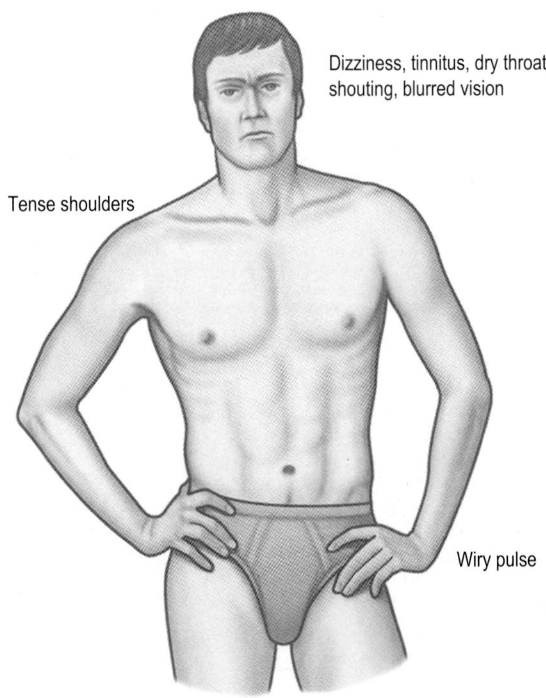

Figure 9.5 Clinical picture of anger.

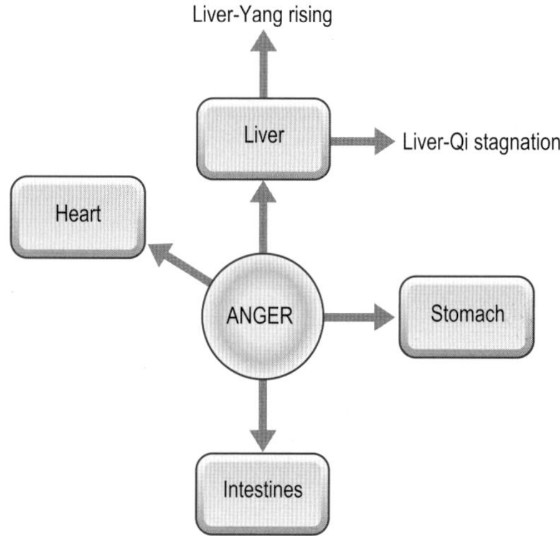

Figure 9.6 Effects of anger.

makes Liver-Qi and Liver-Fire rise and diarrhea because it induces Liver-Qi to invade the Spleen.

Chapter 3 of the *Simple Questions* says: "*Severe anger severs the body and Qi, Blood stagnates in the upper part and the person may suffer from syncope.*"[32]

The effect of anger on the Liver depends, on the one hand, on the person's reaction to the emotional stimulus and, on the other hand, on other concurrent factors. If the anger is bottled up it will cause stagnation of Liver-Qi, whereas if it is expressed it will cause Liver-Yang rising or Liver-Fire blazing (Fig. 9.6). In a woman, stagnation of Liver-Qi may easily lead to stasis of Liver-Blood. If the person also suffers from some Kidney-Yin deficiency (perhaps from overwork), then he or she will develop Liver-Yang rising. If, on the other hand, the person has a tendency to Heat (perhaps from excessive consumption of hot foods), then he or she will tend to develop Liver-Fire blazing.

Anger does not always manifest outwardly with outbursts of anger, irritability, shouting, red face, etc. Some individuals may carry anger inside them for years without ever manifesting it. In particular, long-standing depression may be due to repressed anger or resentment. Because the person is very depressed, he or she may look very subdued and pale, walk slowly and speak with a low voice, all signs which one would associate with a depletion of Qi and Blood deriving from sadness or grief. However, when anger rather than sadness is the cause of disease, the pulse and tongue will clearly show it; the pulse will be Full and Wiry and the tongue will be Red with redder sides and with a dry yellow coating. This type of depression is most probably due to long-standing resentment, often harbored towards a member of that person's family.

In some cases, anger disguises other emotions such as guilt. Some people may harbor guilt inside for many years and may be unable or unwilling to recognize it; they may then use anger as a mask for their guilt.

Moreover, there are some families in which every member is perpetually angry; in these families, anger is used as a mask to hide other emotions such as guilt, fear, dislike of being controlled, weakness or inferiority complex. When this is the case, it is important to be aware of this situation as one needs to treat not the anger, but the underlying psychological and emotional condition.

In some cases anger can affect organs other than the Liver, especially the Stomach. This can be due to stagnant Liver-Qi invading the Stomach. Such a condition is more likely to occur if one gets angry at mealtimes, which may happen if family meals become occasions for regular rows. It also happens when there is a pre-existing weakness of the Stomach, in which case the anger may affect only the Stomach without even affecting the Liver.

If one regularly gets angry an hour or two after meals, then the anger will affect the Intestines rather than the Stomach. This happens, for example, when one goes straight back to a stressful and frustrating job after lunch. In this case, stagnant Liver-Qi invades the Intestines and causes abdominal pain, distension and alternation of constipation with diarrhea.

Finally, anger, like all other emotions, also affects the Heart. This is particularly prone to be affected by anger also because, from a Five-Element perspective, the Liver is the mother of the Heart and often Liver-Fire is transmitted to the Heart giving rise to Heart-Fire. Anger makes the Heart full with blood rushing to it. With time, this leads to Blood-Heat affecting the Heart and therefore the Mind. Anger tends to affect the Heart, particularly when the person does a lot of jogging, hurrying or exercising.

Thus, anger may cause either stagnation of Liver-Qi or Liver-Yang rising. When advising patients on how to deal with their anger, we should note that if anger has caused stagnation of Liver-Qi, expressing the anger may be helpful. However, if anger has given rise to Liver-Yang rising, expressing it will not usually help; it is too late and expressing the anger forcefully may only

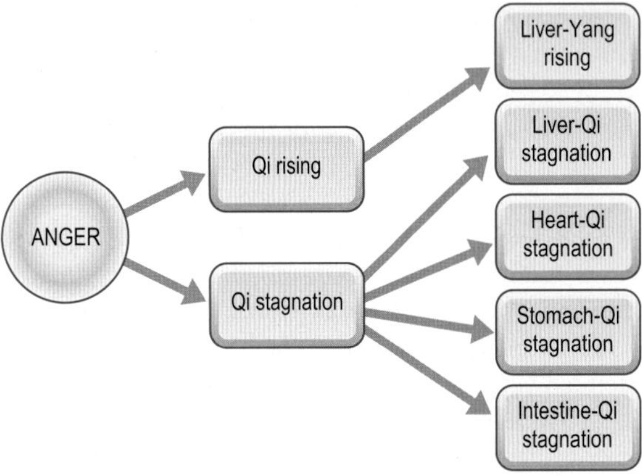

Figure 9.7 Summary of effects of anger.

make Liver-Yang rise even more. Figure 9.7 summarizes the effects of anger and the organs affected by it.

In my opinion, anger is overemphasized as an emotional cause of disease in Chinese books. I feel that this is very much due to the Confucian influence on Chinese medicine. A very important aspect of Confucianism is the emphasis laid on social harmony which, according to them, begins with family harmony which, in turn, is based on the rigid respect of family hierarchy. For example, the younger brother obeys the older brother, the sister obeys the brother, all the children obey the parents, the wife obeys the husband, etc. When every member of the family and society takes his or her proper place and role in the family and social hierarchy, then familial, social and political harmony reigns.

The central place accorded to anger as the most threatening of the emotions is evident from this passage from Zhu Xi (1130–1200), the great Confucian thinker of the Song dynasty:[33]

One's commitments to others should be based on loyalty and honesty; one's conduct should be based on seriousness and watchfulness; a person should control their anger and diminish their desires; a person should correct their mistakes and pay attention to doing good.

> **!**
>
> In my opinion, anger is overemphasized as an emotional cause of disease in Chinese books.

It is easy to see that the emotion that most threatens the established order is anger because this emotion may lead people to rebel. Given the Confucian influence on Chinese medicine, I believe it is for this reason that anger plays such a predominant role among the emotional causes of disease. Cheng Hao (1032–1085), a great Neo-Confucian philosopher of the Song dynasty, says: *"Of all human emotions, anger is the easiest to arouse but the most difficult to control."*[34]

Anger makes Qi "rebel", i.e. go in the wrong direction and it is interesting to note that the Chinese character for "rebellious" Qi is *ni* 逆 which means "rebellious", "contrary", "to counter", "to disobey", "to defy", "to go against"; it is easy to see the "social" nature of this pathological movement of Qi. Indeed, the opposite of *ni* is *shun* 顺 which, in Chinese medicine, denotes Qi going the right, proper way; again it is easy to see the social implication of this term which means "to conform", "in the same direction as", "to obey", "to yield to", "to act in submission to". Indeed, not by chance Mao Ze Dong appealed to the "revolutionary anger" of the Red Guards to overthrow his political opponents.

With regard to Liver-Qi stagnation and anger, there are two issues to consider. First, anger is, in my opinion, overdiagnosed as an emotional cause of disease (see case history below). Second, Qi stagnation does not derive always necessarily from anger and it therefore may affect organs other than the Liver; in emotional problems, Qi stagnation may affect especially the Lungs, Heart and Spleen. It follows that when we diagnose Qi stagnation in a patient we should not assume that it is necessarily due to Liver-Qi stagnation and to anger; worry, sadness, grief and guilt may all cause Qi stagnation in the Lungs and/or Heart. The patterns of Qi stagnation in the Lungs and Heart are mentioned below.

How can we diagnose whether Qi stagnation is due to the Liver or to another organ? Apart from the difference in symptoms, the pulse is an important diagnostic factor. Generally, in Liver-Qi stagnation the pulse is Wiry in all positions. In Qi stagnation due to other organs, the pulse is Wiry only in that organ's position; moreover, it may be Tight rather than Wiry. The Lungs are a good case in point; in Lung-Qi stagnation, the Lung pulse is often very slightly Tight (bearing in mind that the Lung pulse should naturally feel relatively soft and therefore it takes only a very small change to make it "Tight").

CLINICAL NOTE

The points I use for anger are LIV-3 Taichong, G.B.-20 Fengchi, Du-19 Houding, G.B.-13 Benshen and HE-7 Shenmen.

THE PULSE IN ANGER

When anger is the emotional cause of disease, the pulse is Wiry, whether the anger is repressed or not. In Liver-Yang rising the pulse is Wiry and more superficial; in Liver-Qi stagnation, the pulse is Wiry and less superficial than the former. In anger, the pulse is Wiry in all or most positions. If the pulse is relatively Wiry in one position only, the emotion involved may not be anger. For example, worry affecting the Lungs may make the Lung pulse slightly Wiry.

Case history

This case history is presented here to show how, in my opinion, Western therapists also sometimes overemphasize anger as an emotional cause of disease.

A 33-year-old woman complained of a variety of physical symptoms such as some skin eruptions on the arms, a slight breathlessness, some abdominal distension and premenstrual tension.

On an emotional level, she was depressed and her immediate problem was a feeling of sadness deriving from the break-up of a relationship. She found it difficult to keep to a long-term relationship and seemed to go from one unsuitable relationship to another, ending up feeling used by men.

This patient had a history of sexual abuse from her stepfather when she was a teenager. She was under therapy and her therapist suggested that she had repressed anger about the sexual abuse and that she should acknowledge it and manifest it. In my opinion, her pulse and other signs completely contradicted this analysis.

Her pulse was Weak and soft in general and the weakest pulse of all was that of the Lungs; the Heart pulse was very slightly Overflowing. Her complexion was very pale and her voice was very weak.

On the basis of the pulse, complexion and voice, I diagnosed primarily Lung-Qi deficiency and Qi stagnation of the Lungs and Heart. Therefore, in my opinion, in her case, the prevailing emotion deriving from her history of sexual abuse was not anger but sadness and grief.

The counterpart of anger in terms of mental energies is power, dynamism, creativity and generosity. The same energy which is dissipated in outbursts of anger can be harnessed to achieve one's goals in life. It is probably for this reason that the Gall-Bladder (closely related to the Liver) is said to be the source of courage. A strong Gall-Bladder gives one the courage to make decisions and changes in one's life. This aspect of the Gall-Bladder's functions is obviously closely linked to the Liver and the Ethereal Soul. If Liver-Blood is deficient there is fear; therefore if Liver-Blood is abundant the person will be fearless and decisive.

SUMMARY

Anger

- The term "anger" should be interpreted broadly to include resentment, repressed anger, feeling aggrieved, frustration, irritation, rage, indignation, animosity or bitterness.
- Anger makes Qi rise and many of the symptoms and signs will manifest in the head and neck, such as headaches, tinnitus, dizziness, red blotches on the front part of the neck, a red face, thirst, a bitter taste and a Red tongue with red sides.
- If the anger is bottled up it will cause stagnation of Liver-Qi, whereas if it is expressed it will cause Liver-Yang rising or Liver-Fire blazing.
- Anger may sometimes disguise itself as depression.
- Anger may mask guilt.
- Anger can affect organs other than the Liver, e.g. Stomach and Intestines.
- Anger, like all other emotions, also affects the Heart.
- Anger is probably overemphasized as an emotional cause of disease in Chinese books due to the Confucian influence on Chinese medicine.
- Qi stagnation does not derive always necessarily from anger and it may affect organs other than the Liver; in emotional problems, especially the Lungs, Heart and Spleen.

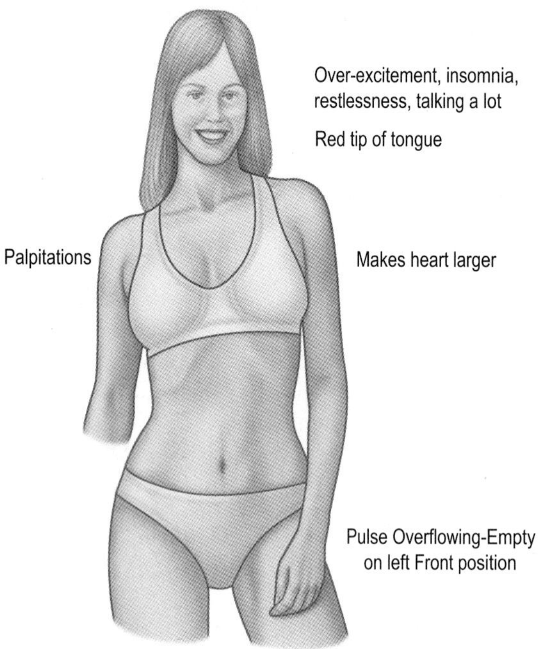

Figure 9.8 Clinical picture of joy.

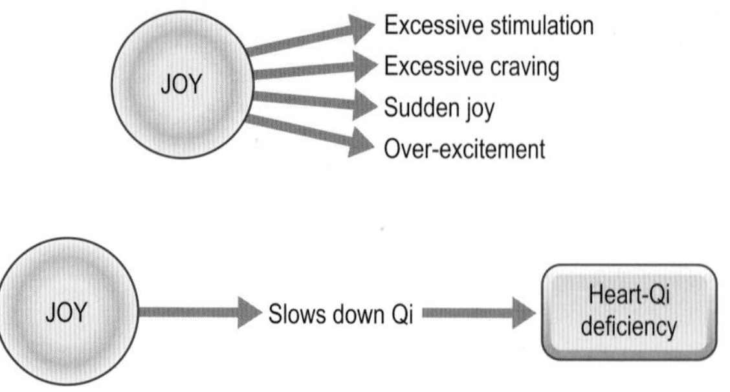

Figure 9.9 Effect of joy.

Joy

A normal state of joy is obviously not in itself a cause of disease; on the contrary, it is a beneficial mental state which promotes a smooth functioning of the Internal Organs and their mental faculties. The *Simple Questions* in Chapter 39 says: "*Joy makes the Mind peaceful and relaxed, it benefits the Nutritive and Defensive Qi and it makes Qi relax and slow down.*"[35] On the other hand, in Chapter 2 the *Simple Questions* says: "*The Heart ... controls joy, joy injures the Heart, fear counteracts joy.*"[36] See Figure 9.8.

What is meant by "joy" as a cause of disease is obviously not a state of healthy contentment but one of excessive excitement and craving which can injure the Heart. This happens to people who live in a state of continuous mental stimulation (however pleasurable) or excessive excitement; in other words, a life of "hard playing".

As indicated above, "desire" or inordinate craving is an aspect of the emotion "joy". "Desire" is considered as a negative emotion by all three main Chinese philosophies, i.e. Daoism, Confucianism and Buddhism. Desire stirs up the Minister Fire which overstimulates the Mind. Craving as an emotional cause of disease is discussed in greater detail below.

Chapter 5 of the *Simple Questions* says: "*Joy injures the Heart.*"[37] Chapter 8 of the *Spiritual Axis* says: "*Joy scatters the Heart and deprives it of its residence.*"[38]

Joy, in the broad sense indicated above, makes the Heart larger. This leads to excessive stimulation of the Heart which, in time, may lead to Heart-related symptoms and signs (Fig. 9.9). These may deviate somewhat from the classic Heart patterns. The main manifestations would be palpitations, over-excitability, insomnia, restlessness, talking a lot and a red tip of the tongue. The pulse would typically be slow, slightly Overflowing but Empty on the left Front position.

> **THE PULSE IN JOY**
>
> Contrary to what one might think, when joy is the emotional cause of disease the pulse becomes Slow; this happens because joy dilates the Heart and therefore slows circulation. In addition, the pulse will be relatively Overflowing but Empty on the Heart position.

Joy may also be marked out as a cause of disease when it is sudden; this happens, for example, on hearing good news unexpectedly. In this situation, "joy" is akin to shock (although the former makes the heart larger and the latter smaller). Fei Bo Xiong (1800–1879) in *Medical Collection of Four Doctors from the Meng He Tradition* says: "*Joy injures the Heart ...* [it causes] *Yang Qi to float and the blood vessels to become too open and dilated ...*"[39]

In these cases of sudden joy and excitement the Heart dilates and slows down and the pulse becomes Slow and slightly Overflowing but Empty. One can understand the effect of sudden joy further if one thinks of situations when a migraine attack is precipitated by the excitement of suddenly hearing good news. Another example of joy as a cause of disease is that of sudden laughter triggering a heart attack; this example also confirms the relationship existing between the Heart and laughter.

One can also understand joy as a cause of disease by observing children; in fact, in children, joy and over-excitement often end in tears.

The best way to understand why "joy" features in Chinese medicine is in relation to the three major Chinese religions, i.e. Confucianism, Buddhism and Daoism. All three religions (or rather philosophies), for different reasons, advocated emotional restraint.

For example, the Daoists shunned social relations and advocated "following the Dao", "absence of desire" (*wu yu*) and "non-action" (*wu wei*). They felt that joy would stop us from following the Dao as much as emotions such as anger.

The Buddhists considered most emotions as the root of human suffering. According to them, our very existence begins out of desire and craving when the mind in the Bardo state (the period after death and before the next reincarnation) is attracted by the warmth of a womb and it reincarnates. Later on in life, desire causes our mind to try to grasp objects like a monkey sways from tree to tree.

Finally, Confucianists believed that the true "gentleman" (a mistranslation of the term *jun zi* that actually applies to both men and women) is not stirred by emotions because these cloud his or her true nature. They used the image of a pond with a muddy bottom. If the water is very still, it becomes clear; if we stir the bottom, the water becomes turbid. The pond is our human nature which is naturally "clear"; if we are stirred by emotions, these will cloud our human nature.

CLINICAL NOTE

The points I use for "excess joy" are HE-7 Shenmen, P-7 Daling, Du-19 Houding and Ren-15 Jiuwei.

SUMMARY

Joy

- A normal state of joy is obviously not in itself a cause of disease.
- What is meant by "joy" as a cause of disease is obviously not a state of healthy contentment but one of excessive excitement and craving which can injure the Heart.
- Joy makes the Heart larger.
- All three major Chinese religions, i.e. Confucianism, Buddhism and Daoism, for different reasons, considered emotions (including "joy") to be disturbing factors clouding our human nature.

Worry

Worry is one of the most common emotional causes of disease in our society. The extremely rapid and radical social changes that have occurred in Western societies in the past decades have created a climate of such insecurity in all spheres of life that very few people are immune to worry (Fig. 9.10).

Of course, there are also people who, because of a pre-existing disharmony of the internal organs, are very prone to worry, even about very minor incidents in life. For example, many people appear to be very tense and worry a lot. On close interrogation about their work and family life, often nothing of note emerges. They simply worry excessively about trivial

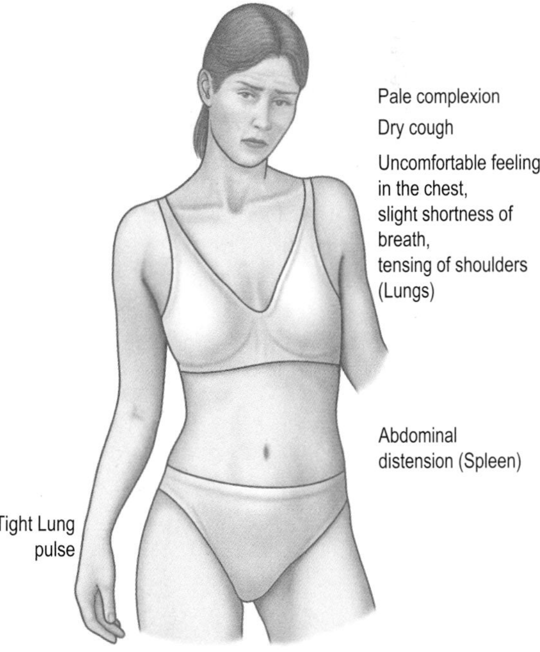

Figure 9.10 Clinical picture of worry.

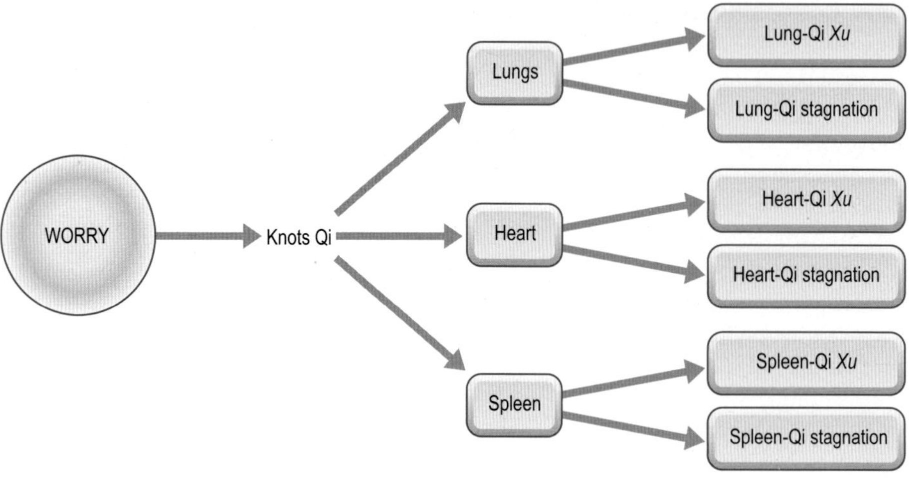

Figure 9.11 Effect of worry.

everyday activities and they tend to do everything in a hurry and be pressed for time. This may be due to a constitutional weakness of the Spleen, Heart or Lungs, or a combination of these.

Chen Wu Ze (1174) says: "*Worry injures the Lungs and makes Qi accumulate.*"[40]

Chapter 8 of the *Spiritual Axis* confirms that worry knots Qi: "*Worry causes obstruction of Qi so that Qi stagnates.*"[41]

Worry knots Qi, which means that it causes stagnation of Qi, and it affects both Lungs and Spleen; the Lungs because when one is worried breathing is shallow, and the Spleen because this organ is responsible for thinking and ideas (Fig. 9.11). Thus, from this point of view, worry is the pathological counterpart of the Spleen's capacity for concentration and focus.

Worry may affect the Spleen as well and Chapter 8 of the *Spiritual Axis* confirms that: "*In the case of the Spleen, excessive worry injures the Intellect [Yi].*"[42] Zhang Jie Bin says: "*Worry is the emotion pertaining to the Lungs but it injures the Spleen too because of the Mother–Child relationship between them.*"[43]

CLINICAL NOTE

Worry knots Lung-Qi and causes Lung-Qi stagnation. LU-7 Lieque is the best point to treat Lung-Qi stagnation deriving from worry.

In many cases, worry may also affect the Liver directly, in my experience causing either Liver-Qi stagnation or Liver-Yang rising. In both cases, when worry affects the Liver, it affects the shoulder muscles, causing a pronounced stiffness and ache of the trapezius muscles. As we have seen above, Zhang Jie Bin did consider that worry affects the Liver.

!

Worry may affect the Liver directly causing either Liver-Qi stagnation or Liver-Yang rising, in both cases resulting in ache and stiffness of the trapezius muscles.

The symptoms and signs caused by worry will vary according to whether it affects the Lungs or the Spleen. If worry affects the Lungs it will cause an uncomfortable feeling of the chest, slight breathlessness, tensing of the shoulders, sometimes a dry cough and a pale complexion.

The right Front pulse position (of the Lungs) may feel slightly Tight or Wiry, indicating the knotting action of worry on Qi. When judging the quality of the Lung pulse, one should bear in mind that, in normal circumstances, this should naturally feel relatively soft (in relation to the other pulse positions). Thus a Lung pulse that feels as hard as a (normal) Liver pulse may well be Tight or Wiry.

If worry affects the Spleen it may cause poor appetite, a slight epigastric discomfort, some abdominal pain and distension, tiredness and a pale complexion. The right Middle pulse position (Spleen) will feel slightly Tight but Weak. If worry also affects the Stomach (which happens if one worries at meal times), the right Middle pulse may be Tight but Empty.

Finally, like all emotions, worry affects the Heart causing stagnation of Heart-Qi. This will cause palpitations, a slight feeling of tightness of the chest and insomnia.

THE PULSE IN WORRY

When worry is the emotional cause of disease, the Lung position may feel slightly Tight or Wiry (bearing in mind that the Lung pulse is naturally relatively soft and it takes a very small hardening to make it "Tight" or "Wiry").

If worry affects the Spleen the Spleen position will feel slightly Tight but Weak. If worry also affects the Stomach, the right Middle pulse may be Tight but Empty.

CLINICAL NOTE

The points I use for worry are LU-7 Lieque, HE-7 Shenmen, L.I.-4 Hegu and Du-24 Shenting.

SUMMARY

Worry

- Worry is one of the most common emotional causes of disease in our society.
- Worry knots Qi, which means that it causes stagnation of Qi, and it affects both Lungs and Spleen.
- In some cases, worry may affect the Liver.
- Like all emotions, worry affects the Heart, causing stagnation of Heart-Qi.

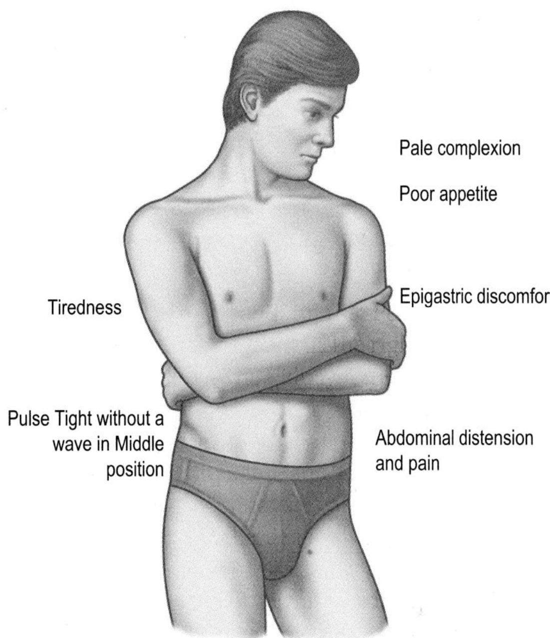

Figure 9.12 Clinical picture of pensiveness.

Pensiveness

Pensiveness is very similar to worry in its character and effect. It consists of brooding, constantly thinking about certain events or people (even though not worrying), nostalgic hankering after the past and generally thinking intensely about life rather than living it. In extreme cases, pensiveness leads to obsessive thoughts. In a different sense, pensiveness also includes excessive mental work in the process of one's work or study (Fig. 9.12).

Some modern Chinese doctors think that "pensiveness" is an umbrella term that includes several different emotions. The modern book *Chinese Medicine Psychology* says that "pensiveness" includes pondering, sadness and resentment.[44] The inclusion of "resentment" under the umbrella of "pensiveness" is interesting as I would associate resentment more with anger. However, it does have elements of both anger and "pensiveness" (intended in the sense of brooding).

The same doctor thinks that "pensiveness" replaced "sadness" in the list of emotions. In fact, Chapter 5 of the *Simple Questions* lists the five emotions as joy, anger, sadness, worry and fear, while later they became joy, anger, pensiveness, worry and fear.[45]

Pensiveness affects the Spleen and, like worry, it knots Qi. Chapter 39 of the *Simple Questions* says: "*Pensiveness makes the Heart* [Qi] *accumulate, causing the Mind to stagnate; the Upright Qi settles and does not move, and therefore Qi stagnates.*"[46]

Chen Wu Ze (1174) says:[47]

Pensiveness injures the Spleen, Qi stagnates and does not move properly, there is accumulation in the Middle

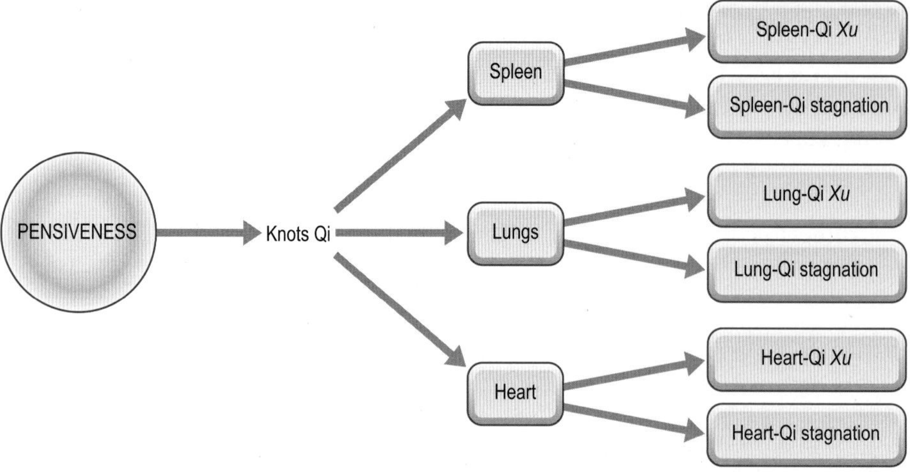

Figure 9.13 Effect of pensiveness.

Burner, food cannot be digested, there is abdominal distension and contraction of the limbs. Pensiveness causes Qi stagnation.

Pensiveness causes similar symptoms as outlined above for worry, i.e. poor appetite, a slight epigastric discomfort, some abdominal pain and distension, tiredness and a pale complexion (Fig. 9.13). The right Middle pulse position (Spleen) will feel slightly Tight but Weak.

The only difference will be that the pulse on the right side will not only feel slightly Tight, but will also have no wave. One can feel the normal pulse as a wave under the fingers moving from the Rear towards the Front position. The pulse without wave lacks this flowing movement from Rear to Front position and it is instead felt as if each individual position were separate from the others (Fig. 9.14). In the case of pensiveness, the pulse will lack a wave only on the right Middle position. A pulse without wave in the Front and Middle positions indicates sadness.

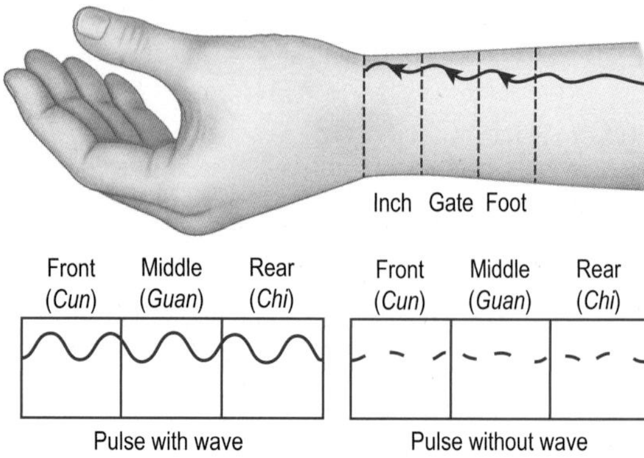

Figure 9.14 Pulse without wave.

THE PULSE IN PENSIVENESS

When pensiveness is the emotional cause of disease, the pulse will be slightly Tight but Weak on the Spleen position. In addition, the pulse of the right Middle position will not only feel slightly Tight, but will also have no wave.

CLINICAL NOTE

The normal pulse should feel like a wave undulating from the Rear towards the Front positions. To feel the wave, one must rest all three fingers on the pulse. A pulse without wave is felt within the individual positions but it does not flow smoothly from one position to the other. A pulse without wave generally indicates sadness. Some pulse qualities by definition refer to a pulse without wave, e.g. Choppy, Short or Scattered.

The positive mental energy corresponding to pensiveness is quiet contemplation and meditation. The same mental energy which makes us capable of meditation and contemplation will, if excessive and misguided, lead to pensiveness, brooding or even obsessive thinking.

CLINICAL NOTE

The points I use for pensiveness are SP-3 Taibai, LU-7 Lieque, Du-24 Shenting, Ren-12 Zhongwan and BL-20 Pishu.

SUMMARY

Pensiveness

- Pensiveness consists of brooding, constantly thinking about certain events or people (even though not worrying), nostalgic hankering after the past and generally thinking intensely about life rather than living it.
- In extreme cases, pensiveness leads to obsessive thoughts.
- Pensiveness also includes excessive mental work in the process of one's work or study.
- Pensiveness affects the Spleen and, like worry, it knots Qi.

Sadness and grief

Sadness and grief are very pervasive emotions in Western patients; in my opinion, they are probably the most common emotional causes of disease in Western patients. Sadness and grief usually derive from loss.

Sadness includes the emotion of regret, as when someone regrets a certain action or decision in the past and the Mind is constantly turned towards that time. Sadness and grief affect the Lungs and Heart (Fig. 9.15).

In fact, according to the *Simple Questions*, sadness affects the Lungs via the Heart. It says in Chapter 39:[48]

Sadness makes the Heart cramped and agitated; this pushes towards the lungs' lobes, the Upper Burner becomes obstructed, Nutritive and Defensive Qi cannot circulate freely, Heat accumulates and dissolves Qi.

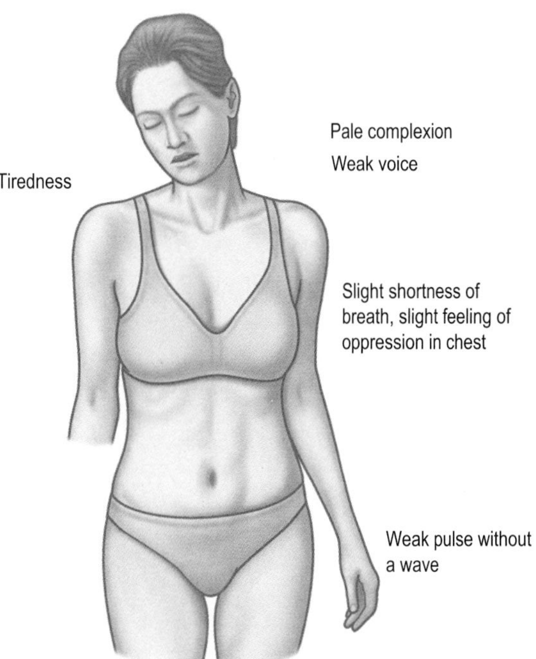

Figure 9.15 Clinical picture of sadness and grief.

According to this passage then, sadness primarily affects the Heart and the Lungs suffer in consequence since they are both situated in the Upper Burner.

A passage in Chapter 44 of the *Simple Questions* confirms this when it says: "*Sadness breaks off the Pericardium channel and agitates Yang inside; this causes bleeding under the heart.*"[49] An English translation of the *Simple Questions* by Chinese doctors translates "bleeding under the heart" as "hematuria".

The Lungs govern Qi and sadness and grief deplete Qi (Fig. 9.16). This is often manifested on the pulse as a Weak quality on both left and right Front positions (Heart and Lungs). In particular, the pulse on both Front positions is Short and has no wave, i.e. it does not flow smoothly towards the thumb.

As indicated above, one can feel the normal pulse as a wave under the fingers moving from the Rear towards the Front position. The pulse without wave lacks this flowing movement from Rear to Front position and it is instead felt as if each individual position were separate from the others. In the case of sadness, the pulse lacks a wave in the Front and Middle positions.

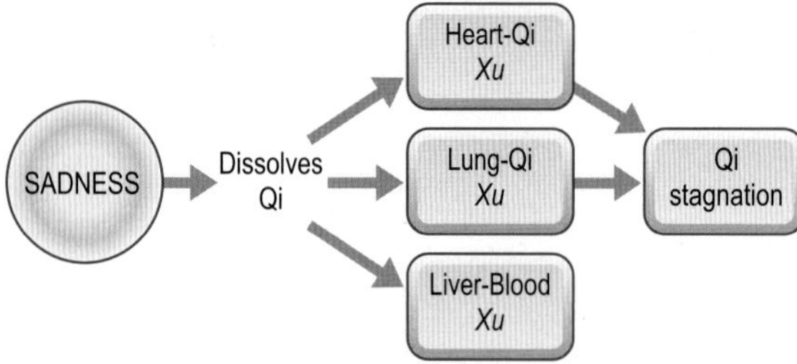

Figure 9.16 Effect of sadness and grief.

THE PULSE IN SADNESS

When sadness is the emotional cause of disease, the pulse is Weak on both left and right Front positions (Heart and Lungs). In particular, the pulse on both Front positions is Short and has no wave, i.e. it does not flow smoothly towards the thumb. In the case of sadness, the pulse lacks a wave in the Front and Middle positions.

Sadness may also cause Qi stagnation in the Heart and Lungs, in which case the pulse would be very slightly Tight on both Front positions.

CLINICAL NOTE

Sadness causes the pulse to lack a "wave"; instead of feeling like a wave flowing from the Rear to the Front position, it feels as if each pulse position were separate. Such a pulse is a very reliable sign of sadness.

Other manifestations deriving from sadness and grief include a weak voice, tiredness, pale complexion, slight breathlessness, weeping and a slight feeling of oppression in the chest. In women, deficiency of Lung-Qi from sadness or grief often leads to Blood deficiency and amenorrhea.

Although sadness and grief deplete Qi and therefore lead to deficiency of Qi, they may also, after some time, lead to stagnation of Qi, because the deficient Lung- and Heart-Qi fail to circulate properly in the chest, in which case the pulse may be slightly Tight on both Front positions.

As mentioned before, each emotion can affect other organs apart from its "specific" one. For example, the *Spiritual Axis* in Chapter 8 mentions injury of the Liver from sadness rather than anger: "*When sadness affects the Liver it injures the Ethereal Soul; this causes mental confusion ... the Yin is damaged, the tendons contract and there is hypochondrial discomfort.*"[50] This shows how organs can be affected by emotions other than their "specific" one. In this case, sadness can naturally affect the Ethereal Soul and therefore Liver-Yin. Sadness has a depleting effect on Qi and it therefore, in some cases, depletes Liver-Yin, leading to mental confusion, depression, lack of a sense of direction in life and inability to plan one's life.

Case history

A 40-year-old woman was under a great deal of stress due to her divorce which caused her great sadness. She often felt weepy. She felt aimless and questioned her role in her relationships with men; she was at a turning point in her life and did not know what direction to take. She slept badly and her pulse was Choppy.

This is a clear example of sadness affecting the Liver and therefore the Ethereal Soul. She was treated, improving tremendously, with the Yin Linking Vessel (*Yin Wei Mai*) points (P-6 Neiguan on the right and SP-4 Gongsun on the left) and BL-23 Shenshu, BL-52 Zhishi and BL-47 Hunmen.

Dr John Shen considers that grief that is unexpressed and borne without tears affects the Kidneys. According to him, when grief is held in without weeping, the fluids cannot come out (in the form of tears) and they upset the fluid metabolism within the Kidneys. This would happen only in situations when grief had been felt for many years.[51]

I personally find that sadness and grief are very common and important causes of disease in Western patients, much more than "anger". As I indicated above, I personally feel that anger as an emotional cause of disease is overemphasized in Chinese books.

What are sadness and grief caused by in Western patients? Apart from the obvious causes due to bereavement, very many Western patients of all ages suffer from sadness and grief deriving from the break-up of relationships or marriage. In other words, sadness and grief are primarily about *loss*, whether it be the loss of a dear one from death or the loss of a partner through separation.

McLean (who elaborated the theory of the triune brain, Chapter 14) suggests that the origins of human language were most likely in infant–mother interaction, babbling based on vowel–consonant combinations beginning about 8 weeks after birth. He singles out the separation cry – a slowly changing tone with a prolonged vowel sound (*aaah*), a distressing cry linked with the most painful emotion, separation.[52] I believe that the grief deriving from separation is probably the most basic and primordial (and therefore most powerful) emotion that plays a huge role in the mental-emotional problems we see in practice.

It is very important to remember that Qi stagnation affects not only the Liver but, especially in emotional problems, also the Heart and Lungs. Sadness, grief and worry are common causes of Qi stagnation affecting the Lungs and Heart. For example, in women, Lung-Qi stagnation affects the chest and breasts and, in the long run, it can give rise to breast lumps (benign or malignant). In my experience, in Western women, this is a more common cause of breast lumps than Liver-Qi stagnation.

Dr Xia Shao Nong thinks that breast lumps and breast cancer are due to sadness and grief deriving from widowhood, breaking of relationships, divorce, death of one's children, and bereavement at a young age from the death of one's spouse. These events, especially if they occur suddenly, upset the Mind and lead to Qi stagnation and Qi depletion. It is interesting to note that all the events mentioned by Dr Xia involve *separation* and *loss*.

CLINICAL NOTE

The points I use for sadness and grief are LU-7 Lieque, Du-24 Shenting, Ren-15 Jiuwei, HE-7 Shenmen, BL-13 Feishu and Du-12 Shenzhu.

SUMMARY

Sadness and grief

- Sadness and grief affect the Lungs and Heart.
- Sadness and grief deplete Qi.
- Sadness often causes a pulse "without wave", i.e. the pulse lacks a flowing movement from Rear to Front position and it is instead felt as if each individual position were separate from the others. In the case of sadness, the pulse lacks a wave in the Front and Middle positions.
- Sadness and grief deplete Qi but, after some time, they also lead to stagnation of Qi.
- In some cases, sadness injures the Liver.
- According to Dr John Shen, grief that is unexpressed and borne without tears affects the Kidneys.
- Sadness and grief often derive from the break-up of relationships or marriage.

Fear

Fear includes a chronic state of fear, anxiety or a sudden fright. Fear depletes Kidney-Qi and it makes Qi descend. The *Simple Questions* in Chapter 39 says: "*Fear depletes the Essence, it blocks the Upper Burner, which makes Qi descend to the Lower Burner.*"[53] Examples of Qi descending are nocturnal enuresis in children and incontinence of urine or diarrhea in adults, following a sudden fright. See Figure 9.17. In fear intended in the sense of fright, the Kidney pulse is Weak.

This statement from the *Simple Questions* is interesting in that it says that fear *blocks* the Upper Burner (resulting in Qi of the Lower Burner to descend); this would imply that fear does not simply "make Qi descend" (as we usually say) but that it also causes some Qi stagnation in the Upper Burner (Fig. 9.18).

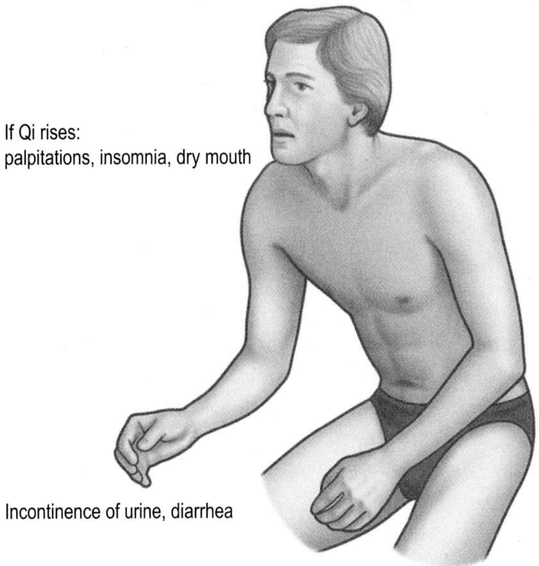

Figure 9.17 Clinical picture of fear.

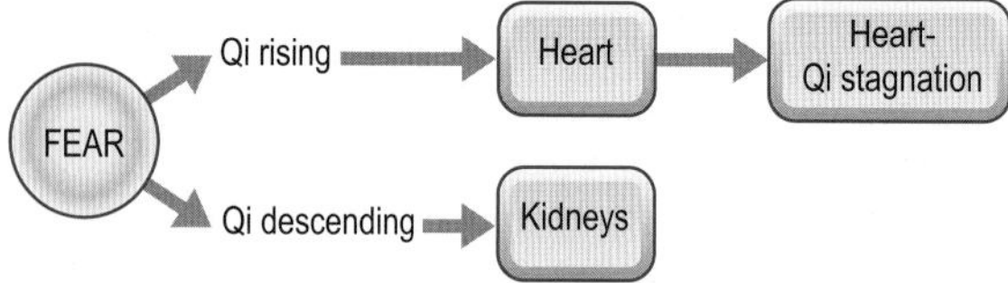

Figure 9.18 Effect of fear.

> **CLINICAL NOTE**
>
> Fear makes Qi descend by *blocking* the Upper Burner. Treatment of fear, therefore, should not consist simply in lifting Qi, e.g. with Du-20 Baihui, but also in unblocking Qi in the Upper Burner with HE-5 Tongli and LU-7 Lieque.

Situations of chronic anxiety and fear will have different effects on Qi depending on the state of the Heart. If the Heart is strong, fear will cause Qi to descend; however, if the Heart is weak, it will cause Qi to rise with such symptoms as palpitations, insomnia, a dry mouth, a malar flush, dizziness and a pulse that is relatively Overflowing on both Front positions and Rapid. In such a situation, the Kidney pulse is Weak and the Heart pulse is relatively Overflowing.

In my opinion, fear (in response to an actual external stimulus) does cause Qi to descend, but a chronic state of anxiety makes Qi rise. Some psychologists make a distinction between fear and anxiety which clarifies their different effect on Qi. Öhman says: "*Fear differs from anxiety primarily in having an identifiable eliciting stimulus. Anxiety is 'pre-stimulus' whereas fear is 'post-stimulus'.*"[54] Epstein thinks that fear is related to coping behavior, particularly escape and avoidance. However, when coping attempts fail, fear is turned into anxiety. Fear is therefore an avoidance motive; anxiety is unresolved fear or a state of undirected arousal following the perception of threat.[55]

In my experience, independently of the patterns involved, in chronic anxiety there is always a disconnection between the Heart and Kidneys. In physiology, Heart- and Kidney-Qi communicate with each other, with Heart-Qi descending towards the Kidneys and Kidney-Qi ascending towards the Heart. Chronic anxiety makes Qi rise towards the Heart and "cramps" it. Heart-Qi cannot descend to the Kidneys and the Kidneys cannot root it (*see Fig. 17.4*).

The correlation between fear and the Kidneys that exists in Chinese medicine is interestingly mirrored in the Western view of our reaction to stress and fear. In fact, when we are subject to fear-causing situations, the adrenal glands (i.e. the "Kidneys" of Chinese medicine) secrete a steroid hormone.

> **THE PULSE IN FEAR**
>
> Fear intended in the sense of fright causes the Kidney pulse to become Weak. In chronic anxiety characterized by a disconnection between Heart and Kidneys, the Kidney pulse is Weak and the Heart pulse is relatively Overflowing.

There are other causes of fear, not related to the Kidneys. Liver-Blood deficiency and a Gall-Bladder deficiency can also make the person fearful. Chapter 8 of the *Spiritual Axis* says: "*If Liver-Qi is deficient there is fear.*"[56]

The positive counterpart of fear within the mental energies of the Kidneys is flexibility, yielding in the face of adversity and quiet endurance of hardship.

> **CLINICAL NOTE**
>
> The points I use for fear are KI-3 Taixi, KI-4 Dazhong, Du-20 Baihui and HE-7 Shenmen.

> **SUMMARY**
>
> **Fear**
>
> - Fear includes a chronic state of fear, anxiety and a sudden fright.
> - Fear depletes Kidney-Qi and it makes Qi descend.
> - Situations of chronic anxiety and fear will have different effects on Qi depending on the state of the Heart; if the Heart is strong, fear will cause Qi to descend, but if the Heart is weak, it will cause Qi to rise in the form of Empty Heat.
> - Liver-Blood deficiency and a Gall-Bladder deficiency can also make the person fearful.

Shock

Mental shock scatters Qi and affects the Heart and Kidneys. It causes a sudden depletion of Heart-Qi, makes the Heart smaller and may lead to palpitations, breathlessness and insomnia. See Figure 9.19.

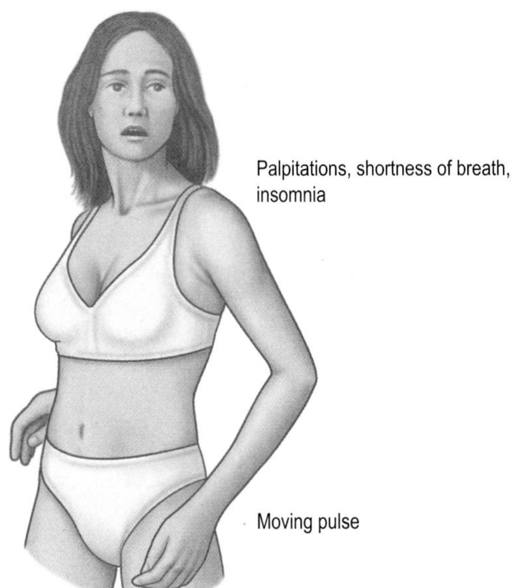

Figure 9.19 Clinical picture of shock.

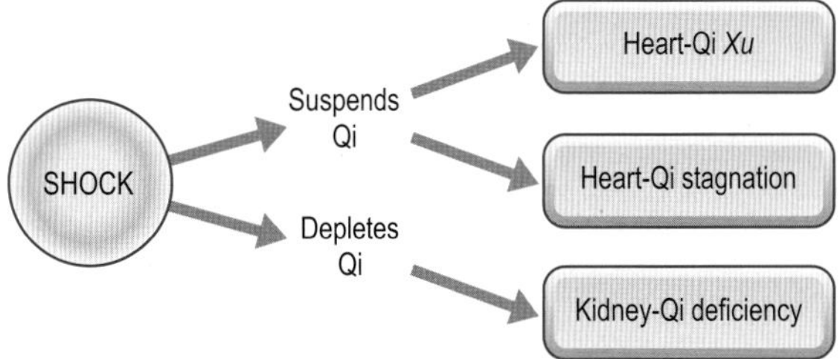

Figure 9.20 Effect of shock.

Shock is often reflected in the pulse with the "Moving" (*Dong*) quality, i.e. a pulse that is short, slippery, shaped like a bean, rapid and giving the impression of vibrating as it pulsates.

The *Simple Questions* in Chapter 39 says: "*Shock affects the Heart, depriving it of residence; the Mind has no shelter and cannot rest, so that Qi becomes chaotic.*"[57]

Shock "closes" the Heart or makes the Heart smaller. This can be observed in a bluish tinge on the forehead and a Heart pulse which is Tight and Fine (Fig. 9.20).

THE PULSE IN SHOCK

When shock is the emotional cause of disease the pulse is "Moving" (*Dong*), i.e. a pulse that is short, slippery, shaped like a bean, rapid and giving the impression of vibrating as it pulsates. The pulse will also be Tight and Fine.

Shock also affects the Kidneys because the body draws on the Kidney-Essence to supplement the sudden depletion of Qi. For this reason, shock can cause such symptoms as night-sweating, a dry mouth, dizziness or tinnitus.

CLINICAL NOTE

The points I use for shock are HE-7 Shenmen, Du-20 Baihui, Ren-15 Jiuwei and KI-4 Dazhong.

SUMMARY

Shock

- Mental shock scatters Qi and affects Heart and Kidneys.
- It causes a sudden depletion of Heart-Qi and makes the Heart smaller.
- Shock also affects the Kidneys because the body draws on the Kidney-Essence to supplement the sudden depletion of Qi.

Love

Here "love" does not refer to the normal affection felt by human beings towards one another, such as, for example, the love of parents for their children and vice-versa, or the affection of a loving couple, but rather obsessive love for a particular person. Love also becomes a cause of disease when it is misdirected as happens, for example, when a person loves someone who persistently hurts them, whether physically or mentally. Obsessive jealousy would also fall under the broad category of "love" (Fig. 9.21).

The inclusion of "love" among disease-causing emotions in Chinese medicine is interesting as it may reflect a totally different attitude and view of love from the one we have in the West. Shaver, Wu and Schwartz interviewed young people in the USA, Italy and the People's Republic of China about their emotional experiences.

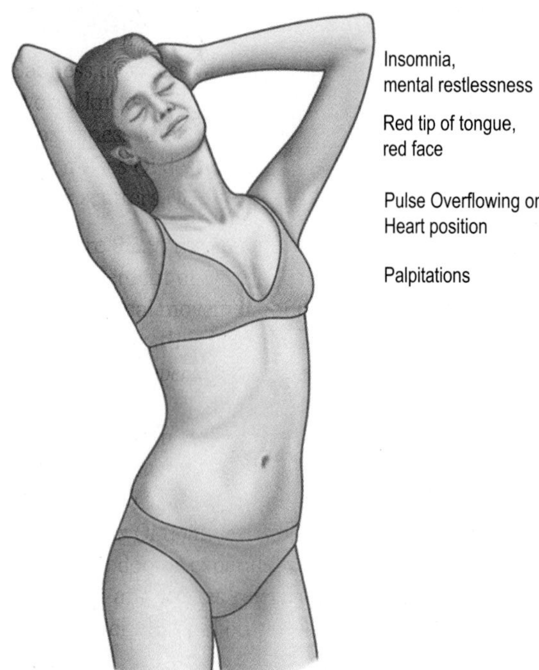

Figure 9.21 Clinical picture of love.

In all cultures, men and women identified the same emotions and they agreed completely except on one emotion, love. The US and Italian subjects equated love with happiness; both passionate and compassionate love were assumed to be intensely positive experiences. Chinese students, however, had a darker view of love. In China, passionate love tended to be associated with such ideographs as "infatuation", "unrequited love", "nostalgia" and "sorrow-love".[58]

"Love" in the sense outlined above affects the Heart and it quickens Qi. This will be felt on the left Front position (Heart) with an Overflowing quality, and the pulse will also be rapid. It may cause Heart-Fire with such symptoms and signs as palpitations, a red tip of the tongue, a red face, insomnia and mental restlessness (Fig. 9.22).

THE PULSE IN LOVE

When "love" is the emotional cause of disease, the Heart pulse is Overflowing and Rapid.

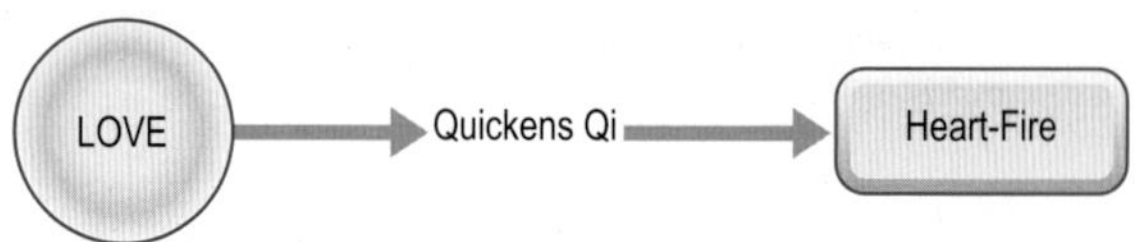

Figure 9.22 Effect of love.

CLINICAL NOTE

The points I use for "love" intended in the sense outlined above are HE-7 Shenmen, Ren-15 Jiuwei and Du-19 Houding.

SUMMARY

Love

- Here "love" does not mean the normal affection felt by human beings towards one another, but rather obsessive love for a particular person.
- Love also becomes a cause of disease when it is misdirected as happens, for example, when a person loves someone who persistently hurts them, whether physically or mentally.
- Obsessive jealousy would also fall under this broad category.
- "Love" affects the Heart and it quickens Qi.

Craving

As explained above, "craving" should be seen in the context of the three major philosophies of China, i.e. Confucianism, Buddhism and Daoism. All these three philosophies considered "craving" and "desire" as the root of mental-emotional suffering. See Figure 9.23.

As mentioned above, the Daoists shunned social relations and advocated "following the Dao", "absence of desire" (*wu yu*) and "non-action" (*wu wei*). They felt that "desire" would stop one from following the Dao. The Buddhists considered "desire" as the root of human suffering. According to them, our very existence begins out of desire and craving when the mind in the Bardo state (the period after death and before the next reincarnation) is attracted by the warmth of a womb and it reincarnates. Later on in life, desire causes our mind to try to grasp objects like a monkey sways from tree to tree.

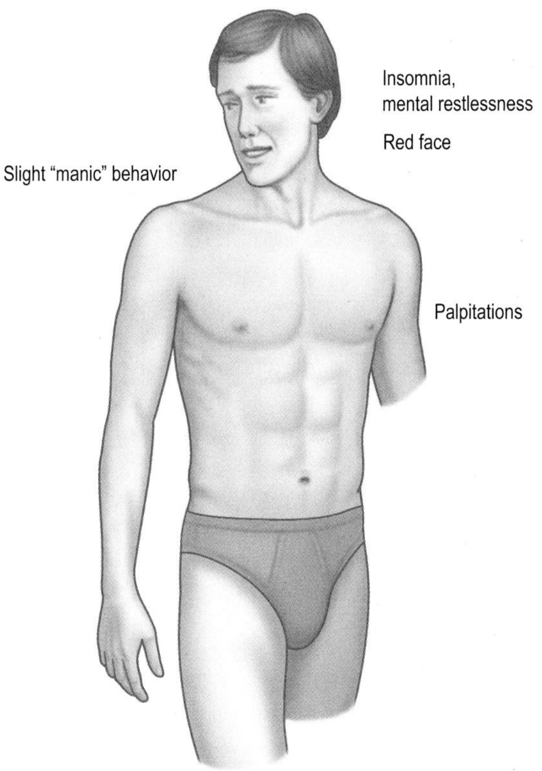

Figure 9.23 Clinical picture of craving.

Finally, Confucianists believed that the true "gentleman" (a mistranslation of the term *jun zi* that actually applies to both men and women) is not stirred by emotions because these cloud his or her true nature.

In the context of Chinese medicine, "craving" indicates a state of constant craving which is never satisfied. This can include craving for material objects or social recognition. Although rooted in the ancient philosophies of China, it is interesting to note that "craving" as an emotional cause of disease is common in our Western consumer societies where not only is there "craving" but where this is also artificially stimulated by advertising.

Craving affects the Heart and it scatters Qi. Craving also affects the Pericardium by stirring the Minister Fire. In disease, Minister Fire refers to a pathological, excessive Empty Fire arising from the Kidneys (Fig. 9.24). It arises from the Kidneys and it affects the Pericardium and therefore the Mind. For this reason "Minister Fire" refers to the physiological or pathological

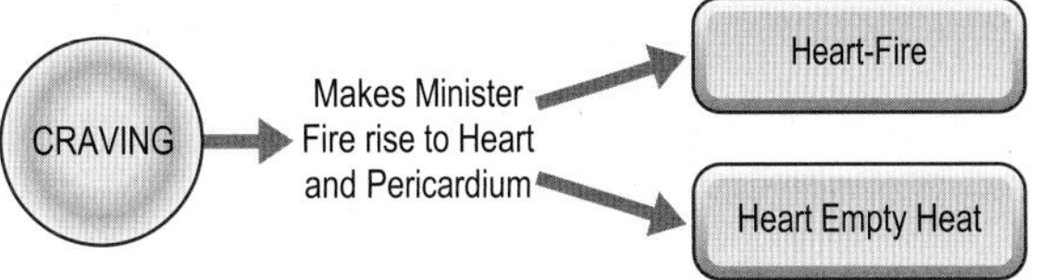

Figure 9.24 Effect of craving.

Fire of the Kidneys and to the Pericardium. This accounts for the assignment of the right Rear position on the pulse, either to the Kidney-Yang by some doctors or to the Pericardium by others.

If the Mind is calm, settled and content, the Pericardium follows its direction and there is a happy and balanced life. If the Mind is weak and dissatisfied, the Pericardium follows the demands of the craving and the person constantly desires new objects or new recognition, which, even when attained, are never satisfying and leave the person more frustrated. It is for these reasons that Confucianism, Daoism and Buddhism put the emphasis on reducing craving to prevent the arousal of Minister Fire which stirs the Mind.

Craving will cause Heart-Fire or Heart Empty Heat depending on the underlying condition of the person. If it causes Heart-Fire, there will be palpitations, a red face, thirst, insomnia, agitation and a slight "manic" behavior. In this case, the Heart pulse is Overflowing and Rapid.

If there is a tendency to Yin deficiency, which is common in people who tend to overwork, it will lead to Heart Empty Heat. This will cause palpitations, a malar flush, a dry throat, insomnia and mental restlessness. In this case, the Heart pulse is Overflowing but Empty and Rapid.

THE PULSE IN CRAVING

When craving is the emotional cause of disease, the Heart pulse is Overflowing and Rapid (in the case of Heart-Fire) or Overflowing-Empty and Rapid (in the case of Heart Empty Heat).

CLINICAL NOTE

The points I use for craving are HE-7 Shenmen, Du-19 Houding, Ren-15 Jiuwei and P-7 Daling.

SUMMARY

Craving

- "Craving" should be seen in the context of the three major philosophies of China, i.e. Confucianism, Buddhism and Daoism.
- All these three philosophies considered "craving" and "desire" as the root of mental-emotional suffering.
- In the context of Chinese medicine, "craving" indicates a state of constant craving which is never satisfied. This can include craving for material objects or social recognition.
- Craving affects the Heart and it scatters Qi. Craving also affects the Pericardium by stirring the Minister Fire.
- Craving will cause Heart-Fire or Heart Empty Heat depending on the underlying condition of the person.

Guilt

For all have sinned and fall short of the glory of God.[59]

Romans 3.23

In Him we have redemption through His blood, the forgiveness of sins, in accordance with the riches of God's grace that He lavished on us with all wisdom and understanding.[60]

Ephesians 1.7

Let us draw near to God with a sincere heart in full assurance of faith, having our hearts sprinkled to cleanse us from a guilty conscience and having our bodies washed with pure water.[61]

Hebrews 10.22

For whoever keeps the whole law and yet stumbles at just one point is guilty of breaking all of it.[62]

James 2.10

Guilt is a pervasive emotion in Western patients. It is completely missing from Chinese medicine books and one could say that it simply does not exist in the Chinese psyche. It could be argued that guilt is intrinsically related to the Judeo-Christian religions and especially the Christian religion with its concept of "original sin".

There are few expressions in Chinese to indicate guilt and all of them refer to "guilt" in a legal sense, rather than a *feeling* of guilt. An everyday expression to indicate a feeling of guilt would be *you zui e gan*, which means "having a guilt feeling", in which *zui* means "guilt" or "crime" in a legal sense.

I have never seen expressions referring to "feeling of guilt" in modern Chinese books. It could be argued that this is due to the fact that in Judeo-Christian societies the feeling of guilt is pervasive, while in Eastern societies such feeling is more or less absent. In fact, the concept of guilt is totally absent in all three major Chinese religions of Confucianism, Daoism and Buddhism. Indeed, Confucius did not even believe in the value of punishment for crimes.

Fingarette concurs that the concept of guilt is absent in the Analects of Confucius.[63] The Analects do mention the word *chi* in several passages but this is shame rather than guilt. Fingarette says:[64]

If we are unaware of the crucial differences in perspective, these texts on chi lend themselves easily to the assimilation of Confucian shame with Western guilt. Although chi is definitely a moral concept, the moral relation to which it corresponds is that of the person to his status and role as defined by li (rituals). Chi looks outward, not inward. It is not, as is guilt, a matter of the inward state, of repugnance at inner corruption, of self-denigration, of the sense that one is as a person, and independently of one's public status and repute, mean or reprehensible. The Confucian concept of shame is a genuinely moral concept, but it is oriented to morality as centering in li, traditionally ceremonially defined social comportment, rather than to an inner core of one's being.

The difference between shame and guilt is discussed further below under "Shame".

It should be stressed that what concerns us here in dealing with emotions is not guilt but the *feeling* of guilt which is totally unrelated to an actual crime or transgression. For example, a person may have committed a crime but feel no guilt at all; conversely, a person may have committed no crime or transgression but feel guilty.

Guilt (and shame) are considered by some to be "moral" emotions as they bear upon morality.[65] Wollheim says:[66]

The role of the moral emotions is to provide the person with an attitude, or orientation. What is distinctive of the moral emotions is that the attitude is reflexive. It is an attitude that the person has towards himself: himself as a person.

Guilt is strongly linked to a sense of self and specifically to a negative sense of self; this is probably an important reason for the absence of guilt in Chinese culture as the self in Chinese culture is not the individualized, psychological self of Western culture, but a socially constructed self. This may also account for the presence of shame in Chinese culture (related to a social sense of self) and the absence of guilt (related to an individual self). This is discussed more at length in Chapter 15.

Guilt can manifest in many different ways and I list some below:

- Feeling of responsibility for negative circumstances that have befallen oneself or others.
- Feeling of regret for real or imagined misdeeds, both past and present.
- Feeling responsible (and guilty) for any negative thing that occurs to members of one's family or one's partner.
- Taking responsibility for someone else's misfortune or problem.

Apart from the above examples of the consequences of a guilt feeling, this may make a person take very important, life-changing steps such as marriage or job. In other words, a subconscious guilty feeling may play a role in the choice of job or life partner. Sadly, when motivated by guilt, such choices often prove to be the wrong ones.

The above are only a few examples of the sort of behavior induced by feelings of guilt. A feeling of guilt may be due to the transgression of social or religious taboos or from having done something "wrong" which is later regretted. However, a feeling of guilt may also be innate and not related to any specific action. This latter feeling is indeed the most destructive one.

Guilt forms the core of Judeo-Christian psychology and theology. Guilt also formed an important cornerstone of Freud's theories.

It is important to distinguish the subjective sense of guilt from its objective counterparts. For example, a person may be found guilty in a court of law, without *feeling* guilty; in a religious context, a person may deem himself to be guilty in front of God but still not *feel* guilty; someone may be guilty of doing something reprehensible, but still not *feel* guilty.

It is therefore the *feeling* of guilt that is all-important. People who are prone to blame themselves for everything that goes wrong may also suffer an unjustified and subjective sense of guilt.

Guilt is self-reproach for some actual misdeeds or an inborn feeling of guilt totally disconnected from any misdeeds. Guilt includes a sense of inadequacy and despair not found in shame (see below). Guilt does not require any particular offence and the doctrine of Original Sin is an example of this. When assailed by a feeling of guilt, a person is one's own judge and a more ruthless and less reasonable judge than any real judge.

Guilt is inwardly-directed and its object is the self; in this sense, it is almost the "opposite" emotion to that of anger, as this latter emotion is usually directed at another person.

Guilt is based on a moral criterion of having broken a law of morality. The "mythology" of guilt is the doctrine of the Original Sin. The "authority" providing the criteria is absolute and unquestionable. Guilt is a "dark" emotion with no redemption; it is a much "darker" emotion than shame.

Guilt can have different effects in different people. First of all, it may lead to Qi stagnation; it affects any organ and especially the Lungs, Heart, Liver and Kidneys (Fig. 9.25). Due to its "dark", "stagnating" character, the Qi stagnation may cause Blood stasis easily. This Blood stasis may be in any part of the body and any organ but particularly in the Lungs, Heart, Spleen and Liver. The pulse is Wiry or Firm.

Under certain conditions, guilt may also cause sinking of Qi and affects the Kidneys, causing some urinary problems or menstrual problems from sinking of Qi (Fig. 9.26). The tongue has a red tip and possibly purple body. The pulse is Deep and Weak on both Kidney positions, and possibly slightly Overflowing on the Heart position and Choppy in general without wave. When guilt results from repressed anger, the pulse will be Wiry.

THE PULSE IN GUILT

When guilt is the emotional cause of disease, the pulse is Wiry or Firm if there is Qi and Blood stagnation. If there is sinking of Qi of the Kidneys, the pulse is Deep and Weak on the Kidney positions, possibly slightly Overflowing on the Heart position and Choppy in general without wave. When guilt results from repressed anger, the pulse will be Wiry.

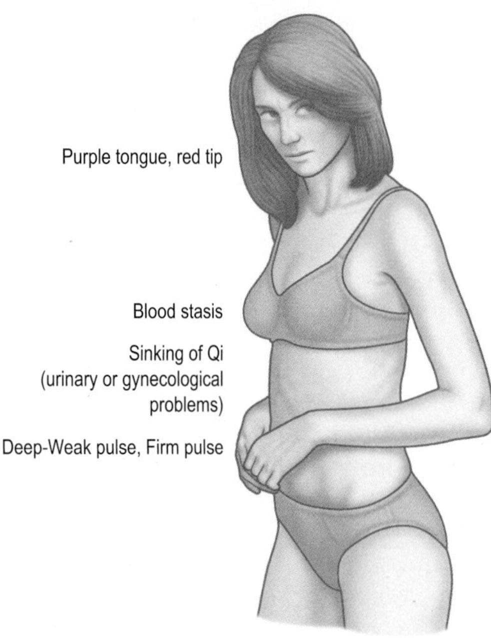

Figure 9.25 Clinical picture of guilt.

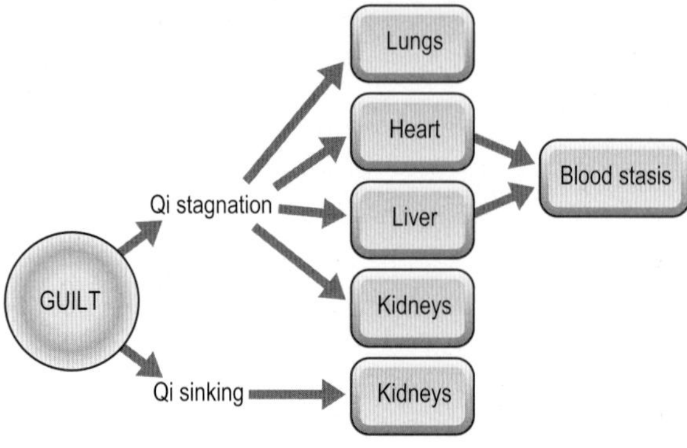

Figure 9.26 Effect of guilt.

CLINICAL NOTE

The points I use for guilt are HE-7 Shenmen, P-7 Daling, LIV-3 Taichong, KI-4 Dazhong, G.B.-13 Benshen and Du-24 Shenting.

SUMMARY

Guilt

- Guilt is a pervasive emotion in Western patients and it is completely missing from Chinese medicine books.
- What concerns us in dealing with emotions is not guilt but the *feeling* of guilt, which is totally unrelated to an actual crime or transgression.
- Guilt forms the core of Judeo-Christian psychology and theology. Guilt also formed an important cornerstone of Freud's theories.
- Guilt is self-reproach for some actual misdeeds or an inborn feeling of guilt totally disconnected from any misdeeds.
- Guilt may lead to Qi stagnation; it affects any organ, especially the Lungs, Heart, Liver and Kidneys.
- Due to its "dark", "stagnating" character, the Qi stagnation may cause Blood stasis (particularly in the Lungs, Heart, Spleen and Liver) easily and quickly.
- Guilt may also cause sinking of Qi and affect the Kidneys, causing some urinary problems or menstrual problems from sinking of Qi.

Shame

Shame is a common emotion in Western patients. It may be caused by a feeling of shame about one's behavior but, more commonly, it is an inborn feeling of shame due to one's upbringing. It is a feeling of worthlessness, an absence of a feeling of self-worth. It is, in a way, the opposite emotion to anger and pride. Anger is outwardly directed ("*I am angry at someone*") while shame is inwardly directed. It is self-accusation; a feeling that one has to *hide* is an important aspect of shame. When affected by shame, one feels *judged* and, most of all, *seen* to be doing something wrong all the time.

According to Solomon, in "small doses" shame may be an affirmation of one's autonomy, a confirmation that one will live by one's standards and accept responsibility. According to him, although opposite to pride, shame is similarly conducive to self-esteem. It is easy to feel good about oneself when one has no values, when one refuses to accept responsibility for one's actions or when one happens not to have done anything wrong. The ability to admit and atone for one's mistakes is as essential to wisdom and personal dignity as the ability to love other people.

Thomas Scheff also concurs that shame (and pride) are "social" emotions which, in small doses, are conducive to social order:[67]

Scheff contends that we are continually in a state of either pride or shame with respect to the judgements of others about our adherence to their and society's moral strictures. When we obey, we experience pride; when we disobey, we experience shame. Since pride is a pleasurable emotion and shame unpleasurable, the effect is to produce conformity in society and hence a high degree of social stability. Pride and shame thus ensure social control without the need for external surveillance and regulation.

This is exactly what Confucius said about the social value of shame (see below).

However, in severe cases (which are the ones that concern us when shame becomes a cause of disease), shame is overwhelming and it is self-demeaning, extremely defensive and impotent.

As a cause of disease, we consider shame that is overwhelming, that is due to one's upbringing and is *not* related to one's actions or to having done anything wrong. A person suffering from this shame will always *feel* as if they had done something wrong and will want to hide.

It is often said that Western societies are "guilt-based" and Eastern ones "shame-based", so it is useful to explore the differences between shame and guilt. Shame is related more to one's place in society, what people think of us, the feeling that one has to hide because one has done something wrong, something that society frowns upon, something "dirty". In other words, as long as we do not do anything that society disapproves of or, most importantly, as long as we are not *seen*, not *found out* to be doing something "wrong", we do not feel shame.

By contrast, in such situations we would feel guilty, even if nobody sees us doing something "wrong". One could say that, with guilt, we *hear* a voice condemning us; with shame, we *see* people condemning us; therefore shame can be avoided if we are not *seen* doing something wrong; guilt is unremitting, we cannot avoid it even if nobody sees us because we hear the voice of the inner judge condemning us.

Wollheim explores the differences between shame and guilt and says:[68]

In the case of shame, the criticism invokes an ideal which we have failed to live up to; in the case of guilt, the criticism invokes a set of injunctions which we have transgressed. In the case of shame, the criticism is based less, and, in the case of guilt, it is based more on identifiable harm or damage that we are supposed to have caused, though not necessarily intentionally. In the case of shame, the criticism can be met and turned only by an attempt on our part to change how we are. In the case of guilt, the criticism can be turned only by an attempt to compensate for what we have done. For this reason, shame will tend to generate the desire to change; guilt will tend to generate the desire to repair. What shame calls for is that others should forget *what we have become; what guilt calls for is that others should* forgive *what we have done. Finally, in the case of shame, the criticism is experienced as being conveyed to us by a look; we feel the eyes of disapproval upon us. In the case of guilt, the criticism is experienced as being conveyed in words; we hear the voice of disapproval.*

What is paramount in shame is how one appears to the other members of the community, not how one feels inside. The more one needs group approval, the more one is vulnerable to shame. Guilt is a "darker" emotion, more inwardly directed, an emotion from which there is no escape; the judgment is there, whether anyone sees us or not. The big difference between guilt and shame is that guilt has no redemption, it "eats" one inside for ever; shame has redemption and repair.

Interestingly, a study of New England colonists of the nineteenth century found that educators deliberately used shame as an educational tool for children and guilt for adults.[69]

It is certainly true that Eastern societies are shame-based, probably due to the strong Confucian influence; however, that does not mean that shame is not a prevalent emotion in the West too.

Shame is very ingrained in Confucianist ethics. It is even something that is considered a beneficial "tool" to keep people in line. Consider this passage from the Analects of Confucius:[70]

The Master said: 'Lead the people with administrative injunctions and keep them orderly with penal law, and they will avoid punishments but will be without a sense of shame. Lead them with morality (de) and keep them orderly through observing ritual propriety (li) and they will develop a sense of shame; and, moreover, will order themselves.

In other words, laws and punishments may keep social order, but even better is to lead by example so that people will regulate themselves due to the sense of shame deriving from not following the social order. Ames captures the primacy of familiar order and the centrality of *li* (ritual propriety) in his claim that "*For Confucius the regulating of society was too important to be left to governments; better would it be to have tradition serve as the binding force of the people.*"[71]

As the Confucian ethics is all about social relationships, and about one's place in society and *conforming* to strict rules of conduct and social hierarchy, it is natural that shame ensues from contravening the established rules of society. Thus, people are worried about not being *seen* to be doing anything that society would frown upon. That is why shame can sometimes produce extreme consequences as when Japanese businessmen commit suicide when they are disgraced socially.

Fingarette clarifies the difference between shame and guilt thus:[72]

Ultimately guilt is an attack upon oneself, whereas shame is an attack upon some specific action or outer condition. Shame is a matter of 'face', of embarrassment, of social status. Shame says 'change your ways, you have lost honour or dignity'. Guilt says 'change yourself, you are infected'. St Augustine speaks of the 'disease of my soul', of its 'wound' or being plucked out of the mire and washed by God, of being soul-sick and monstrous. It takes no demonstration to remind even the casual reader of Confucius that such imagery, or analogous tone, is alien to the Analects.

It is probably also for this reason that anger plays such a prominent role in the emotional causes of disease for the Chinese. Anger is probably the most disruptive of the emotions from the social point of view and an emotion that can potentially challenge and disrupt the social order and hierarchy. The Confucian gentleman never gets angry and it is *shameful* to be seen to be angry.

However, shame is common also in the West and, I would say, more in Protestant countries with a strong Puritan tradition. Kemper says that shame and pride are two emotions that ensure social stability:[73]

We are continually in a state of either pride or shame with respect to the judgement of others about our adherence to their and society's moral strictures. When we obey, we experience pride; when we disobey, we experience shame. Since pride is a pleasurable emotion and shame an unpleasant one, the effect is to produce conformity in society and hence a high degree of social stability.

As in anger, shame involves a courtroom mythology of law and judgment, accusation and punishment. In shame, unlike anger, one casts oneself in the uncomfortable position of defendant rather than judge, but a defendant who has openly admitted to his crime and is willing to accept punishment for it.

Shame is inwardly directed and it therefore makes Qi stagnate but also possibly sink (Fig. 9.27). Indeed, sinking of Qi is a frequent result of shame; Dampness also frequently accompanies shame. When one feels shame, one feels "dirty" and "dirtiness" is characteristic of Dampness. In my experience, shame often manifests with sinking of Qi and Dampness; for example, prolapse of organs, chronic and stubborn vaginal discharge, chronic excessive menstrual bleeding from sinking of Spleen- and Kidney-Qi and chronic slight urinary incontinence (Fig. 9.28). The pulse is Slippery or Soggy.

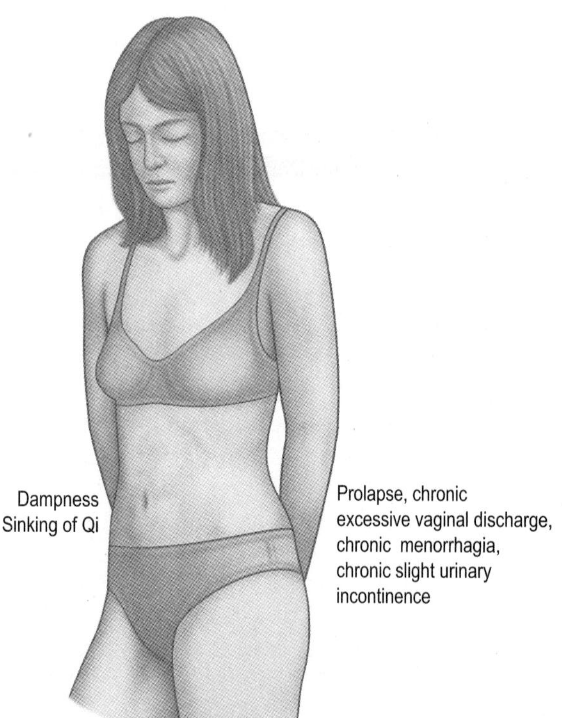

Figure 9.27 Clinical picture of shame.

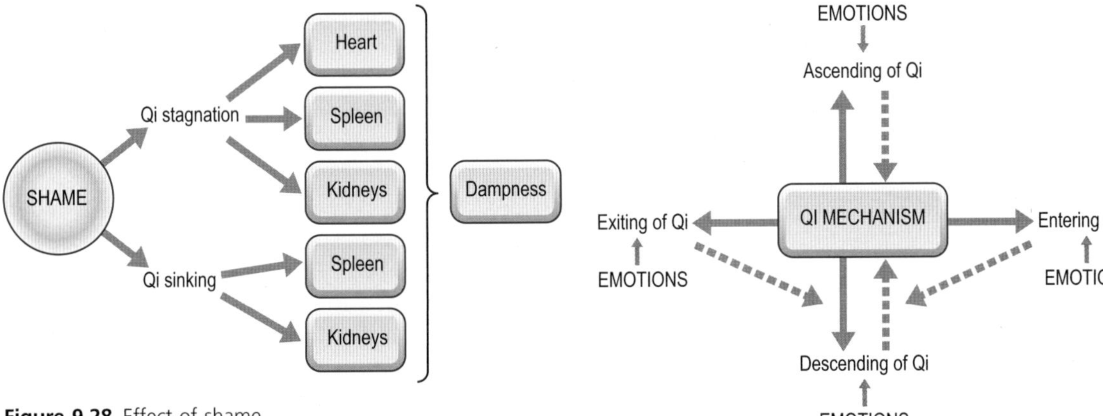

Figure 9.28 Effect of shame.

Figure 9.29 Effect of emotions on Qi Mechanism.

THE PULSE IN SHAME

When shame is the emotional cause of disease, the pulse is Slippery or Soggy.

CLINICAL NOTE

The points I use for shame are HE-7 Shenmen, SP-3 Taibai, Ren-15 Jiuwei, Ren-12 Zhongwan, SP-6 Sanyinjiao and Du-20 Baihui.

SUMMARY

Shame

- Shame is a common emotion in Western patients.
- It may be caused by a feeling of shame about one's behavior but, more commonly, it is an inborn feeling of shame due to one's upbringing.
- Shame is overwhelming and is self-demeaning, extremely defensive and impotent.
- Shame is related more to one's place in society, what people think of us, the feeling that one has to hide because one has done something wrong, something that society frowns upon, something "dirty". By contrast, in such situations we would feel guilty even if nobody sees us doing something "wrong".
- With guilt, we *hear* a voice condemning us; with shame, we *see* people condemning us.
- Shame is inwardly directed and it therefore makes Qi stagnate but also possibly sink. Indeed, sinking of Qi is a frequent result of shame; Dampness also frequently accompanies shame.
- When one feels shame, one feels "dirty" and "dirtiness" is characteristic of Dampness.

THE PATHOLOGY OF QI AND MINISTER FIRE IN EMOTIONAL PROBLEMS

I shall first discuss the effect of emotional stress on the body's Qi and then explore the pathology of the Minister Fire in emotional problems.

The effect of emotions on the body's Qi

Derangement of Qi in emotional problems

The first effect of emotional stress is to affect the circulation of Qi. Qi circulates in the Qi Mechanism in the correct direction in each given pathway. In each part of the body, Qi ascends or descends and enters or exits in the correct direction as appropriate. The correct ascending/descending and entering/exiting of Qi in the Qi Mechanism ensures the smooth flow of Qi.

Emotional stress upsets the ascending/descending and entering/exiting of Qi, and each emotion affects the circulation of Qi in a different way (Fig. 9.29). Chapter 39 of the *Simple Questions* describes the effect of each emotion on Qi as follows.[74]

- Anger makes Qi rise.
- Joy slows Qi down.
- Sadness dissolves Qi.
- Worry knots Qi.
- Pensiveness knots Qi.
- Fear makes Qi descend.
- Shock scatters Qi.

In Figure 9.29, the solid arrows indicate the physiological movement of Qi, while the dotted lines indicate the pathological movement of Qi induced by emotional stress. However, the above are not the only terms used in the *Yellow Emperor's Classic* to describe the effect of the emotions.

Dr Chen Yan in *A Treatise on the Three Categories of Causes of Diseases* (1174) says: "*Joy scatters, anger arouses, worry makes Qi unsmooth, pensiveness knots, sadness makes Qi tight, fear sinks, shock moves.*"[75]

The same doctor expands on the effects of the emotions on Qi and makes reference to the points on the outer Bladder channel on the back:[76]

Joy injures the Heart, scatters Qi and melts the Shentang [BL-44]*; anger injures the Liver, makes Qi rise and loosens the Hunmen* [BL-47]*; worry injures the Lungs, makes Qi accumulate and makes the Pohu* [BL-42] *not shut; pensiveness injures the Spleen, makes Qi stagnate and makes the Yishe* [BL-49] *restless; fear injures the Kidneys, makes Qi descend* [it literally says 'makes Qi timid'] *and makes the Zhishi* [BL-52] *not firm.*

For the sake of readability, I have omitted from the above passage sentences in which Dr Chen postulates that each emotion affects the organ to which it "belongs" (in the Five-Element scheme) but also the organ along the reverse Controlling cycle as follows:[77]

Joy injures the Heart, Fire invades the Kidneys, the pulse becomes Deep and Scattered; anger injures the Liver, Liver-Qi rises and invades the Lungs, the pulse becomes Wiry and Choppy [sic]*; worry injures the Lungs, Lung-Qi accumulates and it invades the Heart, the pulse becomes Overflowing and short; pensiveness injures the Spleen, Earth-Qi accumulates and it invades the Liver, the pulse becomes Wiry and Weak* [sic]*; fear injures the Kidneys, Water-Qi revolves and it invades the Spleen, the pulse becomes Deep and Slowed-Down.*

The effect of each emotion on Qi should not be interpreted too restrictively as, in certain cases, emotional pressure may have a different effect on Qi from the one outlined above. For example, fear is said to make Qi descend and it may cause enuresis, incontinence of urine or diarrhea, since the Kidneys control the two lower orifices (urethra and anus). This is certainly true in cases of extreme and sudden fear which may cause incontinence of urine or diarrhea, or in the case of children when anxiety about a certain family situation may cause enuresis.

However, the effect of fear on Qi depends also on the state of the Heart. If the Heart is strong, it will cause Qi to descend, but if the Heart is weak, it will cause Qi to rise in the form of Empty Heat. This is more common in old people and in women. In such cases, fear and anxiety may weaken Kidney-Yin and give rise to Empty Heat of the Heart with such symptoms as palpitations, insomnia, night-sweating, a dry mouth, red face and a Rapid pulse.

CLINICAL NOTE

The effect of each emotion on the direction of flow of Qi should not be interpreted too rigidly, as occasionally an emotion may have an effect on Qi that is different from the "normal" one. For example, fear may make Qi rise.

Effects of emotions on Internal Organs

As indicated above, each emotion affects one or more organs as follows.

- Anger (including frustration and resentment) affects the Liver.
- Joy affects the Heart.
- Worry affects the Lungs and Spleen.
- Pensiveness affects the Spleen.
- Sadness and grief affect the Lungs and Heart.
- Fear affects the Kidneys.
- Shock affects the Kidneys and Heart.
- Love affects the Heart.
- Craving affects the Heart.
- Guilt affects the Kidneys and Heart.
- Shame affects the Heart and Spleen.

However, just as we discussed for the effects of each emotion on Qi, equally the effect of each emotion on a relevant organ should not be interpreted too restrictively. There are passages from the *Yellow Emperor's Classic* which attribute the effect of emotions to organs other than the ones just mentioned. For example, the *Spiritual Axis* in Chapter 28 says: "*Worry and pensiveness agitate the Heart.*"[78] The *Simple Questions* in Chapter 39 says: "*Sadness agitates the Heart.*"[79]

> **CLINICAL NOTE**
>
> The effect of each emotion on a relevant organ should not be interpreted too restrictively. For example, sadness (usually affecting the Lungs) may affect Liver-Blood, worry (usually affecting the Lungs) may cause Liver-Yang rising, etc.

Indeed, the whole Chapter 216 of the *Classic of Categories* (*Lei Jing*, 1624) is dedicated to the discussion of the influence of each emotion on groups of organs. This passage has already been mentioned above and Zhang Jie Bin lists the following organs affected by the relevant emotion.

Thus, excess joy, anger, pensiveness and worry affect the following organs:

- *Excess joy*: Heart and Lungs
- *Anger*: Liver, Gall-Bladder, Heart and Kidneys
- *Pensiveness*: Spleen and Heart
- *Worry*: Lungs, Heart, Liver and Spleen
- *Fear*: Kidneys, Heart, Liver, Spleen and Stomach.

> **CLINICAL NOTE**
>
> **Multiple organs affected by emotions**
> - *Excess joy*: Heart and Lungs
> - *Anger*: Liver, Gall-Bladder, Heart and Kidneys
> - *Pensiveness*: Spleen and Heart
> - *Worry*: Lungs, Heart, Liver and Spleen
> - *Fear*: Kidneys, Heart, Liver, Spleen and Stomach.

The effect of an emotion on an organ depends also on other circumstances and on whether the emotion is manifested or repressed. For example, anger which is expressed affects the Liver (causing Liver-Yang rising), but anger which is repressed also affects the Heart. If one gets angry at mealtimes (as sadly often happens in certain families), the anger will affect the Stomach and this will be manifested with a Wiry quality on the right Middle position of the pulse.

The effect of an emotion will also depend on the constitutional trait of a person. For example, if a person has a tendency to a constitutional weakness of the Heart (manifested with a midline crack on the tongue extending all the way to the tip), fear will affect the Heart rather than the Kidneys.

Furthermore, all emotions, besides affecting the relevant organ directly, affect the Heart indirectly because the Heart houses the Mind. It alone, being responsible for consciousness and cognition, can recognize and feel the effect of emotional tension. Fei Bo Xiong (1800–1879) put it very clearly when he said:[80]

The seven emotions injure the five Yin organs selectively, but they all affect the Heart. Joy injures the Heart ... Anger injures the Liver, the Liver cannot recognize anger but the Heart can, hence it affects both Liver and Heart. Worry injures the Lungs, the Lungs cannot recognize it but the Heart can, hence it affects both Lungs and Heart. Pensiveness injures the Spleen, the Spleen cannot recognize it but the Heart can, hence it affects both Spleen and Heart.

Yu Chang in *Principles of Medical Practice* (1658) says:[81]

Worry agitates the Heart and has repercussions on the Lungs; pensiveness agitates the Heart and has repercussions on the Spleen; anger agitates the Heart and has repercussions on the Liver; fear agitates the Heart and has repercussions on the Kidneys. Therefore all the five emotions [including joy] *affect the Heart.*

Chapter 28 of the *Spiritual Axis* also says that all emotions affect the Heart:[82]

The Heart is the Master of the five Yin and six Yang organs ... sadness, shock and worry agitate the Heart; when the Heart is agitated the five Yin and six Yang organs are shaken.

Chinese writing clearly bears out the idea that all emotions affect the Heart since the characters for all seven emotions are based on the "heart" radical. This is probably the most important aspect of the Heart functions and the main reason for it being compared to the "monarch".

The way that all emotions afflict the Heart also explains why a red tip of the tongue, indicating Heart-Heat, is so commonly seen even in emotional problems related to other organs.

The main effects of emotional stress are Qi stagnation, Blood stasis, Heat or Fire and Dampness or Phlegm; these are discussed below.

Qi stagnation

The first effect of emotional stress on the body is to affect the proper circulation and direction of Qi. Qi is non-substantial and the Mind with its mental and emotional energies is the most non-material type of Qi. It is therefore natural that emotional stress affecting the Mind impairs the circulation of Qi and disrupts the Qi Mechanism first of all. Although each emotion has a particular effect on Qi, e.g. anger makes it rise, sadness depletes

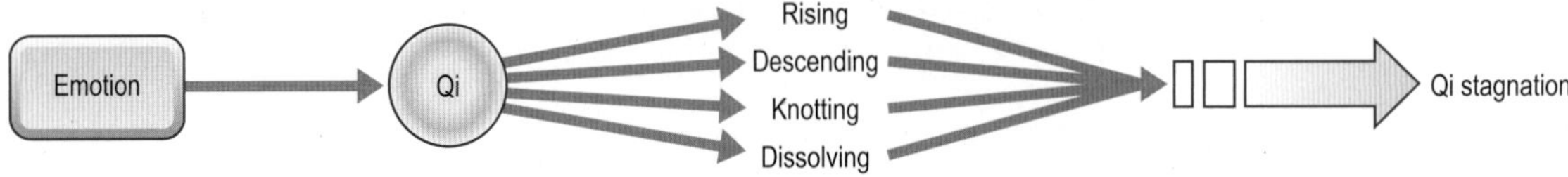

Figure 9.30 Qi stagnation from emotional stress.

it, etc., all emotions have a tendency to cause some stagnation of Qi after some time (Fig. 9.30).

Even the emotions that deplete Qi, such as sadness, may cause some Qi stagnation, because if Qi is deficient it cannot circulate properly and it therefore may tend to stagnate. For example, sadness depletes Lung-Qi in the chest; the deficient Qi in the chest fails to circulate properly and it causes some stagnation of Qi in the chest.

The patterns of Heart-Qi and Lung-Qi stagnation are not often mentioned but they are very common in mental-emotional problems and, for this reason, they are reported below.

Heart-Qi stagnation

Clinical manifestations

Palpitations, a feeling of distension or oppression of the chest, depression, a slight feeling of a lump in the chest, slight shortness of breath, sighing, poor appetite, chest and upper epigastric distension, dislike of lying down, weak and cold limbs, slightly purple lips and pale complexion.

Tongue: slightly Pale-Purple on the sides in the chest area.

Pulse: Empty but very slightly Overflowing on the left Front position.

Acupuncture

Points

HE-5 Tongli, HE-7 Shenmen, P-6 Neiguan, Ren-15 Jiuwei, Ren-17 Shanzhong, LU-7 Lieque, ST-40 Fenglong, L.I.-4 Hegu. Reducing or even method.

Herbal therapy

Prescriptions

MU XIANG LIU QI YIN
Aucklandia Flowing Qi Decoction.
BAN XIA HOU PO TANG
Pinellia-Magnolia Decoction.

Lung-Qi stagnation

Clinical manifestations

A feeling of a lump in the throat, difficulty swallowing, a feeling of oppression or distension of the chest, slight breathlessness, sighing, sadness, slight anxiety, depression.

Tongue: slightly Red on the sides in the chest areas.

Pulse: very slightly Tight on the right Front position.

Acupuncture

Points

LU-7 Lieque, ST-40 Fenglong, Ren-15 Jiuwei, P-6 Neiguan. Reducing or even method.

Herbal therapy

Prescription

BAN XIA HOU PO TANG
Pinella-Magnolia Decoction.

Blood stasis

When Qi stagnates, it may, in time, lead to Blood stasis, especially in women. Blood stasis particularly affects the Heart, Liver and Uterus.

Anger and guilt are particularly prone to lead to Blood stasis after Qi stagnation. However, other emotions such as sadness, grief and worry may also lead to Blood stasis in the chest after a period of Qi stagnation. In women in particular, Qi stagnation in the breasts from sadness and grief may lead to Blood stasis and to breast lumps.

Heat or Fire

Qi stagnation may also lead to Heat, and most of the emotions can, over a long period of time, give rise to

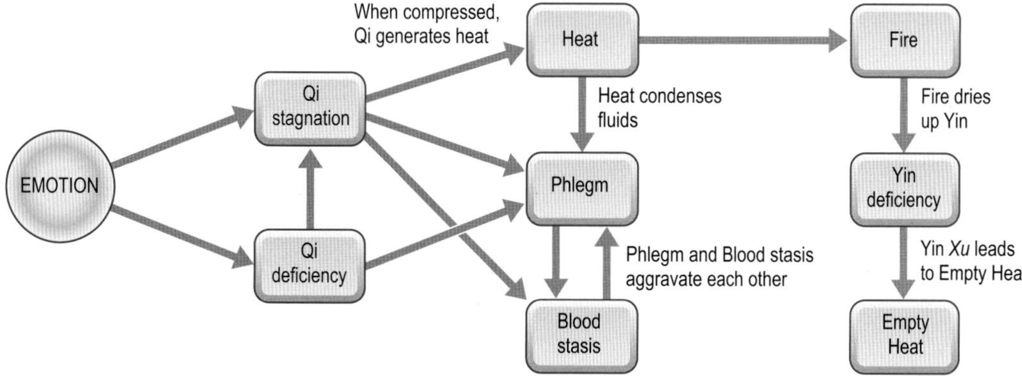

Figure 9.31 Summary of effect of emotions on Qi and Blood.

Heat or Fire. There is a saying in Chinese Medicine: "*The five emotions can turn into Fire.*" This is because most of the emotions can cause stagnation of Qi, and when Qi is compressed in this way over a period of time it creates Heat, just as the temperature of a gas increases when its pressure is increased.

For this reason, when someone has suffered from emotional problems for a long time, there are often signs of Heat, which may be in the Liver, Heart, Lungs or Kidneys (in the case of this last organ, Empty Heat). This often shows on the tongue which becomes red or dark red and dry, and usually has a red tip. A red tip of the tongue is a very common sign in practice which is always a reliable indicator that the patient is subject to some emotional stress.

With time, Heat may turn into Fire which is more intense, more drying and affects the Mind more. Therefore, emotional stress may, in time, cause Fire and this, in turn, harasses the Mind, causing agitation and anxiety.

Dampness or Phlegm

Finally, the disruption of Qi in the Qi Mechanism caused by the emotions may, in time, also lead to the formation of Phlegm. As the proper movement of Qi in the Qi Mechanism is essential to transform, transport and excrete fluids, disruption in the movement of Qi may result in the formation of Dampness or Phlegm. Phlegm, in turn, obstructs the Mind's orifices and becomes a further cause of emotional and mental disturbance.

Figure 9.31 summarizes the effect of emotions on Qi and Blood.

CLINICAL NOTE

Five points to remember:

- Do not interpret the relationship between an organ and an emotion too rigidly (e.g. sadness may affect the Liver).
- Do not interpret the relationship between an emotion and its effect on Qi too rigidly (e.g. fear may make Qi ascend).
- All emotions affect the Heart.
- Other organs besides the Liver suffer from Qi stagnation from emotional stress (e.g. Heart and Lungs).
- Qi stagnation does not derive only from anger but it may also derive from sadness, grief, worry, pensiveness, guilt and shame – in fact, from any emotion.

SUMMARY

The effect of emotions on the body's Qi

- Emotions disrupt the proper direction of movement of Qi (e.g. anger makes Qi rise, fear makes Qi descend, etc.).
- Each emotion affects a given organ, e.g. anger affects the Liver, fear affects the Kidneys, etc.
- All emotions affect the Heart.
- After disrupting the proper direction of flow of Qi, all emotions lead to some Qi stagnation.
- In emotional problems, Qi stagnation affects not only the Liver but other organs too (especially Lungs and Heart).
- Other consequences of the disruption of the Qi Mechanism from emotional stress are Blood stasis, Heat, Dampness and Phlegm.

The pathology of the Minister Fire in emotional problems

The Minister Fire refers to the physiological Fire of the Kidneys. The Minister Fire is the motive force of all functional activities of the body, being the physiological Fire that is essential to life.

The Minister Fire should be "concealed" in its resting place in the Lower Burner. In other words, it carries on its function of heating the body but without the creation of visible Heat signs and symptoms.

The importance of the Fire nature of the Minister Fire is that it provides heat for all our bodily functions and for the Kidney-Essence itself. The Kidneys are unlike any other organ in that they are the origin of Water and Fire of the body, the Primary Yin and Primary Yang (Fig. 9.32). The Minister Fire is the embodiment of the Fire within the Kidneys and it is a special type of Fire in that not only does it not extinguish Water, but it can actually produce Water.

The Minister Fire of the Kidneys complements the Yin quality of the Kidney-Essence (Fig. 9.33).

This "Minister Fire" is quite different from the "Minister Fire" of the Pericardium and these differences will be explored below. In this respect, the theory of the Minister Fire is at variance with the Five-Element theory, according to which the "Minister Fire" is the Triple Burner and Pericardium.

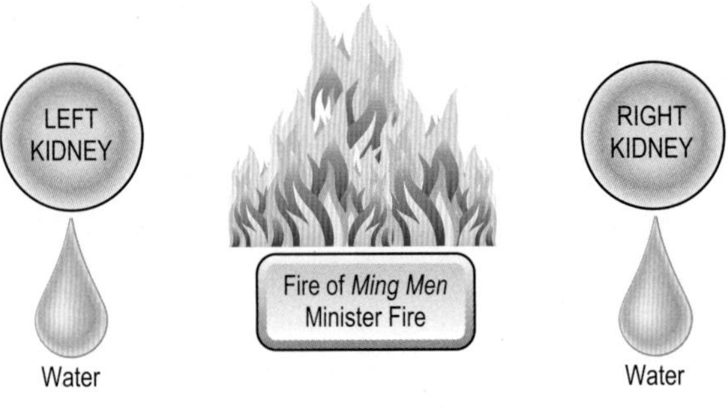

Figure 9.32 The Minister Fire and the Kidneys.

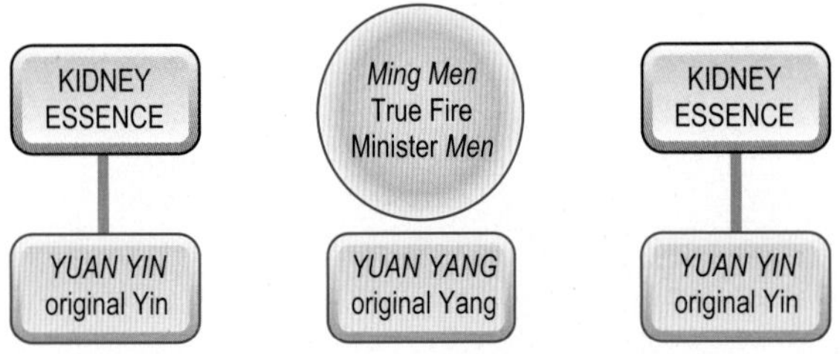

Figure 9.33 The Minister Fire and the Kidney-Essence.

> **CLINICAL NOTE**
>
> The Minister Fire is the physiological Fire of the Kidneys that provides the heat necessary to all physiological processes of the body. It should be "concealed" in the Lower Burner, carrying on its heating function without manifesting itself.
>
> Although the point Du-4 Mingmen is specific to tonify the Fire of the Gate of Life and the Minister Fire (as its name implies), I personally prefer to use the point Ren-4 Guanyuan.

The main functions of the Minister Fire are as follows.

- It is the Root of the Original Qi (*Yuan Qi*).
- It is the Source of (physiological) Fire for all the Internal Organs.
- It warms the Lower Burner and Bladder.
- It warms the Stomach and Spleen to aid digestion.
- It warms the Essence and Uterus and harmonizes the sexual and menstrual functions.
- It assists the Kidney function of reception of Qi.
- It assists the Heart function of housing the Mind.

In the context of mental-emotional problems, the importance of the Minister Fire is that this is frequently and easily "stirred" by emotional stress, with the creation of Heat and an upward movement of Qi which goes up to disturb the Heart and Pericardium. As we have seen in emotional stress, Heat is frequently the result of Qi stagnation; however, in my experience, it may also arise independently, without a preceding Qi stagnation.

> **CLINICAL NOTE**
>
> In mental-emotional problems, the Minister Fire is frequently and easily "stirred" by emotional stress, with the creation of Heat and an upward movement of Qi, which goes up to disturb the Heart and Pericardium.
>
> To subdue the rising Minister Fire in emotional problems, one must use Heart and Pericardium points such as HE-5 Tongli and P-7 Daling. In addition, tonifying the physiological Minister Fire with points such as Ren-4 Guanyuan will also help to bring the Minister Fire back into its place of "concealment" and therefore to calm the Mind.

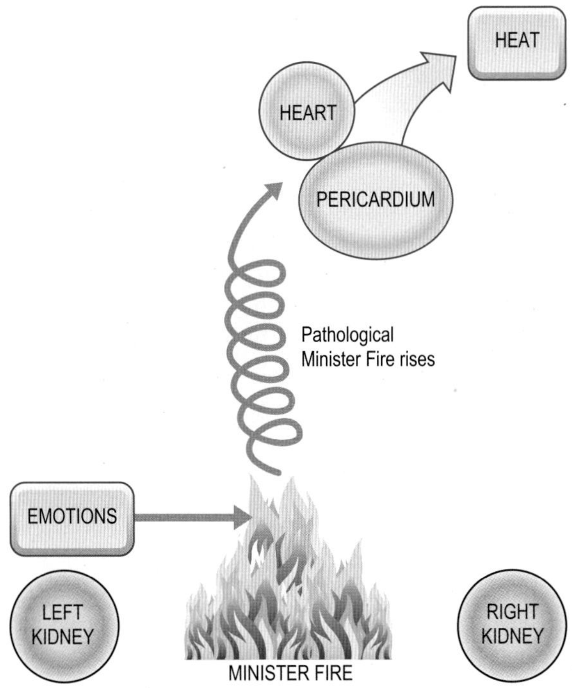

Figure 9.34 Pathological Minister Fire.

When Heat is formed under the influence of emotional stress, the Minister Fire becomes pathological; it is "stirred" out of its residence in the Lower Burner and it flows upwards to the Heart and Pericardium (Fig. 9.34). Some Chinese books actually say that the physiological Minister Fire should be "hidden" in the Lower *Dan Tian* and it should not be seen. When there is Heat, the Minister Fire is seen.

When the Minister Fire is stirred into a pathological state under the influence of emotional stress, three patterns of Heat may appear:

1. Full Heat
2. Empty Heat (from Yin deficiency)
3. Yin Fire.

Full Heat

Full Heat as a result of emotional stress derives usually from long-term Qi stagnation; when Qi stagnates for some time, it may give rise to Heat. However, in emotional stress, Heat may also be formed independently; this may happen, for example, with anger, joy, love or craving.

The main manifestation of Full Heat is the tongue; this is Red and with a yellow coating. If the tongue body is Red and there is a coating with root, there is Full Heat (even if the coating is not yellow).

> **CLINICAL NOTE**
>
> **The tongue in Full Heat**
>
> The tongue in Full Heat is Red or Dark-Red and with a thick and dry yellow coating. The coating may also be dark-yellow, brown or black.

The other important manifestation is the pulse; in Full Heat, the pulse is Full in general (which may include Wiry, Overflowing, Big or Firm). It should also be Rapid, but it frequently is not.

Other clinical manifestations include feeling of heat, thirst, dry mouth, insomnia, agitation, mental restlessness and red face.

Full Heat of any organ may overstimulate the coming and going of the Ethereal Soul and it may therefore lead to "manic" behavior, agitation, mental restlessness, insomnia, hyperactivity and anxiety.

> **SUMMARY**
>
> **Full Heat from emotional problems**
>
> Feeling of heat, thirst, dry mouth, insomnia, agitation, mental restlessness, red face, "manic" behavior, hyperactivity, anxiety, Red tongue with red tip and a yellow coating, Overflowing-Rapid pulse.

Empty Heat

Empty Heat derives from Yin deficiency. It is important to note that, although Empty Heat derives from Yin deficiency eventually, it may occur for many years without Empty Heat.

Empty Heat is seen in emotional stress when this is combined with overwork that leads to Yin deficiency. It is a relatively common situation in Western patients. The combination of overwork with emotional stress leads to Yin deficiency and Empty Heat. Thus, in such cases, the Empty Heat does derive from Yin deficiency but it is aggravated by the emotional stress which, in itself, leads to Heat. Most of all, the emotional stress causes the Empty Heat to rise more, causing agitation, red face and thirst.

In Empty Heat, the tongue is Red but either without a coating (totally or partially) or with a rootless coating. Thus, in Full Heat the tongue is Red with a coating; in Empty Heat it is Red without a coating.

CLINICAL NOTE

The tongue in Empty Heat

The tongue in Empty Heat is Red or Dark-Red and without a coating. The absence of coating indicates Yin deficiency, while the redness of the body indicates Empty Heat.

In Empty Heat, the pulse is Floating-Empty and Rapid. Other clinical manifestations include feeling of heat in the evening, dry mouth with desire to drink in small sips, malar flush, mental restlessness and insomnia.

As Full Heat does, Empty Heat of any organ may also overstimulate the coming and going of the Ethereal Soul and it may therefore lead to "manic" behavior, a vague mental restlessness, insomnia, fidgetiness, hyperactivity and anxiety.

The mental restlessness from Empty Heat manifests differently from that from Full Heat. In Empty Heat, the patient has a vague feeling of anxiety and restlessness that also manifests more in the evening.

SUMMARY

Empty Heat from emotional problems

Feeling of heat in the evening, dry mouth with desire to drink in small sips, malar flush, insomnia, "manic" behavior, a vague mental restlessness, fidgetiness, anxiety, Red tongue without coating (or partially without coating), red tip, Floating-Empty and Rapid pulse.

Yin Fire

The concept of Yin Fire was introduced by Li Dong Yuan in his book *Discussion of Stomach and Spleen* (*Pi Wei Lun*, 1246). Li Dong Yuan says that a dietary irregularity with excessive consumption of cold or warm foods injures the Spleen and Stomach. On the other hand, joy, anger, worry and fright deplete the Original Qi (*Yuan Qi*). As the Spleen and Stomach are weakened, the Original Qi becomes depleted, and Heart-Fire becomes excessive.

Li Dong Yuan says that this excessive Heart-Fire is a "Yin Fire". He introduced the term "Yin Fire" for the first time. This Fire starts from the Lower Burner and links with the Heart. Li Dong Yuan says that "the Heart does not reign by itself"; the Minister Fire is its deputy, just like the Minister serves the Monarch. The Minister Fire is the Fire of the Pericardium arising from the Lower Burner as a result of emotional stress. The Minister Fire leaves its place of "concealment" in the Lower Burner; it flares upwards and manifests itself. Although the patient may feel hot in the face as a result, he or she feels cold in general due to the deficiency of the Original Qi.

Li Dong Yuan defines this Minister Fire arising from the Lower Burner as pathological and a "thief" of the Original Qi. The pathological Minister Fire and the Original Qi are mutually irreconcilable. If one is victorious, the other must be the loser. When Spleen and Stomach become deficient, their Qi sinks down into the Kidneys so that Yin Fire has a chance to overwhelm the Earth element (Fig. 9.35).

The arousal of the pathological Minister Fire upwards causes some Heat symptoms in the upper part of the body, such as a red face and mouth ulcers. This he called "Yin Fire"; Yin Fire is neither Full Heat nor Empty Heat but simply a different kind of Heat that derives from a deficiency of the Original Qi. It follows that Yin Fire is not treated by clearing Heat or draining

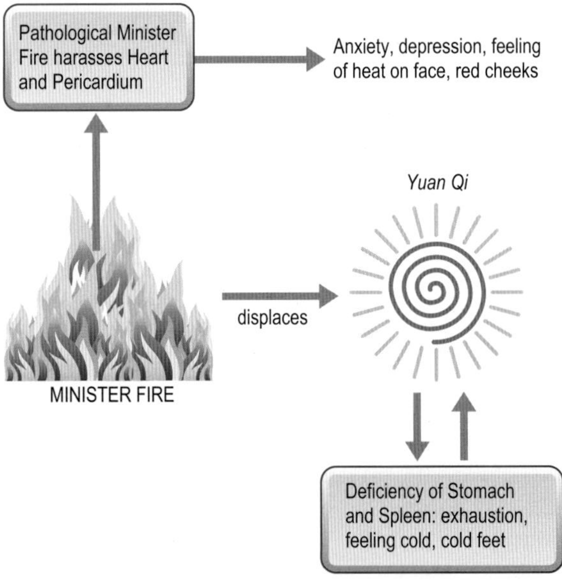

Figure 9.35 Pathology of Yin Fire.

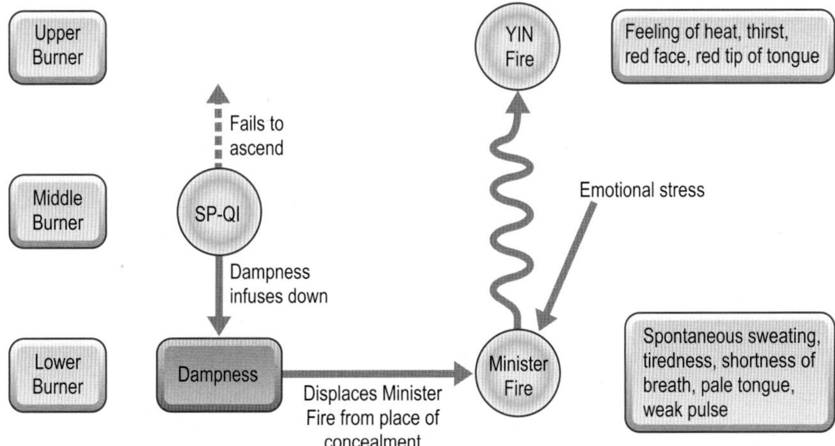

Figure 9.36 Pathology of Yin Fire and Dampness.

Fire but by tonifying the Original Qi and gently clearing Heat upwards.

The pathology of Yin Fire is further complicated by Dampness and by a pathology of the Middle Burner as well (Fig. 9.36). When the Spleen is deficient, Dampness is formed and this infuses down to the Lower Burner. Here it "swamps" the Original Qi and the Minister Fire, displacing the latter from the place (the Lower Burner) where it should be "concealed".

The Middle Burner also has Dampness; Spleen-Qi (or even Spleen-Yang) is deficient and fails to rise. For this reason, Bu Zhong Yi Qi Tang *Tonifying the Center and Benefiting Qi Decoction* is used to raise Spleen-Qi and warm Spleen-Yang so that Dampness no longer infuses downwards to the Lower Burner. When the Lower Burner is opened and unblocked from Dampness, the Minister Fire will return to its place of concealment in the Lower Burner, thus eliminating the symptoms of Yin Fire.

The symptoms of Yin Fire can be very varied as they differ also depending on how much Dampness there is and how deficient is the Original Qi. In general, the main manifestations are:

- red face
- a feeling of heat in the face
- mouth ulcers (with white rim)
- slight thirst
- depression
- anxiety
- tiredness
- abdominal fullness and heaviness (Dampness)
- cold feet
- general cold feeling
- pale tongue
- weak pulse.

These are only the general manifestations; others may vary according to the condition. Indeed, in my experience, Yin Fire plays a role in many modern, difficult diseases such as chronic fatigue syndrome, allergies and autoimmune diseases.

Bu Zhong Yi Qi Tang eliminates Yin Fire by tonifying the Original Qi with Ren Shen *Radix Ginseng* and by lightly clearing Heat upwards with Chai Hu *Radix Bupleuri* and Sheng Ma *Rhizoma Cimicifugae*.

It may seem strange that Dr Li uses Bu Zhong Yi Qi Tang which makes Qi rise while Yin Fire is rising to the top. The use of this formula is necessary to make Spleen-Qi rise, tonify the Original Qi (with Ren Shen) and de-obstruct the Middle Burner of Dampness. The two herbs Chai Hu and Sheng Ma lightly clear Heat upwards and are there to clear the pathological Minister Fire. Moreover, as the pathological Minister Fire and the Original Qi reside in the place in the lower *Dan Tian*, tonifying the Original Qi will automatically reduce the pathological Minister Fire.

Yin Fire is frequently implicated in mental-emotional problems and it is interesting that Li Dong Yuan says specifically that the Yin Fire rises from the Lower Burner under the stimulus of emotional stress. Any emotion can lead to Yin Fire, as all emotions may stir the Minister Fire out of its residing place in the Lower *Dan Tian*.

The situation can be aggravated by the presence of Dampness in the Lower Burner (as happens in shame).

Yin Fire accounts for symptoms of Heat in mental-emotional problems that may defy a classification into Full or Empty Heat; this happens when there are symptoms of Heat above (red face, thirst, feeling of heat in the face) and Cold below (cold feet, general cold feeling) – such a situation is due to Yin Fire.

Emotional stress is more likely to lead to Yin Fire when it is combined with overwork and dietary irregularity, and Yin Fire is frequently a factor in anxiety and depression. Indeed, Bu Zhong Yi Qi Tang may be used for depression when there is Yin Fire; the physical lifting of Spleen-Qi also has a mental lifting effect on the Brain and mood. Moreover, raising Qi also has the effect of stimulating the physiological rising of Liver-Qi. As we have seen in Chapter 3, this physiological rising is a manifestation of the movement of the Ethereal Soul; the movement of the Ethereal Soul is insufficient in depression and the use of Bu Zhong Yi Qi Tang will stimulate that movement and lift depression.

The acupuncture treatment of emotional stress manifesting with Yin Fire should be based on the following steps.

- Tonify the Original (*Yuan*) Qi: Ren-4 Guanyuan.
- Lift Qi: Du-20 Baihui, Ren-6 Qihai.
- Tonify and raise Spleen-Qi: BL-20 Pishu, Ren-12 Zhongwan, ST-36 Zusanli.
- Clear Heat in the upper part of the body: P-8 Laogong, P-7 Daling.
- Calm the Mind: Du-24 Shenting, Du-19 Houding, Ren-15 Jiuwei, HE-5 Tongli.
- Regulate the Triple Burner: T.B.-6 Zhigou, T.B.-5 Waiguan.

SUMMARY

Yin fire from emotional problems

Red face, thirst, feeling of heat in the face, depression, anxiety, general tiredness, cold feet, general cold feeling, red tip of the tongue but Pale tongue body, Weak pulse.

SUMMARY

Tongue manifestation in Heat conditions

- *Full Heat*: Red or Dark-Red with a thick, dry, yellow or brown coating.
- *Empty Heat*: Red or Dark-Red without coating.
- *Yin Fire*: Pale (may have a red tip).

The Pericardium in mental-emotional problems

In the context of mental-emotional problems, it is important to explore the nature of the Pericardium, how it relates to "Minister Fire" and what connection (if any) there is between this "Minister Fire" in a Five-Element context and the Minister Fire of the Kidneys.

The *Simple Questions* in Chapter 8 says: "*The Pericardium is the ambassador and from it joy and happiness derive.*"[83] Like the Heart, the Pericardium houses the Mind and it therefore influences our mental-emotional state deeply. For example, a deficiency of Blood will affect the Pericardium as well as the Heart, making the person depressed and slightly anxious. Heat in the Blood will agitate the Pericardium and make the person agitated and restless. Phlegm obstructing the Pericardium will also obstruct the Mind, causing mental confusion.

The Pericardium's function on the mental-emotional plane could be seen as the psychic equivalent of its physical function of moving Qi and Blood in the chest; just as it does on a physical level, on a mental-emotional level the Pericardium is responsible for "movement" towards others, i.e. in relationships (Fig. 9.37).

Given that the Pericardium is related to the Liver within the Terminal-Yin channels, this "movement" is also related to the "movement" of the Ethereal Soul from the ego towards others in social relationships and

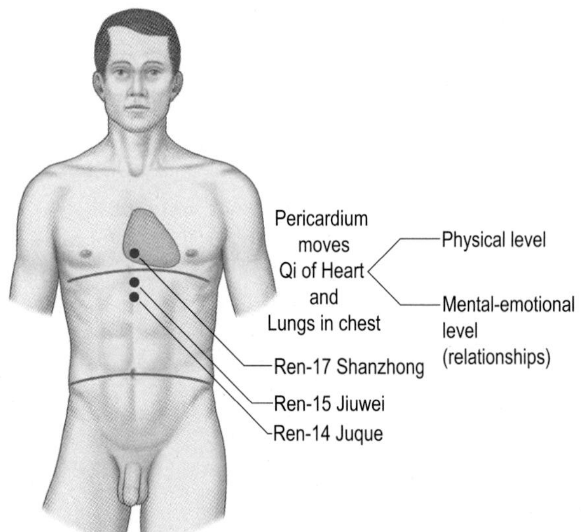

Figure 9.37 The moving action of the Pericardium.

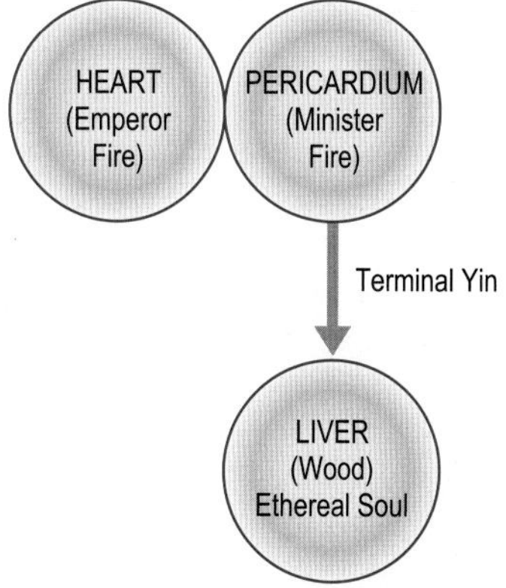

Figure 9.38 The Fire and Wood nature of the Pericardium.

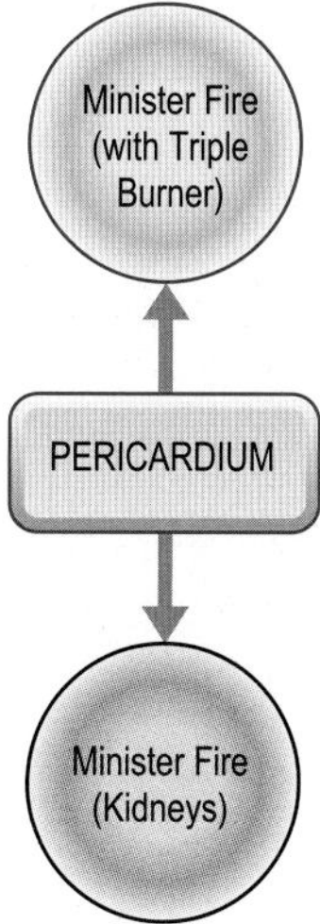

Figure 9.39 Relationship of Pericardium with Heart and Triple Burner.

familial interactions. For this reason, on a mental-emotional level, the Pericardium is particularly responsible for a healthy interaction with other people in social, love and family relationships.

The unique place that the Pericardium occupies in the pathology and treatment of mental-emotional problems is partly due to its partaking of Fire (as it is the "Minister" Fire that assists the Emperor Fire of the Heart) and of Wood (with the Liver within the Terminal Yin). Partaking of Wood and the Ethereal Soul, it gives the Mind "movement" towards others, i.e. it plays an important role in relationships. On a physical level, the Pericardium moves Qi and Blood in the chest. See Figure 9.38.

Moreover, the "moving" nature of the Pericardium is also enhanced by its relationship with the Triple Burner as a channel (within the "Minister Fire" channels). As the Triple Burner is responsible for the free flow of Qi (together with the Liver), the Pericardium's relationship with the Triple Burner accounts for its action in moving Qi and Blood, and its mental-emotional function of "movement" towards others. See Figure 9.39.

The Pericardium houses the Mind (with the Heart) and its pathology includes the following.

- Blood deficiency of the Pericardium will cause depression and slight anxiety.
- Blood Heat of the Pericardium will cause anxiety, insomnia and agitation.
- Phlegm in the Pericardium will cause mental confusion and, in severe cases, mental illness.
- The Pericardium affects emotional problems from relationship difficulties.

The "Minister Fire" is the Fire of the Gate of Life (*Ming Men*). As we have seen above, this Fire is essential to the healthy functioning of the body.

Although many doctors such as Zhu Zhen Heng (1281–1358) identified "Minister Fire" with the Fire of the Gate of Life (*Ming Men*) (and therefore the Kidneys), others, such as Zhang Jie Bin (1563–1640), identified the "Minister Fire" with such internal organs as the Kidney, Liver, Triple Burner, Gall-Bladder and Pericardium.

Thus, purely from a Five-Element perspective, the Pericardium pertains to the Minister Fire (with the Triple Burner) compared to the Emperor Fire of the Heart, while from the perspective of the Internal Organs, the Minister Fire is the Fire of the Gate of Life (*Ming Men*) pertaining to the Kidneys.

However, there is a connection between the two views as the Minister Fire of the Kidneys does flow up to the Liver, Gall-Bladder and Pericardium. In pathology, this has an even greater relevance as the pathological Minister Fire of the Kidneys (driven by emotional stress) flares upwards to harass the Pericardium, causing mental restlessness, agitation, anxiety and insomnia.

Indeed, the Minister Fire and the Original Qi are said to emerge from between the Kidneys through the "intermediary" of the Triple Burner (Fig. 9.40). It is not by chance that the Back-Transporting point of the Triple Burner is on the back at BL-22 Sanjiaoshu, one vertebral space above the Back-Transporting point of

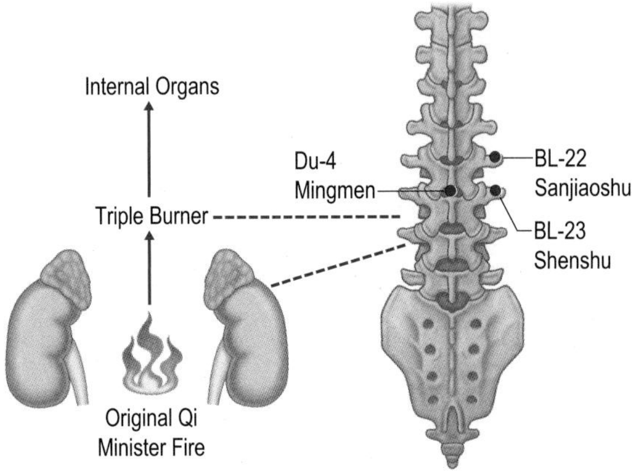

Figure 9.40 Minister Fire and Original Qi emerging through the Triple Burner.

the Kidneys BL-23 Shenshu and the point Du-4 Mingmen: indeed, it reflects the fact that the Minister Fire emerges from the space between the Kidneys through the Triple Burner.

In fact, the Minister Fire of the Kidneys is said to go upwards to the Liver, Gall-Bladder and Pericardium (Fig. 9.41). The Minister Fire going up is compared to the "Fire Dragon flying to the top of a high mountain" and that going down to the Kidneys is compared to the "Fire Dragon immersing in the deep sea" (Fig. 9.42). The fact that the Minister Fire of the Kidneys flows up to the Pericardium could explain the assignment of this organ to "Minister Fire" in the Five-Element relationships.

Many Pericardium channel points have a deep influence on the mental state and are frequently used in mental-emotional problems. In particular, the Pericardium influences a person's relations with other people, and the points on its channel are often used to treat emotional problems caused by relationship difficulties (e.g. P-7 Daling).

CLINICAL NOTE

Action of Pericardium points

- P-6 Neiguan stimulates the coming and going of the Ethereal Soul, lifts mood and treats depression.
- P-7 Daling restrains the coming and going of the Ethereal Soul, settles the Ethereal Soul, calms the Mind and settles anxiety.
- P-5 Jianshi resolves Phlegm from the Pericardium to treat mental confusion.

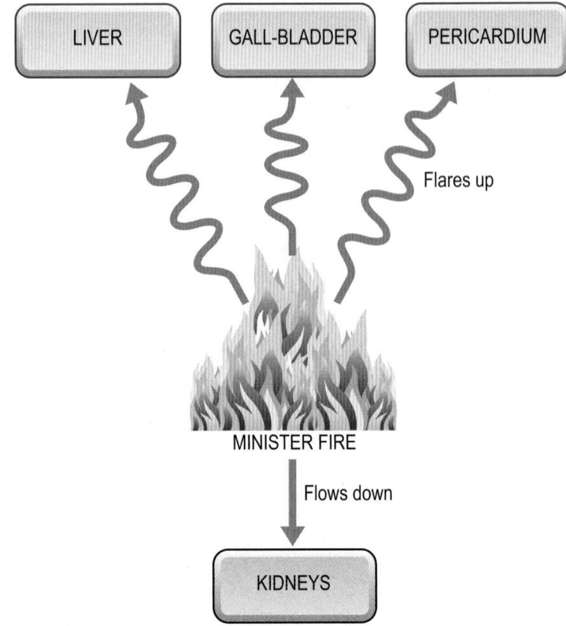

Figure 9.41 Relationship between Minister Fire of the Kidneys and the Pericardium.

It could be said that the protective function of the Pericardium in relation to the Heart so often mentioned is reflected primarily in the mental-emotional sphere where the "Minister Fire" of the Pericardium protects the "Emperor Fire" of the Heart.

The clinical use of the point P-6 Neiguan should be explored further. P-6 Neiguan has a synergistic effect on acupuncture point prescriptions. The addition of P-6 to any prescription increases the therapeutic effect.

Just as P-6 has this effect on a physical level, it has one on a mental-emotional level, i.e. it can bolster the effect of a point combination for mental-emotional problems.

This effect of P-6 is due to various factors. Firstly, it affects the Mind, but how does its effect on the Mind differ from that of the Heart? The Heart is more Yin; it governs Blood which houses the Mind. The Pericardium is more Yang; it is the external covering of the Heart and therefore controls movement of Qi and Blood on a mental-emotional level. This effect on Qi is due also to its relationship with the Liver within the Terminal Yin (*Jue Yin*).

Second, the Pericardium channel, being paired with the Liver channel within the Terminal Yin channels, affects the coming and going of the Ethereal Soul; in

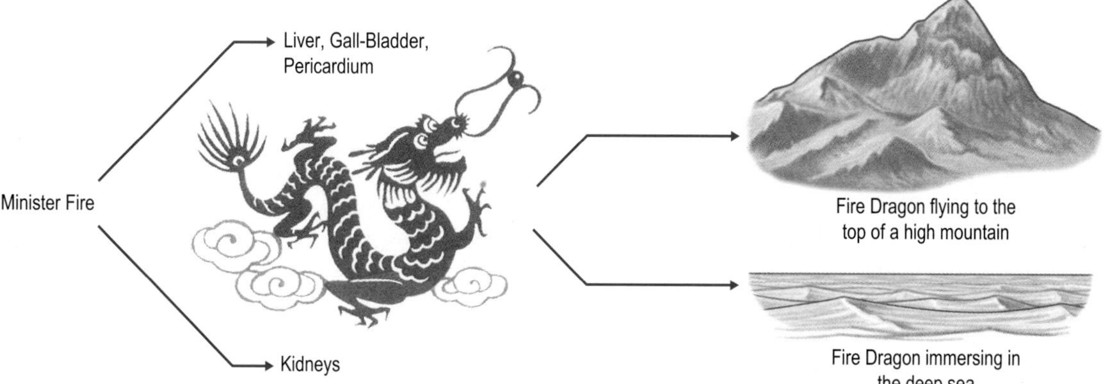

Figure 9.42 Minister Fire flowing up to Liver, Gall-Bladder and Pericardium and down to Kidneys.

particular, P-6 can stimulate the coming and going of the Ethereal Soul and therefore treat depression.

Third, the mental-emotional "moving" effect of P-6 is due also to its being the Connecting (*Luo*) point of the Pericardium channel. As Connecting point, it affects the Triple Burner; it can therefore move Qi of the Triple Burner in all three Burners and this also has a mental-emotional effect.

Fourth, the Pericardium pertains to the Terminal Yin which is the "hinge" of the Yin channels (between the Greater Yin and Lesser Yin). Being the Connecting point and therefore the hinge between Yin and Yang, P-6 is the "hinge" of the Hinge; in its capacity as a "hinge", it connects things. On a mental-emotional level, that means that it regulates our capacity for relationships. Its function of a "hinge" is also related to its being the opening point of the Yin Linking Vessel (*Yin Wei Mai*) which links all the Yin channels.

The use of P-6 in mental-emotional problems is further explored in Chapter 13.

CLINICAL NOTE

P-6 Neiguan

- It has a synergistic effect on acupuncture point prescriptions. The addition of P-6 to any prescription increases the therapeutic effect.
- On a mental-emotional level, P-6 can bolster the effect of a point combination for mental-emotional problems.
- It moves Qi and Blood on an emotional level.
- It stimulates the coming and going of the Ethereal Soul and therefore treats depression.
- It regulates our capacity for relationships.

SUMMARY

The Pericardium in mental-emotional problems

- The Pericardium pertains to the Minister Fire together with the Triple Burner (in terms of channels).
- The Pericardium pertains to the Minister Fire together with the Kidneys as Minister Fire originates there.
- The Minister Fire flares upwards to Liver, Gall-Bladder and Pericardium and flows downwards to the Kidneys.
- From a Five-Element perspective, the Pericardium pertains to the Minister Fire channels with the Triple Burner.
- From an organ perspective, the Minister Fire originates from the Kidneys.
- In emotional problems, the pathological Minister Fire flares upwards to harass the Pericardium.

THE TRIUNE BRAIN AND CHINESE MEDICINE

In the context of emotions as causes of disease, it is interesting to explore the connections between the triune brain theory and Chinese medicine. The subject will be dealt with briefly here as it is discussed more at length in Chapter 14. The triune (meaning "three in one") brain theory was developed by Dr Paul MacLean, Chief of Brain Evolution and Behavior at the National

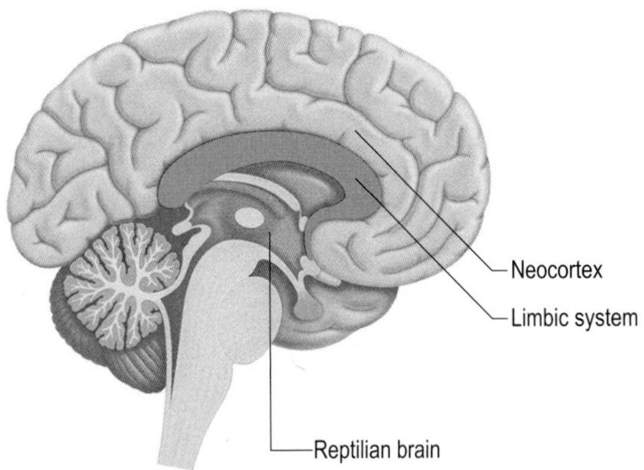

Figure 9.43 The triune brain.

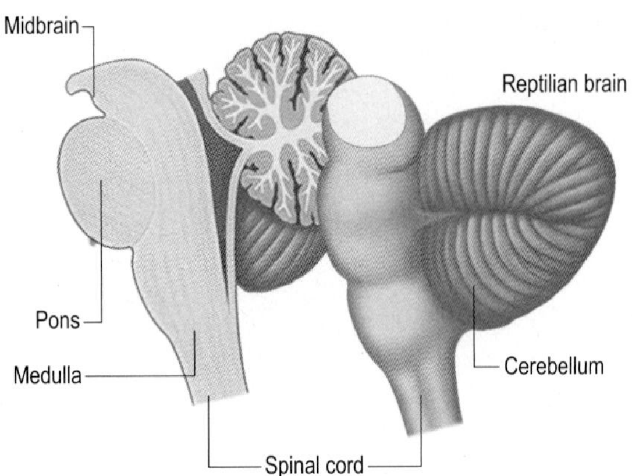

Figure 9.44 Brain stem and cerebellum.

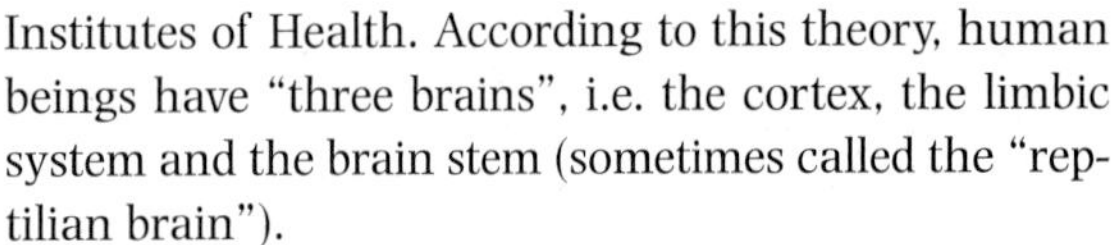

Institutes of Health. According to this theory, human beings have "three brains", i.e. the cortex, the limbic system and the brain stem (sometimes called the "reptilian brain").

The three brains are the neocortex or neomammalian brain, the limbic or paleomammalian system, and the brain stem and cerebellum or reptilian brain. Each of the three brains is connected by nerves to the other two, but each seems to operate as its own brain system with distinct capacities (Fig. 9.43).

MacLean's hypothesis has become a very influential paradigm, which has forced a rethink of how the brain functions. It had previously been assumed that the highest level of the brain, the neocortex, dominates the other, lower levels. MacLean has shown that this is not the case, and that the physically lower limbic system, which rules emotions, can hijack the higher mental functions when it needs to. As we shall see below, and more in depth in Chapter 14, this presents interesting points of contact with the Chinese medicine's view of the relationship between the Mind (*Shen*) and Ethereal Soul (*Hun*).

The brain stem is the "reptilian" brain. It is called that because it is the main brain function of reptiles. We have the brain stem in common with reptiles, some of which are remnants of prehistoric animals. It is a remnant of our prehistoric past.

The reptilian brain acts on stimulus and response. It is useful for quick decisions without thinking. The reptilian brain focuses on survival, and takes over when we are in danger and do not have time to think. In a world of survival of the fittest, the reptilian brain is concerned with getting food and keeping from becoming food. The reptilian brain is fear driven, and takes over when one feels threatened or endangered[84] (Fig. 9.44).

In animals such as reptiles, the brain stem and cerebellum dominate. This brain controls muscles, balance and autonomic functions, such as breathing and heartbeat. This part of the brain is active even in deep sleep. As we shall see below, the reptilian brain resembles the Corporeal Soul of Chinese medicine.

The second brain is the limbic stem or mammalian brain. The limbic system is the root of emotions and feelings. It affects moods and bodily functions. The limbic brain is draped around the reptilian brain. It comprises:

- hippocampus
- fornix
- amygdala
- septum
- cingulate gyrus
- perirhinal and parahippocampal regions (Fig. 9.45).

When this part of the brain is stimulated with a mild electrical current, various emotions (fear, joy, rage, pleasure, pain, etc.) are produced. No emotion has been found to reside in one place for very long. But the limbic system as a whole appears to be the primary seat of emotion, attention and affective (emotion-charged) memories.

The limbic system has vast interconnections with the neocortex, so that brain functions are not either purely limbic or purely cortical, but a mixture of both.

The neocortex is the most evolutionary advanced part of our brain. The cortex, also known as the supe-

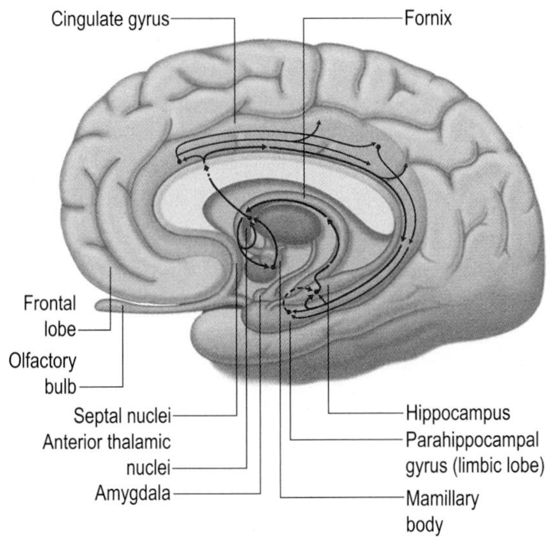

Figure 9.45 The limbic system.

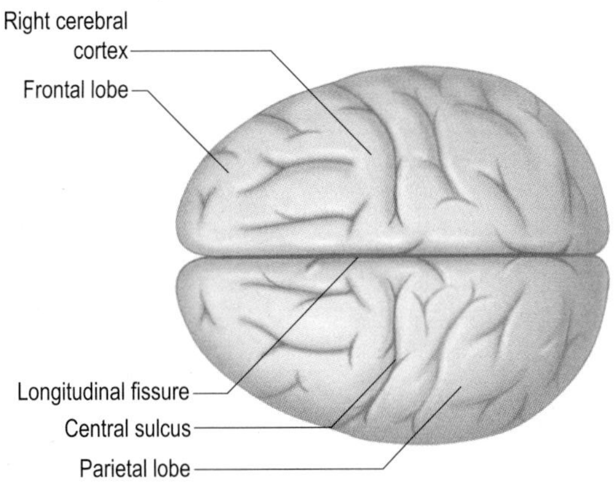

Figure 9.46 The brain hemispheres and cortex.

rior or rational (neomammalian) brain, comprises almost the whole of the hemispheres and some subcortical neuronal groups (Fig. 9.46). It governs our ability to speak, think and solve problems. The neocortex affects our creativity and our ability to learn. The neocortex makes up about 80% of the brain. It corresponds to the brain of the primate mammals and, consequently, the human species. The higher cognitive functions that distinguish humankind from animals are in the cortex.

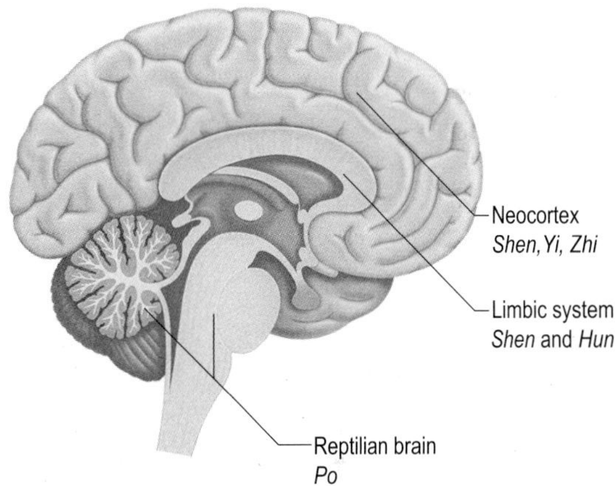

Figure 9.47 The triune brain and the Five Spiritual Aspects of Chinese medicine.

The triune brain, the Mind, Ethereal Soul and Corporeal Soul

There are some interesting connections between the theory of the triune brain and the Mind, Ethereal Soul and Corporeal Soul in Chinese medicine (Fig. 9.47).

The reptilian brain and the Corporeal Soul

As we have seen above, the reptilian brain is responsible for physiological activities such as breathing, heart rate, digestion and body movement. These are the functions that would be attributed to the Corporeal Soul in Chinese medicine. It is interesting also that the reptilian brain's functions are still active when a person is in a vegetative state ("brain dead").

From the Chinese point of view, when the Mind is disabled (and therefore also the Intellect and Will-Power of the Spleen and Kidneys) and the person is in a coma, the person is still alive because the Corporeal Soul is still functioning. This would therefore confirm that the Corporeal Soul is like the reptilian brain.

The limbic system and the Mind and Ethereal Soul

The limbic system developed in mammals and is responsible for our emotional life, family bonding and social bonding. These functions are those of the Mind and Ethereal Soul in Chinese medicine. As we have seen in Chapter 3, the Ethereal Soul is responsible for our outward psychic movement towards others in family, friends and love or work relationships; in other words, the family and social bonding fostered by the limbic brain.

As we have seen above, the limbic system has vast interconnections with the neocortex, so that brain functions are not either purely limbic or purely cortical, but a mixture of both. This mirrors the Chinese view of the inter-relationship between the Mind (*Shen*) and Ethereal Soul (*Hun*); they both pertain to Yang, the Ethereal Soul is the "coming and going" of the Mind, and the two together are responsible not only for our emotional life but also for planning, life dreams, ideas, etc.

There is another interesting connection in that the limbic system, although responsible for emotions, is essential to the development of the cortex in mammals (and humans). One of the physiological processes that limbic regulation directs is the development of the brain itself. The importance of limbic contact for normal brain development shows itself most starkly in the devastating consequences of its omission.[85] Many subsystems of the mammalian brain do not come pre-programmed; maturing mammals need limbic regulation to give coherence to neurodevelopment.[86]

Interestingly, when people are hurting, they turn to affiliations: marriage, family, friends, groups, clubs, pets, massage therapists, etc.[87] These represent relationships modulated by the Ethereal Soul.

The inter-relationship and mutual dependence between the cortex and the limbic system mirrors that between the Mind (*Shen*) and Ethereal Soul (*Hun*) in Chinese medicine.

The cortex and the Mind, Intellect and Memory in Chinese medicine

As we have seen above, the cortex is responsible for thinking, cognition and memory. These are clearly the functions of the Mind (*Shen*), Intellect (*Yi*) and Will-Power (*Zhi*) together. Please remember that, as described in Chapter 6, the *Zhi* of the Kidneys may be translated as "will-power" or as "memory". In this context, some of the cortical activities resonating with Chinese medicine relate to memory.

SUMMARY

The triune brain and Chinese medicine

- Human beings have "three brains", i.e. the cortex, the limbic system and the brain stem.
- Dr MacLean has proposed that our skull holds not one brain, but three, each representing a distinct evolutionary stratum that has formed upon the older layer before it. He calls it the "triune brain".
- The three brains are the neocortex or neomammalian brain, the limbic or paleomammalian system, and the brain stem and cerebellum or reptilian brain. Each of the three brains is connected by nerves to the other two, but each seems to operate as its own brain system with distinct capacities.
- The brain stem is the "reptilian" brain. It is called that because it is the main brain function of reptiles. We have the brain stem in common with reptiles, some of whom are remnants of prehistoric animals. It is a remnant of our prehistoric past.
- In animals such as reptiles, the brain stem and cerebellum dominate.
- The limbic brain is draped around the reptilian brain. It comprises the hippocampus, fornix, amygdala, septum, cingulate gyrus and perirhinal and parahippocampal regions.
- The limbic system is concerned with emotions and instincts: feeding, fighting, fleeing and sexual behavior.
- The limbic system has vast interconnections with the neocortex, so that brain functions are not either purely limbic or purely cortical, but a mixture of both.
- One of the physiological processes that the limbic system directs is development of the brain itself. Many subsystems of the mammalian brain do not come pre-programmed; maturing mammals need limbic regulation to give coherence to neurodevelopment.
- The cortex, also known as the superior or rational (neomammalian) brain, comprises almost the whole of the hemispheres and some subcortical neuronal groups. It corresponds to the brain of primate mammals and, consequently, the human species.
- The higher cognitive functions that distinguish humankind from animals are in the cortex.
- The reptilian brain's functions are those of the Corporeal Soul in Chinese medicine.
- The limbic system developed in mammals and is responsible for our emotional life, family bonding and social bonding. These functions are those of the Mind and Ethereal Soul in Chinese medicine.
- The cortex is responsible for thinking, cognition and memory. These are clearly the functions of the Mind (*Shen*), Intellect (*Yi*) and Will-Power (or Memory) (*Zhi*).

END NOTES

1. Damasio A 1999 The Feeling of What Happens – Body and Emotions in the Making of Consciousness. Harcourt, San Diego, p. 50.
2. Lewis M, Haviland-Jones JM (eds) 2004 Handbook of Emotions. Guilford Press, New York, pp. 258–260.
3. The Feeling of What Happens, p. 136.
4. 1981 Ling Shu Jing 灵枢经 [Spiritual Axis]. People's Health Publishing House, Beijing, pp. 24–25. First published *c.*100 BC.
5. Ibid., p. 25.
6. Ibid., p. 24.
7. Gu Yu Qi 2005 Zhong Yi Xin Li Xue 中医心理学[Chinese Medicine Psychology]. China Medicine Science and Technology Publishing House, Beijing, p. 54.
8. Ibid., p. 54.
9. Ibid., p. 54.
10. Tian Dai Hua 2005 Huang Di Nei Jing Su Wen 黄帝内经素问[The Yellow Emperor's Classic of Internal Medicine – Simple Questions]. People's Health Publishing House, Beijing, pp. 37–41. First published *c.*100 BC.
11. Zhang Jie Bin (also called Zhang Jing Yue) 1982 Lei Jing 类经 [Classic of Categories]. People's Health Publishing House, Beijing, p. 424. First published in 1624.
12. Spiritual Axis, p. 24.
13. 1979 Huang Di Nei Jing Su Wen 黄帝内经素问[The Yellow Emperor's Classic of Internal Medicine – Simple Questions]. People's Health Publishing House, Beijing, pp. 150–151. First published *c.*100 BC.
14. Ibid., p. 339.
15. Spiritual Axis, p. 24.
16. 1979 The Yellow Emperor's Classic of Internal Medicine – Simple Questions, p. 222.
17. Ibid., p. 151.
18. Spiritual Axis, p. 24.
19. Ibid., p. 11.
20. 1979 The Yellow Emperor's Classic of Internal Medicine – Simple Questions, p. 337.
21. Ibid., pp. 124–125.
22. Ibid., p. 150.
23. Classic of Categories, p. 424.
24. Cited in Chinese Medicine Psychology, p. 55.
25. Zhang Yuan Kai 1985 Meng He Si Jia Yi Ji 孟河四家医集 [Medical Collection of Four Doctors from the Meng He Tradition]. Jiangsu Science Publishing House, Nanjing, p. 40.
26. Principles of Medical Practice, cited in Wang Ke Qin 1988 Zhong Yi Shen Zhu Xue Shuo 中医神主学说 [Theory of the Mind in Chinese Medicine]. Ancient Chinese Medical Texts Publishing House, Beijing, p. 34.
27. Spiritual Axis, p. 67.
28. Ibid., p. 23.
29. 1979 The Yellow Emperor's Classic of Internal Medicine – Simple Questions, p. 37.
30. Spiritual Axis, p. 23.
31. 1979 The Yellow Emperor's Classic of Internal Medicine – Simple Questions, p. 221.
32. Ibid., p. 17.
33. Chang C 1977 The Development of Neo-Confucian Thought. Greenwood Press, Westport, Connecticut, p. 67.
34. Huang Siu-chi 1999 Essentials of Neo-Confucianism. Greenwood Press, Westport, Connecticut, p. 91.
35. 1979 The Yellow Emperor's Classic of Internal Medicine – Simple Questions, p. 221.
36. Tian Dai Hua 2005 The Yellow Emperor's Classic of Internal Medicine – Simple Questions, p. 38.
37. Ibid., p. 38.
38. Spiritual Axis, p. 25.
39. Medical Collection of Four Doctors from the Meng He Tradition, p. 40.
40. Cited in Chinese Medicine Psychology, p. 59.
41. Spiritual Axis, p. 24.
42. Ibid., p. 24.
43. Chinese Medicine Psychology, p. 59.
44. Ibid., p. 59.
45. 1979 The Yellow Emperor's Classic of Internal Medicine – Simple Questions, p. 32.
46. Ibid., p. 222.
47. Chinese Medicine Psychology, p. 60.
48. 1979 The Yellow Emperor's Classic of Internal Medicine – Simple Questions, p. 221.
49. Ibid., p. 247.
50. Spiritual Axis, p. 24.
51. Personal communication from Dr John Shen, London, 1982.
52. Trimble M 2007 The Soul in the Brain. Johns Hopkins University Press, Baltimore, p. 189.
53. 1979 The Yellow Emperor's Classic of Internal Medicine – Simple Questions, p. 222.
54. Handbook of Emotions, p. 574.
55. Ibid., p. 574.
56. Spiritual Axis, p. 24.
57. 1979 The Yellow Emperor's Classic of Internal Medicine – Simple Questions, p. 222.
58. Handbook of Emotions, p. 655.
59. Holy Bible, New International Version® 1984 International Bible Society. Online version www.biblegateway.com.
60. Ibid.
61. Ibid.
62. Ibid.
63. Fingarette H 1972 Confucius – The Secular as Sacred. Waveland Press, Prospect Heights, Illinois, p. 28.
64. Ibid., p. 30.
65. Wollheim R 1999 On the Emotions. Yale University Press, New Haven, p. 148.
66. Ibid., p. 149.
67. Handbook of Emotions, p. 50.
68. On the Emotions, pp. 155–156.
69. Handbook of Emotions, p. 21.
70. Ames RT, Rosemont H Jr 1999 The Analects of Confucius – a Philosophical Translation. Ballantine Books, New York, p. 76.
71. Ames RT, Hall D 2001 Focusing the Familiar – A Translation and Philosophical Interpretation of the Zhongyong. University of Hawai'i Press, Honolulu, p. 40.
72. Confucius – The Secular as Sacred, pp. 30–31.
73. Handbook of Emotions, p. 50.
74. 1979 The Yellow Emperor's Classic of Internal Medicine – Simple Questions, p. 221.
75. Chen Yan 1174 San Yin Ji Yi Bing Zheng Fang Lun [A Treatise on the Three Categories of Causes of Diseases], cited in Theory of the Mind in Chinese Medicine, p. 55.
76. Cited in Chinese Medicine Psychology, p. 61.
77. Ibid., p. 61.
78. Spiritual Axis, p. 67.
79. 1979 The Yellow Emperor's Classic of Internal Medicine – Simple Questions, p. 221.
80. Medical Collection of Four Doctors from the Meng He Tradition, p. 40.
81. Principles of Medical Practice, cited in Theory of the Mind in Chinese Medicine, p. 34.
82. Spiritual Axis, p. 67.
83. 1979 The Yellow Emperor's Classic of Internal Medicine – Simple Questions, p. 58.
84. Lewis T, Amini F, Lannon R 2000 A General Theory of Love. Random House, New York, p. 22.
85. Ibid., p. 87.
86. Ibid., p. 88.
87. Ibid., p. 171.

精神病病因

CHAPTER 10

ETIOLOGY OF MENTAL-EMOTIONAL PROBLEMS

CONSTITUTION *162*
Wood type *162*
Fire type *163*
Earth type *164*
Metal type *164*
Water type *165*
DIET *166*
Excessive consumption of hot-energy foods *166*
Excessive consumption of Damp-producing foods *166*
Excessive consumption of cold-energy foods *167*
Irregular eating habits *167*
Insufficient eating *167*
OVERWORK *167*
EXCESSIVE SEXUAL ACTIVITY *167*
DRUGS *167*
Cannabis *168*
Cocaine *168*
Ecstasy *169*
PREVENTION OF MENTAL-EMOTIONAL PROBLEMS *169*

ETIOLOGY OF MENTAL-EMOTIONAL PROBLEMS

In this chapter, I shall discuss the etiology of mental-emotional problems according to the following topics.

- Constitution
- Diet
- Overwork
- Excessive sexual activity
- Drugs
- Prevention of mental-emotional problems

Under etiology, I shall discuss the etiological factors of mental-emotional problems other than emotional stress which was discussed in Chapter 9. Emotional stress is the main cause of mental-emotional problems, and the other etiological factors (e.g. diet) are usually only contributory factors. Although I am discussing etiological factors separately, in practice, they are often combined. In order to formulate an idea of the etiological factors involved, it is useful to divide a person's life into stages.

It is usually the overlap of different causative factors, each originating from different times in one's life, that leads to the development of mental-emotional problems. It is useful to form an idea of the origin of mental-emotional problems in terms of time. To do this, one can divide a person's life into three broad periods, each of which is characterized by its own specific etiological factors.

1. *The period in the womb*: constitution.
2. *Childhood, up until about 18*: childhood patterns.
3. *Adulthood*: emotions, diet, overwork, drugs.

Broadly speaking, inherited traits obviously affect our life in the womb, juvenile development affects our childhood, and emotional problems, diet and overwork affect our adulthood.

Many of the emotional patterns adults fall into are often set during childhood. This may be due to very many different factors such as relations with parents, lack of demonstrative affection from parents, relations with siblings, fighting between parents, emotional strain put on a child by a parent who pours out all his or her troubles to the child, a too strict and rigid upbringing, too many academic demands at school, a parental preference for one child over his or her siblings, pressure on a child to fulfill a parent's failed dreams, a child assuming almost the role of husband or wife after the death of the father or mother respectively, etc.

Table 10.1 The three periods of life

INHERITED OR IN WOMB	CHILDHOOD	ADULT AGE
Weak nervous system	Childhood patterns	Emotions, diet, excessive sexual activity, overwork, drugs

Thus the three stages of life and their causative factors of mental-emotional problems can be summarized as follows (Table 10.1). There is, of course, an interaction among these three periods of life and their respective causes of disease. For example, emotional problems during childhood may also interact with constitutional traits to cause disease later in life. For instance, if a girl has a constitutional imbalance in the Penetrating and Directing Vessels (*Chong* and *Ren Mai*) and she is subject to emotional strain at the time of puberty; this will often cause mental-emotional problems later in life.

It is important to form an idea of the origin of the problem so that we can give the right advice to the patient.

The etiological factors discussed are:

- constitution
- diet
- overwork
- excessive sexual activity
- drugs.

CONSTITUTION

The constitutional make-up of an individual is an extremely important etiological factor in mental-emotional problems. For example, I frequently see patients who are extremely anxious about the smallest things in life and an investigation of their present emotional life and past history does not reveal any cause for this. When this happens, it is generally due to the constitutional make-up of the individual.

"Constitutional" refers to an etiological factor that is either inborn and inherited from the parents, or developed in utero during pregnancy. In either case, the inherited state of the nervous system plays an important role in mental-emotional problems in later life.

For example, a shock to the mother during pregnancy may affect the fetus and cause the newborn baby to sleep fitfully, cry during sleep, open and close the eyes slightly during sleep and sometimes develop fevers of unexplained origin. In such cases, the baby often has a bluish color on the forehead. If not treated, this will have repercussions later in life and affects the Mind and Ethereal Soul.

An inherited weak nervous system is often manifested with a Heart crack on the tongue (*see Fig. 11.6*). Such a crack indicates that the person has an inherited weakness of the Heart which predisposes that person to the development of mental-emotional problems. However, this may never manifest unless other causative factors intervene later in life.

Traditionally, five different constitutional body shapes are described, one for each Element. The Five-Element constitutional types are described below.

Wood type

People of the Wood type have a subtle shade of green in their complexion, a relatively small head and long-shaped face, broad shoulders, straight back, tall, sinewy body and elegant hands and feet.

In terms of personality, they have developed intelligence but their physical strength is poor. They are hard workers, think things over and tend to worry. See Figure 10.1.

From an emotional point of view, people of the Wood type are prone to worry, frustration and repressed anger. These are often the cause of Liver patterns such as Liver-Qi stagnation or Liver-Yang rising.

SUMMARY

Wood type

- Greenish complexion
- Small head
- Long face
- Broad shoulders
- Straight back
- Sinewy body
- Tall
- Elegant hands and feet
- Tendency to worry, frustration and anger

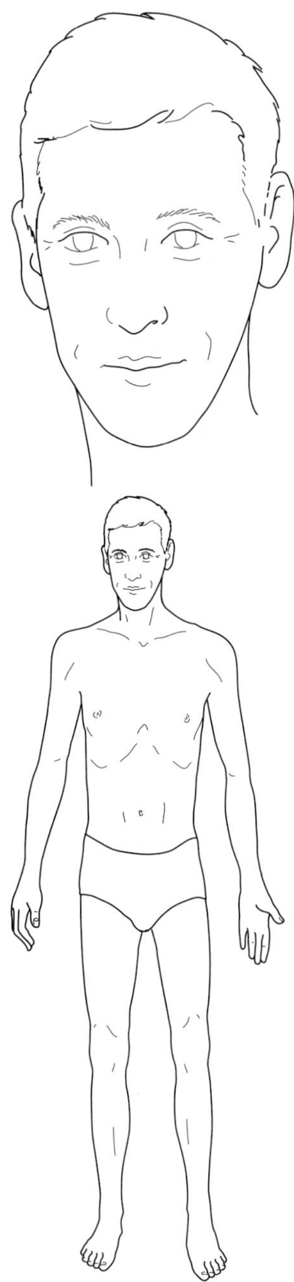

Figure 10.1 Wood type.

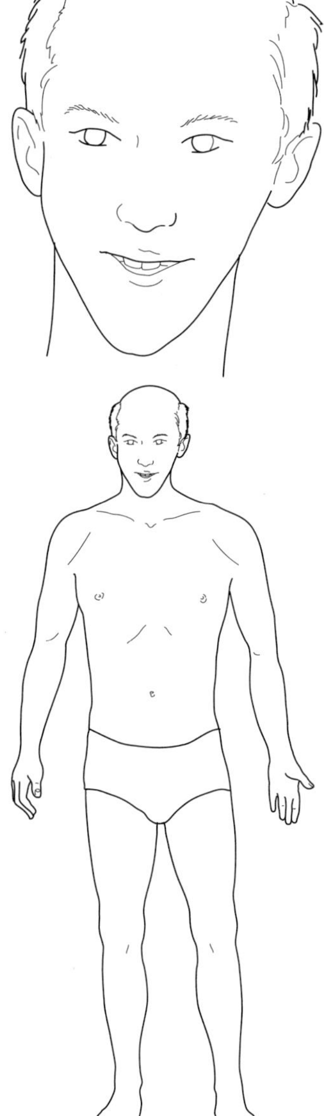

Figure 10.2 Fire type.

Fire type

People of the Fire type have a red, florid complexion, wide teeth, a pointed, small head, possibly with a pointed chin, hair that is either curly or scanty, well-developed muscles of the shoulders, back, hips and head and relatively small hands and feet.

In terms of personality, they are keen thinkers. The Fire type is quick, energetic and active. They are short-tempered. They walk firmly and shake their body while walking. They tend to think too much and often worry. They have a good spirit of observation and they analyze things deeply. See Figure 10.2.

From an emotional point of view, people of the Fire type are very energetic, they laugh a lot and have a tendency to "manic" behavior. However, at the opposite pole, people of the Fire type may be prone to depression and anxiety.

SUMMARY

Fire type
- Red complexion
- Wide teeth
- Pointed, small head
- Well-developed shoulder muscles
- Curly hair or not much hair
- Small hands and feet
- Walking briskly
- Tendency to "manic" behavior

Earth type

People of the Earth type have a yellowish complexion, round-shaped face, relatively big head, wide jaws, well-developed and nice-looking shoulders and back, large abdomen, strong thigh and calf muscles, relatively small hands and feet, and well-built muscles of the whole body. They walk with firm steps without lifting their feet very high.

The Earth type is calm and generous, has a steady character, likes to help people and is not over-ambitious. They are easy to get on with. See Figure 10.3.

From an emotional point of view, people of the Earth type are generous and they like to help others. They give of themselves emotionally; at the opposite pole, they may be the complete opposite and be selfish. They may have a tendency to guilt and shame.

SUMMARY

Earth type
- Yellowish complexion
- Round face
- Wide jaws
- Large head
- Well-developed shoulders and back
- Large abdomen
- Large thighs and calf muscles
- Well-built muscles
- Emotionally giving

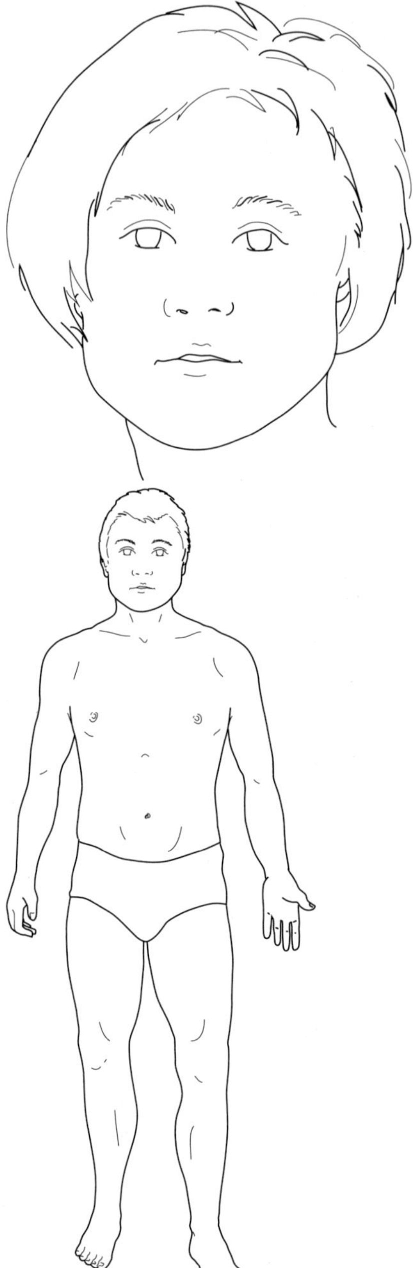

Figure 10.3 Earth type.

Metal type

People of the Metal type have a relatively pale complexion, a square-shaped face, a relatively small head, small shoulders and upper back, a relatively flat abdomen, and small hands and feet. They have a

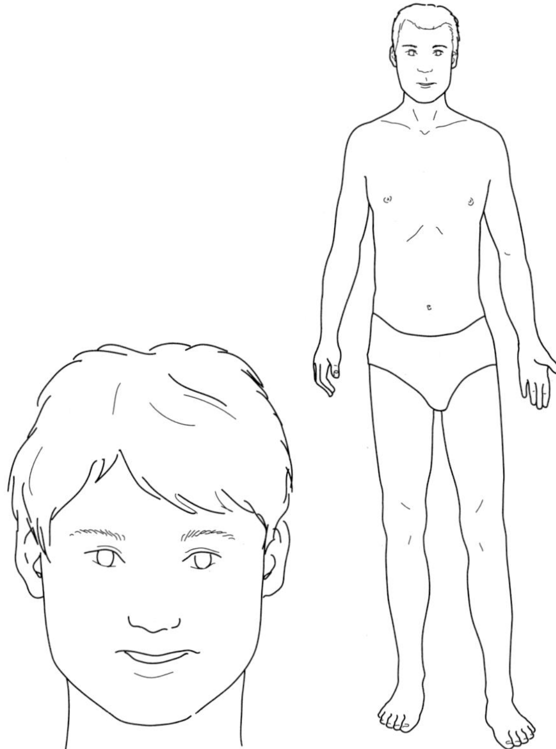

Figure 10.4 Metal type.

strong voice, move swiftly and have keen powers of thought.

They are honest and upright. They are generally quiet and calm in a solid way, but also capable of decisive action when necessary. They have a natural aptitude for leadership and management. See Figure 10.4.

From the emotional point of view, people of the Metal type are prone to worry, sadness and grief and, when under such emotional stress, they tend to weep a lot.

SUMMARY

Metal type

- Pale complexion
- Square face
- Small head
- Small shoulders and upper back
- Flat abdomen
- Strong voice
- Prone to worry, sadness and grief

Water type

People of the Water type have a relatively dark complexion, wrinkles, a relatively large head, a round face and body, broad cheeks, narrow and small shoulders and a large abdomen. They keep their body in motion while walking and find it difficult to keep still. They have a long spine.

The Water type is sympathetic and slightly laid-back. They are good negotiators and loyal to their work colleagues. They are aware and sensitive. See Figure 10.5.

From the emotional point of view, people of the Water type are very sensitive, have a high sex drive and a tendency to guilt.

SUMMARY

Water type

- Dark complexion
- Wrinkly skin
- Large head
- Broad cheeks
- Narrow shoulders
- Large abdomen
- Long spine
- Tendency to guilt

This typology can be used in diagnosis and prognosis. These portraits describe an archetype but, in reality, due to the way people live their lives and other factors, there can be considerable variations from the types. For example, although a Wood type typically has a tall and slender body, if there is a tendency to over-eat, he or she may obviously become fat and deviate from their type.

The Five-Element constitutional body types are useful in practice because they explain inherent differences between people which might otherwise be taken as pathological. For example, the Fire type is active and energetic, and he or she walks fast; if we did not know about the Fire type, we might interpret these characteristics as pathological (i.e. Excess of Yang).

Deviations from the Element type are also significant. For example, to stay with the Fire Element type, if all the characteristics of the body shape point to someone being a Fire type but he or she walks slowly,

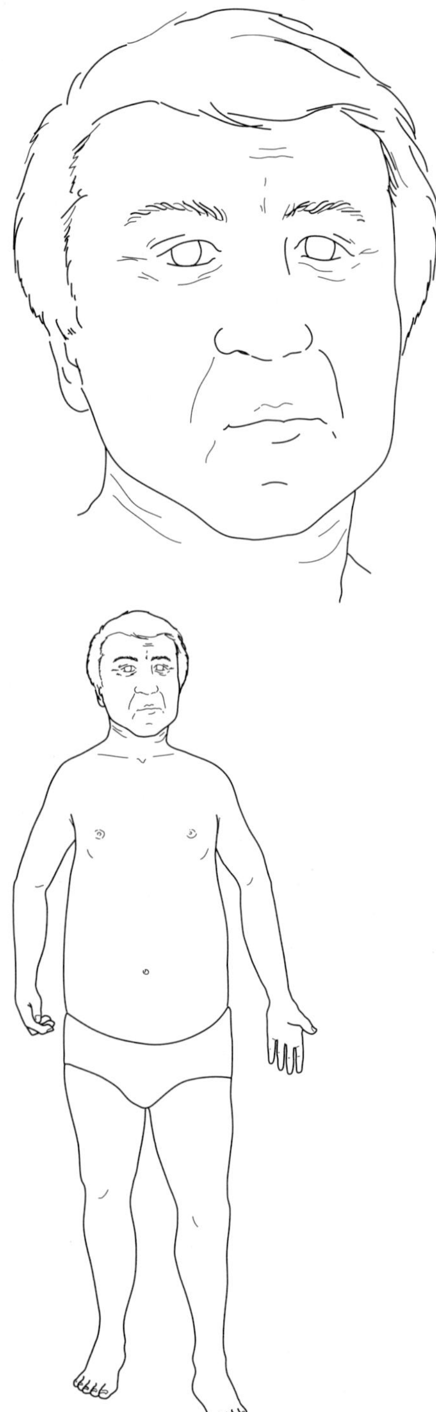

Figure 10.5 Water type.

it indicates a problem. This is useful as this discrepancy may herald a future problem.

It should be borne in mind that a person may be a mixture of two or more types; one can have a mixed Earth–Wood type for example.

Treatment of the constitutional Element type is particularly useful in the case of mental-emotional problems. For example, a Wood type might display some typical emotional traits such as indecision and inability to plan one's life; treatment of the Wood Element would help the person on a mental-emotional level, whatever other disharmony that person might suffer from.

DIET

Diet plays a secondary role in contributing to mental-emotional problems. There are several aspects to "irregular eating" as described in Chinese books. The main ones that apply to Western patients are:

- excessive consumption of hot-energy foods
- excessive consumption of Damp-producing foods
- excessive consumption of cold-energy foods
- irregular eating habits
- insufficient eating.

Excessive consumption of hot-energy foods

An excessive consumption of hot-energy foods (red meat, spices) and drinks (including and especially alcohol) leads to Heat and Fire which may easily harass the Mind. It should be noted that tobacco also has a hot energy and, especially combined with alcohol, it contributes to forming Heat in the body. Indeed, I would say that alcohol and tobacco are the two main "dietary" causes of Heat or Fire.

Heat or Fire harasses the Mind and may therefore cause anxiety, agitation and insomnia. They also overstimulate the Ethereal Soul, leading to a slight "manic" behavior.

Moreover, Fire easily damages Yin and may therefore cause Yin deficiency which, in itself, would aggravate anxiety, agitation and insomnia.

Excessive consumption of Damp-producing foods

An excessive consumption of Damp-producing foods (dairy foods, greasy foods, fats, sugar) leads to the formation of Dampness or Phlegm. Both Dampness and Phlegm may obstruct the Mind but Phlegm more so. Both Dampness and Phlegm are "heavy" pathogenic factors. While on a physical level they cause a feeling of heaviness of the body, on a mental-emotional level, they also "weigh a person down" and aggravate feelings of depression.

In my experience, shame often leads to Dampness. Dampness is a "dirty" pathogenic factor and just as on a physical level it causes turbid discharges, on a mental-emotional level shame makes the person feel "dirty" and unworthy.

Phlegm has a more obstructive effect on the Mind which, in extreme cases, is the cause of serious mental illness. However, it occurs in many degrees of severity and, in mild cases, Phlegm obstructing the Mind causes a certain mental confusion which may aggravate both feelings of depression or feelings of excessive elation and anxiety.

When Phlegm that obstructs the Mind combines with Heat, it leads to agitation, manic behavior and insomnia. In such cases the tongue would be Swollen, with a Stomach–Heart crack with a sticky-yellow coating inside it (*see Fig. 11.8*).

Excessive consumption of cold-energy foods

Excessive consumption of cold-energy foods (fruit, most vegetables, cold drinks) injures Yang and may lead to Yang deficiency of the Spleen and Kidneys. This would aggravate feelings of depression in patients suffering from depression occurring against a background of Kidney-Yang deficiency.

Irregular eating habits

"Irregular eating habits" includes eating late at night, skipping meals, eating on the run, etc. All these habits tend to cause Stomach-Qi and/or Stomach-Yin deficiency. In persons suffering from anxiety occurring against a background of Yin deficiency, the feeling of anxiety would be aggravated by the Stomach-Yin deficiency.

Insufficient eating

It may seem strange to include "insufficient eating" as a cause of disease in affluent Western societies. However, from a Chinese medical perspective, insufficient nourishment may be caused by an injudicious vegetarian diet (especially in women) or by strict slimming diets.

Insufficient eating causes Blood deficiency, and this would aggravate feelings of anxiety and insomnia occurring against a background of Blood deficiency.

OVERWORK

By "overwork" I mean working long hours without adequate rest (often combined with irregular eating); intended in this sense, overwork depletes the Kidneys and especially Kidney-Yin. Overwork would therefore aggravate feelings of depression and/or anxiety occurring against a background of Kidney-Yin deficiency.

Overwork and emotional stress (these two factors often accompany each other) are very common and pervasive etiological factors of mental-emotional problems in Western patients.

EXCESSIVE SEXUAL ACTIVITY

Excessive sexual activity is a cause of disease more in men than in women. This is because sperm is a direct manifestation of Kidney-Essence and, in women, there is no corresponding loss of Kidney-Essence during orgasm. It is difficult to define what is an "excessive" level of sexual activity, as that depends on the age and the physical condition of the man; however, sexual activity could be defined as "excessive" if the man feels very tired after it.

A very rough guide may be provided by dividing the man's age by 5; this gives the recommended frequency of sexual intercourse. For example, for a 50-year-old man, this would be once every 10 days ($50:5 = 10$). By "sexual activity" in men is intended ejaculation, as sexual activity without ejaculation does not deplete the Kidney-Essence.

Excessive sexual activity in men is a cause of Kidney deficiency which may manifest with Yang or Yin deficiency depending on the constitution of the man. Such Kidney-deficiency would aggravate feelings of depression, and Kidney-Yin deficiency would also aggravate feelings of anxiety.

DRUGS

Drugs such as cannabis, cocaine, heroine, LSD and others deeply affect the Mind, the Ethereal Soul and the Corporeal Soul. Prolonged use of such drugs leads to mental confusion and lack of memory and concentration. In combination with other causes of disease, they definitely contribute to mental-emotional problems and cloud the Mind. Indeed, there is considerable and mounting evidence of the link between heavy cannabis use and the development of schizophrenia.[1]

Cannabis

Several studies have shown a correlation between cannabis use and a higher risk of developing schizophrenia. On an individual level, cannabis use confers an overall twofold increase in the relative risk for later schizophrenia. At the population level, elimination of cannabis use would reduce the incidence of schizophrenia by approximately 8%, assuming a causal relationship.[2]

The first evidence that cannabis use might predispose to later psychosis came from a study of Swedish conscripts who were followed up using record-linkage techniques based on inpatient admissions for psychiatric care.

A dose–response relationship was observed between cannabis use at conscription (age 18 years) and schizophrenia diagnosis 15 years later. Self-reported "heavy cannabis users" (i.e. who had used cannabis more than 50 times) were six times more likely than non-users to have been diagnosed with schizophrenia 15 years later. The authors concluded that the findings are consistent with a causal relationship between cannabis use and schizophrenia.[3]

The Dutch Nemesis study examined the effect of cannabis use on self-reported psychotic symptoms among the general population: 4045 psychosis-free individuals and 59 who had a psychotic disorder were assessed at baseline and were administered follow-up assessments 1 year later and again 3 years after the baseline assessment.

Compared with non-users, individuals using cannabis at baseline were nearly three times more likely to manifest psychotic symptoms at follow-up. The highest risk (odds ratio = 6.8) correlated with the highest level of cannabis use.

Lifetime history of cannabis use at baseline, as opposed to use of cannabis at follow-up, was a stronger predictor of psychosis 3 years later. This suggests that the association between cannabis use and psychosis is not merely the result of short-term effects of cannabis use leading to an acute psychotic episode.

The authors concluded that their study confirmed that cannabis use is an independent risk factor for the emergence of psychosis in psychosis-free persons, and that those with an established vulnerability to psychotic disorders are particularly sensitive to its effects, resulting in a poor outcome.[4]

The Christchurch Health and Development Study (New Zealand) examined a general population birth cohort for more than 20 years. The association between cannabis dependence disorder and the presence of psychotic symptoms at ages 18 and 21 years was examined. Findings indicated concurrent associations between cannabis dependence disorder and risk of psychotic symptoms both at ages 18 and 21 years.

Individuals who met the diagnostic criteria for cannabis dependence disorder at age 18 years had a 3.7-fold increased risk of psychotic symptoms than those without cannabis dependence problems. The risk of psychotic symptoms was 2.3 times higher for those with cannabis dependence disorder at age 21 years.

The authors concluded that the findings are clearly consistent with the view that heavy cannabis use may make a causal contribution to the development of psychotic symptoms since they show that, independently of pre-existing psychotic symptoms and a wide range of social and contextual factors, young people who develop cannabis dependence show an elevated rate of psychotic symptoms.[5]

An appreciable proportion of cannabis users report short-lived adverse effects, including psychotic states following heavy consumption, and regular users are at risk of dependence. People with major mental illnesses such as schizophrenia are especially vulnerable in that cannabis generally provokes relapse and aggravates existing symptoms.

The untoward mental effects of cannabis include psychological responses such as panic, anxiety, depression or psychosis. There is good evidence that taking cannabis leads to acute adverse mental effects in a high proportion of regular users. Many of these effects are dose-related, but adverse symptoms may be aggravated by constitutional factors, including youthfulness, personality attributes and vulnerability to serious mental illness.[6]

Cocaine

Studies on cocaine abusers in clinical settings report that more than half of such individuals experience paranoia and hallucinations.[7] Among patients who attend psychiatric emergency services, non-schizophrenic cocaine abusers are reported to have as severe hallucinations as schizophrenic patients who do not abuse cocaine. Believing that their drug-using behavior is being watched and they are being followed, hallucinations, in keeping with these delusions, are typical of cocaine-induced psychosis. This is so typical that it may be used as an important tool to differentiate it from schizophrenia.[8]

Cocaine-induced psychosis shows sensitization, i.e. psychosis becomes more severe and occurs more rapidly with continued cocaine use.[9] Interestingly, sensitization occurs only with psychosis and not with other effects of cocaine.[10]

Ecstasy

Ecstasy (an amfetamine derivative) has become popular with participants in "raves" because it enhances energy, endurance, sociability and sexual arousal. Ecstasy has serious acute and chronic toxic effects that resemble those seen with other amfetamines and are caused by an excess of the same sympathomimetic actions for which the drugs are valued by the users.

Neurotoxicity to the serotonergic system in the brain can also cause permanent physical and psychiatric problems. A review of the literature has revealed over 87 ecstasy-related fatalities, caused by hyperpyrexia, rhabdomyolysis (the destruction of skeletal muscle cells), intravascular coagulopathy, hepatic necrosis, cardiac arrhythmias, cerebrovascular accidents and drug-related accidents or suicide.

Undesired psychological acute effects include:

- hyperactivity, flight of ideas (with a resulting inability to focus one's thoughts in a sustained and useful manner) and insomnia
- hallucinations, depersonalization (a feeling of separation of the self from the body), anxiety, agitation, and bizarre or reckless behavior
- panic attacks
- psychotic episodes.

The long-term adverse effects arise from a neurotoxic action of the methylenedioxy derivatives of the amfetamines. The massive release of serotonin not only gives rise to acute psychotic symptoms but also causes chemical damage to the cells that released it.

Long-term psychiatric problems include:

- impairment of memory, both verbal and visual, with the degree of impairment being roughly proportional to the intensity of the preceding ecstasy use
- impairment of decision-making, information processing, logical reasoning and simple problem solving
- greater impulsivity and lack of self-control
- panic attacks occurring repeatedly when the person is not under the influence of the drug, even after many months of abstinence
- recurrent paranoia, hallucinations, depersonalization, flashbacks and even psychotic episodes, occurring some time after the individual has stopped using ecstasy
- severe depression, which is sometimes resistant to any treatment other than selective serotonin reuptake inhibitors, occasionally accompanied by suicidal thoughts.

PREVENTION OF MENTAL-EMOTIONAL PROBLEMS

Mental activity is the most important aspect of the Mind and this is affected by either excessive thinking or excessive emotional strain. It follows then that the most important measures one can take to prevent mental-emotional problems are to restrain one's mental activity and avoid emotional stress, which, of course, in our modern stressful times, is much easier said than done.

"To restrain one's mental activity" means not only avoiding excessive mental work, but also avoiding thinking too much altogether. These concepts are heavily influenced by Daoist ideas of "nourishing life" by calming the Mind and preventing distracting thoughts. The very first chapter of the *Simple Questions* says:[12]

One should live a quiet life with few desires so that one can preserve one's Qi and guard one's Mind in order to avoid disease. Thus if emotions are absent and craving is curbed, the Heart is peaceful and there is no fear.

Thus, in order to attain a tranquil Mind, the ancient Daoist sages advocated three basic attitudes:

1. avoid excessive thinking
2. avoid excessive craving
3. avoid distracting thoughts.

Restraining craving is particularly applicable to Western industrialized societies where consumerism is rampant and the pressures of advertising contribute to creating ever new "needs". Restraining craving and desire is very important to achieve mental tranquillity, as excessive craving stirs up the Minister Fire which harasses the Heart and Pericardium.

This Daoist ideal is, of course, terribly difficult to attain, but even just barely striving towards parts of it is a step in the right direction.

In the past, some Daoist doctors even formulated "prescriptions", mimicking herbal prescriptions, to calm the Mind, restrain thinking and curb emotions. Two of them will be presented here as examples.

XIANG SUI WAN

"Pill" to the Likeness of Marrow

- **Not thinking too much** = nourishes the Heart (emperor ingredient)
- **Restraining anger** = nourishes the Liver
- **Restraining sexual desire** = nourishes the Kidneys
- **Careful talking** = nourishes the Lungs
- **Regulating diet** = nourishes the Spleen

ZHEN REN YANG ZANG GAO

The Sage's "Paste" to Nourish the Internal Organs

- **Remain indifferent whether granted favors or subjected to humiliation** = makes the Liver balanced
- **Be indifferent whether moving or still** = calms Heart-Fire
- **Regulate diet** = does not overburden the Spleen
- **Regulate breathing and moderate talking** = makes Lungs healthy
- **Calm the Mind and prevent distracting thoughts** = replenishes the Kidneys.

END NOTES

1. Byrne P, Jones S, Williams R 2004 The association between cannabis and alcohol use and the development of mental disorder. Current Opinions in Psychiatry 17: 255–261.
2. Arseneault L, Cannon M, Witton J, Murray RM 2004 Causal association between cannabis and psychosis: examination of the evidence. British Journal of Psychiatry 184: 110–117.
3. Zammit S, Allebeck P, Andreasson S et al. 2002 Self reported cannabis use as a risk factor for schizophrenia in Swedish conscripts of 1969: historical cohort study. British Medical Journal 325: 1199.
4. Os J, Bak M, Hanssen M et al. 2002 Cannabis use and psychosis: a longitudinal population-based study. American Journal of Epidemiology 156: 319–327.
5. Arseneault et al. 2004 British Journal of Psychiatry 184: 110–117.
6. Johns A 2001 Psychiatric effects of cannabis. British Journal of Psychiatry 178. Available from: http://bjp.rcpsych.org/cgi/content/full/178/2/116 [Accessed 8 November 2008].
7. Brady KT, Lydiard RB, Malcolm R, Ballenger JC 1991 Cocaine-induced psychosis. Journal of Clinical Psychiatry 52: 509–512.
8. Serper MR, Chou JC, Allen MH et al. 1999 Symptomatic overlap of cocaine intoxication and acute schizophrenia at emergency presentation. Schizophrenia Bulletin 25: 387–394.
9. Brady et al. 1991 Journal of Clinical Psychiatry 52: 509–512.
10. Bartlett E, Hallin A, Chapman B, Angrist B 1997 Selective sensitization to the psychosis inducing effects of cocaine: a possible marker for addiction relapse vulnerability? Neuropsychopharmacology 16: 77–82.
11. Lieb R, Schuetz CG, Pfister H et al. 2002 Mental disorders in ecstasy users: a prospective-longitudinal investigation. Drug and Alcohol Dependence 68. Available from: http://www.maps.org/research/mdma/litupdates/human/comparisons/09.02/lieb2002-1.html [Accessed 2008].
12. 1979 Huang Di Nei Jing Su Wen 黄帝内经素问 [The Yellow Emperor's Classic of Internal Medicine – Simple Questions]. People's Health Publishing House, Beijing, p. 3. First published *c.*100 BC.

精神病诊断 CHAPTER 11

DIAGNOSIS OF MENTAL-EMOTIONAL PROBLEMS

COMPLEXION *171*

EYES *173*

PULSE *174*
The pulse and the emotions *174*
The Heart pulse *175*
General pulse qualities and the emotions *176*

TONGUE *177*
Red tip *177*
Heart crack *178*
Sides of the tongue *179*
Body shape *179*
Combined Stomach and Heart crack *180*

DIAGNOSIS OF MENTAL-EMOTIONAL PROBLEMS

The diagnosis of mental-emotional problems follows the same lines as diagnosis of other problems, for the body and Mind are an inseparable unit which, when it is disturbed, gives rise to symptoms and signs in both the physical and mental-emotional spheres.

However, some special diagnostic signs in mental-emotional problems will be discussed. The diagnosis of mental-emotional problems will be discussed according to the following topics.

- Complexion
- Eyes
- Pulse
- Tongue

COMPLEXION

All organs can obviously influence the complexion, but, whatever the organ, the complexion shows the state of the Mind and Spirit. Yu Chang in *Principles of Medical Practice* (1658) calls the complexion the "banner of the Mind and Spirit" and he says:[1]

When the Mind and Spirit are flourishing, the complexion is glowing; when the Mind and Spirit are declining, the complexion withers. When the Mind is stable the complexion is florid ...

A healthy Mind and Spirit show most of all in a complexion with *shen*. This indicates an indefinable quality of lustre, glow, glitter and florid state of the complexion which indicates a good prognosis even if the color itself is pathological. Shi Pa Nan in *Origin of Medicine* (1861) says:[2]

The shen of the complexion consists in lustre and body. "Lustre" means that the complexion appears clear and bright from the outside; "body" means that it is moist and with lustre in the inside.

If a complexion has such attributes, even if the color is pathological, it indicates that the Mind and Spirit are stable and unaffected and therefore the prognosis is good.

The *Simple Questions* in Chapter 17 describes the look of pathological colors with or without *shen*:[3]

A red complexion should look like vermilion covered with white, not like ochre. A white complexion should look like feathers of a goose, not like salt. A blue complexion should look like moistened greyish jade, not like indigo. A yellow complexion should look like realgar covered with gauze, not like loess (the soil in North China along the Yellow River basin). A black complexion should look like dark varnish, not like greyish charcoal.

These are summarized in Table 11.1. Therefore, each pathological color may be with *shen* (indicating a

Table 11.1 Good and poor prognosis in pathological complexion colors

COLOR	GOOD PROGNOSIS	POOR PROGNOSIS
Red	Like vermilion covered with white	Like ochre
White	Like goose feathers	Like salt
Blue	Like gray jade	Like indigo
Yellow	Like realgar covered with gauze	Like loess (soil in North China)
Black	Like dark varnish	Like grayish charcoal

good prognosis) or without *shen* (denoting a poor prognosis).

Dr Chen Shi Duo in *Secret Records of the Stone Room* (1687) goes so far as saying:[4]

If the complexion is dark but with shen, the person will live even if the disease is serious. If the complexion is bright but without shen, the person will die even if there is no disease.

Observation of the complexion must be closely linked to the feeling of the pulse. The pulse shows the state of Qi, while the complexion shows the state of the Mind and Spirit. If the pulse shows changes but the complexion is normal, it indicates that the problem is recent. If both the pulse and the complexion show pathological changes, it indicates that the problem is long-standing.

The "*shen*" of the complexion should also be checked against the lustre of the eyes (see below). A change in the complexion always indicates a deeper or more long-standing problem. For example, a sustained period of overwork and inadequate sleep may cause the eyes to lack lustre. If the complexion is not changed, this is not too serious and the person can recover easily by resting. If, however, the eyes lack lustre and the complexion is dull, without lustre or dark, it indicates that the problem is not transient but deeper-rooted.

Various emotions may show on the complexion with specific signs. Anger usually manifests with a greenish tinge on the cheeks, a greenish tinge on the forehead means that Liver-Qi has invaded the Stomach, and a greenish tinge on the tip of the nose indicates that Liver-Qi has invaded the Spleen.

A character prone to anger may also manifest with eyebrows that meet in the center. In some cases, if the anger is bottled up inside as resentment leading to long-standing depression, the complexion may be pale. This is due to the depressing effect of stagnant Liver-Qi on Spleen- or Lung-Qi. In such cases, the Wiry quality of the pulse will betray the existence of anger rather than sadness or grief (indicated by the pale complexion) as a cause of disease.

Excess joy may manifest with a red color on the cheekbones. Worry causes a grayish complexion and a skin without lustre. Worry knots Lung-Qi and affects the Corporeal Soul which manifests on the skin. For this reason, the skin becomes grayish and lustreless.

Pensiveness may manifest with a sallow complexion because it depletes Spleen-Qi.

Fear shows with a bright-white complexion on the cheeks and forehead. If chronic fear causes deficiency of Kidney-Yin and the rising of Empty Heat of the Heart, there will be a malar flush, with the underlying color being bright-white.

Shock also causes a bright-white complexion. Shock early in childhood may manifest with a bluish tinge on the forehead. If there is a bluish tinge on the forehead or around the mouth, it indicates a prenatal shock (whilst in the uterus).

Hatred often shows with a greenish complexion on the cheeks. Craving shows with a reddish color on the cheeks. Guilt shows with a dark-ruddy complexion. Shame manifests with a dull, sallow complexion without lustre.

SUMMARY

The complexion and the emotions

- *Anger*: greenish tinge on the cheeks.
- *Excess joy*: a red color on the cheekbones.
- *Worry*: a grayish complexion and a skin without lustre.
- *Pensiveness*: a sallow complexion.
- *Fear*: a bright-white complexion on the cheeks and forehead.
- *Shock*: a bright-white complexion.
- *Shock early in childhood*: a bluish tinge on the forehead.

- *Prenatal shock*: a bluish tinge on the forehead and around the mouth.
- *Hatred*: a greenish complexion on the cheeks.
- *Craving*: a reddish color on the cheeks.
- *Guilt*: a dark-ruddy complexion.
- *Shame*: a dull, sallow complexion without lustre.

EYES

Observation of the eyes plays an extremely important role in the diagnosis of emotional and mental problems. As soon as the patient sits down, the first thing I observe carefully is the lustre of the eyes. In my experience the lustre (or lack of it) of the eyes reflects very closely and accurately the state of the Mind and Spirit: I have never experienced this sign giving false information.

The eyes reflect the state of the Mind, Spirit and Essence. The *Spiritual Axis* in Chapter 80 says:[5]

The Essence of the five Yin and the six Yang organs ascends to the eyes ... the essence of bones goes to the pupil, the essence of tendons goes to the iris, the essence of Blood goes to the blood vessels in the eyes, the essence of the Lungs goes to the sclera ...

See Figure 11.1.

This shows that the essence of all the Yin organs – and therefore the Mind, Ethereal Soul, Corporeal Soul, Intellect and Will-Power – manifests in the eyes. The same chapter of the *Spiritual Axis* says further on:[6]

The eyes manifest the essence of the five Yin and six Yang organs, the Nutritive and Defensive Qi and they are the place where the Qi of the Mind is generated ... the eyes are the messengers of the Heart which houses the Mind. If the Mind and Essence are not coordinated and not transmitted, one has visual hallucinations. The Mind, Ethereal Soul and Corporeal Soul are scattered so that one has bewildering perceptions.

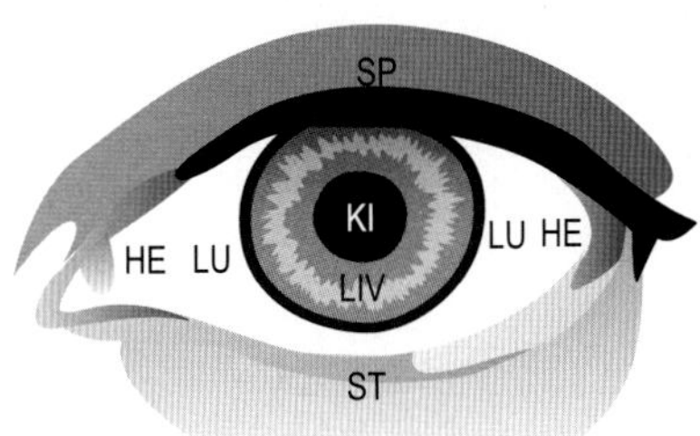

Figure 11.1 The correspondence between parts of the eye and Internal Organs.

Shi Pa Nan in *Origin of Medicine* (1861) says: "*The Qi of the Mind and Spirit dwells in the eyes.*"[7] Zhou Xue Hai in *A Simple Guide to Diagnosis from Body and Color* (1894) says: "*Even if the illness is serious, if the eyes have good shen, the prognosis is good.*"[8]

When looking at the eyes, we need to consider two aspects:

1. whether they have lustre or not
2. whether they are "controlled" or not.

If the eyes are clear, have lustre, sparkle or gleam and are brilliant, it shows that the Mind and Spirit are in a good state of vitality (if the patient is ill). If they are dull as if they were clouded by a mist, it shows that the Mind or Spirit is disturbed by emotional problems. I find that in practice this sign is never wrong and is therefore completely reliable. The duller the eyes, the more severe or long-standing the emotional problems.

"Controlled" look means a fixed, sustained and penetrating look; this indicates a stable and integrated personality. "Uncontrolled" means that the look is shifty or too fixed.

If the eyes look uncontrolled it may indicate that the person is affected by anger. In terms of personality, an uncontrolled look points to a mercurial character, an unreliable person, a person ridden by guilt, fanatical or possibly destructive.

Sadness, grief and shock make the eyes dull and without lustre. Excess joy and guilt make the eyes uncontrolled and slightly too watery. Fear makes the eyes bulge out slightly and shift frequently. Guilt makes the eyes shifty and the eyelids flap shut in rapid movements while talking. Shame makes the eyes dull and "uncontrolled" in the sense that the person is unable to look at others in the eyes.

The lack of lustre of the eyes reflects very accurately the presence of emotional stress, which, however, could also be in the past rather than the present. The intensity of dullness is also directly related to the intensity and duration of the emotional stress; the duller the eyes, the more intense and long-lasting the emotional stress.

SUMMARY

The eyes and the emotions

- The eyes reflect the state of the Mind, Spirit and Essence.
- When looking at the eyes, we need to consider two aspects: whether they have lustre or not and whether they are "controlled" or not.
- Eyes with *shen* are clear, have lustre, sparkle or gleam and are brilliant; Mind and Spirit are in a good state of vitality.
- Eyes without *shen* are dull as if they were clouded by a mist; Mind or Spirit is disturbed by emotional problems.
- "Controlled" look refers to a fixed, sustained and penetrating look: stable and integrated personality.
- "Uncontrolled" look refers to a look that is shifty or too fixed: the person is affected by anger, mercurial character, guilt, fanatical.
- *Sadness, grief and shock*: eyes dull and without lustre.
- *Excess joy and guilt*: eyes uncontrolled and slightly too watery.
- *Fear*: eyes bulging out slightly and shifting frequently.
- *Guilt*: eyes shifty and eyelids flapping shut in rapid movements while talking.
- *Shame*: eyes dull and "uncontrolled" in the sense that the person is unable to look at others in the eyes.

PULSE

The pulse reflects the state of Qi while the eyes directly reflect the state of the Mind and Spirit. Of course, by reflecting Qi, the pulse also reflects the state of the Mind and Spirit but, when confronted with a pulse sign, it is often very difficult to determine (from the pulse alone) whether that is due to emotional problems or to other causative factors.

For example, sadness and grief can render the eyes dull and without lustre, which definitely indicates a disturbance of the Spirit. The same emotions can make the Lung pulse Weak, but this can be caused by very many other factors too. Thus the pulse, tongue and complexion should always be closely integrated in order to diagnose mental-emotional problems correctly. It is only after some years of clinical experience that one can draw conclusions about the relation between certain pulse qualities and mental-emotional problems.

The pulse and the emotions

Anger makes the pulse Wiry, sometimes only on the left side. A Wiry quality of the pulse is always a reliable pointer to problems from anger when other signs (such as a pale face and weak voice) seem to point to sadness and grief.

If anger occurs at mealtimes, it manifests with a Wiry quality on the Stomach position. Repressed anger and resentment make the pulse "stagnant", a quality which is not one of the traditional 28 pulse qualities. A stagnant pulse is somewhat tight, but not as hard as the Tight pulse, and it seems to flow reluctantly.

I find that a Wiry pulse is a reliable indication of emotions such as anger, repressed anger, frustration, hatred or resentment. Indeed, I would go as far as to say that if the pulse is not Wiry (at least in one position), then the problem is not from anger.

However, please remember that a Wiry pulse is the necessary, but not sufficient, factor to diagnose anger. In other words, it is important to remember that a Wiry pulse does *not* always indicate anger (whether repressed or not). For example, a Wiry pulse may also sometimes reflect guilt. Moreover, I find that a Wiry pulse often reflects emotional stress that may derive from a range of emotions, e.g. guilt, worry, fear. This is particularly so when the pulse is Wiry in a position other than the Liver position.

For example, a Wiry pulse in the Heart position may reflect guilt, worry or fear; a Wiry pulse on the Lung position may indicate worry; a Wiry quality on the Kidney position may also point to guilt (or fear).

It is important to remember also that, in the elderly, the pulse often becomes Wiry because the arteries harden, so we cannot necessarily draw the conclusion that they are suffering from anger or repressed anger.

Sadness and grief make the pulse Choppy or Short and it characteristically flows without a wave. The pulse without wave seems to flow distally towards each pulse position separately, rather than flowing smoothly from the rear towards the Front position (Fig. 11.2).

The sad pulse quality occurs only in the Front and Middle position, seldom on the Rear position. If only one position is affected (e.g. only the Lung position),

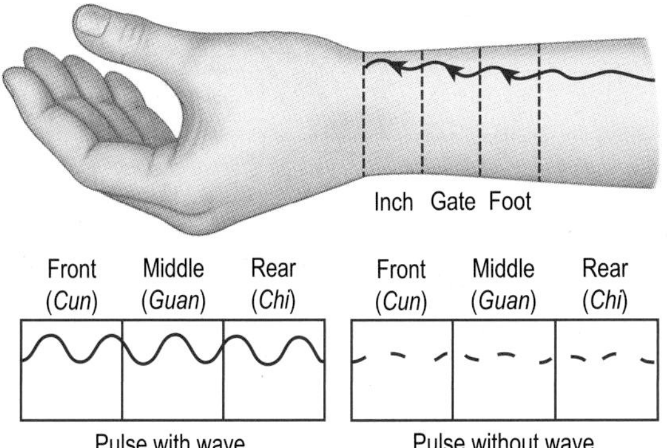

Figure 11.2 Pulse without wave.

the sadness has not lasted for over a year. If both the Front and Middle positions of left and right have the sad quality, the sadness is long-standing.

Sometimes sadness and grief manifest with a very Weak quality on both Lung and Heart positions. Again, this finding should be checked against others, since such a pulse configuration can also be caused by an accident to the chest.

Excessive joy makes the pulse slow and slightly Hollow or Overflowing-Empty on the Heart position.

Fear and shock render the pulse rapid. In severe cases they can give the pulse a Moving quality, i.e. a pulse that is short and shaped like a bean, and which gives the impression of vibrating rather than pulsating. Shock also makes the Heart pulse Tight and Fine.

Guilt makes the pulse rapid; the pulse also gives the impression of shaking as it pulsates. Shame makes the pulse Slippery and without a wave.

SUMMARY

The pulse and the emotions

- *Anger*: Wiry, sometimes only on the left side.
- *Repressed anger and resentment*: "stagnant", i.e. somewhat tight, but not as hard as the Tight pulse, flowing reluctantly.
- *Sadness and grief*: Choppy or Short, without wave; also very Weak on both Lung and Heart positions.
- *Excessive joy*: Slow and slightly Hollow or Overflowing-Empty on the Heart position.
- *Fear*: Rapid.
- *Shock*: Moving; also makes the Heart pulse Tight and Fine.
- *Guilt*: Rapid; also gives the impression of shaking as it pulsates.
- *Shame*: Slippery and without a wave.

The Heart pulse

The Heart pulse is, of course, very important in the diagnosis of mental-emotional problems because the Heart houses the Mind; its pulse qualities and significance often differ from the traditional ones. The following are some Heart-pulse qualities and their emotional significance according to my experience.

An *Overflowing* quality on the Heart pulse often indicates emotional problems of most kinds (sadness, grief, anger, guilt, etc.). Please note that I use the word "Overflowing" in a different sense from the true Overflowing quality. "Overflowing" here means that the Heart pulse is slightly more superficial (and relatively Full) *in relation* to other positions; thus, it is not really Overflowing as the true Overflowing pulse but it is bigger and more superficial than the other pulses.

In some cases, it may be that the pulse is all Weak and Choppy and the only position that stands out is the Heart one. One might be inclined to think that, in such a picture, only the Heart position is normal while it is, in fact, the opposite. When all positions are Weak and Choppy and only the Heart pulse can be felt clearly, I consider that Heart-pulse quality as relatively "Overflowing", and such a picture usually indicates deep emotional problems.

A *Rounded* quality of the Heart pulse refers to a pulse that feels rounder than normal, somewhat like a small ball, but at the same time, rather short. This quality indicates stagnation of Qi in the Heart, together with a deficiency of Heart-Qi. Therefore it is associated with emotions such as sadness and grief, especially when unexpressed.

A *Choppy* Heart-pulse quality indicates Heart-Blood deficiency from sadness, grief or worry. It is very common in women and it may also indicate unexpressed emotions.

An *Empty* Heart-pulse quality indicates Heart-Qi deficiency from sadness and grief.

The Pericardium pulse is also felt on the Heart position, especially in emotional problems. A Pericardium pathology is reflected especially in Full types of Heart

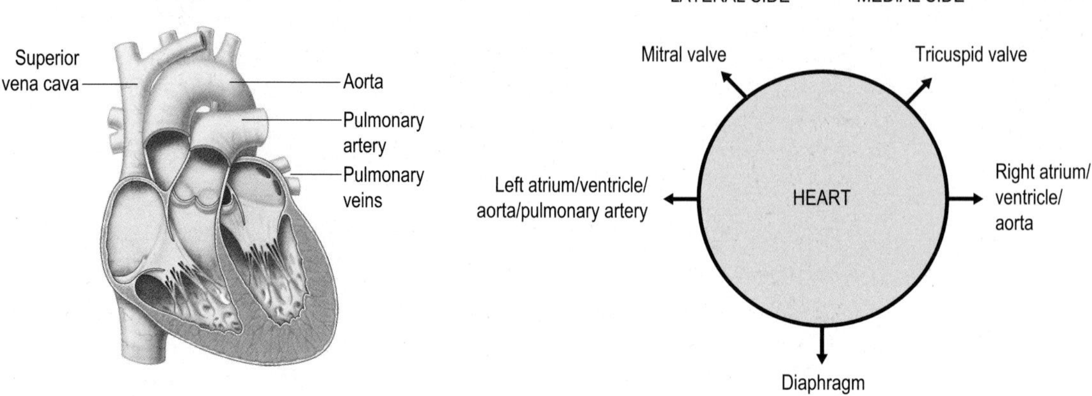

Figure 11.3 Heart pulse in actual heart problems.

pulse and particularly when there are chest symptoms (oppression, stuffiness, tightness, discomfort, pain).

When we feel a pathological quality on the Heart pulse, how do we know that that particular quality reflects emotional problems rather than an actual heart problem of Western medicine?

Generally, an actual heart problem is often indicated by an abnormal pulse quality in the peripheral pulse positions, felt by rolling the finger proximally, distally, laterally and medially from the Heart position itself. These qualities are usually Slippery and/or Wiry. These peripheral pulse positions are related to the heart valves, aorta and pulmonary vein. A Slippery or Wiry quality of such peripheral pulse positions may indicate aortic aneurysm, hypertension, arteriosclerosis or valve problems (Fig. 11.3).

However, in some cases, a congenital valve problem may be indicated by a Deep, Weak and Choppy Heart pulse, combined with a pulse that is Weak and Choppy in general.

SUMMARY

The Heart pulse

- *Overflowing*: emotional problems of most kinds (sadness, grief, anger, guilt, etc.).
- *Rounded*: stagnation of Qi in the Heart, together with a deficiency of Heart-Qi; sadness and grief, especially when unexpressed.
- *Choppy*: Heart-Blood deficiency from sadness, grief, worry.
- *Empty*: Heart-Qi deficiency from sadness and grief.

General pulse qualities and the emotions

The following is a discussion of general pulse qualities in emotional problems.

Choppy

The Choppy pulse feels, weak, "jagged", soft, empty and without wave. In the context of mental-emotional problems, the Choppy pulse indicates sadness primarily (usually against a background of Blood deficiency). Indeed, one of the characteristics of the Choppy pulse is that it lacks a "wave", as what Dr Shen calls the Sad pulse does (see below).

Sad

The "Sad" pulse was described by Dr J.H.F. Shen. It is similar to the Choppy pulse in that it has no wave; however, it is not necessarily Choppy. The Sad pulse would appear before the pulse becomes Choppy. The normal pulse should flow smoothly like a wave from the Rear to the Front position. The Sad pulse has no such wave and it flows reluctantly and "sadly" (see Fig. 11.2).

The Sad pulse is also similar to the Short pulse as it does not fill the pulse position. The Sad pulse indicates sadness. According to Dr Shen, one can judge the severity and duration of the sadness according to how many pulse positions have the Sad quality. Generally, only the first or first and second positions show the Sad quality; if all three positions have this quality, it indicates that the sadness the patient is suffering from is severe and of long duration.

Wiry

A pulse that is Wiry all over is a clear indication of stagnation (of Qi or Blood) and it is usually related to anger and other allied emotional states (frustration, resentment, hatred, fury) and also to guilt. The Wiry pulse may also reflect Liver-Yang rising or Liver-Fire, also deriving from such emotions.

However, Qi stagnation may affect other organs besides the Liver (e.g. Lungs, Heart, Stomach, Spleen, Intestines). When it does, the pulse may be Wiry in a specific position, for example on the right Front, left Front, right Middle and both Rear positions respectively. Please bear in mind that a "Wiry" Lung pulse will never be as Wiry as a Wiry Liver pulse. As the normal Lung pulse is soft, it takes only a small change in quality to make it "Wiry".

In emotional problems, a Wiry quality on the Lung pulse usually indicates worry, while on the Heart pulse it may indicate various emotions such as worry, fear, guilt, shame or anger.

SUMMARY

General pulse qualities and the emotions

- *Choppy*: sadness (usually against a background of Blood deficiency).
- *Sad*: sadness.
- *Wiry*: stagnation (of Qi or Blood), usually related to anger and other allied emotional states (frustration, resentment, hatred, fury).
- *Wiry on Lung position*: worry.
- *Wiry on Heart position*: worry, fear, guilt, shame, anger.

TONGUE

Red tip

One of the tongue's most reliable indicators of emotional problems is a red tip (Plate 11.1). However, although this is a sure sign of emotional or mental problems, it is not very specific since it can arise from almost any emotion.

Why is the tip of the tongue affected and why is it red? First of all, the tip of the tongue is affected because it corresponds to the Heart and this organ, as mentioned above, is affected by all emotions. This is because the Heart is the seat of insight and feelings, and although each emotion affects its relevant organ, it also affects the Heart which alone feels it.

Second, the tip becomes red because every emotion, after some time, causes some stagnation of Qi and this, in turn, often produces Heat. Hence the Chinese medicine saying: "*All emotions lead to Heat*".

It is important to remember that "tip" here means the very tip of the tongue. If a larger area in the front part of the tongue is red, it usually indicates Lung-Heat (Fig. 11.4).

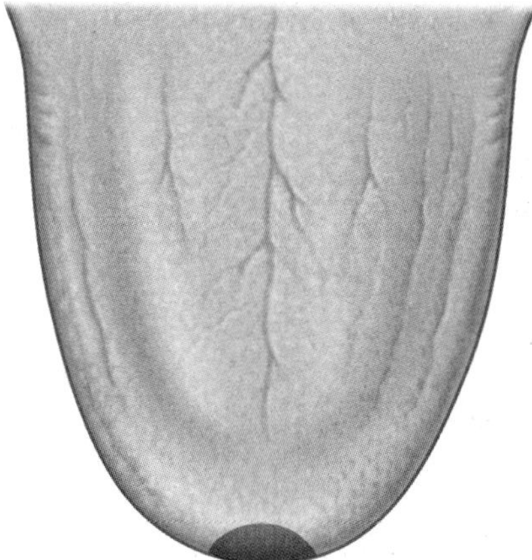

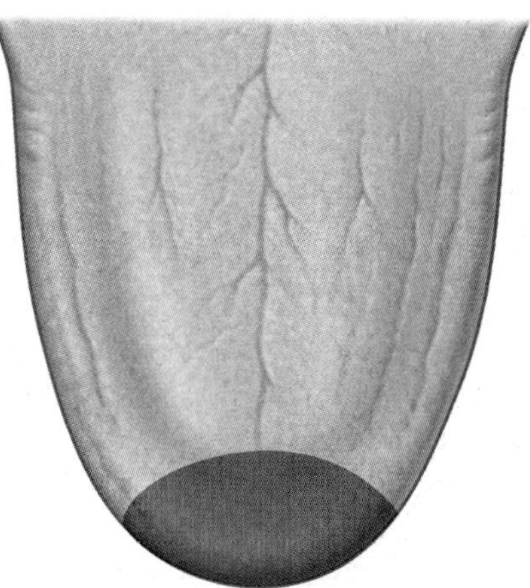

Figure 11.4 Comparison of Heart and Lung areas on the tongue.

If the tip of the tongue is Red, how do we know that this is due to Heart-Heat deriving from emotional problems and not from an actual heart disease in a Western medical sense? In my experience, the tip of the tongue reflects the condition of the Heart specifically in the sense of the Mind (*Shen*) and not really the heart itself. I find that pathologies of the actual heart in a Western sense are reflected on the chest/breast areas of the tongue (Fig. 11.5).

For example, when there is Blood stasis in the Heart and a Western heart pathology (such as coronary heart disease), I find that the chest areas on the tongue become Purple, never the tip. Thus, we can say that the tip of the tongue reflects the condition of the Mind (*Shen*) while the chest areas on the tongue reflect the condition of the actual heart.

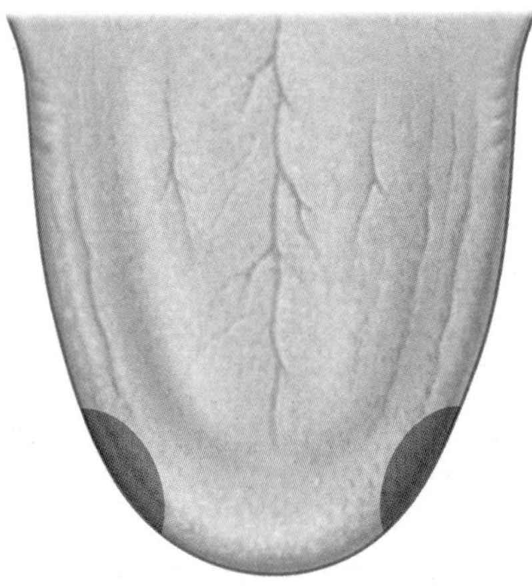

Figure 11.5 Chest/breast areas.

!

The tip of the tongue reflects the condition of the Mind (*Shen*) while the chest areas on the tongue reflect the condition of the actual heart.

It is interesting to note that this situation does not apply to other areas of the tongue; for example, the sides of the tongue reflect the condition of the Liver both in a Chinese and in a Western sense. If the sides of the tongue are Red, it may indicate both an emotional problem deriving from anger and a condition of Heat in the liver organ itself.

Heart crack

A Heart crack is in the midline; it is relatively narrow and it extends from the border of the root of the tongue to edge of the tip (Fig. 11.6 shows a Heart crack on the left and compares it to a Stomach crack). See Plate 11.2.

If the Heart crack is shallow and the body color normal, it simply indicates a constitutional tendency to Heart patterns and to emotional problems but it does not have a specific clinical significance. However, if a person has such a crack, any emotional stress from which he or she might suffer will have deeper repercus-

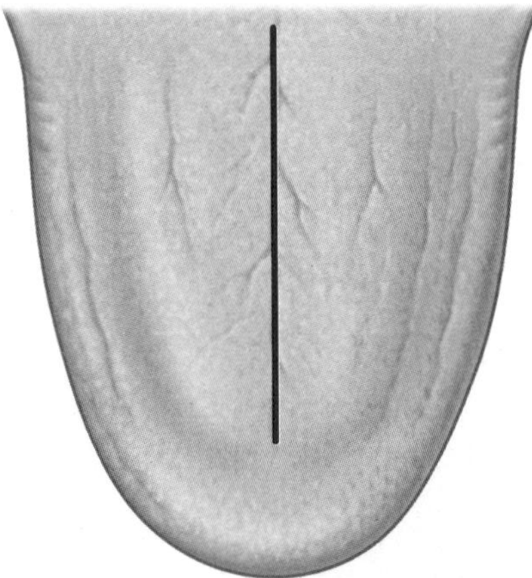

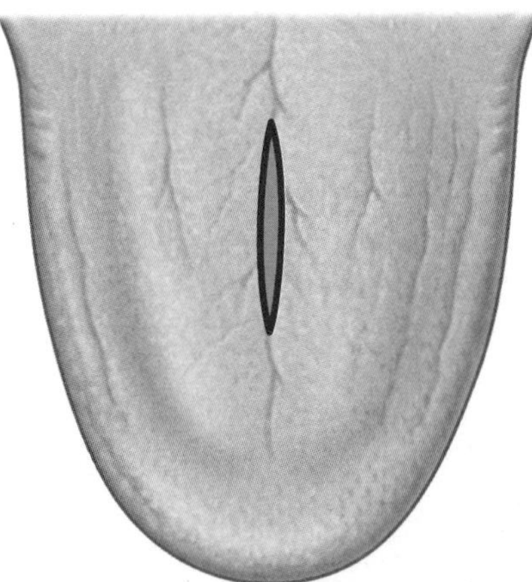

Figure 11.6 Comparison of Heart crack and Stomach crack.

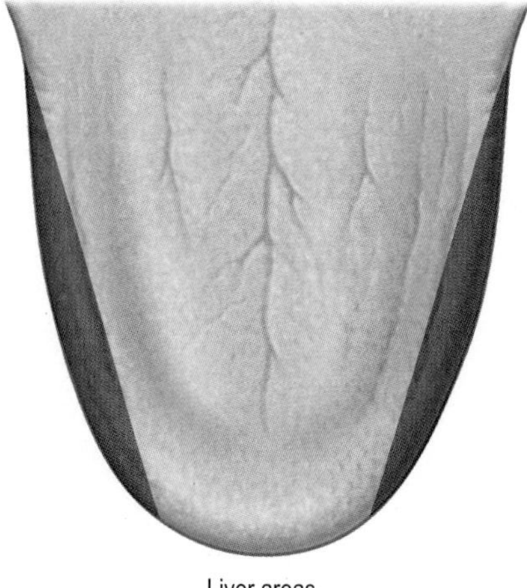

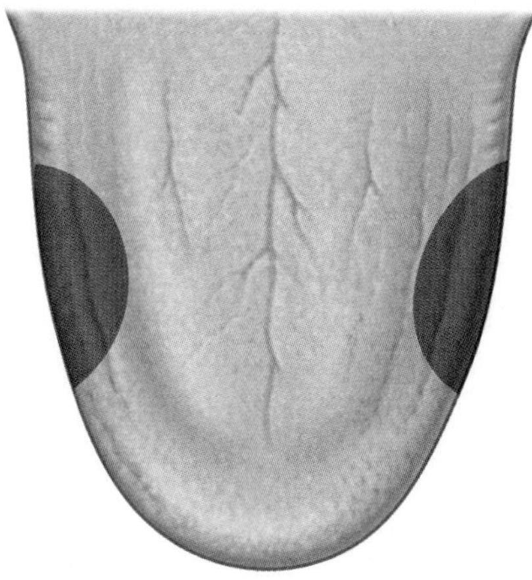

Figure 11.7 Comparison of Liver and Stomach/Spleen areas.

sions than in someone without a Heart crack. According to Dr Shen, a shallow Heart crack on a normal body color may also indicate heart disease in the parents or even grandparents.

The clinical significance of the Heart crack depends on its depth and on the color of the tongue body. If the Heart crack is accompanied by a change in the tongue-body color and a red tip, it then indicates actual mental-emotional problems. If the Heart crack is deep, it indicates that the person may suffer from a Heart pattern due to emotional stress, all the more so if the tip is also Red; the deeper the crack, the more severe the emotional problem.

One could describe different situations of emotional stress in order of increasing severity as manifested on the tongue as follows:

- shallow Heart crack, normal body color
- no Heart crack, Red tip
- deep Heart crack, normal body color
- shallow Heart crack, Red tip
- deep Heart crack, Red tip
- deep Heart crack, Red tip with red points
- deep Heart crack, Red tongue with redder tip and red points
- deep Heart crack, Red tongue with redder and swollen tip and red points.

I personally find that a Heart crack on the tongue is a very reliable sign of either a tendency to emotional stress (as indicated above) or an actual severe emotional stress.

Sides of the tongue

The sides of the tongue reflect the state of the Liver. With regard to the sides of the tongue, we should differentiate clearly between the areas that reflect the condition of the Liver and those that reflect that of the Spleen (Fig. 11.7). The areas on the edge of the tongue extending from the edge of the root to the edge of the tip reflect the condition of the Liver; the areas on the tongue in the middle section of it and extending more towards the center of the tongue reflect the condition of the Spleen and Stomach.

Anger very often manifests with red sides of the tongue, indicating severe Liver-Qi stagnation, Liver-Yang rising or Liver-Fire (Plate 11.3). If both sides and tip are red, it usually indicates severe emotional problems from anger and frustration affecting both the Liver and Heart (Plate 11.4).

Please remember that when the sides of the tongue (in the Liver area) are Purple, in women they may indicate Blood stasis in the Uterus.

Body shape

There are a few other body-shape signs on the tongue which show emotional or mental problems. For example, severe mental problems such as manic-depression or psychosis can manifest with a grossly abnormal shape of the tongue as in shown in Figure 11.8 and Plate 11.5. This consists of a large swelling of the front third of the tongue.

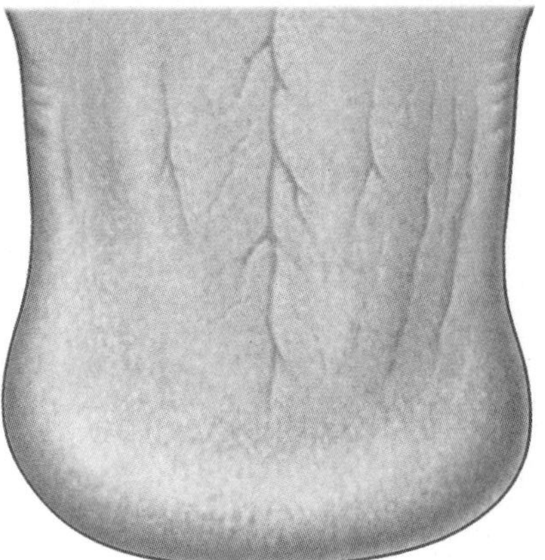

Figure 11.8 Tongue swelling indicating tendency to mental illness.

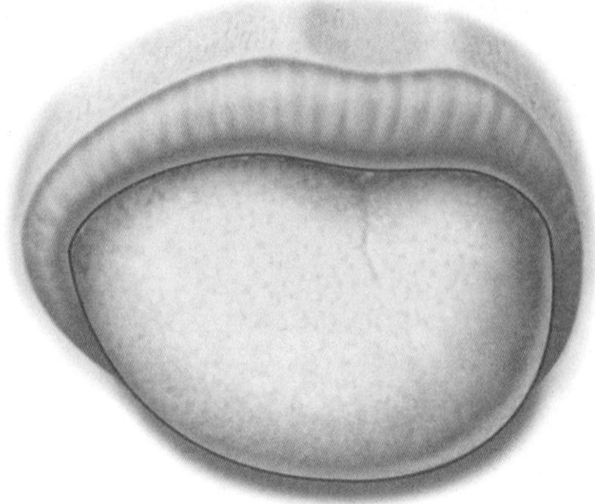

Figure 11.9 Gross swelling of the tongue indicating tendency to mental illness.

If such a shape is seen in people who do not apparently have any mental problems, it indicates that they have a tendency to develop such problems if the inner balance is suddenly upset, such as by a shock or by a traumatic childbirth. These people are nearly always sad; even if they do experience happiness, it only lasts a few minutes. If such a tongue is combined with very dull eyes, this is a very bad sign, indicating the possibility of severe mental illness.

Another sign in the tongue-body shape indicating the tendency to severe mental problems is a tongue that is grossly Swollen almost to the point of being round (Fig. 11.9).

Combined Stomach and Heart crack

Yet another tongue sign in mental-emotional problems is a combined Stomach and Heart crack. As indicated in Figure 11.6, the Heart crack is narrow and extends almost the whole length of the tongue, while the Stomach crack is wide and is concentrated in the middle section of the tongue (Plate 11.6).

A combined Stomach and Heart crack extends the whole length of the tongue and is wide in the middle section (Fig. 11.10). Such a crack usually indicates severe emotional stress which may derive from sadness, grief, worry, guilt or shame.

If there is a sticky, rough, brush-like yellow coating inside the crack, it indicates the presence of Phlegm clouding the Mind. If, in addition, the tongue body is Red, it denotes the presence of Phlegm and Fire obstructing the Stomach and the Heart, and misting the Mind. It is often seen in bipolar disorder (Plate 11.7).

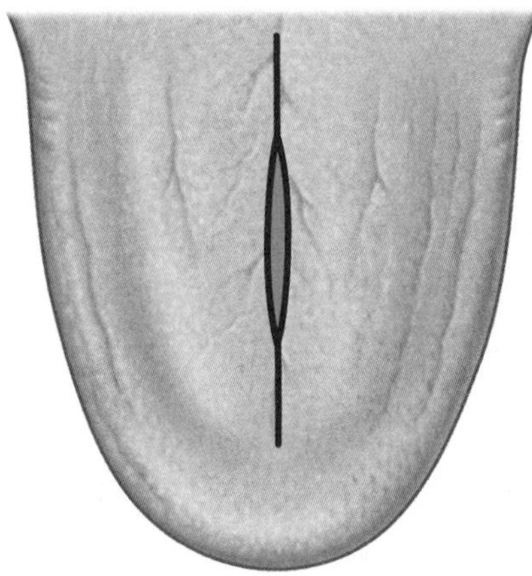

Figure 11.10 Combined Stomach/Heart crack.

SUMMARY

The tongue and the emotions

Red tip

- Red tip of the tongue: emotional stress giving rise to Heat.

Heart crack

- A Heart crack is in the midline; it is relatively narrow and it extends from the border of the root of the tongue to edge of the tip.
- Heart crack shallow and body color normal: constitutional tendency to Heart patterns and to emotional problems.

- Heart crack with a change in tongue-body color and a red tip: actual mental-emotional problems.
- The deeper the crack, the more severe the emotional problem.

Sides of the tongue

- The sides of the tongue reflect the state of the Liver.
- Anger often manifests with red sides of the tongue, indicating severe Liver-Qi stagnation, Liver-Yang rising or Liver-Fire.
- Both sides and tip red: severe emotional problems from anger and frustration affecting both the Liver and Heart.

Body shape

- Grossly abnormal shape of the tongue with a large swelling of the front third of the tongue: tendency to mental problems.
- Grossly Swollen tongue almost to the point of being round: tendency to mental problems, obstruction of the Mind.

Combined Stomach and Heart crack

- Combined Stomach and Heart crack: severe emotional stress which may derive from sadness, grief, worry, guilt or shame.
- Combined Stomach and Heart crack with a sticky, rough, brush-like yellow coating inside the crack: Phlegm clouding the Mind.
- Combined Stomach and Heart crack with a sticky, rough, brush-like yellow coating inside the crack, red tongue body: Phlegm and Fire obstructing the Stomach and the Heart and misting the Mind; manic-depression.

END NOTES

1. Yi Men Fa Yu [Principles of Medical Practice], cited in Wang Ke Qin 1988 Zhong Yi Shen Zhu Xue Shuo 中医神主学说 [Theory of the Mind in Chinese Medicine]. Ancient Chinese Medical Texts Publishing House, Beijing, p. 56.
2. Shi Pa Nan 1861 Yi Yuan [Origin of Medicine], cited in Theory of the Mind in Chinese Medicine, p. 55.
3. 1979 Huang Di Nei Jing Su Wen 黄帝内经素问 [The Yellow Emperor's Classic of Internal Medicine – Simple Questions]. People's Health Publishing House, Beijing, p. 99. First published *c.*100 BC.
4. Chen Shi Duo 1687 Shi Shi Mi Lu [Secret Records of the Stone Room], cited in Theory of the Mind in Chinese Medicine, p. 56.
5. 1981 Ling Shu Jing 灵枢经 [Spiritual Axis]. People's Health Publishing House, Beijing, pp. 151–152. First published *c.*100 BC.
6. Ibid., pp. 151–152.
7. Shi Pa Nan 1861 Yi Yuan [Origin of Medicine], cited in Guo Zhen Qiu 1985 Zhong Yi Zhen Duan Xue 中医诊断学 [Diagnosis in Chinese Medicine]. Hunan Science Publishing House, Changsha, p. 33.
8. Zhou Xue Hai 1894 Xing Se Wai Zhen Jian Mo [A Simple Guide to Diagnosis from Body and Color], cited in Diagnosis in Chinese Medicine, p. 33.

精神病辨证与针药治疗

CHAPTER 12

PATTERNS IN MENTAL-EMOTIONAL PROBLEMS AND THEIR TREATMENT WITH HERBAL MEDICINE AND ACUPUNCTURE

THE EFFECT OF MENTAL-EMOTIONAL PROBLEMS ON QI, BLOOD, YIN AND PATHOGENIC FACTORS *183*

Effects on Qi *184*

Effects on Blood *185*

Effects on Yin *188*

Pathogenic factors in mental-emotional problems *190*

MIND OBSTRUCTED, UNSETTLED, WEAKENED *196*

Mind Obstructed *196*

Mind Unsettled *196*

Mind Weakened *197*

Herbal treatment methods for Mind Obstructed, Unsettled or Weakened *198*

Treatment principles *199*

MIND OBSTRUCTED *200*

Qi stagnation *200*

Blood stasis *205*

Phlegm misting the Mind *208*

MIND UNSETTLED *212*

Blood deficiency *212*

Yin deficiency *213*

Yin deficiency with Empty Heat *217*

Qi stagnation *221*

Blood stasis *221*

Fire *221*

Phlegm-Fire *226*

MIND WEAKENED *228*

Qi and Blood deficiency *228*

Yang deficiency *232*

Blood deficiency *234*

Yin deficiency *234*

PATTERNS IN MENTAL-EMOTIONAL PROBLEMS AND THEIR TREATMENT WITH HERBAL MEDICINE AND ACUPUNCTURE

In this chapter, we turn our attention to differentiating mental-emotional problems and their treatment according to patterns. I will discuss first the pathology of mental-emotional problems in terms of their effects on Qi, Blood, Yin and pathogenic factors.

I will then classify mental-emotional patterns in the three broad categories of Mind Obstructed, Mind Unsettled and Mind Weakened.

The discussion will be conducted according to the following topics.

- The effect of mental-emotional problems on Qi, Blood, Yin and pathogenic factors
- Mind Obstructed, Unsettled, Weakened
- Mind Obstructed
- Mind Unsettled
- Mind Weakened

THE EFFECT OF MENTAL-EMOTIONAL PROBLEMS ON QI, BLOOD, YIN AND PATHOGENIC FACTORS

The effects of the various etiological factors in mental-emotional problems can be classified into four broad categories:

1. Effects on Qi
2. Effects on Blood
3. Effects on Yin
4. Generation of pathogenic factors.

Given the indissoluble link between body and mind in Chinese medicine, it should be remembered that, just as emotional problems have an effect on Qi, Blood or Yin, a disharmony of Qi, Blood or Yin (from causes other than emotional) will affect the Mind. The following discussion of conditions arising from emotional stress applies equally to mental-emotional problems deriving from a disharmony of Qi, Blood and Yin of the internal organs.

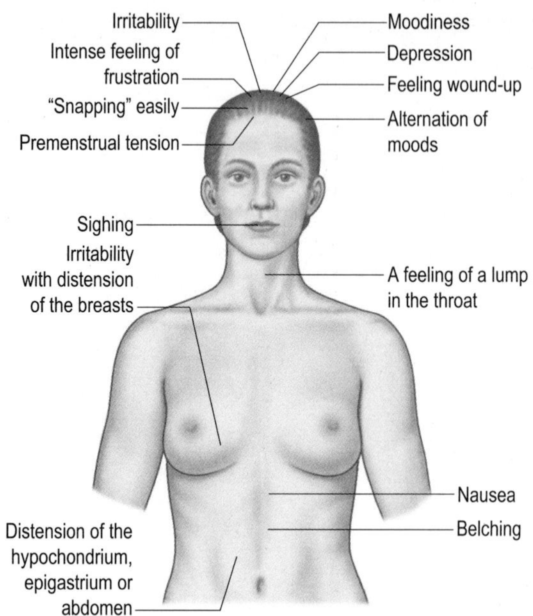

Figure 12.1 Liver-Qi stagnation.

Effects on Qi

The Mind and Spirit are a form of Qi in its subtlest state. Therefore the very first effect of emotional causative factors is to upset the movement and transformation of Qi. As we have seen, each emotion has a certain effect on Qi by raising it, depleting it, knotting it, scattering it or making it descend.

Hence, injury to the Mind or Spirit by emotions causes either Qi-deficiency or rebellious Qi. Rebellious Qi, it will be remembered, indicates a counterflow movement of Qi, i.e. Qi rising when it should descend (as in the case of Stomach-Qi) or Qi descending when it should rise (as in the case of Spleen-Qi). Ultimately, however, both deficient and rebellious Qi may lead to stagnation of Qi. This happens because, especially in emotional problems, deficient or rebellious Qi impairs the proper circulation and movement of Qi, leading to stagnation. Stagnation of Qi from emotional problems affects various organs but the Liver, Heart and Lungs most of all.

Liver-Qi stagnation

This is the most common effect of emotional stress on the Liver. It derives from anger, resentment, frustration, worry and guilt. Anger causes Liver-Qi stagnation, especially if it is held in and not manifested.

The main manifestations of Liver-Qi stagnation are distension of the hypochondrium, epigastrium or abdomen, belching, sighing, nausea, depression, moodiness, feeling wound-up, a feeling of a lump in the throat, premenstrual tension, irritability with distension of the breasts and a Wiry pulse (Fig. 12.1).

From an emotional perspective the most characteristic and common signs are mental depression, alternation of moods, irritability, "snapping" easily and an intense feeling of frustration. Liver-Qi stagnation affects the movement of the Ethereal Soul (*Hun*), restraining its "coming and going"; this causes a lack of movement of the Ethereal Soul towards the Mind (*Shen*) with the resulting lack of ideas, plans, inspiration, creativity, life dreams, etc. In short, this leads to some mental depression.

Heart- and Lung-Qi stagnation

Heart- and Lung-Qi stagnation derive either from worry which knots Qi or from sadness and grief which deplete Qi and lead to Qi-stagnation in the chest after some time.

Heart- and Lung-Qi stagnation are characterized by a feeling of distension and tightness in the chest, palpitations, sighing, slight breathlessness, a feeling of a lump in the throat with difficulty in swallowing, a weak voice, a pale complexion and a pulse which may be slightly Overflowing or Tight in both Heart and Lung positions and is without wave (Fig. 12.2).

From an emotional point of view, a person will feel very sad and depressed and will tend to weep. This state is due to the constriction of the Corporeal Soul by the stagnation of Qi. The person will also be very sensitive to outside psychic influences.

The effects of emotional causative factors are confined to Qi only in the early stages. After some time, disruption in the movement and transformation of Qi eventually lead to the formation of pathogenic factors such as Dampness, Phlegm, stasis of Blood, Fire or Wind, all of which further affect and disturb the Mind and Spirit (Fig. 12.3).

Effects on Blood

The effects of emotional problems on Blood are more important than those on Qi, for Blood provides the material foundation for the Mind and Spirit. Blood, which is Yin, houses and anchors the Mind and Spirit, which are Yang in nature. It embraces the Mind and Spirit, providing the harbor within which they can flourish. In particular, Heart-Blood houses the Mind (*Shen*) and Liver-Blood the Ethereal Soul (*Hun*). See Figure 12.4.

The *Simple Questions* in Chapter 26 says: "*Blood is the Mind of a person.*"[1] The *Spiritual Axis* says in Chapter 32: "*When Blood is harmonized, the Mind has a residence.*"[2]

Blood is also closely related to Mind and Spirit because of its relation with the Heart and Liver. The Heart, which houses the Mind, also governs Blood, and the

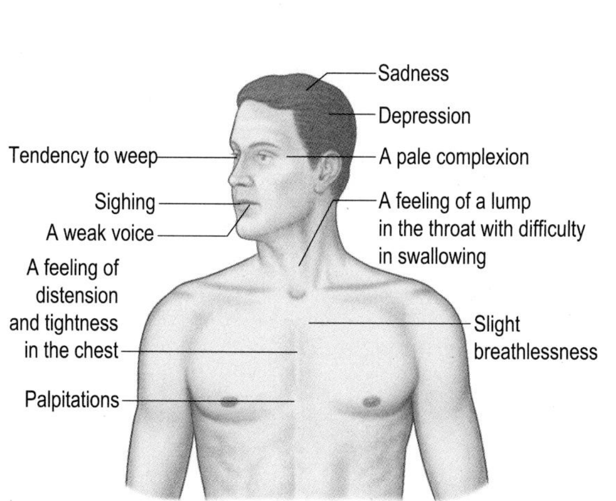

Figure 12.2 Heart- and Lung-Qi stagnation.

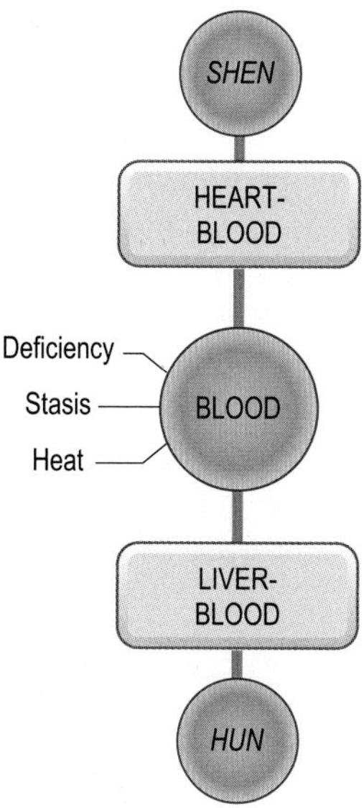

Figure 12.4 Heart-Blood and Liver-Blood.

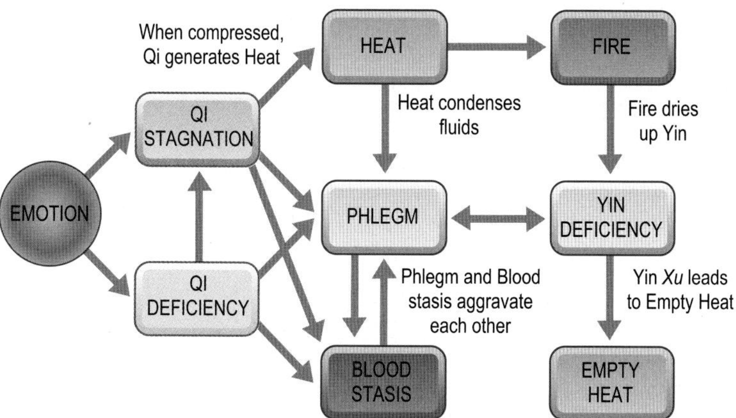

Figure 12.3 Consequences of emotional stress.

Liver, which houses the Ethereal Soul, also stores Blood. Any emotional stress that affects the Heart or Liver would influence Heart-Blood or Liver-Blood and therefore the Mind or Ethereal Soul.

The Blood can be affected by emotional problems in three ways: it can become deficient, stagnant or hot.

Blood deficiency

Blood deficiency is one of the most common consequences of emotional problems. Its manifestations will vary according to whether the Heart or Liver is more affected.

Heart-Blood deficiency

If the Heart is affected (as it is by sadness and grief) there will be palpitations, mild anxiety, insomnia (inability to fall asleep), poor memory, mild dizziness, a propensity to be startled, a dull-pale complexion, a Pale-Thin tongue and a Choppy pulse (Fig. 12.5).

From a mental-emotional point of view, such a person may feel depressed, anxious and tired, and the Mind may be confused and lack concentration. This is due to a weakness of the Mind, it being deprived of its residence and therefore failing to direct all the mental activities.

Liver-Blood deficiency

If Liver-Blood is affected, there will be mild dizziness, numbness of the limbs, insomnia (inability to fall asleep), blurred vision, floaters in eyes, scanty menstruation or amenorrhea, a dull-pale complexion, muscle cramps, brittle nails, a Pale-Thin tongue and a Choppy pulse (Fig. 12.6).

From a mental-emotional point of view, the person may feel anxious and tired, and not sleep well. This is due to the Ethereal Soul not being rooted in Liver-Blood and therefore leading to anxiety and insomnia.

Both these conditions of Blood deficiency are more frequent in women.

Blood stasis

Blood stasis also affects the Mind, albeit in a different way. Blood stasis may agitate the Mind and Spirit causing anxiety and insomnia; Blood stasis also obstructs the Mind and it may lead to some loss of insight causing mental confusion.

Heart-Blood stasis

If Blood stasis affects the Heart it will cause chest pain, a feeling of tightness in the chest, anxiety, insomnia,

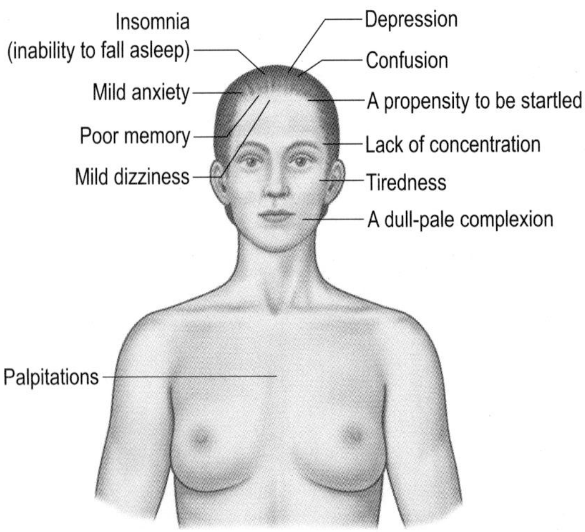

Figure 12.5 Heart-Blood deficiency.

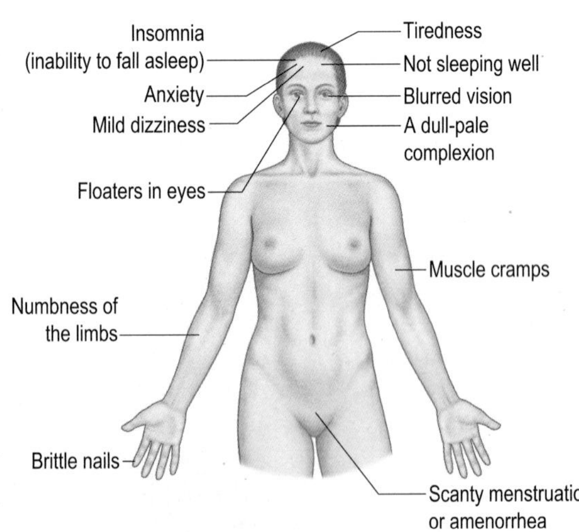

Figure 12.6 Liver-Blood deficiency.

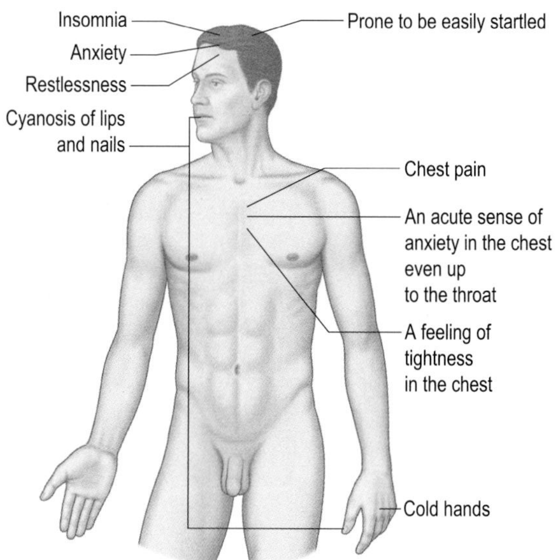

Figure 12.7 Heart-Blood stasis.

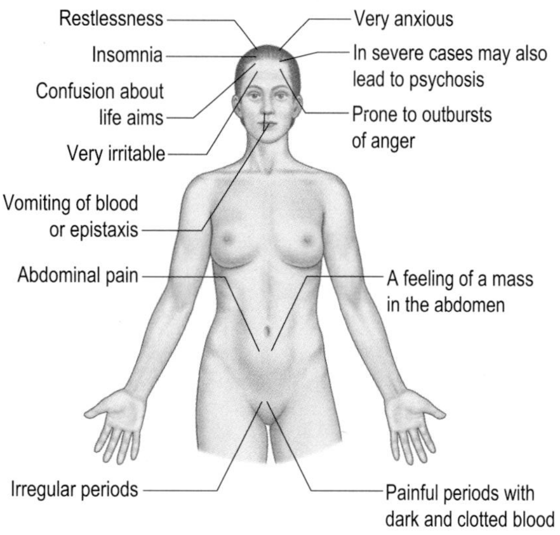

Figure 12.8 Liver-Blood stasis.

cold hands, cyanosis of lips and nails, a Purple tongue and a Knotted or Choppy pulse (Fig. 12.7).

From a mental-emotional point of view, this person will feel very anxious with an acute sense of anxiety in the chest, and even up to the throat. The person will be restless and prone to be easily startled. This condition is due to stagnant Blood agitating and confusing the Mind. In severe cases, if the Mind is obstructed the person may lose insight and become psychotic. The postnatal psychosis occurring when there is Blood stasis after childbirth is an example of such a condition.

Liver-Blood stasis

If Liver-Blood is stagnant, there may be vomiting of blood or epistaxis, painful periods with dark and clotted blood, irregular periods, abdominal pain, a feeling of a mass in the abdomen, insomnia, a tongue which is Purple on the sides and a Wiry pulse (Fig. 12.8).

From a mental-emotional point of view, the person will be very anxious, restless and confused about his or her aims in life. He or she will also be very irritable and prone to outbursts of anger. This condition is due to the Ethereal Soul being agitated and confused by the stasis of Blood. In severe cases, this may also lead to psychosis.

Blood-Heat

Blood-Heat is the third possible effect of emotional problems affecting Blood; Blood-Heat affects the Mind and Spirit by agitating and harassing them. Blood-Heat also mostly affects the Heart or Liver.

Heart-Blood Heat

If Blood-Heat affects the Heart, there will be palpitations, insomnia (inability to stay asleep), anxiety, mental restlessness, thirst, tongue ulcers, a feeling of heat, a red face, a bitter taste, a Red tongue and a Rapid and Overflowing pulse (Fig. 12.9).

This person will be extremely anxious and agitated, and in some cases may be very impulsive and restless. All these symptoms and signs are due to Blood-Heat agitating the Mind.

Liver-Blood Heat

If Blood-Heat affects the Liver, there will be irritability, propensity to outbursts of anger, thirst, a bitter taste, dizziness, tinnitus, insomnia, dream-disturbed sleep, headache, red face and eyes, dark urine, dry stools, a

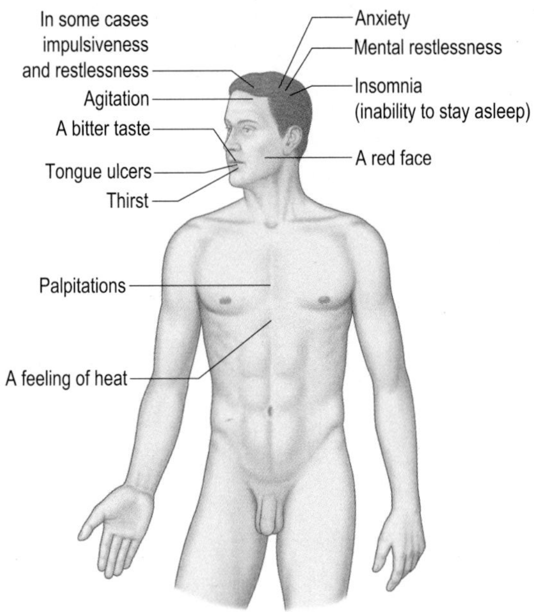

Figure 12.9 Heart-Blood Heat.

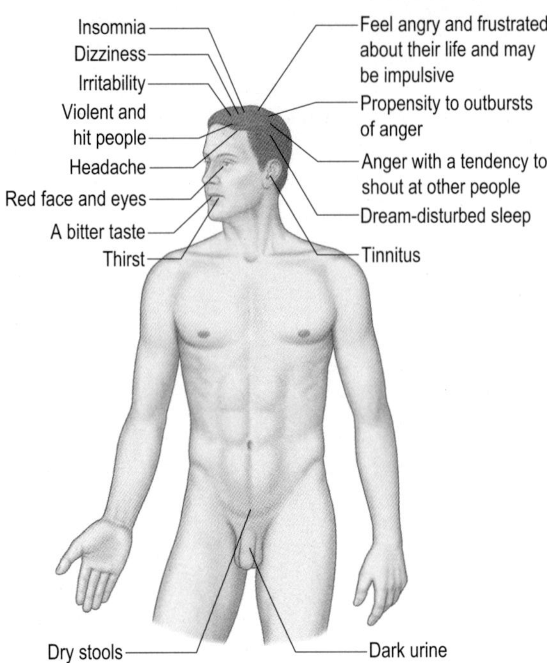

Figure 12.10 Liver-Blood Heat.

Red tongue which is redder on the sides and a Rapid-Wiry pulse (Fig. 12.10).

The person will be very angry and tend to shout at other people. He or she may also be violent and hit people, and may also feel angry and frustrated about their life and may tend to be impulsive. All this is due to Blood-Heat disturbing the Ethereal Soul and over-accentuating its essential character of movement towards the outer world and relations with other people (Fig. 12.11).

Effects on Yin

Blood is part of Yin and the effects of emotional stress on Yin are similar to those on Blood. Affection of Yin may, however, be considered as a deeper level of problem than affliction of Blood.

Yin, like Blood, is the residence and anchor of the Mind and Spirit. Emotional problems can affect the Yin of different organs, especially the Heart, Liver, Kidneys, Lungs and Spleen. The effect depends on whether Yin deficiency gives rise to Empty Heat or not. If there is Yin deficiency only, without Empty Heat, the Mind and Spirit become weakened and the person feels

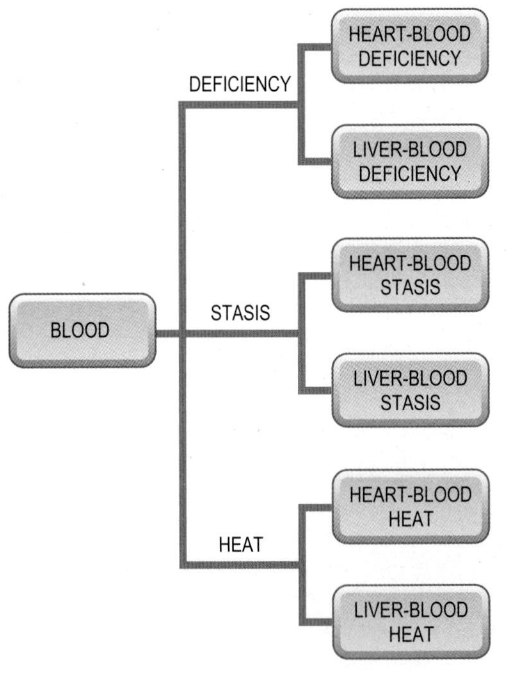

Figure 12.11 Pathology of Heart- and Liver-Blood.

depressed, tired and dispirited; the Mind is confused and the memory and concentration poor. If Yin deficiency gives rise to Empty Heat, this unsettles the Mind and Spirit, causing anxiety, insomnia and mental restlessness.

Heart-Yin deficiency with Empty Heat

Heart-Yin is readily affected by emotional stress since it is the residence of the Mind. Heart-Yin deficiency deprives the Mind of residence and there will be palpitations, insomnia (inability to stay asleep), propensity to be startled, poor memory, anxiety, mental restlessness, a malar flush, night-sweating, a dry mouth, five-palm heat, a Red tongue (with redder tip) without coating and a Rapid-Thin or Floating-Empty pulse (Fig. 12.12).

The person will feel very anxious, particularly in the evening, with a vague and fidgety sense of anxiety, uneasy without knowing why. "Mental restlessness" is a loose translation of a typical Chinese expression (*xin fan*), which always refers to this pattern and literally means "heart feels vexed". The person will also feel dispirited, depressed and tired. Memory and concentration will be poor. The sleep will be disturbed and, typically, the person wakes up frequently during the night. All this is due to the Mind being deprived of its residence.

If the Empty Heat is pronounced, the effects on the Mind will be more pronounced; the patient will feel extremely restless and anxious.

Liver-Yin deficiency with Empty Heat

Liver-Yin is the residence of the Ethereal Soul, and when emotional stress depletes Liver-Yin it may cause anxiety, insomnia and mental restlessness. On a physical level this may cause poor memory, dizziness, dry eyes, skin and hair, scanty periods, insomnia, five-palm heat, night-sweating, a red tongue without coating and a Floating-Empty pulse (Fig. 12.13).

On a mental-emotional level, the patient may suffer from anxiety, insomnia with many dreams and mental restlessness. He or she may also have a floating sensation immediately before falling asleep.

Both a deficiency of Liver-Yin and the resulting Empty Heat affect the Ethereal Soul. A deficiency of Liver-Yin will render the Ethereal Soul rootless, resulting in anxiety and insomnia. The Empty Heat, on the

Figure 12.12 Heart-Yin deficiency with Empty Heat.

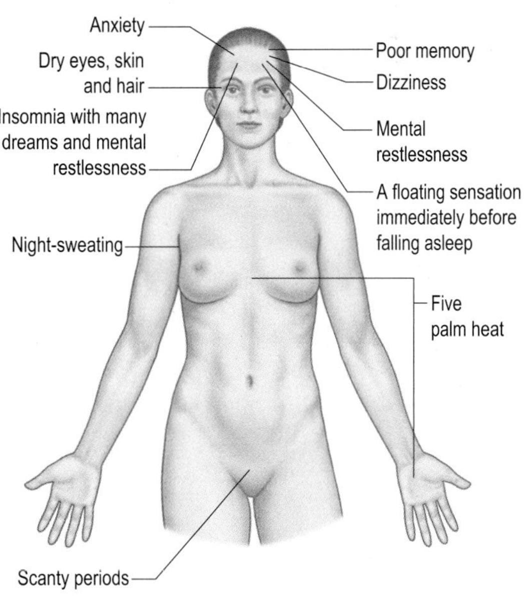

Figure 12.13 Liver-Yin deficiency with Empty Heat.

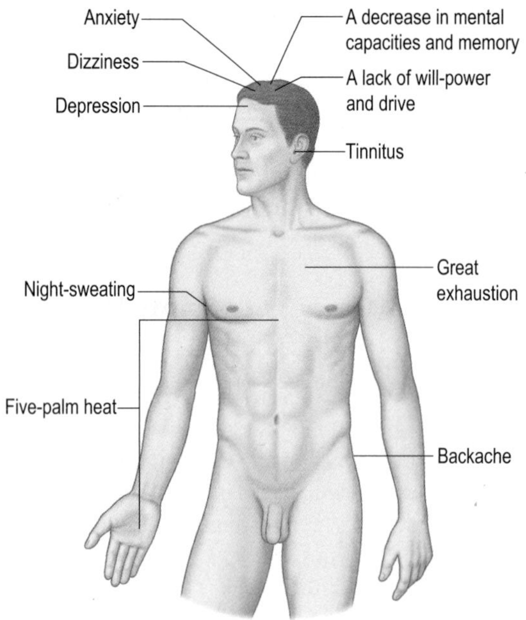

Figure 12.14 Kidney-Yin deficiency with Empty Heat.

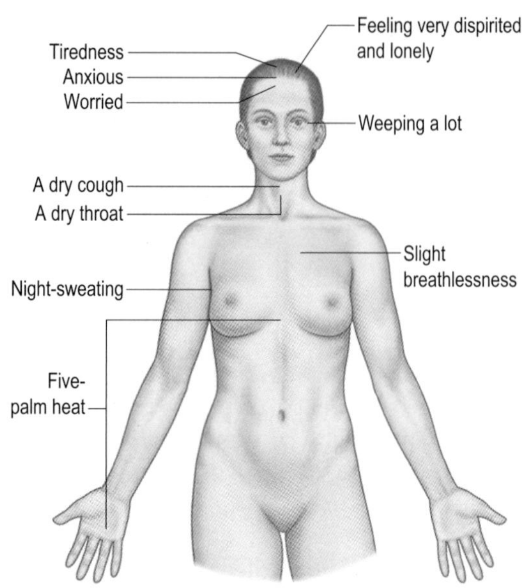

Figure 12.15 Lung-Yin deficiency with Empty Heat.

other hand, will agitate the Ethereal Soul and, if the Heat is pronounced, this may even cause slight manic behavior.

Kidney-Yin deficiency with Empty Heat

Kidney-Yin is the residence of Will-Power and memory. Emotional stress that affects Kidney-Yin will cause great exhaustion, a lack of will-power and drive, depression, anxiety and a decrease in mental capacities and memory. On a physical level, it will cause dizziness, tinnitus, night-sweating, five-palm heat, backache, a Red tongue without coating and a Floating-Empty pulse (Fig. 12.14).

The Empty Heat from Kidney-Yin deficiency will affect the Mind, causing insomnia and pronounced anxiety.

Lung-Yin deficiency with Empty Heat

Lung-Yin is the residence of the Corporeal Soul (*Po*). Emotional problems that affect Lung-Yin will cause tiredness, a dry cough, slight breathlessness, night-sweating, five-palm heat, a dry throat, a Red tongue without coating and a Floating-Empty pulse (Fig. 12.15).

On a mental-emotional level, the patient may be anxious and worried. They will tend to weep a lot and will feel very dispirited and lonely.

Spleen-Yin deficiency with Empty Heat

Spleen-Yin is the residence of the Intellect (*Yi*) and Spleen-Yin deficiency may cause a dry mouth with no desire to drink, dry lips, dry stools, poor appetite, a slight abdominal pain, a tongue without coating in the center and a Floating-Empty pulse in the right Middle position (Fig. 12.16).

From a mental-emotional point of view, these people will suffer from poor memory and concentration, and will find it very difficult to apply themselves to study. The imbalance may also work in the opposite way and may lead to anxiety, overthinking and obsessive ideas.

Pathogenic factors in mental-emotional problems

The effects of emotional stress on the body's vital substances are summarized in Table 12.1, which shows

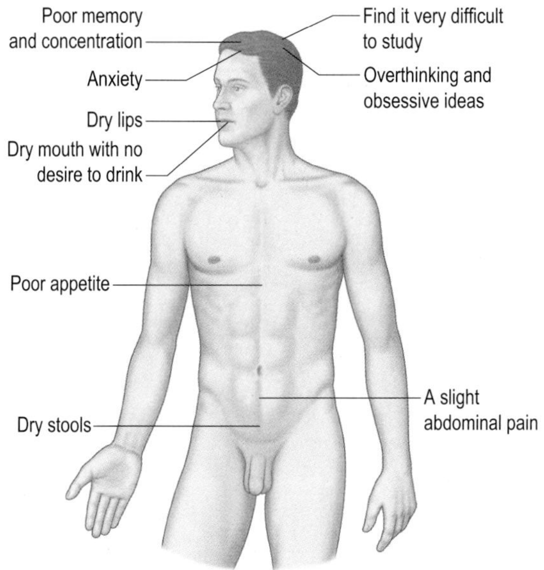

Figure 12.16 Spleen-Yin deficiency with Empty Heat.

Table 12.1 The effect of emotional stress on vital substances

VITAL SUBSTANCE	EFFECT	CONSEQUENCE
Qi	Deficiency Stagnation	Phlegm Blood stasis
Blood	Deficiency Heat Stasis	– Phlegm-Fire Heat
Yin	Deficiency	Empty Heat Internal Wind

the effects of emotional stress on the vital substances under the column headed "Effect". These conditions themselves, with time, become a cause of further disharmony and the effects are in the column headed "Consequence". For example, Blood-Heat may easily lead to the formation of Phlegm-Heat because Heat condenses the body fluids into Phlegm.

Qi deficiency of the Spleen, Lungs or Kidneys easily leads to the formation of Phlegm as Qi fails to transform, move and excrete fluids, which therefore accumulate into Phlegm. Qi stagnation easily leads to Blood stasis and Yin deficiency may lead to Empty Heat or internal Wind. Blood stasis may lead to Heat.

All these pathogenic factors – Phlegm, Phlegm-Heat, Empty Heat and internal Wind – further disturb the Mind. We shall now discuss their effects and symptomatology. Blood stasis has already been discussed above.

Phlegm

Phlegm obstructs the Mind (the Heart's orifices) and may cause dullness of thought, a fuzzy head, a confused mind and dizziness. In the mental-emotional field, Phlegm obstructing the Mind causes a certain loss of insight which, in extreme degrees, gives rise to serious mental illnesses such as psychosis, schizophrenia or bipolar disorder.

However, it is important to note that there are many different degrees of obstruction of the Mind by Phlegm. In mild degrees, obstruction of the Mind by Phlegm will manifest with mental confusion, a slight "manic" behavior if there is also Heat, and irrational behavior.

Phlegm obstructs the Mind and thinking but it does not agitate the Mind (unless it is combined with Heat). Thus the person will not be restless but, on the contrary, tired, subdued, depressed and quiet.

Phlegm shows with a Swollen tongue body, a sticky coating and a Slippery pulse. In particular, I relate the swelling of the tongue body more to Phlegm than Dampness (Fig. 12.17).

Fire or Heat

In the context of mental-emotional problems, the Minister Fire is frequently and easily "stirred" by emotional stress, with the creation of Heat and an upward movement of Qi which goes up to disturb the Heart and Pericardium. In emotional stress, Heat is frequently the result of Qi stagnation; however, it may also arise independently, without a preceding Qi stagnation.

When Heat is formed under the influence of emotional stress, the Minister Fire becomes pathological; it is "stirred" out of its residence in the Lower Burner and it flows upwards to the Heart and Pericardium. Chinese books say that the physiological Minister Fire should

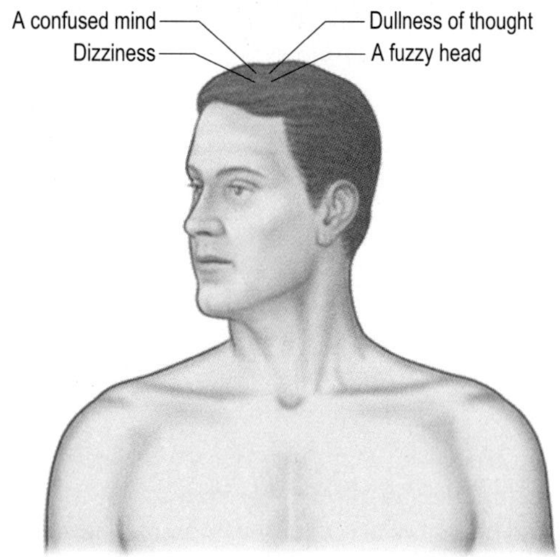

Figure 12.17 Phlegm.

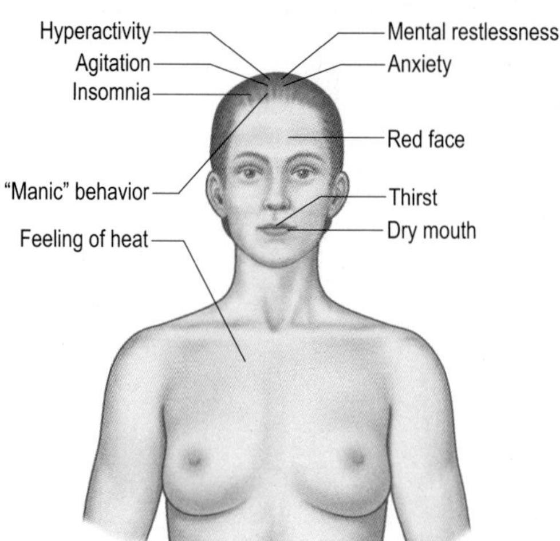

Figure 12.18 Fire or Heat.

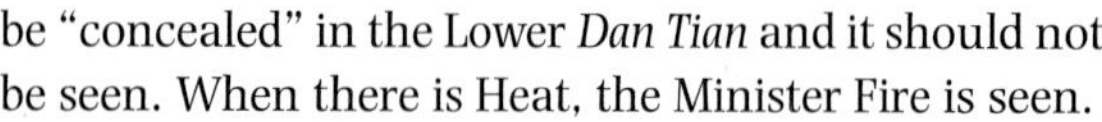

be "concealed" in the Lower *Dan Tian* and it should not be seen. When there is Heat, the Minister Fire is seen.

When the Minister Fire is stirred into a pathological state under the influence of emotional stress, three patterns of Heat may appear:

1. Full Heat (or Fire)
2. Empty Heat (from Yin deficiency)
3. Yin Fire.

Empty Heat and Yin Fire are discussed below.

Full Heat as a result of emotional stress derives usually from long-term Qi stagnation; when Qi stagnates for some time, it may give rise to Heat. However, in emotional stress, Heat may also be formed independently; this may happen, for example, with anger, joy, love, guilt or craving.

The tongue provides a crucial indication of Full Heat; in this condition, it is Red and with a yellow coating. If the tongue body is Red and there is a coating with root, there is Full Heat (even if the coating is not yellow). If the tongue is Red but without coating (totally or partially), it is Empty Heat (see below).

The other important manifestation is the pulse; in Full Heat, this is Full in general (which may include Wiry, Overflowing, Big or Firm). It should also be Rapid, but it frequently is not.

Other clinical manifestations include feeling of heat, thirst, dry mouth, insomnia, agitation, mental restlessness and a red face.

Full Heat of any organ may overstimulate the coming and going of the Ethereal Soul, and it may therefore lead to "manic" behavior, agitation, mental restlessness, insomnia, hyperactivity and anxiety (Fig. 12.18).

Fire or Heat agitates the Mind and Spirit. Fire and Heat are the same in nature but there are some differences between the two. Fire is a more "solid" pathogenic factor and more intense than Heat. It differs from Heat in the following respects.

- It is more intense (pronounced feeling of heat, Deep-Red tongue, Rapid pulse).
- It dries up fluids more (thirst, scanty urine, dry stools).
- It affects the Mind more (pronounced anxiety, insomnia).
- It easily causes bleeding.
- It is located in deeper energetic layers (Fig. 12.19).

Therefore, Fire affects and agitates the Mind more than Heat. In treatment, Heat is cleared with pungent-cold herbs; Fire is drained with bitter-cold herbs.

Phlegm-Fire

In Phlegm-Fire, Phlegm obstructs the Mind and Fire agitates it. Phlegm-Fire therefore makes the person agitated, restless and anxious. In some cases, the person may alternate between periods of depression and confusion (due to Phlegm) and periods of abnor-

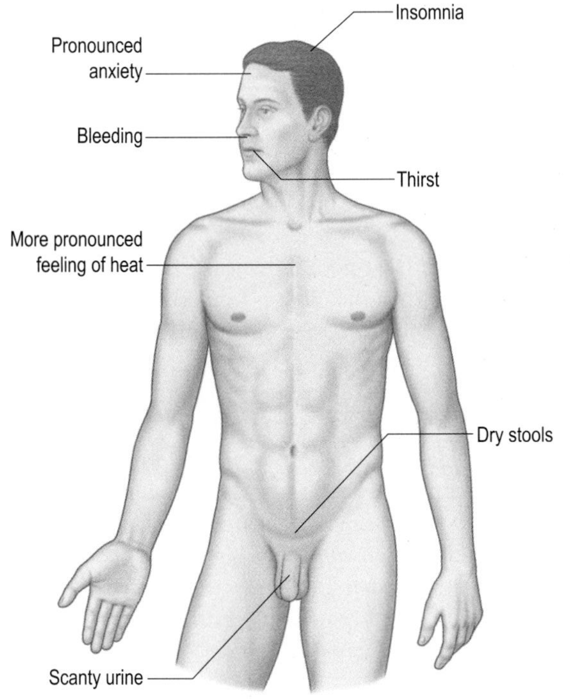

Figure 12.19 Fire.

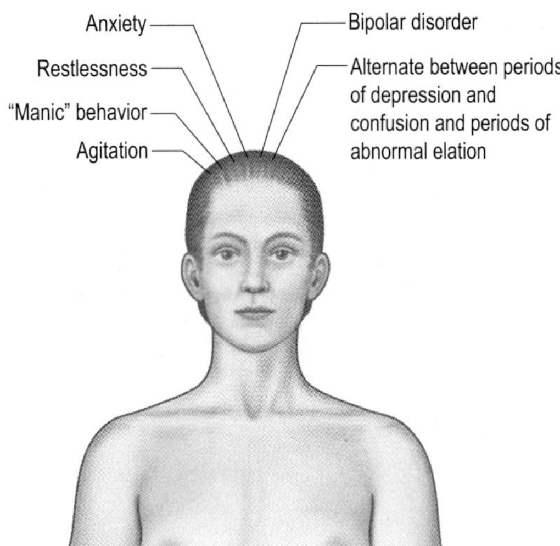

Figure 12.20 Phlegm-Fire.

mal elation, agitation and manic behavior (due to Fire). In severe cases this leads to bipolar disorder (Fig. 12.20).

Chinese books always describe this condition as alternation of periods of severe depression (the depressive phase called *Dian*) and periods of manic behavior (the manic phase called *Kuang*). The manic phase is usually described as shouting, scolding or hitting people, climbing mountains, taking off clothes, crying or laughing uncontrollably.

It is important to realize that, in practice, much milder versions of this condition appear fairly frequently, and one should not always expect such violent symptomatology in order to diagnose this condition.

Phlegm-Fire manifests with a Slippery and Rapid pulse and a Red-Swollen tongue with a sticky yellow coating and a Heart crack in the midline.

Empty Heat

Empty Heat derives from Yin deficiency. It is important to note that, although Empty Heat derives from Yin deficiency eventually, Yin deficiency may occur for many years without Empty Heat. In such cases, the tongue lacks a coating (indicating Yin deficiency) but it is not Red (because there is no Empty Heat). See Figure 12.21.

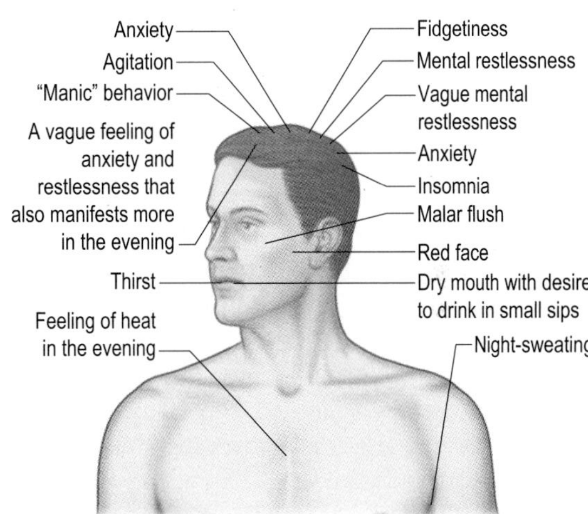

Figure 12.21 Empty Heat.

Empty Heat is seen in emotional stress when this is combined with overwork which leads to Yin deficiency;

the Yin deficiency caused by overwork is the fertile ground that gives rise to Empty Heat under the stimulation of emotional stress. This stress often derives from excess joy, craving, anger, worry, guilt or jealousy.

Thus, in such cases, the Empty Heat does derive from Yin deficiency but it is aggravated by the emotional stress which, in itself, leads to Heat. Most of all, the emotional stress causes the Empty Heat to rise more, causing agitation, anxiety, a red face and thirst.

In Empty Heat, the tongue is Red but either without a coating (totally or partially) or with a rootless coating. In Empty Heat, the pulse is Floating-Empty and Rapid.

Other clinical manifestations include feeling of heat in the evening, night-sweating, dry mouth with desire to drink in small sips, malar flush, mental restlessness and insomnia.

Empty Heat of any organ may overstimulate the coming and going of the Ethereal Soul, and it may therefore lead to "manic" behavior, a vague mental restlessness, insomnia, fidgetiness and anxiety.

The mental restlessness from Empty Heat manifests differently from that from Full Heat. In Empty Heat, the patient has a vague feeling of anxiety and restlessness that also manifests more in the evening.

Empty Heat may agitate the Heart and Pericardium (and therefore the Mind), the Liver (and therefore the Ethereal Soul) and the Kidneys (which also affects the Mind). We should not make the mistake of thinking that Empty Heat is not "real" Heat; it is "real" Heat which heats the body and affects the Mind as much as Full Heat does. Indeed, in the mental-emotional sphere, the effect of Empty Heat may be even more pronounced than that of Heat, because the Yin deficiency (from which Empty Heat derives) deprives the Mind and the Ethereal Soul of their residence. This agitates the Mind and the Ethereal Soul even more.

Yin Fire

Yin Fire was discussed also in Chapter 9. The concept of Yin Fire was introduced by Li Dong Yuan in his book *Discussion of Stomach and Spleen* (*Pi Wei Lun*, 1246). Dr Li says that, as a result of improper diet and overwork, the Original Qi (*Yuan Qi*) becomes weak in the Lower Burner. This causes the patient to feel tired and often cold. When the patient is also subject to emotional stress, the Minister Fire is stirred, it becomes pathological and it leaves its place of "concealment" in the Lower *Dan Tian*.

As the Minister Fire and the Original Qi reside in the same place in the Lower *Dan Tian*, the pathological Minister Fire displaces and weakens the Original Qi even more. Dr Li said that the pathological Minister Fire becomes a "thief" of the Original Qi. The arousal of the pathological Minister Fire upwards causes some Heat symptoms in the upper part of the body such as a red face and thirst. This he called "Yin Fire"; Yin Fire is neither Full Heat nor Empty Heat, but simply a different kind of Heat that derives from a deficiency of the Original Qi. It follows that Yin Fire is not treated by clearing Heat or draining Fire but by tonifying the Original Qi and gently clearing Heat upwards (Fig. 12.22).

The pathology of Yin Fire is further complicated by Dampness and by a pathology of the Middle Burner as well. When the Spleen is deficient, Dampness is formed and this infuses down to the Lower Burner. Here it "swamps" the Original Qi and the Minister Fire, displacing the latter from the place (the Lower Burner) where it should be "concealed". See Figures 12.23 and 12.24.

The Middle Burner has Dampness too; Spleen-Qi (or even Spleen-Yang) is deficient and fails to rise. For this reason, Bu Zhong Yi Qi Tang *Tonifying the Center and Benefiting Qi Decoction* is used to raise Spleen-Qi and warm Spleen-Yang so that Dampness no longer infuses downwards to the Lower Burner. When the Lower Burner is opened and unblocked from Dampness, the Minister Fire will return to its place of concealment in the Lower Burner, thus eliminating the symptoms of Yin Fire.

Bu Zhong Yi Qi Tang eliminates Yin Fire by tonifying the Original Qi with Ren Shen *Radix Ginseng* and by

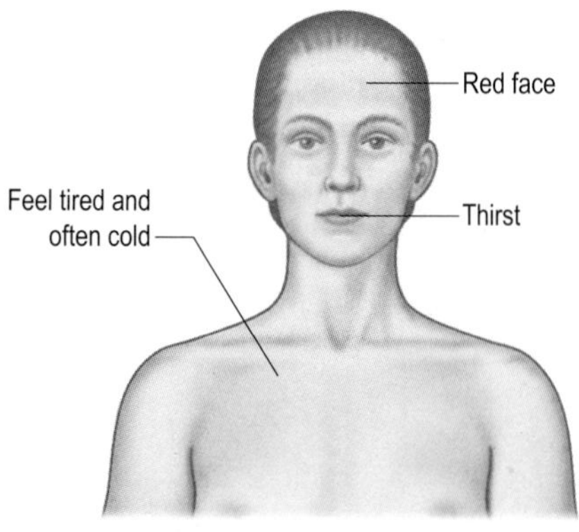

Figure 12.22 Yin Fire symptoms.

lightly clearing Heat upwards with Chai Hu *Radix Bupleuri* and Sheng Ma *Rhizoma Cimicifugae*.

Any emotion can lead to Yin Fire as all emotions may stir the Minister Fire out of its residing place in the Lower *Dan Tian*. All emotions lead to Qi stagnation which, in turn, eventually leads to some Heat. The situation can be aggravated by the presence of Dampness in the Lower Burner (as happens in shame).

Yin Fire accounts for symptoms of Heat in mental-emotional problems that may defy a classification into Full or Empty Heat; this happens when there are symptoms of Heat above (red face, thirst, feeling of heat in the face) and Cold below (cold feet, general cold feeling): such situation is due to Yin Fire.

Emotional stress is more likely to lead to Yin Fire when it is combined with overwork and dietary irregularity.

With acupuncture, the following are the treatment principles and points.

- Tonify the Original (*Yuan*) Qi: Ren-4 Guanyuan.
- Lift Qi: Du-20 Baihui, Ren-6 Qihai.
- Tonify and raise Spleen-Qi: BL-20 Pishu, Ren-12 Zhongwan, ST-36 Zusanli.
- Calm the Mind: Du-24 Shenting, Du-19 Houding, Ren-15 Jiuwei, HE-5 Tongli.
- Clear Heat upwards: P-8 Laogong, P-7 Daling.
- Regulate the Triple Burner: T.B.-6 Zhigou, T.B.-5 Waiguan.

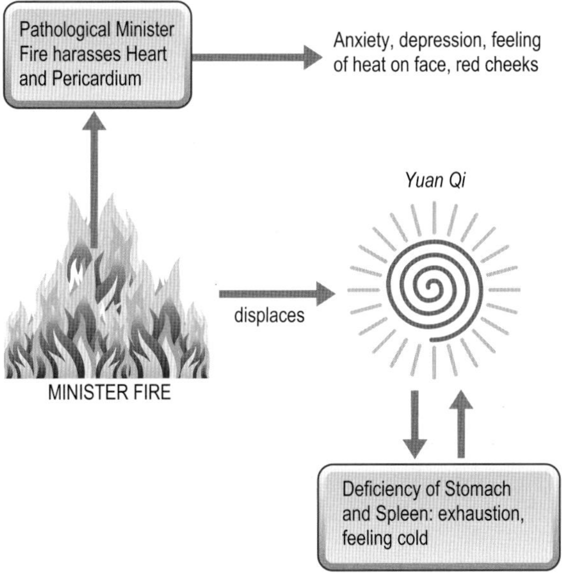

Figure 12.23 Pathology of Yin Fire.

Internal Wind

Internal Wind agitates the Mind in a similar way as Liver-Yang rising does and causes nervous tics and tremors (Fig. 12.25).

> **SUMMARY**
>
> **Effects of mental-emotional problems**
>
> ***Effects on Qi***
>
> - Liver-Qi stagnation
> - Heart- and Lung-Qi stagnation

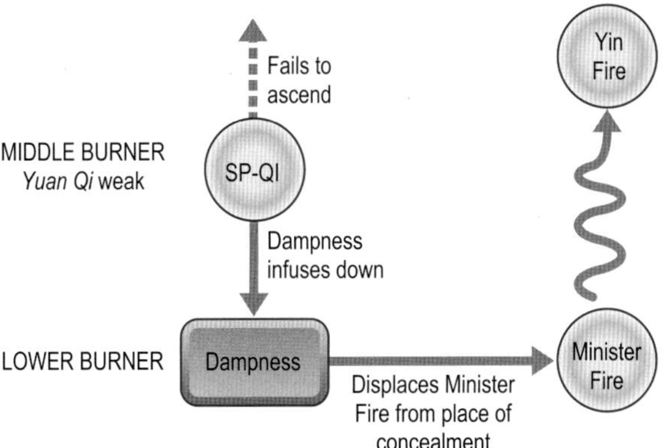

Figure 12.24 Pathology of Yin Fire with Dampness.

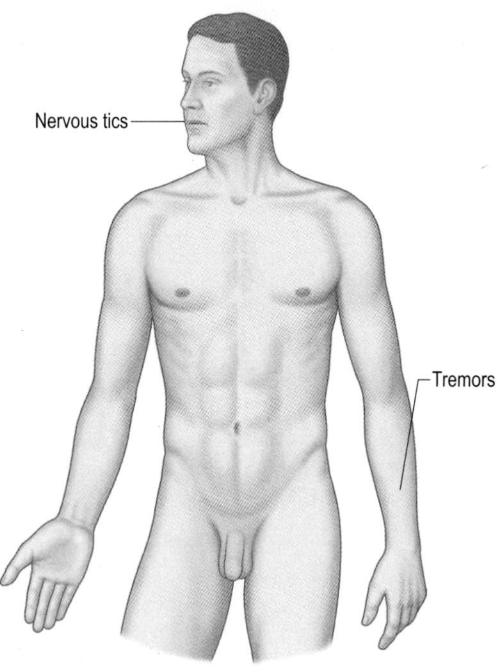

Figure 12.25 Internal Wind.

Effects on Blood

- Blood deficiency
  - Heart-Blood deficiency
  - Liver-Blood deficiency
- Blood stasis
  - Heart-Blood stasis
  - Liver-Blood stasis
- Blood-Heat
  - Heart-Blood Heat
  - Liver-Blood Heat

Effects on Yin

- Heart-Yin deficiency with Empty Heat
- Liver-Yin deficiency with Empty Heat
- Kidney-Yin deficiency with Empty Heat
- Lung-Yin deficiency with Empty Heat
- Spleen-Yin deficiency with Empty Heat

Pathogenic factors in mental-emotional problems

- Phlegm
- Fire or Heat
- Phlegm-Fire
- Empty Heat
- Internal Wind

MIND OBSTRUCTED, UNSETTLED, WEAKENED

The mental-emotional effects of emotions and other pathogenic factors may be summarized in three broad types.

1. *Mind Obstructed*: characterized by confused thinking, irrational behavior, clouding of the Mind and, in severe cases, complete loss of insight resulting in mental illness.
2. *Mind Unsettled*: characterized by insomnia, agitation, mental restlessness and anxiety.
3. *Mind Weakened*: characterized by depression, melancholy, mental exhaustion and physical tiredness.

Mind Obstructed

When the Mind is obstructed, there is a certain loss of insight, resulting in confused thinking, irrational thinking and behavior, and, if there is also Heat, manic behavior. In extreme cases, obstruction of the Mind leads to the psychosis seen in bipolar disorder or schizophrenia (Fig. 12.26). However, it is important to realize that obstruction of the Mind occurs in a wide variety of degrees, and having the Mind obstructed does not by any means mean mental illness in every case (Fig. 12.27).

The Mind is obstructed by Phlegm or by Blood stasis. In mild cases it may be obstructed by severe stagnation of Qi (Fig. 12.28). The etiology of Mind Obstructed is illustrated in Figure 12.29.

Mind Unsettled

If the Mind is unsettled, there is no loss of insight as there is when the Mind is obstructed, but the person suffers from insomnia, anxiety and worry. A good example of the difference between Mind Obstructed and Mind Unsettled can be seen in anxiety and panic attacks. Anxiety and panic attacks are a clear sign of Mind Unsettled; however, if the person has very severe panic attacks to the point of having an irrational fear of dying, then we can say that the Mind is slightly obstructed (Fig. 12.30).

The Mind is unsettled by deficiency of Blood or Yin (mild cases), Qi stagnation, Blood stasis, Fire, Empty Heat, Phlegm-Fire and internal Wind (Fig. 12.31).

Mind Weakened

The Mind is weakened by a deficiency of Qi (intended here in a general sense and to include deficiency of Qi, Yang, Blood or Yin); the patient becomes physically and mentally tired, depressed, dispirited and lacking initiative and motivation (Fig. 12.32).

Of course, there can be combinations of these three conditions. For example, a deficiency of Yin may lead to Mind Weakened causing tiredness and depression,

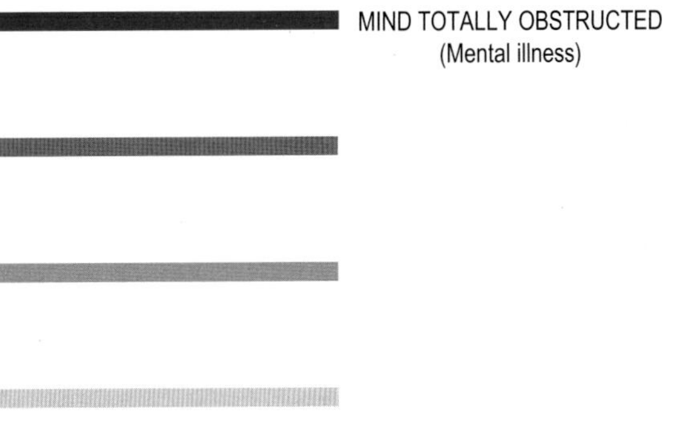

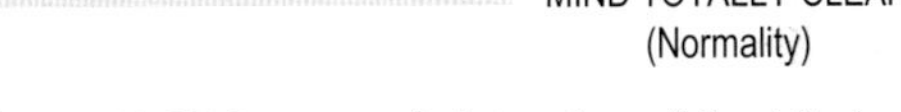

Figure 12.27 Degrees of obstruction of the Mind.

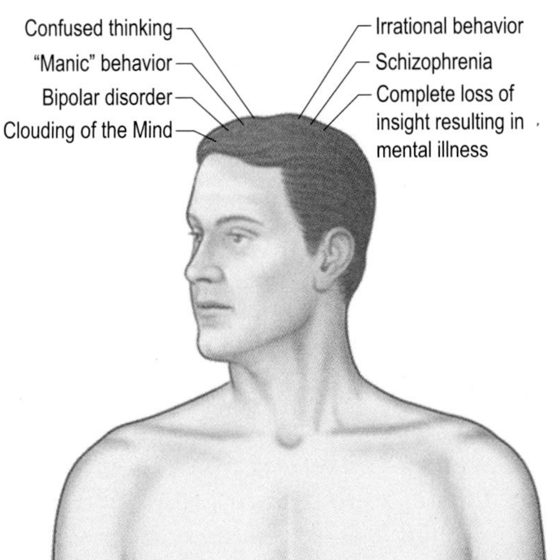

Figure 12.26 Symptoms of Mind Obstructed.

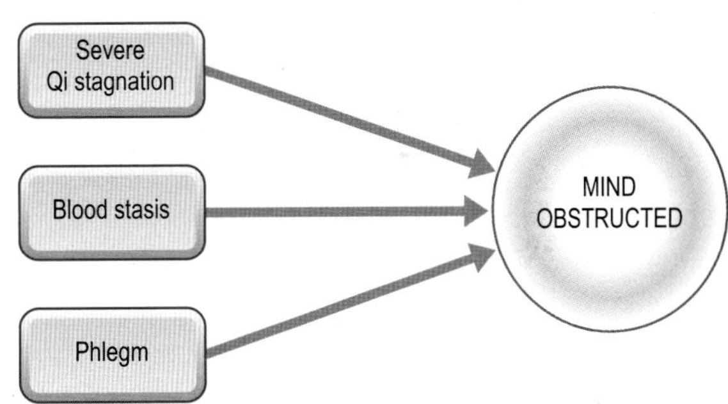

Figure 12.28 Patterns in Mind Obstructed.

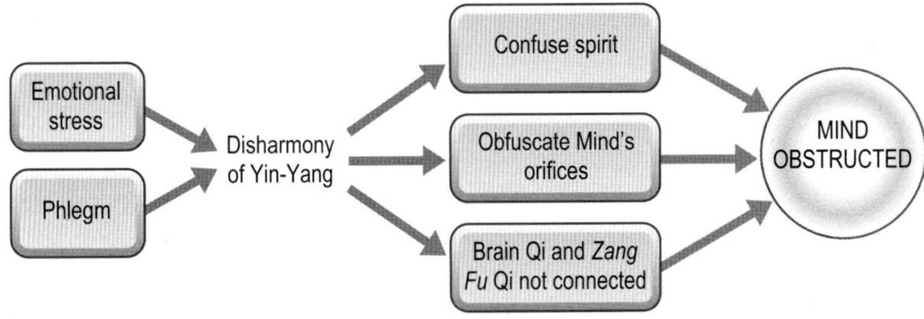

Figure 12.29 Etiology of Mind Obstructed.

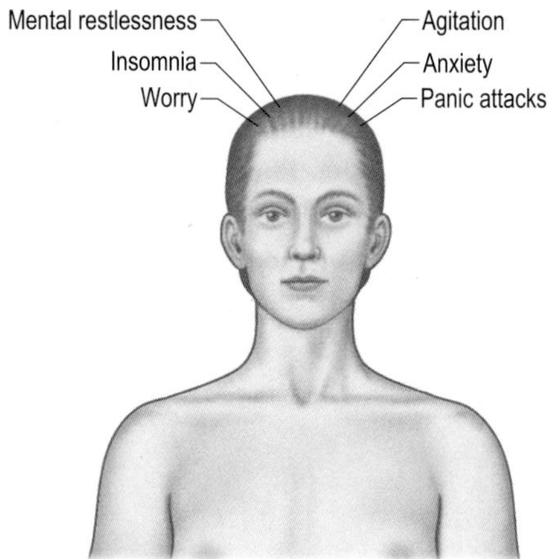

Figure 12.30 Mind Unsettled.

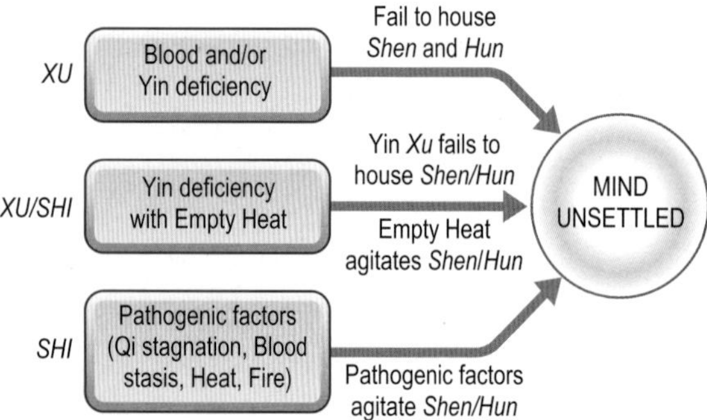

Figure 12.31 Patterns in Mind Unsettled.

and Empty Heat may lead to Mind Unsettled (insomnia and anxiety).

A combination of Mind Obstructed and Mind Unsettled is also common as when, for example, Blood stasis affects the Mind, causing some loss of insight (obstruction) and anxiety. The Mind may also be Obstructed and Weakened at the same time, and anorexia is an example of this. In fact, in anorexia, the Mind is obviously Weakened, resulting in physical tiredness and depression; however, the Spleen deficiency may lead to Phlegm which may obstruct the Mind so that the person's mind is obfuscated. Indeed, a person suffering from severe anorexia may look at themselves in the mirror and genuinely see themselves as fat. This is a good example of mental hallucination that indicates obstruction of the Mind.

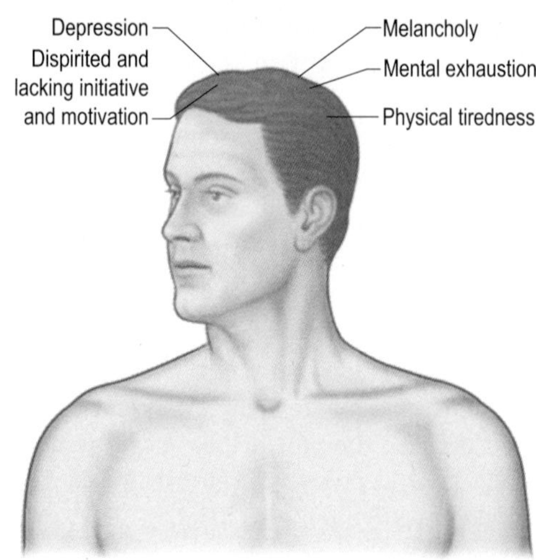

Figure 12.32 Mind Weakened.

Case history

A 51-year-old man sought treatment for atopic asthma and eczema. For 10 years from the age of 32 he drank a lot of alcohol and used amfetamines regularly and heavily. His eyes were dull and lacked lustre, and he complained of poor memory and concentration. When spoken to, he always looked like he was slightly absent and he found it difficult to find words. His tongue was Swollen and had a Stomach–Heart crack with a sticky-yellow coating (Plate 12.1), and his pulse was slightly Slippery.

This is given here as an example of a mild case of obstruction of the Mind, in his case by Phlegm.

Herbal treatment methods for Mind Obstructed, Unsettled or Weakened

The principle of treatment for mental-emotional problems follows the above classification closely and must be based, as usual, on a clear distinction between Deficiency and Excess and between the Root and the Manifestation. Such distinction is very important to choose the correct herbal formula.

When selecting a herbal formula in mental-emotional problems, I always keep in mind the distinction between Mind Obstructed, Mind Unsettled and Mind Weakened. I do this because I attach great importance to the taste of the herbs (and therefore the predominant taste of the prescription). Although a formula contains several herbs with different tastes, I still expect the resulting decoction to have a predominant taste according to the desired effect.

The taste I aim for depends on my classification of mental-emotional problems in the three broad categories of Mind Obstructed, Mind Unsettled and Mind Weakened.

In Mind Obstructed, I aim for the decoction (or powdered formula) to have a predominantly pungent and also fragrant taste. The pungent and fragrant taste moves Qi and opens the Mind's orifices. It is therefore absolutely essential for the prescription to have that taste predominantly.

In Mind Unsettled, one needs to make Qi descend with herbs that have a sinking movement (as many minerals do). If there is Heat, herbs with a bitter taste, which also makes Qi descend, should be employed. Of course, Mind Unsettled may also derive from a deficiency of Blood and/or Yin and therefore one needs herbs that are sweet and sour (to absorb Yin).

In Mind Weakened, one needs to tonify Qi, Blood or Yin, and one must rely primarily on the sweet taste (sweet and warm in case of Qi and Yang deficiency, and sweet and cold in case of Yin deficiency).

Treatment principles

In more detail, the main principles of treatment in mental-emotional problems are five.

1. *Nourish the Heart and calm the Mind*: this is applicable to Deficiency conditions, i.e. Qi, Blood or Yin deficiency causing Mind Weakened or Mind Unsettled.
2. *Clear pathogenic factors and calm the Mind*: this is applicable to Excess conditions such as stagnation of Qi or Blood, Phlegm-Fire and Fire, causing Mind Obstructed or Mind Unsettled.
3. *Clear pathogenic factors, nourish the Heart and calm the Mind*: this is applicable to deficiency of Yin leading to Empty Heat, causing Mind Unsettled and/or Mind Weakened.
4. *Resolve Phlegm, open the orifices and calm the Mind*: this is applicable to Phlegm or Phlegm-Fire, causing Mind Obstructed.
5. *Sink and calm the Mind*: this consists of the use of heavy minerals to sink rising Qi and is used as an addition to other methods of treatment to treat the Manifestation when the Mind is very unsettled. Please note that the use of minerals in herbal prescriptions is not allowed in Europe.

It should be noted that "calm the Mind" in the context of herbal treatment methods is an expression that recurs, as a method of treatment, in all cases of mental-emotional problems. It should be interpreted broadly to include not only the strict sense of calming the Mind (as in anxiety), but also the broader sense of lifting mood (as in depression).

The various pathologies and relevant methods of treatment may be summarized in tabular form (Table 12.2).

The actions of some of the most frequently used points in mental-emotional problems are shown in Chapter 13.

We can now discuss the acupuncture and herbal treatment for each of the patterns discussed above.

The mental-emotional pattern for each of the syndromes will be mentioned after the relevant herbal prescription; those who use only acupuncture are invited to read them as they obviously apply whether one uses acupuncture or herbs. Figure 12.33 clarifies

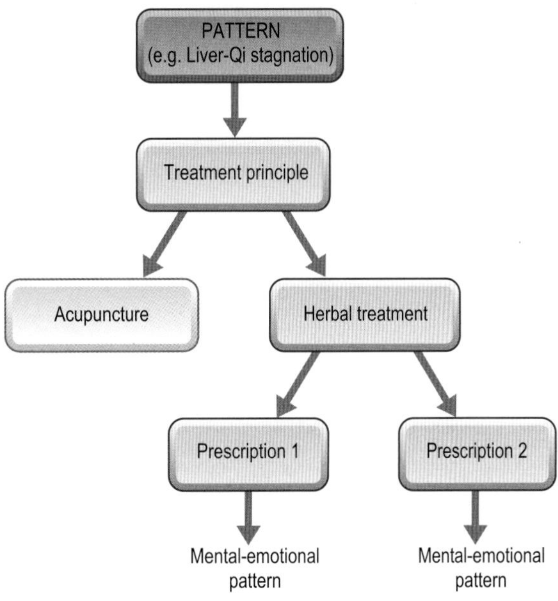

Figure 12.33 Structure of patterns' treatment discussion.

Table 12.2 Mind pathologies and methods of treatment

AFFLICTION OF MIND	PATHOLOGY	METHOD OF TREATMENT
Obstructed	Stagnation of Qi Stasis of Blood Phlegm	Move Qi, calm the Mind Invigorate Blood, calm the Mind Resolve Phlegm, open the orifices, calm the Mind
Unsettled	Blood-Yin deficiency Yin deficiency with Empty Heat Qi stagnation Blood stasis Fire Phlegm-Fire	Nourish Blood or Yin, nourish the Heart and calm the Mind Nourish Yin, clear Empty Heat and calm the Mind Move Qi and calm the Mind Invigorate Blood and calm the Mind Drain Fire and calm the Mind Drain Fire, resolve Phlegm, open the orifices and calm the Mind
Weakened	Qi deficiency Yang deficiency Blood deficiency Yin deficiency	Tonify Qi, calm and clear the Mind Tonify Yang, calm and clear the Mind Nourish Blood and calm the Mind Nourish Yin and calm the Mind

how the discussion of the treatment for each pattern is structured.

MIND OBSTRUCTED

The Mind may be obstructed or "misted" by stagnation of Qi, stasis of Blood or Phlegm. It may also be obstructed by Heat during an acute febrile disease, such as in the pattern "Heat in Pericardium" at the Nutritive Qi level, but this is a special case which does not concern us here.

Obstruction of the Mind causes mental confusion because the obstructing factor impairs the Mind's activity of thinking, memory, insight, conceptualization, application and understanding. Thus the person will suffer from mental confusion, poor memory, dizziness, poor concentration, inability to find the right words and slow thinking. In severe cases, there may be a complete loss of insight causing mental illness.

On an emotional level, when the Mind is obstructed there is a certain loss of insight, the person will feel mentally confused and behave somewhat irrationally. Obstruction of the Mind can occur in many different degrees, ranging from very mild and manifesting with a slight mental confusion, to very severe in which case there may be complete loss of insight in conditions such as manic-depression, psychosis or schizophrenia.

Of course there is a difference of degree in obstruction of the Mind by stagnation of Qi, stasis of Blood or Phlegm, stagnation of Qi being the mildest and Phlegm the most severe.

The treatment principle in obstruction of the Mind is to eliminate the pathogenic factors, open the Mind's orifices and calm the Mind. As indicated above, a herbal formula should have a predominantly pungent and fragrant taste.

Herbs to open the orifices in mental-emotional problems include:

- Shi Chang Pu *Rhizoma Acori tatarinowii*
- Yu Jin *Radix Curcumae*
- Yuan Zhi *Radix Polygalae*
- He Huan Pi *Cortex Albiziae*
- Su He *Xiang Styrax*
- Hu Po *Succinum*.

Acupuncture points that open the Mind's orifices include P-5 Jianshi, Du-20 Baihui, Du-24 Shenting, Du-26 Renzhong, ST-40 Fenglong, ST-25 Tianshu, all the Well points, G.B.-17 Zhengying, G.B.-18 Chengling, Du-19 Houding and G.B.-13 Benshen.

Qi stagnation

Stagnation of Liver-Qi

Treatment principle
Move Qi, pacify the Liver, settle the Ethereal Soul and calm the Mind.

Acupuncture

Points

LIV-3 Taichong, L.I.-4 Hegu, LIV-14 Qimen, P-6 Neiguan, T.B.-6 Zhigou, Du-24 Shenting, G.B.-13 Benshen. Reducing or even method.

Explanation

- LIV-3 is the main point to simultaneously move Liver-Qi and calm the Mind. In combination with L.I.-4 (the "Four Gates"), it has a very powerful calming effect on the Mind.
- LIV-14, Front-Collecting point of the Liver, moves Liver-Qi.
- P-6, indirectly connected to the Liver via the Terminal Yin channels, moves Liver-Qi and calms the Mind.
- T.B.-6 moves Liver-Qi.
- Du-24 and G.B.-13 powerfully calm the Mind in Liver patterns.

Special formula

ST-30 Qichong, KI-14 Siman, KI-13 Qixue, LIV-3 Taichong, P-6 Neiguan, BL-15 Xinshu, BL-18 Ganshu, SP-6 Sanyinjiao.

Explanation

This formula is used for Liver-Qi stagnating in the lower abdomen and Qi of the Penetrating Vessel (*Chong Mai*) rebelling upwards to disturb the Heart. This condition arises from shock, anger, guilt or prolonged worry and pensiveness, which cause stagnation of Qi. Combined with other causes of disease (such as, for example, excessive lifting, loss of blood in childbirth, or declining Blood and Yin during the menopause), this may cause stagnation of Liver-Qi and rebellious Qi in the Penetrating Vessel.

The Liver channel courses through the lower abdomen, the stomach, diaphragm, lungs and throat; the Kidney channel goes through the liver, diaphragm, lungs and throat. Thus they both go up to the throat where they may cause a feeling of constriction of the throat. They both also go to the chest where, with stagnation of Qi, they may cause a feeling of oppression and tightness of the chest. In the chest, they affect the Heart and Lungs and therefore Mind and Corporeal Soul, giving rise to anxiety, palpitations and unhappiness.

The *Spiritual Axis* in Chapter 65 says: "*The Penetrating and Directing Vessels originate from the uterus, go up through the spine and form the Sea of channels ... from the abdomen, they go up to the throat.*"[3] The *Simple Questions* in Chapter 60 says: "*The Penetrating Vessel rises through ST-30 Qichong, follows the Kidney channel to the umbilicus and chest, where it scatters.*"[4] Thus, rebellious Qi in the Penetrating Vessel affects the Heart, causing anxiety, palpitations and mental confusion.

- ST-30 is an important point of the Penetrating Vessel which emerges at this point, coming from the perineum. The point name means "rushing Qi" or "penetrating Qi", and the *chong* in its name refers to the *Chong Mai*, i.e. the Penetrating Vessel. This vessel is also related to the Bright Yang and the connection takes place through this point. ST-30 is therefore used to subdue rebellious Qi in the Penetrating Vessel affecting not only the lower abdomen, but the whole length of this vessel.
- KI-14 also subdues rebellious Qi in the Penetrating Vessel when this affects the lower abdomen. The name of this point means "four fullnesses", which may refer to a feeling of fullness of the lower abdomen radiating in all four directions; this feeling of fullness derives from stagnation of Qi in the Penetrating Vessel. Another meaning of its name is that the point treats four fullnesses deriving from stagnation of Qi, Blood, food and Dampness.
- KI-13 is another point along the Penetrating Vessel, and it also regulates its Qi by strengthening its root in the lower abdomen.
- LIV-3 subdues rebellious Qi in the Liver channel and settles the Ethereal Soul.
- P-6 also subdues rebellious Qi in the Liver channel, relaxes the chest, calms the Mind, settles the Ethereal Soul and relieves unhappiness.
- BL-15 and BL-18 regulate Qi of the Heart and Liver channel, move Qi, calm the Mind and settle the Ethereal Soul.
- SP-6 helps to subdue rebellious Qi by strengthening the root, i.e. Liver and Kidneys.

Herbal therapy

Prescription

YUE JU WAN

Gardenia-Chuanxiong Pill

Explanation

This formula is primarily for Liver-Qi stagnation, although it also treats stasis of Blood, retention of Food, stagnation of Phlegm and Dampness and knotted Heat. For this reason it is called the "formula for the six stagnations". It is, however, extremely effective in moving Qi, pacifying the Liver and calming the Mind. It is especially effective in opening the Mind's orifices and lifting mental depression deriving from stagnation of Liver-Qi.

Mental-emotional pattern

This formula addresses the emotional and mental manifestations of stagnation of Liver-Qi when it causes the Mind to be obstructed: moodiness, mental depression, severe premenstrual tension, irritability, frustration, irrational behavior, annoyance and impatience. On a physical level, there would be a feeling of distension, sighing, belching, tiredness, hypochondrial pain, a feeling of tightness in the chest, irregular periods, clumsiness, breast distension and a Wiry pulse (which may be Wiry only on the left side). In most cases, the tongue may not change, whilst in severe cases it may be slightly red on the sides.

The three most important signs for the use of this formula are tiredness, depression and a Wiry pulse.

Modifications

- For the Mind obstruction of this condition add Shi Chang Pu *Rhizoma Acori tatarinowii* to open the Mind's orifices and Yu Jin *Radix Curcumae* to open orifices and move Qi. Yu Jin, in particular, is extremely effective for mental depression because its strongly moving nature provides the necessary "push" to unblock the set patterns established by chronic depression.
- If there is pronounced stagnation of Qi, increase the dosage of Xiang Fu and, if necessary, add Mu Xiang *Radix Aucklandiae* and Fo Shou *Fructus Citri sarcodactylis*.
- If there is pronounced depression, add He Huan Pi *Cortex Albiziae*.
- If Dampness is pronounced, increase the dosage of Cang Zhu and, if necessary, add Fu Ling *Poria*, Ze Xie *Rhizoma Alismatis* and Hou Po *Cortex Magnoliae officinalis*.
- If stasis of Blood is pronounced, increase the dosage of Chuan Xiong and, if necessary, add Hong Hua *Flos Carthami tinctorii* and Tao Ren *Semen Armeniacae*.
- If Fire is pronounced, increase the dosage of Zhi Zi and, if necessary, add Huang Lian *Rhizoma Coptidis*.
- If Phlegm is pronounced, add Ban Xia *Rhizoma Pinelliae preparatum*.
- If retention of food is pronounced, increase the dosage of Shen Qu and, if necessary, add Mai Ya *Fructus Hordei germinatus*, Shan Zha *Fructus Crataegi* and Sha Ren *Fructus Amomi*.
- If there is emotional confusion, add Shi Chang Pu *Rhizoma Acori tatarinowii*.

SUMMARY

Mind Obstructed – Qi stagnation, stagnation of Liver-Qi

Treatment principle

Move Qi, pacify the Liver, settle the Ethereal Soul and calm the Mind.

Points

LIV-3 Taichong, L.I.-4 Hegu, LIV-14 Qimen, P-6 Neiguan, T.B.-6 Zhigou, Du-24 Shenting, G.B.-13 Benshen. Reducing or even method.

Herbal therapy

Prescription

YUE JU WAN
Gardenia-Chuanxiong Pill

Case history

A 38-year-old woman sought treatment for primary infertility. She had been trying to conceive for 2 years. The gynecologist had diagnosed endometriosis and adhesions in the fallopian tubes for which she had had laser treatment. Her periods were quite normal and regular, except for being rather scanty (lasting 3 days). She suffered from very pronounced abdominal distension and fullness. She had panic attacks and experienced a feeling of oppression of the chest and palpitations. During such attacks she also had a suffocating feeling in the throat. Her eyes had an unstable look as if she were scared. Her tongue had a Red tip and sides, but apart from that it was quite normal. Her pulse was Slippery, Short and Moving (the Moving pulse is short, shaped like a bean and vibrating).

During the consultation, on asking her about any shocks she might have had, she said she had been raped when she was 22.

Diagnosis This is a condition of stagnation of Qi in the Liver channel and the Penetrating Vessel affecting the Heart. Shock affects the Heart, but also the Kidneys; in women, this often causes stagnation of Qi in the Penetrating Vessel and the Liver channel. Rebellious Qi in the lower abdomen rises upwards to harass the Heart and the Mind causing, in her case, palpitations, a feeling of oppression in the chest and anxiety. The stagnation of Qi in the Penetrating Vessel in the lower abdomen caused the feeling of fullness and distension there. Her eyes and her pulse clearly showed the strong possibility of shock in the past, and this was the reason for me asking her about this. The tongue also showed stagnation in the Liver and Heart. In this case, therefore, infertility was not due to a deficiency, but to stagnation of Qi in the Penetrating and Directing Vessels preventing conception.

Treatment She was treated with both acupuncture and herbs. The acupuncture treatment was quite infrequent as she lived over 100 miles away. Whenever I saw her I used the special formula indicated above, more or less unchanged, i.e. ST-30 Qichong, KI-14 Siman, KI-13 Qixue, LIV-3 Taichong, P-6 Neiguan, BL-15 Xinshu, BL-18 Ganshu and SP-6 Sanyinjiao. This formula was explained above under *Stagnation of Liver-Qi*.

The herbal decoction used was a variation of two formulae together: Yue Ju Wan *Gardenia-Chuanxiong Pill* and An Shen Ding Zhi Wan *Calming the Mind and Settling the Spirit Pill*.

- **Xiang Fu** *Rhizoma Cyperi* 9 g
- **Shan Zhi Zi** *Fructus Gardeniae* 4 g
- **Chuan Xiong** *Radix Chuanxiong* 4 g
- **Shen Qu** *Massa Fermentata Medicinalis* 4 g
- **Cang Zhu** *Rhizoma Atractylodis* 4 g
- **Dang Shen** *Radix Codonopsis* 6 g
- **Fu Shen** *Sclerotium Poriae cocos pararadicis* 6 g
- **Yuan Zhi** *Radix Polygalae* 6 g
- **Shi Chang Pu** *Rhizoma Acori tatarinowii* 4 g
- **Dang Gui** *Radix Angelicae sinensis* 6 g
- **Chen Xiang** *Lignum Aquilariae* 4 g
- **Suan Zao Ren** *Semen Ziziphi spinosae* 4 g
- **Bai Zi Ren** *Semen Platycladi* 6 g
- **Zhi Gan Cao** *Radix Glycyrrhizae uralensis preparata* 3 g

Explanation

- The first five herbs constitute the Yue Ju Wan *Gardenia-Chuanxiong Pill* which pacifies the Liver and eliminates stagnation. The emphasis is on Xiang Fu (hence with a higher dose) to eliminate stagnation and subdue rebellious Qi in the Penetrating Vessel.
- The next four herbs make the An Shen Ding Zhi Wan *Calming the Mind and Settling the Spirit Pill* (without Long Chi *Fossilia Dentis Mastodi*), which tonifies the Heart and calms the Mind, especially after shock.
- Dang Gui was added to nourish and root the Penetrating Vessel in the lower abdomen; this will help to root it and subdue rebellious Qi.
- Chen Xiang was added to subdue rebellious Qi in the Penetrating Vessel, a function also attributed to it by Li Shi Zhen in his book on the Extraordinary Vessels.[5]
- Suan Zao Ren and Bai Zi Ren were added to settle the Ethereal Soul and calm the Mind.

After 6 months of this treatment she conceived, but unfortunately she miscarried in the second month. She re-started the treatment and again she became pregnant after 6 months. This time, I prescribed a decoction to take as soon as she became pregnant to prevent miscarriage:

- **Tu Si Zi** *Semen Cuscutae* 6 g
- **Du Zhong** *Cortex Eucommiae ulmoidis* 6 g
- **Sha Ren** *Fructus Amomi* 4 g
- **Zi Su Ye** *Folium Perillae* 4 g
- **Bai Zhu** *Rhizoma Atractylodis macrocephalae* 6 g

All these herbs prevent miscarriage and, this time, she was able to continue her pregnancy to full term and give birth to a baby.

Stagnation of Heart- and Lung-Qi

Treatment principle

Move Qi, stimulate the descending of Heart- and Lung-Qi and calm the Mind, settle the Corporeal Soul.

Acupuncture

Points

LU-7 Lieque, HE-7 Shenmen, P-6 Neiguan, Ren-15 Jiuwei, Ren-17 Shanzhong, ST-40 Fenglong, L.I.-4 Hegu. Reducing or even method if the condition is chronic.

Explanation

- LU-7 stimulates the descending of Lung-Qi and calms the Corporeal Soul. It has a strong mental effect and it relieves stagnation of Qi in the chest. According to *An Explanation of Acupuncture Points* (1654), this point is used when the person is sad and cries a lot.[6]
- HE-7 nourishes the Heart and calms the Mind.
- P-6 stimulates the descending of Heart-Qi, opens the chest, relieves fullness and stagnation and calms the Mind.
- Ren-15 has a powerful calming effect on the Mind. It also relieves fullness in the chest.
- Ren-17 stimulates the descending of Lung-Qi and relieves fullness and stagnation in the chest.
- ST-40 harmonizes the Stomach, opens the chest and calms the Mind.
- L.I.-4 harmonizes the ascending and descending of Qi in the Middle Burner, relieves fullness and calms the Mind.

Herbal therapy

Prescription

BAN XIA HOU PO TANG
Pinellia-Magnolia Decoction

Explanation

This formula, from the *Discussion of Cold-Induced Diseases*, is normally used for the plum-stone pattern characterized by a feeling of obstruction in the throat, mental depression and irritability. In modern times this pattern is related to stagnation of Liver-Qi, for which this formula is used. An analysis of the formula, however, reveals that it contains no herbs that move Liver-Qi or even enter the Liver. The main emphasis of the formula is to move stagnant Heart- and Lung-Qi.

Stagnation of Heart- and Lung-Qi derives from sadness and grief over a long period of time. These emotions first deplete Heart-Qi and Lung-Qi and depress the Mind and Corporeal Soul. The depletion of Lung-Qi from sadness and grief leads to shallow breathing and poor circulation of Qi in the chest and, eventually, to stagnation of Lung-Qi in the chest. The simultaneous weakness and stagnation of Lung-Qi may also lead to Phlegm. The Lung channel influences the throat and its stagnation can cause a feeling of obstruction in the throat. Other manifestations include sighing, difficulty in swallowing, slight breathlessness, tightness of the chest, nausea and vomiting. The pulse will be Weak on both Front positions.

Mental-emotional pattern

Stagnation of Heart- and Lung-Qi derives from long-term sadness and grief, with the resulting depletion of the Mind and Corporeal Soul. This resides in the Lungs and it therefore affects breathing. The person becomes anxious as well as sad, sighs frequently and has the typical feeling of obstruction in the throat and chest. This is caused by the constriction of the Corporeal Soul in the throat and chest. The chronic stagnation of Heart-Qi obstructs the Mind and causes severe confusion.

When this pattern causes obstruction of the Mind, the patient will feel confused and experience mental cloudiness. He or she may also suffer from severe panic attacks with fear of death.

Modifications

- Similarly as for stagnation of Liver-Qi, Shi Chang Pu *Rhizoma Acori tatarinowii* should be added to open the Mind's orifices.
- If there is a pronounced feeling of oppression of the chest from Qi stagnation (slightly Wiry pulse), add Qing Pi *Pericarpium Citri reticulatae viride* and Mu Xiang *Radix Aucklandiae*.
- If there is vomiting, increase Ban Xia *Rhizoma Pinelliae preparatum* and Sheng Jiang *Rhizoma Zingiberis recens*.
- If there is a feeling of heaviness under the heart, add Zhi Shi *Fructus Aurantii immaturus*.
- If there is epigastric pain, add Sha Ren *Fructus Amomi*.
- If there is sour regurgitation with a yellow tongue coating, add Huang Lian *Rhizoma Coptidis*.
- If there is sour regurgitation with a Pale tongue, add Wu Zei Gu *Os Sepiae*.
- If there is a bitter taste, add Huang Qin *Radix Scutellariae*.

- If mental restlessness and irritability are pronounced, add He Huan Pi *Cortex Albiziae*.

Associated prescription
SI QI TANG
Four Seasons Decoction for the Seven Emotions

This consists of Ban Xia Hou Po Tang plus Da Zao *Fructus Jujubae*.

This formula has the same use and indications as Ban Xia Hou Po Tang, except that its effect on the Mind is even stronger. "Seven" in the name of the formula stands for the seven emotions and "Four" stands for the four seasons, indicating an emotional condition that spans at least four seasons, i.e. a chronic condition.

SUMMARY

Mind Obstructed – Qi stagnation, stagnation of Heart- and Lung-Qi

Treatment principle

Move Qi, stimulate the descending of Heart- and Lung-Qi and calm the Mind, settle the Corporeal Soul.

Points

LU-7 Lieque, HE-7 Shenmen, P-6 Neiguan, Ren-15 Jiuwei, Ren-17 Shanzhong, ST-40 Fenglong, L.I.-4 Hegu. Reducing or even method if the condition is chronic.

Herbal therapy

Prescription

BAN XIA HOU PO TANG
Pinellia-Magnolia Decoction

Associated prescription

SI QI TANG
Four Seasons Decoction for the Seven Emotions

Blood stasis

Heart-Blood stasis

Treatment principle
Invigorate Blood, eliminate stasis, clear the Heart, calm the Mind.

Acupuncture

Points
P-6 Neiguan, P-5 Jianshi, Ren-14 Juque, BL-14 Jueyinshu, BL-15 Xinshu, Ren-17 Shanzhong, HE-7 Shenmen, SP-6 Sanyinjiao, BL-17 Geshu, BL-44 Shentang, G.B.-18 Chenling. Reducing or even method if the condition is chronic.

Explanation
- P-6 invigorates Heart-Blood, opens the chest and calms the Mind.
- P-5 opens the Mind's orifices.
- Ren-14, Front-Collecting point of the Heart, invigorates Heart-Blood and calms the Mind.
- BL-14 and BL-15, Back-Transporting points of the Pericardium and Heart, respectively, invigorate Blood and calm the Mind.
- Ren-17 moves Qi in the chest; moving Qi will help to invigorate Blood.
- HE-7 calms the Mind.
- SP-6 invigorates Blood and calms the Mind.
- BL-17, Gathering point for Blood, invigorates Blood (if needled with reducing or even method).
- BL-44 clears the Heart and calms the Mind.
- G.B.-18 opens the Mind's orifices.

Herbal therapy

Prescription
XUE FU ZHU YU TANG
Blood-Mansion Eliminating Stasis Decoction

Explanation
This formula is very widely used for stasis of Blood in the Upper Burner causing chest pain. The tongue is Purple and the pulse is Wiry or Choppy.

Mental-emotional pattern
Since Blood is the residence of the Mind, any Blood pathology can affect the Mind. Blood stasis agitates and obstructs the Mind. It agitates the Mind because Qi and Blood cannot flow smoothly and this is reflected on the mental-emotional level with anxiety, mental restlessness and insomnia. It obstructs the Mind because the impeded flow of Blood retards the circulation of Blood to the Mind and thus obfuscates its orifices.

Anger, frustration, resentment, excess joy, shock, craving and guilt can all lead to Heart-Blood stasis.

This usually occurs only after a long period of time, going through the stage of Qi stagnation first.

When stagnant Blood in the Heart affects the Mind, it may cause depression, anxiety, palpitations, insomnia, a suffocating sensation in the chest, irritability, mood swings and, in severe cases, manic behavior. Sleep is very disturbed, the patient waking up frequently at night, tossing and turning and with nightmares.

Modifications

- Shi Chang Pu *Rhizoma Acori tatarinowii* and Yu Jin *Radix Curcumae* should be added to open the Mind's orifices and invigorate Blood.

SUMMARY

Mind Obstructed – Blood stasis, Heart-Blood stasis

Treatment principle

Invigorate Blood, eliminate stasis, clear the Heart, calm the Mind.

Points

P-6 Neiguan, P-5 Jianshi, Ren-14 Juque, BL-14 Jueyinshu, BL-15 Xinshu, Ren-17 Shanzhong, HE-7 Shenmen, SP-6 Sanyinjiao, BL-17 Geshu, BL-44 Shentang, G.B.-18 Chenling. Reducing or even method if the condition is chronic.

Herbal therapy

Prescription

XUE FU ZHU YU TANG

Blood-Mansion Eliminating Stasis Decoction

Liver-Blood stasis

Treatment principle

Invigorate Blood, pacify the Liver, calm the Mind and settle the Ethereal Soul.

Acupuncture

Points

LIV-3 Taichong, LIV-14 Qimen, BL-18 Ganshu, BL-17 Geshu, BL-47 Hunmen, P-6 Neiguan, P-7 Daling, SP-6 Sanyinjiao, Du-24 Shenting and G.B.-13 Benshen, G.B.-18 Chengling. Reducing or even method if the condition is chronic, except for BL-47 which should be reinforced.

Explanation

- LIV-3 invigorates Liver-Blood and calms the Mind and Ethereal Soul.
- LIV-14 and BL-18, Front-Collecting and Back-Transporting point, respectively, invigorate Liver-Blood.
- BL-17 invigorates Blood.
- BL-47 settles the Ethereal Soul and regulates its coming and going.
- P-6 invigorates Blood, pacifies the Liver and calms the Mind.
- P-7 invigorates Blood, opens the Mind orifices and calms the Mind.
- SP-6 invigorates Blood and calms the Mind.
- Du-24 and G.B.-13 calm the Mind in Liver patterns.
- G.B.-18 opens the Mind's orifices.

Herbal therapy

Prescription

YUE JU WAN

Gardenia-Chuanxiong Pill

Explanation

This formula has already been discussed under Liver-Qi stagnation. It can be adapted to treat Liver-Blood stasis by increasing the dosage of Chuan Xiong.

Mental-emotional pattern

Anger, resentment, frustration, jealousy, guilt and hatred may all lead to Liver-Blood stasis. This will cause extreme depression, severe mood swings, intense irritability, propensity to violent outbursts of anger, obsessive jealousy and, in severe cases, manic behavior.

Modifications

- Yu Jin *Radix Curcumae* should be added to invigorate Liver-Blood, open the Mind's orifices and relieve depression.
- In cases of severe depression, add He Huan Pi *Cortex Albiziae*.
- In cases of violent outbursts of anger, add Suan Zao Ren *Semen Ziziphi spinosae*.

SUMMARY

Mind Obstructed – Blood stasis, Liver-Blood stasis

Treatment principle

Invigorate Blood, pacify the Liver, calm the Mind and settle the Ethereal Soul.

Points

LIV-3 Taichong, LIV-14 Qimen, BL-18 Ganshu, BL-17 Geshu, BL-47 Hunmen, P-6 Neiguan, P-7 Daling, SP-6 Sanyinjiao, Du-24 Shenting and G.B.-13 Benshen, G.B.-18 Chengling. Reducing or even method if the condition is chronic, except for BL-47 which should be reinforced.

Herbal therapy

Prescription

YUE JU WAN
Gardenia-Chuanxiong Pill

Stasis of Blood in the Lower Burner

Treatment principle

Invigorate Blood, harmonize the Penetrating and Directing vessels, eliminate stasis and calm the Mind.

Acupuncture

Points

SP-10 Xuehai, SP-6 Sanyinjiao, SP-4 Gongsun and P-6 Neiguan, Ren-6 Qihai, KI-14 Siman, ST-29 Guilai, BL-18 Ganshu, BL-17 Geshu, SP-1 Yinbai, Du-18 Qiangjian. Reducing method.

Explanation

- SP-10 invigorates Blood in the uterus.
- SP-6 invigorates Blood and calms the Mind.
- SP-4 and P-6 in combination regulate the Penetrating Vessel and invigorate Blood.
- Ren-6 moves Qi in order to invigorate Blood.
- KI-14 is a point of the Penetrating Vessel which invigorates Blood.
- ST-29 invigorates Blood in the uterus.
- BL-18 and BL-17 in combination invigorate Blood.
- SP-1 invigorates Blood in the uterus and calms the Mind.
- Du-18 opens the Mind's orifices, calms the Mind and regulates Liver-Blood. It is a strong head point for mental restlessness, manic behavior and agitation.

Herbal therapy

Prescription

TAO HE CHENG QI TANG
Persica Conducting Qi Decoction

Explanation

This formula is for Blood stasis in the Lower Burner. It is from the *Discussion of Cold-Induced Diseases* and it invigorates Blood in the Lower Burner by moving downwards with Da Huang *Radix et Rhizoma Rhei* and Mang Xiao *Natrii Sulfas*.

Mental-emotional pattern

This prescription is from the *Discussion of Cold-Induced Diseases* and it refers to the Greater Yang-organ pattern from accumulation of Blood. This consists of accumulation of Blood in the hypogastrium following an invasion of Cold. It manifests with fever at night, delirium, severe lower abdominal pain, mental restlessness and manic behavior. This is the original use of the formula. It can be used for mental-emotional problems deriving from (or causing) stasis of Blood in the Lower Burner.

Anger, frustration, hatred, resentment and guilt may all lead to this condition over a long period of time. Guilt frequently leads to stasis of Blood in the Lower Burner, especially in women. Why do these emotions in this case lead to stasis of Blood in the Lower Burner and not somewhere else? First of all, it is obviously more common in women who are prone to stasis of Blood in the uterus. However, it may also be due to other concurrent causes of disease such as excessive lifting which leads to stagnation in the Lower Burner.

A special use of this formula is for psychosis from stasis of Blood in the uterus following childbirth.

SUMMARY

Mind Obstructed – Blood stasis, stasis of blood in the Lower Burner

Treatment principle

Invigorate Blood, harmonize the Penetrating and Directing vessels, eliminate stasis and calm the Mind.

Points

SP-10 Xuehai, SP-6 Sanyinjiao, SP-4 Gongsun and P-6 Neiguan, Ren-6 Qihai, KI-14 Siman, ST-29 Guilai, BL-18 Ganshu, BL-17 Geshu, SP-1 Yinbai, Du-18 Qiangjian. Reducing method.

Herbal therapy

Prescription

TAO HE CHENG QI TANG
Persica Conducting Qi Decoction

Phlegm misting the Mind

Phlegm-Heat harassing the Mind

Treatment principle
Resolve Phlegm, open the orifices and calm the Mind.

Acupuncture

Points
ST-40 Fenglong, P-7 Daling, P-6 Neiguan, P-5 Jianshi, Du-14 Dazhui, BL-15 Xinshu, BL-44 Shentang, Du-20 Baihui, L.I.-4 Hegu, LU-7 Lieque, Ren-12 Zhongwan, ST-36 Zusanli, BL-20 Pishu, L.I.-7 Wenliu, ST-25 Tianshu. Reducing or even method, except for Du-14, Du-20, Ren-12, ST-36, BL-20, BL-15 and BL-44, which should be reinforced.

Explanation
- ST-40 resolves Phlegm.
- P-7 resolves Phlegm from the Heart and calms the Mind.
- P-6 opens the Mind's orifices.
- P-5 resolves Phlegm from the Heart.
- Du-14, with reducing method, clears Heart-Heat.
- BL-15 and BL-44 tonify the Heart and clear the Mind.
- Du-20 clears the Mind.
- L.I.-4 and LU-7 regulate the ascending of clear Qi and descending of turbid Qi in the head, thus clearing the Mind.
- Ren-12, ST-36 and BL-20 tonify the Spleen to resolve Phlegm.
- L.I.-7 opens the Mind's orifices. The book *An Explanation of Acupuncture Points* (1654) says this point is for "*madness and seeing ghosts*".[7]
- ST-25 is an important point for mental-emotional problems from Phlegm misting the Mind. It regulates the Stomach and opens the Mind's orifices. The book *An Explanation of Acupuncture Points* says this point is used when "*Ethereal Soul and Corporeal Soul have no residence.*"[8]

Herbal therapy

Prescription
WEN DAN TANG
Warming the Gall-Bladder Decoction

Explanation
This interesting formula (dating from 1174) has two main interpretations. Originally it was used for a Gall-Bladder deficiency following a severe acute disease, the Gall-Bladder deficiency manifesting with timidity, jumpiness, insomnia (waking up early in the morning) and mental restlessness. From this point of view, its action was exactly that described by its name, i.e. "Warming the Gall-Bladder": it tonifies the Gall-Bladder and stimulates the *physiological* rise of Liver-Qi.

In more recent times, it is more frequently used for Phlegm-Heat affecting Stomach, Heart or Lungs. The main manifestations for which it is used in this context are mental restlessness, jumpiness, insomnia, a bitter and sticky taste, a flustered feeling in the heart region, mental confusion, irritability, manic behavior, nausea, vomiting, palpitations, dizziness, a Swollen tongue with a sticky-yellow coating and a Wiry or Slippery pulse.

Two characteristic pulse and tongue configurations strongly indicate the use of this formula. One is a tongue that is Swollen and has a combination of Heart and Stomach crack with a rough, brush-like yellow coating inside the Stomach crack. A combined Heart and Stomach crack extends all the way to the tip, as a Heart crack would do, but it is wide and shallow in the center, as a Stomach crack would be (see Fig. 12.34).

The other sign is a pulse which is Big, Slippery and Wiry on both Middle positions of left and right.

Mental-emotional pattern
Phlegm-Heat disturbs the Mind in two ways: Phlegm obstructs the Mind's orifices and Heat agitates the Mind. The combination of these two factors will cause mental restlessness, slightly "manic" behavior, mental confusion, irrational behavior, talking a lot, laughing a lot, staying up late at night to work and insomnia. In

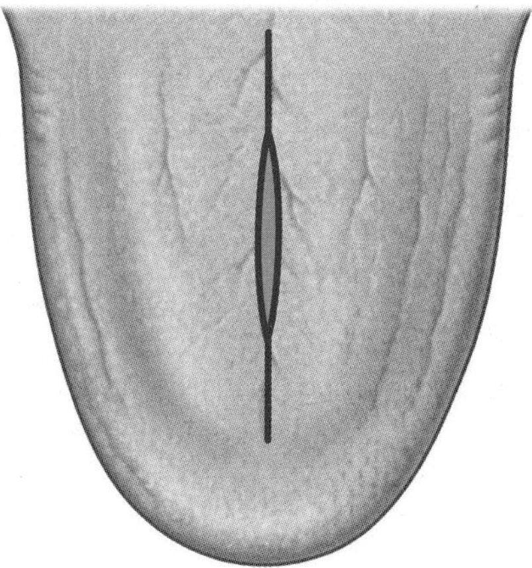

Figure 12.34 Combined Stomach and Heart crack.

severe cases, this corresponds to bipolar disorder or schizophrenia.

Prescription
GUI SHEN TANG
Restoring the Mind Decoction

Explanation
This formula combines opening the Mind's orifices and resolving Phlegm with tonifying the Spleen, Heart and Kidneys. It is therefore suitable in chronic conditions when Phlegm mists the Mind on a background of Qi and Yang deficiency.

Mental-emotional pattern
From a mental-emotional viewpoint, the patient will be calmer than in the previous two cases. He or she will feel very confused mentally, exhausted and depressed. The obstruction of the Mind by Phlegm, combined with the deficient Heart and Kidneys not nourishing the Mind, will make this person very forgetful and disorientated.

SUMMARY

Mind Obstructed – Phlegm misting the Mind, Phlegm-Heat harassing the Mind

Treatment principle

Resolve Phlegm, open the orifices and calm the Mind.

Points

ST-40 Fenglong, P-7 Daling, P-6 Neiguan, P-5 Jianshi, Du-14 Dazhui, BL-15 Xinshu, BL-44 Shentang, Du-20 Baihui, L.I.-4 Hegu, LU-7 Lieque, Ren-12 Zhongwan, ST-36 Zusanli, BL-20 Pishu, L.I.-7 Wenliu, ST-25 Tianshu. Reducing or even method, except for Du-14, Du-20, Ren-12, ST-36, BL-20, BL-15 and BL-44 which should be reinforced.

Herbal therapy

Prescription

WEN DAN TANG
Warming the Gall-Bladder Decoction

Prescription

GUI SHEN TANG
Restoring the Mind Decoction

Case history

A 39-year-old man had been suffering from what was labeled as "phobic anxiety" for 8 years. His history was quite complex and many factors contributed to his problem, so rather than starting from his presenting symptoms, it might be better to describe his history from the beginning. His childhood had been very troubled, most of all because his mother was very unloving towards him and she constantly reproached him. At the age of 28 he worked in Belfast at the time of a very tense political and military situation which caused a great deal of anxiety to him. He suffered a shock when he found a bomb under his car. When he was 30 he had a car accident and had concussion. Nine months after that he contracted an extremely severe case of influenza that was nearly fatal. He was in bed for a month with a constant temperature. A few months after that he collapsed crying hysterically, he was unable to speak, could not move and could not bear to look at a light. His GP thought he had a brain hemorrhage but this was not the case. After that collapse he continued to be extremely anxious, lost all confidence in himself, lacked self-esteem, felt extremely insecure and was prone to bouts of crying. At this time he started seeing a psychotherapist and then a psychiatrist who prescribed tranquillizers (diazepam and temazepam) and antidepressants of the monoamine oxidase kind.

He started having acupuncture with a colleague who referred him to me for herbal treatment.

His main symptoms when he came to me were epigastric pain, alternation of constipation and diarrhea, ache in the joints, burning eyes and a hot feeling at the back of the head.

On a mental level his main manifestations were severe anxiety, insomnia, bouts of crying, poor memory and concentration, depression and a lack of confidence and self-esteem.

His eyes lacked glitter and looked scared, his body was overweight and his complexion was very dull and sallow.

His tongue was dark-Red, Swollen, with a Heart crack, without coating and dry. The tip of the tongue was redder and the root had no spirit (Plate 12.2). His pulse, however, was slightly Rapid, quite Full and Slippery.

Diagnosis This is an extremely complex condition. As far as patterns are concerned, there are basically two main patterns: severe Yin deficiency of the Heart and Kidneys (Red-peeled tongue with red tip and root without spirit, mental restlessness, anxiety, insomnia, burning eyes, a hot feeling on the occiput, lack of confidence and self-esteem) and Phlegm-Heat misting the Mind (crying without reason, poor memory and concentration). There are a few other patterns but these can be considered secondary. For example, there is Stomach-Yin deficiency causing the epigastric pain, Damp Heat causing the joint pain, some stagnation of Liver-Qi causing the alternation of constipation and diarrhea, and some Spleen deficiency causing him to be overweight and generally tired. It is this underlying Spleen deficiency which, over the years, led to the formation of Phlegm, later transformed into Phlegm-Heat.

If there is Phlegm, why does the tongue not have a thick-sticky coating? This is because there is an underlying severe deficiency of Yin which caused the coating to fall off. Thus, although not shown on the tongue-body color, Phlegm does manifest in the swelling of the tongue body (which in such a severe case of Yin deficiency should have been Thin) and in the symptoms and the pulse which is Full and Slippery.

The Yin deficiency obviously derived from the time of his severe influenza. A constant temperature for a month burned the body fluids and injured Yin. The deficiency of Yin over the years led to the formation of Empty Heat which harasses the Mind. On the other hand, the deficiency of Yin itself deprives the Mind and Ethereal Soul of their root and causes lack of confidence and self-esteem. Phlegm-Heat, conversely, obstructs the Mind and causes the bouts of crying.

Obviously all this is affected by his childhood experiences which formed the basis for the development of his condition later on in life especially, causing his lack of confidence and self-esteem, having never received love from his mother. Other etiological factors also played a role. The concussion suffered following the car accident could have affected his brain and therefore contributed to his illness.

Thus we can summarize his causes of disease in three stages (Fig. 12.35).

Treatment principle Treatment was focused on the two main patterns of Yin deficiency and Phlegm-Heat; the treatment principles were to nourish Heart- and Kidney-Yin, clear Empty Heat, open the Mind's orifices, calm the Mind, root the Ethereal Soul and Corporeal Soul and strengthen Will-Power.

Herbal therapy This patient was treated for 4 years and is still under treatment; therefore the formula used was obviously modified very many times. The formula used most frequently was a variation of three prescriptions.

1. Wen Dan Tang *Warming the Gall-Bladder Decoction*
2. Tian Wang Bu Xin Dan *Heavenly Emperor Tonifying the Heart Pill*
3. Gan Mai Da Zao Tang *Glycyrrhiza-Triticum-Jujuba Decoction*

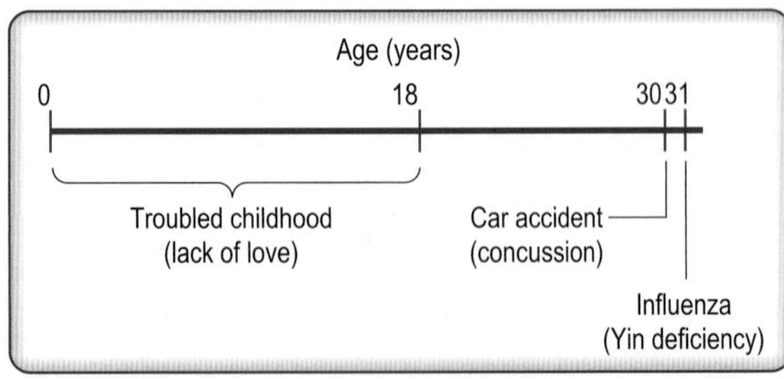

Figure 12.35 Causes of disease in a patient diagnosed with "phobic anxiety".

An example of a formula used is as follows.

- **Zhu Ru** *Caulis Bambusae in Taeniam* 6 g
- **Zhi Shi** *Fructus Aurantii immaturus* 4 g
- **Ban Xia** *Rhizoma Pinelliae preparatum* 6 g
- **Fu Ling** *Poria* 6 g
- **Chen Pi** *Pericarpium Citri reticulatae* 3 g
- **Sheng Di Huang** *Radix Rehmanniae glutinosae* 9 g
- **Mai Men Dong** *Radix Ophiopogonis* 6 g
- **Xuan Shen** *Radix Scrophulariae* 4 g
- **Ren Shen** *Radix Ginseng* 6 g
- **Bai Zi Ren** *Semen Platycladi* 6 g
- **Suan Zao Ren** *Semen Ziziphi spinosae* 6 g
- **Wu Wei Zi** *Fructus Schisandrae* 4 g
- **Yuan Zhi** *Radix Polygalae* 9 g
- **Shi Chang Pu** *Rhizoma Acori tatarinowii* 4 g
- **Yu Jin** *Radix Curcumae* 4 g
- **Fu Xiao Mai** *Fructus Tritici levis* 6 g
- **Zhi Gan Cao** *Radix Glycyrrhizae uralensis preparata* 9 g
- **Da Zao** *Fructus Jujubae* 10 dates

Explanation

This is a variation of the three formulae listed above. The main additions are Shi Chang Pu and Yu Jin to open the Mind's orifices. These two herbs were not used every time as they are pungent and therefore injure Yin.

Modifications Modifications used at different times according to the patient's condition were:

- Du Zhong *Cortex Eucommiae ulmoidis* to strengthen the Kidneys, the Will-Power and his sense of self-confidence and self-esteem. Although this herb tonifies Kidney-Yang, it can be added to the prescription in combination with the many herbs that nourish Yin.
- He Huan Pi *Cortex Albiziae* to open the Mind's orifices and lift depression.
- Bai He *Bulbus Lilii* to nourish Lung-Yin and relieve sadness and crying.
- Ju Hua *Flos Chrysanthemi* to relieve burning eyes.
- Ye Jiao Teng *Caulis Polygoni multiflori* to promote sleep.
- Mu Xiang *Radix Aucklandiae* to move Qi to help resolve Phlegm.
- Tai Zi Shen *Radix Pseudostellariae* and Shan Yao *Rhizoma Dioscoreae* to nourish Stomach-Yin.

Recently this patient had a consultation with Professor Zhou Zhong Ying, one of my teachers from Nanjing, and he confirmed the diagnosis of Phlegm-Heat misting the Mind and Yin deficiency. He suggested a prescription which incorporates the formula Bai He Zhi Mu Tang *Lilium-Anemarrhena Decoction* from the *Essential Prescriptions from the Golden Chest*.[9] A mental condition similar to this patient's was described in this old classic and was called "Lilium syndrome". The book says:[10]

Symptoms and signs [of the Lilium syndrome] *include the patient wants to eat but he cannot swallow and cannot speak. He wants to lie in bed yet he cannot lie quietly as he is restless. He wants to walk but soon becomes tired. Sometimes he likes eating, at other times he cannot tolerate the smell of food. He feels sometimes hot and sometimes cold, but without fever or chill. He has a bitter taste and the urine is dark. The patient looks as if he was possessed and his pulse is rapid.*

The treatment suggested for this condition is a decoction of Bai He *Bulbus Lilii* and Zhi Mu *Radix Anemarrhenae asphodeloidis*.

Thus the formula suggested by Professor Zhou was as follows.

- **Huang Lian** *Rhizoma Coptidis* 4 g
- **Ban Xia** *Rhizoma Pinelliae preparatum* 6 g
- **Dan Nan Xing** *Rhizoma Arisaematis preparatum* 4 g
- **Fu Ling** *Poria* 9 g
- **Zhi Gan Cao** *Radix Glycyrrhizae uralensis preparata* 3 g
- **Chen Pi** *Pericarpium Citri reticulatae* 4 g
- **Zhu Ru** *Caulis Bambusae in Taeniam* 6 g
- **Dan Shen** *Radix Salviae miltiorrhizae* 6 g
- **Mai Men Dong** *Radix Ophiopogonis* 9 g
- **Zhi Mu** *Radix Anemarrhenae* 9 g
- **Bai He** *Bulbus Lilii* 9 g
- **Mu Li** *Concha Ostreae* 15 g

Explanation

- The first seven herbs are a variation of Wen Dan Tang *Warming the Gall-Bladder Decoction*, eliminating Zhi Shi *Fructus Aurantii immaturus* and adding Huang Lian and Nan Xing to resolve Phlegm-Heat.
- Dan Shen enters the Heart and calms the Mind.
- Mai Dong nourishes Heart-Yin.
- Zhi Mu nourishes Yin and clears Empty Heat.

- Bai He nourishes Yin and relieves sadness and crying.
- Mu Li nourishes Yin.

After 4 years of treatment, this patient has improved considerably, although there is still a way to go. On a physical level, he has lost all his symptoms and his tongue is considerably less Red and now has a thin coating. On a mental level, his memory and concentration have improved, and his self-confidence and self-esteem are much better. He is less anxious and is off all medication.

MIND UNSETTLED

The Mind (*Shen*), Ethereal Soul (*Hun*) and Corporeal Soul (*Po*) may be unsettled, either because of a deficiency of Blood-Yin or because of the presence of a pathogenic factor that disturbs the Mind. Such pathogenic factors may be stagnation of Qi, stasis of Blood, Fire, Phlegm-Fire or Empty Heat. The manifestations will be similar in both cases, except that they will be milder if they are due purely to a deficiency without a pathogenic factor.

The main manifestations of unsettled Mind are anxiety, mental restlessness, insomnia and agitation. In case of unsettled Ethereal Soul, there will be, in addition, nightmares, irritability and absent-mindedness. In cases of unsettled Corporeal Soul, there will be anxiety with breathlessness and a feeling of tightness of the chest, worrying a lot and some somatization of the emotions on the skin such as itchy rashes.

The treatment principle for an unsettled Mind is to nourish Blood or Yin, eliminate pathogenic factors and calm the Mind.

Blood deficiency

Heart-Blood deficiency

Treatment principle

Tonify the Heart, nourish Blood and calm the Mind.

Acupuncture

Points

BL-15 Xinshu, BL-44 Shentang, Ren-14 Juque, HE-7 Shenmen, Ren-4 Guanyuan, ST-36 Zusanli, SP-6 Sanyinjiao, P-6 Neiguan and SP-4 Gongsun. Reinforcing method; moxa may be applied.

Explanation

- BL-15, Back-Transporting point of the Heart, tonifies the Heart. It can be used with direct moxa cones only.
- BL-44 tonifies the Heart and calms the Mind.
- Ren-14, Front-Collecting point of the Heart, and HE-7 calm the Mind.
- Ren-4 nourishes Blood and calms the Mind.
- ST-36 nourishes Blood.
- SP-6 nourishes Blood and calms the Mind. It is effective for insomnia from Blood deficiency.
- P-6 and SP-4 open the Yin Linking Vessel (*Yin Wei Mai*), which nourishes Blood and calms the Mind.

Herbal therapy

Prescription

YANG XIN TANG (I)

Nourishing the Heart Decoction

Explanation

This formula is specific to treat any mental and emotional effect of Heart-Blood deficiency, such as insomnia (difficulty in falling asleep), palpitations, mild anxiety and poor memory. Other manifestations would include a dull-pale complexion, a Pale-Thin tongue and a Choppy pulse.

Mental-emotional pattern

Fear, sadness, grief and worry may weaken Heart-Blood and cause this condition. This person would be pale with a dull complexion, the eyes would look anxious and rather dull, and he or she would be fearful, mildly anxious and vaguely depressed. In this case, the manifestations of an unsettled Mind (anxiety and agitation) would be rather mild as there is only deficiency of Blood with no Empty Heat.

He or she would also be very eager to please other people and members of his or her family. Due to women's propensity for Blood deficiency, this condition is much more common in women. In fact, it may also arise from loss of Blood in childbirth. The loss of Blood from the Directing and Penetrating Vessels during childbirth may affect the Heart due to its connection with the uterus via the Uterus Vessel (*Bao-Mai*). When Heart-Blood is weakened, the Mind is deprived of its residence and becomes fearful and anxious.

Modifications

- If there is severe insomnia, add Long Yan Rou *Arillus Longan*, which nourishes Heart-Blood and calms the Mind.

SUMMARY

Mind Unsettled – Blood deficiency, Heart-Blood deficiency

Treatment principle

Tonify the Heart, nourish Blood and calm the Mind.

Points

BL-15 Xinshu, BL-44 Shentang, Ren-14 Juque, HE-7 Shenmen, Ren-4 Guanyuan, ST-36 Zusanli, SP-6 Sanyinjiao, P-6 Neiguan and SP-4 Gongsun. Reinforcing method; moxa may be applied.

Herbal therapy

Prescription

YANG XIN TANG (I)
Nourishing the Heart Decoction

Yin deficiency

Heart-Yin deficiency

Treatment principle

Tonify the Heart, nourish Yin and calm the Mind.

Acupuncture

Points

BL-15 Xinshu, BL-44 Shentang, Ren-14 Juque, HE-7 Shenmen, HE-6 Yinxi, Ren-15 Jiuwei, Ren-4 Guanyuan, ST-36 Zusanli, SP-6 Sanyinjiao. Reinforcing method, no moxa.

Explanation

- BL-15, Back-Transporting point of the Heart, tonifies the Heart.
- BL-44 tonifies the Heart and calms the Mind.
- Ren-14, Front-Collecting point of the Heart, and HE-7 calm the Mind.
- HE-6 nourishes Heart-Yin.
- Ren-15 calms the Mind and relieves anxiety.
- Ren-4 nourishes Yin and calms the Mind. It nourishes Kidney-Yin which is often at the basis of Heart-Yin deficiency.
- ST-36 nourishes Stomach-Yin.
- SP-6 nourishes Yin and calms the Mind.

Herbal therapy

Prescription

BAI ZI YANG XIN WAN
Platycladum Nourishing the Heart Pill

Explanation

This formula is similar to the previous one as it also nourishes Heart-Blood; it differs from it in so far as it nourishes Heart-Yin. The configuration of symptoms and signs would therefore be different as there would be more Yin-deficiency manifestations: insomnia (waking up at night frequently), a feeling of heat in the evening, a dry mouth and throat, night-sweating, more pronounced anxiety and mental restlessness, a malar flush, palpitations, a Red tongue without coating with a redder tip and a Floating-Empty pulse.

Mental-emotional pattern

Fear, sadness, grief and worry, combined with overwork over many years, may lead to Heart-Yin deficiency. Yin deficiency is a deeper level of deficiency than Blood deficiency, and when it affects the Heart, the Mind is deprived of its residence. This makes the person fearful, very anxious and restless. These symptoms would be more severe than in Heart-Blood deficiency. Another difference is that they would be more pronounced in the evening. Please note that Yin deficiency makes the Mind unsettled even without Empty Heat.

A person suffering from this condition would tend to be depressed and dispirited, lacking will-power and drive, and the body would probably be thin.

SUMMARY

Mind Unsettled – Yin deficiency, Heart-Yin deficiency

Treatment principle

Tonify the Heart, nourish Yin and calm the Mind.

Points

BL-15 Xinshu, BL-44 Shentang, Ren-14 Juque, HE-7 Shenmen, HE-6 Yinxi, Ren-15 Jiuwei, Ren-4 Guanyuan, ST-36 Zusanli, SP-6 Sanyinjiao. Reinforcing method, no moxa.

Herbal therapy

Prescription

BAI ZI YANG XIN WAN
Platycladum Nourishing the Heart Pill

Case history

A 28-year-old man complained of nervousness with shaking of the hands. He said he felt nearly always very nervous, especially at work, and found the shaking of his hands very distressing. He also complained of dryness of the mouth, sweating, shortness of breath and insomnia (waking up during the night). He also lacked confidence and felt insecure, worried and anxious most of the time.

His tongue was unremarkable, being only slightly Swollen. His pulse was Moving; this is a pulse which is Rapid, Short, shaped like a bean and giving the impression of vibrating rather than pulsating.

Diagnosis This man's symptoms fall somewhat outside the scope of regular patterns. Some of the symptoms seem to point to Yin deficiency (waking up at night and feeling hot), but they are not severe enough to warrant such a diagnosis and the tongue does not show any Yin deficiency. There are, on the other hand, some signs of Qi deficiency (sweating, shortness of breath).

This is a problem caused by fear and worry over many years; fear affected the Heart and the Mind and worry affected the Lungs and Corporeal Soul. Affliction of the Mind caused the insomnia and affliction of the Corporeal Soul caused the breathlessness, sweating and shaking of the hands.

When asked about his childhood, he said that it was quite troubled and insecure due to his father's open preference for his sister. His father constantly praised his sister for being quite brilliant at school and blamed him for not being up to his sister's standards. The unyielding censure by his father over several years of childhood development instilled a deep feeling of insecurity in him which led to fear and worry.

Treatment principle Tonify Qi and Yin of Lungs and Heart, nourish and calm the Mind and settle the Corporeal Soul.

Acupuncture The following points were reinforced.

- HE-7 Shenmen, SP-6 Sanyinjiao, BL-15 Xinshu, BL-44 Shentang and Ren-15 Jiuwei nourish the Heart and calm the Mind.
- LU-9 Taiyuan, BL-13 Feishu and BL-42 Pohu tonify the Lungs and settle the Corporeal Soul.

After 6 months of weekly treatments, all his symptoms disappeared and his hands stopped shaking. In conjunction with counseling which I recommended, he explored the behavioral patterns developed in his childhood and gained much self-confidence and self-assurance.

Liver-Yin deficiency

Treatment principle

Tonify the Liver, nourish Yin, calm the Mind and settle the Ethereal Soul.

Acupuncture

Points

LIV-8 Ququan, SP-6 Sanyinjiao, KI-3 Taixi, Ren-4 Guanyuan, Du-24 Shenting, G.B.-13 Benshen, BL-18 Ganshu, BL-47 Hunmen. Reinforcing method, no moxa.

Explanation

- LIV-8 nourishes Liver-Yin.
- SP-6 nourishes Yin and strengthens Liver, Spleen and Kidneys.
- KI-3 and Ren-4 nourish Kidney-Yin. As this is the mother of Liver-Yin, it will indirectly nourish Liver-Yin. Ren-4 has also a strong grounding effect and it calms the Mind and settles the Ethereal Soul.
- Du-24 and G.B.-13 calm the Mind, especially in Liver disharmonies.
- BL-18 and BL-47 root the Ethereal Soul.

Herbal therapy

Prescription

SUAN ZAO REN TANG
Ziziphus Decoction

Explanation

This formula nourishes Liver-Yin, calms the Mind and settles the Ethereal Soul. It has a sweet and sour taste that nourishes Yin and "absorbs" the Ethereal Soul back into Liver-Yin.

Mental-emotional pattern

Anger, frustration and resentment, combined with overwork and/or excessive sexual activity, over many years may lead to this condition. In women, a contributory factor is excessive loss of blood at childbirth or a prolonged, excessive loss of blood if the periods are heavy.

Liver-Yin deficiency deprives the Ethereal Soul of its residence and it necessarily affects the Mind as well since Liver-Yin is the mother of Heart-Yin. Those suffering from this condition will feel depressed, lack a sense of direction in life and be mentally restless. Their sleep will be broken and they may wake up frequently during the night. They may also have restless dreams due to the wandering of the unrooted Ethereal Soul at night.

Prescription

ZHEN ZHU MU WAN

Concha Margaritiferae Pill

Explanation

This formula sinks Liver-Yang, calms the Mind and settles the Ethereal Soul. Please note that Zhu Sha is a toxic substance and should therefore be removed from the formula. The use of Zhen Zhu Mu and Long Chi is not allowed in Europe.

This formula, originally for the pattern of Liver-Wind at the Blood level of the Four Levels, nourishes Liver-Yin, subdues Liver-Yang, calms the Mind and settles the Ethereal Soul. It has a similar action to the previous one, but it differs in so far as the emphasis is on subduing Liver-Yang and calming the Mind, whereas in the previous one the emphasis was more on nourishing Yin and clearing Heat.

The main manifestations leading to the use of this prescription are dizziness, tinnitus, headache, insomnia, propensity to outbursts of anger, poor memory, dry hair and eyes, numbness of the limbs, a tongue with red sides and a Wiry-Fine pulse.

Mental-emotional pattern

Anger, frustration, resentment and hatred can cause this condition. In particular, anger will cause Liver-Yang or Liver-Wind to rise, for which condition this prescription is indicated. This person would therefore be very angry and be prone to outbursts of anger. His or her sleep would be very restless and filled with unpleasant dreams.

Prescription

YIN MEI TANG

Attracting Sleep Decoction

Explanation

This formula restores Liver-Blood and Liver-Yin to allow the Ethereal Soul to settle and the person to sleep peacefully. When Liver-Yin is deficient, the Ethereal Soul has no residence and there is insomnia. This formula makes the Ethereal Soul peaceful so that it does not wander. It tonifies Liver- and Heart-Yin, calms the Mind and settles the Ethereal Soul. The tongue presentation appropriate to this formula is a Red body without coating.

The original text says that this formula makes the Ethereal Soul peaceful so that it cannot "jump over".

Mental-emotional pattern

Frustration, resentment, old grudges and sometimes sadness can cause Liver-Yin to become deficient. This person's Liver-Yin would have been consumed by repressed anger over many years; he or she would feel very tense, anxious and sleep very badly, with the sleep being disturbed by unpleasant dreams. The pulse would be Fine but also slightly Wiry on the left side.

In some cases, sadness depletes Liver-Yin; in this case the person would feel very depressed, sad and sleep badly, but without too many dreams. The pulse would be Choppy or Fine.

SUMMARY

Mind Unsettled – Yin deficiency, Liver-Yin deficiency

Treatment principle

Tonify the Liver, nourish Yin, calm the Mind and settle the Ethereal Soul.

Points

LIV-8 Ququan, SP-6 Sanyinjiao, KI-3 Taixi, Ren-4 Guanyuan, Du-24 Shenting, G.B.-13 Benshen, BL-18 Ganshu, BL-47 Hunmen. Reinforcing method, no moxa.

Herbal therapy

Prescription

SUAN ZAO REN TANG
Ziziphus Decoction

Prescription

ZHEN ZHU MU WAN
Concha Margaritiferae Pill

Prescription

YIN MEI TANG
Attracting Sleep Decoction

Kidney-Yin deficiency

Treatment principle
Tonify the Kidneys, nourish Yin, calm the Mind and strengthen the Will-Power (*Zhi*).

Acupuncture

Points
KI-3 Taixi, KI-6 Zhaohai, Ren-4 Guanyuan, BL-23 Shenshu, BL-52 Zhishi, HE-6 Yinxi, Ren-15 Jiuwei. Reinforcing method except for HE-6, which is either reduced or needled with even method according to how chronic the condition is.

Explanation
- KI-3 and KI-6 nourish Kidney-Yin.
- Ren-4 nourishes Kidney-Yin and calms the Mind.
- BL-23 strengthens the Kidneys.
- BL-52 strengthens the Will-Power.
- HE-6 clears Heart Empty Heat.
- Ren-15 calms the Mind.

Herbal therapy

Prescription
GUI ZHI GAN CAO LONG GU MU LI TANG
Cinnamomum-Glycyrrhiza-Mastodi Ossis fossilia-Concha Ostreae Decoction

Explanation
This formula warms and tonifies the Heart, calms the Mind, nourishes Kidney-Yin and strengthens Will-Power. Long Gu and Mu Li also help timidity. Being astringent, on a physical level they stop sweating, whilst on a mental level they "absorb" the Mind and the Ethereal Soul into the Yin.

The main manifestations are palpitations, mental restlessness, propensity to be startled, sweating, cold limbs and a Pale tongue.

Although it contains Mu Li which primarily strengthens Kidney-Yin, this formula can be adapted to treat both Kidney-Yin and Kidney-Yang deficiency. In fact, its primary aim is to strengthen Heart-Yang with Gui Zhi and Zhi Gan Cao (hence the Pale tongue) and calm the Mind with the sinking substances Long Gu and Mu Li.

Please note that the use of minerals in herbal prescriptions is not allowed in the European Union countries at the time of writing (2008). Although Long Gu and Mu Li are an important part of the prescriptions, substitutes can be found and these are listed in Appendix 2.

Mental-emotional pattern
This formula is suitable, with adaptations, to treat the mental restlessness deriving from Kidney-Yin deficiency and Heart deficiency. Fear, guilt and shock, perhaps combined with overwork and/or excessive sexual activity, may lead to this condition, which guilt is especially liable to cause. This emotion, when suffered for a long time, weakens the Kidneys and the Will-Power, and it gnaws away at the Mind, thus depleting the Heart. Such patients are very anxious and mentally restless, and they sleep fitfully. They tend to be thin (indicating Yin deficiency), are tired, depressed and lack will-power.

Prescription
ZHEN ZHONG DAN
Bedside Pill

Explanation
This formula nourishes Kidney-Yin, clears Empty Heat, calms the Mind, opens the Mind's orifices and harmonizes the Heart and Kidneys.

This formula differs from the previous one in so far as it is slightly more directed at opening the Mind's orifices and clearing the Heart, whilst the previous one tonifies the Heart.

On a physical level, the manifestations corresponding to this prescription would include insomnia, anxiety, backache, night-sweating, dizziness, tinnitus, poor memory, a Red tongue without coating and a Floating-Empty pulse.

Mental-emotional pattern

A person with this condition would suffer from a confused Mind and would be unable to see clearly what needs to be done. He or she would also be anxious, depressed and lack will-power, and would sleep badly and sweat at night. This condition would also be caused by fear or guilt.

SUMMARY

Mind Unsettled – Yin deficiency, Kidney-Yin deficiency

Treatment principle

Tonify the Kidneys, nourish Yin, calm the Mind and strengthen the Will-Power.

Points

KI-3 Taixi, KI-6 Zhaohai, Ren-4 Guanyuan, BL-23 Shenshu, BL-52 Zhishi, HE-6 Yinxi, Ren-15 Jiuwei. Reinforcing method except for HE-6, which is either reduced or needled with even method according to how chronic the condition is.

Herbal therapy

Prescription

GUI ZHI GAN CAO LONG GU MU LI TANG

Cinnamomum-Glycyrrhiza-Mastodi Ossis fossilia-Concha Ostreae Decoction

Prescription

ZHEN ZHONG DAN

Bedside Pill

Yin deficiency with Empty Heat

Heart- and Kidney-Yin deficiency with Heart Empty Heat

Treatment principle

Nourish Heart- and Kidney-Yin, strengthen the Will-Power and calm the Mind.

Acupuncture

Points

HE-7 Shenmen, HE-6 Yinxi, P-7 Daling, Yintang, Ren-15 Jiuwei, Du-19 Houding, KI-3 Taixi, KI-6 Zhaohai, KI-10 Yingu, KI-9 Zhubin, Ren-4 Guanyuan, SP-6 Sanyinjiao. The first three with reducing or even method; Yintang, Ren-15 and Du-19 with even method; all the others with reinforcing method. No moxa.

Explanation

- HE-7, HE-6 and P-7 can all calm the Mind. In combination with KI-7 Fuliu, HE-6 also stops night-sweating.
- Yintang, Ren-15 and Du-19 calm the Mind.
- KI-3 Source point, nourishes the Kidneys.
- KI-6 nourishes Kidney-Yin, benefits the throat, promotes fluids and helps sleep.
- KI-10 nourishes Kidney-Yin.
- KI-9 tonifies the Kidneys, calms the Mind and opens the chest.
- Ren-4 nourishes Kidney-Yin and roots the Mind.
- SP-6 nourishes Yin, calms the Mind and promotes sleep.

Herbal therapy

Prescription

TIAN WANG BU XIN DAN

Heavenly Emperor Tonifying the Heart Pill

Explanation

This is the most widely used formula to nourish Heart- and Kidney-Yin (also called "harmonizing Heart and Kidneys"), clear Empty Heat and calm the Mind. The main manifestations are night-sweating, backache, dizziness, tinnitus, a malar flush, feeling of heat in the evening, palpitations, insomnia, restless sleep, dry mouth and throat, poor memory, dry stools, a Red tongue without coating with a redder tip and a Rapid-Fine pulse. Such a condition is common in menopause so it can be used with modifications; also, if there is some Kidney-Yang deficiency in addition to Kidney-Yin deficiency, modify with the addition of a small dose (1.5 g) of Rou Gui *Cortex Cinnamomi*.

Mental-emotional pattern

Fear, guilt and shock can all cause this condition. Since there is a deficiency of Kidney-Yin, there usually are concurrent causes of disease such as overwork, irregular diet and excessive sexual activity. It is also a common pattern appearing in menopausal problems.

This person would be very anxious, especially in the evening, and he or she would sleep very badly, waking up several times. There might be dreams of fires or flying. He or she would be unable to relax and there would be palpitations.

Prescription
LIU WEI DI HUANG WAN Variation
Six-Ingredient Rehmannia Pill Variation

Explanation
This formula is used for mental restlessness and insomnia from Yin deficiency and Empty Heat, especially in the elderly. It is specific to restore the connection between Heart-Fire and Kidney-Water; the Heart fluids rely on the nourishment of the Kidney-Essence. Thus one needs to nourish Kidney-Water in order to subdue Heart Empty Heat.

Mental-emotional pattern
This is almost the same as for the previous formula, except that the emphasis is on Yin deficiency, with the consequent depression and lack of will-power, in addition to anxiety and insomnia. Also, because of its emphasis on the Liver, it is suitable for mental-emotional problems deriving from resentment and bitterness harbored for many years.

SUMMARY

Mind Unsettled – Yin deficiency with Empty Heat, Heart- and Kidney-Yin deficiency with Heart Empty Heat

Treatment principle

Nourish Heart- and Kidney-Yin, strengthen the Will-Power and calm the Mind.

Points

HE-7 Shenmen, HE-6 Yinxi, P-7 Daling, Yintang, Ren-15 Jiuwei, Du-19 Houding, KI-3 Taixi, KI-6 Zhaohai, KI-10 Yingu, KI-9 Zhubin, Ren-4 Guanyuan, SP-6 Sanyinjiao. The first three with reducing or even method; Yintang, Ren-15 and Du-19 with even method; all the others with reinforcing method. No moxa.

Herbal therapy

Prescription

TIAN WANG BU XIN DAN
Heavenly Emperor Tonifying the Heart Pill

Prescription
LIU WEI DI HUANG WAN Variation
Six-Ingredient Rehmannia Pill Variation

Case history

A 52-year-old woman sought treatment for persistent night-sweating and hot flushes. She also complained of abdominal distension and water retention. Her periods had stopped the year before and she had been worse since then. Apart from the above symptoms, she often felt anxious in the evening and experienced palpitations. Her sleep was disturbed by the hot flushes and she felt mentally restless. She was overweight, her cheekbones were slightly red, and her eyes had no glitter and looked scared.

Her tongue was slightly Red, Swollen on the sides (Spleen-type of swelling), cracked and with a rootless coating; it also had a Heart crack in the middle (Plate 12.3). Her pulse was Weak on both Rear positions, the Heart position was Weak and Short, and the whole pulse had no wave.

She had been treated with acupuncture elsewhere (tonifying Spleen and resolving Dampness) without much result. Her acupuncturist referred her to me.

Diagnosis This patient obviously has a Spleen deficiency, manifesting with being overweight, water retention and a swelling on the sides of the tongue. However, there are other factors involved. The hot flushes, red cheekbones, insomnia, mental restlessness, Red tongue with rootless coating and Weak pulse on both Kidney positions clearly indicate Kidney-Yin deficiency. Besides this, there is also a Heart deficiency as evidenced by the palpitations and the eyes without glitter, indicating that the Mind is disturbed.

When asked about it, she confirmed that she had been under tremendous strain when she lived in East Africa, having to manage a large farm for 2 years after being widowed suddenly. Thus the main causes of disease were sadness and shock (from bereavement) and fear. The sadness showed in her eyes' lack of glitter and the fear in their scared look.

Treatment principle Nourish Kidney-Yin and Heart-Yin, subdue Empty Heat, calm the Mind and strengthen Will-Power.

Herbal therapy She was treated with herbs only. The main formula used was a variation of Tian Wang Bu Xin Dan *Heavenly Emperor Tonifying the Heart Pill*.

- **Sheng Di Huang** *Radix Rehmanniae* 12 g
- **Mai Men Dong** *Radix Ophiopogonis* 6 g
- **Tian Men Dong** *Radix Asparagi* 6 g
- **Ren Shen** *Radix Ginseng* 6 g
- **Fu Ling** *Poria* 6 g
- **Wu Wei Zi** *Fructus Schisandrae* 6 g
- **Dang Gui** *Radix Angelicae sinensis* 6 g
- **Dan Shen** *Radix Salviae miltiorrhizae* 6 g
- **Bai Zi Ren** *Semen Platycladi* 6 g
- **Suan Zao Ren** *Semen Ziziphi spinosae* 6 g
- **Yuan Zhi** *Radix Polygalae* 6 g
- **Jie Geng** *Radix Platycodi* 3 g
- **Ze Xie** *Rhizoma Alismatis* 4 g
- **Qing Hao** *Herba Artemisiae annuae* 3 g
- **Qin Jiao** *Radix Gentianae macrophyllae* 3 g
- **Zhi Gan Cao** *Radix Glycyrrhizae uralensis preparata* 3 g

Explanation

The first 12 herbs constitute the original formula which nourishes Kidney-Yin and Heart-Yin, clears Empty Heat and calms the Mind. Xuan Shen was eliminated from the formula as Yin deficiency is not too pronounced yet.

- Ze Xie, Qing Hao and Qin Jiao were added to clear Empty Heat and treat the hot flushes.
- Gan Cao harmonizes.

This formula, repeated several times, produced a dramatic improvement in her mental state from the beginning, feeling much more relaxed, calmer and happier. Her eyes gradually changed too, acquiring more lustre.

Liver-Yin deficiency with Empty Heat

Treatment principle

Nourish Liver-Yin, clear Empty Heat, calm the Mind and settle the Ethereal Soul.

Acupuncture

Points

LIV-8 Ququan, SP-6 Sanyinjiao, KI-3 Taixi, Ren-4 Guanyuan, Du-24 Shenting, G.B.-13 Benshen, Du-18 Qiangjian, BL-18 Ganshu, BL-47 Hunmen, KI-2 Rangu, LIV-3 Taichong. Reinforcing method, except for the last two points which should be reduced.

Explanation

- LIV-8 nourishes Liver-Yin.
- SP-6 nourishes Yin and strengthens Liver, Spleen and Kidneys.
- KI-3 and Ren-4 nourish Kidney-Yin. As this is the mother of Liver-Yin, it will indirectly nourish Liver-Yin. Ren-4 has also a strong grounding effect and it calms the Mind.
- Du-24 and G.B.-13 calm the Mind, especially in Liver disharmonies.
- Du-18 calms the Mind and settles the Ethereal Soul. It is indicated for mental restlessness, agitation and manic behavior.
- BL-18 and BL-47 root the Ethereal Soul.
- KI-2 and LIV-3 would be used only if there is Empty Heat.

Herbal therapy

Prescription

SUAN ZAO REN TANG

Ziziphus Decoction

Explanation

This formula nourishes Liver-Yin, calms the Mind, settles the Ethereal Soul and clears Empty Heat.

Mental-emotional pattern

This formula is specific for Liver-Yin deficiency with its associated symptoms and signs, such as insomnia, waking up frequently at night, dry throat, blurred vision, dry eyes, mental restlessness, night-sweating, a Red tongue without coating and a Floating-Empty pulse.

This situation can arise in two ways. Emotional stress, such as anger, resentment or frustration, may lead to the rising of Minister Fire which agitates the Heart and the Liver. Fire injures Yin so that the Ethereal Soul is deprived of its residence. Alternatively, it may start with a reverse process; overwork combined with irregular diet and excessive sexual activity (and in women too many childbirths or chronic menorrhagia) may deplete Liver-Yin and therefore deprive the Ethereal Soul of its residence.

No matter how this situation arises, the end result is a condition characterized most of all by insomnia. The person may also be depressed and lack any sense of vision in life. The mental restlessness in this condition derives from Yin deficiency and typically manifests with a vague feeling of anxiety, restlessness and fidgetiness which is worse in the evening.

The Liver is a harmonizing organ and its harmony derives from a proper balance between its Yang (the free flow of Liver-Qi) and its Yin aspect (Blood and Yin). Mental irritation from emotional stress stirs up Liver-Yang and injures Liver-Yin, thus altering the balance of Yin and Yang within the Liver.

This formula is also applicable to some women's problems such as premenstrual tension with breast distension or breast lumps from stagnation of Liver-Qi on a background of Liver-Yin deficiency. In women, Liver-Yin deficiency is even more likely to happen due to the monthly loss of menstrual blood which depletes Liver-Blood. In these cases, stagnation of Liver-Qi, with its associated emotional consequences, is very often secondary to a deficiency of Liver-Yin. The Yin and Yang aspects of the Liver need to be harmonized and coordinated. If Liver-Yin is deficient, the Yang aspect of the Liver gets out of control and this may lead to both stagnation of Liver-Qi and Liver-Yang rising. Thus, this formula can be used for premenstrual tension if it presents with the above configuration.

Finally, although this formula is specific for Liver-Yin deficiency with Empty Heat, it can also be used for Liver-Yin deficiency without Empty Heat. It is therefore applicable also to Mind Unsettled or Mind Weakened from Yin deficiency.

Modifications

- If Empty Heat manifestations are severe (malar flush and feeling of heat), decrease the amount of Chuan Xiong and add Sheng Di Huang *Radix Rehmanniae*, Nu Zhen Zi *Fructus Ligustri lucidi* and Han Lian Cao *Herba Ecliptae*.
- If night-sweating is profuse, add Di Gu Pi *Cortex Lycii* and Wu Wei Zi *Fructus Schisandrae*.
- If insomnia is difficult to treat, add Ye Jiao Teng *Caulis Polygoni multiflori*.
- If the person is very depressed, add He Huan Pi *Cortex Albiziae*.

SUMMARY

Mind Unsettled – Yin deficiency with Empty Heat, Liver-Yin deficiency with Empty Heat

Treatment principle

Nourish Liver-Yin, clear Empty Heat, calm the Mind and settle the Ethereal Soul.

Points

LIV-8 Ququan, SP-6 Sanyinjiao, KI-3 Taixi, Ren-4 Guanyuan, Du-24 Shenting, G.B.-13 Benshen, Du-18 Qiangjian, BL-18 Ganshu, BL-47 Hunmen, KI-2 Rangu, LIV-3 Taichong. Reinforcing method, except for the last two points which should be reduced.

Herbal therapy

Prescription

SUAN ZAO REN TANG
Ziziphus Decoction

Case history

A 63-year-old woman sought treatment for hypertension. The systolic blood pressure, which oscillated between 200 and 150, was more of a problem than the diastolic one, which was always 95. Her main physical symptoms included a stiff neck, a feeling of pressure in the head, throbbing headaches on the vertex, dizziness, tinnitus, blurred vision, dry eyes, insomnia (waking up frequently during the night) and a feeling of heat in the evening.

Her complexion was dull with red patches on both cheekbones and her eyes were rather dull and without glitter.

Her tongue was Red, redder on the sides, slightly Stiff and the coating was too thin. Her pulse was Wiry but Fine.

Diagnosis The blurred vision, dry eyes, insomnia, Fine pulse and Stiff tongue with insufficient tongue coating indicate Liver-Yin deficiency, while the feeling of heat in the evening, red cheekbones and Red tongue with insufficient coating denote Empty Heat.

Due to the deficiency of Liver-Yin, there was also Liver-Yang rising, as manifested by the stiff neck, throbbing vertical headaches, dizziness, tinnitus, a feeling of pressure in the head and a Wiry pulse.

Her hypertension, which was the reason for seeking treatment, was due to the rising of Liver-Yang. When the systolic pressure is high while the diastolic one is near to normal, it usually indicates the rising of Liver-Yang. Furthermore, when the systolic reading oscillates considerably from day to day, it indicates that nervous stress, rather than a hardening of the arteries, is the cause of the problem. This is usually due to emotional strain affecting the Liver. In this patient's case, this was very obvious from the dullness of her complexion (lack of *shen*) and eyes which indicate long-standing affliction of the Mind and/or Ethereal Soul by emotional strain. When asked about emotional strain, she confirmed that she had been under great stress about her daughter's marital problems. Due to financial problems, her daughter was trapped in a marriage to a very cruel husband and suffered a great deal; this made her mother very angry towards her son-in-law and, over the years, caused the rising of Liver-Yang and deficiency of Liver-Yin.

Treatment principle Nourish Liver-Yin, clear Empty Heat, subdue Liver-Yang, calm the Mind and root the Ethereal Soul.

Acupuncture Reinforce LIV-8 Ququan, Ren-4 Guanyuan, SP-6 Sanyinjiao, KI-3 Taixi. Even method: LIV-3 Taichong, KI-2 Rangu, Du-24 Shenting, G.B.-13 Benshen, P-7 Daling.

Explanation

- LIV-8, Ren-4, SP-6 and KI-3 nourish Liver-Yin.
- LIV-3 subdues Liver-Yang.
- KI-2, in combination with LIV-3, clears Empty Heat from Liver-Yin deficiency.
- Du-24 and G.B.-13 calm the Mind and root the Ethereal Soul.
- P-7 calms the Mind and indirectly subdues Liver-Yang.

Herbal therapy No herbs were prescribed but only the patent remedy Suan Zao Ren Tang Pian *Tablet of Ziziphus Decoction*, which fit her symptoms quite well.

After 20 weekly treatments, most of her symptoms had cleared up or decreased in intensity, and she was able to react more calmly to her daughter's plight and not to allow her anger to dominate her life.

Qi stagnation

This has already been discussed under *Mind Obstructed* above. The manifestations of Qi stagnation when it causes the Mind to be unsettled are similar. The main difference is that, instead of mental confusion, the predominant manifestations will be anxiety, irritability and mental restlessness.

Treatment principle

Move Qi, eliminate stagnation and calm the Mind.

The same prescriptions and acupuncture points indicated for Stagnation of Qi under *Mind Obstructed* are applicable.

Blood stasis

Again, the manifestations of this condition are similar to those discussed under *Mind Obstructed* from Blood stasis. The main difference is that, when stasis of Blood causes the Mind to become unsettled, there will be severe anxiety and mental restlessness.

Treatment principle

Invigorate Blood, eliminate stasis and calm the Mind.

The same prescriptions and acupuncture points indicated under *Mind Obstructed* from Blood stasis are applicable.

Fire

Heart-Fire

Treatment principle

Clear the Heart, drain Fire and calm the Mind.

Acupuncture

Points

HE-8 Shaofu, HE-7 Shenmen, P-7 Daling, Ren-15 Jiuwei, SP-6 Sanyinjiao, G.B.-15 Toulinqi. Reducing method on all points.

Explanation

- HE-8 clears Heart-Fire and calms the Mind.
- HE-7 calms the Mind.
- P-7 clears Heart-Heat and calms the Mind.
- Ren-15 calms the Mind.
- SP-6 nourishes Yin which helps to cool Fire and it calms the Mind.
- G.B.-15 clears Heat and calms the Mind. It balances moods when they oscillate violently. It is particularly indicated if the eyes are red.

Herbal therapy

Prescription

DAO CHI SAN

Eliminating Redness Powder

Explanation

This formula drains Heart-Fire causing such symptoms as a sensation of heat in the chest, thirst, red face, tongue ulcers, mental restlessness, red eyes, scanty-dark urine, burning on urination, a Red tongue with a redder tip and yellow coating and an Overflowing pulse.

Please note that this formula contains Mu Tong *Caulis Akebiae trifoliatae*, the use of which is not allowed. It can be replaced by Tong Cao *Medulla Tetrapanacis*.

Mental-emotional pattern

Excess joy, worry, anger, guilt and craving may lead to this pattern. These emotions agitate the Mind and create an implosion of Qi which leads to Fire. Fire agitates the Mind and the person will be very agitated, restless, impatient and unable to sleep well. The sleep will be very restless and disturbed by violent dreams, which may involve flying, fires and killings.

The mental restlessness deriving from Fire is quite different from that deriving from Empty Heat. A person with Empty Heat will feel restless and anxious, especially in the evening, but will, by and large, endure it in silence. A person with Fire will feel restless all the time and will project it outwards towards other people or will always be doing something in a compulsive way. These people may be quite creative and artistic.

Modifications

- In case of severe anxiety add Bai Zi Ren *Semen Platycladi*, Suan Zao Ren *Semen Ziziphi spinosae* and Yuan Zhi *Radix Polygalae*.

SUMMARY

Mind Unsettled – Fire, Heart-Fire

Treatment principle

Clear the Heart, drain Fire and calm the Mind.

Points

HE-8 Shaofu, HE-7 Shenmen, P-7 Daling, Ren-15 Jiuwei, SP-6 Sanyinjiao, G.B.-15 Toulinqi. Reducing method on all points.

Herbal therapy

Prescription

DAO CHI SAN

Eliminating Redness Powder

Case history

A 33-year-old woman sought treatment for infertility. She had been trying to become pregnant for 8 years and there was no abnormality in her hormone levels or fallopian tubes. Her periods were always late (from a 32- to a 44-day cycle), the menstrual blood was bright-red but with dark clots and the periods were painful. She also felt cold during the period and liked to have a hot water bottle on her abdomen.

She suffered from lower backache, loose stools and general exhaustion. The backache started after a fall 10 years before. Her memory was poor and she dreamt a lot every night. Her dreams were always unpleasant and she regularly dreamed of burning buildings, often waking up crying or laughing. She occasionally experienced palpitations.

In her teenage years, from 13 to 18, she had been very nervous, frequently had palpitations and often fainted.

Facial diagnosis revealed an uneven, blemished surface on the forehead in the area corresponding to the teenage years between 16 and 19 (Fig. 12.36) and rather dull eyes.

Her tongue was Pale but with a Red tip. Her pulse was Weak on the right side and on both Rear positions, and the Heart pulse was relatively Overflowing and very slightly Moving, i.e. it was

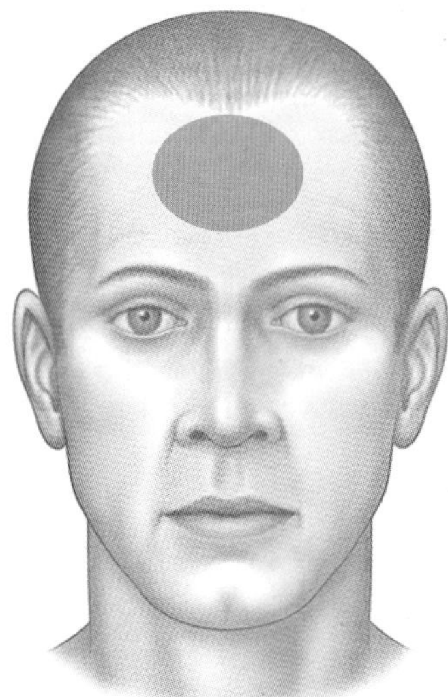

Figure 12.36 Area corresponding to parents' influence and years from 16 to 19.

Overflowing in relation to all the other pulse positions, which were Weak.

Diagnosis At first observation, all her symptoms would seem to point to Spleen- and Kidney-Yang deficiency. Whilst there certainly was a Spleen-Yang deficiency (tiredness, loose stools, Pale tongue and pulse Weak on the right side), there was not much Kidney-Yang deficiency. The symptoms which would seem to point to Kidney-Yang deficiency are a late menstrual cycle, feeling cold during the period, infertility, backache and poor memory. However, on closer analysis, although there was some Kidney-Yang deficiency, some of these symptoms could be explained differently. First of all, the backache started only after the fall and was therefore due to a structural rather than an energetic Kidney problem.

As for the other symptoms, they are also partially due to the Heart's influence on the Kidneys. The Fire of the Heart (in a Five-Element sense) needs to communicate with Kidney-Water; Kidney-Water needs to flow upwards to nourish Heart-Yin, while the Fire of the Heart needs to flow downwards to the Kidneys and the Lower Burner. In this case, this patient had been affected by deep emotional problems during her teenage years. This was probably a mixture of shock and sadness which caused Heart-Fire (in a pathological sense). This was deduced from the Heart pulse's Overflowing and Moving quality, from the blemished area on her forehead, dull eyes and her dreams. The shock and sadness had obviously affected the Heart (causing dreams of fire and waking up laughing) and Lungs (causing dreams of buildings and waking up crying). When asked about it, she confirmed this was true but she did not wish to discuss it further. Thus, Heart-Fire was blocked upwards, unable to communicate downwards with the Kidneys and Lower Burner, which became cold. This was the cause of the infertility, delayed menstrual cycle, blood clots and cold feeling.

Treatment principle The main treatment principle adopted was to calm the Mind, and conduct Heart-Fire downwards to communicate with the Kidneys. In this case, it was not a matter of "clearing" Heart-Fire so as to establish a communication between the Fire of the Heart and the Kidneys. Shock "closes" the Heart and makes it smaller, while sadness depletes Heart- and Lung-Qi. The formula therefore needs some herbs with a pungent taste to open the Heart's orifices, some with a sour taste to nourish the Heart and calm the Mind and some sinking substances to calm the Mind and make Heart-Qi descend to the Lower Burner.

Herbal therapy She was already receiving acupuncture from another practitioner who referred her to me for herbal treatment. The prescription used was not a classic one but one I formulated for this particular case. This was as follows.

- **Dang Shen** *Radix Codonopsis* 9 g
- **Fu Shen** *Sclerotium Poriae cocos pararadicis* 6 g
- **Yuan Zhi** *Radix Polygalae* 9 g
- **Bai Zi Ren** *Semen Platycladi* 6 g
- **Suan Zao Ren** *Semen Ziziphi spinosae* 3 g
- **Bai He** *Bulbus Lilii* 6 g
- **Shi Chang Pu** *Rhizoma Acori tatrinowii* 4 g
- **Huang Qin** *Radix Scutellariae* 3 g
- **Rou Gui** *Cortex Cinnamomi* 1.5 g
- **Zhi Gan Cao** *Radix Glycyrrhizae uralensis preparata* 2 g
- **Hong Zao** *Fructus Jujubae* 3 dates

Explanation

- Dang Shen and Fu Shen tonify the Spleen. Fu Shen also calms the Mind.
- Yuan Zhi, Bai Zi Ren and Suan Zao Ren calm the Mind and nourish the Heart. Yuan Zhi is pungent and opens the Heart's orifices, while

Bai Zi Ren and Suan Zao Ren are sweet and sour, respectively, and therefore nourish the Heart and calm the Mind.

- Bai He nourishes the Lungs, especially when they are affected by sadness.
- Chang Pu opens the Mind's orifices and counteracts the effects of shock.
- Huang Qin clears Heart-Heat and calms the Mind. It is used in a very small dose, more to enter the Heart than to clear it.
- Rou Gui was used to warm the Fire of the Gate of Vitality, attract the Fire of the Heart downwards and re-establish the communication between the Kidneys and Heart.
- Zhi Gan Cao and Hong Zao harmonize.

This formula was repeated with minor modifications over a period of 4 months, producing a marked improvement in the mental state of this patient. Her dreams of fire stopped and the menstrual blood became normal.

Liver-Fire

Treatment principle

Drain Liver-Fire, calm the Mind and settle the Ethereal Soul.

Acupuncture

Points

LIV-2 Xingjian, LIV-3 Taichong, L.I.-4 Hegu, BL-18 Ganshu, SP-6 Sanyinjiao, Du-18 Qiangjian, Du-24 Shenting, G.B.-13 Benshen, G.B.-15 Toulinqi, HE-7 Shenmen, P-7 Daling, LU-3 Tianfu. All with reducing or even method.

Explanation

- LIV-2 clears Liver-Fire.
- LIV-3 pacifies the Liver and calms the Mind. In combination with L.I.-4 it strongly calms the Mind and settles the Ethereal Soul.
- BL-18, Back-Transporting point of the Liver, clears Liver-Fire.
- SP-6 nourishes Yin and calms the Mind.
- Du-18 calms the Mind, regulates the Liver and settles the Ethereal Soul.
- Du-24 and G.B.-13 calm the Mind and settle the Ethereal Soul in Liver disharmonies. G.B.-13 also treats jealousy and suspicion.
- G.B.-15 clears Heat, brightens the eyes and settles the Ethereal Soul.
- HE-7 and P-7 calm the Mind. P-7 is related to the Liver via the Terminal Yin channels.
- LU-3 harmonizes Liver and Lungs and, according to *An Explanation of Acupuncture Points* (1654), is particularly indicated when Liver-Fire obstructs the Lungs causing forgetfulness. The book also says this point is indicated when the person "*talks to ghosts*".[11]

Herbal therapy

Prescription

XIE GAN AN SHEN WAN

Draining the Liver and Calming the Mind Pill

Explanation

This formula (a variation of Long Dan Xie Gan Tang *Gentiana Draining the Liver Decoction*) specifically drains Liver-Fire and calms the Mind. It addresses the mental restlessness and irritability deriving from Liver-Fire. The main manifestations are dizziness, tinnitus, red face and eyes, thirst, scanty-dark urine, dry stools, insomnia, dream-disturbed sleep, propensity to outbursts of anger, headache, a Red tongue with redder sides and yellow coating and a Wiry and Rapid pulse.

Please note that this formula contains three minerals, the use of which is not allowed in European Union countries. Please consult Appendix 2 to find substitutions.

Mental-emotional pattern

Anger, frustration, resentment and hatred can all cause rising of Liver-Yang and, over a long period of time, Liver-Fire. This especially happens if the person eats very greasy food and drinks alcohol. These people would be very angry, prone to outbursts of anger, impatient, mentally restless and irritable, and their sleep would be very disturbed by violent dreams of fights. In this condition, Fire harasses the Ethereal Soul and makes the person destructive and restless.

At times, this situation may lead to depression, especially if the anger (usually towards a member of the family) is harbored inside for many years. In these cases, the appearance of the person – depressed, subdued and speaking in a low voice – may disguise the true origin of the problem and look as if sadness and grief were the cause of the disease. However, the Red tongue with redder sides and the Wiry and Rapid pulse clearly point to the true origin of the problem, i.e. anger.

SUMMARY

Mind Unsettled – Fire, Liver-Fire

Treatment principle

Drain Liver-Fire, calm the Mind and settle the Ethereal Soul.

Points

LIV-2 Xingjian, LIV-3 Taichong, L.I.-4 Hegu, BL-18 Ganshu, SP-6 Sanyinjiao, Du-18 Qiangjian, Du-24 Shenting, G.B.-13 Benshen, G.B.-15 Toulinqi, HE-7 Shenmen, P-7 Daling, LU-3 Tianfu. All with reducing or even method.

Herbal therapy

Prescription

XIE GAN AN SHEN WAN
Draining the Liver and Calming the Mind Pill

Case history

A 40-year-old woman complained of asthma which had started in her early twenties from "emotional trauma" as she herself described it. She used Ventolin and Becotide inhalers every day as well as tablets of prednisolone. Her attacks were clearly elicited by emotional strain and the asthma did not have an allergic basis.

She felt very tense and irritable, and often had a pain under the right rib cage. She also suffered from premenstrual tension.

Her tongue was Red, redder on the sides, with a yellow coating (Plate 12.4). Her pulse was Weak on the right and Wiry on the left.

Diagnosis The main problem in this case is Liver-Qi stagnation leading to Liver-Fire. Prolonged stagnation of Qi over many years often leads to Fire. Liver-Fire can overflow into the chest and obstruct the descending of Lung-Qi, causing asthma. This type of asthma starts later in life (i.e. not during childhood) and is clearly related to emotional strain as it is in this case. Liver-Fire is evident from the Red sides of the tongue but not many other symptoms; this is because it did not arise independently but from stagnation of Liver-Qi. Hence the symptoms of stagnation of Liver-Qi, such as the hypochondrial pain, the irritability, the premenstrual tension and the Wiry pulse on the left.

Treatment principle When Liver-Fire develops from Liver-Qi stagnation, it does not require draining with bitter-cold herbs or purging, but only clearing with a combination of pungent herbs to open and move Qi and some light-bitter herbs to clear.

Hence the treatment principle is to move Qi, clear Liver-Fire, restore the descending of Lung-Qi, calm the Mind and settle the Ethereal Soul.

Acupuncture LU-7 Lieque, LU-1 Zhongfu, G.B.-34 Yanglingquan, LIV-3 Taichong, LIV-14 Qimen, P-7 Daling, P-6 Neiguan, ST-40 Fenglong. All with even method.

Explanation
- LU-7 and LU-1 restore the descending of Lung-Qi.
- G.B.-34, LIV-3 and LIV-14 move Liver-Qi. LIV-14, in particular, will move Liver-Qi in the chest.
- P-7 and P-6 calm the Mind, settle the Ethereal Soul, indirectly move Liver-Qi, restore the descending of Lung-Qi and open the chest.
- ST-40, especially in combination with P-6, opens the chest and eases breathing.

Herbal therapy The formula used was a variation of Si Ni San *Four Rebellious Powder*.
- **Chai Hu** *Radix Bupleuri* 6 g
- **Bai Shao** *Radix Paeoniae alba* 9 g
- **Zhi Shi** *Fructus Aurantii immaturus* 6 g
- **Zhi Gan Cao** *Radix Glycyrrhizae uralensis preparata* 6 g
- **Huang Qin** *Radix Scutellariae* 3 g
- **Shan Zhi Zi** *Fructus Gardeniae* 3 g
- **Xing Ren** *Semen Armeniacae* 6 g
- **Su Zi** *Fructus Perillae* 6 g
- **Suan Zao Ren** *Semen Ziziphi spinosae* 4 g
- **He Huan Pi** *Cortex Albiziae* 6 g

Explanation The first four herbs constitute Si Ni San.

- Huang Qin and Zhi Zi lightly clear Heat. In combination with the pungent herbs to move Qi, they clear Liver-Fire from stagnation of Liver-Qi.
- Xing Ren and Su Zi restore the descending of Lung-Qi and ease asthma.
- Suan Zao Ren and He Huan Pi calm the Mind and settle the Ethereal Soul.

This patient was off all medication after 6 months of treatment and felt much less irritable and depressed.

Phlegm-Fire

Stomach and Heart Phlegm-Fire

Treatment principle
Resolve Phlegm, harmonize the Stomach, open the Mind's orifices, clear the Heart and calm the Mind.

Acupuncture

Points
ST-40 Fenglong, Ren-12 Zhongwan, Ren-9 Shuifen, ST-25 Tianshu, G.B.-13 Benshen, ST-8 Touwei, G.B.-18 Chengling, G.B.-15 Toulinqi, G.B.-17 Zhengying, BL-20 Pishu, BL-49 Yishe, P-7 Daling, Du-20 Baihui. ST-40 and P-7 with reducing method, Ren-12, BL-20 and BL-49 with reinforcing method and all the others with even method.

Explanation
- ST-40 resolves Phlegm, harmonizes the Stomach and calms the Mind.
- Ren-12 and Ren-9 tonify the Spleen to resolve Phlegm.
- ST-25 calms the Mind, opens the Mind's orifices and settles the Ethereal Soul and Corporeal Soul. It is an important point for mental-emotional problems occurring against a background of Stomach-Fire or Stomach Phlegm-Fire.
- G.B.-13 clears the Mind's orifices and calms mental restlessness.
- ST-8 is a local point to resolve Phlegm affecting the head.
- G.B.-18 calms the Mind, stops obsessive ideas and relieves dizziness.
- G.B.-15 calms the Mind, settles the Ethereal Soul and clears Heat.
- G.B.-17 calms the Mind and stimulates concentration. It combines with ST-40 to clear Phlegm from the head and clear the Mind.
- BL-20 tonifies the Spleen to resolve Phlegm.
- BL-49 strengthens the Intellect and clears the Mind.
- P-7 calms the Mind and resolves Phlegm-Fire from the Heart.
- Du-20 clears the Mind.

Herbal therapy

Prescription
WEN DAN TANG
Warming the Gall-Bladder Decoction

Explanation
This formula, already discussed above under *Mind Obstructed*, resolves Phlegm-Heat from the Stomach and Heart.

Mental-emotional pattern
Worry and pensiveness knot Qi and, after a long time, the impaired Qi movement leads to the formation of Phlegm. On the other hand, knotted Qi easily turns into Fire after a long time. Fire, in turn, may lead to the formation of more Phlegm as it burns and condenses fluids.

Phlegm-Fire both mists and agitates the Mind. The Phlegm aspect of it causes mental confusion, poor memory, dizziness and, in severe cases, total mental confusion with loss of insight. The Fire aspect of it causes agitation, mental restlessness, insomnia, a flustered feeling in the chest, anxiety and, in severe cases, manic behavior. Nowadays this formula is widely used for manic-depression.

Phlegm-Fire in this case affects Stomach, Heart and Gall-Bladder. In the Heart, it mists the Mind and causes mental confusion. In the Gall-Bladder, it prevents the Ethereal Soul from returning to the Liver at night, hence the insomnia. Disturbance of the Ethereal Soul also causes depression and a lack of direction in life.

Obviously, irregular eating plays an important role in the development of this pattern. These people are often busy executives who eat at irregular times or in a hurry while working or late at night.

Modifications
- If Heart-Fire is evident, add Huang Lian *Rhizoma Coptidis*.

- If obstruction of the Mind by Phlegm is pronounced, add Shi Chang Pu *Rhizoma Acori tatarinowii* and Yuan Zhi *Radix Polygalae*.
- If there is pronounced mental restlessness and anxiety, add Suan Zao Ren *Semen Ziziphi spinosae*.
- If insomnia is pronounced, add Ye Jiao Teng *Caulis Polygoni multiflori*.

SUMMARY

Mind Unsettled – Phlegm-Fire, Stomach and Heart Phlegm-Fire

Treatment principle

Resolve Phlegm, harmonize the Stomach, open the Mind's orifices, clear the Heart and calm the Mind.

Points

ST-40 Fenglong, Ren-12 Zhongwan, Ren-9 Shuifen, ST-25 Tianshu, G.B.-13 Benshen, ST-8 Touwei, G.B.-18 Chengling, G.B.-15 Toulinqi, G.B.-17 Zhengying, BL-20 Pishu, BL-49 Yishe, P-7 Daling, Du-20 Baihui. ST-40 and P-7 with reducing method, Ren-12, BL-20 and BL-49 with reinforcing method and all the others with even method.

Herbal therapy

Prescription

WEN DAN TANG
Warming the Gall-Bladder Decoction

Case history

A 54-year-old woman complained of long-standing depression and anxiety since she was 10. She had had a very unhappy childhood and harbored deep feelings of resentment towards her father. She had been on antidepressants (tricyclics) for several years and she had just recently come off tranquillizers (Valium). In spite of the antidepressants, she still felt very depressed and she described her condition as a "black cloud hanging over her". She also felt extremely anxious and her sleep was very restless. She also suffered from severe stabbing headaches on the forehead and was prone to a lot of catarrh. Her tongue was Reddish-Purple, Stiff, Swollen, with a Stomach crack in the center, and a thick-sticky-yellow coating (Plate 12.5). Her pulse was Wiry, Slippery and Full.

Diagnosis This patient suffered from two main conditions: Phlegm-Fire affecting Stomach and Heart and stasis of Blood. Both Phlegm-Fire and stasis of Blood agitate the Mind and the Ethereal Soul, leading to depression and anxiety.

Treatment The principle of treatment adopted was to resolve Phlegm, drain Fire, invigorate Blood, calm the Mind, and settle the Ethereal Soul. She was treated with herbs only and the formula used was a variation of Wen Dan Tang *Warming the Gall-Bladder Decoction*:

- **Ban Xia** *Rhizoma Pinelliae preparatum* 6 g
- **Fu Ling** *Poria* 5 g
- **Chen Pi** *Pericarpium Citri reticulatae* 9 g
- **Zhu Ru** *Caulis Bambusae in Taeniam* 6 g
- **Zhi Shi** *Fructus Aurantii immaturus* 6 g
- **Zhi Gan Cao** *Radix Glycyrrhizae uralensis preparata* 3 g
- **Sheng Jiang** *Rhizoma Zingiberis recens* 5 slices
- **Da Zao** *Fructus Jujubae* 1 date
- **Yuan Zhi** *Radix Polygalae* 6 g
- **Suan Zao Ren** *Semen Ziziphi spinosae* 4 g
- **He Huan Pi** *Cortex Albiziae* 6 g
- **Yu Jin** *Radix Curcumae* 6 g

Explanation

- The first 8 herbs constitute the root formula, which resolves Phlegm-Heat from the Stomach and Heart.
- Yuan Zhi and Suan Zao Ren calm the Mind and open the Mind's orifices. These two herbs blend particularly well together as one is pungent and the other sour.
- He Huan Pi and Yu Jin invigorate Blood, open the Mind's orifices and lift depression.

The patient was treated with modifications of the above prescription for 9 months, after which she felt a lot better and was able to come off the antidepressants completely.

MIND WEAKENED

This is characterized by physical and mental exhaustion, depression, lack of will-power and initiative, insomnia (waking up early), mild anxiety, poor memory, dislike to speak and pessimism.

More than the conditions associated with Unsettled Mind and Obstructed Mind, the conditions of Weakened Mind are often the result rather than the cause of a disharmony of the internal organs, Qi and Blood. For example, the Mind can easily become weakened after a long chronic disease, after many childbirths too close together or after a lifetime of overwork that has severely depleted Qi and Essence.

The conditions causing a weakened Mind are Qi deficiency, Blood deficiency or Yin deficiency.

The treatment principle for weakened Mind is to nourish Qi, Blood or Yin, calm the Mind and strengthen Will-Power.

Qi and Blood deficiency

Qi deficiency

Treatment principle

Tonify Qi, strengthen the Mind.

Acupuncture

Points

ST-36 Zusanli, SP-3 Taibai, Ren-6 Qihai, BL-20 Pishu, BL-21 Weishu, Du-20 Baihui, HE-7 Shenmen, LU-3 Tianfu, BL-15 Xinshu, BL-13 Feishu, BL-44 Shentang, BL-42 Pohu. All with reinforcing method. Moxa is applicable.

Explanation

- ST-36, SP-3, BL-20 and BL-21 tonify Stomach- and Spleen-Qi. As the Stomach and Spleen are the source of the Postnatal Qi, they should always be tonified in Qi deficiency.
- Ren-6 tonifies Original Qi.
- Du-20 clears the Mind and lifts mood.
- HE-7 calms the Mind.
- LU-3 tonifies Lung-Qi and stimulates the ascending of clear Qi to the brain.
- BL-15, with direct moxa, tonifies Heart-Qi, clears the Mind and lifts mood.
- BL-13 tonifies Lung-Qi and is selected if there is Lung deficiency, as there would be when sadness is the cause of this pattern.
- BL-44 tonifies the Heart and calms and clears the Mind.
- BL-42 tonifies the Lungs and settles the Corporeal Soul that suffers from sadness and grief.

Herbal therapy

Prescription

AN SHEN DING ZHI WAN

Calming the Mind and Settling the Spirit Pill

Explanation

This formula tonifies Qi, strengthens the Original Qi, calms and clears the Mind, and lifts mood. It is used for chronic Qi deficiency affecting the Mind, making it, on the one hand, restless and, on the other hand, confused and depressed. The main manifestations would be extreme tiredness, dislike to speak, slight breathlessness, no appetite, restless sleep with unpleasant dreams, palpitations, a weak voice, a Pale tongue and an Empty or Weak pulse.

Please note that this formula contains a mineral substance (Long Chi *Fossilia Dentis Mastodi*), the use of which is not allowed in European Union countries. Please consult Appendix 2 to find substitutions.

Mental-emotional pattern

This pattern either arises from a depletion of Qi due to a chronic disease or from emotional problems affecting Qi. Sadness, grief and regret are the most likely causes of this condition, as they deplete Qi of the Lungs and Heart. This person would feel very tired, be depressed and not sleep well. He or she would also lack motivation.

Prescription

DING ZHI WAN

Settling the Spirit Pill

Explanation

This formula is very similar to the previous one. It differs from it in so far as it does not have as strong a calming effect on the Mind due to the omission of Long Chi *Fossilia Dentis Mastodi*. This formula tonifies Qi, strengthens the Original Qi, calms and clears the Mind, and lifts mood. It is used for chronic Qi deficiency affecting the Mind, making it confused and depressed. The main manifestations would be extreme tiredness, dislike to speak, slight breathlessness, no appetite, palpitations, a weak voice, a Pale tongue and an Empty or Weak pulse.

Mental-emotional pattern

As in the previous case, this pattern arises either from a depletion of Qi due to a chronic disease or from emotional problems affecting Qi. Sadness, grief and regret are the most likely causes of this condition, as they deplete Qi of the Lungs and Heart. This person would feel very tired, depressed and would also lack motivation.

SUMMARY

Mind Weakened – Qi and Blood deficiency, Qi deficiency

Treatment principle

Tonify Qi, strengthen the Mind.

Points

ST-36 Zusanli, SP-3 Taibai, Ren-6 Qihai, BL-20 Pishu, BL-21 Weishu, Du-20 Baihui, HE-7 Shenmen, LU-3 Tianfu, BL-15 Xinshu, BL-13 Feishu, BL-44 Shentang, BL-42 Pohu. All with reinforcing method. Moxa is applicable.

Herbal therapy

Prescription

AN SHEN DING ZHI WAN
Calming the Mind and Settling the Spirit Pill

Prescription

DING ZHI WAN
Settling the Spirit Pill.

Case history

A 41-year-old woman suffered from abdominal distension, belching, constipation and hypochondrial pain. Her periods started hesitantly and were painful. The menstrual blood was dark with some clots. She also complained of premenstrual tension and irritability.

She had a feeling of vague anxiety at night with a sensation of tightness of the chest. Some years before, she had gone through a difficult period emotionally and experienced great sadness. Her complexion was pale and her eyes were slightly dull. Her tongue-body color was normal with teethmarks. Her pulse was very Weak and Fine on the Lung position and slightly Wiry on the left side.

Diagnosis Most of the symptoms and signs point to stagnation of Liver-Qi and Liver-Blood: abdominal distension, belching, hypochondrial pain, painful periods with dark blood and premenstrual tension. However, the very Fine Lung pulse, the feeling of anxiety at night, the pale complexion and the teethmarks on the tongue point to Lung-Qi deficiency. This, combined with the absence of a Red color on the sides of the tongue, indicated that the main problem lay in deficient Lung-Qi not controlling the Liver (Metal insulting Wood from a Five-Element perspective) and leading to stagnation of Liver-Qi. The feeling of vague anxiety at night was due to agitation of the Corporeal Soul from Lung-Qi deficiency. The deficiency of Lung-Qi was obviously due to the period of great sadness years before.

Treatment principle Tonify Lung-Qi, settle the Corporeal Soul and Ethereal Soul and move Liver-Qi.

Herbal therapy The prescription used was not a classic one but one I formulated for this patient.

- **Bai He** *Bulbus Lilii* 9 g
- **Mai Men Dong** *Radix Ophiopogonis* 6 g
- **Bei Sha Shen** *Radix Glehniae* 6 g
- **Huang Qi** *Radix Astragali* 6 g
- **Dang Shen** *Radix Codonopsis* 9 g
- **Wu Wei Zi** *Fructus Schisandrae* 4 g
- **Shu Di Huang** *Radix Rehmanniae preparata* 9 g
- **Bai Shao** *Radix Paeoniae alba* 9 g
- **Yi Mu Cao** *Herba Leonuri* 4 g
- **Yu Jin** *Radix Curcumae* 6 g
- **Zhi Gan Cao** *Radix Glycyrrhizae uralensis preparata* 6 g

Explanation

- Bai He, Mai Men Dong and Bei Sha Shen nourish Lung-Yin. Although she does not suffer from Lung-Yin deficiency, these herbs are used to nourish and settle the Corporeal Soul and relieve sadness.
- Huang Qi and Dang Shen tonify Lung- and Spleen-Qi. It is necessary to tonify Spleen-Qi

according to the principle of reinforcing Earth to strengthen Metal.
- Wu Wei Zi tonifies Lung-Qi and Lung-Yin and settles the Corporeal Soul.
- Shu Di, Bai Shao and Yi Mu Cao harmonize Liver-Blood. Bai Shao is sour and absorbing and, in combination with Gan Cao, it stops pain, calms the Mind and moderates urgency.
- Yu Jin invigorates Liver-Blood, opens the Mind's orifices and lifts depression.
- Zhi Gan Cao, in a larger dose than normal, is combined with Bai Shao as indicated above.

After taking this prescription for 2 weeks, the patient experienced less abdominal distension, less belching and no constipation. She felt calmer in the evening and brighter in herself but also more moody and more up and down emotionally. I attributed this to Yu Jin *Radix Curcumae* within the prescription; this herb is pungent and hot and powerfully moves Liver-Qi and Liver-Blood. The second prescription was:
- **Bai He** *Bulbus Lilii* 9 g
- **Bei Sha Shen** *Radix Glehniae* 6 g
- **Mai Men Dong** *Radix Ophiopogonis* 6 g
- **Dang Shen** *Radix Codonopsis* 6 g
- **Hou Po** *Cortex Magnoliae officinalis* 6 g
- **Ban Xia** *Rhizoma Pinelliae preparatum* 6 g
- **Su Ye** *Folium Perillae* 6 g
- **Fu Ling** *Poria* 4 g
- **Xiang Fu** *Rhizoma Cyperi* 4 g
- **Suan Zao Ren** *Semen Ziziphi spinosae* 3 g
- **Zhi Gan Cao** *Radix Glycyrrhizae uralensis preparata* 6 g
- **Bai Shao** *Radix Paeoniae alba* 6 g
- **Da Zao** *Fructus Jujubae* 5 dates

Explanation
- The first four herbs have already been discussed above.
- Hou Po, Ban Xia, Su Ye and Fu Ling constitute Ban Xia Hou Po Tang *Pinellia-Magnolia Decoction* which moves Liver-Qi in the chest and makes Lung-Qi and Stomach-Qi descend. It particularly relieves depression, moodiness and sadness associated with the Lungs.
- Xiang Fu and Suan Zao Ren move Liver-Qi and settle the Ethereal Soul. They are coordinated, as one is pungent and moves, the other is sour and absorbs.
- Zhi Gan Cao and Bai Shao stop pain, harmonize the Liver and moderate urgency.
- Da Zao harmonizes.

After repeating this prescription three times, she was much better and her periods became painless.

Qi and Blood deficiency

Treatment principle
Tonify Qi, nourish Blood and calm the Mind.

Acupuncture

Points
ST-36 Zusanli, SP-6 Sanyinjiao, Ren-4 Guanyuan, BL-20 Pishu, BL-21 Weishu, Du-20 Baihui, HE-7 Shenmen, Ren-15 Jiuwei, BL-15 Xinshu, BL-44 Shentang. All with reinforcing method. Moxa is applicable.

Explanation
- ST-36, SP-6, BL-20 and BL-21 tonify Stomach- and Spleen-Qi. As the Stomach and Spleen are the source of the Postnatal Qi, they should always be tonified in Qi deficiency. SP-6 also nourishes Blood, calms the Mind and promotes sleep.
- Ren-4 tonifies Original Qi and nourishes Blood.
- Du-20 clears the Mind and lifts mood.
- HE-7 calms the Mind.
- Ren-15 calms the Mind and nourishes Heart-Blood.
- BL-15, with direct moxa, tonifies Heart-Qi, clears the Mind and lifts mood.
- BL-44 tonifies the Heart and calms and clears the Mind.

Herbal therapy

Prescription
GUI PI TANG
Tonifying the Spleen Decoction

Explanation
This well-tested prescription is excellent to tonify Spleen-Qi and Heart-Blood and calm the Mind. Besides calming the Mind, it also clears and stimulates it, helping memory, thinking and concentration. The main manifestations are palpitations, tiredness, a pale complexion, insomnia (difficulty in falling asleep), poor memory, poor appetite, menorrhagia in women (from

Spleen-Qi not holding Blood), a Pale tongue and a Weak or Choppy pulse.

Mental-emotional pattern

Worry, pensiveness or shame over a long period of time injure the Spleen and Heart and lead to Spleen-Qi deficiency and Heart-Blood deficiency. This weakens the Mind, which is deprived of its residence. Thus the patient becomes tired and depressed and finds sleep difficult. The Mind controls memory and thinking, and therefore there is a poor memory, poor concentration and slow thinking. Another feature of this pattern is obsessive thinking or phobias, which are due to Spleen and Blood deficiency. The Spleen controls thinking, intelligence and concentration and, when in disharmony, these same qualities may generate obsessive thinking or phobias.

Modifications

- If Blood deficiency is pronounced, add Shu Di Huang *Radix Rehmanniae preparata*. With the addition of this herb, this formula is called Hei Gui Pi Tang *Black Tonifying the Spleen Decoction*.

Prescription

SHI WEI WEN DAN TANG

Ten-Ingredient Warming the Gall-Bladder Decoction

Explanation

This formula is a variation of Wen Dan Tang *Warming the Gall-Bladder Decoction*; like the original prescription, it resolves Phlegm, but it does not clear Heat. In addition, this formula tonifies Qi and Blood. The main manifestations are tiredness, poor appetite, poor memory, timidity, insomnia, palpitations, mild anxiety, propensity to be startled, a Pale tongue and a Weak or Choppy pulse.

This formula, contrary to the previous one, also addresses any sweating that may derive from Empty Heat developing from Blood deficiency. This is quite possible and it happens more frequently in women. In the prescription, Wu Wei Zi and Suan Zao Ren have this function.

Another important difference from the previous formula is that this one resolves Phlegm as well. It is therefore suited to treat mental confusion as well as anxiety and restlessness.

Mental-emotional pattern

Worry, pensiveness or shame depletes the Spleen and the Heart, and this leads to deficiency of Qi and Blood. The Mind is deprived of its residence and the person feels exhausted, depressed and anxious. The Spleen-Qi deficiency leads to the formation of Phlegm, which mists the Mind, causing confused thinking and obsessive thoughts. The Blood deficiency causes insomnia, poor memory, timidity and the propensity to be startled.

Prescription

GAN MAI DA ZAO TANG

Glycyrrhiza-Triticum-Jujuba Decoction

Explanation

This interesting formula has been the subject of much speculation and different interpretations. Essentially, it tonifies Heart-Qi and calms the Mind. It can also be used for deficiency of Heart-Yin with Empty Heat, only when the Empty Heat is not such that it requires the use of bitter-cold herbs because these would further injure Qi. On the other hand, the deficiency of Qi is not such that it requires strong tonifying herbs, hence the gentle tonification of these three herbs.

The hallmark of this prescription then is that it provides enough tonification but not so much that it would make any Empty Heat worse. All the herbs in it are sweet and this taste soothes the Liver. For this reason, this formula is also said to treat Liver-Qi stagnation which may be associated with Heart-Qi deficiency.

I personally use this formula very frequently to nourish the Heart and tonify Qi, not only in cases of Mind Weakened, but also of Mind Unsettled and Mind Obstructed. As it contains only three herbs, I may often combine this formula with other ones to nourish the Heart and calm the Mind. However, it can be used in both anxiety and depression.

Mental-emotional pattern

All the manifestations normally relevant to this formula are of mental or emotional character. Worry, excess joy, craving, love, guilt and pensiveness may all injure Heart-Qi and lead to this condition. The main manifestations are worrying, anxiety, sadness, weeping, insomnia, depression, inability to control oneself, yawning, moaning, speaking to oneself, disorientation, a Weak pulse and a Pale tongue. The tongue may be Red without coating if there is Heart-Yin deficiency. In severe cases, this corresponds to the depressive phase of manic-depression.

This formula is often added as a whole to other prescriptions to treat the above manifestations.

SUMMARY

Mind Weakened – Qi and Blood deficiency, Qi and Blood deficiency

Treatment principle

Tonify Qi, nourish Blood and calm the Mind.

Points

ST-36 Zusanli, SP-6 Sanyinjiao, Ren-4 Guanyuan, BL-20 Pishu, BL-21 Weishu, Du-20 Baihui, HE-7 Shenmen, Ren-15 Jiuwei, BL-15 Xinshu, BL-44 Shentang. All with reinforcing method. Moxa is applicable.

Herbal therapy

Prescription

GUI PI TANG
Tonifying the Spleen Decoction

Prescription

SHI WEI WEN DAN TANG
Ten-Ingredient Warming the Gall-Bladder Decoction

Prescription

GAN MAI DA ZAO TANG
Glycyrrhiza-Triticum-Jujuba Decoction

Yang deficiency

Kidney-Yang deficiency

Treatment principle
Tonify and warm Yang, strengthen the Kidneys, calm the Mind and lift mood.

Acupuncture

Points
BL-23 Shenshu, BL-52 Zhishi, Du-4 Mingmen, Du-14 Dazhui, Ren-4 Guanyuan, KI-3 Taixi, KI-7 Fuliu, ST-36 Zusanli, SP-6 Sanyinjiao, Du-20 Baihui, BL-8 Luoque, BL-10 Tianzhu. All with reinforcing method except for the points in the head, which are usually needled with even method. Moxa should be used.

Explanation
- BL-23 tonifies Kidney-Yang.
- BL-52 tonifies the Kidneys and strengthens the Will-Power.
- Du-4, with direct moxa, strongly tonifies the Fire of the Gate of Vitality and lifts mood.
- Du-14, with direct moxa, tonifies Yang and lifts mood.
- Ren-4 nourishes the Kidneys and calms the Mind.
- KI-3 and KI-7 tonify Kidney-Yang. KI-7 in particular would resolve edema, a possible consequence of Kidney-Yang deficiency.
- ST-36 and SP-6 tonify the Stomach and Spleen to raise vitality in general. In particular, SP-6 also nourishes Yin and is therefore indicated in complicated cases of deficiency of both Yang and Yin of the Kidneys.
- Du-20 raises Yang, improves memory and concentration and lifts mood.
- BL-8 calms the Mind, lifts mood and strengthens memory.
- BL-10 clears the Mind.

Herbal therapy

Prescription
YOU GUI WAN
Restoring the Right [Kidney] *Pill*

Explanation
This formula is excellent to tonify Kidney-Yang and the Fire of the Gate of Life (*Ming Men*) with its associated mental manifestations. The main physical manifestations are lower backache, weak knees, poor memory, exhaustion, cold legs and back, frequent-pale urination, a Pale and Swollen tongue and a Weak-Deep pulse.

I personally prefer this formula to Jin Gui Shen Qi Wan *Golden Chest Kidney-Qi Pill* for two reasons: first of all, it also nourishes Blood, which makes it more suitable for women (due to the inclusion of Gou Qi Zi *Fructus Lycii chinensis* and Dang Gui *Radix Angelicae sinensis*), and second, because it is better for the mental aspects of Kidney-Yang deficiency (due to the inclusion of Du Zhong *Cortex Eucommiae ulmoidis* and Lu Jiao Jiao *Gelatinum Cornu Cervi*).

Please note that this formula contains Fu Zi *Radix Aconiti lateralis preparata* and Lu Jiao Jiao *Gelatinum Cornu Cervi*, the use of which is not allowed in European Union countries. Fu Zi can be simply eliminated from the prescription by increasing the dosage of Rou Gui *Cortex Cinnamomi*. Lu Jiao Jiao can be eliminated from the formula without altering it substantially.

Mental-emotional pattern

Fear, shock and guilt may injure the Kidneys and cause this condition. However, it is often the result rather than the cause of Kidney-Yang deficiency. Kidney-Yang may be depleted by chronic disease, overwork, excessive physical work and lifting, and excessive sexual activity.

This person will feel mentally and physically exhausted, will be depressed, lack will-power and spirit of initiative. He or she will have almost given up any hope of getting better, of starting or changing anything in life. Everything is too much effort.

This condition is characterized not only by Kidney-Yang deficiency but also by Essence depletion. The Kidney-Essence is the material basis for all the Kidney's physiological activities. The Essence has a Yin and a Yang aspect and, in this case, its Yang aspect is deficient. Because the Essence is the foundation for the Three Treasures – the Essence, Qi and Mind – a deficiency of its Yang aspect causes extreme exhaustion and low spirits.

Modifications

- In cases of mixed Yin and Yang deficiency symptoms of the Kidneys (a very frequent occurrence), halve the dosage of Fu Zi and Rou Gui to 1.5 g each, and replace Shu Di Huang with Sheng Di Huang *Radix Rehmanniae*.

SUMMARY

Mind Weakened – Yang deficiency, Kidney-Yang deficiency

Treatment principle

Tonify and warm Yang, strengthen the Kidneys, calm the Mind and lift mood.

Points

BL-23 Shenshu, BL-52 Zhishi, Du-4 Mingmen, Du-14 Dazhui, Ren-4 Guanyuan, KI-3 Taixi, KI-7 Fuliu, ST-36 Zusanli, SP-6 Sanyinjiao, Du-20 Baihui, BL-8 Luoque, BL-10 Tianzhu. All with reinforcing method except for the points in the head, which are usually needled with even method. Moxa should be used.

Herbal therapy

Prescription

YOU GUI WAN
Restoring the Right [Kidney] *Pill*

Case history

A 46-year-old woman complained of nocturia; she woke to urinate up to seven times a night. Her urine was generally pale and she experienced a dry mouth at night. She had a lower backache and felt generally cold, although she occasionally also felt hot in the face.

Her tongue was slightly Pale with a Red tip with red points (Plate 12.6). Her pulse was Weak on both Kidney positions of left and right.

Diagnosis This is a clear pattern of Kidney-Yang deficiency. Although this is the predominant condition, there is also the very beginning of some Kidney-Yin deficiency, manifesting with a dry mouth at night and the occasional hot flush.

When asked about her earlier life and how the condition might have developed, she said that as a child she was evacuated during the war to stay with a family who did not treat her well. She was with them from the age of 4 to 8. She was intimidated by her foster parents and was often scared. At that time she developed nocturnal enuresis that did not disappear until she was 13. This is a very clear example of the effect of fear on the Kidneys in children, producing a deficiency of Kidney-Yang which persisted throughout her life.

Treatment principle Tonify Kidney-Yang, astringe the Essence, strengthen Will-Power and calm the Mind.

Acupuncture The following points were reinforced.

- BL-23 Shenshu, Du-4 Mingmen (with moxa), Ren-4 Guanyuan (moxa) and KI-3 to tonify Kidney-Yang and strengthen Will-Power.
- P-7 Daling and Ren-15 to calm the Mind.

Herbal therapy No herbs were used but only the patent remedy Jin Suo Gu Jing Wan *Metal Lock Consolidating the Essence Pill*.

- **Qian Shi** *Semen Euryales*
- **Lian Xu** *Stamen Nelumbinis*
- **Long Gu** *Mastodi Ossis fossilia* (calcined)
- **Mu Li** *Concha Ostreae* (calcined)
- **Lian Zi** *Semen Nelumbinis*
- **Sha Yuan Ji Li** *Semen Astragali complanati*

This remedy is mostly astringent rather than tonifying. It treats the Manifestation by astringing the urine but not the Root, i.e. Kidney-Yang deficiency. It is therefore suitable to be used in conjunction with the acupuncture treatment which is aimed at treating the Root.

Blood deficiency

Treatment principle

Nourish Blood and calm the Mind.

Herbal therapy

The same prescriptions used for Blood deficiency under *Mind Unsettled* are applicable here.

Yin deficiency

Kidney-Yin deficiency

Treatment principle
Nourish Yin, calm the Mind and lift mood.

Acupuncture

Points
KI-3 Taixi, KI-6 Zhaohai, SP-6 Sanyinjiao, Ren-4 Guanyuan, BL-23 Shenshu, BL-52 Zhishi, Du-20 Baihui. Reinforcing method.

Explanation
- KI-3, KI-6, SP-6 and Ren-4 nourish Kidney-Yin and calm the Mind.
- BL-23 and BL-52 tonify the Kidneys and strengthen Will-Power. Although BL-23 is better to tonify Kidney-Yang, it is added here for its mental effect in lifting mood.
- Du-20 lifts mood and relieves depression.

Herbal therapy

All the prescriptions mentioned for Yin deficiency causing unsettled Mind are applicable here. However, the emphasis of those prescriptions was on calming the Mind, whilst in the case of weakened Mind, the emphasis should be on clearing the Mind and lifting mood. They should therefore be suitably adapted by the addition of more Yin-nourishing herbs, such as Sheng Di Huang *Radix Rehmanniae*, Mai Men Dong *Radix Ophiopogonis* or Tian Men Dong *Radix Asparagi*.

The following are formulae that nourish Yin, with the emphasis on lifting mood rather than calming the Mind.

Prescription
LIU WEI DI HUANG WAN
Six-Ingredient Rehmannia Pill

Explanation
This is the most famous Yin-nourishing formula. Fear, guilt and shock can deplete the Kidneys. A feeling of guilt, especially when harbored for many years, is very destructive and may lead to Kidney deficiency. The main manifestations that apply to this formula are dizziness, tinnitus, backache, night-sweating, a dry mouth, five-palm heat, exhaustion, a dark complexion, a thin body, dry hair, a Red tongue without coating and a Floating-Empty pulse.

Mental-emotional pattern
Again, this condition can arise either as a consequence of emotional problems due to shock, fear or guilt, or, vice versa, as a result of depletion of Kidney-Yin and Kidney Essence.

This person will feel very exhausted and depressed, lacking in will-power and spirit of initiative. Unlike those who suffer from Kidney-Yang deficiency with similar mental characteristics, those who suffer from Kidney-Yin deficiency are slightly more restless, uneasy and fidgety. They may also tend to complain more.

The Essence is the foundation of the Three Treasures – Essence, Qi and Mind – and when it is depleted, the Mind and the Will-Power suffer, causing exhaustion, depression and despair.

SUMMARY

Mind Weakened – Yin deficiency, Kidney-Yin deficiency

Treatment principle

Nourish Yin, calm the Mind and lift mood.

Points

KI-3 Taixi, KI-6 Zhaohai, SP-6 Sanyinjiao, Ren-4 Guanyuan, BL-23 Shenshu, BL-52 Zhishi, Du-20 Baihui. Reinforcing method.

Herbal therapy

Prescription

LIU WEI DI HUANG WAN

Six-Ingredient Rehmannia Pill

Lung- and Kidney-Yin deficiency

Treatment principle

Nourish Lung- and Kidney-Yin, strengthen Will-Power and settle the Corporeal Soul.

Acupuncture

Points

LU-9 Taiyuan, LU-5 Chize, KI-3 Taixi, Ren-4 Guanyuan, LU-7 Lieque and KI-6 Zhaohai, BL-23 Shenshu, BL-52 Zhishi, BL-42 Pohu. Reinforcing method.

Explanation

- LU-9 tonifies Lung-Yin.
- LU-5 nourishes the Water of the Lungs and, according to the book *An Explanation of Acupuncture Points* (1654), when sadness has affected the Lungs, causing dryness of this organ, the person cries a lot.[12]
- KI-3 and Ren-4 nourish Kidney-Yin and calm the Mind.
- LU-7 and KI-6 open the Directing Vessel, nourish Lung- and Kidney-Yin and benefit the throat.
- BL-23 and BL-52 tonify the Kidneys and strengthen Will-Power.
- BL-42 tonifies the Lungs and settles the Corporeal Soul.

Herbal therapy

Prescription

MAI WEI DI HUANG WAN

Ophiopogon-Schisandra-Rehmannia Pill

Explanation

This is a variation of the previous formula with the addition of Mai Men Dong *Radix Ophiopogonis* and Wu Wei Zi *Fructus Schisandrae*, which nourish Lung-Yin. The main physical manifestations, in addition to those of Liu Wei Di Huang Wan, are therefore a dry cough, a dry throat, slight breathlessness and possibly blood-flecked sputum.

Mental-emotional pattern

All the mental-emotional characteristics of the previous case apply here. The main difference is that, in this case, the Corporeal Soul is affected and this condition may be caused by emotions that injure the Lungs such as sadness, worry and grief.

In terms of mental-emotional manifestations, this person will probably somatize the emotions on the skin, which will be dry with skin rashes.

This person will also tend to be more melancholic, sad and apt to hanker nostalgically after the past.

Prescription

DI PO TANG

Earth Corporeal Soul Decoction

Explanation

This formula nourishes Lung-Yin, roots the Corporeal Soul into the Lungs and subdues rebellious Lung-Qi.

Mental-emotional pattern

This formula is from the *Discussion on Blood Diseases* (1884) and is for mental confusion and restlessness resulting from an unsettled Corporeal Soul.

The patient is mildly restless, depressed, slightly confused and has palpitations, symptoms occurring against a background of deficient Lung-Yin not rooting the Corporeal Soul.

Please note that Mu Li *Concha Ostreae* can be replaced by Suan Zao Ren *Semen Ziziphi spinosae*.

SUMMARY

Mind Weakened – Yin deficiency, Lung- and Kidney-Yin deficiency

Treatment principle

Nourish Lung- and Kidney-Yin, strengthen Will-Power and settle the Corporeal Soul.

Points

LU-9 Taiyuan, LU-5 Chize, KI-3 Taixi, Ren-4 Guanyuan, LU-7 Lieque and KI-6 Zhaohai, BL-23 Shenshu, BL-52 Zhishi, BL-42 Pohu. Reinforcing method.

Herbal therapy

Prescription

MAI WEI DI HUANG WAN
Ophiopogon-Schisandra-Rehmannia Pill

Prescription

DI PO TANG
Earth Corporeal Soul Decoction.

Case history

A 35-year-old man presented with insomnia (waking up during the night), slight anxiety, depression, lack of concentration, numbness of the hands at night, a dry mouth, a feeling of heat in the evening and palpitations.

His eyes lacked glitter and were unstable, his tongue was Red, with a Heart crack and without enough coating (Plate 12.7), and his pulse was Rapid and Moving.

Diagnosis The pattern is Heart-Yin deficiency and his eyes and pulse (Moving quality) clearly point to shock as the cause of the disease. When asked about it, he confirmed that he had suffered a tremendous shock when his brother was murdered a few years before.

Treatment principle Nourish the Heart, tonify Yin, open the Heart's orifices and calm the Mind. It is necessary to open the Heart's orifices as shock "closes" the Heart.

Acupuncture The main points used (with reinforcing method) were as follows.

- HE-7 Shenmen, SP-6 Sanyinjiao and Ren-14 Juque to nourish the Heart and calm the Mind.
- Ren-15 Jiuwei and BL-15 Xinshu to open the Heart's orifices.
- Ren-4 Guanyuan to nourish Yin and root the Mind.

Herbal therapy The formula used was a variation of Mai Wei Di Huang Wan *Ophiopogon-Schisandra-Rehmannia Pill.*

- **Shu Di Huang** *Radix Rehmanniae preparata* 12 g
- **Ren Shen** *Radix Ginseng* 6 g
- **Ze Xie** *Rhizoma Alismatis* 6 g
- **Fu Shen** *Sclerotium Poriae cocos pararadicis* 6 g
- **Mai Men Dong** *Radix Ophiopogonis* 9 g
- **Wu Wei Zi** *Fructus Schisandrae* 6 g
- **Yuan Zhi** *Radix Polygalae* 6 g
- **Shi Chang Pu** *Rhizoma Acori tatarinowii* 6 g
- **Zhi Gan Cao** *Radix Glycyrrhizae uralensis preparata* 3 g

Explanation The original formula nourishes Lung- and Kidney-Yin but, modified as above, it can nourish Heart-Yin and calm the Mind.

- Shu Di Huang, besides tonifying the Kidneys, also enters the Heart and therefore settles the Mind.
- Shan Zhu Yu and Mu Dan Pi were eliminated; they are in the original formula to nourish the Liver which is not deficient in this case.
- Shan Yao was replaced by Ren Shen as this enters the Heart. Also, in combination with Wu Wei Zi and Mai Men Dong (see below), it makes the Sheng Mai Tang which nourishes Qi and Yin of the Heart.
- Ze Xie combines with Shu Di Huang to clear any Empty Heat.
- Fu Ling was replaced with Fu Shen to calm the Mind.
- Mai Dong and Wu Wei Zi are part of the original prescription and they both enter the Heart.
- Yuan Zhi and Chang Pu open the Heart's orifices. They are both pungent, and therefore scattering, and are coordinated with Wu Wei Zi, which is sour and absorbing.
- Zhi Gan Cao harmonizes.

This patient was treated for 9 months, producing an all-round improvement in his physical and mental symptoms.

Kidney- and Liver-Yin deficiency

Treatment principle

Nourish Kidney- and Liver-Yin, strengthen the Will-Power and settle the Ethereal Soul.

Acupuncture

Points

KI-3 Taixi, KI-6 Zhaohai, SP-6 Sanyinjiao, Ren-4 Guanyuan, LIV-8 Ququan, BL-23 Shenshu, BL-52 Zhishi, BL-47 Hunmen. Reinforcing method.

Explanation

- KI-3, KI-6, SP-6, Ren-4 and LIV-8 nourish Kidney- and Liver-Yin.
- BL-23 and BL-52 strengthen the Kidneys and Will-Power.
- BL-47 settles the Ethereal Soul. The combination of BL-47, BL-23 and BL-52 is excellent to relieve mental depression deriving from a deficiency of Liver and Kidneys.

Herbal therapy

Prescription

DA BU YIN JIAN

Great Tonifying Yin Decoction

Explanation

This formula is for deficiency of Kidney- and Liver-Yin. The main manifestations are dizziness, tinnitus, backache, weak knees, blurred vision, dry eyes, night-sweating, five-palm heat, headache, a Red tongue without coating and a Floating-Empty pulse.

Mental-emotional pattern

Fear, shock and guilt may cause a deficiency of Kidney- and Liver-Yin in the same way as mentioned above. In this case, the Mind, Ethereal Soul and Will-Power are all affected.

This person may feel exhausted and depressed and lack will-power. As the Ethereal Soul is deprived of its residence, he or she will also feel aimless and sleep badly.

Prescription

ZUO GUI WAN

Restoring the Left [Kidney] *Pill*

Explanation

This formula nourishes Liver- and Kidney-Yin. Its emphasis is on strengthening the tendons and bones, tissues related to Liver and Kidneys, respectively. Niu Xi and Lu Jiao have this function in the prescription. There is a correlation between the physical aspect of strengthening tendons and bones with herbs, which act on the Liver and Kidneys, and the strengthening of the Ethereal Soul and Will-Power related to these organs.

The main physical manifestations for this formula are, apart from other Yin-deficiency symptoms as above, weakness, stiffness and ache of the lower back and knees, a cold sensation of legs, knees and lower back, dizziness and a headache with a feeling of emptiness of the head.

Please note that this formula contains Lu Jiao *Cornu Cervi*, the use of which is not allowed in European Union countries. It can be removed from the formula without altering it substantially.

Mental-emotional pattern

The same emotions mentioned for the previous two formulae may lead to this condition. Alternatively, a weakness of the Liver and Kidneys from overwork and excessive sexual activity, or simply from old age, may cause this condition.

This person will feel exhausted, depressed and will lack will-power. In the same way that there is physical stiffness in the back, this person may tend to be rather rigid in his or her mental attitude.

SUMMARY

Mind Weakened – Yin deficiency, Kidney- and Liver-Yin deficiency

Treatment principle

Nourish Kidney- and Liver-Yin, strengthen the Will-Power and settle the Ethereal Soul.

Points

KI-3 Taixi, KI-6 Zhaohai, SP-6 Sanyinjiao, Ren-4 Guanyuan, LIV-8 Ququan, BL-23 Shenshu, BL-52 Zhishi, BL-47 Hunmen. Reinforcing method.

Herbal therapy

Prescription

DA BU YIN JIAN

Great Tonifying Yin Decoction

Prescription

ZUO GUI WAN

Restoring the Left [Kidney] *Pill*

Case history

A 39-year-old woman complained of an irregular menstrual cycle (always late) with some premenstrual tension, a lack of will-power and insomnia (waking up during the night). Her eyes often felt very dry. She also felt generally very tired, both physically and mentally. She had had a lot of stress in the past due to a difficult divorce and she now felt aimless, was undecided about her current relationship and did not know what direction to take in her life.

Her tongue was Red, with a Heart crack, almost entirely without coating (Plate 12.8), and her pulse was Empty on the deep level on the left side and Choppy on the right. The pulse also completely lacked any wave.

Diagnosis This is a clear pattern of Liver-Yin deficiency, even though there are not many symptoms. However, the pulse and tongue clearly indicate Yin deficiency and the insomnia, late menstrual cycle and dry eyes allow us to locate the Yin deficiency in the Liver. Most of all, the feeling of being aimless, the indecision and lack of direction in life clearly point to the Ethereal Soul being deprived of its root in Liver-Yin. Secondary to Liver-Yin deficiency, there was some Liver-Qi stagnation, manifested in the premenstrual tension.

The lack of wave in the pulse points to sadness as the emotion at the root of the problem. Different individuals react in different ways to the stresses of life. When going through a painful and stressful divorce, some may feel angry, some worried, some discouraged, etc. This woman reacted by feeling very sad about the breaking up of her marriage, and sadness weakened Liver-Blood and Liver-Yin.

Treatment principle Nourish Yin, strengthen the Liver and root the Ethereal Soul.

Acupuncture This patient was treated only four times with very good results.

The first treatment consisted only in the opening points of the Yin Linking Vessel, i.e. P-6 Neiguan on the right and SP-4 Gongsun on the left. This Extraordinary Vessel nourishes Yin and roots the Ethereal Soul.

In the second treatment, the opening points of the Yin Linking Vessel were repeated, with the addition of SP-6 Sanyinjiao and Ren-15 Jiuwei (both reinforced) to help to nourish Yin and root the Ethereal Soul. In the third and fourth treatments, the above points were needled again with the addition of the following points.

- ST-36 Zusanli and LIV-8 Ququan to nourish the Liver.
- BL-23 Shenshu, BL-52 Zhishi and BL-47 Hunmen to nourish the Kidneys and Liver and root the Ethereal Soul. The Kidneys were treated not because there was any Kidney deficiency but because Liver and Kidneys share a common root, and the points BL-52 and BL-42, combined with BL-23, strengthen the Will-Power, root the Ethereal Soul and help a person find a sense of direction.

After these four treatments she felt much better, more positive and decisive, so much so that she decided to break off her current troubled relationship, which she felt very good about.

Case history

A 32-year-old woman complained of fatigue, hypochondrial pain, a feeling of oppression of the chest and an ache behind the eyes. Her periods were always late and painful and the menstrual blood was dark with clots. Her sleep was restless and disturbed by many dreams, she felt hot in the evenings and her vision was sometimes blurred.

She felt aimless and lacked a sense of direction in her life. She was at a crossroads in both her work and a personal relationship, and she often felt that she "did not see the point of it all". Her tongue was Red and without coating. Her pulse was Floating-Empty and Fine but also slightly Wiry on the left side.

Diagnosis This is another clear example of Liver-Yin deficiency as in the previous patient. In this case, however, there is a much more pronounced stagnation of Liver-Qi and Liver-Blood (hypochondrial pain, feeling of oppression of the chest, painful periods with dark blood). In this case too, stagnation of Liver-Qi is secondary to Liver-Yin deficiency.

The deficient Liver-Yin fails to root the Ethereal Soul and this causes the feeling of aimlessness in her life and dream-disturbed sleep.

Treatment principle Nourish Liver-Yin, move Liver-Qi and Liver-Blood and root the Ethereal Soul.

Acupuncture The main points used were as follows.

- LIV-8 Ququan, ST-36 Zusanli, Ren-4 Guanyuan and SP-6 Sanyinjiao, reinforced, to nourish Liver-Yin.
- LIV-3 Taichong and G.B.-34 Yanglingquan, with even method, to move Liver-Qi and Liver-Blood.
- Ren-15 Jiuwei and BL-47 Hunmen to root the Ethereal Soul.

Herbal therapy The formula used was a variation of Da Bu Yin Jian *Great Tonifying Yin Decoction*.

- **Shu Di Huang** *Radix Rehmanniae preparata* 12 g
- **Shan Yao** *Radix Dioscoreae* 9 g
- **Shan Zhu Yu** *Fructus Corni* 4 g
- **Gou Qi Zi** *Fructus Lycii chinensis* 9 g
- **Dang Gui** *Radix Angelicae sinensis* 6 g
- **Dang Shen** *Radix Codonopsis* 6 g
- **Du Zhong** *Cortex Eucommiae* 6 g
- **Zhi Gan Cao** *Radix Glycyrrhizae uralensis preparata* 3 g
- **Chuan Lian Zi** *Fructus Toosendan* 4 g
- **Mei Gui Hua** *Flos Rosae rugosae* 3 g
- **Yi Mu Cao** *Herba Leonuri* 4 g
- **Suan Zao Ren** *Semen Ziziphi spinosae* 4 g

Explanation The formula was left unchanged, apart from the dosages which were reduced. Du Zhong could have been eliminated as there is no Kidney-deficiency, but it was left in for its mental effect of strengthening the Will-Power and providing a strong basis for the Ethereal Soul.

- Chuan Lian Zi and Mei Gui Hua move Liver-Qi without injuring Yin.
- Yi Mu Cao invigorates Liver-Blood.
- Suan Zao Ren, sour and astringent, roots the Ethereal Soul and calms the Mind.

Apart from an improvement in her menstrual cycle, this patient felt a lot stronger, more focused and determined after 3 months' treatment.

Kidney-Essence deficiency

Treatment principle

Nourish the Kidneys, tonify the Essence and strengthen Will-Power.

Acupuncture

Points

Ren-4 Guanyuan, Ren-7 Yinjiao, BL-23 Shenshu, BL-52 Zhishi, KI-3 Taixi, SP-6 Sanyinjiao, G.B.-13 Benshen, Du-20 Baihui. Reinforcing method. These points are suitable to treat both Kidney-Yang and Kidney-Yin deficiency, depending on whether one uses moxa or not.

Explanation

- Ren-4 and Ren-7 nourish the Essence.
- BL-23 and BL-52 tonify the Kidneys and strengthen Will-Power.
- KI-3 and SP-6 nourish Kidney-Yin.
- G.B.-13 gathers Essence to the brain.
- Du-20 raises clear Qi and lifts depression.

Herbal therapy

Prescription

HE CHE DA ZAO WAN
Placenta Great Fortifying Pill

Explanation

This formula's emphasis is on tonification of the Essence. Zi He Che, Wu Wei Zi, Gou Qi Zi and Suo Yang all benefit the Essence. Its secondary therapeutic aim is also to tonify Kidney-Yang. This formula is therefore well adapted to treat complicated cases of deficiency of all aspects of the Kidneys: Yin, Essence and Yang.

It should be noted that the doses are to make a quantity of pills, not for individual daily decoctions. The daily dosages of a decoction can be adapted according to proportions.

The main manifestations for this prescription would be exhaustion, depression, weak back and knees, weak sexual function (lack of desire or impotence), nocturnal emissions, weak teeth, prematurely gray or falling hair, dizziness, tinnitus, night-sweating, a thin body, a Red tongue without coating and a Floating-Empty pulse.

Please note that the use of placenta is not allowed in European Union countries; it can be removed from the formula.

Mental-emotional pattern

Fear, shock and guilt may cause a deficiency of Kidney-Yin and Kidney-Essence or, vice versa, may be the result of overwork and excessive sexual activity. In women it may result from too many childbirths or prolonged loss of blood with the periods over many years.

This person will feel mentally and physically exhausted and depressed, and lack will-power and initiative. He or she may also suffer from some deficiency in sexual function, such as lack of desire or impotence.

Modifications

The following are modifications which apply to all four formulae above. It should, first of all, be noted that, when nourishing Kidney-Yin in mental-emotional problems, it is advisable to add one or two Kidney-Yang tonics in a small dosage. This is necessary to make the formula more moving and dynamic, and thus affect the Mind and Will-Power more readily.

In chronic depression especially, one of the clear features of the condition is the way the patient is "stuck" in a mental-emotional pattern from which it is very difficult to break out. A certain resistance to treatment, hopelessness and despair are typical of chronic depression. In such cases, assuming they present with a configuration of Yin deficiency, it is important to add some Kidney-Yang tonics to invigorate Yang and provide movement to the prescription.

In particular, one would choose those Kidney-Yang tonics that are pungent in taste as this taste moves and invigorates. Two examples are Du Zhong *Cortex Eucommiae ulmoidis* and Ba Ji Tian *Radix Morindae officinalis*. Of course, some of the above prescriptions already contain some Kidney-Yang tonics.

Another frequent addition to the above Yin-nourishing prescriptions is Shi Chang Pu *Rhizoma Acori tatarinowii* to open the Mind's orifices, clear the Mind and lift mood. This would be an essential addition to all four previous prescriptions. It is also pungent in taste and would therefore also have a beneficial moving effect as the Yang tonics mentioned above.

SUMMARY

Mind Weakened – Yin deficiency, Kidney-Essence deficiency

Treatment principle

Nourish the Kidneys, tonify the Essence and strengthen Will-Power.

Points

Ren-4 Guanyuan, Ren-7 Yinjiao, BL-23 Shenshu, BL-52 Zhishi, KI-3 Taixi, SP-6 Sanyinjiao, G.B.-13 Benshen, Du-20 Baihui. Reinforcing method. These points are suitable to treat both Kidney-Yang and Kidney-Yin deficiency, depending on whether one uses moxa or not.

Herbal therapy

Prescription

HE CHE DA ZAO WAN
Placenta Great Fortifying Pill

NOTE

As will be remembered, the main treatment methods used in mental-emotional problems were five:

1. nourish the Heart and calm the Mind
2. clear pathogenic factors and calm the Mind
3. clear pathogenic factors, nourish the Heart and calm the Mind
4. resolve Phlegm, open the orifices and calm the Mind
5. sink and calm the Mind.

The first four have all been discussed when dealing with the various patterns of mental-emotional problems. We should now discuss the fifth method of treatment and that is to sink and calm the Mind. This consists of the use of minerals and shells which have a high density and are heavy. The traditional idea is that they weigh upon the Heart to sink the Mind, thus relieving anxiety, agitation and insomnia when these are caused by rebellious Qi. This is usually either Liver-Yang or Liver-Wind rising or Heart Empty Heat.

These substances may be added to any of the formulae we discussed to treat the Manifestation whenever the symptoms are severe, i.e. very severe agitation, intractable insomnia, intense anxiety and, in serious cases, violent behavior.

All these substances have side-effects because they are indigestible and therefore their prolonged use may injure the Stomach and Spleen. For this reason, they are usually combined with digestive herbs.

Please note that the use of minerals is not allowed in European Union countries.

The main sinking substances that calm the Mind are:

- Long Gu *Mastodi Ossis fossilia*
- Long Chi *Fossilia Dentis Mastodi*
- Mu Li *Concha Ostreae*
- Ci Shi *Magnetitum*
- Zhen Zhu Mu *Concha Margaritiferae usta*
- Hu Po *Succinum*.

Long Gu, Long Chi and Mu Li are all astringent and therefore also nourish Yin. Mu Li is especially good at nourishing Yin, while Long Chi is the best of the three to sink and calm the Mind.

Ci Shi and Zhen Zhu Mu both sink Liver-Yang and Liver-Wind.

Hu Po, besides sinking and calming the Mind, also invigorates Blood and enters the Liver; this makes it useful to treat depression and anxiety from Liver-Qi or Liver-Blood stagnation.

As for sinking and calming the Mind prescriptions, these have not been mentioned because many of them contain many indigestible and often toxic minerals. Their use is not often necessary. Most mental-emotional problems can be treated by the prescriptions discussed above, with the addition of one or two sinking substances if the manifestations call for it.

END NOTES

1. 1979 Huang Di Nei Jing Su Wen 黄帝内经素问 [The Yellow Emperor's Classic of Internal Medicine – Simple Questions]. People's Health Publishing House, Beijing, p. 168. First published *c*.100 BC.
2. 1981 Ling Shu Jing 灵枢经 [Spiritual Axis]. People's Health Publishing House, Beijing, p. 72. First published *c*.100 BC.
3. Ibid., p. 120.
4. Simple Questions, p. 319.
5. Wang Luo Zhen 1985 Qi Jing Ba Mai Kao Jiao Zhu 奇经八脉考校注 [A Compilation of the Study of the Eight Extraordinary Vessels]. Shanghai Science Publishing House, Shanghai, p. 129. The *Study of the Eight Extraordinary Vessels* was written by Li Shi Zhen and first published in 1578.
6. Shan Chang Hua 1990 Jing Xue Jie 经学解 [An Explanation of the Acupuncture Points]. People's Health Publishing House, Beijing, p. 31. An *Explanation of the Acupuncture Points* was written by Yue Han Zhen and first published in 1654.
7. Ibid., p. 45.
8. Ibid., p. 88.
9. 1981 Jin Gui Yao Lue Fang Xin Jie 金匮要略方新解 [A New Explanation of the Essential Prescriptions of the Golden Chest]. Zhejiang Scientific Publishing House, Zhejiang, p. 24. The *Essential Prescriptions of the Golden Chest* was written by Zhang Zhong Jing and first published *c*.AD 220.
10. Ibid., p. 24.
11. An Explanation of Acupuncture Points, pp. 26–27.
12. Ibid., p. 28.

针灸治疗精神情志疾病

CHAPTER 13

ACUPUNCTURE IN THE TREATMENT OF MENTAL-EMOTIONAL PROBLEMS

LUNG CHANNEL *245*
LU-3 Tianfu *245*
LU-7 Lieque *246*
LU-10 Yuji *246*

LARGE INTESTINE CHANNEL *247*
L.I.-4 Hegu *247*
L.I.-5 Yangxi *247*
L.I.-7 Wenliu *247*

STOMACH CHANNEL *248*
ST-25 Tianshu *248*
ST-40 Fenglong *249*
ST-41 Jiexi *249*
ST-42 Chongyang *249*
ST-45 Lidui *249*

SPLEEN CHANNEL *250*
SP-1 Yinbai *250*
SP-3 Taibai *250*
SP-4 Gongsun *251*
SP-5 Shangqiu *251*
SP-6 Sanyinjiao *251*

HEART CHANNEL *252*
HE-3 Shaohai *252*
HE-4 Lingdao *252*
HE-5 Tongli *252*
HE-7 Shenmen *253*
HE-8 Shaofu *253*
HE-9 Shaochong *253*

SMALL INTESTINE CHANNEL *254*
S.I.-5 Yanggu *254*
S.I.-7 Zhizheng *255*
S.I.-16 Tianchuang *255*

BLADDER CHANNEL *255*
BL-10 Tianzhu *255*
BL-13 Feishu *256*
BL-15 Xinshu *256*
BL-23 Shenshu *257*
BL-42 Pohu *257*
BL-44 Shentang *258*
BL-47 Hunmen *258*
BL-49 Yishe *259*
BL-52 Zhishi *259*
BL-62 Shenmai *259*

KIDNEY CHANNEL *260*
KI-1 Yongquan *260*
KI-3 Taixi *261*
KI-4 Dazhong *261*
KI-6 Zhaohai *261*
KI-9 Zhubin *261*
KI-16 Huangshu *262*

PERICARDIUM CHANNEL *263*
P-3 Quze *264*
P-4 Ximen *264*
P-5 Jianshi *264*
P-6 Neiguan *264*
P-7 Daling *266*
P-8 Laogong *267*

TRIPLE BURNER CHANNEL *268*
T.B.-3 Zhongzhu *268*
T.B.-10 Tianjing *268*

GALL-BLADDER CHANNEL *268*
G.B.-9 Tianchong *268*
G.B.-12 Wangu *268*

G.B.-13 Benshen *268*
G.B.-15 Linqi *270*
G.B.-17 Zhengying *270*
G.B.-18 Chengling *270*
G.B.-19 Naokong *270*
G.B.-40 Qiuxu *270*
G.B.-44 Zuqiaoyin *270*

LIVER CHANNEL *271*
LIV-2 Xingjian *271*
LIV-3 Taichong *271*

DIRECTING VESSEL (*REN MAI*) *272*
Ren-4 Guanyuan *272*
Ren-8 Shenque *272*
Ren-12 Zhongwan *273*
Ren-14 Juque *273*
Ren-15 Jiuwei *275*

GOVERNING VESSEL (*DU MAI*) *276*
Du-4 Mingmen *276*
Du-10 Lingtai *277*
Du-11 Shendao *277*
Du-12 Shenzhu *277*
Du-14 Dazhui *278*
Du-16 Fengfu *278*
Du-17 Naohu *278*
Du-18 Qiangjian *278*
Du-19 Houding *278*
Du-20 Baihui *278*
Du-24 Shenting *278*

EXTRA POINTS *280*
Hunshe *280*
Yintang *280*

POINTS FOR MENTAL PROBLEMS FROM NANJING AFFILIATED HOSPITAL *281*

EXAMPLES OF POINT COMBINATIONS FOR MENTAL-EMOTIONAL PROBLEMS *281*

ACUPUNCTURE IN THE TREATMENT OF MENTAL-EMOTIONAL PROBLEMS

After discussing the acupuncture and herbal treatment of each pattern in mental-emotional problems (Chapter 12), it is worth mentioning the action of some of the most frequently used points in mental-emotional problems.

For each point I give the traditional indications with their explanation but I also highlight my own use of the point in mental-emotional problems. Over the years, I have come to appreciate the importance of a good combination of points for an effective therapeutic result. I have come to the conclusion that a balanced combination of points is an important part of the therapeutic process. As I see it, there are three main steps to a successful point choice:

1. select the appropriate points according to both indications and actions
2. use the correct needling technique
3. use a balanced combination of points.

For this reason, I highlight some of my favorite point combinations for mental-emotional problems at the end of this chapter.

The main points used for depression are also discussed in Chapter 16. The discussion of the points for mental-emotional problems will be conducted according to the following topics.

- Lung channel
- Large Intestine channel
- Stomach channel
- Spleen channel
- Heart channel
- Small Intestine channel
- Bladder channel
- Kidney channel
- Pericardium channel
- Triple Burner channel
- Gall-Bladder channel
- Liver channel
- Directing Vessel (*Ren Mai*)
- Governing Vessel (*Du Mai*)
- Extra points
- Points for mental problems from Nanjing Affiliated Hospital
- Examples of point combinations for mental-emotional problems

Unless otherwise indicated, the mental-emotional indications of the points are taken from Deadman and Al Khafaji.[1] Please note that many of the points contain the indication of *Dian Kuang* (or only one of these two). I translate the disease of *Dian Kuang* as "Dullness and Mania" to preserve the original Chinese meaning of the term and to avoid direct connections with Western-defined diseases of "manic-depression" or "bipolar disorder". As we shall see in Chapter 19, there is no direct and exclusive correspondence between *Dian Kuang* and bipolar disorder.

When *Kuang* appears on its own (and therefore as a symptom rather than as a disease), I translate it as "mania" or "manic behavior". When *Dian* appears on its own (and therefore as a symptom rather than as a disease), I translate it as "dullness". Please note that I deliberately do not translate *Dian* as "depression" because what we call "depression" in a Western clinical setting is very different from the condition of *Dian*. This is explained in the chapters on depression (Chapter 16) and on bipolar disorder (Chapter 19).

LUNG CHANNEL

The Lung channel points for emotional problems are illustrated in Figure 13.1.

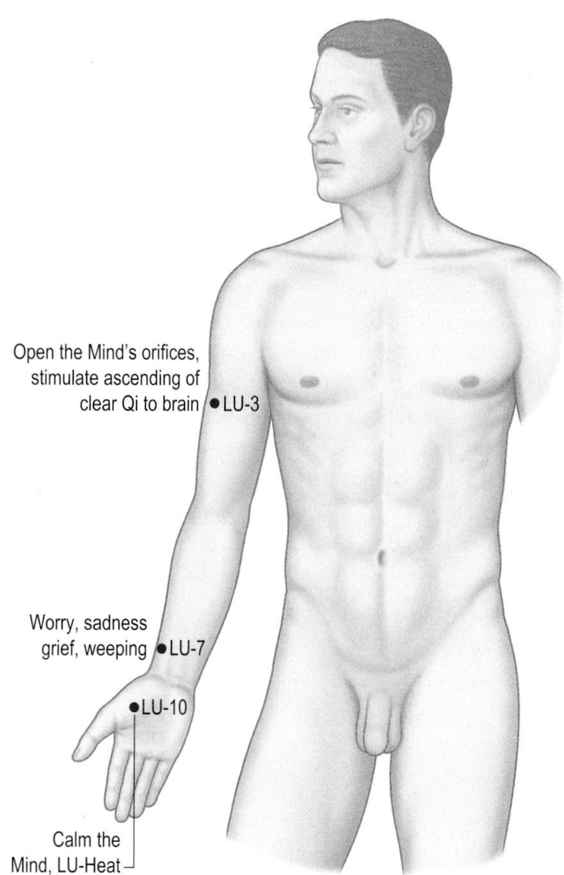

Figure 13.1 Lung channel points.

LU-3 Tianfu *Heavenly Palace*

LU-3 opens the Mind's orifices and soothes the Corporeal Soul (*Po*). Among its indications are somnolence, insomnia, sadness, weeping, forgetfulness and "talking to ghosts".

Among the mental indications, the *Great Compendium of Acupuncture* (*Zhen Jiu Da Cheng*, 1601) has only "talking to ghosts".[2] As mentioned before, whenever the indications of a point refer to "ghosts", it generally refers to a serious mental condition with loss of insight.

The *Gatherings from Eminent Acupuncturists* (*Zhen Jiu Ju Ying*, 1529) lists "talking to ghosts and corpses flying" among the indications of LU-3.[3] Other books do not mention "corpses flying" for this point. "Three corpses" refers to a Daoist belief in haunting of the body by three female ghosts: a green female ghost attacking the upper part causes eye problems, a white female ghost attacking the center part causes problems in the Internal Organs, and a blood-colored female ghost attacking the lower part of the body causes death.

The reference to "corpses" should be seen in the context of the Corporeal Soul, which has a centripetal movement ending in fragmentation and death, hence the association of this soul with death. This is discussed in more detail under the points BL-13 Feishu, BL-42 Pohu and Du-12 Shenzhu.

The actions and indications of this point are closely related to its being a Window of Heaven point. One of the characteristics of these points is that they regulate the ascending and descending of Qi from the body to and from the head; they do so in the crucial neck area (the gateway between the body and the head).

On a mental-emotional level, regulating the ascending and descending of Qi to and from the head can have the effect of calming the Mind or opening the Mind's orifices as required. In fact, insomnia is due to Qi ascending too much to the head (or not descending from it), while somnolence and forgetfulness are due to clear Qi not ascending to the head (or to turbid Qi not descending from the head).

The *Explanation of the Acupuncture Points* (*Zhen Jiu Xue Jie*) says that LU-3 can make Qi rise to treat forgetfulness, sadness and weeping due to Qi not rising to the head.[4] Forgetfulness is an important indication for this point; this is forgetfulness due to clear Qi not rising to the head. According to the *Explanation of the Acupuncture Points*, this point treats forgetfulness by stimulating the ascending of Qi of both Lungs and Heart.[5]

The *Gatherings from Eminent Acupuncturists* (1529) lists "blurred vision" under the indications for LU-3.[6] This confirms this point's action in promoting the ascending of clear Qi to the head (a function of Window of Heaven points) to brighten the eyes and promote clear vision. This is exactly the same way in which this point treats forgetfulness (see above).

> !
>
> Forgetfulness is an important indication for the point LU-3 Tianfu.

Finally, "talking to ghosts" features heavily in this point's indications. Generally speaking, when ancient books mention such symptoms as talking or seeing ghosts among the indications of a point, it means that the point is indicated for relatively serious mental-emotional problems, in particular when the Mind is obstructed. Obstruction of the Mind can potentially cause serious mental problems such as bipolar disorder, psychosis or schizophrenia. Again, this point can open the Mind's orifices, i.e. de-obstruct the Mind by regulating the ascending and descending of Qi to and from the head; it opens the Mind's orifices by promoting the descending of turbid Qi from the head and the ascending of clear Qi to the head.

It is interesting to compare the names and their implications of LU-3 Tianfu and LU-1 Zhongfu. "Fu" means "palace"; this usually confers importance to a point, indicating that it is at the center of an important directing and governing structure as a palace is. LU-1 is a "central" while LU-3 is a "heavenly" palace. LU-1 is a central palace because, although it is located in the upper chest, the Lung channel originates from the Middle Burner and emerges at this point. For this reason, this point can also promote the descending of Stomach-Qi, it has a certain effect on the Middle Burner and it does not have an effect on the head. By contrast, LU-3 is a "heavenly" palace, which means that its sphere of action is very much the head as indicated above.

LU-7 Lieque *Branching Cleft*

LU-7 settles and opens up the Corporeal Soul. Among its indications are poor memory, palpitations, propensity to (inappropriate) laughter and frequent yawning.

In my experience, LU-7 is a very important point from the psychological and emotional point of view, and can be used in emotional problems caused by worry, grief or sadness. LU-7 is particularly indicated in cases in which the person bears his or her problems in silence and keeps them inside. LU-7 tends to stimulate a beneficial outpouring of repressed emotions.

Weeping is the sound associated with the Lungs according to the Five Elements, and those who have been suppressing their emotions may burst out crying when this point is used or shortly after. Interestingly, "tendency to crying" is listed as a prominent indication for LU-7 in the Qing dynasty's *Explanation of the Acupuncture Points* (but not in modern books).[7]

The Lungs are the residence of the Corporeal Soul (*Po*) and this point will release the emotional tensions of the Corporeal Soul, manifesting on a physical level with tense shoulders, shallow breathing and a feeling of oppression in the chest. These symptoms are often due to excessive worrying over a long period of time, preventing the free breathing of the Corporeal Soul and constraining the Lung energy. LU-7 will calm the Mind, settle the Corporeal Soul, open the chest and release tension.

LU-10 Yuji *Fish Border*

LU-10 calms the Mind and is generally used when the Mind, Corporeal Soul and Ethereal Soul are agitated by Heat. Among its indications are sadness, fear, mental restlessness, anger, manic behavior and fright.

It clears Heat from the Heart and Lungs and treats mental-emotional symptoms deriving from Heart-Heat and Lung-Heat, such as fear, mental restlessness, anger, manic behavior and fright.

> **SUMMARY**
>
> **Lung channel points for emotional problems**
>
> - The Lungs are affected by sadness, worry and grief and many of its points treat these emotions
> - The Lungs govern Qi and its points can bring pure Qi to the Brain and therefore clear the Mind.

LU-3 Tianfu **Heavenly Palace**

LU-3 opens the Mind's orifices and soothes the Corporeal Soul (*Po*). Among its indications are somnolence, insomnia, sadness, weeping, forgetfulness and "talking to ghosts".

LU-7 Lieque **Branching Cleft**

LU-7 settles and opens up the Corporeal Soul. Among its indications are poor memory, palpitations, propensity to (inappropriate) laughter and frequent yawning. This is a very important point from the psychological and emotional point of view that can be used in emotional problems caused by worry, grief or sadness.

LU-10 Yuji **Fish Border**

LU-10 calms the Mind and is generally used when the Mind, Corporeal Soul and Ethereal Soul are agitated by Heat. Among its indications are sadness, fear, mental restlessness, anger, manic behavior and fright.

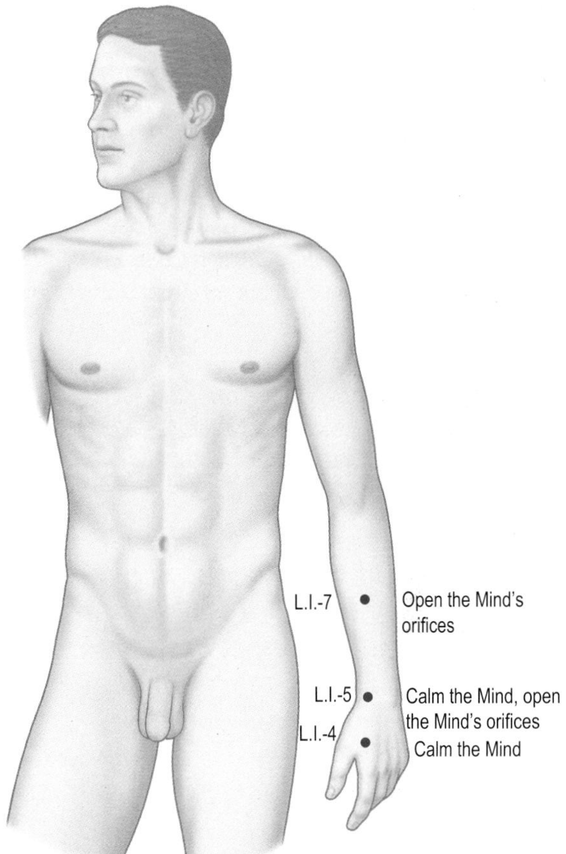

Figure 13.2 Large Intestine channel points.

LARGE INTESTINE CHANNEL

The Large Intestine channel points for emotional problems are illustrated in Figure 13.2.

L.I.-4 Hegu *Enclosed Valley*

L.I.-4 calms the Mind and subdues rebellious Qi from the head. Combined with LIV-3 Taichong (the "Four Gates"), L.I.-4 calms the Mind and settles the Ethereal Soul.

In my experience, L.I.-4 has a strong calming influence on the Mind and can be used to soothe the Mind and allay anxiety, particularly if combined with LIV-3 Taichong and with Du-24 Shenting and G.B.-13 Benshen.

L.I.-4 also promotes the descending of Qi from the head; this action is reinforced if L.I.-4 is combined with LU-7 Lieque. As these two points promote the descending of Qi from the head, this combination is widely used to treat headaches. From an emotional point of view, the combination of L.I.-4 and LU-7 calms the Mind and settles the Corporeal Soul by promoting the descending of Qi.

L.I.-5 Yangxi *Yang Stream*

L.I.-5 calms the Mind and opens the Mind's orifices. Among its indications are manic behavior, propensity to (inappropriate) laughter, "seeing ghosts" and fright.

The *Gatherings from Eminent Acupuncturists* (1529) lists "manic talking, inappropriate laughter and seeing ghosts" among the indications for L.I.-5.[8]

This point calms the Mind and opens the Mind's orifices when there is Fire in the Bright Yang causing manic behavior, propensity to (inappropriate) laughter and fright. It is appropriate to treat such manic behavior deriving from Fire in the Stomach and Large Intestine.

L.I.-7 Wenliu *Warm Gathering*

L.I.-7 opens the Mind's orifices. Among its indications are "inappropriate laughter, manic behavior and seeing ghosts".[9] Similarly to L.I.-5 Yangxi, L.I.-7 can be used to treat manic behavior occurring against a background of Fire in the Stomach and Large Intestine.

As mentioned before, whenever ancient books mention "seeing ghosts" or "talking to ghosts", it usually means that the point is indicated in serious mental conditions such as psychosis.

The *Great Compendium of Acupuncture* (1601) lists among the indications "inappropriate laughter, incoherent speech and seeing ghosts".[10]

SUMMARY

Large Intestine channel points for emotional problems

- Most Large Intestine points for emotional problems are used for Heat patterns.
- L.I.-4 calms the Mind.

L.I.-4 Hegu Enclosed Valley

L.I.-4 calms the Mind and subdues rebellious Qi from the head. Particularly effective if combined with LIV-3 Taichong and with Du-24 Shenting and G.B.-13 Benshen.

L.I.-5 Yangxi Yang Stream

L.I.-5 calms the Mind and opens the Mind's orifices when there is Heat in the Bright Yang. Among its indications are manic behavior, propensity to (inappropriate) laughter, "seeing ghosts" and fright.

L.I.-7 Wenliu Warm Gathering

L.I.-7 opens the Mind's orifices. Among its indications are inappropriate laughter, manic behavior and "seeing ghosts". Similarly to L.I.-5 Yangxi, L.I.-7 can be used to treat manic behavior occurring against a background of Heat in the Stomach and Large Intestine.

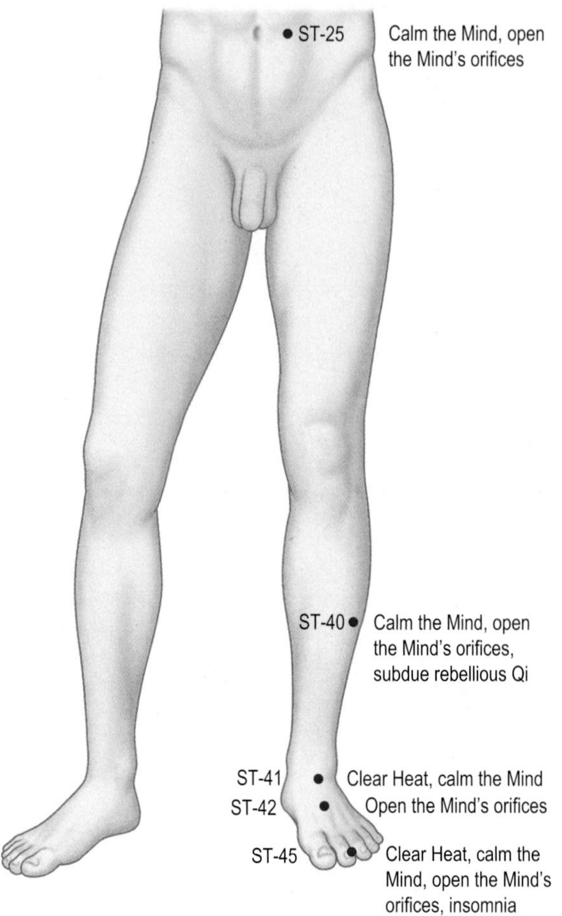

Figure 13.3 Stomach channel points.

STOMACH CHANNEL

The Stomach channel points for emotional problems are illustrated in Figure 13.3.

ST-25 Tianshu *Heavenly Pivot*

ST-25 calms the Mind and opens the Mind's orifices. From a psychological point of view, it is effective in mental restlessness, anxiety, schizophrenia and mania, when these are due to a Stomach disharmony, particularly Full patterns of the Stomach such as Phlegm-Fire in the Stomach.

The *Gatherings from Eminent Acupuncturists* (1529) lists "manic talking", among the indications for ST-25.[11]

The Qing dynasty's *An Explanation of the Acupuncture Points* reports Sun Si Miao as saying that ST-25 is the abode of the Corporeal Soul and Ethereal Soul; this would explain the mental effect of this point that is actually not reported by modern books.[12] It is interesting that Sun Si Miao considers ST-25 to be the abode of both the Ethereal Soul and Corporeal Soul. There may be various reasons why ST-25 would be the abode of the Ethereal Soul: it is on the lower abdomen where the Essence resides and close to the extra point Hunshe

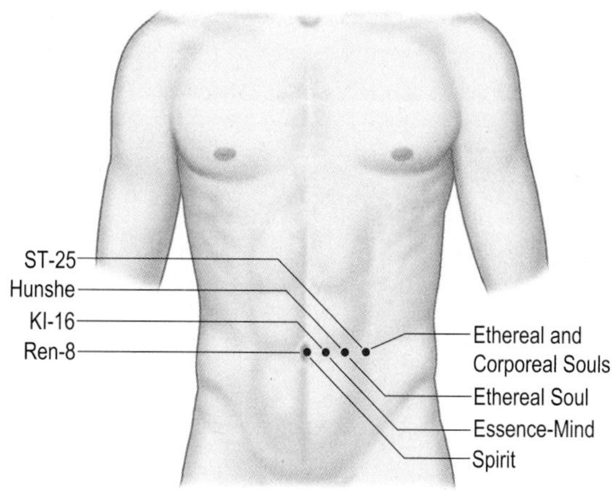

Figure 13.4 Points level with the umbilicus and spiritual aspects.

(level with the umbilicus and 1 *cun* lateral to it) and Ren-8 where the Ethereal Soul and Spirit reside. On a physical level, the Stomach is the root of the Postnatal Essence that nourishes the body; for this reason, it is close to the Corporeal Soul.

It is interesting that several points that are aligned with the umbilicus (or in the umbilicus itself) have a profound effect on the Mind and the Ethereal Soul, i.e. Ren-8 Shenque (see below), KI-16 Huangshu (see below), Hunshe extra point (see below) and ST-25 Tianshu.

Thus, Ren-8 is the abode of the Spirit, KI-16 connects the Essence (Kidneys) with the Mind (Heart), Hunshe is the abode of the Ethereal Soul and ST-25 is the abode of Ethereal Soul and Corporeal Soul (Fig. 13.4).

ST-40 Fenglong *Abundant Bulge*

ST-40 calms the Mind and opens the Mind's orifices. Among its indications are:[13]

"*Dullness and Mania*" [*Dian Kuang*], *inappropriate laughter, inappropriate elation, desire to ascend to high places and sing, undress and run around, mental restlessness, and seeing ghosts.*

The *Gatherings from Eminent Acupuncturists* (1529) lists similar indications: "*Ascends to high places, sings and discards clothes, seeing ghosts, inappropriate laughter.*"[14] It also says: "*In Full conditions,* [ST-40 is for] *Dullness and Mania (Dian Kuang).*"[15]

This point calms the Mind and opens the Mind's orifices. It can be used in all cases of anxiety, fears and phobias, not only if they are caused by misting of the Mind by Phlegm but also if they are caused by rebellious Qi.

In my opinion, the Phlegm-resolving action of this point is overemphasized. ST-40 has many other important actions apart from its Phlegm-resolving one. Moreover, the Phlegm-resolving effect of ST-40 is specific for Phlegm clouding the Mind. From the mental-emotional point of view, ST-40 has a strong "calming the Mind" action. I use this point very frequently to calm the Mind (whether there is Phlegm or not) in anxiety, insomnia, worry or mental restlessness. Interestingly, the very first indication listed by the *Gatherings from Eminent Acupuncturists* for ST-40 is "rebellious Qi".[16]

ST-40 also subdues rebellious Qi rising up the abdomen, chest and throat. In the mental-emotional sphere, rebellious Qi causes anxiety and panic attacks. This point calms the Mind when this is agitated by rebellious Qi; this also includes rebellious Qi of the Penetrating Vessel.

ST-41 Jiexi *Dispersing Stream*

ST-41 clears Heat and calms the Mind. Among its indications are "manic behavior, agitation, weeping, fright and 'seeing ghosts'". It calms the Mind and conducts Heat downwards away from the head. The *Explanation of Acupuncture Points* (1654) lists "mental restlessness and sadness" among the indications for ST-41.[17]

ST-42 Chongyang *Penetrating Yang*

ST-42 opens the Mind's orifices. Among its indications are "manic-depression, desire to ascend to high places and sing, discarding clothes and running around". This point opens the Mind's orifices and is used for mental illness occurring against a background of Phlegm obstructing the Mind and Heat in the Stomach and Large Intestine agitating the Mind.

ST-45 Lidui *Sick mouth*

ST-45 clears Stomach-Heat, calms the Mind and opens the Mind's orifices. Among its indications are "excessive dreaming, fright, insomnia, dizziness, Dullness and Mania, desire to ascend to high places, sing, discard clothes and run around".[18]

This point is frequently used to calm the Mind when this is disturbed in the context of a Stomach-Heat pattern, such as Stomach-Fire being transmitted to the Heart and giving rise to Heart-Fire. The use of this point can, at the same time, sedate the Stomach, calm the Mind and open the Mind's orifices. In this context, it is often used for insomnia.

One particular use of this point is to drain Heart-Fire, in which case it is used with direct moxa cones.

SUMMARY

Stomach channel points for emotional problems

- Many Stomach points for mental-emotional indications are used in the presence of Heat patterns.
- ST-40 is the most important point to calm the Mind and open the Mind's orifices.

ST-25 Tianshu Heavenly Pivot

ST-25 calms the Mind and opens the Mind's orifices. Effective for mental restlessness, anxiety, schizophrenia and mania, when these are due to a Stomach disharmony, particularly Excess patterns of the Stomach such as Phlegm-Fire in the Stomach.

ST-40 Fenglong Abundant Bulge

ST-40 calms the Mind and opens the Mind's orifices. Among its indications are "manic-depression, inappropriate laughter, inappropriate elation, desire to ascend to high places and sing, undress and run around, mental restlessness, and seeing ghosts".

ST-41 Jiexi Dispersing Stream

ST-41 clears Heat and calms the Mind. Among its indications are "manic behavior, agitation, weeping, fright and 'seeing ghosts' ". It calms the Mind and conducts Heat downwards away from the head.

ST-42 Chongyang Penetrating Yang

ST-42 opens the Mind's orifices. Among its indications are "manic-depression, desire to ascend to high places and sing, discard clothes and run around". This point opens the Mind's orifices and is used for mental illness occurring against a background of Phlegm obstructing the Mind and Heat in the Stomach and Large Intestine agitating the Mind.

ST-45 Lidui Sick mouth

ST-45 clears Stomach-Heat, calms the Mind and opens the Mind's orifices. Among its indications are "excessive dreaming, fright, insomnia, dizziness, Dullness and Mania, desire to ascend high places, sing, discard clothes and run around".

SPLEEN CHANNEL

The Spleen channel points for emotional problems are illustrated in Figure 13.5.

SP-1 Yinbai *Hidden White*

One of Sun Si Miao's 13 Ghost points, SP-1 calms the Mind. Among its indications are "agitation, sighing, sadness, manic-depression, excessive dreaming and insomnia".

This point is used for mental restlessness and depression in Excess patterns, resulting from stasis of Blood. In such conditions it calms the Mind and stops excessive dreaming.

SP-3 Taibai *Supreme White*

In my experience, SP-3 stimulates the Intellect (*Yi*) housed in the Spleen. It can therefore be used for poor memory, confused thinking, muzziness of the head and difficulty in concentrating.

SP-3 stimulates the mental faculties pertaining to the Intellect (*Yi*) that are associated with the Spleen and it can be used in cases when Spleen-Qi has been weakened by excessive mental work. The use of SP-3 can then stimulate the brain, promote memory and induce mental clarity. This point is useful to stimulate mental powers in patients suffering from post-viral, chronic fatigue syndrome.

Although the above symptoms are not mentioned in Chinese books, the Qing dynasty's *An Explanation of the Acupuncture Points* does say that SP-3 can treat both the Spleen and the Heart (and therefore Intellect and Mind).[19]

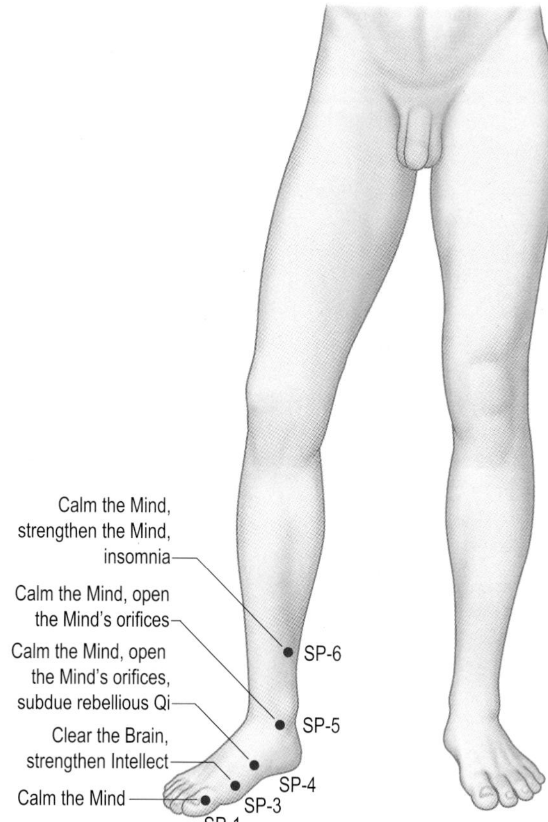

Figure 13.5 Spleen channel points.

SP-4 Gongsun *Minute Connecting Channels*

SP-4 calms the Mind and opens the Mind's orifices. Among its indications are "Dullness and Mania, anxiety, insomnia, and mental restlessness with chest pain".[20]

The *Gatherings from Eminent Acupuncturists* (1529) lists "mental restlessness and manic talking" among the indications from SP-4.[21]

The Penetrating Vessel (*Chong Mai*) goes through the heart and its syndrome of rebellious Qi affects the Heart and Mind; for this reason, this point can be used for anxiety, mental restlessness, chest tightness and pain, and insomnia. It is therefore specific for the anxiety occurring against a background of rebellious Qi of the Penetrating Vessel.

SP-5 Shangqiu *Metal Mound*

SP-5 calms the Mind and opens the Mind's orifices. Among its indications are "manic-depression, agitation, excessive pensiveness, inappropriate laughter, nightmares and melancholy".

Although this point is not frequently mentioned in the context of mental-emotional problems, it does have a powerful effect in calming the Mind and opening the Mind's orifices.

SP-5 is a River (*Jing*) point and, interestingly, many such points seem to have a strong mental-emotional effect (e.g. L.I.-5 Yangxi, S.I.-5 Yanggu, ST-41 Jiexi, etc.).

SP-6 Sanyinjiao *Three Yin Meeting*

SP-6 moves Liver-Qi and calms the Mind. Among its indications are "palpitations, insomnia and Gall-Bladder deficiency timidity".

From the emotional point of view, it helps to smooth Liver-Qi, thus calming the Mind, settling the Ethereal Soul and allaying irritability. SP-6 has a strong calming action on the Mind, and is often used for insomnia, particularly if from Blood or Yin deficiency.

In particular, it is used for Spleen- and Heart- Blood deficiency. When the Spleen is not making enough Blood, the Heart is not supplied with enough Blood and the Mind lacks residence and floats at night, so that insomnia ensues. SP-6 is the point to use in this case, as it will simultaneously tonify the Spleen, nourish Blood and calm the Mind.

Therefore, SP-6 affects the Mind and the Ethereal Soul in two major ways: on the one hand, it can promote the free flow of Qi and therefore the "movement" of the Ethereal Soul, the lack of which makes a person depressed; on the other hand, SP-6 nourishes Blood and it treats anxiety and insomnia from Heart-, Spleen- and Liver-Blood deficiency.

SUMMARY

Spleen channel points for emotional problems

- Spleen channel points can clear the Mind and stimulate the Intellect (*Yi*).
- SP-3 is the best point to stimulate the Intellect.
- SP-6 is the best point to calm and nourish the Mind.

SP-1 Yinbai Hidden White

One of Sun Si Miao's 13 Ghost points, SP-1 calms the Mind. Among its indications are "agitation, sighing, sadness, manic-depression, excessive dreaming and insomnia".

SP-3 Taibai Supreme White

SP-3 stimulates the Intellect (*Yi*) housed in the Spleen. It can therefore be used for poor memory, confused thinking, muzziness of the head and difficulty in concentrating. Useful to stimulate mental powers in patients suffering from post-viral, chronic fatigue syndrome.

SP-4 Gongsun Minute Connecting Channels

SP-4 calms the Mind and opens the Mind's orifices. Among its indications are "manic-depression, anxiety, insomnia and mental restlessness with chest pain". For anxiety occurring against a background of rebellious Qi of the Penetrating Vessel.

SP-5 Shangqiu Metal Mound

SP-5 calms the Mind and opens the Mind's orifices. Among its indications are "manic-depression, agitation, excessive pensiveness, inappropriate laughter, nightmares and melancholy".

SP-6 Sanyinjiao Three Yin Meeting

SP-6 moves Liver-Qi and calms the Mind. Among its indications are "palpitations, insomnia and Gall-Bladder deficiency timidity". From the emotional point of view, it helps to smooth Liver-Qi to calm the Mind and allay irritability. SP-6 has a strong calming action on the Mind, and is often used for insomnia, particularly if from Blood or Yin deficiency.

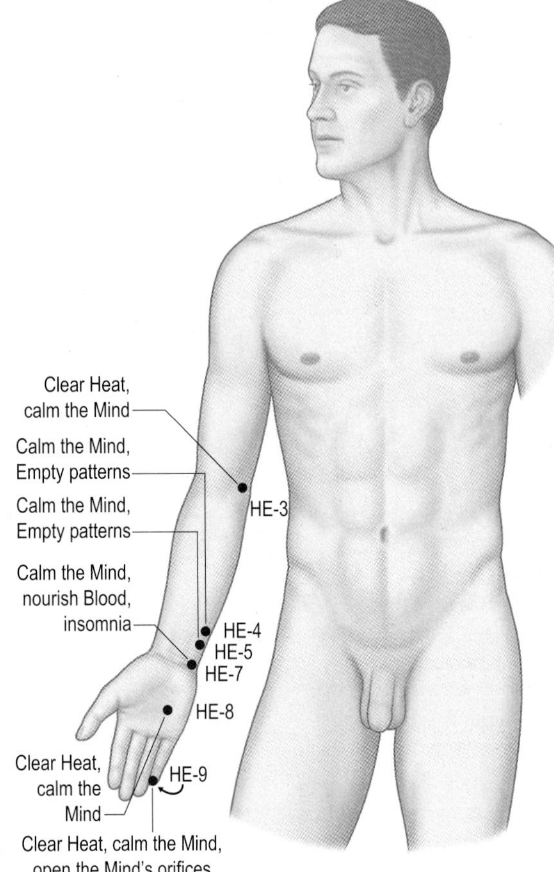

Figure 13.6 Heart channel points.

HEART CHANNEL

The Heart channel points for emotional problems are illustrated in Figure 13.6.

Obviously all points of the Heart channel affect the Mind in one way or another: some are better to nourish the Mind in Deficiency patterns (e.g. HE-7 Shenmen), some are better to calm the Mind in Full patterns (e.g. HE-8 Shaofu) and others are better to open the Mind's orifices (e.g. HE-9 Shaochong).

I shall list below the points I use most frequently.

HE-3 Shaohai *Lesser-Yin Sea*

HE-3 clears Heat and calms the Mind. Among its indications are "manic behavior, inappropriate laughter, mental restlessness and anxiety".

This point is used mostly to drain Heart-Fire or clear Heart Empty Heat. It has an important calming action on the mental level (by clearing Heart-Fire), and is indicated for anxiety and mental restlessness.

HE-4 Lingdao *Spirit Path*

HE-4, a River (*Jing*) point, calms the Mind and is used especially in Empty patterns of the Heart. Among its indications are "sadness, fear, anxiety and mental restlessness".

The Qing dynasty's *An Explanation of the Acupuncture Points* confirms that this point is used primarily for Empty patterns when it says that HE-4 is used for "*sadness and fear from Heart-Qi deficiency*".[22]

HE-5 Tongli *Inner Communication*

HE-5 calms the Mind, especially in Empty patterns of the Heart. Among its indications are "sadness, mental restlessness, anger, fright, depression and agitation". I use this point frequently to tonify Heart-Qi in mental-emotional problems, and especially depression.

Being a Connecting (*Luo*) point, this point has a dynamic effect; as such it can stimulate the movement of the Ethereal Soul when one is depressed.

HE-7 Shenmen *Mind Door*

HE-7 nourishes Heart-Blood, calms the Mind and opens the Mind's orifices. Among its indications are "insomnia, poor memory, Dullness and Mania, inappropriate laughter, shouting at people, sadness, fear, mental restlessness, agitation and palpitations".

The *Great Compendium of Acupuncture* (1601) lists "inappropriate laughter and mental retardation" among the indications for this point.[23]

An Explanation of Acupuncture Points (1654) lists "manic behavior, sadness, inappropriate laughter, poor memory and fear" among the indications for HE-7.[24] The *Gatherings from Eminent Acupuncturists* lists "mania, inappropriate laughter and sadness" among the indications for this point.[25]

HE-7 can be used in virtually any Heart pattern in order to calm the Mind, which is its main action. However, in my opinion, it primarily nourishes Heart-Blood and is the point of choice for Heart-Blood deficiency causing the Mind to be deprived of its "residence", resulting in anxiety, insomnia, poor memory, palpitations and a Pale tongue.

In my experience, it is a "gentle" point and therefore not the choice point in Full patterns of the Heart (although the classic indications do suggest that it can be used in Full mental-emotional patterns), for which other points would be better indicated (such as P-5 Jianshi or HE-8 Shaofu). It is, however, the best point to calm the Mind when there is great anxiety and worrying under stressful situations.

As the Heart is the residence for the Mind, which in Chinese medicine includes mental activity, thinking, memory and consciousness, this point has an effect not only on emotional problems such as anxiety, but also on memory and mental capacity. In fact, this point can be used for mental retardation in children.[26]

HE-7 is a good point to use in the syndrome of Gall-Bladder Qi deficiency manifesting with timidity, fearfulness, indecision and depression; for this syndrome I use HE-7 with G.B.-40 Qiuxu.

Interestingly, the ancient classics do not always stress the use of this point for emotional or mental problems. For example, the *ABC of Acupuncture* (*Zhen Jiu Jia Yi Jing*, AD 282) by Huang Fu Mi, says only that this point is used for cold hands, vomiting of blood and rebellious Qi.[27] The *Thousand Ducat Prescriptions* (*Qian Jin Yao Fang*, AD 652) by Sun Si Miao, says that this point can be used for contraction of the arm.[28]

A comparison between the functions of HE-7 and P-7 Daling is given below under the latter point.

HE-8 Shaofu *Lesser-Yin Mansion*

HE-8 drains Heart-Fire and clears Heart Empty Heat. It calms the Mind, and among its indications are "palpitations, sadness, worry, chest pain, agitation and mental restlessness".

HE-8 Shaofu is a stronger point than HE-7 Shenmen. Its main action is to clear Heat in the Heart, whether it is Full Heat, Empty Heat or Heat with Phlegm. Its main range of action is therefore mental-emotional problems occurring against a background of Full patterns of the Heart. The main symptoms would be insomnia with restless dreams, mental restlessness or manic behavior.

HE-9 Shaochong *Lesser-Yin Penetrating*

HE-9 clears Heat, calms the Mind and opens the Mind's orifices. Among its indications are "manic-depression, fright, sadness, agitation and mental restlessness".

HE-9 Shaochong is mostly used in Excess patterns with Heat in the Heart. It is similar in action to HE-8 Shaofu in so far as it clears Heat.

Table 13.1 compares and contrasts the Heart channel points.

Table 13.1 Comparison of emotional effect of Heart channel points

POINT	PATTERN	SYMPTOMS
HE-3 Shaohai	Heat	Anxiety, insomnia
HE-4 Lingdao	Deficiency	Sadness, fear, depression
HE-5 Tongli	Deficiency	Depression, sadness
HE-7 Shenmen	Deficiency of Blood	Insomnia, depression
HE-8 Shaofu	Heat	Anxiety, mental restlessness, insomnia
HE-9 Shaochong	Phlegm, Heat	Agitation, mental restlessness, manic behavior

SUMMARY

Heart channel points for emotional problems

- All Heart channel points affect the Mind.
- HE-4, HE-5 and HE-7: better to nourish the Mind in Deficiency patterns.
- HE-8 and HE-9: better to calm the Mind in Full patterns.

HE-3 Shaohai Lesser-Yin Sea

HE-3 clears Heat and calms the Mind. Among its indications are "manic behavior, inappropriate laughter, mental restlessness and anxiety". This point is used mostly to drain Heart-Fire or clear Heart Empty Heat.

HE-4 Lingdao Spirit Path

HE-4 calms the Mind and is used especially in Empty patterns of the Heart. Among its indications are "sadness, fear, anxiety and mental restlessness".

HE-5 Tongli Inner Communication

HE-5 calms the Mind, especially in Empty patterns of the Heart. Among its indications are "sadness, mental restlessness, anger, fright, depression and agitation".

HE-7 Shenmen Mind Door

HE-7 nourishes Heart-Blood, calms the Mind and opens the Mind's orifices. Among its indications are "insomnia, poor memory, manic-depression, inappropriate laughter, shouting at people, sadness, fear, mental restlessness, agitation and palpitations".

HE-8 Shaofu Lesser-Yin Mansion

HE-8 drains Heart-Fire and clears Heart Empty Heat. It calms the Mind and among its indications are "palpitations, sadness, worry, chest pain, agitation and mental restlessness".

HE-9 Shaochong Lesser-Yin Penetrating

HE-9 clears Heat, calms the Mind and opens the Mind's orifices. Among its indications are "manic-depression, fright, sadness, agitation and mental restlessness". HE-9 Shaochong is mostly used in Excess patterns with Heat in the Heart.

SMALL INTESTINE CHANNEL

The Small Intestine channel points for emotional problems are illustrated in Figure 13.7.

S.I.-5 Yanggu *Yang Valley*

S.I.-5 clears Heat and calms the Mind. Its indications include "manic behavior". Although Chinese books indicate "manic behavior" as this point's chief mental symptom, in my experience S.I.-5 is very useful to "clear the Mind". It helps the person to gain mental clarity and distinguish the right path to take amongst several. It can help a person at difficult times to distinguish what is right to do at a particular moment in life.

Both the *Great Compendium of Acupuncture* (1601)[29] and the *Explanation of Acupuncture Points* (1654)[30] list

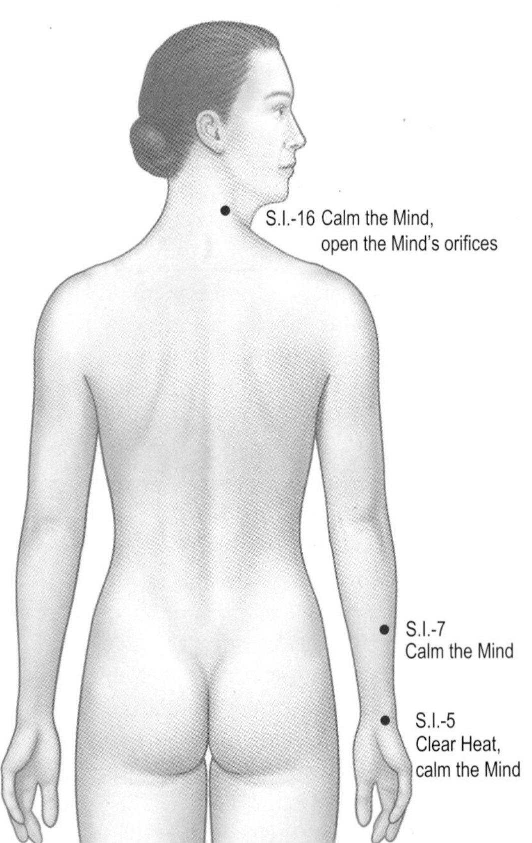

Figure 13.7 Small Intestine channel points.

"Dullness and Mania (*Dian Kuang*) and incoherent speech" among the indications for S.I.-5.

The *Gatherings from Eminent Acupuncturists* also lists "Dullness and Mania (*Dian Kuang*)" among the indications of this point.[31]

S.I.-7 Zhizheng *Branch to Heart Channel*

S.I.-7 calms the Mind and opens the Mind's orifices; among its indications are "Dullness and Mania, fright, sadness, anxiety and mental restlessness".

The *Great Compendium of Acupuncture* (1601) lists "shock, fear, sadness, worry and Dullness and Mania (*Dian Kuang*)" among the indications for S.I.-7.[32] The *Gatherings from Eminent Acupuncturists* lists the same symptoms.[33]

The *Explanation of the Acupuncture Points* (1654) lists "manic behavior, sadness and worry" among the indications for S.I.-7.[34]

Being the Connecting point, it connects with the Heart channel and, because of this connection, it can be used to calm the Mind in severe anxiety and mental restlessness.

S.I.-16 Tianchuang *Heavenly Window*

S.I.-16 calms the Mind and opens the Mind's orifices; among its indications are "manic behavior, Dullness and Mania, and talking with ghosts".[35]

S.I.-16 is one of the Window of Heaven points; as such, it subdues rebellious Qi from the head, it regulates the ascending and descending of Qi to and from the head, and it calms the Mind.

In my experience, this point has an important mental effect, related partly to its being a Small Intestine point and partly to its being a Window of Heaven point. The psychic equivalent of the Small Intestine's physical action of separating clear from turbid fluids is the capacity to discriminate between issues with clarity. As we have seen, S.I.-5 has this particular effect of stimulating the capacity to discriminate between issues. S.I.-16 has the same effect but in an even stronger way due to its nature as a Window of Heaven point. I therefore use this point when the person is confused about life's issues, unable to distinguish the right path and is depressed.

SUMMARY

Small Intestine channel points for emotional problems

- Most important mental-emotional function of Small Intestine channel points is that of stimulating the capacity to discriminate between issues with clarity.

S.I.-5 Yanggu Yang Valley

S.I.-5 clears Heat and calms the Mind. Its indications include "manic behavior". S.I.-5 is very useful to "clear the Mind" in the sense that it helps the person to gain mental clarity and distinguish the right path to take amongst several.

S.I.-7 Zhizheng Branch to Heart Channel

S.I.-7 calms the Mind and opens the Mind's orifices; among its indications are "manic-depression, fright, sadness, anxiety and mental restlessness".

S.I.-16 Tianchuang Heavenly Window

S.I.-16 calms the Mind; among its indications are "manic behavior, manic-depression and talking with ghosts". Stimulates capacity to discriminate between issues with clarity.

BLADDER CHANNEL

The Bladder channel points for emotional problems are illustrated in Figure 13.8.

BL-10 Tianzhu *Heaven Pillar*

BL-10 clears the brain and opens the Mind's orifices. Indications include "mental confusion, difficulty in concentrating and poor memory" and "manic behavior, incessant talking and 'seeing ghosts' ".

Being Yang in nature due to its channel polarity and position, BL-10 treats mental problems from excess of Yang ("incessant talking, seeing ghosts, manic behavior").

As a Window of Heaven point, BL-10 regulates the ascending and descending of Qi to and from the head and subdues rebellious Qi; this is another reason why it can be used for mental-emotional problems characterized by Excess of Yang in the head.

However, BL-10 can also have the opposite action, i.e. promote the ascending of clear Qi to the head to

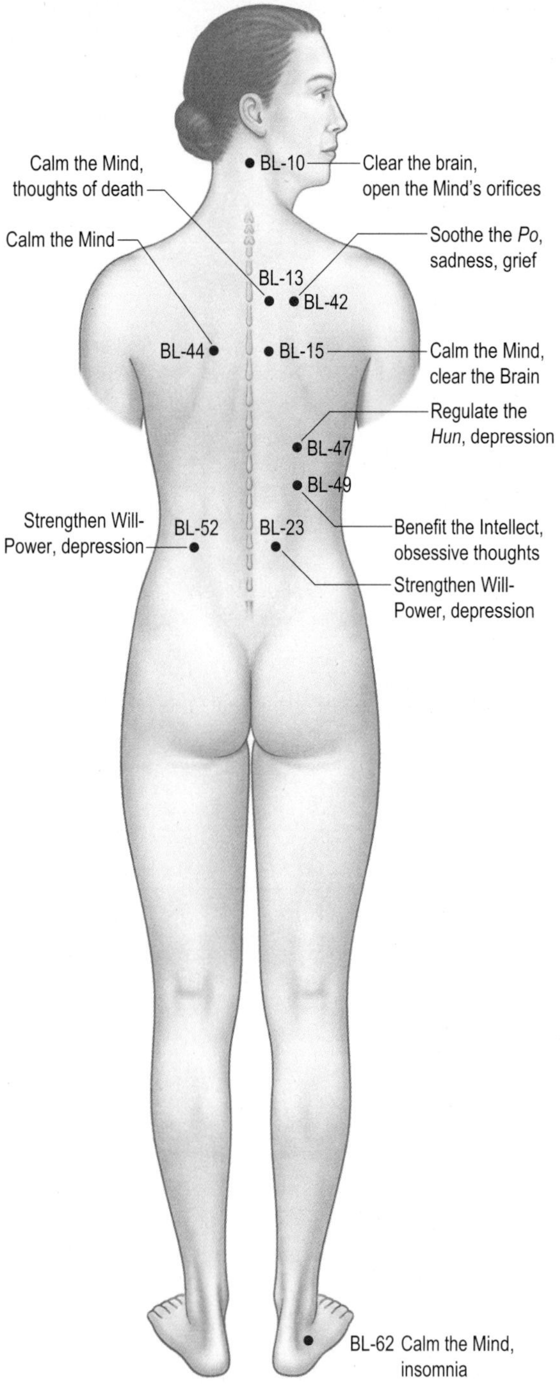

Figure 13.8 Bladder channel points.

treat "mental confusion, difficulty in concentrating and poor memory".

BL-13 Feishu *Lung Back-Transporting Point*

BL-13 calms the Mind. Among its indications are "manic behavior, desire to commit suicide".[36] The *Gatherings from Eminent Acupuncturists* reports the same symptoms.[37]

The indication "desire to commit suicide" must be seen in the context of the Corporeal Soul (*Po*) which is housed in the Lungs. The Corporeal Soul is a physical soul with a centripetal movement, constantly materializing and constantly separating into different constituent aspects. The Corporeal Soul is in relation with *gui,* i.e. ghosts or spirits (of dead people). Confucius said: "*Qi is the fullness of the Mind (Shen); the Corporeal Soul (Po) is the fullness of Gui.*"[38]

The centripetal forces of *gui* within the Corporeal Soul, constantly fragmenting are, eventually, the germ of death. With regard to fragmenting, there is a resonance between *gui* and *kuai* (*gui* with "earth" in front) which means "pieces" (*see Chapter 7*).

Because of the connection between the Corporeal Soul and death, points associated with the Corporeal Soul (such as BL-13 Feishu) are indicated for suicidal thoughts. As we shall see below, the point BL-42 Pohu (that is on the outer Bladder line level with BL-13 Feishu) is also indicated for suicidal thoughts. Du-12 Shenzhu, level with BL-13 and BL-42, has also indications to do with death ("desire to kill people").

BL-15 Xinshu *Heart Back-Transporting Point*

BL-15 calms the Mind, nourishes the Heart and stimulates the Brain. Its indications include "anxiety, weeping, fright, insomnia, excessive dreaming and Dullness and Mania" and "disorientation, delayed speech development, poor memory, poor concentration, mental confusion and Heart-Qi deficiency in children".[39]

The *Gatherings from Eminent Acupuncturists* (1529) reports the symptom of "disorientation from Heart-Qi being scattered" for BL-15.[40]

BL-15 is a very important point for many mental-emotional problems. It calms the Mind and can be used for nervous anxiety and insomnia mostly deriving from Full conditions of the Heart, such as Heart-Fire or Heart Empty Heat. In these cases it is needled with reducing method.

It also calms the Mind by nourishing the Heart and, for this reason, it is used for poor memory and insomnia. At the same time as calming the Mind, it also stimulates the brain if used with reinforcing method or with direct moxibustion. In particular, used with direct moxibustion, it has a good effect in stimulating the brain and is effective for depression, mental confusion and poor concentration in adults and slow development in children.

BL-23 Shenshu *Kidney Back-Transporting Point*

BL-23 does not have any mental-emotional indications in Chinese books, but I use it frequently to strengthen the Will-Power (*Zhi*) in patients who are depressed against a background of Deficiency; when I do so, I usually combine this point with BL-52 Zhishi. In order to strengthen will-power, drive and enthusiasm in depression, I often use these two points even in the absence of Kidney patterns.

BL-42 Pohu *Door of the Corporeal Soul*

BL-42 Pohu is the first of the five points on the outer Bladder line (3 *cun* from the spine), which are level with the five Back-Transporting points of the five Yin organs (Lungs, Heart, Liver, Spleen and Kidneys, in descending order).

Each of the five points on the outer Bladder line corresponds to the spiritual aspect housed in the related Yin organs and take their names from such spiritual aspects, i.e. the Corporeal Soul (*Po*) for the Lungs, the Mind (*Shen*) for the Heart, the Ethereal Soul (*Hun*) for the Liver, the Intellect (*Yi*) for the Spleen and the Will-Power (*Zhi*) for the Kidneys. The names of the points are as follows.

ORGAN	INNER BLADDER LINE	OUTER BLADDER LINE
Lungs	BL-13 Feishu	BL-42 Pohu
Heart	BL-15 Xinshu	BL-44 Shentang
Liver	BL-18 Ganshu	BL-47 Hunmen
Spleen	BL-20 Pishu	BL-49 Yishe
Kidneys	BL-23 Shenshu	BL-52 Zhishi

If we analyze the names of the above five points we get the following pattern (Fig. 13.9).

- BL-42 Pohu (*hu* means "window") = "Window of Po"
- BL-44 Shentang (*tang* means "hall") = "Hall of Shen"
- BL-47 Hunmen (*men* means "door") = "Door of Hun"
- BL-49 Yishe (*she* means "abode") = "Abode of Yi"
- BL-52 Zhishi (*shi* means "room") = "Room of Zhi"

We can detect a pattern as the points correspond to a house – in dreams, an image for the psyche – with the Mind (*Shen*), Will-Power (*Zhi*) and Intellect (*Yi*) corresponding to "hall", "room" and "abode", respectively, and the Ethereal Soul (*Hun*) and Corporeal Soul (*Po*) corresponding to a "door" and "window", respectively.

The images of door and window fit well the nature of the Ethereal Soul and Corporeal Soul, which provide

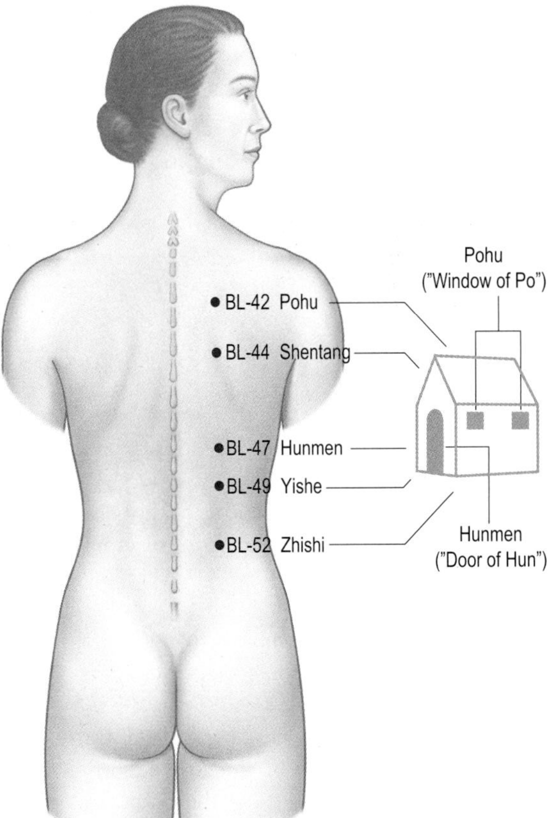

Figure 13.9 The points for the Five Spiritual Aspects on the Bladder channel.

movement to the psyche, the former providing the "coming and going of the Mind" on a psychic level and the latter the "entering and exiting of the Essence" on a physical level.

The correspondence of the Heart to a hall also fits in with old Chinese customs, according to which the hall is the most important room of the house as it is the one that gives the first impression to visitors; for this reason, it was always kept scrupulously clean.

The *Explanation of the Acupuncture Points* confirms the image of a house in the names of these five points (although it makes reference to a "gate" that is not in these points' names and not to the "hall"): "*There is a door, a gate* [hall, tang], *a window, an abode and a room: the image of a house.*"[41]

BL-42 soothes the Corporeal Soul (*Po*) and its indications include "sadness, grief, feeling of oppression of the chest, depression, suicidal thoughts and 'three corpses flowing' ".[42] The *Gatherings from Eminent Acupuncturists* (1529) also includes the symptom of "three corpses flowing" for this point.[43]

On a psychological level, it is related to the Corporeal Soul (*Po*), which is the mental-spiritual aspect residing in the Lungs (*see Chapter 4*). BL-42 strengthens and roots the Corporeal Soul in the Lungs. It frees breathing when the Corporeal Soul is constricted by worry, sadness or grief. It calms the Mind and settles the Corporeal Soul to make the person turn inwards and be comfortable with oneself. It is therefore used for emotional problems related to the Lungs, particularly sadness, grief and worry. It has a very soothing effect on the spirit and it nourishes Qi when this is dispersed by a prolonged period of sadness or grief.

The *Explanation of the Acupuncture Points* reports the interesting indication "three corpses flowing" for this point.[44] The *Great Compendium of Acupuncture* also reports the same symptom.[45] "Three corpses flowing" refers to a Daoist belief in haunting of the body by three female ghosts: a green female ghost attacking the upper part causes eye problems, a white female ghost attacking the center part causes problems in the Internal Organs, and a blood-colored female ghost attacking the lower part of the body causes death.

The association of BL-42 with these three ghosts is interesting as, on the one hand, it confirms the relation between the Corporeal Soul and gui and, on the other hand, it confirms the nature of the Corporeal Soul as the soul of the body.

The association with corpses and death should be interpreted so that this point is indicated for suicidal thought. As we have seen above when discussing the indications for BL-13 Feishu, the Corporeal Soul is associated with *gui* (ghosts, spirits) and with a centripetal movement, eventually ending in death. For this reason, these two points are indicated for suicidal thoughts.

BL-44 Shentang *Mind Hall*

BL-44 calms the Mind. Its indications include "depression, insomnia, anxiety, mental restlessness, sadness, grief and worry".

BL-44 is mostly used for emotional and psychological problems related to the Heart. It is best used in conjunction with BL-15 Xinshu for anxiety, insomnia and depression. BL-44 can also stimulate the Mind's clarity and intelligence.

BL-47 Hunmen *Door of the Ethereal Soul*

BL-47 roots the Ethereal Soul into the Liver, promotes the free flow of Liver-Qi and regulates the "coming and going" of the Ethereal Soul. Its indications include "fear, depression, insomnia, excessive dreaming, lack of sense of direction in life and 'possession by corpse' ".[46]

Interestingly, the very first symptom the *Gatherings from Eminent Acupuncturists* reports is "chronic fevers from Summer-Heat in children due to corpse rebellious flowing".[47]

BL-47 is used for emotional problems related to the Liver, such as depression, frustration and resentment over a long period of time. This point settles and roots the Ethereal Soul in the Liver. It strengthens the Ethereal Soul's capacity of planning, sense of aim in life, life dreams and projects. It is a "door", so this point regulates the "coming and going" of the Ethereal Soul and Mind, i.e. relationships with other people and the world in general. It has an outward movement which could be compared and contrasted with the inward movement of BL-42 Pohu.

The *Explanation of Acupuncture Points* (1654) confirms that, due to this point's nature of "window", "gate" or "door", the Ethereal Soul goes in and out through it. This confirms the dynamic nature of this point in stimulating the movement of the Ethereal Soul and Mind; however, it can also work the other way, i.e. to calm down the excessive movement of the Ethereal Soul when the person is slightly manic.

In my experience, when used in conjunction with BL-18 Ganshu, it has a profound influence on a person's capacity to plan his or her life by rooting and steadying the Ethereal Soul. It can help a person find a sense of direction and purpose in life. This point will also help to lift mental depression associated with such difficulties.

Because it roots the Ethereal Soul, it can be used for a vague feeling of fear occurring at night in persons suffering from severe deficiency of Yin. When used to calm down the excessive movement of the Ethereal Soul, this point can be used for slightly manic behavior and mental confusion.

In depression, BL-47 can stimulate the coming and going of the Ethereal Soul to unblock situations when people feel emotionally "stuck".

The *Explanation of the Acupuncture Points* (1654) points out that BL-47 treats the Liver and Lungs and it should be used when Liver-Qi (or Liver-Yang or Liver-Fire) rebels upwards to invade the Lungs, causing cough and breathlessness.[48] From an emotional point of view, this point can be used when anger affects the Liver and causes its Qi to rebel upwards to the Lungs, causing sadness. Thus, the patient may appear sad, but the root of the problem is in the Liver and in anger. This situation will be reflected on the pulse that will be Wiry on the Liver position and Weak on the Lung position.

BL-49 Yishe *Intellect Abode*

BL-49 benefits the Intellect (*Yi*) and its indications include "poor memory, poor concentration, worry, pensiveness and obsessive thinking".

BL-49 strengthens the Intellect (*Yi*), clears the Mind (*Shen*) and stimulates memory and concentration. It also relieves the Mind and Intellect of obsessive thoughts, brooding, worry and pensiveness. It can also be used for obsessive thoughts that are often related to a Spleen deficiency and are like the pathological correspondent of this organ's mental activity of memorization and concentration.

BL-52 Zhishi *Room of Will-Power*

BL-52 tonifies the Kidneys and strengthens the Will-Power (*Zhi*). Its indications include "depression, lack of motivation, lack of drive, and lack of will-power".

This point strengthens will-power and determination, which are the mental-spiritual phenomena pertaining to the Kidneys. It is a very useful point in the treatment of certain types of depression, when the person lacks motivation, drive, will-power and the mental strength to make an effort to get out of the spiral of depression. Needling this point with reinforcing method, especially if combined with BL-23 Shenshu, will stimulate the will-power and lift the spirit.

BL-52 strengthens will-power, drive, determination, the capacity of pursuing one's goals with single-mindedness, spirit of initiative and steadfastness. I often use this point if there is a Kidney deficiency, in combination with one of the other four points affecting the Spiritual Aspects of the Yin organs, i.e. BL-42 Pohu, BL-44 Shentang, BL-47 Hunmen and BL-49 Yishe, as a solid mental-emotional foundation for the other aspects of the psyche.

The following are some examples of such combinations.

- BL-23 Shenshu, BL-52 Zhishi and BL-47 Hunmen to strengthen will-power and drive, and to instill a sense of direction and aim in one's life. This combination is excellent to treat the mental exhaustion, lack of drive and aimlessness and confusion that is typical of chronic depression.
- BL-23 Shenshu, BL-52 Zhishi and BL-49 Yishe to strengthen will-power and drive, and to empty the Mind (*Shen*) and Intellect (*Yi*) of obsessive thoughts, worries and confused thinking.
- BL-23 Shenshu, BL-52 Zhishi and BL-42 Pohu to strengthen will-power and drive, settle the Corporeal Soul and release emotions constrained in the chest and diaphragm.
- BL-23 Shenshu, BL-52 Zhishi and BL-44 Shentang to strengthen will-power and drive, calm the Mind and relieve anxiety, depression, mental restlessness and insomnia. This combination harmonizes Kidneys and Heart (and therefore Will-Power and Mind) on a mental-emotional level.

BL-62 Shenmai *Ninth Channel*

One of Sun Si Miao's 13 Ghost points, BL-62 calms the Mind. Its indications include "insomnia and manic behavior".

BL-62 can be used in combination with KI-6 Zhaohai for the treatment of insomnia; in which case BL-62 is reduced and KI-6 reinforced, and vice versa for somnolence.

BL-62 is the starting and opening point of the Yang Stepping Vessel (*Yang Qiao Mai*) and one of its pathologies is Excess of Yang in the head; from a mental-emotional perspective, this means that this point can be used in Full patterns causing insomnia, agitation, anxiety and manic behavior.

SUMMARY

Bladder channel points for emotional problems

- The five points on the outer line of the Bladder channel, in line with the Back-Transporting points of the five Yin organs, are very important to treat mental-emotional problems.
- Some Bladder points are for Full conditions (e.g. BL-62 Shenmai) and others for Empty conditions (e.g. BL-23 Shenshu).

BL-10 Tianzhu Heaven Pillar

BL-10 clears the brain and opens the Mind's orifices. Indications include "mental confusion, difficulty in concentrating and poor memory" and "manic behavior, incessant talking and 'seeing ghosts' ".

BL-13 Feishu Lung Back-Transporting Point

BL-13 calms the Mind. Among its indications are "manic behavior, desire to commit suicide".

BL-15 Xinshu Heart Back-Transporting Point

BL-15 calms the Mind, nourishes the Heart and stimulates the Brain. Its indications include "anxiety, weeping, fright, insomnia, excessive dreaming and manic-depression" and "disorientation, delayed speech development, poor memory, poor concentration, mental confusion and Heart-Qi deficiency in children".

BL-23 Shenshu Kidney Back-Transporting Point

Strengthen the Will-Power (*Zhi*) in patients who are depressed against a background of Deficiency; usually combined with BL-52 Zhishi.

BL-42 Pohu Door of the Corporeal Soul

BL-42 soothes the Corporeal Soul (*Po*). Its indications include "sadness, grief, feeling of oppression of the chest, depression, suicidal thoughts, and 'three corpses flowing' ". It strengthens and roots the Corporeal Soul in the Lungs. It frees breathing when the Corporeal Soul is constricted by worry, sadness or grief. It calms the Mind and settles the Corporeal Soul to make the person turn inwards and be comfortable with oneself.

BL-44 Shentang Mind Hall

BL-44 calms the Mind. Its indications include "depression, insomnia, anxiety, mental restlessness, sadness, grief and worry". BL-44 is mostly used for emotional and psychological problems related to the Heart.

BL-47 Hunmen Door of the Ethereal Soul

BL-47 roots the Ethereal Soul into the Liver, promotes the free flow of Liver-Qi and regulates the "coming and going" of the Ethereal Soul. Its indications include "fear, depression, insomnia, excessive dreaming, lack of sense of direction in life and 'possession by corpse' ". BL-47 is used for emotional problems related to the Liver, such as depression, frustration and resentment over a long period of time.

BL-49 Yishe Intellect Abode

BL-49 benefits the Intellect (*Yi*). Its indications include "poor memory, poor concentration, worry, pensiveness and obsessive thinking". BL-49 strengthens the Intellect (*Yi*), clears the Mind (*Shen*) and stimulates memory and concentration.

BL-52 Zhishi Room of Will-Power

BL-52 tonifies the Kidneys and strengthens the Will-Power (*Zhi*). Its indications include "depression, lack of motivation, lack of drive and lack of will-power".

BL-62 Shenmai Ninth Channel

One of Sun Si Miao's 13 Ghost points, BL-62 calms the Mind. Its indications include "insomnia and manic behavior".

KIDNEY CHANNEL

The Kidney channel points for emotional problems are illustrated in Figure 13.10.

KI-1 Yongquan *Bubbling Spring*

KI-1 calms the Mind and settles the Ethereal Soul. Its indications include "agitation, insomnia, poor memory, fear, rage with desire to kill people and manic behavior".

KI-1 has a very strong calming effect on the Mind, and is used in severe anxiety or mental illness such as

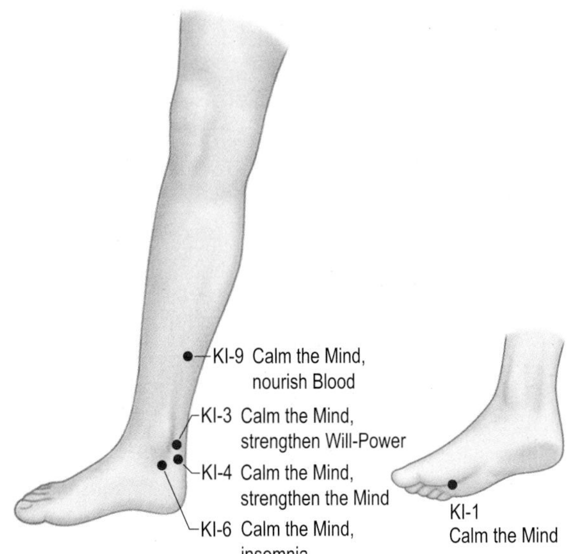

Figure 13.10 Kidney channel points.

manic behavior. Its calming effect is also partially due to its capacity of subduing rebellious Qi from the head.

KI-1 is particularly indicated to treat mental restlessness occurring against a background of Deficiency of Yin with Empty Heat rising to the head.

KI-3 Taixi *Greater Stream*

KI-3 calms the Mind. Its indications include "insomnia, excessive dreaming and poor memory".

KI-3 is an extremely important point used to tonify the Kidneys and strengthen the Will-Power (*Zhi*) in any deficiency pattern of Kidney-Yin or Kidney-Yang. Being the Source point, it is in contact with the Original Qi (*Yuan Qi*) of the Kidney channel, and since the Kidneys are the foundation of all the Qi of the body and the seat of the Original Qi, this point goes straight to the core of the Original Qi. As the Kidneys also store Essence, this point can tonify the Essence, bones and Marrow.

Although some of the indications for KI-3 are the same as for KI-1 (e.g. insomnia), they are used for two very different situations. While KI-1 is used for Empty Heat deriving from Yin deficiency, KI-3 is used to tonify the Kidneys, both Kidney-Yang and Kidney-Yin.

I usually use KI-3 in combination with Ren-4 Guanyuan or BL-23 Shenshu, or both.

KI-4 Dazhong *Big Bell*

KI-4 calms and strengthens the Mind. Its indications include "palpitations, agitation, mental retardation, manic behavior, propensity to anger, somnolence, fright, unhappiness and desire to close doors and remain at home".

KI-4, in common with other Yin Connecting points, has a marked effect on the Mind, and can be used both to calm the Mind and to "lift" the spirit when the person is exhausted and depressed from a chronic Kidney deficiency.

KI-6 Zhaohai *Shining Sea*

KI-6 calms the Mind. Its indications include "insomnia, sadness, fright and nightmares".

By nourishing Yin and carrying Yin up to the head and eyes, KI-6, opening and starting point of the Yin Stepping Vessel (*Yin Qiao Mai*), calms the Mind in cases of anxiety and restlessness deriving from Yin deficiency. Furthermore, it is used to treat insomnia, as its use brings Yin energy to the eyes and makes them close at night.

KI-9 Zhubin *Guest House*

KI-9 calms the Mind and opens the Mind's orifices. Its indications include "anxiety, insomnia, palpitations and manic behavior". The *Great Compendium of Acupuncture* lists "Dullness and Mania (*Dian Kuang*), incoherent speech and angry shouting" among the indications of this point.[49] The *Gatherings from Eminent Acupuncturists* (1529) reports exactly the same symptoms.[50]

The *Explanation of the Acupuncture Points* (1654) lists "Dullness and Mania (*Dian Kuang*), incoherent speech and angry shouting" among the indications of KI-9.[51]

KI-9 is an excellent point to calm the Mind in cases of deep anxiety and mental restlessness deriving from Kidney-Yin deficiency. It has a profound calming effect and it tonifies Kidney-Yin at the same time.

It also relaxes any tension or feeling of oppression felt in the chest, often with palpitations. Because it tonifies Kidney-Yin, calms the Mind and treats palpitations, this point is particularly indicated in the pattern of "Heart and Kidneys not harmonized".

The name of this point ("Guest House") refers precisely to this point's action in connecting Kidneys and Heart, and therefore Essence and Mind (the "guest" is the Heart being received by the Kidneys).

I often use this point, the Accumulation point of the Yin Linking Vessel (*Yin Wei Mai*), with the opening points of this vessel, i.e. P-6 Neiguan and SP-4 Gongsun.

KI-16 Huangshu *Membranes Transporting Point*

KI-16 is related to *Gaohuang*, i.e. the space between the heart and the diaphragm. Kidney Qi goes through this point to connect upwards with the diaphragm and the Heart, hence the name of this point (*Gaohuang* refers to the space between and the heart and the diaphragm). According to the *Explanation of the Acupuncture Points*, KI-16 Huangshu should be seen in connection with BL-17 Geshu.[52]

This point, the Back-Transporting point of the diaphragm, influences the *Gaohuang* region which is above the diaphragm. BL-17 is situated either side of the Governing Vessel (*Du Mai*), which governs all Yang, and KI-16 is either side of the Directing Vessel (*Ren Mai*), which governs all Yin (Fig. 13.11). It is because of the connection between KI-16 and the diaphragm that it can affect both Heart and Lungs. I use KI-16 to calm the Heart and relieve anxiety deriving from rebellious Qi of the Penetrating Vessel.

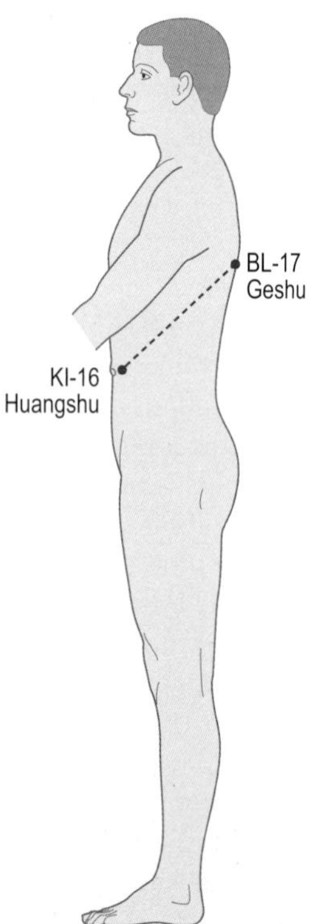

Figure 13.11 Connection between KI-16 and BL-17.

It is worth noting that KI-16 is called *Huangshu*, which means "Transporting point for Huang". *Shu* is a character that refers usually to points on the back of the body, such as in the Back-Transporting (*Shu*) points. The fact that KI-16 is called a *Shu* point would seem to confirm the idea that it is in relation with BL-17 on the back.

Huang in the name of this point refers also to the Membranes (*Huang*). The membranes run inside the abdomen (corresponding to the superficial and deep fascia, mesentery and omentum) and penetrate upwards in the chest and diaphragm. KI-16, being near the umbilicus, controls the origin of Membranes. Because of its connection with the Membranes, I use KI-16 to subdue rebellious Qi of the Penetrating Vessel. Being in the center of the abdomen, this point is in connection with the Membranes extending to the Kidneys below and to the Heart above; because of this, this point can be used to harmonize Kidneys and Heart.

This means that this point can be used to tonify the Kidneys, and, at the same time, tonify the Heart and calm the Mind. It is therefore useful when Kidney-Yin is deficient and fails to nourish the Heart.

KI-16 is a point of the Penetrating Vessel. From a mental-emotional point of view, its most important characteristic is that of connecting the Heart above with the Kidneys below. The Penetrating Vessel originates from the Kidneys and flows past the heart: because of this, this point facilitates the connection between Heart and Kidneys. This characteristic is also due to its being in the middle of the body, thus facilitating the connecting between Above and Below.

KI-16 subdues rebellious Qi of the Penetrating Vessel; this pattern is characterized by a series of symptoms in the abdomen, chest and throat, and a feeling of anxiety. By subduing rebellious Qi, KI-16 calms the Mind and settles the Ethereal Soul.

Moreover, this point is very close to the umbilicus where the Spirit resides; this is an added reason for its influence on the Heart.

SUMMARY

Kidney channel points for emotional problems

- The Kidney channel points are mostly used in two ways in mental-emotional problems: some calm the Mind by bringing Qi down (e.g. KI-1 Yongquan), others lift spirits by tonifying the Kidneys (e.g. KI-3 Taixi).

- Some Kidney points are for Full conditions (e.g. KI-1 Yongquan), others for Empty conditions (e.g. KI-3 Taixi, KI-4 Dazhong, KI-6 Zhaohai, KI-9 Zhubin).

KI-1 Yongquan Bubbling Spring

KI-1 calms the Mind and settles the Ethereal Soul. Its indications include "agitation, insomnia, poor memory, fear, rage with desire to kill people and manic behavior". KI-1 is particularly indicated to treat mental restlessness occurring against a background of Deficiency of Yin with Empty Heat rising to the head.

KI-3 Taixi Greater Stream

KI-3 calms the Mind. Its indications include "insomnia, excessive dreaming and poor memory". KI-3 is an extremely important point used to tonify the Kidneys and strengthen the Will-Power (*Zhi*) in any deficiency pattern of Kidney-Yin or Kidney-Yang.

KI-4 Dazhong Big Bell

KI-4 calms and lifts the Mind. Its indications include "palpitations, agitation, mental retardation, manic behavior, propensity to anger, somnolence, fright, unhappiness and desire to close doors and remain at home".

KI-6 Zhaohai Shining Sea

KI-6 calms the Mind. Its indications include "insomnia, sadness, fright and nightmares". By nourishing Yin and carrying Yin up to the head and eyes, KI-6, opening and starting point of the Yin Stepping Vessel (*Yin Qiao Mai*), calms the Mind in cases of anxiety and insomnia deriving from Yin deficiency.

KI-9 Zhubin Guest House

KI-9 calms the Mind and opens the Mind's orifices. Its indications include "anxiety, insomnia, palpitations and manic behavior". KI-9 is an excellent point to calm the Mind in cases of deep anxiety and mental restlessness deriving from Kidney-Yin deficiency. It has a profound calming effect and it tonifies Kidney-Yin at the same time.

KI-16 Huangshu Membranes Transporting Point

KI-16 is connected to the diaphragm and it affects both Heart and Lungs. I use KI-16 to calm the Heart and relieve anxiety deriving from rebellious Qi of the Penetrating Vessel.

Being in the center of the abdomen, this point is in connection with the Membranes extending to the Kidneys below and to the Heart above; because of this, this point can be used to harmonize Kidneys and Heart. This means that this point can be used to tonify the Kidneys, and, at the same time, tonify the Heart and calm the Mind. It is therefore useful when Kidney-Yin is deficient and fails to nourish the Heart.

By subduing rebellious Qi, KI-16 calms the Mind and settles the Ethereal Soul.

PERICARDIUM CHANNEL

The Pericardium channel points for emotional problems are illustrated in Figure 13.12.

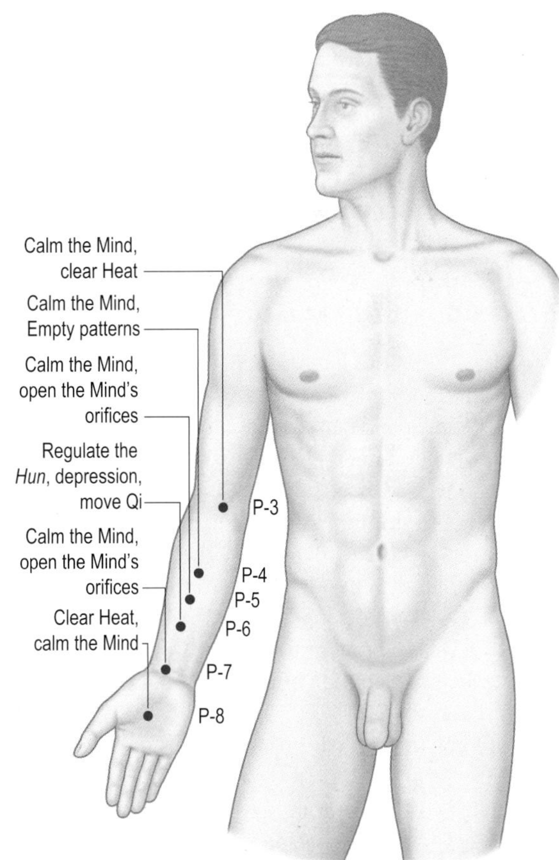

Figure 13.12 Pericardium channel points.

P-3 Quze *Marsh on Bend*

P-3 calms the Mind. Its indications include "fright, anxiety and mental restlessness".

P-3 calms the Mind when there is severe anxiety caused by Heart-Fire.

P-4 Ximen *Cleft Door*

P-4 calms the Mind. Its indications include "agitation, anxiety, insomnia, mental restlessness, depression and fright".

P-4 strengthens the Mind in cases of Heart deficiency, which may give rise to fear, anxiety, insomnia and depression.

P-5 Jianshi *Intermediary*

P-5 calms the Mind, opens the Mind's orifices and resolves Phlegm in the Heart. Its indications include "palpitations, agitation, feeling of oppression of the chest, manic behavior, fright, mental restlessness, poor memory and 'seeing ghosts'".

P-5 is a very important point to resolve Phlegm obstructing the Mind's orifices. This is non-substantial Phlegm obstructing the Heart and "misting" the mental faculties. In chronic cases, Phlegm obstructing the Heart can cause mental illness, such as manic-depression, with periods of deep depression alternating with periods of manic behavior with incessant talking, uncontrolled activity and reckless behavior.

P-6 Neiguan *Inner Gate*

P-6 calms the Mind, lifts the spirit, promotes the free flow of Liver-Qi and stimulates the movement of the Ethereal Soul. Its indications include "insomnia, manic behavior, poor memory, anxiety, fright, sadness and depression".

The Pericardium function on the mental-emotional plane is the psychic equivalent of the function of the Pericardium in the chest with regard to moving Qi and Blood of Heart and Lungs; just as it does that on a physical level, on a mental-emotional level, the Pericardium is responsible for "movement" towards others, i.e. in relationships.

Given that the Pericardium is related to the Liver within the Terminal-Yin channels, this "movement" is also related to the "movement" of the Ethereal Soul from the ego towards others in social relationships and familial interactions. For this reason, on a mental-emotional level, the Pericardium is particularly responsible for a healthy interaction with other people in social, love and family relationships (Fig. 13.13).

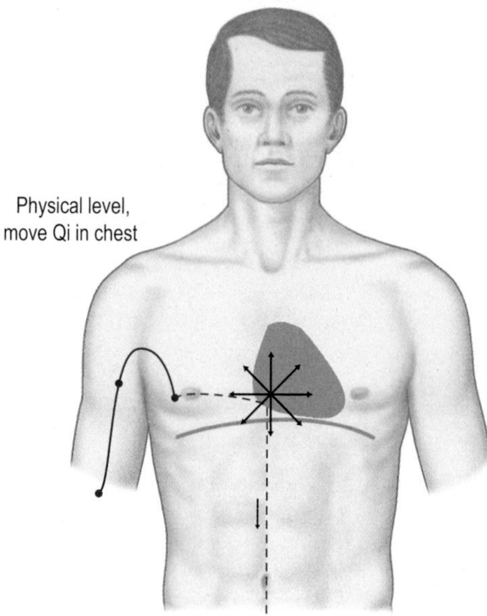

Figure 13.13 Physical and emotional effect of P-6 Neiguan.

Moreover, the "moving" nature of the Pericardium is also enhanced by its relationship with the Triple Burner as a channel (within the "Minister Fire" channels). As the Triple Burner is responsible for the free flow of Qi (together with the Liver), the Pericardium's relationship with the Triple Burner accounts for its action in moving Qi and Blood, and its mental-emotional function of "movement" towards others (Fig. 13.14).

From a Five-Element perspective, the Pericardium pertains to the Minister Fire (with the Triple Burner), compared to the Emperor Fire of the Heart, while from the perspective of the Internal Organs, the Minister Fire is the Fire of the Gate of Life (*Ming Men*) pertaining to the Kidneys (Figs 13.15, 13.16 and 13.17). However, there is a connection between the two views as the Minister Fire does flow up to the Liver, Gall-Bladder and Pericardium. In pathology, this has an even greater relevance as the pathological Minister Fire (driven by emotional stress) flares upwards to harass the Pericardium, causing mental restlessness, agitation, anxiety and insomnia.

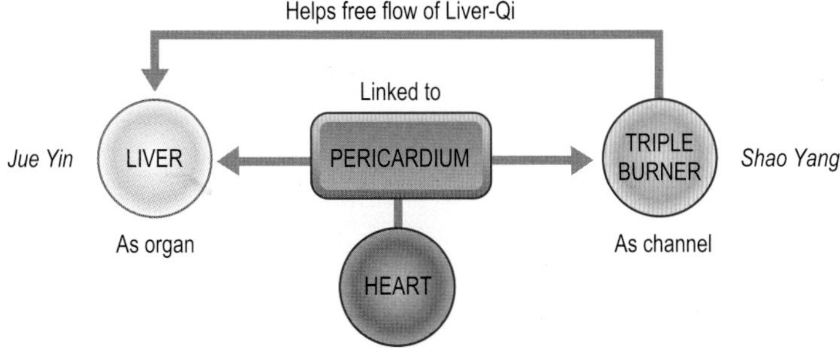

Figure 13.14 Connection of Pericardium with Liver and Triple Burner.

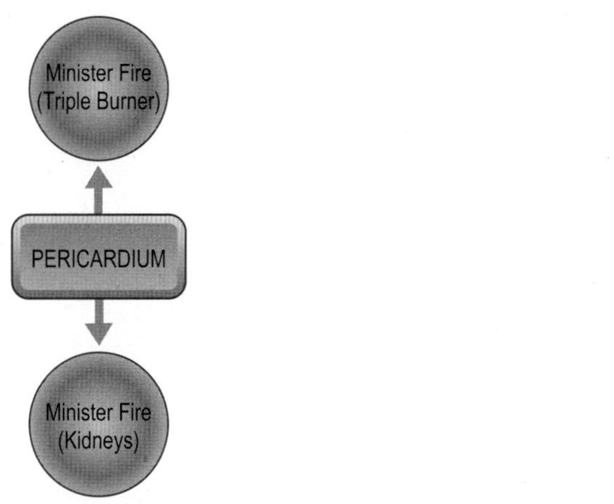

Figure 13.15 Connection of Pericardium with Minister Fire.

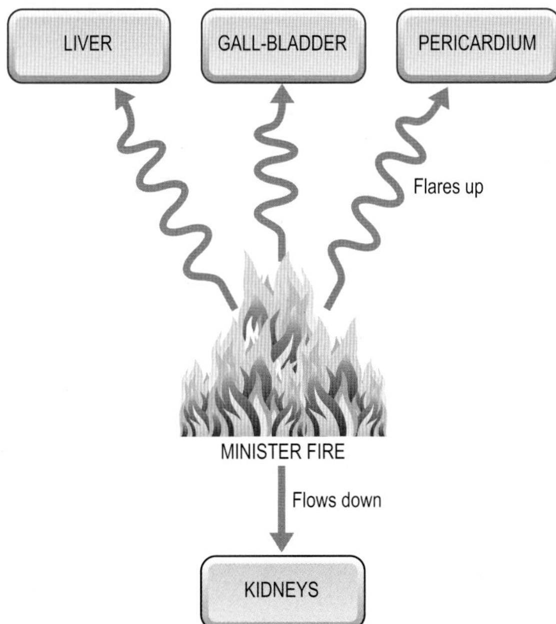

Figure 13.16 Minister Fire flowing up to Pericardium and down to Kidneys.

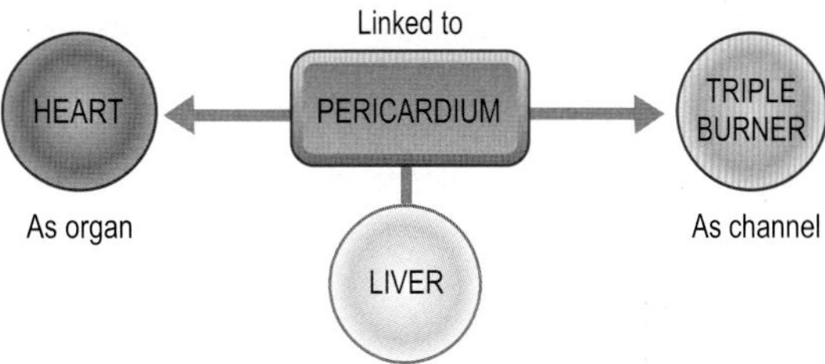

Figure 13.17 Connection of Pericardium with Heart, Liver and Triple Burner.

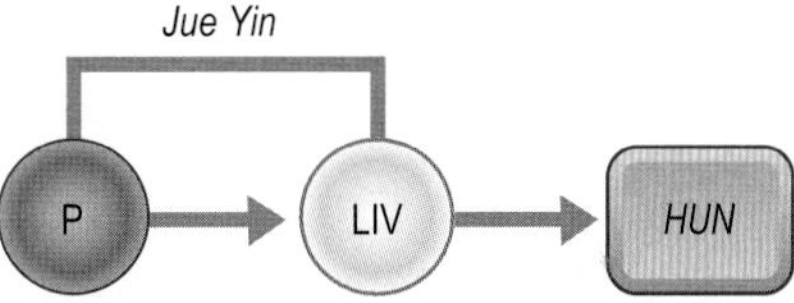

Figure 13.18 Relationship between Pericardium, Liver and Ethereal Soul.

P-6 has a powerful calming action on the Mind and can be used in anxiety caused by any of the Heart patterns. It also calms the Mind by its indirect action on the Liver (to which the Pericardium is related within the Terminal Yin). It can therefore be used for irritability due to stagnation of Liver-Qi, particularly if combined with anxiety from a Heart pattern (Fig. 13.18).

It is particularly effective in women and is most useful to calm the Mind in women suffering from premenstrual depression and irritability. It also promotes sleep.

Besides calming the Mind, it lifts the spirit by promoting the free flow of Liver-Qi and stimulating the "coming and going" of the Ethereal Soul. For this reason, it is a very important point to use in depression from Liver-Qi stagnation with insufficient "movement" of the Ethereal Soul.

CLINICAL NOTE

- P-6 Neiguan lifts mood and treats depression.
- P-7 Daling calms the *Shen* and settles anxiety.
- P-5 Jianshi resolves Phlegm from the Pericardium to treat mental confusion.

P-6 Neiguan has a synergistic effect on acupuncture point prescriptions. The addition of P-6 to any prescription increases the therapeutic effect. Just as P-6 has this effect on a physical level, it has one on a mental-emotional level, i.e. it can bolster the effect of a point combination for mental-emotional problems.

This effect of P-6 is due to various factors. It affects the Mind (*Shen*), but how does its effect on the Mind differ from that of the Heart? The Heart is more Yin, it governs Blood which houses the Mind. The Pericardium is more Yang, it is the external covering of the Heart and therefore controls movement of Qi on a mental-emotional level. This effect on Qi is due also to its relationship with the Liver within the Terminal Yin (*Jue Yin*).

The moving effect of P-6 is also due to other factors.

1. The mental-emotional "moving" effect of P-6 is partly due to its being the Connecting (*Luo*) point of the Pericardium channel. As Connecting point, it affects the Triple Burner; it can therefore move Qi of the Triple Burner in all three Burners and this also has a mental-emotional effect.
2. The Pericardium channel, being paired with the Liver channel within the Terminal Yin channels, affects the coming and going of the Ethereal Soul; in particular, P-6 can stimulate the coming and going of the Ethereal Soul and therefore treat depression.
3. The Pericardium pertains to the Terminal Yin which is the "hinge" of the Yin channels (between the Greater Yin and Lesser Yin). Being the Connecting point, and therefore the hinge between Yin and Yang, P-6 is the "hinge" of the Hinge; in its capacity as a "hinge" it connects things. On a mental-emotional level, that means that it regulates our capacity for relationships. Its function of a "hinge" is also related to its being the opening point of the Yin Linking Vessel (*Yin Wei Mai*) that links all the Yin channels.

To compare and contrast P-6 with P-7, the former has an "outward", centrifugal movement, it moves Qi, resolves stagnation and stimulates the "coming and going" of the Ethereal Soul, whilst the latter has an "inward", centripetal movement, calms the Mind and restrains the movement of the Ethereal Soul (see below under P-7 Daling).

P-6 combines well with:

- SP-4 Gongsun to open the Yin Linking Vessel, nourish Blood, relax the chest, calm the Mind and settle the Ethereal Soul
- LIV-3 Taichong to strengthen its Qi-moving action in emotional problems from repressed anger
- G.B.-40 Qiuxu to stimulate the movement of the Ethereal Soul in depression
- Du-20 Baihui to lift mood, clear the Mind and relieve depression
- Du-26 Renzhong to lift mood, clear the Mind, open the Mind's orifices and relieve depression
- ST-40 Fenglong to calm the Mind, open the chest to relieve it of constrained emotions, and open the Mind's orifices.

P-7 Daling *Great Hill*

One of Sun Si Miao's 13 Ghost points, P-7 calms the Mind and opens the Mind's orifices. Its indications include "insomnia, manic behavior, palpitations, agitation, mental restlessness, sadness and fright".

The *Explanation of the Acupuncture Points* (1654) lists "manic incessant talking, inappropriate laughter and mental restlessness" among the indications for P-7.[53] The *Gatherings from Eminent Acupuncturists* (1529) lists "manic talking, sadness, fright and fear" among the indications for this point.[54]

P-7 has an important function in calming the Mind. In this respect, it has all the same functions as HE-7 Shenmen. As a matter of fact, historically, P-7 Daling was used as the Source (*Yuan*) point of the Heart channel. The first chapter of the *Spiritual Axis* lists P-7 as the Source point of the Heart.[55]

In my experience, P-7 is better than HE-7 to deal with the emotional consequences of the breaking up of relationships.

P-7 also clears Heart-Fire and is particularly important to use when Heart-Fire causes mental problems, such as great anxiety and mental restlessness or even manic behavior.

It is useful to compare and contrast the actions of HE-7 Shenmen and P-7 Daling (both of which can nourish Heart-Blood and calm the Mind), and also of P-6 Neiguan and P-7 Dahling.

HE-7 SHENMEN	P-7 DALING
More for Empty patterns	More for Full patterns
Not for Warm diseases	Important for Warm diseases, Heat in Pericardium (Nutritive-Qi level)
Gentle action in calming the Mind	Better for severe anxiety and mania
Not so strong in opening the Mind's orifices	Opens Mind's orifices. Especially indicated for emotional upsets deriving from the breaking of relationships

P-6 NEIGUAN	P-7 DALING
Outward, centrifugal movement	Inward, centripetal movement
Moves Qi	Calms the Mind
Resolves stagnation	Clears Heat
Lifts the spirit	Allays anxiety
Stimulates the coming and going of the Ethereal Soul	Restrains the coming and going of the Ethereal Soul

P-8 Laogong *Labor Palace*

One of Sun Si Miao's 13 Ghost points, P-8 calms the Mind. Its indications include "insomnia, agitation, manic behavior, fright, anxiety and mental restlessness".

The *Great Compendium of Acupuncture* (1601) lists "anger, sadness and inappropriate laughter" among the indications for P-8.[56]

The following is a comparison between P-3 Quze, P-4 Ximen, P-5 Jianshi, P-6 Neiguan, P-7 Daling and P-8 Laogong, specifically in relation to their mental-emotional effect. They can all calm the Mind.

- P-3 clears Heat and cools Blood. It is indicated for emotional problems from Heart-Fire.
- P-4 is better for emotional problems occurring against a background of Deficiency.
- P-5 resolves Phlegm from the Heart for symptoms of Phlegm misting the Heart and Mind.
- P-6 opens the chest, calms the Mind and regulates Liver-Qi. It is the best point to lift the Spirit and stimulate the coming and going of the Ethereal Soul in depression.
- P-7 calms the Mind, particularly for emotional problems deriving from difficult relationships.
- P-8 Laogong is specific for mental-emotional problems from Heart-Fire.

SUMMARY

Pericardium channel points for emotional problems

- Pericardium channel points are particularly indicated for mental-emotional problems occurring against a background of Heat.
- P-4 Ximen is better for mental-emotional problems from Deficiency.
- P-6 is a very important point to move Liver-Qi, stimulate the coming and going of the Ethereal Soul and treat depression from Liver-Qi stagnation.

P-3 Quze Marsh on Bend

P-3 calms the Mind in Heart-Fire. Its indications include "fright, anxiety and mental restlessness".

P-4 Ximen Cleft Door

P-4 calms the Mind. Its indications include "agitation, anxiety, insomnia, mental restlessness, depression and fright". P-4 strengthens the Mind in cases of Heart deficiency which may give rise to fear, anxiety, insomnia and depression.

P-5 Jianshi Intermediary

P-5 calms the Mind, opens the Mind's orifices and resolves Phlegm in the Heart. Its indications include "palpitations, agitation, feeling of oppression of the chest, manic behavior, fright, mental restlessness, poor memory and 'seeing ghosts' ".

P-6 Neiguan Inner Gate

P-6 calms the Mind, lifts the spirit, promotes the free flow of Liver-Qi and stimulates the movement of the Ethereal Soul. Its indications include "insomnia, manic behavior, poor memory, anxiety, fright, sadness and depression".

P-7 Daling Great Hill

One of Sun Si Miao's 13 Ghost points, P-7 calms the Mind and opens the Mind's orifices. Its indications include "insomnia, manic behavior, palpitations, agitation, mental restlessness, sadness and fright".

P-8 Laogong Labor Palace

One of Sun Si Miao's 13 Ghost points, P-8 calms the Mind. Its indications include "insomnia, agitation, manic behavior, fright, anxiety and mental restlessness".

TRIPLE BURNER CHANNEL

The Triple Burner channel points for emotional problems are illustrated in Figure 13.19.

T.B.-3 Zhongzhu *Middle Islet*

Although Chinese books do not mention any emotional indication for this point, in my experience, T.B.-3 promotes the free flow of Qi, lifts the spirit and stimulates the coming and going of the Ethereal Soul.

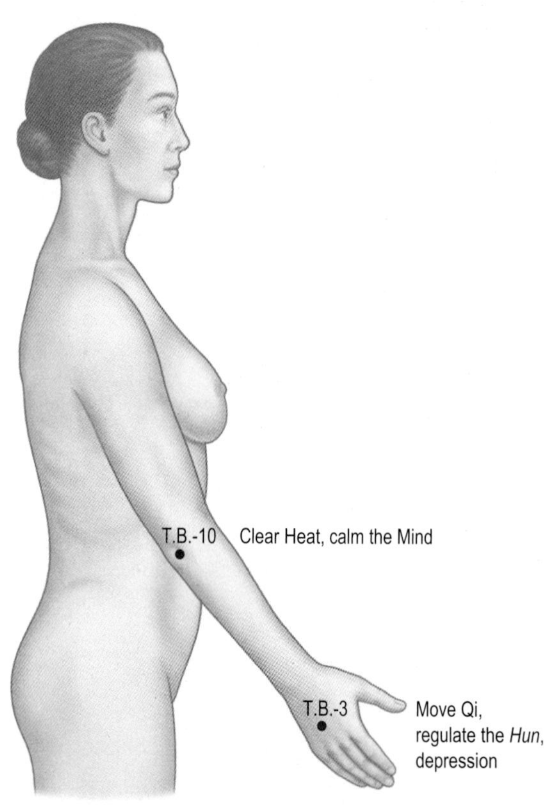

Figure 13.19 Triple Burner channel points.

T.B.-10 Tianjing *Heavenly Well*

T.B.-10 calms the Mind. Its indications include "manic behavior, sadness, fright and palpitations".

T.B.-10 calms the Mind when there are mental-emotional problems occurring against a background of Heart-Heat. It is similar in action to P-7 Daling.

SUMMARY

Triple Burner channel points for emotional problems

T.B.-3 Zhongzhu Middle Islet

T.B.-3 promotes the free flow of Qi, lifts the spirit and stimulates the coming and going of the Ethereal Soul.

T.B.-10 Tianjing Heavenly Well

T.B.-10 calms the Mind in patterns with Heat. Its indications include "manic behavior, sadness, fright and palpitations".

GALL-BLADDER CHANNEL

The Gall-Bladder channel points for emotional problems are illustrated in Figure 13.20.

G.B.-9 Tianchong *Penetrating Heaven*

G.B.-9 calms the Mind. Its indications include "fright, fear, palpitations and manic behavior".

G.B.-9 has a powerful mental effect, and is used to calm the Mind. In serious mental disorders such as hypomania, it is an important adjuvant to the treatment with distal points.

G.B.-12 Wangu *Whole Bone*

G.B.-12 calms the Mind. Its indications include "manic behavior, agitation and insomnia".

This point is frequently used for insomnia from rising of Liver-Yang or Liver-Fire, combined with BL-18 Ganshu and BL-19 Danshu.

G.B.-13 Benshen *Mind Root*

G.B.-13 calms the Mind, clears the Brain and gathers Essence (*Jing*) to the head. Its indications include "manic behavior and fright". The *Gatherings from*

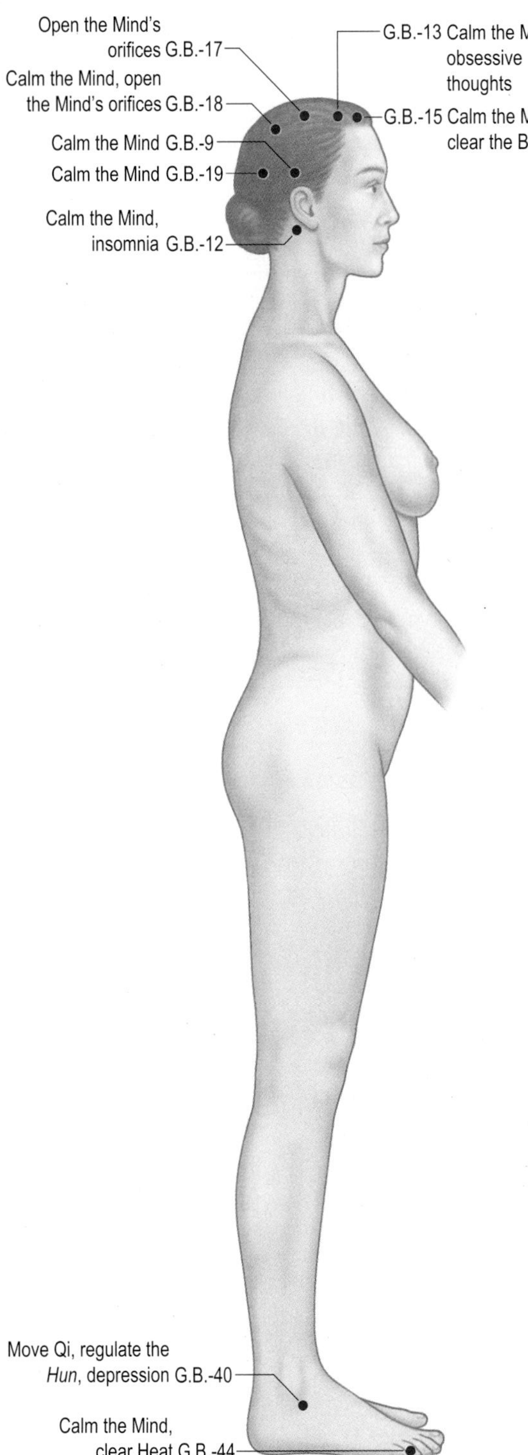

Figure 13.20 Gall-Bladder channel points.

Eminent Acupuncturists (1529) lists "Dullness (*Dian*)" among the indications of G.B.-13.[57]

G.B.-13 is a very important point for mental and emotional problems. It is very much used in psychiatric practice for schizophrenia and split personality, combined with HE-5 Tongli and G.B.-38 Yangfu.[58] It is also indicated when the person has persistent and unreasonable feelings of jealousy and suspicion.

Apart from these mental traits, it has a powerful effect in calming the Mind and relieving anxiety deriving from constant worry and fixed thoughts. Its effect is enhanced if it is combined with Du-24 Shenting.

Its deep mental and emotional effect is also due to its action of "gathering" Essence to the head. The Kidney-Essence is the root of our Pre-Heaven Qi and is the foundation for our mental and emotional life. A strong Essence is the fundamental prerequisite for a clear Mind (*Shen*) and a balanced emotional life. This is the meaning of this point's name "Root of the Mind", i.e. this point gathers the Essence which is the root of the Mind (*Shen*).

The Kidney-Essence is the source of Marrow which fills up the Brain (called Sea of Marrow); G.B.-13 is a point where Essence and Marrow "gather". The *Great Dictionary of Acupuncture* says that this point "*makes the Mind [Shen] return to its root*":[59] the "root" of the Mind is the Essence, hence this point "gathers" the Essence to the Brain and affects the Mind. As it connects the Mind and the Essence, it also treats both the Heart and the Kidneys, and therefore the Mind (*Shen*) and Will-Power (*Zhi*); for this reason, it is an important point in the treatment of depression.

When combined with other points to nourish Essence (such as Ren-4 Guanyuan), G.B.-13 attracts Essence towards the head with the effect of calming the Mind, clearing the Brain and strengthening clarity of mind, memory and will-power. The connection between G.B.-13 and the Essence is confirmed by the text *An Enquiry into Chinese Acupuncture* which has, among the indications of this point: "*excessive menstrual bleeding, impotence and seminal emissions.*"[60]

The *Complete Book of Jing Yue (Jing Yue Quan Shu*, 1624) says that this point is for lack of clarity of the Mind deriving from injury of the Ethereal Soul by sadness.[61]

Finally, G.B.-13 resolves Phlegm in the context of mental-emotional disorders or epilepsy, i.e. it opens the Mind's orifices when these are clouded by Phlegm. The *Explanation of the Acupuncture Points* says:[62]

The indications of G.B.-13 show that it eliminates the three pathogenic factors of Wind, Fire and Phlegm from the Lesser Yang, in which cases this point should be reduced.

This point can be combined with:

- *Du-24 Shenting to enhance its calming effect*: the combination of these two points has a powerful calming effect on the Mind and Ethereal Soul, and they are particularly useful in Liver disharmonies.
- *HE-7 Shenmen to calm the Mind in severe anxiety*, occurring against a background of Heart disharmonies.

G.B.-15 Linqi *Falling Tears*

G.B.-15 calms the Mind. Its indications include "obsessive thoughts, pensiveness and oscillation of moods".

G.B.-15 has a deep effect on the mental-emotional life, and is particularly indicated to balance the moods when the person oscillates between periods of low spirits and periods of elation.[63] In my experience, this point is effective to stop obsessive thoughts and pensiveness.

G.B.-17 Zhengying *Top Convergence*

G.B.-17 resolves Phlegm and opens the Mind's orifices. Among its indications are "obsessive thoughts, pensiveness and manic behavior".

G.B.-17 has a strong mental-emotional effect in opening the Mind's orifices and resolving Phlegm. In my experience, it is effective to eliminate Phlegm from the head when this obstructs the Mind, causing obsessive thoughts, pensiveness and mild manic behavior.

According to *An Enquiry into Chinese Acupuncture*, G.B.-17 can be used for schizophrenia and hysteria.[64]

G.B.-18 Chengling *Spirit Receiver*

G.B.-18 calms the Mind and opens the Mind's orifices. Its indications include "obsessive thoughts and pensiveness".

G.B.-18 has a deep effect on mental problems such as obsessional thoughts and dementia.[65]

G.B.-19 Naokong *Brain Cavity*

G.B.-19 calms the Mind. Among its indications are "Dullness and Mania, fright and palpitations".

G.B.-40 Qiuxu *Mound Ruins*

G.B.-40 promotes the free flow of Liver-Qi, lifts the spirit, stimulates the coming and going of the Ethereal Soul and strengthens decisiveness. Among its indications are "depression and moodiness".

The *Great Compendium of Acupuncture* (1601) lists "*Dian*" among the indications for G.B.-40; this would confirm its use to stimulate the movement of the Ethereal Soul in depression.[66]

In my experience, G.B.-40 can be used to strengthen the Gall-Bladder mental aspect, i.e. the strength of character that allows one to take difficult decisions. It is also the best point to use to strengthen the Gall-Bladder and Heart in the syndrome of "Deficiency of the Gall-Bladder", characterized by timidity, lack of initiative, difficulty in making decisions and depression.

On a mental level, the Gall-Bladder channel can be used to stimulate the "coming and going" of the Ethereal Soul when the person is depressed and lacks a sense of direction and purpose in life. In my experience, G.B.-40 is the best point to stimulate this aspect of the Gall-Bladder.

G.B.-44 Zuqiaoyin (*Foot*) *Yin Orifice*

G.B.-44 calms the Mind. Its indications include "insomnia, nightmares, somnolence, agitation and anxiety".

G.B.-44 calms the Mind in cases of insomnia and agitation deriving from Liver-Fire.

SUMMARY

Gall-Bladder channel points for emotional problems

- Gall-Bladder points on the head are very important for serious mental-emotional problems.
- Most of them open the Mind's orifices.

G.B.-9 *Tianchong* Penetrating Heaven

G.B.-9 calms the Mind. Its indications include "fright, fear, palpitations and manic behavior".

G.B.-12 *Wangu* Whole Bone

G.B.-12 calms the Mind. Its indications include "manic behavior, agitation and insomnia". Frequently used for insomnia from rising of Liver-Yang or Liver-Fire, combined with BL-18 Ganshu and BL-19 Danshu.

G.B.-13 Benshen Mind Root

G.B.-13 calms the Mind, clears the Brain and gathers Essence (*Jing*) to the head. Its indications include "manic behavior and fright". G.B.-13 is a very important point for mental and emotional problems.

G.B.-15 Linqi Falling Tears

G.B.-15 calms the Mind. Its indications include "obsessive thoughts, pensiveness and oscillation of moods". Particularly indicated to balance the moods when the person oscillates between periods of low spirits and periods of elation.

G.B.-17 Zhengying Top Convergence

G.B.-17 resolves Phlegm and opens the Mind's orifices. Among its indications are "obsessive thoughts, pensiveness and manic behavior". G.B.-17 has a strong mental-emotional effect in opening the Mind's orifices and resolving Phlegm.

G.B.-18 Chengling Spirit Receiver

G.B.-18 calms the Mind and opens the Mind's orifices. Its indications include "obsessive thoughts and pensiveness".

G.B.-19 Naokong Brain Cavity

G.B.-19 calms the Mind. Among its indications are "manic-depression, fright and palpitations".

G.B.-40 Qiuxu Mound Ruins

G.B.-40 promotes the free flow of Liver-Qi, lifts the spirit, stimulates the coming and going of the Ethereal Soul and strengthens decisiveness. Among its indications are "depression and moodiness". In my experience, G.B.-40 point can be used to strengthen the Gall-Bladder mental aspect, i.e. the strength of character which allows one to take difficult decisions.

*G.B.-44 Zuqiaoyin (*Foot*)* Yin Orifice

G.B.-44 calms the Mind. Its indications include "insomnia, nightmares, somnolence, agitation and anxiety". G.B.-44 calms the Mind in cases of insomnia and agitation deriving from Liver-Fire.

LIVER CHANNEL

The Liver channel points for emotional problems are illustrated in Figure 13.21.

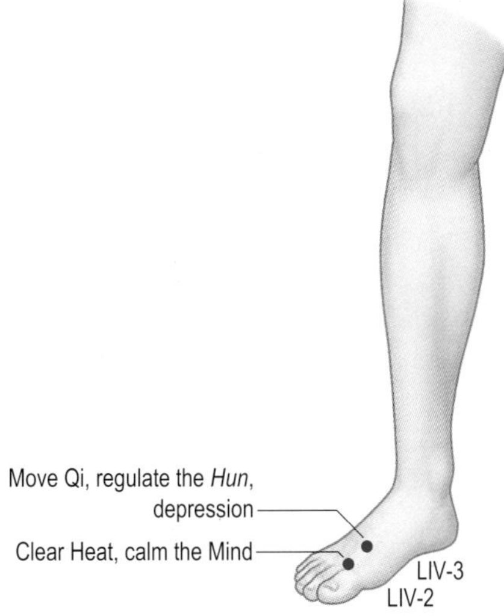

Figure 13.21 Liver channel points.

LIV-2 Xingjian *Temporary In-between*

LIV-2 calms the Mind. Among its indications are "propensity to outbursts of anger, sadness, fright, 'seeing ghosts', manic behavior, insomnia and palpitations".

LIV-2 calms the Mind and settles the Ethereal Soul when these are agitated by Fire.

LIV-3 Taichong *Bigger Penetrating*

LIV-3 calms the Mind, settles the Ethereal Soul and regulates the coming and going of the Ethereal Soul. Its indications include "propensity to outbursts of anger, irritability, insomnia and worrying".

LIV-3 has a profound calming effect on the Mind, and is effective in calming very tense people who are prone to short temper or experience feelings of deep frustration and repressed anger. However, its calming action is not limited to its action on feelings of anger, which are typical of a Liver disharmony, as it is also effective in general irritability and tendency to worry from emotional stress. Its calming action is enhanced when combined with L.I.-4 Hegu (the "Four Gates").

Besides a calming action, LIV-3 also stimulates the coming and going of the Ethereal Soul when this is restrained by Liver-Qi stagnation, making the person depressed and aimless. However, LIV-3 has a regulating action on the Ethereal Soul and can also restrain its movement in people who are slightly manic.

SUMMARY

Liver channel points for emotional problems

LIV-2 Xingjian Temporary In-between

LIV-2 calms the Mind. Among its indications are "propensity to outbursts of anger, sadness, fright, 'seeing ghosts', manic behavior, insomnia and palpitations". LIV-2 calms the Mind and settles the Ethereal Soul when these are agitated by Fire.

LIV-3 Taichong Bigger Penetrating

LIV-3 calms the Mind, settles the Ethereal Soul and regulates the coming and going of the Ethereal Soul. Its indications include "propensity to outbursts of anger, irritability, insomnia and worrying". Besides a calming action, LIV-3 also stimulates the coming and going of the Ethereal Soul when this is restrained by Liver-Qi stagnation, making the person depressed and aimless.

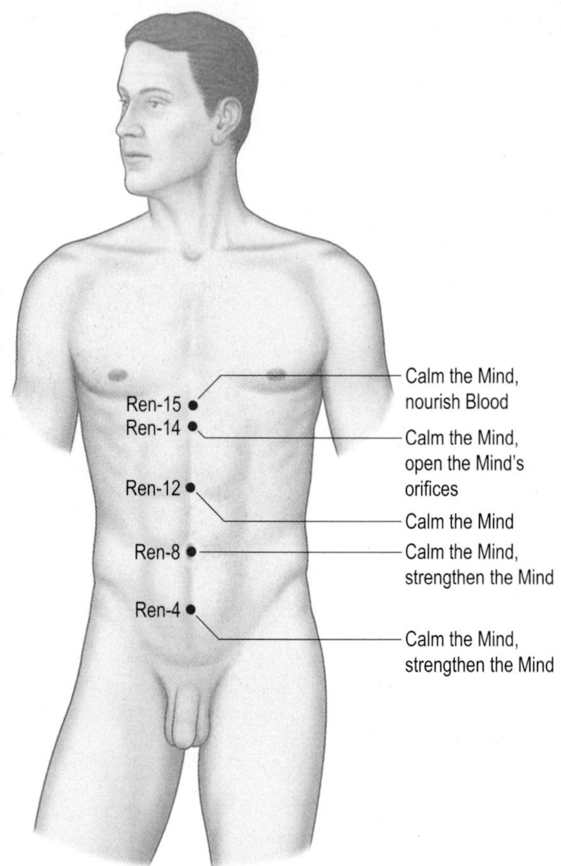

Figure 13.22 Directing Vessel points.

DIRECTING VESSEL (*REN MAI*)

The Directing Vessel channel points for emotional problems are illustrated in Figure 13.22.

Ren-4 Guanyuan *Gate to the Original Qi*

Ren-4 calms the Mind and settles the Ethereal Soul. Its indications include "fear, fright and insomnia".

Ren-4 is a meeting point of the three leg Yin channels that converge at this point and penetrate deeply in the Directing Vessel; this point is the "gate" that keeps the Qi of these three channels in the Lower Burner. This point's mental-emotional effect is due to this function, i.e. by rooting the Qi of the leg Yin channels – Liver, Spleen and Kidney – it gives the Heart a "foundation", so that its Qi does not escape upwards. Therefore, Ren-4 calms the Mind by rooting it into the Yin in the Lower Burner.

Ren-4 calms the Mind by strengthening the Kidneys and the Original Qi (*Yuan Qi*) and "rooting" the Mind (*Shen*) and the Ethereal Soul (*Hun*) in the Lower Burner. I use it specifically for anxiety occurring against a background of Deficiency. This point tonifies the Qi of the Lower Burner, thus rooting Qi downwards and subduing the rising of Qi to the head, which happens in severe anxiety. In this way it has a powerful calming effect.

Ren-8 Shenque *Spirit Palace*

Ren-8 calms the Mind and lifts the Spirit. Although its indications do not include many mental-emotional symptoms, I personally use this point to calm the Mind and lift the Spirit when the person is depressed against a background of Deficiency of the Original Qi (*Yuan Qi*). Remember that it is used only with moxa cones on salt, not needling.

It is worth exploring the meaning of this point's name as it sheds light on its nature and functions. The *Great Dictionary of Chinese Acupuncture* reports an explanation of the meaning of this point from an old text:[67]

Ren-8 is the Abode of the Spirit [Shen She]. Heaven is above, Earth is below, Person is in the Middle; on both sides there is KI-13 Qixue and KI-16 Huangshu. Above there is Ren-9 Shuifen and Ren-10 Xiawan; below there is Ren-4 Guanyuan [here called Bao Men] *and Ren-3 Zhongji. The umbilicus is in the centre like an opening of a door through which the Spirit communicates with the Pre-Heaven Jing. When mother and father unite, a fetus is formed, the umbilical cord is formed linking the fetus to the mother's Ming Men like a lotus stem. The Pre-Heaven Jing generates Water and the Kidneys: like an unopened lotus flower, the Five Elements come into being and the mother's Qi is transferred. In 10 months when the fetus is fully formed, the Spirit infuses through the centre of the umbilicus and forms a new human being.*

According to this image, Ren-8 is at the center of an energetic vortex with three levels: Heaven above (Ren-9 and Ren-10), Earth below (Ren-4 and Ren-7) and Person in the center (Ren-8), with KI-13 Qixue and KI-16 Huangshu on either side, like watchtowers guarding the entrance to the Imperial Palace. I translated the word *que* in this point's name as "Palace" (rather than "gate" or "gateway" as most authors do) to indicate the energetic importance of this point, i.e. like an Imperial Palace that is the residence of the Spirit (Figs 13.23 and 13.24).

The word *que* also implies the idea of an open space, something empty. This is the space through which the fetus was connected to the mother's Gate of Life (*Ming Men*), the space through which the Spirit entered the fetus and was nourished by the mother. Because of this association, Ren-8 is the point that most affects our Pre-Heaven Jing. However, this "space" is not like a "gate" (*guan*) or "door" (*men*) through which Qi moves in and out, and this point therefore does not have the function that most points with *guan* or *men* in their name have, i.e. that of promoting the movement and entering/exiting of Qi. This "space" is rather like the entrance to a palace, a "space" that is the residence of the Spirit, and that is why I translate the word *que* in this point's name as "palace".

The connection between the fetus and the mother through Ren-8 is also shown by one of the many alternative names for this point, *Ming Di*, which means "Life's Stem", the "stem" being the umbilical cord and "Life" referring to the mother's Gate of Life (*Ming Men*).

For these reasons, I use this point in patients who are depressed and whose depression revolves around issues of mothering.

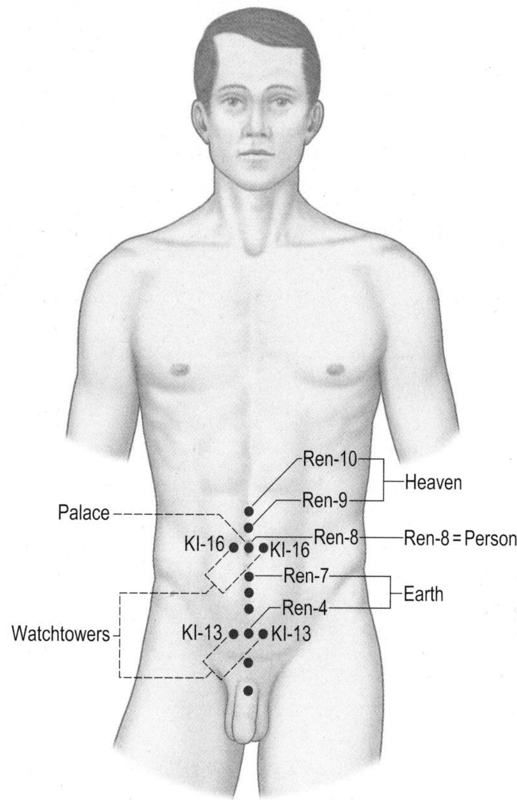

Figure 13.23 Ren-8 Shenque.

Ren-12 Zhongwan *Middle of Epigastrium*

Ren-12 calms the Mind. Its indications include "worry, anxiety and pensiveness".

It is interesting that the traditional indications for this point include "worry, anxiety and pensiveness". I personally find Ren-12 very effective in calming the Mind in patients who suffer from digestive problems caused by emotional strain. For this action, I usually combine Ren-12 with Ren-15 Jiuwei and Du-24 Shenting.

I personally use Ren-12 to calm the Mind and stop pensiveness when the person is affected by emotions that damage the Spleen (such as pensiveness, worry and shame).

Ren-14 Juque *Great Palace*

Ren-14 calms the Mind and opens the Mind's orifices. Its indications include "anxiety, insomnia, Dullness and Mania, shouting, anger, disorientation and

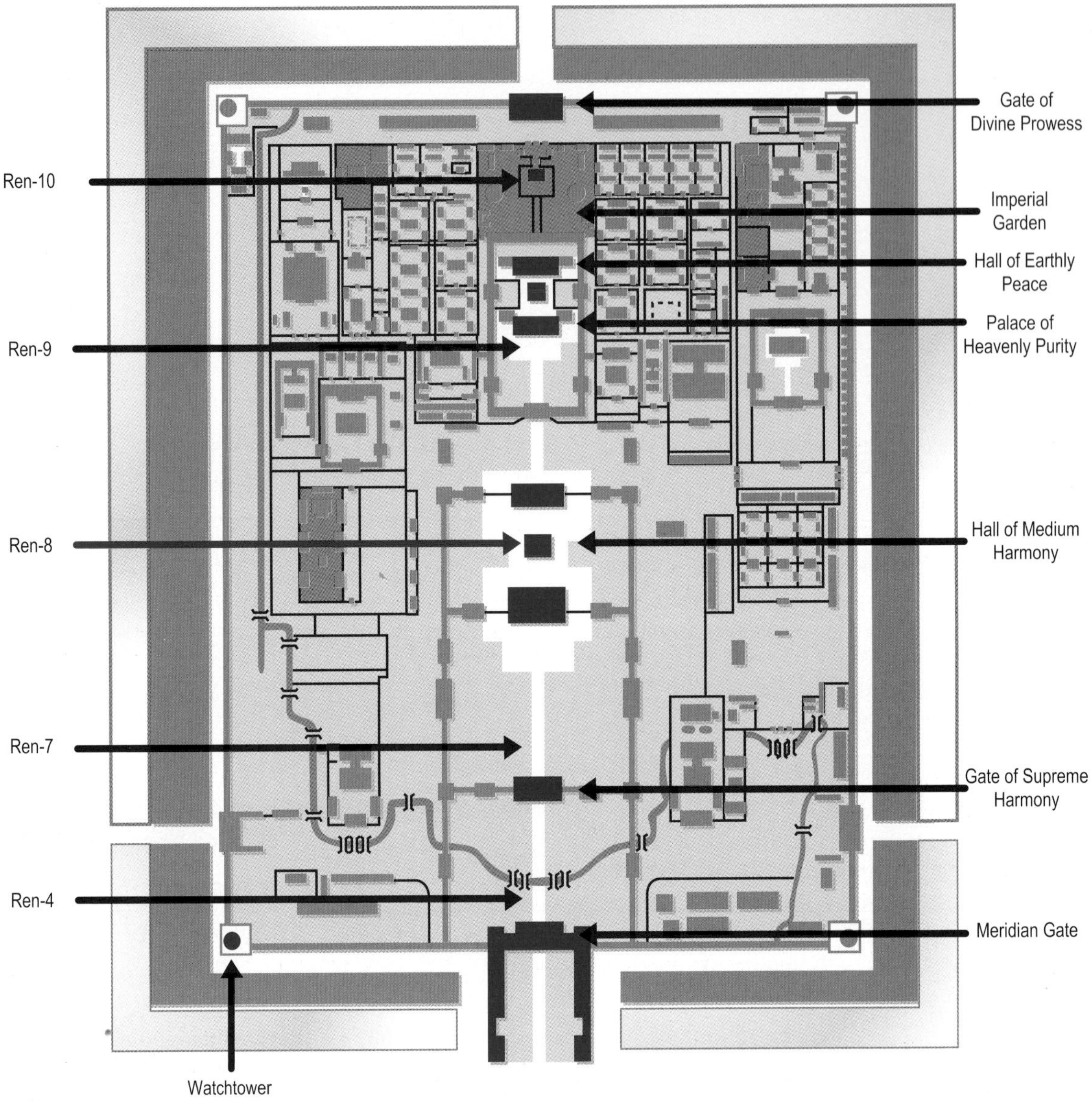

Figure 13.24 The Directing Vessel points comparison to the Forbidden City.

agitation". The *Great Compendium of Acupuncture* (1601) lists "disorientation and manic behavior" among the indications for Ren-14.[68] The *Gatherings from Eminent Acupuncturists* also lists Mania (*Kuang*) among its indications.[69]

Ren-14 calms the Mind and is frequently used for the pattern of Phlegm-Heat misting the Heart and leading to mental symptoms or for the pattern of Heart-Fire leading to insomnia, agitation and anxiety. This does not mean that Ren-14 cannot be used for mental-emotional symptoms occurring against a background of Heart deficiency. However, in this latter case, I personally tend to use Ren-15 Jiuwei more.

The character *que* in this point's name is the same as that in *Shen Que* for Ren-8; for this reason, I have translated it as "Palace" in accordance with "Spirit Palace" of Ren-8. There is therefore a correspondence between these two points. The Spirit (*Shen*) relies on the Essence of the Kidneys as its foundation. Therefore, Ren-8 affects the Spirit through the Essence and Ren-14 through the Mind (*Shen*) of the Heart (Fig. 13.25).

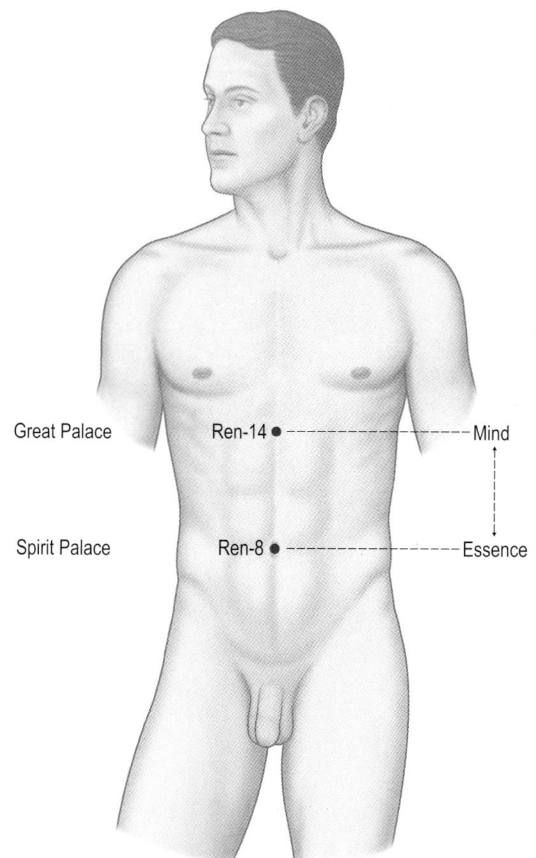

Figure 13.25 Relationship between Ren-8 Shenque and Ren-14 Juque.

Ren-15 Jiuwei *Dove Tail*

Ren-15 calms the Mind, settles the Corporeal Soul and opens the Mind's orifices. Its indications include "manic-depression, palpitations, anxiety and insomnia". The *Great Compendium of Acupuncture* lists "mania, incessant talking and intolerance of other people talking" among the indications for Ren-15.[70]

The *Explanation of the Acupuncture Points* (1654) lists "incessant talking and intolerance to other people's talking" among the indications for Ren-15.[71]

Ren-15 is a very important and powerful point to calm the Mind. According to Chapter 1 of the *Spiritual Axis*, it is the Source point of all the Yin organs, which means that it affects the Original Qi (*Yuan Qi*) of all Yin organs.[72]

This point nourishes all Yin organs and it calms the Mind, particularly in Deficiency of Yin and/or Blood. It has a very powerful calming action in severe anxiety, worry, emotional upsets, fears or obsessions. Although its indications show that it can be used to open the Mind's orifices in serious mental disorders from a Full condition, I personally use this point in mental-emotional states occurring against a background of Deficiency of Blood or Yin.

It is especially indicated to release emotions constraining the Corporeal Soul in the chest and manifesting with a feeling of oppression or tightness of the chest.

In emotional problems occurring against a background of Kidney deficiency, I frequently use this point in combination with Ren-4 Guanyuan and Du-24 Shenting.

This point also combines well with Du-19 Houding to calm the Mind and relieve anxiety, insomnia and mental restlessness.

The book *An Explanation of Acupuncture Points* (1654) says that this point affects the Lungs, Heart, Liver and Kidneys; it therefore affects four of the five Yin organs. This is another way in which this point calms the Mind. When listing the indications pertaining to the Heart, it gives "epilepsy, aphasia, feeling of oppression in the heart region, cannot stand hearing people talk, palpitations, spirit scattered".

SUMMARY

Directing Vessel channel points for emotional problems

- Directing Vessel points are particularly indicated to treat mental-emotional problems arising against a background of Deficiency.

Ren-4 Guanyuan **Gate to the Original Qi**

Ren-4 calms the Mind and settles the Ethereal Soul. Its indications include "fear, fright and insomnia". Ren-4 calms the Mind by strengthening the Kidneys and the Original Qi (*Yuan Qi*) and "rooting" the Mind (*Shen*) and the Ethereal Soul (*Hun*) in the Lower Burner. I use it specifically for anxiety occurring against a background of Deficiency.

Ren-8 Shenque **Spirit Palace**

Ren-8 calms the Mind and lifts the Spirit. Although its indications do not include many mental-emotional symptoms, I personally use this point to calm the Mind and lift the Spirit when the person is depressed against a background of Deficiency of the Original Qi (*Yuan Qi*). Ren-8 is the space through which the fetus was connected to the mother's Gate of Life (*Ming Men*), the space through which the Spirit entered the fetus and was nourished by the mother. Because of this association, Ren-8 is the point that most affects our Pre-Heaven Jing.

Ren-12 Zhongwan Middle of Epigastrium

Ren-12 calms the Mind. Its indications include "worry, anxiety and pensiveness".

Ren-14 Juque Great Palace

Ren-14 calms the Mind and opens the Mind's orifices. Its indications include "anxiety, insomnia, manic-depression, shouting, anger, disorientation and agitation".

Ren-15 Jiuwei Dove Tail

Ren-15 calms the Mind, settles the Corporeal Soul and opens the Mind's orifices. Its indications include "manic-depression, palpitations, anxiety and insomnia". Ren-15 is a very important and powerful point to calm the Mind.

GOVERNING VESSEL (*DU MAI*)

The Governing Vessel channel points for emotional problems are illustrated in Figure 13.26.

Du-4 Mingmen *Gate of Life*

Du-4 clears the Mind, lifts the spirit and strengthens Will-Power. Its indications include "depression, lack of will-power and mental confusion".

The Fire of the Gate of Life (*Ming Men*) is closely linked to the Pre-Heaven Essence. Situated in between the Kidneys, the Fire of the Gate of Life is the physiological Fire of the body which provides the warmth that is essential for all physiological processes of the body and for all the internal organs. The Fire of the Gate of Life is already present from birth and, indeed, from conception. The Pre-Heaven Essence is also present from conception and birth but it then "matures" into the Kidney-Essence (with the help of the warmth of the Fire of the Gate of Life) at puberty, when it generates menstrual blood and ova in women and sperm in men.

Thus, the Fire of the Gate of Life can be said to represent the Yang aspect of the Pre-Heaven Essence, while the Pre-Heaven Essence proper (transforming into Kidney-Essence at puberty) represents the Yin aspect. Du-4's alternative name, *Jing Gong*, i.e. "Palace of Essence [*Jing*]", clearly shows the connection of the Gate of Life with the Essence, i.e. it is the Yang aspect of the Essence.

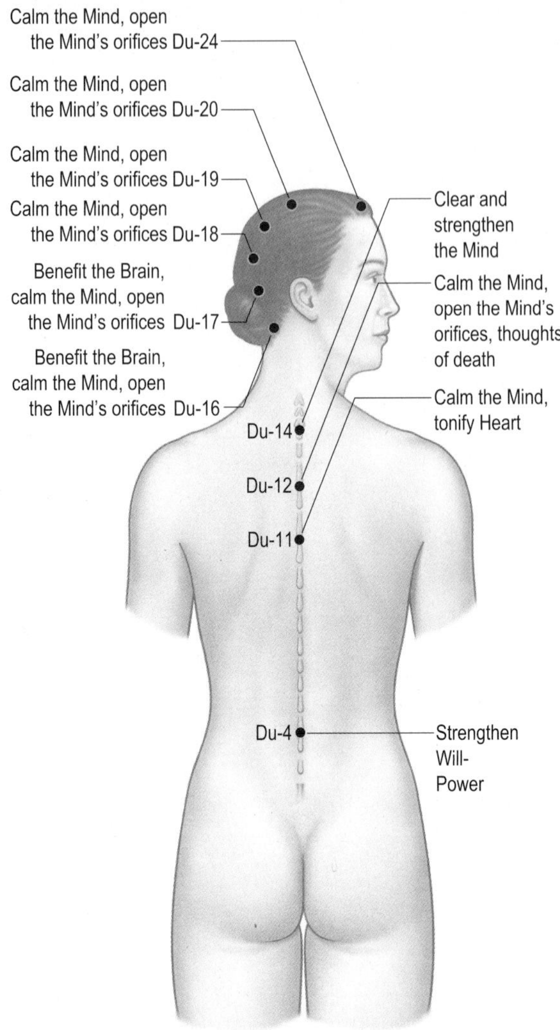

Figure 13.26 Governing Vessel points.

The Fire of the Gate of Life accumulates at the point Du-4 Mingmen on the spine at conception, while the Pre-Heaven Essence concentrates at the point Ren-4 Guanyuan, also at conception. This correlates with the Uterus (where menstrual blood is stored) in women and with the Room of Sperm in men.[73] Chapter 36 of the *Classic of Difficulties* says:[74]

The Gate of Life is the residence of the Mind and Essence and it is connected to the Original Qi [Yuan Qi]: in men it houses the Sperm; in women, the Uterus.

The Governing Vessel has a strong influence on the Mind (*Shen*) because it affects it in three different ways. First, the Governing Vessel emanates from the space between the kidneys and is related to the Essence (in particular, the Yang aspect of the Essence). The Essence (*Jing*) is the foundation of Qi and Mind (*Shen*) and the residence of Will-Power (*Zhi*); a strong Essence, therefore, will create the basis for a strong Mind and Will-Power.

Second, the Governing Vessel flows through the heart and it therefore affects the Mind through the Heart. Third, the Governing Vessel enters the Brain which, according to some doctors, is the residence of the Mind. For these reasons, the Governing Vessel, and in particular Du-4, affects the Mind; it clears the Mind and lifts moods and is an important point to treat depression occurring against a background of Kidney-Yang deficiency (Fig. 13.27).

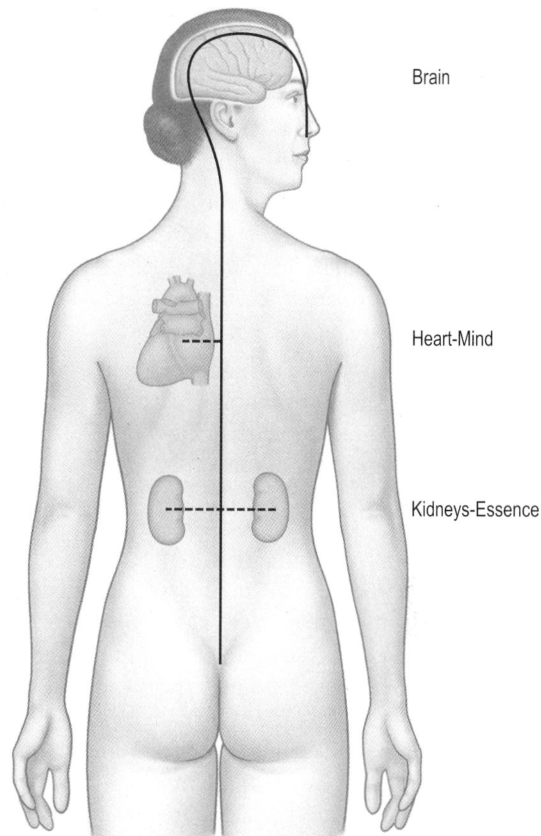

Figure 13.27 Influence of Governing Vessel on Essence, Mind and Brain.

Du-10 Lingtai *Spirit Platform*

This point is below the spinous process of the sixth dorsal vertebra, level with Du-16 Dushu. It is therefore one vertebral space below BL-15 Xinshu, hence its name – it is the platform below the Heart.

The *Gatherings from Eminent Acupuncturists* emphasizes the connection of this point to the Heart. It says that this point is the connection between the Heart and the Governing Vessel and it combines well with HE-7 Shenmen.[75]

I use this point primarily in Deficiency conditions underlying emotional problems. I use it to strengthen the Heart to treat depression or anxiety.

Du-11 Shendao *Mind Way*

Du-11 strengthens the Heart and calms the Mind. Its indications include "sadness, anxiety, poor memory, palpitations, disorientation and timidity". The *Great Compendium of Acupuncture* (1601) lists "disorientation, sadness, worry and poor memory" among the indications for Du-11.[76]

The *Gatherings from Eminent Acupuncturists* (1529) lists "disorientation, sadness, worry and palpitations from shock" for the indications of this point.[77]

Du-11 is on the same level as BL-15 Xinshu, the Back-Transporting point of the Heart, and its action mostly extends to the Heart. It nourishes the Heart and calms the Mind, and therefore treats depression, sadness, and anxiety.

Du-12 Shenzhu *Body Pillar*

Du-12 calms the Mind and opens the Mind's orifices. Among its indications are "manic behavior, 'seeing ghosts' and rage with desire to kill people". The *Great Compendium of Acupuncture* (1601) lists "incoherent speech, Dullness and Mania (*Dian Kuang*), 'seeing ghosts' and desire to kill people" among the indications for Du-12.[78]

The indication "desire to kill people" for this point is interesting. As discussed above under the points BL-13 Feishu and BL-42 Pohu, the indication "desire to commit suicide" for BL-13 Feishu must be seen in the context of the Corporeal Soul (*Po*), which is housed in the Lungs. The Corporeal Soul is a physical soul with a centripetal movement, constantly materializing and constantly separating into different constituent aspects. The Corporeal Soul is in relation with *gui*, i.e. ghosts or spirits (of dead people). The centripetal forces of *gui* within the Corporeal Soul, constantly fragmenting, are, eventually, the germ of death.

It is therefore interesting that the three points related to the Lungs (which house the Corporeal Soul), all aligned on the back, are indicated either for desire to commit suicide or desire to kill, i.e. they are related to thoughts of death. The indications are as follows.

- Du-12 Shenzhu: "desire to kill people".
- BL-13 Feishu: "desire to commit suicide".
- BL-42 Pohu: "three corpses flowing".

Du-14 Dazhui *Big Vertebra*

Du-14 clears and strengthens the Mind. Among its indications are "depression, tiredness, poor memory and poor concentration".

If used with reinforcing method and, in particular, with direct moxa, Du-14 tonifies the Yang and can be used in any interior pattern of Yang deficiency. In particular, it tonifies Heart- and Kidney-Yang.

Since it is also the meeting point of all the Yang channels that transport clear Yang upwards to the head, it is a point of the Sea of Qi and where the Governing Vessel enters the brain. Du-14 can also clear the Mind and stimulate the brain when the person is depressed and confused. Thus, Du-14 acts on the Spirit in three ways: first by tonifying Heart-Yang and therefore the Mind, second by tonifying Kidney-Yang and therefore the Will-Power (*Zhi*) and third by clearing the Brain.

Du-16 Fengfu *Wind Palace*

One of Sun Si Miao's 13 Ghost points, Du-16 nourishes Marrow, benefits the Brain, calms the Mind and opens the Mind's orifices. Among its indications are "manic behavior, desire to commit suicide, sadness and fear".

Du-16 is a point of the Sea of Marrow. Marrow fills up the brain, and this point can clear the Mind and stimulate the brain.

Du-17 Naohu *Brain Window*

Du-17 benefits the Brain, calms the Mind and opens the Mind's orifices. Its indications include "manic behavior".

Du-18 Qiangjian *Unyielding Space*

Du-18 opens the Mind's orifices and calms the Mind. Among its indications are "mad walking, insomnia, and Dullness and Mania".

Du-18 also regulates Liver-Blood and is therefore indicated for severe mental restlessness, agitation, mental confusion and obsessive thoughts from Mind Obstructed occurring against a background of Blood stasis.

Du-19 Houding *Posterior Vertex*

Du-19 calms the Mind and opens the Mind's orifices. Its indications include "manic behavior, anxiety, mental restlessness and insomnia".

The *Explanation of the Acupuncture Points* (1654) lists "manic walking without rest and dullness (*Dian*)" among the indications for Du-19.[79] The *Gatherings from Eminent Acupuncturists* lists the same symptoms.[80]

Du-19 has a powerful calming effect on the Mind and is very often used in severe anxiety, especially in combination with Ren-15 Jiuwei.

Du-20 Baihui *Hundred Meetings*

Du-20 benefits the Brain, clears the Mind and lifts the spirits. The *Explanation of the Acupuncture Points* (1654) lists "mental restlessness, poor memory, disorientation, crying a lot and incoherent speech" among the indications for Du-20.[81]

The *Gatherings from Eminent Acupuncturists* (1529) lists "fright, palpitations, poor memory, crying and confused speech" among the indications for Du-20.[82]

I use Du-20 in all cases of depression, whether occurring against a background of an Empty or a Full pattern. It is particularly indicated in depression from Deficiency.

This point's lifting action on Yang has a mental effect, promoting the rising of clear Yang to the Brain and the Mind. In my experience, Du-20 has a powerful effect in lifting depression and clearing the Mind.

When using this point with moxa to raise the Yang, caution must be exercised to make sure that there are no Heat symptoms. Also, this point should not be stimulated with moxa if the person suffers from high blood pressure.

Du-24 Shenting *Mind Courtyard*

Du-24 calms and lifts the Mind and opens the Mind's orifices. Among its indications are "Dullness and

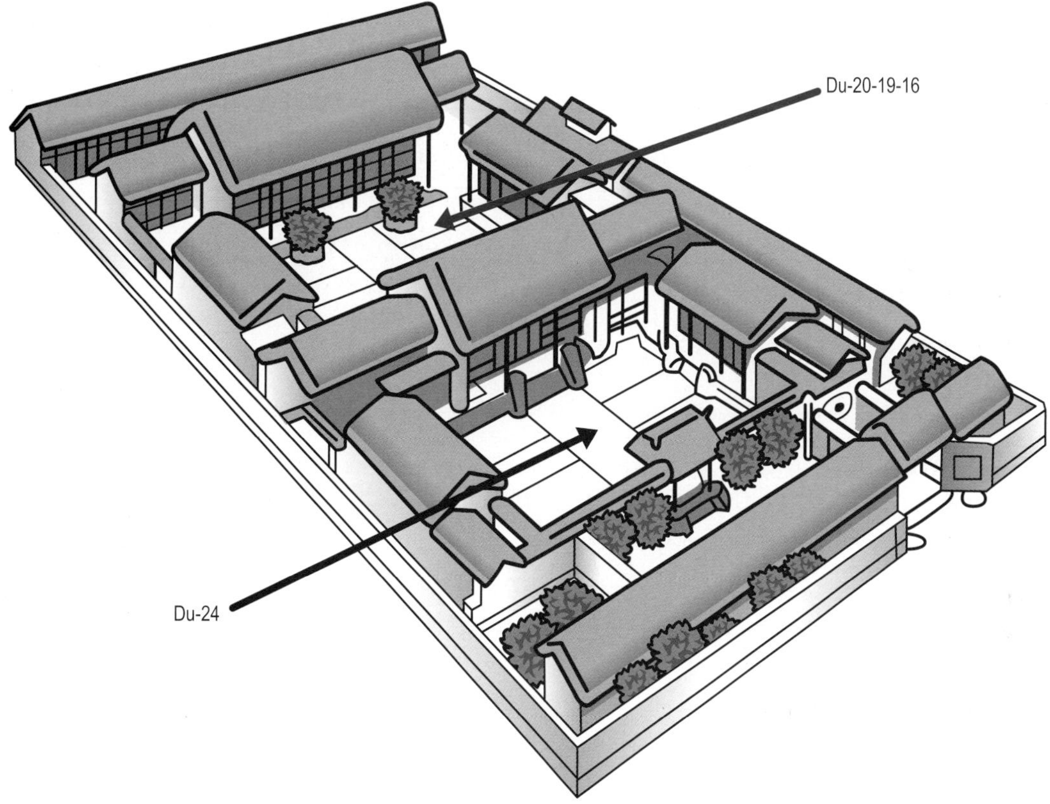

Figure 13.28 Energetic action of Du-24 Shenting.

Mania, depression, anxiety, poor memory and insomnia". The *Explanation of the Acupuncture Points* lists "dreaming, manic behavior, ascending to high places, singing and discarding clothes" among its indications.[83]

The *Gatherings from Eminent Acupuncturists* lists "ascending to high places, singing and discarding clothes, fright, palpitations and insomnia" among the indications for Du-24.[84]

The most important aspect of Du-24's energetic action is its downward movement; it makes Qi descend and subdues rebellious Yang. This is a very important and powerful point to calm the Mind. It is frequently combined with G.B.-13 Benshen for severe anxiety and fears.

Another important feature of this point which makes it particularly useful is that it can both calm and lift the Mind; therefore, it is used not only for anxiety and insomnia but also for depression and sadness. It is also used in psychiatric practice for schizophrenia and split personality.[85]

The name of this point refers to its strong influence on the Mind and Spirit. The courtyard was traditionally considered to be a very important part of the house as it was the one that gave the first impression to visitors; it is the entrance. Thus, this point could be said to be the "entrance" to the Mind and Spirit, and its being a courtyard highlights its importance (Fig. 13.28).

SUMMARY

Governing Vessel channel points for emotional problems

- With the exception of Du-4, Governing Vessel points are especially indicated for mental-emotional problems occurring against a background of Full patterns.
- Governing Vessel points on the head are very important in the treatment of mental-emotional problems.

Du-4 Mingmen Gate of Life

Du-4 clears the Mind, lifts the spirit and strengthens Will-Power. Its indications include "depression, lack of will-power and mental confusion".

Du-10 Lingtai Spirit Platform

Du-10 is the connection between the Heart and the Governing Vessel. I use this point primarily in Deficiency conditions underlying emotional problems.

Du-11 Shendao Mind Way

Du-11 strengthens the Heart and calms the Mind. Its indications include "sadness, anxiety, poor memory, palpitations, disorientation and timidity".

Du-12 Shenzhu Body Pillar

Du-12 calms the Mind and opens the Mind's orifices. Among its indications are "manic behavior, 'seeing ghosts' and rage with desire to kill people".

Du-14 Dazhui Big Vertebra

Du-14 clears and strengthens the Mind. Among its indications are "depression, tiredness, poor memory and poor concentration".

Du-16 Fengfu Wind Palace

One of Sun Si Miao's 13 Ghost points, Du-16 nourishes Marrow, benefits the Brain, calms the Mind and opens the Mind's orifices. Among its indications are "manic behavior, desire to commit suicide, sadness, and fear".

Du-17 Naohu Brain Window

Du-17 benefits the Brain, calms the Mind and opens the Mind's orifices. Its indications include "manic behavior".

Du-18 Qiangjian Unyielding Space

Du-18 opens the Mind's orifices and calms the Mind. Among its indications are "mad walking, insomnia and manic-depression".

Du-19 Houding Posterior Vertex

Du-19 calms the Mind and opens the Mind's orifices. Its indications include "manic behavior, anxiety, mental restlessness and insomnia". Often used in combination with Ren-15 Jiuwei.

Du-20 Baihui Hundred Meetings

Du-20 benefits the Brain, clears the Mind and lifts the spirits. I use Du-20 in all cases of depression, whether occurring against a background of an Empty or a Full pattern. It is particularly indicated in depression from a Deficiency.

Du-24 Shenting Mind Courtyard

Du-24 calms and lifts the Mind and opens the Mind's orifices. Among its indications are "manic-depression, depression, anxiety, poor memory and insomnia".

EXTRA POINTS

Hunshe *House of the Ethereal Soul*

The extra point Hunshe is situated on the abdomen, level with the umbilicus and 1 *cun* lateral to it; it is therefore between the Kidney and the Stomach channels. The name "Hunshe" means "house of the Ethereal Soul".

The location of this point and its reference to the Ethereal Soul is significant. Ren-8 Shenque means "Palace of the Spirit" and the location of the "house of the Ethereal Soul" next to it illustrates the close connection between the Spirit and the Ethereal Soul. As we have seen in Chapter 3, the Ethereal Soul provides movement to the Mind and Spirit in the form of ideas, intuition, inspiration, plans, projects and life dreams.

Modern books report only physical indications for this point, such as "diarrhea with pus and blood and constipation". In my experience, this point has actions that are similar to those of BL-47 Hunmen, i.e. it regulates the movement of the Ethereal Soul. It can be used to stimulate the movement of the Ethereal Soul when the person is depressed or to restrain it when the person is manic.

For this purpose, I frequently use this point together with Ren-8 Shenque, especially when I want to stimulate the movement of the Ethereal Soul against a background of a Deficiency condition.

Yintang *Seal Hall*

This extra point is in between the eyebrows, on the Governing Vessel. It has a long history of use for convulsions, especially in children. However, it is also used to calm the Mind and especially to promote sleep in insomnia.

POINTS FOR MENTAL PROBLEMS FROM NANJING AFFILIATED HOSPITAL

The following are point combinations used in the Provincial Psychiatric Hospital in Nanjing.[86]

- *Dreamy state*: Du-14 Dazhui, L.I.-11 Quchi, G.B.-34 Yanglingquan, Ren-8 Shenque and Ren-4 Guanyuan.
- *Forgetting words*: Du-20 Baihui, BL-8 Luoque, HE-5 Tongli, KI-4 Dazhong.
- *Obsessive ideas*: Du-18 Qiangjian, S.I.-3 Houxi, G.B.-39 Xuanzhong.
- *Jealousy*: P-7 Daling and G.B.-43 Xiaxi.
- *Difficulty in concentrating*: G.B.-17 Zhengying, P-5 Jianshi, Yintang, ST-40 Fenglong.
- *Poor memory*: Du-20 Baihui, HE-7 Shenmen, KI-3 Taixi, G.B.-18 Chengling.
- *Lack of will-power*: Du-19 Houding, G.B.-6 Xuanli, P-6 Neiguan, SP-10 Xuehai.
- *Emotionally up and down*: G.B.-15 Toulinqi, Du-20 Baihui, P-8 Laogong, KI-1 Yongquan, Du-25 Suliao.

EXAMPLES OF POINT COMBINATIONS FOR MENTAL-EMOTIONAL PROBLEMS

The following are combinations of points for mental-emotional problems that I use frequently. I often use points unilaterally and crossed over, i.e. one point on one side and the other on the opposite side.

- *LU-7 Lieque and LIV-3*: harmonize Left-Right, settle the Ethereal Soul and Corporeal Soul, harmonize Liver and Lungs, calm anxiety, worry and agitation, lift depression, regulate the coming and going of the Ethereal Soul.
- *LU-7 Lieque and ST-40 Fenglong*: make Lung-Qi descend, calm the Mind, settle the Corporeal Soul, open the chest, treat worry, depression and anxiety from Lung-Qi stagnation and Phlegm.
- *LU-7 Lieque and P-6 Neiguan*: make Lung- and Heart-Qi descend, calm the Mind, settle the Corporeal Soul, stimulate the coming and going of the Ethereal Soul, treat problems from relationships, worry and depression, occurring against a background of Qi stagnation (of Lungs and/or Liver and/or Heart).
- *LI-4 Hegu and LIV-3 Taichong*: calm the Mind, settle the Ethereal Soul, subdue Liver-Qi and Liver-Yang, treat worry, depression, irritability and anger.
- *T.B.-3 Zhongzhu and G.B.-40 Qiuxu*: move Liver-Qi, regulate the Triple Burner, stimulate the coming and going of the Ethereal Soul, treat depression, moodiness, indecision and lack of courage occurring against a background of Liver-Qi stagnation.
- *P-6 Neiguan and LIV-3 Taichong*: move Liver-Qi, stimulate the movement of the Ethereal Soul in depression, calm the Mind and settle the Ethereal Soul.
- *P-7 Daling and LIV-3 Taichong*: calm the Mind, settle the Ethereal Soul, restrain the movement of the Ethereal Soul when the person is slightly manic.
- *P-6 Neiguan and G.B.-40 Qiuxu*: these two points stimulate the movement of the Ethereal Soul when the person is depressed.
- *Du-20 Baihui and Ren-15 Jiuwei*: these two points lift mood in depression but also calm the Mind if the person is anxious. They are especially indicated for Empty patterns.
- *Du-24 Shenting and Ren-15 Jiuwei*: calm the Mind and nourish the Heart. This combination is used for depression, anxiety and mental-emotional problems occurring against a background of Deficiency. Du-24 can both lift mood in depression and calm the Mind in anxiety. It also improves memory.
- *Du-24 Shenting and Ren-4 Guanyuan*: calm the Spirit by nourishing the Kidneys and strengthening the Original Qi. It is suitable for severe anxiety occurring against a background of Kidney deficiency. It is particularly indicated for anxiety as it roots Qi in the Lower Burner and draws it downwards away from the head and the Heart where it harasses the Mind.
- *Du-20 Baihui and Ren-4 Guanyuan*: calm the Spirit, nourish the Kidneys and strengthen Original Qi. This relieves depression by nourishing the Kidneys and strengthening the Original Qi.
- *Du-19 Houding and Ren-15 Jiuwei*: calm the Spirit and allay anxiety. Du-19 calms the Spirit while Ren-15 calms the Spirit and nourishes the Heart. This combination has a powerful calming effect. Ren-15 will also relieve anxiety manifesting with a feeling of oppression in the chest.

END NOTES

1. Deadman P, Al-Khafaji M 1998 A Manual of Acupuncture. Journal of Chinese Medicine Publications, Hove, England.
2. Heilongjiang Province National Medical Research Group 1984 Zhen Jiu Da Cheng Jiao Shi 针灸大成教释 [An Explanation of the Great Compendium of Acupuncture]. People's Health Publishing House, Beijing, p. 716. The *Great Compendium of Acupuncture* itself, by Yang Ji Zhou, was first published in 1601.
3. 1991 Zhen Jiu Ju Ying 针灸聚英 [Gatherings from Eminent Acupuncturists]. Shanghai Science and Technology Publishing House, Shanghai, p. 12. The *Gatherings from Eminent Acupuncturists* was written by Gao Wu and first published in 1529.
4. Shan Chang Hua 1990 Jing Xue Jie 经穴解 [An Explanation of the Acupuncture Points]. People's Health Publishing House, Beijing, pp. 26–27. An *Explanation of the Acupuncture Points* was written by Yue Han Zhen and first published in 1654.
5. Ibid., p. 27.
6. Gatherings from Eminent Acupuncturists, p. 12.
7. An Explanation of the Acupuncture Points, p. 31.
8. Gatherings from Eminent Acupuncturists, p. 19.
9. An Explanation of the Acupuncture Points, p. 50.
10. Great Compendium of Acupuncture, p. 734.
11. Gatherings from Eminent Acupuncturists, p. 30.
12. An Explanation of the Acupuncture Points, p. 88.
13. Ibid., p. 102.
14. Gatherings from Eminent Acupuncturists, p. 85.
15. Ibid., p. 85.
16. Ibid., p. 84.
17. An Explanation of the Acupuncture Points, p. 103.
18. Ibid., p. 106.
19. Ibid., p. 116.
20. Ibid., p. 117.
21. Gatherings from Eminent Acupuncturists, p. 40.
22. An Explanation of the Acupuncture Points, p. 138.
23. Great Compendium of Acupuncture, p. 808.
24. An Explanation of the Acupuncture Points, p. 141.
25. Gatherings from Eminent Acupuncturists, p. 47.
26. Ji Jie Yin 1984 Tai Yi Shen Zhen Jiu Lin Zheng Lu 太已神针灸临证录 [Clinical Records of Tai Yi Shen Acupuncture]. Shanxi Province Scientific Publishing House, Shanxi, p. 23.
27. Zhang Shan Chen 1982 Zhen Jiu Jia Yi Jing Shu Xue Zhong Ji 针灸甲已经输穴中集 [Essential Collection of Acupuncture Points from the ABC of Acupuncture]. Shandong Scientific Publishing House, Shandong, p. 112. First published AD 282.
28. Sun Si Miao AD 652 Thousand Ducat Prescriptions, cited in Anwei College of Traditional Chinese Medicine-Shanghai College of Traditional Chinese Medicine 1987 Zhen Jiu Xue Ci Dian 针灸学辞典 [Dictionary of Acupuncture]. Shanghai Scientific Publishing House, Shanghai, p. 477.
29. Great Compendium of Acupuncture, p. 816.
30. An Explanation of the Acupuncture Points, p. 152.
31. Gatherings from Eminent Acupuncturists, p. 51.
32. Great Compendium of Acupuncture, p. 817.
33. Gatherings from Eminent Acupuncturists, p. 52.
34. An Explanation of the Acupuncture Points, p. 153.
35. Ibid., p. 158.
36. Ibid., p. 182.
37. Gatherings from Eminent Acupuncturists, p. 61.
38. Eyssalet J-M 1990 Le Secret de la Maison des Ancêtres. Guy Trédaniel Editeur, Paris, p. 30.
39. An Explanation of the Acupuncture Points, p. 184.
40. Gatherings from Eminent Acupuncturists, p. 61.
41. An Explanation of the Acupuncture Points, p. 211.
42. Ibid., p. 206.
43. Gatherings from Eminent Acupuncturists, p. 67.
44. An Explanation of the Acupuncture Points, p. 207.
45. Great Compendium of Acupuncture, p. 843.
46. An Explanation of the Acupuncture Points, p. 211.
47. Gatherings from Eminent Acupuncturists, p. 69.
48. An Explanation of the Acupuncture Points, p. 211.
49. The Great Compendium of Acupuncture, p. 871.
50. Gatherings from Eminent Acupuncturists, p. 81.
51. An Explanation of the Acupuncture Points, p. 259.
52. Ibid., p. 266.
53. Ibid., 287.
54. Gatherings from Eminent Acupuncturists, p. 88.
55. 1981 Ling Shu Jing 灵枢经 [Spiritual Axis]. People's Health Publishing House, Beijing, p. 3. First published *c.*100 BC.
56. The Great Compendium of Acupuncture, p. 886.
57. Gatherings from Eminent Acupuncturists, p. 101.
58. Dr Zhang Ming Jiu, personal communication, Nanjing 1982.
59. Cheng Bao Shu 1988 Zhen Jiu Da Ci Dian 针灸大辞典 [Great Dictionary of Acupuncture]. Beijing Science Publishing House, Beijing, p. 11.
60. Jiao Shun Fa 1987 Zhong Guo Zhen Jiu Qiu Zheng 中国针灸求证 [An Enquiry into Chinese Acupuncture]. Shanxi Science Publishing House, Shanxi, p. 52.
61. Zhang Jie Bin 1986 Jing Yue Quan Shu 京岳全书 [The Complete Book of Jing Yue]. Shanghai Science Publishing House, Shanghai, p. 573. First published in 1624.
62. An Explanation of the Acupuncture Points, p. 334.
63. Dr Zhang Ming Jiu, personal communication, Nanjing 1982.
64. Jiao Shun Fa 1987 An Enquiry into Chinese Acupuncture, p. 52.
65. Dr Zhang Ming Jiu, personal communication, Nanjing 1982.
66. The Great Compendium of Acupuncture, p. 923.
67. Cheng Bao Shu 1988 Zhen Jiu Da Ci Dian 针灸大辞典 [Great Dictionary of Chinese Acupuncture]. Beijing Science and Technology Press, Beijing, p. 219.
68. The Great Compendium of Acupuncture, p. 960.
69. Gatherings from Eminent Acupuncturists, p. 129.
70. The Great Compendium of Acupuncture, p. 961.
71. An Explanation of the Acupuncture Points, p. 443.
72. Spiritual Axis, p. 3.
73. The "Room of Sperm" is not an anatomical, physical structure but simply indicates the Lower *Dan Tian* in a man where sperm was thought to be made by the Kidneys.
74. Nanjing College of Traditional Chinese Medicine 1979 Nan Jing Jiao Shi 难经教释 [A Revised Explanation of the Classic of Difficulties]. People's Health Publishing House, Beijing, p. 90. First published *c.*AD 100.
75. Gatherings from Eminent Acupuncturists, p. 117.
76. The Great Compendium of Acupuncture, p. 972.
77. Gatherings from Eminent Acupuncturists, p. 119.
78. The Great Compendium of Acupuncture, p. 973.
79. An Explanation of the Acupuncture Points, p. 411.
80. Gatherings from Eminent Acupuncturists, p. 121.
81. An Explanation of the Acupuncture Points, p. 412.
82. Gatherings from Eminent Acupuncturists, p. 122.
83. An Explanation of the Acupuncture Points, p. 415.
84. Gatherings from Eminent Acupuncturists, p. 123.
85. Dr Zhang Ming Jiu, personal communication, Nanjing 1982.
86. Course notes, Advanced Acupuncture Course at the Nanjing University of Traditional Chinese Medicine, 1981–1982.

西方哲学中的情志和自我概念

CHAPTER 14

EMOTIONS AND CONCEPT OF SELF IN WESTERN PHILOSOPHY

ANCIENT THEORIES ON EMOTIONS *285*
Pythagoras *285*
Heraclitus *285*
Socrates *286*
Plato *286*
Aristotle *286*
Stoics *287*
Middle Ages and Christianity *288*
St Augustine *288*
Thomas Aquinas *288*
Descartes *290*
Thomas Willis *290*
Spinoza *291*
Hume *291*
Kant *291*
EARLY MODERN THEORIES ABOUT EMOTIONS *291*
THE JAMES–LANGE THEORY OF EMOTIONS *292*
MODERN THEORIES ABOUT EMOTIONS *294*
Sartre *295*
Solomon's theory of emotions *295*
Bockover's theory of emotions *297*
Damasio's theory of emotions *297*
FREUD, JUNG AND BOWLBY *299*
Freud *299*
Jung *300*
Bowlby *302*
MODERN NEUROPHYSIOLOGICAL VIEW ON EMOTIONS *303*
Neurophysiology of emotions *303*
The triune brain *306*
SUMMARY *309*

EMOTIONS AND CONCEPT OF SELF IN WESTERN PHILOSOPHY

In this chapter, I will discuss the Western view of emotions as described by various Western philosophers, ancient and modern, by modern Western psychologists and by neurophysiologists. I personally think it is important to do this in order to balance the view of emotions in Chinese medicine with that of emotions in Western culture. This is important for two reasons.

First, we should not look at the Chinese medicine view of emotions as the only possible one; there is much more to the emotions than their being merely causes of disease as they are in Chinese medicine. As we shall see, although some Western philosophers do look upon the emotions as causes of disease (as Chinese medicine does), others consider them an essential way in which our mind works.

Second, it is important to explore the emotions as seen by Western philosophers and psychologists because their view stems from Western concepts of Self. As we shall see in the next chapter (Chapter 15), the concept of Self in Chinese society differs greatly from that in Western societies. This has an important relevance in the exploration of how the Chinese medicine's view of emotions applies to Western patients.

A constant theme in all of Western philosophy, ancient and modern (with few exceptions), has been that the emotions (or passions) are factors that cloud Reason. As we have seen in Chapter 9, this point of view is similar to that of the three main Chinese philosophies, i.e. Daoism, Confucianism and Buddhism. According to this view, emotions are blind forces that sweep reason away and lead us into trouble. The metaphor of describing emotions as overwhelming natural events is very common in Western philosophical literature, and many Western philosophers do see emotions as causes of disease in a similar way to that of Chinese medicine.

James reports from ancient writers:[1]

Images of civil strife within the soul are matched by a view of the passions as natural disorders – as storms, torrents, tempest. They are winds that put the mind in tumult, sweeping us along like ships in a gale. In these metaphors, passion is understood as motion. The passions are turbulent, they are furious reboundings, they are violent and rash sallies. As such, they are often portrayed in addition as diseases, pathological states in which we easily succumb and of which we need to be cured. The passions induce blindness of understanding, perversion of the will, alteration of the humours.

As we saw in Chapter 9, this view of emotions accords with that of Chinese medicine in which the action of emotions is described as a "surge" like the surge of a wave.

!

Most Western philosophers regarded emotions as factors which disturb and cloud Reason.

The Cartesian philosopher Malebranche (1638–1715) expressed a disdain of emotions in the strongest terms: "*Impose silence on your senses, your imagination and your passions, and you will hear the pure voice of inner truth.*"[2] From this perspective, the intellect provides accurate information, while emotion clouds our minds with disinformation. Young even went so far as saying that emotions have no conscious purpose and cause a "*complete loss of cerebral control*".[3]

Over the course of centuries, various Western philosophers have advocated different strategies for achieving release from emotional turmoil, e.g. the *euthumia* advocated by Democritus, the *tranquillitas* of Seneca, the *ataraxia* of the Epicureans, etc.[4]

However, there have been dissenting voices over the centuries, especially from Hume, Spinoza, Nietzsche and Sartre. In modern times, Solomon strongly makes the case for emotions being judgments and he disagrees with what he calls the "Myth of passions", i.e. that emotions are factors that cloud our reason and mind.

Greenfield thinks that emotions are the building blocks of consciousness; she says that one cannot understand consciousness without understanding emotions and that consciousness is not purely rational or cognitive.[5]

As we shall see below, emotions are far from being simply psychic factors that cloud reason; indeed, they are an essential way in which our mind (and "reason") develops. Lewis mapped out the emotional development of babies from 3 months to 3 years old. Newborn babies display a bipolar emotional life; on the one hand, there is distress marked by crying and, on the other, there is pleasure marked by satiation and attention.

By 3 months, joy emerges; infants start to smile and appear to show excitement and happiness. Also by 3 months, sadness emerges around the withdrawal of positive stimulus events.[6] Anger has been reported to emerge between 4 and 6 months. Anger is manifested when children are frustrated, in particular when their hands and feet are pinned down.

Fearfulness emerges later and it reflects a further cognitive development. Schaffer says: "*In order for children to show fearfulness, they have to be capable of comparing the event that causes them fearfulness with some other event.*"[7] Cognitive processes play an important role in the emergence of the early emotions. By the time the baby is over 2 years old, a new cognitive capacity emerges; the emergence of consciousness or objective self-awareness gives rise to a new class of emotions. These have been called the "self-conscious emotions" and include embarrassment, empathy and envy.

The emotional development of a baby mirrors the Chinese medicine's view, according to which the Mind (*Shen*) is immature in babies and it gradually matures to reach more or less full maturity at 7 years old.

Modern neuroscientists confirm that the limbic system (seat of emotions) is *essential* to the development of the cortex; in other words, emotions, far from being factors that disturb "reason", are an essential way in which "reason" develops. Lewis, Amini and Lannon say:[8]

One of the physiological processes that limbic regulation directs is the development of the brain itself – and that means attachment determines the ultimate nature of a child's mind. Many subsystems of the mammalian brain do not come pre-programmed; maturing mammals need limbic regulation to give coherence to neurodevelopment.

> !
>
> Maturing mammals need limbic regulation to give coherence to neurodevelopment.

Lewis, Amini and Lannon point out that emotions are much more ancient than cortical development. They say:[9]

Emotions reach back 100 million years while cognition is a few hundred thousands years old. Despite their youth, the prominent capacities of the neocortical brain dazzled the Western world and eclipsed the mind's quieter limbic inhabitant. Because logic and deduction accomplish so plainly, they have been presumed the master keys that open all doors.

They continue by saying:[10]

Limbic resonance, regulation and revision define our emotional existence; they are the walls and towers of the neural edifice that evolution has built for mammals to live in. Our intellect is largely blind to them. Within the heart's true edifice, those who allow themselves to be guided by Reason blunder into walls and stumble over sills. Our culture teems with experts who propose to tell us how to think our way to a better future, as if that could be done. They capitalize on the ease of credibly presuming that intellect is running the show. Not so. Reason's last step – wrote Pascal – is recognizing that an infinity of things surpass it.

We know that emotions played an important evolutionary role in our development and, besides becoming causes of disease under certain circumstances, they can also perform positive roles. For example, sadness can strengthen social bonds. In the course of evolution, by strengthening social bonds, grief increased the probability of surviving.[11]

Anger allows us to mobilize and sustain energy at high levels; shame ensures social order and stability; fear motivates escape from dangerous situations.[12]

The discussion of emotions and concepts of self in modern philosophy will be conducted according to the following topics.

- Ancient theories on emotions
- Early modern theories about emotions
- The James–Lange theory of emotions
- Modern theories about emotions
- Freud, Jung and Bowlby
- Modern neurophysiological view on emotions

ANCIENT THEORIES ON EMOTIONS

Most of the ancient philosophers discussed the nature and function of emotions. Solomon presents a summary of the view on emotions by ancient philosophers.[13] By the times of Pythagoras, Heraclitus and Plato, the soul was established as residing in the brain.

The soul was variously divided. In one version, the spirit (*spiritus naturalis*), which originates in the liver, is carried to the heart and lungs and is converted into the essential life spirit (*spiritus vitalis*), which is then distilled in the brain to become the animal spirit (*spiritus animalis*), the conveyer of thought, judgment and memory.[14] The embodied soul is in the brain. This view presents some interesting similarities with that of Chinese medicine in which the Ethereal Soul (in the Liver) interacts with the Mind of the Heart to produce judgment, cognition and volition.

Pythagoras

Pythagoras (570–490 BC) thought that plants have souls, and that human souls, for instance, can come to animate plants. Some think that the very term "soul" (*psyche* φυχη) was coined by Pythagoras for the first time. The philosophy of Pythagoras was concerned with the continued existence of the person (or something suitably person-like) after death.

Against the Homeric background, "soul" was an appropriate word to use so as to denote the person, or quasi-person, that continued to exist after death. Pythagoras conceived of the "transmigration" of souls after that, a concept similar to the Buddhist view on reincarnation. This belief is well illustrated by a story about Pythagoras, reported by Xenophanes:[15]

Once, they say, he was passing by when a puppy was being whipped, and he took pity and said: 'Stop, do not beat it; it is the soul of a friend that I recognized when I heard its soul's voice.'

Heraclitus

Heraclitus (535–475 BC) is credited by some to being the first Greek philosopher who conceived of a soul.

Heraclitus attributes wisdom to the soul, provided that it is in the right state or condition; he considered "a dry soul" as the best. He may have been the first thinker to articulate a connection between soul and motor functions. He thought that a man who is drunk resembles a boy stumbling and not knowing where he goes, and that this is due to his soul being "moist".

Heraclitus thought that the soul was bodily, but composed of an unusually fine or rare kind of matter, e.g. air or fire. Soul and body were not thought to be radically different in kind; their difference seemed just to consist of a difference in degree of properties such as fineness and mobility.

Heraclitus's views present some similarity to the Chinese views of the body and mind/soul, since they are both manifestations of Qi in different states of condensation.

Socrates

Socrates (469–399 BC) presented arguments for the immortality of the soul. Apart from the question of immortality or otherwise, there is the further question of whether the soul, if it does have some form of existence after the person has died, still possesses some power and wisdom. Answering both questions, Socrates says not only that the soul is immortal, but also that it contemplates truths after its separation from the body at the time of death.

Plato

Plato (429–347 BC) conceives the soul as possessing cognitive and intellectual features: it is something that reasons; something that regulates and controls the body and its desires and affections; and something that has virtues such as temperance, justice and courage. The soul as conceived by Plato is not simply the mind. It is broader in that Plato retains the traditional idea of soul as distinguishing the animate from the inanimate.

Like many philosophers after him will do, Plato considers that we are good when reason rules and bad when we are dominated by our desires. To be master of oneself means to have the higher part of the soul rule over the lower, to have reason rule over desires.

Plato considered also the irrational forces of the soul, creating the image of a charioteer (reason, the rational side of the soul) riding a chariot pulled by two horses, one representing anger and domination, the other the lower appetites. Plato described the "tugging" between the charioteer and the horses. This is an image that influenced Freud's theory of the ego and the id.

According to Plato, the rational side of the soul is not fully developed until the child becomes 14. He says:[16]

This rational element is small and weak at first but finishes large and strong around the 14th year, by when it is right for it, like the charioteer, to take control and rule over the pair of horses naturally conjoined with it, appetite and anger.

Aristotle

Aristotle (384–322 BC) discussed emotions at length. He said:[17]

Emotion is that which leads one's condition to become so transformed that his judgement is affected, and which is accompanied by pleasure and pain. Examples of emotion include anger, fear, pity and the like, as well as the opposite of these.

To Aristotle, they are not only feelings but also judgments of the mind. To Aristotle, an emotion is a state of mind, directed at a certain object, on certain grounds. In the example of anger, this is a desire for revenge, directed at a particular person, on the grounds that he or she has insulted me.[18]

An interesting aspect of Aristotle's ideas on emotions is their physical manifestation, which presents interesting analogies with Chinese medicine. Aristotle said that angry people are hot around the heart, and because in anger this heat moves upwards, they become "*red in the face and full of breath*".[19] The important and interesting thing is that these are not just metaphors but describe a physical process that takes place under the influence of emotions (as Chinese medicine describes).

Aristotle thought that the cognitive element of emotions constitutes its "form" and the underlying physiological changes brought about by feelings constitute its "matter". This view opens the way to two separate ways of treating emotions: emotions might be calmed either by addressing the physiological process or by addressing the cognitions.

Aristotle thought that the soul resides in the heart rather than the brain. He thought that the function of the brain is to cool the blood but that the heart was the prime organ of the soul – hence, in Shakespeare's *Mer-*

chant of Venice: "Where is fancy bred, or in the heart or in the head?"

Interestingly, Aristotle believed in the existence of three souls: a vegetative one which animated the vegetable world; a sensitive one which animated animals; and an intellectual one which animated human beings.[20] Therefore, human beings have two souls in common with the animal world and one in common with the vegetable world. This view is very similar to the Chinese one of three types of Ethereal Soul.

Stoics

The Stoics had a very negative view of emotions, considering them psychic factors conducive to misery. The Stoics considered emotions to be judgments about the world and one's place in it.[21] However, as they considered the world to be out of control, emotions were therefore misguided judgments; consequently, emotions make us miserable and frustrated.

The Stoics made a careful study of the component judgments that comprise the emotions – the presumptuousness of moral judgment in anger, the vulnerability of love, the self-absorption of security in fear.

Chrysippus (280–206 BC) developed the standard Stoic view on the nature of emotions. In his view, all emotions consist of two judgments: the judgment that there is benefit or harm at hand from a situation, and the judgment that it is appropriate to react.[22] The Stoics made a clear distinction between the emotion, which involves a judgment, and the corresponding feeling which does not. The feeling may precede the emotion, in which case the Stoics called it "first movements". Interestingly, Chrysippus put the command center of the soul in the heart.

In the Stoics' view, emotions can be "treated" since they are not involuntary reactions (the Stoics discounted the "first movements") but judgments which can be suspended. It is interesting that such training is remarkably close to modern cognitive behavioral therapy.

Seneca (4 BC–AD 65) distinguished three stages in emotions: the first stage is the feeling stage (which he called "first movements"), the second stage is the emotion proper when a judgment is made, and the third stage is when the emotion is uncontrolled and "floods" our mind.

The Stoics' position on emotions differed from that of Aristotle. For Aristotle, emotions are useful in moderation; he called this *metriopatheia*. The Stoics thought that all emotions are pernicious and should be eradicated; they called this state *apatheia* (from which, with a change of meaning, our word "apathy" derives).

Chrysippus describes four basic emotions:

- *distress* is the judgment that there is bad at hand and it is appropriate to feel a contraction
- *pleasure* is the judgment that there is good at hand and that it is appropriate to feel an expansion
- *fear* is the judgment that there is bad at hand and that it is appropriate to avoid it
- *appetite* is the judgment that there is good at hand and that it is appropriate to reach for it.

The reaction to fear and appetite is behavioral and voluntary. The reaction to distress and pleasure is involuntary and it involves contraction and expansion, respectively. Sorabji says: "*What contracts and expands is said to be the mind (animus), and the mind is a physical spirit for the Stoic materialists.*"[23] This is very interesting as it resonates with the Chinese view of expansion (called *shen*) and contraction (called *gui*) of our mind (*see Chapter 7*).

Posidonius (1st century BC) considered also the irrational aspects of the soul, referring back to Plato's views of the charioteer (reason) driving a chariot pulled by two horses, one being the irascible part of the soul, the other the lower appetites. From this, Posidonius concludes that two types of training are needed for the control of emotions:[24]

> *The education of this rational element is the understanding of the nature of things, as that of the charioteer is understanding of the instructions for driving chariots. For understanding does not get generated in the non-rational capacities of the soul, any more than in the horses. For these, the proper virtue accrues from a kind of non-rational habituation; for charioteers, from rational instruction.*

Modern neurophysiology validates Seneca's views on "first movements" as the first stirrings of a feeling before it acquires a cognitive nature and becomes an emotion; it also validates Posidonius's views on the lower, autonomous, irrational sides of the soul (the two horses).

Modern neurophysiology shows that when we perceive a sound associated with danger, this perception travels to the brain via two routes. The first is through the amygdala and this is a fast route that occurs even before the feeling enters consciousness. After the amygdala has been alerted, it takes about twice the time for the cortical regions to be alerted.

Sorabji says:[25]

The reactions of the amygdala system provide the modern counterpart of Posidonius' horses. We no longer believe, like him, in spatial movements of a physical soul, but Posidonius' instinct was right. Important as judgements are to many instances of emotion, there is another factor to be considered: the physical reactions of the amygdala and our awareness of those reactions.

The fast stirrings of the amygdala from stimuli correspond also to Seneca's "first movements".

Middle Ages and Christianity

During the Middle Ages, the philosophical study of emotions was linked with ethics, so that some emotions came to be considered "sinful" and some pure and "higher". The sinful emotions were notably greed, gluttony, lust, anger, envy and pride; the higher emotions were love, hope and faith, so much so that St Thomas of Aquino equated these with reason itself.

As was common in previous centuries, emotions in the Middle Ages were seen as factors that sway the mind and spirit away from Divine Grace. They therefore had to be firmly controlled by Reason (Fig. 14.1).

St Augustine

The Western concept of self developed over many centuries and Christian religion played a role in the formation of this concept. The most influential Christian thinkers in this respect were Thomas Aquinas and St Augustine (AD 354–430). St Augustine thought that the self is inward. He says: "*Do not go outward; return within yourself. In the inward man dwells truth.*"[26] According to him, this inward movement gets us in touch with God because God is within. It is the light of the soul. God is to be found in the intimacy of self presence. According to Taylor, "*It is hardly an exaggeration to say that it was Augustine who introduced the inwardness of radical reflexivity and bequeathed it to the Western tradition of thought.*"[27]

St Augustine was the first to establish the first-person standpoint (later taken by Descartes) of "I think, therefore I am" and he was the first to make this standpoint fundamental to our search for the truth. Taylor says of St Augustine's thought: "*I am certain of my existence: the certainty is contingent on the fact that knower and known are the same. It is a certainty of self-presence.*"[28] According to St Augustine, nothing is superior to reason in human nature.

As Taylor says:[29]

St Augustine's path leads from the exterior to the interior and from the interior to the superior. The language of inwardness for St Augustine represents a radical new doctrine of moral resources, one where the route to the higher passes within. In this doctrine, radical reflexivity takes on a new status because it is the space where we come to encounter God, in which we effect the turning from lower to higher.

St Augustine used the term *anima* (i.e. feminine) for "soul" and *animus* (i.e. masculine) for "mind".

Thomas Aquinas

Thomas Aquinas (1225–1274) saw passions as being extremely sensitive to an agent's perception of the world. He thinks that passions modulate around one main kind of perception, i.e. whether the object of passion is easy or difficult to fend off or attain.

Aquinas distinguishes the passions according to two of what he calls "appetites", i.e. a striving of the individual towards something. Under the *concupiscible* appetite are passions that can be easily attained (whether good or evil). Under these he includes love, desire and joy for the positive ones, and hatred, avoidance and sorrow among the negative ones.

If the objects are difficult to attain (or avoid), five other passions are generated and this is called *irascible* appetite. The five passions are hope, despair, audacity, fear and anger.

Thomas Aquinas concerned himself with emotions at length. He lists the basic emotions in couples of opposites as follows:

- love and hatred
- desire and aversion
- sadness and joy
- hope and despair
- fear and daring
- anger (this is the only passion that has no contrary).

Aquinas placed the seat of consciousness and emotions in the heart. Interestingly, both the Old and New Testaments firmly place consciousness in the heart.[30] The heart is the seat of memory, consciousness,

The VSE of
PASSIONS
Writen in French by
J.F. Senault.
And
put into English
by
Henry Earle of
Monmouth
1649.
Divine Grace
Reason
Joy
Sorrow
Choller
Feare
Despaire
Hope
Boldnesse
Love
Eschewing
Hatred
Desire
Passions araing'd by Reason here you see,
As shee's Advis'd therein by Grace Divine:
But this,(yowll say)'s but in Effigie!
Peruse this Booke, and you in ev'ry line
(Thereof will finde this truth so prov'd, that yow
Must Reason contradict, or grant it True.

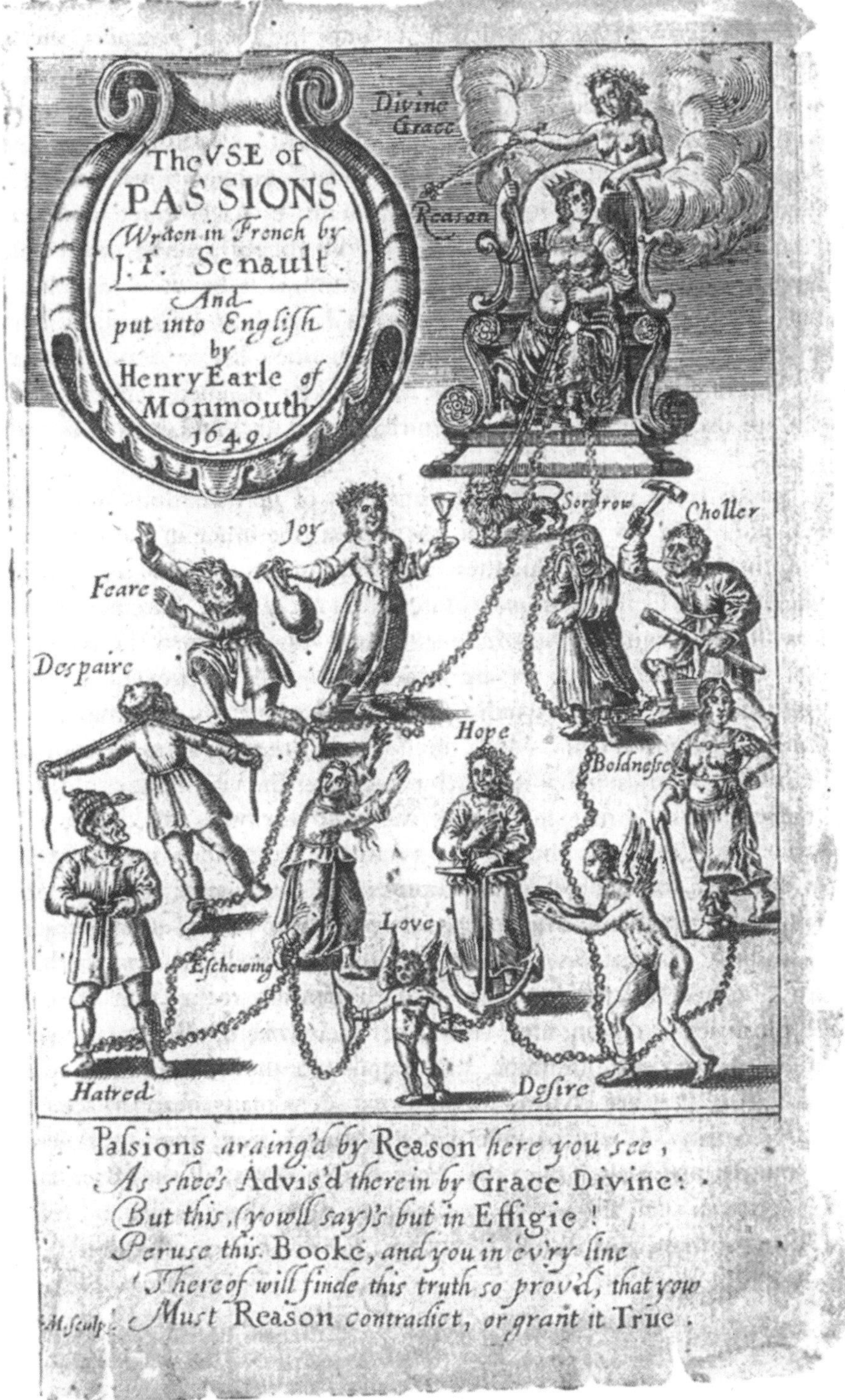

Figure 14.1 The control of emotions by Reason. (Reproduced with permission from James S 2003 Passion and Action. Clarendon Press, Oxford. This is itself reproduced from Senault JF The Use of Passions, trans. Henry Early of Monmouth (1649). Cambridge University Library.)

thought, wisdom and intelligence as it is in Chinese medicine.

Descartes

René Descartes (1596–1650) discussed emotions at length in his works and wrote a book entitled *On the Passions of the Soul.* Descartes assigned an absolute supremacy to the mind and he disdained the "animal" side of man. He considered the mind to have a separate "substance" from that of the body. Indeed, Descartes's philosophy is the clearest example of the separation of body and mind in Western philosophy. Such separation created a problem for him in explaining the emotions as these clearly involve a participation of both the mind and the body (because of the physiological changes brought about by the emotions).

Damasio says:[31]

In spite of Descartes' sophisticated views of mental and physiological body processes, which he separately considered, he either left the mutual connections of mind and body unspecified or made them implausible.

In order to explain this, Descartes thought that body and mind come together in a gland at the base of the brain (the pineal gland) and that the body affects the mind by the agitation of "animal spirits" (minute particles of blood) which bring about the emotions and their physical effects in various parts of the body.[32] Solomon explains Descartes's thinking:[33]

The emotions involve not only sensations caused by this physical agitation, but perceptions, desires and beliefs. Accordingly, it is not as if an emotion is merely a perception of the body; it may also be, as Descartes put it, a perception of the soul and some perceptions may be of things that do not exist at all.

Descartes defined passions as "*the perceptions, feelings or emotions of the soul which we relate specifically to it, and which are caused, maintained and fortified by some movement of the animal spirits*".[34] According to him, the passions render judgment confused and obscure.

Descartes played a huge role in developing the concept of self in the West as a center of reason. "*I am certain that I have no knowledge of what is outside me except by means of the ideas I have within me.*"[35] Ideas are intrapsychic contents related to the self. Descartes identified cognition and consciousness with the mind. Incidentally, Descartes was also the first to change the terminology of Western psychology from "soul" to "mind".[36]

According to Descartes, passions are functional devices that the Creator has designed for us to help preserve the body–soul substantial union. Passions are emotions in the soul, caused by the movement of the animal spirits, which have as their function to strengthen the response which the survival or well-being of the organism requires in a given situation.

Interestingly, Descartes sees three parts to an emotion: the first is a reflex reaction, the second is a cognitive process which brings about a rational recognition of the emotional stimulus, and the third is the passion which has the effect of strengthening the response. The first is brought about by the Corporeal Soul, the second by the Mind, and the third by the Ethereal Soul.

That is why Descartes does not call on us to get rid of our passions. On the contrary, he admires the "*great souls whose reasoning powers are strong and powerful, that although they also have passions, and often even more violent than is common, nonetheless their reason remains sovereign*".[37]

Descartes did say that mind and body influenced each other but he never proposed plausible means for those mutual influences to exert themselves. Damasio says:[38]

In a bizarre twist, Descartes proposed that mind and body interacted, but never explained how the interaction might take place beyond saying that the pineal gland was the conduit for such interactions.

In spite of Descartes's sophisticated views of mental and physiological body processes, which he considered separate, he either left the mutual connections of mind and body unspecified or made them implausible.[39]

Thomas Willis

Thomas Willis (1621–1675) thought the human being to be a double-souled animal, possessing a *sensitive soul*, found in lower animals as well, and a *rational soul*. The rational soul, placed in the brain by God, was thought to be immaterial and immortal. He thought this resided in the corpus callosum.[40]

Willis's idea of a double soul presents some similarities with the Chinese view of three Ethereal Souls: the "sensitive" soul being similar to the second Ethereal

Soul which we share with plants and animals, and the "rational" being similar to the third Ethereal Soul which pertains only to human beings.

Spinoza

Baruch Spinoza (1632–1677) saw emotions as a form of "thoughts" that misunderstand the world and make us miserable and frustrated (as the Stoics thought). Spinoza thought that most emotions are unwarranted expectations of the world; there are, however, also positive emotions that emanate from our true nature and heighten our awareness. He considered only three emotions as being fundamental: pleasure, pain and desire. All other emotions can be explained as arising out of these three.

Spinoza avoided the dualism of body and mind of Descartes. He thought that all substance is one and mind and body are aspects of the same being. Damasio says:[41]

Spinoza's solution no longer required mind and body to integrate or interact; mind and body would spring in parallel from the same substance, fully and mutually mimicking each other in their different manifestations. In a strict sense, the mind did not cause the body and the body did not cause the mind.

Spinoza's view of the human mind presents interesting connections with modern neurophysiology. Spinoza says: "*The object of the idea constituting the human Mind is the Body.*"[43]

Spinoza's greatest insight is that "*mind and body are parallel and mutually correlated processes, mimicking each other at every crossroad, as two faces of the same thing*".[43]

Hume

David Hume (1711–1776) wrote about the passions in his work *Treatise of Human Nature*. Hume is rather like a lone voice among the Western philosophers in assigning an important and central role to emotions as an essential part of our psychic life and not as factors that cloud our reason. Hume considered that emotions involved not only a perception and a bodily change (the "animal spirits" of Descartes) but also ideas. Thus, there are three dimensions to emotions: the perception, a bodily change and an idea (what we would call nowadays the cognitive part).

Hume considered emotions to be not factors that cloud our reason but the very essence of human social existence and morality. They should not be unfavorably contrasted and opposed to reason; on the contrary, they should be celebrated and defended along with it.[44]

Hume argued that emotional impulses motivate all action. He believed that reason does nothing more than consider facts and generate inferences about the world relevant to achieving and prioritizing the agendas set by the passions.[45]

Hume considered all emotions to derive from pleasure or pain. Those that require other factors to derive from pleasure or pain are called *indirect* passions and they are pride, humility, love and hate. Pride and its opposite, humility, require a sense of self to be experienced.

The *direct* passions derive directly from pleasure or pain and they are desire, aversion, grief, joy, hope, fear, despair and security.

Kant

Immanuel Kant (1724–1804) was an uncompromising champion of Reason. Kant made a distinction between reason and what he called the "inclinations" (emotions, moods and desires) and dismissed the latter as inessentials to morals, intrusive at best and disruptive at worst.[46]

However, Kant was not entirely dismissive of emotions and he actually said that "nothing great is ever achieved without passion".

EARLY MODERN THEORIES ABOUT EMOTIONS

Charles Darwin, the British scientist who developed the theory of natural selection, also studied emotions. In his book *The Expression of the Emotions in Man and Animals* (1872), Darwin said that emotional behavior originally served both as an aid to survival and as a method of communicating intentions. For example, angry people show their teeth because they have inherited behavior patterns that their prehistoric ancestors needed for fighting. Bared teeth also signal an intention to attack.

Darwin showed that emotions serve two purposes. First, they energize adaptive behavior such as flight (in response to fear) and procreation (in response to lust). Second, emotions give rise to a signalling and communication system that confers a significant survival advantage to entire species as well as individuals.

Friederich Nietzsche (1844–1900) had a view of emotions that contrasted sharply with the general view of emotions as factors that disturb and cloud reason. Nietzsche celebrated the darker, more instinctual and less rational motives of the human mind, which he called "dyonisian" as opposed to the rational "apollonian" side. Nietzsche praised the passions and described them as having more reason than Reason.[47]

!

Nietzsche praised the passions and described them as having more reason than Reason.

John B. Watson, an American psychologist who helped found the school of psychology called behaviorism, believed emotions were psycho-physical reactions to specific events. He observed that babies stimulated by certain events, such as falling, having their arms held tightly or being stroked, showed three basic emotions. He labeled these emotions fear, anger and love. Watson's view that there are only three basic emotions has been challenged frequently since he proposed it in 1919.

In 1927, the American physiologist Walter B. Cannon and his associate Philip Bard proposed the Cannon–Bard theory of emotions. Cannon and Bard thought emotions arose only when the hypothalamus was stimulated. They believed the hypothalamus was the "seat" of emotions. Several researchers have since shown that stimulation of different parts of the brain, especially the limbic system, triggers emotions.

According to Cannon and Bard, external emotional stimuli processed by the thalamus are routed to the cerebral cortex and to the hypothalamus simultaneously. The hypothalamus, in turn, sends messages to both the muscles and organs and to the cortex. The interaction of messages in the cortex about what the stimulus is and about its emotional significance results in the conscious experience of emotion.[48] As we can see, this view accords with the Chinese view of emotions as simultaneous physical and psychic movement of Qi.

According to Papez, sensory messages reaching the thalamus are directed to both the cerebral cortex and the hypothalamus: the outputs of the hypothalamus to the body control emotional responses; outputs to the cortex give rise to emotional feelings. He calls the paths to the cortex "streams of thinking" and those to the thalamus "streams of feeling".

Papez proposed a series of connections from the hypothalamus to the anterior thalamus, to the cingulate cortex. Emotional experiences occur when the cingulate cortex integrates signals from the sensory cortex and the hypothalamus.[49]

THE JAMES–LANGE THEORY OF EMOTIONS

I shall discuss the James–Lange theory of emotions more in depth as it presents interesting similarities to the Chinese medicine's view of emotions. The James–Lange theory refers to a hypothesis on the origin and nature of emotions developed independently by two 19th century doctors, William James (1842–1910) and Carl Lange (1834–1900). The theory states that, as a response to experiences in the world, the autonomic nervous system creates physiological events such as muscular tension, a rise in heart rate, perspiration and dryness of the mouth.

James and Lange proposed that emotions are feelings which come about as a *result* of these physiological changes, rather than being their cause. Lange even stated that the vasomotor changes occurring when we have an emotion *are* the emotion. Figure 14.2 shows the traditional view of emotions as causes of physiological changes on the top and the James–Lange view at the bottom.

William James described it thus:[50]

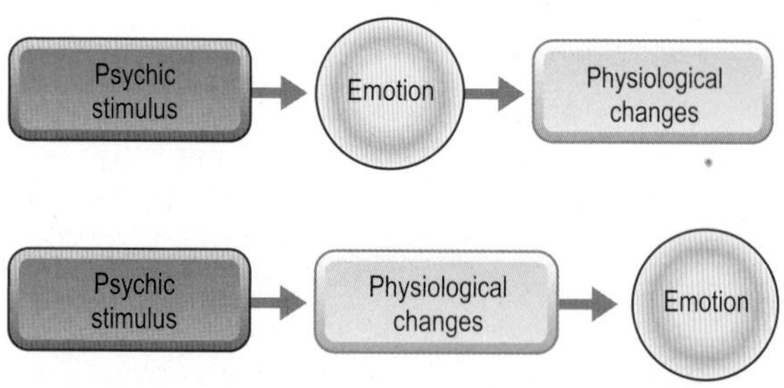

Figure 14.2 The traditional view of emotions compared to the James–Lange view.

My theory ... is that the bodily changes follow directly the perception of the exciting fact, and that our feeling of the same changes as they occur is the emotion. Common sense says, we lose our fortune, are sorry and weep; we meet a bear, are frightened and run; we are insulted by a rival, are angry and strike. The hypothesis here to be defended says that this order of sequence is incorrect ... and that the more rational statement is that we feel sorry because we cry, angry because we strike, afraid because we tremble ... Without the bodily states following on the perception, the latter would be purely cognitive in form, pale, colourless, destitute of emotional warmth. We might then see the bear, and judge it best to run, receive the insult and deem it right to strike, but we should not actually feel afraid or angry.

Therefore, one could say that a person feels sad because he weeps, not that he weeps because he feels sad. James says: "*We feel sorry because we cry, angry because we strike, afraid because we tremble.*"[51]

James also says:[52]

Why do we run away if we notice that we are in danger? Because we are afraid of what will happen if we don't. This obvious (and incorrect) answer to a seemingly trivial question has been the central concern of a century-old debate about the nature of our emotions.

James makes his point clearly when he says:[53]

If we fancy [imagine] *some strong emotion and then try to abstract from our consciousness of it all the feelings of its bodily symptoms, we find we have nothing left behind, no 'mind-stuff' out of which the emotion can be constituted, and that a cold and neutral state of intellectual perception is all that remains.*

James strengthens his point by saying:[54]

What kind of an emotion of fear would be left if the feeling neither of quickened heart beats nor of shallow breathing, neither of trembling lips nor of weakened limbs, neither of goose-flesh nor of visceral stirrings were present, it is quite impossible for me to think. Can one fancy [imagine] *the state of rage and picture no ebullition in the chest, no flushing of the face, no dilatation of the nostrils, no clenching of the teeth, no impulse to vigorous action, but in their stead limp muscles, calm breathing and a placid face?*

In 1884 William James published an article entitled "What Is an Emotion?". In the article, he conceived of an emotion in terms of a sequence of events that starts with the occurrence of an arousing stimulus (the sympathetic or parasympathetic nervous system) and ends with a passionate feeling, a conscious emotional experience.[55]

James asked: "*Do we run from a bear because we are afraid or are we afraid because we run?*" He proposed that the obvious answer, that we run because we are afraid, was *wrong*, and instead argued that we are afraid because we run.

Our natural way of thinking about emotions is that the mental perception of some fact excites the mental affection called emotion, and that this latter state of mind gives rise to the bodily expression. James's theory, on the contrary, is that the bodily changes follow directly the perception of the exciting fact, and that our feeling of the same changes as they occur is the emotion (called "feeling" by Damasio).

The essence of James's proposal was simple. It was premised on the fact that emotions are accompanied by bodily responses (racing heart, tight stomach, sweaty palms, tense muscles, and so on) and that we can sense what is going on inside our body much the same as we can sense what is going on in the outside world. According to James, emotions feel different from other states of mind because they have these bodily responses that give rise to internal sensations, and different emotions feel different from one another because they are accompanied by different bodily responses and sensations.

For example, when we see "James's bear", we run away. During this act of escape, the body goes through a physiological upheaval: blood pressure rises, heart rate increases, pupils dilate, palms sweat, muscles contract in certain ways. Other kinds of emotional situations will result in different bodily upheavals. In each case, the physiological responses return to the brain in the form of bodily sensations, and the unique pattern of sensory feedback gives each emotion its unique quality. Fear feels different from anger or love because it has a different physiological signature. The mental aspect of emotion, the feeling, is a slave to its physiology, not vice versa: we do not tremble because we are afraid or cry because we feel sad; we are afraid because we tremble and are sad because we cry.

To James and Lange, the physical changes occurring with an emotion are an essential part of it; without

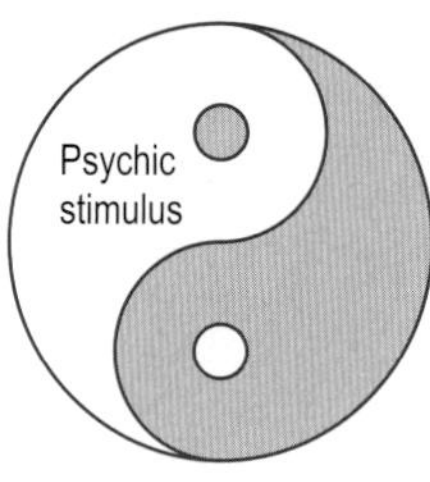

Figure 14.3 The Chinese medicine's view of emotions.

them, there is no emotion. This theory presents interesting parallels with Chinese medicine that views the psychic energy of an emotion as inseparable and just another manifestation of a pathological change in Qi (anger makes Qi rise, fear makes it descend, etc.). Figure 14.3 shows the Chinese view of emotions in which an emotion is *simultaneously* a psychic and physical change.

Indeed, several passages from James provide a glimpse of interesting connections with Chinese medicine. For example, in one passage, James describes the heart and circulatory system as a "sounding board" of emotions. He says:[56]

Not only the heart, but the entire circulatory system forms a sort of sounding board, which every change of our consciousness, however slight, may make reverberate. Hardly a sensation comes to us without sending waves of alternate constriction and dilatation down the arteries of our arms.

This presents a fascinating parallel with the Chinese medicine view of the Heart governing Blood and housing the Mind (*Shen*).

The same view is held by Lange, who gives a description of the consequences of sorrow that is uncannily like the pattern of Heart-Blood deficiency:[57]

The deficient blood supply to the brain is manifested by mental lassitude, dullness, a feeling of mental fatigue and effort, by an indisposition for mental work and frequently by sleeplessness.

Of course, the James–Lange theory of emotions has some loopholes and is open to criticism. Although the James–Lange view of the bodily changes *being* the emotion is an interesting one, emotions must also clearly involve a cognitive aspect.

MODERN THEORIES ABOUT EMOTIONS

In 1962, the American psychologist Stanley Schachter proposed a two-factor theory of emotion, based on an experiment he conducted with Jerome E. Singer. The two factors that determine different emotions, he claimed, are physical changes in a person's body, plus the reason the individual gives for those changes. This theory states that emotions result from people's interpretations of their situations after they have been physiologically stimulated.

The most widely accepted view is that emotions occur as a complex sequence of events. The sequence begins when a person encounters an important event or thought. The person then interprets the meaning of the encounter, and the interpretation determines the feeling that is likely to follow. For example, someone who encounters a grizzly bear would probably interpret the event as dangerous. The sense of danger would cause the individual to feel fear. Each feeling is followed by a series of physical changes and impulses to action, which are responses to the event that started the sequence. Thus, the person who met the bear would probably run away, increasing the person's chances of survival.

Izard and Ackerman propose that emotions have social and human functions. For example, they say that sadness can strengthen social bonds:[58]

The breaking of a tie from death is a compelling reminder of the value of family, friendships and community. A unique function of sadness is its capacity to slow the cognitive and motor systems. The sadness-induced slowing of mental and motor activity can have adaptive effects. The slowing of cognitive processes may enable a more careful look for the source of trouble. This slower and more deliberate scrutiny of the self and the circumstances may help the individual to gain a new perspective – one that facilitates plans for a better performance in the future.

As for anger, a unique function of this emotion is that of mobilizing and sustaining energy at high levels. No other emotion can equal the consistency and vigor of anger in increasing and sustaining extremely high levels of motor activity.[59]

Shame can act as a force for social conformity and social cohesion, and the anticipation of shame motivates the individual to accept his or her share of responsibility for the welfare of the community. According to Izard and Ackerman, no other emotion is as effective as shame in calling attention to failures and weaknesses in the functioning of the self.[60]

The unique function of fear is to motivate escape from dangerous situations.

Sartre

Jean-Paul Sartre (1905–1980) wrote extensively about emotions in his book *Sketch for a Theory of the Emotions* (1939). To Sartre, emotions are a specific way of apprehending the world, of making sense of our life. He thinks that emotions are a "magical" way of apprehending the world. Warnock says in the preface of the above book:[61]

When the obstacles become too great, we pretend that we can get what we need by magic instead of by the proper, natural means. This effort to change the world by magical means is not an object of consciousness, it is part of the consciousness. The new apprehension of the world produces new behaviour, but ineffectual and would-be-magical behaviour. We aim to change the world, but if we cannot do this we change ourselves. In extreme cases, we may even faint, thus magically annihilating the world for ourselves by severing our connection with it for the time being.

To Sartre, emotions are an indissoluble part of consciousness, not factors that disturb it. He says:[62]

In emotion, we can rediscover the whole of human reality, for emotion is the human reality assuming itself and 'emotionally directing' itself towards the world. Can one conceive of consciousnesses that do not include emotions among their potentialities or must we indeed regard it as an indispensable constituent of consciousness?

Sartre continues:[63]

An emotion signifies in its own manner the whole of the consciousness, or, if we take our stand on the existential plane, of the human reality. It is that human reality itself, realizing itself in the form of 'emotion'. Hence it is impossible to regard emotion as a psycho-physiological disorder. It has its own essence, its peculiar structures, its laws of appearance, its meaning. It cannot possibly come from outside human reality. It is man, on the contrary, who assumes his emotion, and emotion is therefore an organized form of human existence.

Sartre sees emotions as a way of coping with life. He says:[64]

Emotional behaviour is not a disorder at all; it is an organized pattern of means directed to an end. And these means are summoned up in order to mask, replace or reject a line of conduct that one cannot or will not pursue. Emotions represent, each of them, a different way of eluding a difficulty, a particular way of escaping, a special trick.

Solomon's theory of emotions

According to Solomon (1942–2007), emotions (which he calls passions) are "value judgments" and evaluations. He disagrees with the general view of emotions as factors that disturb our Reason. He says:[65]

The thesis in this book is quite simply stated: it is to return to the passions the central and defining roles in our lives that they have so long and persistently been denied, to limit the pretensions of 'objectivity' and self-demeaning reason which have exclusively ruled Western philosophy, religion and science since the days of Socrates.

One of the central themes of Solomon's book is what he calls the "Myth of the Passions", i.e. the idea that has pervaded the whole of Western philosophy (with few exceptions) that Reason is supreme and constitutes our true Self, and that if only we could get rid of our emotions we would be true to our nature. As we shall see in Chapter 15, this is actually also the view of the three main philosophies of China, i.e. Confucianism, Daoism and Buddhism.

The very terms we use seem to confirm the existence of what Solomon calls the "Myth of Passions", i.e. that emotions are psychic forces which cloud our mind, our reason and, in Confucian terms, our very human nature: we "fall" in love, we are "overwhelmed" by joy, "consumed" by envy, "paralyzed" with fear, "beside ourselves" with anger.

Solomon says of the Myth of the Passions:[66]

It is the myth of passivity; the self-serving half truth is the fact that we often suffer from our passions, submit ourselves to them, find ourselves carried away and foolishly behaving because of them.

In fact, expressions we use confirm the view that emotions are blind forces that sweep us away or enslave us.

Solomon says:[67]

We 'fall' in love, much as one might fall into a tiger trap or a swamp. We find ourselves 'paralyzed' with fear, as if we had been inoculated with a powerful drug; we are 'plagued' with remorse, as if by flies or mosquitoes; we are 'struck' by jealousy, as if by a Buick; 'felled' by shame, as a tree by an axe; 'distracted' by grief, as if by a trombone in the kitchen; 'haunted' by guilt, as if by a ghost; and 'driven' by anger, as if pushed by a prod. Our richest poetic metaphors, grown trite with overuse, are images of passivity. We are 'heartbroken', 'crushed', 'smitten', 'overwhelmed', 'carried away' and 'undone' by passion.

As we saw in Chapter 9, the Chinese expression most Chinese books use to describe the "stimulation" or "excitation" produced by the emotions is *ci ji* where "*ji*" contains the radical for "water" and means to "swash, surge" as a wave does, i.e. it denotes the surge of emotions like a wave that carries us away.

Solomon thinks that, far from being factors that disturb Reason with a blind irrationality, emotions give meaning to our life, they are the life force of the soul and they, not Reason, actually constitute our Self. He says that the role of Reason is not to react against passions but to distinguish between them, and that wisdom is not opposite of passions (as is also in Confucianism, Buddhism and Daoism).

!

Far from being factors that disturb Reason with a blind irrationality, emotions give meaning to our life, they are the life force of the soul and they, not Reason, actually constitute our Self.

Solomon says:[68]

The passions are the very soul of our existence; it is not they who require the controls and rationalizations of Reason. Rather, it is Reason that requires the anchorage and earthly wisdom of the passions. The passions are not irrational; they are in their very essence 'rational'.

Tomkins says:[69]

Out of the marriage of reason with affect there issues clarity with passion. Reason without affect would be impotent, affect without reason would be blind.

Solomon therefore thinks that emotions are evaluative judgments. He says:[70]

Through our passions, we constitute our subjective world, render it meaningful, and with it our lives and our Selves. The passions are not occurrences but activities; they are not inside our minds but rather the structures we place in our world. My anger, even that simmering suppressed anger that is allowed no expression, is my projection into the world, my silent indictment of someone who has wronged me, my judgement of the offensive state of the world.

This is how Solomon explains that the emotions are judgments:[71]

An emotion is a judgement, something we do. An emotion is a basic judgement about our Selves and our place in the world, the projection of values and ideas, structures and mythologies, according to which we live and through which we experience our lives. Anger involves a moral judgement; my anger is that set of judgements. My shame is my judgement to the effect that I am responsible for an untoward situation or incident. My sadness, my sorrow and my grief are judgements of various severity to the effect that I have suffered a loss. An emotion is an evaluative judgement, a judgement about my situation and about myself and/or about other people.

According to Solomon, the ultimate object of our emotional judgments is always our own sense of self-esteem and personal dignity.

Solomon points out another important "function" (if it may be called that) of emotions; they create a "mythology" in our life, and a set of heroes and villains, and mythology is central to our life. Anger involves a courtroom mythology and a moral judgment towards the person who has wronged me; shame and guilt also involve a courtroom mythology, but one in which the person himself or herself is the accused. Through our passions we mythologize the world, an essential part of our Self.

Emotions have another important role in that, as Hume says, they alone "move" us; Reason does not "move" us. Hume uses "move" not in the sense of being moved, i.e. feeling emotional about something. He means that emotions "move" Reason in that they provide an essential direction in life in the form of plans, ideas, projects and life dreams. This is exactly the same as the role of the Ethereal Soul towards the Mind (*Shen*) in Chinese medicine.

Bockover's theory of emotions

Bockover considers emotions as psychic events that are at the same time intentional and affective. She says:[72]

My claim is that the concept of emotion entails a different kind of feeling but one that cannot be equated with felt bodily occurrences (as James holds). Unlike bodily feeling, 'emotionally relevant feeling' (ERF) is inherently and irreducibly intentional and affective in nature. Emotion is a kind of intentional event which forms an irreducibly unity which is affective in itself.

She then explains the difference between beliefs and emotions thus:[73]

The difference between beliefs and emotions is that emotions entail distinctly affective ways of being conscious about things. We have been conditioned to think that all 'feelings' are unintentional, like felt bodily disturbances, and that the only intentional events are thoughts, beliefs and judgements. A more accurate analysis of emotions cannot ignore their distinctively intentional and affective characters.

Bockover disagrees with Solomon's view of emotions as evaluative judgments. She thinks that seeing emotions as evaluative judgments is too general and fails to account for the differences among various emotions.

Damasio's theory of emotions

Damasio also thinks that, far from being psychic factors that merely cloud the mind, emotions are actually integral to the process of reasoning and decision-making. Studies that have been conducted on individuals with brain lesions in the limbic system confirm this. Damasio says:[74]

These findings suggest that selective reduction of emotions is at least as prejudicial for rationality as excessive emotions. It certainly does not seem true that reason stands to gain from operating without the leverage of emotions. On the contrary, probably emotions assist reasoning, especially when it comes to personal and social matters involving risk and conflict.

Indeed, Damasio says that:[75]

Absence of emotion is a reliable correlate of defective core consciousness, perhaps as much as the presence of some degree of continuous emoting is virtually always associated with the conscious state.

Damasio proposed the "somatic marker hypothesis". According to this theory, emotions *mark* certain aspects of a situation or certain outcomes of possible actions. Damasio says:[76]

Emotions achieve this marking overtly as in a 'gut feeling', or covertly via signals occurring below the radar of our awareness (examples of covert signals would be neuromodulator responses, such as those of dopamine or oxytocin, which can change the behaviour of neuron groups that represent a certain choice).

According to Damasio, "*The brain systems that are jointly engaged in emotion and decision-making are generally involved in the management of social cognition and behaviour.*"[77] In other words, from the Chinese point of view, the intuition and creativity deriving from the Ethereal Soul are coordinated with the activity of the Mind to produce thinking and social behavior. Salk (the originator of the polio vaccine) says something that could apply exactly to the relationship between the Ethereal Soul and the Mind: "*Creativity rests on a merging of intuition and reason.*"[78]

According to Damasio, emotions are an integral component of the machinery of reasons. He reached this conclusion after many years of clinical observation in patients whose cognitive faculties were absolutely intact but who had brain lesions in centers that control emotions. Although their "reason" was absolutely intact, these patients made a succession of mistakes in daily life, in a perpetual violation of what would be considered socially appropriate and personally advantageous.[79]

Damasio acknowledges that, under certain circumstances, emotions may play havoc with our reasoning but, he says, *absence* of emotion and feeling is no less damaging.[80] He says:[81]

At their best, feelings point us in the proper direction, take us to the appropriate place in a decision-making space, where we may put the instruments of logic to good use. We are faced by uncertainty when we have to make a moral judgement, decide on the course of a personal relationship. Emotion and feeling, along with the covert physiological machinery underlying them, assist us with the daunting task of predicting an uncertain future and planning our actions accordingly.

Damasio goes further and says that feelings are just as cognitive as reason:[82]

Feelings, along with the emotions they come from, are not a luxury. They serve as internal guides and they help us communicate to others signals that can also guide them. And feelings are neither intangible nor elusive. Contrary to traditional scientific opinion, feelings are just as cognitive as other percepts. They are the result of the most curious physiological arrangement that has turned the brain into the body's captive audience.

Interestingly, Damasio also sees the same close integration between body and mind that Chinese medicine sees:[83]

The body, as represented in the brain, constitutes the indispensable frame of reference for the neural processes that we experience as the mind; our very organism is used as the ground reference for the constructions we make of the world around us and for the construction of the ever present sense of subjectivity that is part and parcel of our experiences; our most refined thoughts and best actions, our greatest joys and deepest sorrows, use the body as a yardstick.

Damasio is very clear about the role of so-called lower centers of the brain in the reasoning process:[84]

The apparatus of rationality, traditionally presumed to be neocortical, does not seem to work without that of biological regulation, traditionally presumed to be subcortical. Nature appears to have built the apparatus of rationality not just on top of the apparatus of biological regulation, but also from *it and* with *it.*

The difference between deep sleep (in which consciousness is temporarily suspended) and dream sleep illustrates how emotions accompany consciousness. Damasio says: "*Deep sleep is not accompanied by emotional expression, but in dream sleep during which consciousness returns in its odd way, emotional expressions are easily detectable in humans and animals.*"[85] He then says: "*In other words, emotions and core consciousness tend to go together in the literal sense by being present together or absent together.*"[86]

The above presents interesting connections with Chinese medicine as core consciousness is akin to the Corporeal Soul and, as we know, the Corporeal Soul modulates all emotions and feelings at a deep, autonomic and automatic level.

Far from being factors which merely cloud reason, emotions are the result of a long history of evolutionary fine-tuning. Emotions are part of the bioregulatory system with which we come equipped to survive. Darwin studied emotional responses the world over and, beyond some cultural differences, found a remarkable similarity.

According to Damasio, the biological function of emotions is twofold: (1) they produce a specific reaction to an inducing situation; (2) they regulate the internal state of the organism so that it can be prepared for the specific reaction. Damasio says: "*In other words, the biological purpose of emotions is clear and they are not a dispensable luxury.*"[87] Damasio says concisively: "*Emotion is devoted to an organism's survival, and so is consciousness.*"[88]

This is Damasio's definition of an emotion:[89]

1. Emotions are complicated collections of chemical and neural responses, forming a pattern: all emotions have some kind of regulatory role to play, leading to the creation of circumstances advantageous to the organism. 2. Emotions are biologically determined processes depending on innately set brain devices, laid down by a long evolutionary history. 3. The devices that produce emotions occupy a fairly restricted ensemble of subcortical regions, beginning at the level of the brain stem and moving up to the higher brain. 4. All the devices can be engaged automatically without conscious deliberation. The fact that culture plays a role in shaping some inducers does not deny the fundamental stereotypicity, automaticity and regulatory purpose of the emotions. 5. All emotions use the body as their theatre but emotions also affect the mode of operation of numerous brain circuits.

Interestingly, Damasio makes a distinction between *feeling* and *emotion*. He says that feelings are inwardly directed and private, while emotions are outwardly directed and public. Damasio maintains that there are feelings we are conscious of and feelings that we are not. He says:[90]

An organism may represent in mental and neural patterns the state that we conscious creatures call a feeling without ever knowing that the feeling is taking place.

Damasio further clarifies this distinction thus:[91]

Although some feelings relate to emotions, there are many that do not; all emotions generate feelings if you are awake and alert, but not all feelings originate from emotions. I call background feelings those that do not originate in emotions.

Clarifying the difference between emotion and feeling, Damasio says:[92]

In our attempt to understand the complex chain of events that begins with emotion and ends up in feeling, we can be helped by a principled separation between the part of the process that is made public and the part that remains private. For the purpose of my work, I call the former part emotion *and the latter part* feeling.

Damasio thinks that feelings follow emotions and not the other way round. Feelings can occur outside our field of consciousness; these are the feelings originating from the Corporeal Soul from the Chinese point of view. Damasio says: "*How many times do we notice at a certain time of a given day that we are feeling especially well and filled with energy and hope, but don't know the reason? Or, on the contrary, that we are feeling blue and edgy?*"[93] In such cases feelings are being processed outside our field of consciousness.

This is Damasio's definition of feeling: "*A feeling is the perception of a certain state of the body along with the perception of a certain mode of thinking and of thoughts with certain themes.*"[94] This view partly echoes that of James and Lange, according to which a feeling is inseparable from the physical changes out of which it arises.

Damasio says that feelings are not merely clusters of thought. He attaches importance to the physical manifestation of feelings:[95]

My view is that feelings are functionally distinctive because their essence consists of the thoughts that represent the body involved in a reactive process. Remove that essence and the notion of feeling vanishes. Remove that essence and one should never again be allowed to say 'I feel' happy, but rather 'I think' happy.

The distinction between emotions and feelings is interesting, and it is one that presents intriguing similarities with Chinese medicine. In fact, we could say that the feelings we are not conscious of are the Corporeal Soul (*Po*) while emotions involve the Mind (*Shen*) and Ethereal Soul (*Hun*).

FREUD, JUNG AND BOWLBY

Freud (1856–1939)

The end of the 19th and the beginning of the 20th centuries saw the emergence of psychoanalysis and the theory of the unconscious. Freud was the first to introduce the concept of the unconscious mind.

The unconscious

The concept of the unconscious as proposed by Freud was revolutionary in that he proposed that awareness existed in layers and that some thoughts occurred "below the surface", i.e. in a layer of the mind that we are not conscious of, i.e. the unconscious.

Freud was led to the discovery of the unconscious by the analysis of dreams and what we call "slips of the tongue". Freud believed that dreams are a symbolic expression of unconscious desires or fears; as these are by definition unconscious, they can surface only in a symbolic way in dreams.

Dreams, which he called the "royal road to the unconscious", provided the best access to our unconscious life and the best illustration of its "logic", which was different from the logic of conscious thought. Freud developed his first topology of the psyche in *The Interpretation of Dreams* (1899), in which he proposed the argument that the unconscious exists and described a method for gaining access to it.

The everyday phenomenon of "slips of the tongue" was also considered a manifestation of unconscious desires or fears. Such a thought has become so much part of everyday language that we refer to these slips as "Freudian slips".

Crucial to the operation of the unconscious is "repression". According to Freud, people experience thoughts and feelings that are so painful that they cannot be acknowledged (the Oedipus complex, i.e. the incestuous impulse of a son for his mother and/or a daughter for her father being one of them). According to Freud, such thoughts and feelings – and associated memories – cannot be banished from the mind, but can be banished from consciousness. Thus they come to constitute the unconscious.

Freud observed that the process of repression is itself a non-conscious act (in other words, it did not occur through people willing away certain thoughts or feelings). Freud supposed that what people repressed was in part determined by their unconscious. In other words, the unconscious was, for Freud, both a cause and an effect of repression.

Freud named his new theory of unconscious incestuous desires the Oedipus complex after the famous Greek tragedy *Oedipus Rex* by Sophocles. He used the Oedipus conflict to point out how much he believed that people have incestuous desires and must repress them.

The id, ego and super-ego

In his later work, Freud proposed that the psyche could be divided into three parts: ego, super-ego and id. The id is known as the child-like portion of the psyche that is very impulsive and takes into account only what it wants and disregards all consequences. The super-ego is the moral code of the psyche that solely follows right and wrong. Finally, the ego is the balance between the two. After the super-ego and id are balanced, the ego acts in a way that takes both impulses and morality into consideration.

The threefold structure of id, ego and super-ego offers some similarities to the Chinese view of the psyche. We could, for example, posit that the Ethereal and Corporeal Souls are like the id, the former on a psychic and the latter on a physical level. As we have seen in Chapters 3 and 4, an essential characteristic of the Ethereal and Corporeal Souls are their *independent* existence from that of the Mind (*Shen* of the Heart).

Freud believed that humans were driven by two conflicting central desires: the life drive (libido, responsible for survival, propagation, hunger, thirst and sex) and the death drive (Thanatos). Freud's description of libido (which he also called cathexis) included not merely sexual libido but all creative, life-producing drives.

The death drive, whose energy is known as anticathexis, represented an urge inherent in all living things to return to a state of calm; in other words, an inorganic or dead state. Freud's view of the death drive has some similarities with the activity of the Corporeal Soul. As we have seen in Chapter 4, the Corporeal Soul has a centripetal movement towards fragmentation, eventually ending in death.

Jung (1875–1961)

The collective unconscious

Jung's analytical psychology differs from Freud's psychology in many respects. An important one is the concept of the unconscious. While Freud conceived only of a personal unconscious as the depository of all unwanted (or removed) psychological material, Jung conceived also of a universal unconscious as the depository of universal symbols, ideas and archetypes common to all mankind. Thus, the symbols coming up in our dreams may be manifestations of our repressed unconscious material but also of universal symbols or archetypes. It follows that Jungian psychology has much more of a spiritual dimension than that of Freud.

The collective unconscious contains archetypes common to all human beings. That is, individuation may bring to the surface symbols that do not relate to the life experiences of a single person. This content is more easily viewed as answers to the more fundamental questions of humanity: life, death, meaning, happiness, fear. Among these, more spiritual concepts may arise and be integrated into the personality.

The archetypes of the collective unconscious could be thought of as ideas common to all mankind. All humans have innate psychological predispositions in the form of archetypes, which compose the collective unconscious.

Archetypes can be revealed through an examination of the symbolic communication of the human psyche – in art, dreams, religion, myths. Jung theorized that certain symbolic themes exist across all cultures, all epochs and in every individual.

The shadow

An important part of Jungian psychology is the concept of *shadow*. The shadow is an unconscious complex that is defined as the repressed and suppressed aspects of the conscious self. There are constructive and destructive types of shadow. On the destructive side, it often represents everything that the conscious person does not wish to acknowledge within themselves. For instance, someone who identifies as being kind has a shadow that is harsh or unkind. Conversely, an individual who is brutal may have a kind shadow.

Jung emphasized the importance of being aware of shadow material and incorporating it into conscious awareness, lest one project these attributes on others. The shadow in dreams is often represented by dark figures of the same gender as the dreamer. According to Jung, we deal with the shadow in four ways: denial, projection, integration and/or transmutation.

I personally feel that the Jungian concept of shadow is somewhat akin to that of *gui* in Chinese medicine. As discussed in Chapter 7, the Chinese concept of *gui* could be interpreted as a metaphor for the shadow: it is the "dark" aspect that is part of the Ethereal Soul and Corporeal Soul, but an essential part of our being in providing "movement" to these two souls, the former on a psychic level, the latter on a physical one. Without *gui*, there is no movement from the Ethereal Soul and Corporeal Soul; just as without shadow, the self would lack originality and movement.

The animus and anima

The concepts of *animus* and *anima* are two other fundamental aspects of Jungian psychology. Jung identified the anima as being the unconscious feminine component of men's psyche and the animus as the unconscious masculine component in women's. However, this is rarely taken literally; many modern Jungian practitioners believe that every person has both an anima and an animus. Jung stated that the anima and animus act as guides to the unconscious unified Self, and that forming an awareness and a connection with the anima or animus is one of the most difficult and rewarding steps in psychological growth. Jung reported that he identified his anima as she spoke to him, as an inner voice, unexpectedly one day.

Often, when people ignore the anima or animus complexes, the anima or animus vies for attention by projecting itself on others. This explains, according to Jung, why we are sometimes immediately attracted to certain strangers: we see our anima or animus in them. Love at first sight is an example of anima and animus projection. Moreover, people who strongly identify with their gender role (e.g. a man who acts aggressively and never cries) have not actively recognized or engaged their anima or animus.

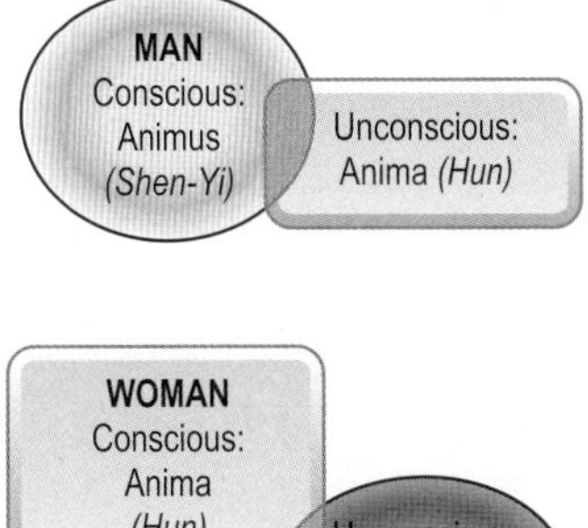

Figure 14.4 Connections between animus and anima and Ethereal Soul, Mind and Intellect.

Jung thinks that the animus is responsible for rational thinking while the anima is responsible for intuition and creativity. What Jung is defining here are our unconscious tendencies as, consciously, of course both men and women are equally capable of rational thinking and intuition and creativity (albeit in different degrees in different individuals).

Thus, the anima is the unconscious part of men and the animus that of women. The animus and anima often "possess" us and manifest with their negative qualities. When a man is possessed by his negative anima, he becomes moody, irritable and uncommunicative; when a woman is possessed by her negative animus, she becomes hypercritical and judgmental.

We could postulate some connections between the Jungian view of the animus and anima and Chinese medicine. In a way, the qualities of the anima are similar to that of the Ethereal Soul, while those of the animus would correspond to those of the Mind (*Shen*) and Intellect (*Yi*). See Figure 14.4.

Psychological types

Analytical psychology distinguishes several psychological types or temperaments.

First, *extrovert* and *introvert* refer to the flow of libido (psychic energy); the introvert's flow is directed inward toward concepts and ideas, the extrovert's is directed outward towards people and objects. Everyone has both the introversion and the extroversion mechanisms, and the collectively dominant type determines whether an individual is introvert or extrovert.

According to Jung, the conscious psyche consists of four basic functions:

- *sensing* – perception by means of the sense organs
- *intuition* – perceiving in unconscious way or perception of unconscious contents
- *thinking* – function of intellectual cognition; the forming of logical conclusions
- *feeling* – function of subjective estimation.

Thinking and feeling functions are *rational*, while sensing and intuition are *non-rational*. According to Jung, rationality consists of figurative thoughts, feelings or actions with reason – a point of view based on objective value, which is set by practical experience. In any person, the degree of introversion/extroversion of one function can be quite different from that of another function.

Generally, we tend to favor our most developed, *superior* function, while we can broaden our personality by developing the others. Related to this, Jung noted that the unconscious often tends to reveal itself most easily through a person's least developed, *inferior* function. The encounter with the unconscious and development of the underdeveloped function(s) thus tend to progress together.

Again, parallels could be found with Chinese medicine. We could postulate that the *thinking* and *feeling* function is a function of the Mind (*Shen*), Will-Power (*Zhi*) and Intellect (*Yi*), the *sensing* function a function of the Corporeal Soul and the *intuitive* function a function of the Ethereal Soul.

Bowlby

The limbic system and our emotional life throw an interesting light on the nature of emotions. As mentioned above, the limbic system modulates the cortex and the latter cannot develop without the former. Thus, far from being psychic factors that "disturb" our mind and cloud our human nature (as Chinese medicine maintains, especially under the influence of a Confucian or Daoist view of the emotions), emotions are an essential way in which our psyche functions. Without emotional bonding, children simply die.

In the 1940s, the psychoanalyst Spitz reported on the fate of orphaned children brought up in homes or institutions, as well as babies separated from young mothers in prisons. In deference to the new germ theory of disease, institutionalized children were fed and clothed, kept warm and clean, but they were not played with, held or handled.[96] Many children became withdrawn, sickly and lost weight, and many died. In an interesting paradox, the children fell ill with the very infections their isolation was trying to avoid. Interestingly, 40% of the institutionalized children who contracted measles died as opposed to 0.5% of the children outside. Quite simply, a lack of human interaction (handling, cooing, talking, stroking, playing) is fatal to infants.

The British psychoanalyst John Bowlby (1907–1990) conducted pioneering work on the theory of attachment and baby bonding. Bowlby theorized that human infants are born with a brain system that promotes safety by establishing an instinctive behavioral bond with their mothers. That bond leads to distress when the mother is absent, as well as the drive for the two to seek each other when the child is frightened or in pain.[97]

Although Bowlby's ideas are now mainstream, they were surprisingly revolutionary in the 1950s. For example, the founder of the behaviorism school, John Watson (1878–1958), wrote: "*Mother love is a dangerous instrument. Never hug and kiss children, never let them sit on your lap. If you must, kiss them once on the forehead when they say goodnight.*"[98] Bowlby attracted the wrath of both psychiatrists and psychoanalysts.

In Bowlby's view, an infant is born with few motor skills and so, when his mother strays, he can keep her near by crying. As a baby develops muscular coordination, attachment behaviors become more sophisticated: the baby reaches, grasps, beckons, crawls to bring his mother close.[99] As we have seen in Chapter 4, these activities of the baby are manifestations of the Corporeal Soul.

There is an interesting parallel between Bowlby's mother–baby bonding and the Chinese view of the Corporeal Soul. As we have seen in Chapter 4, being the closest to the Essence, the Corporeal Soul is responsible for the first physiological processes after birth. Zhang Jie Bin says: "*In the beginning of life, ears, eyes and Heart perceive, hands and feet move and breathing starts: all this is due to the sharpness of the Corporeal Soul.*"[100]

It is said that, in the first month of life especially, the baby is "all Corporeal Soul". As it resides in the Lungs, the Corporeal Soul is responsible for touch and skin sensations, and it is nourished by the mother's Corporeal Soul through breast feeding and touching. This explains the importance of touching in a baby's life; it not only establishes a bonding between mother and baby but it also physically nourishes the Corporeal Soul and therefore the Lungs.

MODERN NEUROPHYSIOLOGICAL VIEW ON EMOTIONS

Neurophysiology of emotions

The neurobiological explanation of human emotion is that emotion is a pleasant or unpleasant mental state organized in the limbic system of the mammalian brain. Unlike reptiles, emotions are mammalian elaborations of feelings in which neurotransmitters – for example, dopamine, noradrenaline (norepinephrine) and serotonin – step-up or step-down the brain's activity level, as visible in body movements, gestures and postures. In mammals, primates and human beings, feelings are displayed as emotion cues.

For example, the human emotion of love is thought to have evolved from paleocircuits of the mammalian brain (specifically, modules of the cingulate gyrus) designed for the care, feeding and grooming of offspring.

Before the mammalian brain, life was automatic, preconscious and predictable. The motor centers of reptiles react to sensory cues of vision, sound, touch, chemical, gravity and motion with pre-set body movements and programmed postures. With the arrival of night-active mammals, circa 180 million years ago, smell replaced vision as the dominant sense, and a different way of responding arose from the olfactory sense, which is thought to have developed into mammalian emotion and emotional memory.

In the Jurassic Period, the mammalian brain invested heavily in olfaction to succeed at night as reptiles slept – one explanation for why olfactory lobes in mammalian brains are proportionally larger than in reptiles. These odour pathways gradually formed the neural blueprint for what was later to become our limbic brain.

Emotions are related to activity in brain areas that direct our attention, motivate our behavior and determine the significance of what is going on around us. Pioneering work by Broca, Papez and MacLean suggested that emotion is related to a group of structures in the center of the brain called the limbic system; this includes the hypothalamus, cingulate cortex, amygdala, hippocampus, fornix, septum, ventral striatum, insula, perirhinal and parahippocampal regions, as well as other structures (Fig. 14.5). More recent research has shown that some of these limbic structures are not as directly related to emotion as are others, while some non-limbic structures have been found to be of greater emotional relevance.

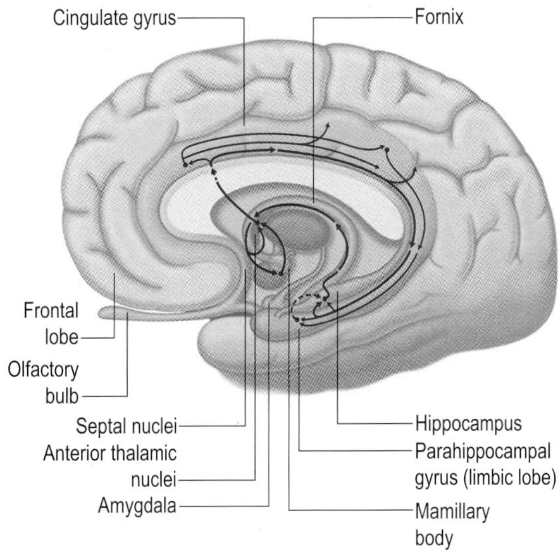

Figure 14.5 The limbic system.

The following brain structures are currently thought to be most involved in emotion.

- *Amygdala*: The amygdala is a small, round structure located anterior to the hippocampus near the temporal poles. The amygdala is involved in detecting and learning what parts of our surroundings are important and have emotional significance. They are critical for the production of emotion, and may be particularly so for negative emotions, especially fear (Fig. 14.6). The amygdala is involved in emotional learning.[101]
- *Prefrontal cortex*: The term prefrontal cortex refers to the very front of the brain, behind the forehead and above the eyes. It appears to play a critical role in the regulation of emotion and behavior by anticipating the consequences of our actions. The prefrontal cortex may play an important role in delayed gratification by maintaining emotions over time and organizing behavior toward specific goals (Fig. 14.7).

  The prefrontal cortex is responsible for the executive functions, which include mediating conflicting thoughts, making choices between right and wrong or good and bad, predicting future events and governing social control – such

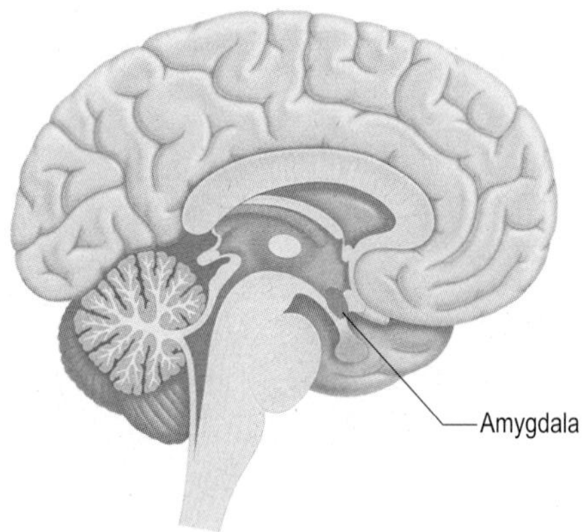

Figure 14.6 The amygdala.

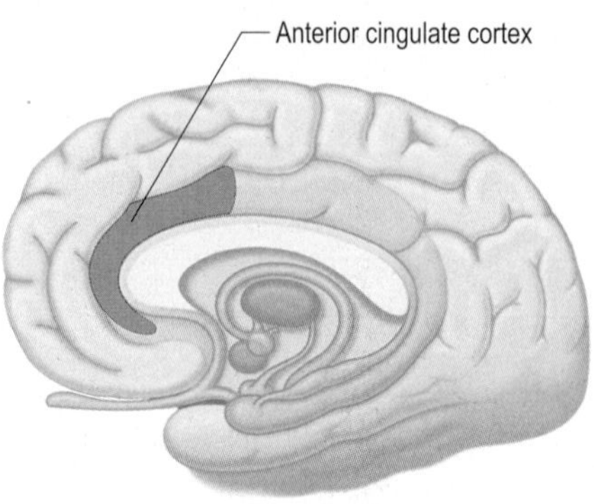

Figure 14.8 Anterior cingulate cortex.

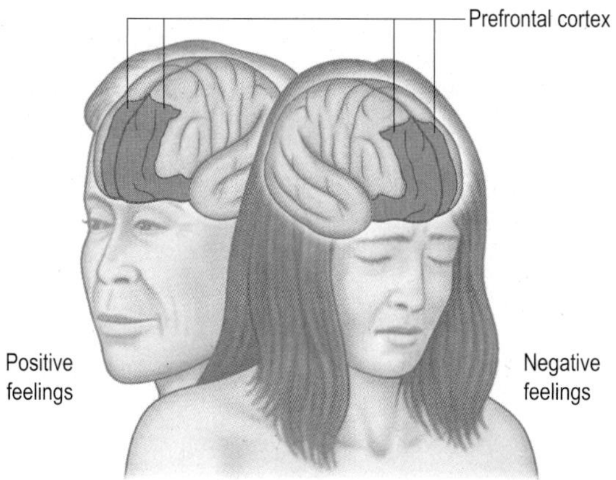

Figure 14.7 Prefrontal cortex.

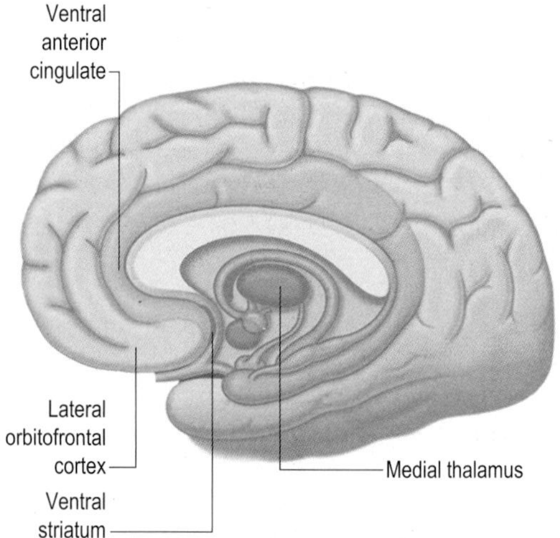

Figure 14.9 Ventral striatum.

as suppressing emotional or sexual urges. The basic activity of this brain region is considered to be orchestration of thoughts and actions in accordance with internal goals. An interesting feature of the prefrontal cortex is that its left side is activated when positive emotions are experienced and its right side is activated when negative emotions are experienced.[102] Indeed, a left-sided injury of the prefrontal cortex such as that which happens in stroke results in depression.[103] Even in neurologically intact depressed patients, measurements of regional brain activity showed a pattern of left prefrontal hypoactivation.[104]

- *Anterior cingulate cortex*: The anterior cingulate cortex (ACC) is located in the middle of the brain, just behind the prefrontal cortex. The ACC is thought to play a central role in attention, and may be particularly important with regard to conscious, subjective emotional awareness. This region of the brain may also play an important role in the initiation of motivated behavior (Fig. 14.8).
- *Ventral striatum*: The ventral striatum is a group of subcortical structures thought to play an important role in emotion and behavior. One part of the ventral striatum, the nucleus accumbens, is thought to be involved in the experience of goal-directed positive emotion. Individuals with addictions experience increased activity in this area when they encounter the object of their addiction (Fig. 14.9).
- *Insula*: The insular cortex is thought to play a critical role in the bodily experience of emotion, as it is connected to other brain structures that regulate the body's autonomic functions (heart

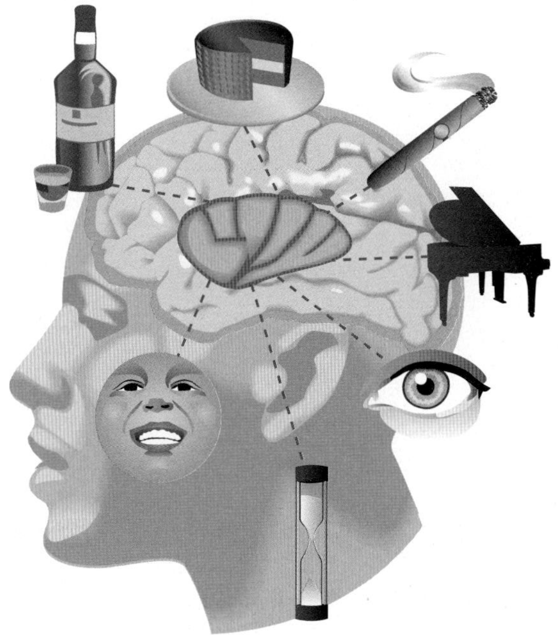

Figure 14.10 Insula.

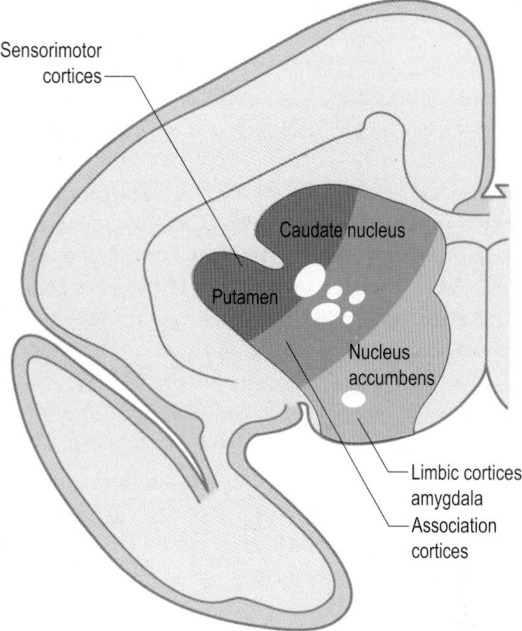

Figure 14.11 Interaction between basal ganglia and limbic system.

rate, breathing, digestion, etc.). This region also processes taste information and is thought to play an important role in experiencing the emotion of disgust (Fig. 14.10).

The insula is a brain region that has emerged as crucial to understanding what it feels like to be human. It is the wellspring of social emotions, things like lust and disgust, pride and humiliation, guilt and atonement. It helps to give rise to moral intuition, empathy and the capacity to respond emotionally to music. Its anatomy and evolution shed light on the profound differences between humans and other animals. The insula also reads body states like hunger and craving, and may play a role in addictions.

There is an interesting correlation between certain areas of the brain circuitry and a specific emotion (up to a certain point). Positron emission tomography (PET) and functional magnetic resonance imaging (fMRI) has shown that:[105]

... the induction and experience of sadness, anger, fear and happiness lead to activation in several sites, but the pattern for each emotion is distinctive. For instance, sadness activates the ventromedial prefrontal cortex, hypothalamus and brain stem, while anger or fear activates neither the prefrontal cortex nor the hypothalamus. Brain-stem activation is shared by all three emotions [sadness, anger, fear], *but intense hypothalamic and ventromedial prefrontal activation appears specific to sadness. The amygdala is indispensable to recognizing fear in facial expressions, to being conditioned to fear and even to express fear.*

An important new realization about the interaction between the cortex and the limbic system has emerged in recent times. Until recently, it was thought that the cortex is responsible for cognition and the limbic system for emotions. However, as described also below, the cortex depends on the limbic system for its early development in babies. Moreover, it has recently come to light that the rostral parts of the basal ganglia, far from being exclusively motor in function, are actually innervated by the limbic system (Fig. 14.11). In fact, limbic structures exhibit a stronger connectivity with the basal ganglia than with the hypothalamus, overthrowing entirely the idea that the limbic system is a discrete system dedicated to the hypothalamus and unable to influence the basal ganglia.[106]

As Trimble says:[107]

It is becoming increasingly evident that the limbic system and therefore our emotions play a role in cognition and personal knowledge. Emotion is no longer seen as a counterpart to reason in human cognition but rather as a collaborator, and indeed constructor of our reasons and thinking.

Such views are in stark contrast to the views of the three philosophies of China (Daoism, Confucianism and Buddhism), according to which emotions are factors that cloud our reasoning and indeed, our human nature. According to such a view, emotions are merely causes of disease but, as we have seen above, emotions are far more than that, as they are essential to our functioning as human beings and indeed even for our cognition.

Language itself may have derived initially from emotions rather than reason. Language in its earliest form was probably an expression of emotions. Rousseau says: "*It seems that need dictated the first gestures while the passions* [emotions] *stimulated the first words.*"[108] Indeed, it may be that music itself developed in conjunction with the first guttural sounds dictated by the emotions.

The study of the physical manifestations of various emotions presents interesting parallels (or sometimes differences) with Chinese medicine.

- *Fear* is felt as a heightened heartbeat, increased "flinch" response and increased muscle tension. This description is interesting as it confirms my view that chronic fear affects the Heart more than the Kidneys.
- *Anger*, based on sensation, seems indistinguishable from fear.
- *Happiness* is often felt as an expansive or swelling feeling in the chest and the sensation of lightness or buoyancy, as if standing under water. The "swelling" feeling seems to resonate with the Chinese view, according to which excess joy makes the heart larger.
- *Sadness* is often experienced as a feeling of tightness in the throat and eyes, and relaxation in the arms and legs. The tightness in the throat is a sign of Qi stagnation in the Lung channels (which are affected by sadness).
- *Shame* can be felt as heat in the upper chest and face. This indicates that shame affects the Heart.
- *Desire* can be accompanied by a dry throat, heavy breathing and increased heart rate. This confirms the Chinese view, according to which excessive desire leads to Heart Heat.

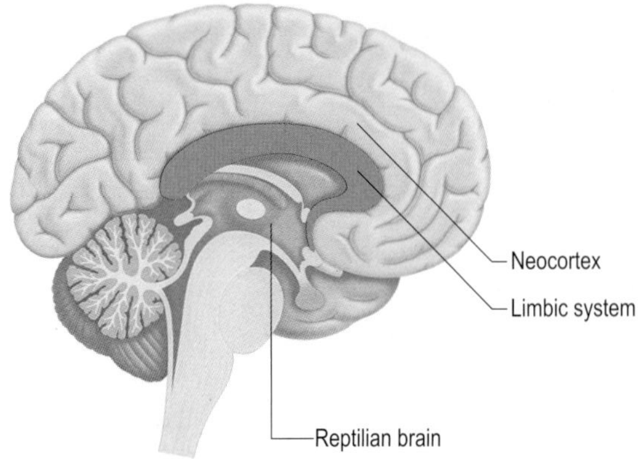

Figure 14.12 The triune brain.

The triune brain

According to the triune brain theory developed by Dr Paul MacLean (1913–2007), former Chief of Brain Evolution and Behavior at the National Institutes of Health, we have "three brains" (Fig. 14.12).

The brain stem is the *reptilian brain*. It is a remnant of our prehistoric past. The reptilian brain acts on stimulus and response. It is useful for quick decisions without thinking. The reptilian brain focuses on survival, and takes over when we are in danger and we do not have time to think. In a world of survival of the fittest, the reptilian brain is concerned with getting food and keeping from becoming food. The reptilian brain is fear driven, and takes over when one feels threatened or endangered.

A second part of the brain is the *limbic system* or *mammalian brain*. The limbic system is the root of emotions and feelings. It affects moods and bodily functions.

The *neocortex* is the most evolutionary advanced part of our brain. It governs our ability to speak, think and solve problems. The neocortex affects our creativity and our ability to learn. The neocortex makes up about 80% of the brain.

The neurologist Paul MacLean has proposed that each of our three brains represents a distinct evolutionary stratum that has formed upon the older layer before it, like an archaeological site. He calls it the "triune brain". MacLean says that the three brains operate like "three interconnected biological computers, [each] with its own special intelligence, its own subjectivity, its own sense of time and space and its own memory". He refers to these three brains as the neocortex or *neo-*

mammalian brain, the limbic or *paleomammalian* system, and the reptilian brain, consisting of the brain stem and cerebellum.

Each of the three brains is connected by nerves to the other two, but each seems to operate as its own brain system with distinct capacities.

This hypothesis has become a very influential paradigm, which has forced a rethink of how the brain functions. It had previously been assumed that the highest level of the brain, the neocortex, dominates the other, lower levels. MacLean has shown that this is not the case, and that the physically lower limbic system, which rules emotions, can hijack the higher mental functions when it needs to.

The reptilian brain

The reptilian brain includes the brain stem and cerebellum (Fig. 14.13). The brain stem is the oldest and smallest region in the evolving human brain. It evolved hundreds of millions of years ago and is more like the entire brain of present-day reptiles. For this reason, it is often called the "reptilian brain". Various clumps of cells in the brain stem determine the brain's general level of alertness and regulate the vegetative processes of the body, such as breathing and heartbeat.

It is similar to the brain possessed by the hardy reptiles that preceded mammals, roughly 200 million years ago. It is "preverbal", but it controls life functions such as autonomic brain, breathing, heart rate and the fight-or-flight mechanism. Lacking language, its impulses are instinctual and ritualistic. It is concerned with fundamental needs such as survival, physical maintenance, hoarding, dominance, preening and mating. It is also found in lower life forms such as lizards, crocodiles and birds. It is at the base of the skull, emerging from the spinal column.

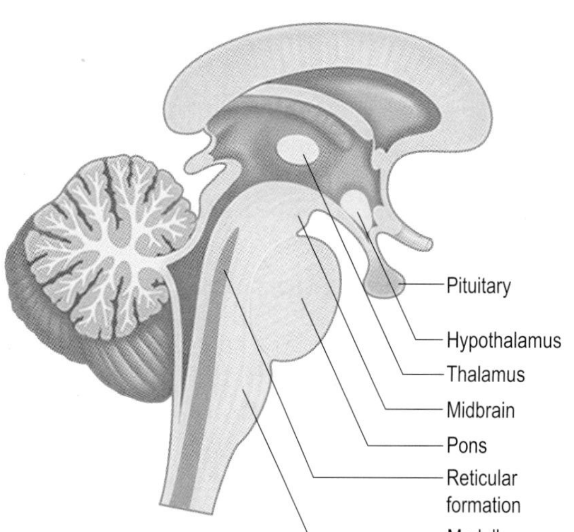

Figure 14.13 The reptilian brain.

The reptilian brain has the same type of archaic behavioral programs as snakes and lizards. It is rigid, obsessive, compulsive, ritualistic and paranoid; it is "filled with ancestral memories". It keeps repeating the same behaviors over and over again, never learning from past mistakes. This part of the brain is active even in deep sleep.

The brain stem is composed of three parts: the mesencephalon, medulla oblongata and pons.

- The brain stem, which contains most of the cranial nerves, is responsible for:
  - alertness
  - arousal
  - breathing
  - blood pressure
  - digestion
  - heart rate
  - relaying information between the peripheral nerves and spinal cord to the upper parts of the brain
  - other autonomic functions.
- The mesencephalon is responsible for:
  - control of responses to sight
  - eye movement
  - pupil dilation
  - body movement
  - hearing.
- The medulla oblongata is responsible for:
  - control of autonomic functions
  - relaying nerve signals between the brain and spinal cord.
- The pons is responsible for:
  - arousal
  - assisting in controlling autonomic functions
  - relaying sensory information between the cerebrum and cerebellum
  - sleep.

The paleomammalian brain

The limbic brain is draped around the reptilian brain. It comprises:

- hippocampus
- fornix
- amygdala
- septum
- cingulate gyrus
- ventral striatum
- insula
- perirhinal and parahippocampal regions (see Fig. 14.5).

In 1952 MacLean first coined the name "limbic system" for the middle part of the brain. It can also be termed the paleopallium or intermediate (old mammalian) brain. It corresponds to the brain of most mammals. The old mammalian brain residing in the limbic system is concerned with emotions and instincts, feeding, fighting, fleeing and sexual behavior. Everything in this emotional system is either "agreeable or disagreeable". Survival depends on avoidance of pain and repetition of pleasure.

When this part of the brain is stimulated with a mild electrical current, various emotions (fear, joy, rage, pleasure, pain, etc.) are produced. Although no emotion has been found to reside in one place for very long, the limbic system as a whole appears to be the primary seat of emotion, attention and affective (emotion-charged) memories.

The limbic system helps to determine valence (e.g. whether we feel positive or negative toward something; in Buddhism referred to as *vedena* – "feeling") and salience (e.g. what gets our attention), unpredictability and creative behavior. It has vast interconnections with the neocortex, so that brain functions are not either purely limbic or purely cortical but a mixture of both.

As mammals split off from the reptilian line, a fresh neural structure blossomed. This new brain transformed the organismic orientation towards offspring. Detachment and disinterest mark the parental attitude of the typical reptile, while mammals can enter into subtle and elaborate interactions with their young. Mammals bear their young live; they nurse, defend and rear them while immature. Mammals *take care of their own.*[109] Mammals form close-knit, mutually nurturing social groups – *families* – in which members spend time touching and caring for one another. The emotional and relational function of the limbic system resembles the functions and attributes of the Ethereal Soul.

McLean considers the three cardinal mammalian behaviors associated with the limbic system to be nursing and maternal care, maternal–infant audio-vocal communication, and play. McLean further suggests that the origins of human language were most likely in infant–mother interaction, babbling based on vowel–consonant combinations beginning about 8 weeks after birth. He singles out the separation cry – a slowly changing tone with a prolonged vowel sound (*aaah*), a distressing cry linked with the most painful emotion, separation.[110]

Mammals can *play* with one another, an activity unique to mammals with limbic functions. Anyone who has joined a dog in a tug-of-war with an old shoe and has let the shoe go, knows that the dog will trot back. What he desires is *playing*, not the shoe itself.

Why is the dog playing? The play fulfills a need of the limbic system. Remove a mother hamster's whole cortex and she can still raise her pups, but even slight limbic damage devastates her maternal abilities.[111]

Limbic lesions in monkeys can obliterate the entire *awareness of others*. After a limbic lobotomy, one impaired monkey stepped on its outraged peers as if they were logs and took food out of their hands with the nonchalance of one oblivious to their very existence.[112]

Children with Asperger's syndrome can be bright and intelligent but they are emotionally clumsy, tone-deaf to social subtleties in others and sometimes to their own emotions.

One of the physiological processes that the limbic system directs is development of the brain itself. The importance of limbic contact for normal human brain development shows itself most starkly in the devastating consequences of its omission. Feed and clothe a human baby but deprive him of emotional contact and he will die.

Many subsystems of the mammalian brain do not come pre-programmed; maturing mammals need limbic regulation to give coherence to neurodevelopment.

The cortex (neomammalian brain)

The neocortex, cerebrum, the cortex or neopallium, also known as the superior or rational (neomammalian) brain, comprises almost the whole of the hemispheres (made up of a more recent type of cortex, called neocortex) and some subcortical neuronal groups (Fig. 14.14). It corresponds to the brain of the primate mammals and, consequently, the human species. The higher cognitive functions that distinguish human

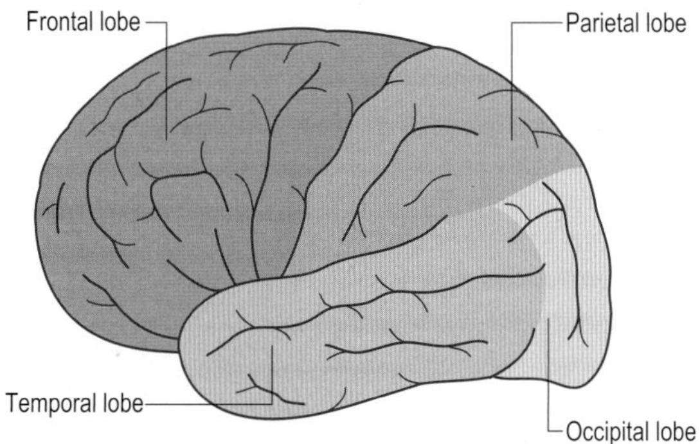

Figure 14.14 The cortex of the brain.

beings from other mammals are in the cortex. MacLean refers to the cortex as "the mother of invention and father of abstract thought". In human beings, the neocortex takes up two-thirds of the total brain mass. Although all animals also have a neocortex, it is relatively small, with few or no folds (indicating surface area and complexity and development). A mouse without a cortex can act in fairly normal way (at least to superficial appearance), whereas a human without a cortex is a vegetable.

The cortex is divided into left and right hemispheres. The left hemisphere controls the right side of the body and the right hemisphere the left side of the body. Also, the right hemisphere is more spatial, abstract, musical and artistic, while the left is more linear, rational and verbal.

In conclusion, we can postulate the following correspondences between the triune brain and the Chinese view of the psyche:

- Reptilian brain = Corporeal Soul (*Po*)
- Limbic system = Ethereal Soul (*Hun*) and Mind (*Shen*)
- Cortex = Mind (*Shen*), Intellect (*Yi*) and Will-Power or Memory (*Zhi*).

SUMMARY

I consider it important to look at the theory of the emotions, self and consciousness in the West for several reasons which have been highlighted above. These are the main conclusions from what has been discussed above.

- All philosophers in the West have discussed the emotions from the times of Socrates and Plato right down to modern philosophers. What emerges clearly from their discussions is that emotions are far more than just causes of disease as Chinese medicine sees them. Not only do emotions have a cognitive, judgmental value, they also play a vital role in the development of the cortex.
- Some of the Western philosophers hold the same view as the ancient Confucianists, Buddhists and Daoists, i.e. that emotions cloud reason.
- However, many of the Western philosophers do not share the view that emotions cloud human reason. First, emotions are considered to be value judgments by many philosophers, from the ancient Stoics, through Hume and right down to the contemporary American philosopher Robert Solomon. Damasio proposed the "somatic marker hypothesis", according to which emotions *mark* certain aspects of a situation or certain outcomes of possible actions. According to Damasio, the brain systems that are jointly engaged in emotion and decision-making are generally involved in the management of social cognition and behavior. According to Damasio, emotions are an integral component of the machinery of reasons.
- The development of the cortex relies partly on the limbic system. Thus, from a neurophysiological point of view, far from being factors that "cloud reason", they play a vital role in coordinating our social life with the cortex. This is the equivalent of the Chinese view of the relationship between the Mind and the Ethereal Soul.
- Emotions are an essential way in which mammals developed. As the theory of the triune brain shows, the limbic system played an essential role in the evolution of mammals and it continues to do so by interacting with the cortex to modulate thought and behavior.
- Crucially, the Western concept of self is completely different from that in the Confucian philosophy. I single out the Confucian philosophy because I maintain that it had a profound influence on Chinese medicine. The Western concept of self of an individualized, inward-looking, autonomous center of consciousness is completely different from the Confucian self that is family- and society-defined.
- The implications of this difference are many-fold. First, emotions in Confucian philosophy and in Chinese medicine are seen as pathologies of Qi, almost outside the self; they are objective disharmonies of Qi which generate physical and emotional symptoms simultaneously.

Second, the absence of an individual, inward-looking center of consciousness means that, although Chinese medicine looks at emotions as causes of disease, it does not delve into the root of those emotions, i.e. the influence of childhood experience with its emotional nurturing or lack of it, defences, projections and complexes.

- Emotions in Chinese medicine are objective disharmonies of Qi, almost like exterior forces that cloud our Mind; they are not the passions of the individual, inner-directed self. Emotions need healing, not to heal the individual but to ensure the "harmony" of the individual, because this reflects on the family and society and even the whole State. Dealing with our emotions is an ethical, social issue rather than a psychological one.

END NOTES

1. James S 2003 Passion and Action – the Emotions in Seventeenth-Century Philosophy. Clarendon Press, Oxford, p. 13.
2. Lewis M, Haviland-Jones JM (eds) 2004 Handbook of Emotions. Guilford Press, New York, p. 505.
3. Ibid., p. 505.
4. Sorabji R 2002 Emotion and Peace of Mind – From Stoic Agitation to Christian Temptation. Oxford University Press, Oxford, p. 182.
5. Greenfield S 2000 The Private Life of the Brain. Penguin Books, London, p. 21.
6. Handbook of Emotions, p. 276.
7. Ibid., p. 277.
8. Lewis T, Amini F, Lannon R 2000 A General Theory of Love. Random House, New York, p. 86.
9. Ibid., p. 228.
10. Ibid., p. 229.
11. Handbook of Emotions, p. 258.
12. Ibid., p. 259.
13. Ibid., p. 276.
14. Trimble MR 2007 The Soul in the Brain. Johns Hopkins University Press, Baltimore, p. 26.
15. Stanford Encyclopedia of Philosophy (online). http://plato.stanford.edu/entries/ancient-soul/ [Accessed 2008].
16. Emotion and Peace of Mind, p. 96.
17. Handbook of Emotions, p. 4.
18. Passion and Action, p. 41.
19. Ibid., p. 42.
20. Crabbe J (ed) 1999 From Soul to Self. Routledge, London, pp. 33–34.
21. Handbook of Emotions, p. 5.
22. Emotion and Peace of Mind, pp. 2-4.
23. Ibid., p. 31.
24. Ibid., p. 96.
25. Ibid., p. 97.
26. Taylor C 2003 Sources of the Self – The Making of the Modern Identity. Cambridge University Press, Cambridge, p. 129.
27. Ibid., p. 131.
28. Ibid., p. 133.
29. Ibid., p. 136.
30. Crabbe J (ed) 1999 From Soul to Self. Routledge, London, p. 56.
31. Damasio A 2003 Looking for Spinoza – Joy, Sorrow and the Feeling Brain. Harcourt, San Diego, p. 188.
32. Handbook of Emotions, p. 6.
33. Ibid., p. 6.
34. Ibid., p. 6.
35. Sources of the Self, p. 144.
36. Crabbe J (ed) 1999 From Soul to Self. Routledge, London, p. 8.
37. Sources of the Self, p. 150.
38. Looking for Spinoza, p. 188.
39. Ibid., p. 188.
40. The Soul in the Brain, p. 27.
41. Looking for Spinoza, p. 209.
42. Ibid., p. 211.
43. Ibid., p. 217.
44. Handbook of Emotions, p. 8.
45. Ibid., p. 505.
46. Ibid., p. 8.
47. Ibid., p. 8.
48. LeDoux J 1996 The Emotional Brain. Simon and Schuster, New York, p. 84.
49. Ibid., p. 89.
50. Lange CG, James W 1922 The Emotions, Vol. 1. Williams and Wilkins, Baltimore, p. 13.
51. Cited in Emotion and Peace of Mind, p. 160.
52. James W 1884 What is an Emotion? *Mind* 9: 188–205.
53. Damasio A 1994 Descartes' Error – Emotion, Reason and the Human Brain. Penguin Books, London, p. 129.
54. Ibid., p. 129.
55. *Mind*, pp. 188–205.
56. The Emotions, p. 15.
57. Ibid., p. 43.
58. Handbook of Emotions, pp. 258–259.
59. Ibid., p. 259.
60. Ibid., p. 260.
61. Sartre JP 2004 Sketch for a Theory of the Emotions. Routledge, London, pp. xiii–xiv.
62. Ibid., p. 10.
63. Ibid., p. 12.
64. Ibid., p. 22.
65. Solomon RC 1993 The Passions – Emotions and the Meaning of Life. Hackett, Indianapolis, p. xiv.
66. Ibid., p. xv.
67. Ibid., p. xv.
68. Ibid., p. xvii.
69. Handbook of Emotions, p. 506.
70. The Passions, p. 108.
71. Ibid., p. 126.
72. Bockover M 1995 The concept of emotion revisited In: Marks J, Ames RT (eds) Emotions in Asian Thought. State University of New York Press, New York, p. 173.
73. Ibid., p. 174.
74. Damasio A 1999 The Feeling of What Happens – Body and Emotion in the Making of Consciousness. Harcourt, San Diego, p. 41.
75. Ibid., p. 100.
76. Damasio A 1994 Descartes' Error – Emotion, Reason and the Human Brain. Penguin Books, London, p. xii.
77. Ibid., p. xiii.
78. Ibid., p. 189.
79. Ibid., p. xv.
80. Ibid., p. xvi.
81. Ibid., p. xvii.
82. Ibid., p. xix.
83. Ibid., p. xx.
84. Ibid., p. 128.
85. The Feeling of What Happens, p. 100.
86. Ibid., p. 100.
87. Ibid., p. 54.
88. Ibid., p. 56.
89. Ibid., p. 50.
90. Ibid., p. 136.
91. Descartes' Error, p. 143.
92. Looking for Spinoza, p. 27.

93. Ibid., p. 72.
94. Ibid., p. 86.
95. Ibid., pp. 86–87.
96. Ibid., p. 69.
97. Ibid., p. 70.
98. Ibid., p. 71.
99. Ibid., p. 72.
100. 1982 Lei Jing 类经 [Classic of Categories]. People's Health Publishing House, Beijing, p. 63. The *Classic of Categories* was written by Zhang Jie Bing (also called Zhang Jing Yue) and first published in 1624.
101. Davidson R, Harrington A 2002 Visions of Compassion – Western Scientists and Tibetan Buddhists Examine Human Nature. Oxford University Press, Oxford, p. 121.
102. Ibid., pp. 111–112.
103. Ibid., p. 112.
104. Ibid., p. 112.
105. The Feeling of What Happens, pp. 60–61.
106. The Soul in the Brain, p. 46.
107. Ibid., p. 50.
108. Ibid., p. 73.
109. A General Theory of Love, p. 25.
110. The Soul in the Brain, p. 189.
111. A General Theory of Love, p. 26.
112. Ibid., p. 27.

儒学理论对于中国人神和意志观念的影响

CHAPTER 15

THE INFLUENCE OF CONFUCIANISM ON THE CHINESE VIEW OF THE MIND AND SPIRIT

CONFUCIANISM *315*

Confucius *315*

Tian (Heaven) *316*

Confucian ethics *317*

Confucian ethics, society and state *320*

NEO-CONFUCIANISM *323*

Human nature (*Xing*) *325*

Li (Principle) *326*

THE CONCEPT OF SELF IN WESTERN AND CHINESE PHILOSOPHY *327*

EMOTIONS IN NEO-CONFUCIANISM *332*

INFLUENCE OF NEO-CONFUCIANISM ON CHINESE MEDICINE *336*

CONCLUSIONS *339*

THE INFLUENCE OF CONFUCIANISM ON THE CHINESE VIEW OF THE MIND AND SPIRIT

In this chapter I shall explore first the nature and teachings of Confucianism and Neo-Confucianism and then the differences between the concept of self in Western and Chinese philosophy. I shall then examine the Confucian view of emotions to see whether this applies to a Western notion of self.

I discuss Confucianism at length because it is my opinion that Confucianism had the strongest influence on Chinese medicine, particularly with regard to its view of emotions. Certainly, there are two other important philosophical strands running through Chinese medicine, i.e. the school of Yin-Yang (and Five Elements) and the school of *Dao* (or Daoist school).

However, the point that is often missed is that some of the thoughts and ideas from these two schools were integrated into Chinese medicine relatively late by the Neo-Confucianist philosophers of the Song and Ming dynasties. For example, many of Chinese medicine's ideas on Qi, and especially on its condensation and dispersal, giving rise at the same time to material and subtle phenomena of the universe, are derived from the Neo-Confucianist philosopher Zhang Zai (1020–1077).

Something else that is not often remembered is that the Legalist School also had an influence on Chinese medicine, at least in the beginning, i.e. during the Warring States period (475–221 BC) and the Qin dynasty (221–206 BC).

The Legalist School was called the School of Law (*Fa Jia*) in ancient China. The Legalist School flourished during the Warring States period and, although it did not leave deep roots in Chinese culture as the Confucianists or Daoists did, it did prevail during the Qin dynasty (221–206 BC), a brief dynasty started by the first emperor Qin Shi Huang Di who enthusiastically adopted the principles of government advocated by the

Legalist School. The most famous representative of the Legalist School was Han Fei Zi.

According to the Legalists, neither the wisdom of ancient kings nor an ethical code (as the Confucians advocated) would make a state strong. Instead "good" and "bad" were defined by whatever the self-interest of the ruler demanded. A system of harsh punishments and rewards, regulated through strict laws and enforced without exceptions, should guarantee good behavior within the state. The Legalists considered military service and agriculture as the only occupations beneficial to the welfare of the state and discouraged all scholarship. Indeed, Qin Shi Huang Di, the first emperor who unified China and a devoted follower of the Legalist School, had all books burned (except those on agriculture and medicine) and had many Confucian scholars buried alive.

The state of Qin in Western China was the first to adopt Legalist doctrines. The Qin were so successful that by 221 BC they had conquered the other Chinese states and unified the empire after centuries of war. Legalist ideas on human nature, society and government could not be further from those of Confucius; the Legalists thought that human nature is essentially unruly and order in society can be kept only by strict laws and harsh punishments, not through ethical behavior as the Confucians thought.

What is interesting about the Legalist School from the Chinese medicine point of view is the fact that the Qin dynasty (which adopted Legalist ideas) was the first to unify China. They established irrigation, unified weights, coins, Chinese script, measures and other things, such as the gauge of wheel axles throughout China. The first Qin emperor also initiated a huge program of road building and canal digging. Another important innovation of the Qin dynasty was the fostering of trade among various regions of China on a huge scale.

The Qin dynasty therefore provided the first model of a unified state with an emperor, a central government, local officials, a unified economy and a state-wide irrigation system. This provided the first metaphor of Chinese medicine in which the Heart is the emperor, the other Internal Organs are the officials, the body's physiology is the unified economy and the acupuncture channels are the irrigation canals.

Unschuld says:[1]

One may well conclude that all these structural changes that accompanied the unification of China were sufficiently innovative to supply intellectuals of that time with the concept of an integrated complex system, the individual parts of which can function only as long as their relations with the remaining parts are not disturbed. The symbolic value of the newly structured social and economic environment may have been significant enough to have been transferred by thinkers concerned with health and illness to an understanding of structure and function of the human organism; hence the physiological and pathological basis of the medicine of systematic correspondence accurately reflected these structural innovations.

In another passage, Unschuld says:[2]

The structure of the human organism and the functions assigned to its individual elements reflect a complex social organism founded on the wide-scale movement of goods. They further reflect the bureaucratic apparatus of a state in which a wide variety of tasks have been delegated to a responsible ruler and his many civil servants. This is no longer the small feudal state and principality of the waning Zhou period, but rather the Confucian-Legalist administration system of the united empire.

There is, however, another interesting possible influence of the Legalist School on Chinese medicine. If Chinese medicine had been influenced primarily by Daoism (what I call a "romantic" view of Chinese medicine that the West often purports), one would expect a philosophy of treatment similar to that of the modern naturopathic philosophy, with its belief in the healing power of a life force and therefore its belief in letting Nature take its course.

But this is not the therapeutic approach of Chinese medicine which directly "attacks" and expels pathogenic factors, counteracts Cold with Heat and vice versa, and uses sweating, purging and vomiting as treatment methods. Indeed, quite a proportion of the terminology of Chinese medicine uses military analogies – for example, the character *wei* for Defensive Qi evokes the idea of "patrolling sentinels"; the character *ying* for Nutritive Qi conveys the idea of "army camps"; the Controlling cycle of the Five Elements is called *ke*, which means "to subdue".

One can therefore see an influence of the Legalist School in this therapeutic approach, i.e. just as human nature cannot be relied upon and must be "straightened" with strict laws and harsh punishments, the body's Qi must be regulated by attacking pathogenic factors decisively and by making sure that the "ruler" and officials do their jobs properly.

> **!**
>
> The Legalist School of Han Fei Zi did have some influence on the development of some of Chinese medicine's ideas.

Of course, one part of Chinese medicine is strongly influenced by Daoism, and does stress harmony with the Dao and the seasons and regulation of one's life as a key to health maintenance. The Daoist influence on Chinese medicine can also be seen clearly in breathing exercises and sexual practices.

The discussion in this chapter will be conducted according to the following topics.

- Confucianism
- Neo-Confucianism
- The concept of self in Western and Chinese philosophy
- Emotions in Neo-Confucianism
- Influence of Neo-Confucianism on Chinese medicine
- Conclusions

CONFUCIANISM

Confucius

Confucius (551–479 BC) was a thinker, political figure and educator born during the Spring and Autumn Annals period (770–476 BC). He was the founder of the Ru (scholar) School of thought. Confucius is the Latinized name of Kong Zi or "Master Kong". His family name was Kong and his personal name was Jiu. He was born in the state of Lu, in southern Shandong. His ancestors had been members of the ducal house of the state of Song which was descended from the royal house of Shang, the dynasty that preceded the Zhou.

The Six Confucian Classics were the *Yi Jing* (Book of Changes), *Shi Jing* (Book of Odes), *Shu Jing* (Book of History), *Li Jing* (Book of Rites), *Yue Jing* (Book of Music) and *Chun Qiu Jing* (Spring and Autumn Annals). As feudalism began to disintegrate in the Warring States period, the tutors of the aristocrats began to scatter among the people. They made their living by teaching the Classics or by acting as skilled "assistants", well versed in the rituals, on the occasion of funerals, sacrifices, weddings and other ceremonies. This class of men was known as the *ru* or literati and the Confucian school was known as the School of Literati (*Ru*).

This school was one of the main schools of thought during the Warring States period (475–221 BC). Other major schools at that time were the School of *Dao* (Daoists), the School of Yin-Yang and the Legalist School. Although Confucius did not succeed in implementing his ideas in his lifetime, his school of thought became the official state philosophy during the Han dynasty (206 BC–AD 220) and remained so for 2000 years.

The original Confucian philosophy was firmly based on ethics and was not concerned much with ontological questions. It was a philosophy that advocated a social order based on duties and responsibilities according to rigid hierarchical rules. This system became the foundation of Chinese society to this day. Confucius stressed the importance of social order and dignity based on responsibilities inherent in human relationships in an ever growing pyramid; the younger brother respects the elder brother, the children respect the parents, the wife respects the husband, the pupils respect the teacher, all the subjects respect the emperor. Confucius thought that the only way to have order in society is for everyone to recognize and fulfill his or her proper place. The rigidity of family relationships and hierarchical order within a family is well illustrated by the fact that every member of the family has a specific name (Fig. 15.1).

Confucius's teachings, preserved in the *Lunyu* or *Analects*, form the foundation of much of subsequent Chinese thought on the education and behavior of the ideal person. The ideas of Confucius truly shaped Chinese family, society and state for 2000 years, and they formed the basis of ethics and ethical government until modern times (and indeed, in my opinion, even during the Communist era).

With its emphasis on tradition, rituals, filial obligations and ancestor reverence, Confucianism truly became the soul of the Chinese people down to the present day. Most Chinese people are followers of Confucianism, even without any first-hand knowledge of the Analects of Confucius. Indeed, in my opinion, very many aspects of Chinese family, society and government today do not reflect a Marxist outlook but a Confucianist one.

Confucianism became, during the Han dynasty, the official doctrine of the bureaucratic society, erroneously defined by the modern Communist Chinese as

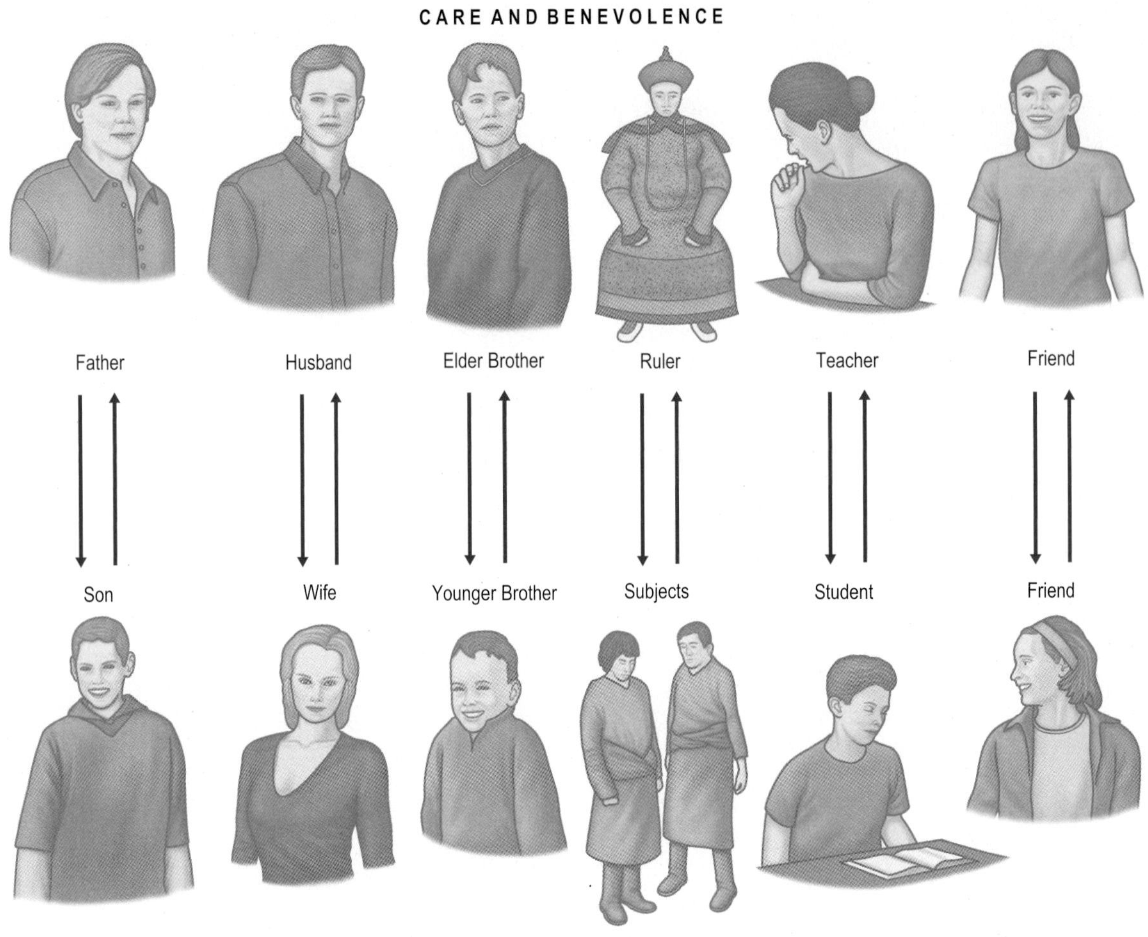

Figure 15.1 The six relationships in Confucian ethics.

"feudal society". It was not feudal because rulers did not get power by birth as in a feudal society, but acceded to power through examinations based on the Confucian Classics; thus, for those times, it was meritocratic.

Tian (Heaven)

Confucius frequently talked about Heaven (*Tian* 天) and the Will of Heaven. He believed that people live their lives within parameters firmly established by "Heaven", but he argued that people are responsible for their actions and especially for their treatment of others. Although we cannot influence our destiny as shaped by "Heaven", we can make a difference in this world by behaving in an ethical manner as Confucius advocated.

Hall and Ames list three main meanings of *Tian*.

1. *Tian* is both *what* our world is and *how* it is. *Tian* is both creator and the field of creatures. There is no apparent distinction between the order itself and what orders it.
2. *Tian* is self-so-ing (*zi ran*, which most people translate as "Nature").
3. *Tian* is anthropomorphic, suggesting its intimate relationship with the process of euhemerization that grounds Chinese ancestor worship.

It is probably this common foundation in ancestor worship that allowed for the conflation of the Shang dynasty's *Di* with the notion of *Tian* imported with the Zhou tribes. *Tian* does not speak but communicates effectively, although not always clearly, through oracles, through perturbations in the climate and through alterations in the natural conditions of the human world.[3]

As the term "Heaven" recurs very frequently in Chinese medicine, it is useful to try to describe its meaning. Ames opts not to translate the Chinese term *Tian* as, according to him, the word "Heaven" would immediately give it Judeo-Christian connotations. He also rejects the translation of *Tian* as "Nature".[4] Ames says:[5]

The God of the Bible, often referred to metonymically as "Heaven", created the world, but Tian in classical Chinese is *the world. Tian is both* what *our world is and* how *it is.*

But there is also another meaning of *Tian* that is important from the point of view of Chinese medicine and that is that *Tian* is also the collective community of the dead (and that is why the Ethereal Soul goes to "Heaven" after death). Ames says:[6]

In the absence of some transcendent creator deity as the repository of truth, beauty and goodness, Tian would seem to stand for a cumulative and continuing cultural legacy focused in the spirits of those who have come before. Tian is anthropomorphic, suggesting its intimate relationship with the process of euhemerization – historical human beings becoming gods – that grounds Chinese ancestor reverence.

The Daoist Classic *Huai Nan Zi*, often quoted by Zhu Xi, describes clearly the origin of Heaven and Earth:[7]

When Heaven and Earth did not yet have physical form, there was only undifferentiated formlessness. Therefore it is called the great beginning. The Dao began from the empty extensiveness and this empty extensiveness produced the universe. The universe produced Qi. Qi had limits. That which was clear and light drifted upwards and became Heaven; that which was heavy and turbid congealed and became the Earth. The union of the clear and refined is especially easy, whereas the congelation of the heavy and turbid is extremely difficult. Therefore, Heaven was formed first and then the Earth was formed later.

Confucian ethics

The Confucian ideal is a person who cultivates *li* (rites), *yi* (righteousness) and *ren* (humanity, benevolence, compassion). All these terms are very difficult, if not impossible, to translate. In fact, whatever expression we use for translating these terms, it inevitably gives them a Western cultural connotation.

In order to shed light on Confucius's philosophy, I will explain the meaning of the main qualities a human being should have according to him. These are:

- *ren* 仁
- *yi* 義
- *zhong* 忠
- *shu* 恕
- *li* 礼

Ren

Ren is essentially impossible to translate. It may be variously translated as "benevolence", "kindness", "compassion", "humanity", "human-heartedness", "altruism", "love" or "goodness", but none of these terms accurately expresses the Confucian view of *ren*.

The Chinese character for *ren* shows a "person" and the number "two" (Fig. 15.2). Ames says:[8]

This etymological analysis underscores the Confucian assumption that one cannot become a person by oneself – we are, from our inchoate beginnings, irreducibly social. Fingarette has stated the matter concisely: 'For Confucius, unless there are at least two human beings, there can be no human beings'.

Any translation of the term *ren* as "benevolence" or "compassion" would give it a Christian or Buddhist slant. The essential feature of *ren* is that it is not a description of a psychological state but of a socially determined state.

Ames describes *ren* as follows:[9]

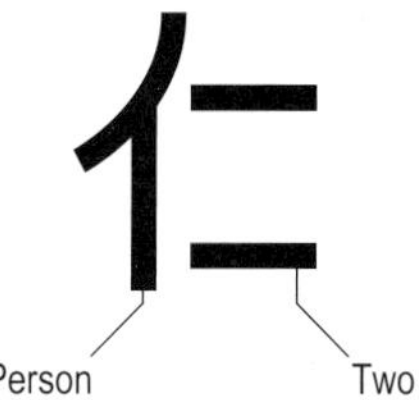

Figure 15.2 Chinese character for "Ren".

Ren is one's entire person: one's cultivated cognitive, esthetic, moral and religious sensibilities as they are expressed in one's ritualized roles and relationships. It is one's 'field of selves', the sum of significant relationships, which constitute one as a resolutely social person. Hence, translating 'ren' as 'benevolence' is to psychologize it in a tradition that does not rely upon the notion of psyche as a way of defining the human experience.

Ames further says about *ren*:[10]

As these renderings [translations of 'ren'] *clearly indicate, there has been a tendency for scholars to psychologize ren as a subjective feeling made manifest in objective social norms or mores which we submit to or accord with ritual conduct.*

Ames therefore clearly thinks that *ren* is not a psychological disposition of an individual self, which simply does not exist in Confucian philosophy. Fingarette states very clearly:[11]

Ren seems to emphasize the individual, the subjective: it seems in short a psychological notion. The problem of interpreting ren thus becomes particularly acute if one thinks, as I do, that it is of the essence of the Analects that the thought expressed in it is not based on psychological notions. And, indeed, one of the chief results of the present analysis of ren will be to reveal how Confucius could handle in a non-psychological way basic issues which we in the West naturally cast in psychological terms.

Fingarette is even more explicit when explaining the meaning of *ren*:[12]

I must emphasize that my point is not that Confucius' words are intended to exclude reference to the inner psyche. He could have done this if he had such a basic metaphor in mind, had seen its plausibility, but on reflection, had decided to reject it. But this is not what I am arguing here. My thesis is that the entire notion never entered his head. The metaphor of an inner psychic life, in all its ramifications so familiar to us, simply is not present in the Analects, not even as a rejected possibility. Hence when I say that in the above passages using Yu (the opposite of ren indicating anxiety, worry, unhappiness) there is no reference to the inner, subjective states, I do not mean that these passages clearly and explicitly exclude such elaboration, but that they make no use of it and do not require it for intelligibility or validity.

> **!**
>
> The concept of a psychological, individual self is totally absent in the Analects of Confucius.

Thus *ren* is a socially constructed ethical behavior consisting of fulfilling one's duties according to one's status in the family and society. The father acts according to the way a father should act out of love. Confucius said: "*Ren consist in loving others.*" The practice of *ren* leads to the carrying out of one's responsibilities and duties in society, in which is comprised the quality of *yi* (see below). Filial piety and fraternal love were aspects of *ren* and the cornerstone of the social structure. The formal essence of duties is *yi* but the material essence of these duties is *ren*, "loving others" (Fig. 15.3).

Therefore *ren* has to do with relatedness and social relations and has nothing to do with the individual *feeling* of "compassion" or "love" by an individual psyche. In the Confucian world, there are no essences of things or persons, but only inter-relationships or correlation. This is an intrinsic as opposed to an extrinsic correlation (Fig. 15.4); a breakdown of this intrinsic correlation diminishes both. Figure 15.5 attempts to illustrate the difference between the self in the West (top part) and the self in China (bottom part).

Ames stresses very much that *ren* does not stem from a Western notion of self and "altruism". He says:[13]

When we translate ren as "benevolence", we psychologize and make altruistic a term which originally had a radically different range of sociological service of others. But this "self-sacrifice" implicitly entails a notion of

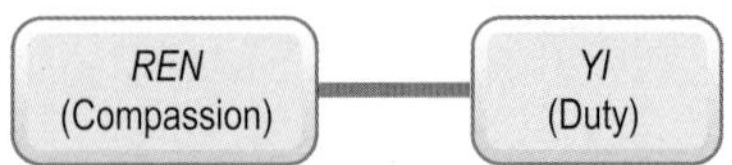

Figure 15.3 Relationship between *yi* and *ren*.

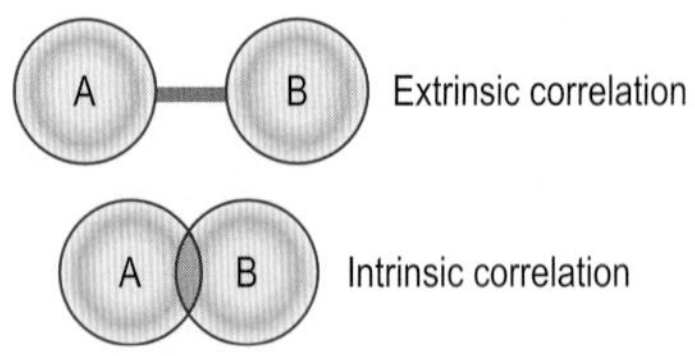

Figure 15.4 Extrinsic and intrinsic correlation of selves.

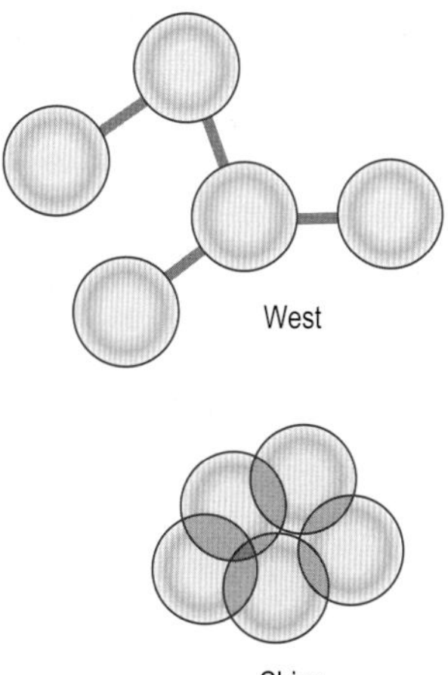

Figure 15.5 The self in the West and China.

"self" which exists independently of others and that can be surrendered – a notion of self which we believe is alien to the world of the Analects: indeed, such a reading transforms what is fundamentally a strategy for self-realization into one of self-abnegation.

> **!**
>
> When we translate *ren* as "benevolence", we psychologize and make altruistic a term which originally had a radically different meaning. "Benevolence" or "compassion" implies a notion of "self" which exists independently of others and that can be surrendered – a notion of self which we believe is alien to the world of Confucius. Indeed, such a reading transforms what is fundamentally a strategy for self-realization into one of self-abnegation.

According to Cheng Hao (1032–1085), *ren* is also the realization that Heaven, Earth and the myriad things are all one substance and all part of the self. He also makes an interesting parallel with numbness of the hands and feet, which is called *bu ren*, i.e. "lack of *ren*" in Chinese medicine, another example of the influence of Confucianism in Chinese medicine.

Cheng Hao says:[14]

In medical writing the term 'lack of humanity' [bu ren] is used for numbness of the hands and feet. This is an excellent description of the point. A man of ren regards Heaven, Earth and the myriad things as one substance, and there is nothing that is not himself. Recognizing all things in himself, will there be any boundary for him? If things are not parts of the self, naturally there will be no connection between them and himself, just as in the case of numbness of the four limbs, the Qi will not circulate through them and they no longer belong to the self.

In other words, a person of *ren* is someone who regards others as extensions of himself, like his limbs. Such a person is naturally sensitive to the needs and feelings of others, since to be insensitive of their feelings is to be insensitive of one's own limbs.

In a practical sense, for Confucius, *ren* begins in the family, which is the first unit where one is exposed to social relationships. Gardner says:[15]

In a model family, one comes to know how to behave with propriety as a child, as a parent, as a younger sibling or as an older sibling. Moving outside the family to the larger society, the child of such a family is sure to show respect and obedience to superiors; the parent is sure to treat subordinates with compassion and empathy; the younger sibling is sure to be dutiful towards elders; the older sibling is sure to be considerate and caring towards the young.

Yi

Yi is, again, impossible to translate. Any translation such as "duty" or "morality" does not convey the complex meaning of the term. Ames thinks that "appropriate" or "fitting" is a better translation of *yi*. He says:[16]

Yi, then, is one's sense of appropriateness that enables one to act in a proper and fitting manner, given the specific situation. By extension, it is also the meaning invested by a cumulative tradition in the forms of ritual propriety that define it.

Yi is righteousness; it is the "oughtness" of a situation; it is a categorical imperative. Everyone in society has to do certain things for their own sake, because they are morally right; if, however, they do them only out of duty or for non-moral considerations, then even though they do what they ought to do, their action is no longer a righteous one.

Zhong

Zhong indicates the state of mind when one is completely honest with oneself; it also means "doing one's utmost". It is composed of the radical for "heart" and "center". With one's heart at the center of one's being, one is true to oneself.

Shu

Shu indicates the state of mind when one is in complete understanding and empathy with the outside world and other people. It has the meaning "as one's heart" or "putting oneself in the other's place", i.e. "do unto others as your heart prompts you".

The two states of *zhong* and *shu* are correlated with each other. A passage from the *Doctrine of the Mean* (*Zhong Yong*), however, gives away the social meaning of these two behaviors:

Zhong and shu are not far from the Way (Dao). What you do not like done to yourself, do not do to others ... Serve your father as you would require your son to serve you ... serve your ruler as you would require your subordinate to serve you ... serve your elder brother as you would require your younger brother to serve you ... set the example in behaving to your friends as you would require them to behave to you.

This statement clearly shows that the Confucian concept of "altruism" is very different from the compassion advocated by the Buddhists or Christians.

Li

Li may be translated as "rituals". Please note that this is a different word from *Li* (Principle) described below with which it shares the same sound. To Confucius, rituals are not simply the formal repetitions of certain ceremonies but part of everyday life. Confucius thought that rituals are what distinguish human beings from animals. *Li* may also be translated as "propriety"; when every person assumes his or her proper role in the family and society, this will be expressed with certain rituals. Although this idea may at first seem strange to a Westerner, in fact we also have rituals in our daily life; shaking hands when meeting someone is a ritual.

Li, or rituals, were a very formal and important part of living a distinctive human life. In fact, *li* is described as the essence of living a life in dignified harmony with others. According to Bockover: "*Most crucially, li is relational, in the sense that it provides patterns of conduct with others that are also essential to defining the person.*"[17]

Ames stresses the social dimension of "rituals" in Chinese culture:[18]

The centrality of ritual practice in Confucianism is clear when we begin from Confucius's premise that a person is irreducibly social, measurable in terms of the quality of the relationships that one is able to effect. It is ritual practice, taken in its broadest sense, that enables persons to assume roles and, literally, to find their appropriate place in relationship to others. It is a social syntax that enables them to communicate with others and, in so doing, to constitute themselves as a matrix of relationships.

Li and *ren* are indissolubly linked: *li* are the forms of conduct done with the right spirit; *ren* tells us what that spirit is, i.e. to approach others empathetically. Fingarette says:[19]

Thus li and ren are two aspects of the same thing. Li directs our attention to the traditional social pattern of conduct and relationships; ren directs our attention to the person as the one who pursues that pattern of conduct and thus maintains those relationships.

It would be a mistake to think that Confucius advocated a blind and mechanical adherence to codified rituals and ceremonies – far from it. Confucius repeatedly said that the significance of the ritual does not lie in the ritual itself but in the feeling and meaning one invests in it.

Confucian ethics, society and state

An important feature of Confucian ethics is also the idea that ethical personal conduct influences our family, society and the state, and vice versa. How much personal conduct and social order are intertwined is obvious from this passage from Confucius:[20]

Ancient kings first regulated the government of the State
To do that, first they put order in their family
To do that, first they regulated their own person
To do that, first they controlled their emotions
To do that, first they controlled their desires
To do that, first they sharpened their knowledge

To do that, first they penetrated the nature of things.
Having penetrated the nature of things, their knowledge was sharpened;
Having done that, their desires were controlled
Having done that, they controlled their emotions
Having done that, they regulated their person
Having done that they put order in their family
Having done that, the State was governed well
The Empire therefore enjoyed peace (Tai Ping)
Therefore from the Emperor down to the humblest commoner, everyone must regulate their behaviour.

Figures 15.6 and 15.7 illustrate this concept.

With time, Confucianism rigidly codified all areas of human behavior in the family, society and state so that every person had to behave according to rigid rules and every person had to assume his or her proper role in the family and society. For example, the following are ethical rules of behavior by Zhu Xi (1130–1200):[21]

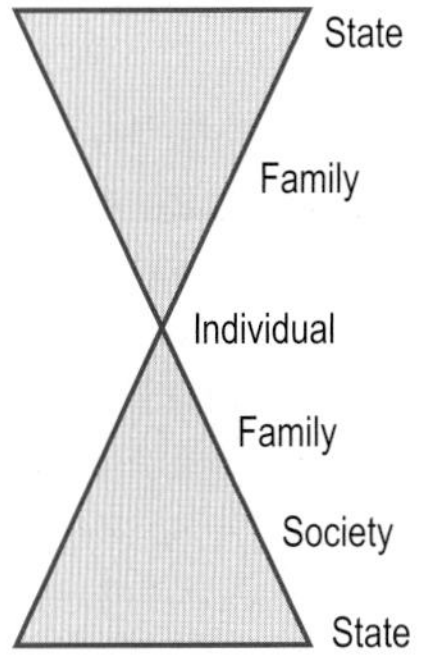

Figure 15.6 Relationship among individual, family, society and state.

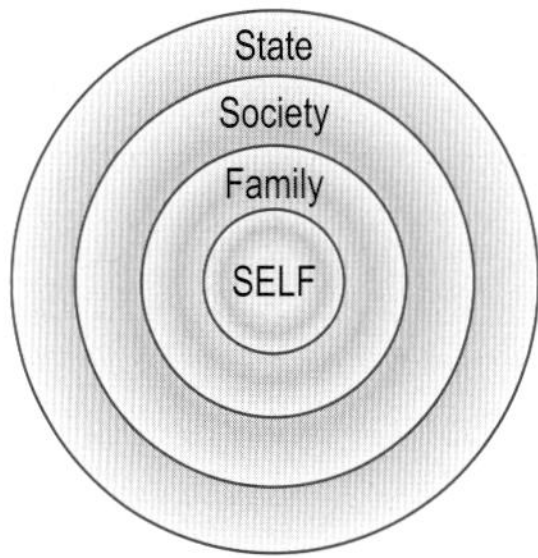

Figure 15.7 Relationship among self, family, society and state.

Between parents and children there should be love
Between the emperor and his subjects there should be a proper sense of duties
Between husband and wife there should be a separation in regard to work
Between elder and younger persons there should be order and harmony
Between friends there should be mutual confidence.

He then went on to explain how this is achieved:[22]

One's commitments to others should be based on loyalty and honesty
One's conduct should be based on seriousness and watchfulness
A person should control their anger and diminish their desires
A person should correct their mistakes and pay attention to doing good.

The following quote by a Confucian thinker, reported by Needham, is probably the best illustration of how much the Chinese medicine theory of the Internal Organs as "officials" reflects Neo-Confucian views on personal ethics, on assuming proper roles and on society and government. Ko Hong in *Bao Pu Zi*:[23]

Thus the body of a person is the image of a State. The thorax and abdomen correspond to the palaces (Yin organs) and offices (Yang organs). The four limbs correspond to the frontiers and boundaries. The divisions of the bones and sinews correspond to the functional distinctions of the inherited officials. The pores of the flesh correspond to the four thoroughfares. The spirit [shen] corresponds to the prince. The blood corresponds to the ministers, and Qi to the people. Thus we see that he who can govern his body can control a kingdom. Loving his people, he will bring peace to the country; nourishing Qi, he will preserve his body. If the people are alienated the country is lost; if Qi is exhausted the body dies.

Unschuld confirms that Confucianism influenced Chinese medicine very early on during the Han dynasty:[24]

During the course of the last three centuries BC, *unknown authors began to develop a system of healing whose theoretical principles corresponded closely to the socio-political order advocated during the same period by Confucian political ideology. As a consequence, this system of healing was continuously dependent on the interests and fate of Confucianism itself. With the elevation of Confucianism to orthodox political doctrine by the Emperor Wu, the Han period theoretical foundations of this ideology remained fixed for a long span of time.*

!

Under Confucian influence, Chinese medicine compared the Internal Organs to ministers of a government and the body's physiology to the running of government.

Many chapters of the *Yellow Emperor's Classic of Internal Medicine* show a clear Confucian influence, deriving from later centuries when Confucianism had been established as the orthodoxy. Consider these two statements reported by Unschuld. The first is by a Confucian scholar Xun Xi: "*The true ruler begins to put his state in order while order prevails. He does not wait until insurrections have already erupted.*" The second statement is from Chapter 1 of the *Nei Jing*: "*The sages do not treat those who have already fallen ill, but rather those who are not yet ill. They do not put their state in order only when revolt is under way, but before an insurrection occurs.*"[25] These two statements clearly show a strong Confucian influence on the concept of health in Chinese medicine and the allegory of Internal Organs as the minister of a government.

Another can be found in Chapter 29 of the *Spiritual Axis*, which says:[26]

To govern the people and one's own body, to govern here and there, to govern on a small or large scale, to govern the state or a family, it has never been achieved by not following the rules [*ni*, rebelling]. *It is only by following the rules* [*shun*, conforming] *that success can be achieved. To 'follow the rules'* [*shun*] *does not apply only to following* [*shun*] *or going against* [*ni*] *Qi and Yin-Yang channels; it applies also to the entire population whose intention* [*zhi*] *one must follow.*

The Sui dynasty commentary called *An Elucidation of the Yellow Emperor's Classic of Internal Medicine*, written by Yang Shang Shan (AD 581–618), comments on this passage:[27]

The Way [Dao] *of dealing with the state, the family and the body all have their Li* [Principle]. *It is not possible to have order in one's body without following* [its] *Li. The reason one must make enquiries in all these situations is to find out the Li of each and conform* [*shun*] *to it.*

Both passages from Chapter 29 of the *Spiritual Axis* and the commentary by Yang Shang Shan are a clear reflection of Confucian thinking in many respects. First, there is the Confucian concept of equivalence between the body, a family and the whole state. "Order" in one's body reflects order in the family and the whole state, and vice versa.

Second, there is a strong emphasis on the concepts of "conforming" or "following the rules" (*shun*) and its opposite "rebelling" or "not following the rules" (*ni*). As we have seen, these two terms are used in Chinese medicine to denote "rebellious Qi" (*ni*) or Qi that goes the right way (*shun*). Third, the passages reflect the Confucian idea that the body must be "governed" like the family and the state. As we have seen above, this idea is also influenced by Legalist thinking.

From the Song dynasty onward, Neo-Confucianism encouraged a strictly authoritarian form of government, including the establishment of censorship, thought control and other authoritarian features. In Ming and Qing times, the charge of heterodoxy (*bu-jing*) supplied the authorities with a convenient excuse for ridding themselves of political opponents and other people whose thoughts were considered dangerous to the security of the State – exactly as under Communism. Thus, Marxism, far from being the antithesis of Confucianism, grafted onto it perfectly to continue the political subjugation of the Chinese people which started with Neo-Confucianism. Indeed, I would say that the Marxist ideology and the Communist social–political–administrative structure is the logical and most consistent continuation of the Neo-Confucianist tradition.

!

Marxism, far from being the antithesis of Confucianism, grafted onto it perfectly to continue the political subjugation of the Chinese people which started with Neo-Confucianism. The Marxist ideology and the Communist social–political–administrative structure is the logical and most consistent continuation of the Neo-Confucianist tradition.

During the Yuan dynasty, Buddhism underwent a revival; however, with the Ming dynasty, Neo-Confucianism (and particularly the philosophy of Zhu Xi) was established as the undisputed dominant ideology. The authorities came to view any non-Confucian thought with suspicion and at various times exercised censorship and took measures for thought control. In the later years of the Ming dynasty the Chinese state became very oppressive.

Confucian ethics and views on family and society are strongly at variance with those of Daoism. The Daoists did not believe in conforming to rules but believed in spontaneity, in following nature and practicing non-action (*wu wei*). Graham says:[28]

Daoism represents everything that is spontaneous, imaginative, private, unconventional in Chinese society. Confucianism represents everything that is controlled, prosaic, public, conventional, respectable.

The following passage from Chuang Zi could not be a starker rejection of Confucianist ethical views on family and society:[29]

Your life is not your possession; it is harmony between your forces, granted for a time by Heaven and Earth. Your nature and destiny are not your possession; they are the course laid down for you by Heaven and Earth. Therefore you travel without knowing where you go, stay without knowing what you cling to, are fed without knowing how. You are the breath of Heaven and Earth which goes to and fro: how can you ever possess it?

NEO-CONFUCIANISM

"Neo-Confucianism" is a Western term that was not used in China at the time or in later times. It broadly indicates the new schools of Confucianism that were developed during the Song and Ming dynasties (particularly former) and which were based on an absorption of Buddhist and Daoist concepts into Confucianism. It was at this time that Confucianism developed from a philosophy primarily concerned with ethics to one concerned with ontology and metaphysics. The schools of thought called "Neo-Confucianism" were actually three: the School of Principle (*Li*), School of Mind (*Xin*) and School of Names (*Ming*).

In order to counteract the Buddhist theories of impermanence and emptiness, the Neo-Confucianists had to construct a new philosophy based on Confucianism. The sponsors of this new philosophy had to build a system that would contain a cosmology to account for the creation of the Universe, an ethics treating humankind as a unity and affirming the value of human effort, and an epistemology to determine the basis of knowledge.

The seeds of this movement were sown by Han Yu in the Tang dynasty and then developed in the Song dynasty with Zhou Dun Yi, the Cheng brothers, Zhang Zai and especially Zhu Xi.

The first cosmological philosopher was Zhou Dun Yi (1017–1073), the author of the famous *Tai Ji* diagram that was the object of discussion by many later Neo-Confucian philosophers. Neo-Confucianism then declined and its influence waned during the late Qing dynasty; however, inertia kept it going as China's dominant ideology until 1949 (and I would say beyond that). Neo-Confucianism thus dominated Chinese thought, society, politics, ethics and medicine for 1000 years (and Confucianism for 2200 years).

During the Yuan dynasty, Buddhism underwent a revival and Confucianist philosophers were at pains to create a new, all-encompassing philosophy that could compete with Buddhism. With the Ming dynasty, Neo-Confucianism (and particularly the philosophy of Zhu Xi) was established as the undisputed dominant ideology. The authorities came to view any non-Confucianist thought with suspicion and at various times exercised censorship and took measures for thought control.

In its later years, government during the Ming dynasty became very oppressive. Patronized by the government, the Confucian principles began to work through the daily life of the people. The separation of the sexes began and the seclusion of women was practiced in earnest. The chastity of women became a veritable cult, the remarrying of widows was frowned upon (and still is now) and divorce was considered a disgrace for a woman whatever the reason.

Interestingly, whereas men in general were interested in Confucianism, Daoism and Buddhism alike, women favored nearly exclusively Buddhism. The Buddhist creed of universal love and compassion, preaching equality of all beings, answered women's spiritual needs, while the dazzling ceremonies centering around beautiful female deities, like the deity of compassion, Kuan Yin, who helps people in distress and grants children to the childless, lent color to the rather monotonous daily life.

The Neo-Confucianists exerted a profound influence on Chinese medicine; indeed, in my opinion, more important than that exerted by Daoism. When reading the *Yellow Emperor's Classic of Internal Medicine* we should be very careful not to assume that reference to "Dao" always reflects a Daoist influence. We should be very clear that Confucius and all other Confucianist (and especially Neo-Confucianist) thinkers talk about the Dao. Indeed, even the Legalists talked about Dao.

For example, the Neo-Confucianist Wang Ming Sheng (1722–1798) said that "*The classics are employed to understand the Dao.*"[30] Dai Zhen claimed that "*The classics provide the route to Dao.*"[31] Ng says explicitly: "*The Dao that Wang and Dai celebrated and sought was not the Buddhist or Daoist Dao; it was the same Confucian Dao that the Song-Ming Confucians honoured.*"[32]

For each school the term "Dao" has different connotations. To the Daoists, "Dao" denotes Dao, i.e. an unfathomable force or principle that works in the universe without effort and without trying. To the Confucianists, Dao was synonymous with *ren*. To the Neo-Confucianists, Dao was equivalent to *Li* (Principle); to the Legalists, Dao was the source of laws to govern the State. Consider this passage in a Ma Wang Dui text of Legalist inspiration: "*It is out of Dao that the law comes into being.*"[33] A very "un-Daoist" statement indeed, but one that uses the term "Dao".

The influence of Neo-Confucian thought in the field of emotions is discussed below. Besides that, there are many examples of a superimposition of a Confucian view on old Chinese medicine concepts as detailed below.

As we know, Confucianism was preoccupied with the establishment of clear rules of ethics and behavior so that there would be harmony in the individual, family, society and state. Every individual had to abide to the principles of benevolence (*ren*), righteousness (*yi*), propriety (*li*), altruism (*shun*), honesty (*zhong*) and wisdom (*zhi*) for harmony to prevail at every level of society. Indeed, the emperor himself (and therefore government officials) had to abide by the same rules and their ethical behavior would influence all of society. Even natural calamities were sometimes attributed to the emperor not following the "mandate of Heaven".

These views are very much reflected in Chinese medicine where the Internal Organs are compared to government officials with an emperor in the form of the Heart. Each internal organ is compared to a Minister and health depends on good "governance" by the Internal Organs. Ill health is not so much a medical problem as an ethical problem stemming from not abiding by the rules of behavior.

It is also interesting to note that a large part of the acupuncture vocabulary is influenced by the metaphor of water irrigation systems. For example, the main channels are compared to canals and the eight extraordinary vessels to reservoirs or lakes that absorb the excess water from the canals in case of heavy rain. The Lower Burner is an "irrigation ditch".

This metaphor probably reflects the fact that, in ancient China, the largest irrigation systems were controlled directly by the central government. This metaphor is carried on in Chinese medicine, where there is a monarch (the Heart) and 11 other officials.

This is very apparent in the writing of Dong Zhong Shu (179–104 BC), a Confucian scholar who actively criticized and opposed modes of government and rulership that were inspired by Daoism. How much the view of the body and mind in Chinese medicine reflected Confucian political view on government is apparent from this passage by Dong:[34]

Heaven's ordinance is called Mandate and this cannot be put in operation except by sages. The natural quality of human beings is called human nature (Xing 性) and this cannot be fulfilled save by moral education and transformation. Human desires are called emotions (qing) and these cannot be regulated except by institution and rules. This is why the human sovereign carefully receives the intention of Heaven from above, so that he may conform with the Mandate. Down below he strives to educate and transform his norms for law and institutions, distinguishing between the upper and the lower orders of society to preclude desire. If he achieves these three aims, the fundamental basis will be established.

Incidentally, it was Dong Zhong Shu who suggested to emperor Wu (141–87 BC) to disband and proscribe all other schools of thought (the "hundred schools") in favor of Confucianism in 139 BC. His suggestion was greatly appreciated by the emperor, though not fully implemented until the reign of emperor Yuan (48–33 BC) who established Confucianism as the official ideology of imperial China until 1911 (and, I would say, beyond).

There are passages that show how the Confucians placed an ethical emphasis even on things like Qi, Yin-Yang and the Five Elements. For example, Zhu Xi often talks about "good Qi" and "bad Qi", and Qi was directly invested with moral qualities. He also mentioned "wicked Qi" and "evil Qi".[35]

As for Yin-Yang, even these were invested with moral qualities, listing "good", "virtue" and "noble" under Yang qualities and "bad", "evil" and "humble" as the corresponding Yin qualities. For example, Cheng Hao said: "*Everything comes in opposites. Yin has Yang as its counterpart. Good has evil as the entity opposed to it. When Yang grows, Yin declines. When good increases, evil decreases.*"[36] Of course, the philosophy of Yin-Yang developed by Zou Yen in the Warring States period was a naturalist philosophy that had nothing to do with ethical considerations.[37]

Zhu Xi attributed moral qualities also to the Five Elements, listing the Five Virtues corresponding to them as follows:[38]

- Wood: benevolence (*ren*)
- Fire: propriety (*li*)
- Metal: righteousness (*yi*)
- Water: wisdom (*zhi*)
- Earth: trustworthiness (*xin*).

!

Under the Neo-Confucianist influence, there was an arbitrary superimposition of Confucian ideas onto ancient Chinese medicine ideas.

Of course, the Five Elements are a philosophy of Nature that explains natural phenomena; superimposing an ethical dimension on them is, therefore, totally arbitrary.

Confucian scholars gave a Confucian interpretation to Chinese medicine concepts which, developed by the Yin-Yang School, essentially had nothing to do with ethical considerations. This happened from very early on in the history of Chinese medicine. For example the Confucian scholar Lu Jia (206–180 BC) says of Yin-Yang:[39]

Yang Qi is generated by benevolence (ren) and the regulation of Yin is descended by righteousness (yi). Heaven and Earth come together with benevolence, the eight trigrams follow one another with righteousness.

Human nature (*Xing*)

The concept of human nature is central to Neo-Confucianist preoccupations. To them, human nature is what defines us as human beings; it is the pure nature that is part of "Heaven" (*Tian*), bearing in mind the essentially immanent and not transcendental nature of Heaven (see above).

The Confucianists distinguished two types of human nature: one is the "Heaven-Earth human nature" (*tian-di zhi xing*) which, as a manifestation of Principle (*Li*) is inherently good; the other is human Mind (*ren xin*) which is prone to error. This is because, in human beings, human nature is influenced by the nature of Qi and it is the variations of the quality of Qi of human beings that accounts for good and evil.

Ng calls the former "prior human nature" and the latter "posterior human nature" and says:[40]

Some are given a pure, clear and brilliant Qi, while others receive an impure, turbid and cloudy one. It is only in the realm of Qi that evil arises. The prior human nature is always good; the posterior human nature is the repository of both good and evil.

Confucianists see human nature as essentially pure and untainted. Emotions are factors that disturb and cloud our human nature; indeed they make us lose our human nature.

The great Neo-Confucian philosopher Zhang Zai (1020–1077) said:[41]

The term Xing [human nature] *is derived from the combination of Void (Xu) and Qi. Where there is form, there is the physical nature. One should return to the goodness of heavenly nature so that the nature of Heaven and Earth may be preserved. Therefore, the physical nature is that to which the sage does not allow himself to be attached. There is no evil in the nature of man; it depends on whether or not one returns to the heavenly nature. The nature of Heaven in the nature of a human being is truly like the nature of water in ice. Although freezing and thawing are different, their nature is the same.*

The very concept of Mind is closely bound with that of human nature (although they do not coincide with one another). Please note that in the quotations that follow I use the term "*Xin*" (Heart) as synonymous with "Mind". Zhang Zai said: "*The name of Mind (Xin) is derived from the union of nature (Xing) and consciousness.*"[42] The Mind of a human being enables him or her to develop his or her nature and partake of "Heaven"; however, when the Mind is clouded by emotions, we lose our human nature.

Both Cheng Hao and Cheng Yi identified human nature with *Li* (see below). They considered that man's *Li* lies in his human nature and this latter consists of the four virtues of benevolence (*ren*), propriety (*li*), righteousness (*yi*) and wisdom (*zhi*). Cheng Yi said:[43]

What is ordained by Heaven is the heavenly Mandate. What persists in things is Li. What makes a person is human nature. What acts as the determining factor in a person is Mind (Xin). When Mind operates, the resultant thoughts may be good or bad. After Mind has ceased operating, the thoughts that remain are the work of the emotions rather than of the Mind.

Li (Principle)

The concept of *Li* is central to Neo-Confucian philosophy and particularly in the thought of the great Neo-Confucian philosopher Zhu Xi (1130–1200). The concept of *Li* occupies a central place in the ontology of Neo-Confucian thought. One of the main thrusts of Neo-Confucian philosophy, as we have seen, was the elaboration of an ontology and epistemology; this was done primarily to fight the rising Buddhist influence on Chinese society and government.

Li 理 is, as usual with Chinese words, difficult to translate. It literally means "grain" (of wood), "truth" or "principle". Most Western authors translate it as "Principle" or leave it untranslated. *Li* is the nature, principle or essence underlying everything in the world; it has a metaphysical aspect.

Everything is made of Qi and every change in the world is due to transformations of Qi. But if everything is made of Qi, what distinguishes one thing from another, especially across species? If everything is made of Qi, what makes a human being different from a rock or a rhinoceros? It is *Li* that accounts for the difference among species. In spite of the endless variations in human beings, variations that are due to Qi, every human being carries the imprint of a human being's *Li*, while a rhino carries the imprint of a rhino's *Li*.

!

Qi is responsible for all changes in all things, while *Li* is responsible for the variation among species. For example, Qi accounts for the endless variations among individuals of the human species but the human *Li* is what distinguishes human beings from apes (or any other animals). Human beings have the *Li* of a human being; apes have the *Li* of an ape.

Cheng Yi (1033–1107) says:[44]

All things in the universe can be understood in light of the Principle (Li). Since there is a thing, there must be a rule for it. Every single thing must have its own principle. All things have principles, such as that by which fire is hot, and that by which water is cold.

In typical Confucian fashion (as Confucianism was preoccupied with ethics and social order), Cheng Yi then relates *Li* to social relationships:[45]

If there is a thing there must be a rule for it. A father rests in paternal affections, a son in filial piety, a ruler in benevolence, and a subject in respectfulness. Every single thing or activity has its own proper place. Getting this place, there is peace; losing it, there is disorder.

It is often said that Chinese philosophy never developed a metaphysical view that is so typical of much of Western philosophy. However, this is not entirely true. For example, Cheng Yi talked about a world of "above form" (*xing er shang*) being a metaphysical world, independent of the physical world, and a world of "below form" (*xing er xia*) being the physical form. He said that *Li* pertains to the "above form" world and Qi to the "below form" world.[46] See Figure 15.8.

Zhu Xi (1130–1220), the greatest Neo-Confucian philosopher, said:[47]

What is above form refers to Li; what is below form refers to things and events. The things and events can be seen, but Li are difficult to know.

Ng says:[48]

Although Li does not exist in the absence of Qi, it is only in the realm of Qi that evil arises. Principle is prior to Qi. Thus the Li-Qi metaphysical world is animated by a sense of duality.

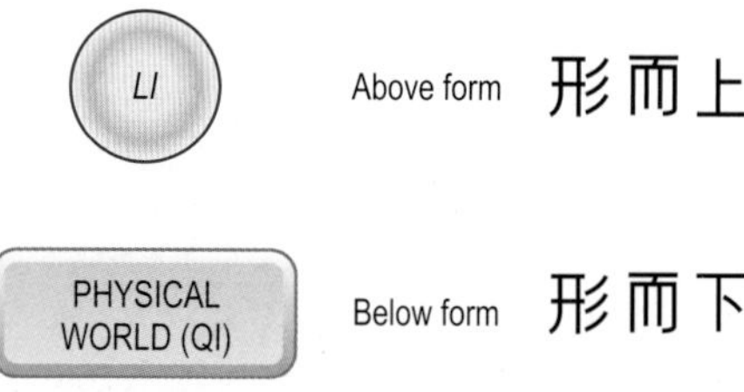

Figure 15.8 Relationship between Li and Qi.

However, there were dissenting views on this matter. For example, Liu Zong Zhou says: "*Li is the principle of Qi and it is definitely not prior to and outside of Qi.*"[49] Liu Guang Di says: "*Li is not a separate entity which depends on Qi in order to exist or which attaches to Qi in order to operate.*"[50] He also says simply: "*Li is Qi and Qi is Li.*"[51]

!

Chinese philosophy did develop a metaphysics with a dualism between the metaphysical and the physical. *Li* is "above form" and things are "below form".

Zhu Xi also developed further the relationship between *Li* and Qi. He said:[52]

Before Heaven and Earth existed, there was only Principle (Li). As there was this Principle, this Heaven and Earth then came into existence. If there were no Principle, then there would be no Heaven and Earth, no man and no things: none of these would have anything to contain it. As there is Principle, there is Qi which prevails everywhere, develops and nourishes the myriad things.

He also said:[53]

Only after there is Principle, there is Qi. When there is Qi, then Principle has a place to settle. Whether they are as large as Heaven and Earth or as small as ants, this is the process by which all things are produced.

It can therefore be said in a Kantian sense that *Li* pertains to the noumenal world and Qi to the phenomenal world. This dualism has led some philosophers to equate the philosophy of Zhu Xi with that of Plato and Aristotle. However, Needham disagrees and says:[54]

I believe that Li was not in any strict sense metaphysical, as were Platonic ideas or Aristotelian forms, but rather the invisible organizing fields or forces existing in all levels within the natural world ... attempt should be made to reappraise Zhu Xi's philosophy in light of the philosophy of organism.

However, the duality of a metaphysical and physical world seems apparent in this passage from Zhu Xi:[55]

Which comes first, Li or Qi? Li is never separable from Qi. However, Li belongs to what is above form whereas Qi belongs to what is below form. Hence, speaking in terms of what is above form and what is below form, how can there not be before and after? How about your statement that there must first be Li, then there can be Qi afterwards? Fundamentally, they cannot be spoken of in terms of priority and posteriority. However, if it is necessary to trace their origin, one is obliged to admit that Li has priority.

Therefore, according to Huang Siu-chi, *Li* is universal, transcendent, unchanging and beyond time and space, while Qi is particular, immanent, forever changing and with temporal and spatial limitations.[56] Qi is the actualization and manifestation of *Li* in individualized things.

However, other philosophers disagreed with this view and held a unified view of the universe. For example, Wang Yang Ming (1472–1529) held that there is only one level of reality as opposed to Zhu Xi's view of "above form" and "below form" worlds. Wang maintained that there is no distinction between what is above and what is below, and that the Mind and Principle are identical. Wang said:[57]

The Mind is the same as Principle. The substance of the Mind is human nature and this is the same as Principle. Consequently, as there is the Mind of filial piety, then there is the principle of filial piety. If there is no mind of filial piety, there will be no principle of filial piety.

With Dai Dong Yuan (1728–1777) of the Qing dynasty, this discussion comes full circle as this philosopher gives a distinctly "materialistic" view of *Li*. Dai Dong Yuan said that there is no difference between *Li* and Qi. He criticizes the dualism of a metaphysical *Li* and physical Qi. The notion of *Li* as the ultimate cosmic reality of previous schools is now interpreted by Dai Dong Yuan in terms of *tiao-li*, i.e. orderly principle or pattern as the fiber of every physical thing.

THE CONCEPT OF SELF IN WESTERN AND CHINESE PHILOSOPHY

The concepts of self in Western and Chinese philosophy are very different and that raises the question of how to interpret the Chinese medicine view of emotions. We should be careful not to attribute to Chinese medicine (and philosophy) a psychological view of the self which has actually never been there.

Lau and Ames investigate the differences between the self in Western philosophy and that in Chinese philosophy. They say:[58]

If Western notions of 'self' are typically framed in terms of the consciousness of an autonomous will or reason, such a self can only refer to the one's individuated consciousness in relation to itself. The self, in other words, is self-consciousness. But self-consciousness requires that one is able to objectify one's thoughts, feelings and so on. Hyper self-consciousness of this sort is a modern Western invention that does not play a role in classical Chinese concern about personal development.

Lau and Ames correctly say in the above statement that "*hyper self-consciousness is a modern Western invention*". Indeed, the concept of an individual, autonomous, inner-directed self with an inner life is a concept that arose in the West over the course of many centuries from Plato down to Freud and Jung. As Taylor says, "*Our modern sense of self is related to, one might say constituted by, a certain sense in inwardness.*"[59]

According to Taylor, the Western notion of the self is inseparably linked to a sense of inwardness. He says:[60]

In our language of self-understanding, the opposition inside-outside plays an important role. We think of our thoughts, ideas and feelings as being 'within' us. When a given constellation of self, moral sources and localization is ours, that means it is the one from within which we experience and deliberate about our moral situation.

Taylor continues: "*We think of our thoughts, feelings and ideas as being 'within' us, while the objects in the world which these mental states bear on are 'without'.*"[61] As Taylor says, "*We are creatures with inner depths, with partly unexplored and dark interiors.*"[62]

The Western concept of self developed over many centuries, starting especially with Plato. In later centuries, Christian thinkers contributed to forming a concept of self. In particular, Taylor says, "*It is hardly an exaggeration to say that it was St Augustine who introduced the inwardness of radical reflexivity and bequeathed it to the Western tradition of thought.*"[63] Christian thinkers developed the concept of self in relation to God. St Augustine's concern was to show that God is to be found, not just in the world but also, and more importantly, at the very foundation of the person; God was to be found in the intimacy of self-presence. In the Christian doctrine, the inner self takes on a new status because it is the space in which we come to encounter God.

A definition of consciousness and therefore self by Damasio is a good illustration of the Western concepts of self and how they differ from Confucian concepts of self. Damasio says: "*Consciousness is an entirely private, first-person phenomenon which occurs as part of the private, first-person process we call mind.*"[64] The use of the word "private" twice is an interesting illustration of the Western concept of a private, individual, inner-directed self. Any Confucian philosopher would not recognize the above statement as a description of consciousness or self because, in Confucian philosophy, the self is socially constructed.

Damasio's definition of *core* and *extended consciousness* presents interesting similarities with Chinese medicine. He calls *core consciousness* the one that provides the organism with a sense of self about one moment – now – and about one place – here. The scope of core consciousness is here and now. This is similar to the function of the Corporeal Soul.

He calls *extended consciousness* the one that provides "*the organism with an elaborate sense of self and places the person at a point in individual historical time, richly aware of the lived past and of the anticipated future.*"[65] This is a function of the Mind (*Shen* of the Heart) in Chinese medicine.

These two types of consciousness correspond to two types of self, the *core self* and what Damasio calls the *autobiographical self* which he describes so:[66]

The autobiographical self depends on systematical memories of situations in which core consciousness was involved in the knowing, who you were born to, where, when, your likes and dislikes, the way you usually react to a problem or a conflict, and so on.

Again, the core self corresponds to the Corporeal Soul (*Po*) while the autobiographical self corresponds to the Mind of the Heart (*Shen*).

According to Taylor, modern individualism is based on the two pillars of the *independence* of the self and that of the *particularity* of the self, two concepts totally alien to the Confucian view of the self.[67]

Confucianism sees the self as indissolubly part of a society without the individuality typical of Western societies. Jones says:[68]

The Chinese traditionally have viewed society as being the source for the circumscribing characteristics of the individual. Consequently, society becomes a repository of values of the dead ancestors and is not seen as an arena for actualizing human potential as it is in the West. Typically, Westerners will foreground individuality and background their belonging to communities. The Chinese are more inclined to reverse this process.

Ames says:[69]

In the Confucian model of constitutive relations, we are not individuals who associate in community, but rather because we associate effectively in community, we become distinguished as individuals.

Suleski says:[70]

In emphasizing the social roles played by individuals, Mencius (an important Confucian philosopher) deflects concern away from the development of the inner personal emotional growth. For Mencius, the correct conduct acted out in visible social roles was important because it was the clearest way the individual could express an inner maturity.

Crabbe lists nine attributes of the self and it is interesting to note from this list that they are almost all diametrically opposed to a Confucian vision of the self. Crabbe's nine attributes of the self are as follows.[71]

- The self is a *thing*
- The self is *mental*
- The self is *single*
- at a time
- and through time
- The self is ontologically distinct from its thoughts, experiences
- The self is the *subject of experience*, a conscious feeler, thinker, decider, chooser
- The self is thought of as an *agent*
- The self has a *personality*

The Chinese concept of self is quite different from the one in the West. As Fingarette said of Confucius's Analects: "*The metaphor of an inner psychic life, in all its ramifications so familiar to us, simply is not present in the Analects, not even as a rejected possibility.*"[72] In other words, the self as the individual center on consciousness in Western psychology is very different from the self in Chinese philosophy and medicine. In China, the self is an ethical, socially constructed consciousness and the introspective self of Western philosophy and psychology plays no role in Chinese philosophy. Personal accomplishment is measurable in terms of the quality of relationships that one is able to establish.[73]

Lau and Ames express clearly what the path to self-realization is in Chinese philosophy, in the process highlighting the concept of self in China:[74]

If agitation is not referenced primarily within one's soul, it can only be a disturbance in the relationships *which constitute the self in its interactions with external things. Said another way, if a person is not in fact constituted by some essential, partitioned 'soul' but is rather seen as a dynamic pattern of personal, social and natural relationships, agitation must arise as a consequence of poor management of these constitutive roles and relationships. Hence, agitation in the heart and mind is not narrowly 'psychological', but more properly of broad ethical concern.*

Hume said reason is slave to the passions. Freud saw the individual psyche as the battleground of the struggle between ego, id and super-ego. The main reason that the Chinese self is not internally conflicted is that there is nothing strictly internal to the self. The Daoist self is a function of its relationships with the world. The Confucian self is determined by deferential activity (*shu*), guided by ritually structured roles and relationships.[75]

It can be argued that Chinese understandings of self do not entail a strong notion of "individuality". The Western notion of a separate, distinct individual in its various forms is anathema to the Chinese. Hall and Ames observe:[76]

In the Confucian model, the self is contextual; it is a shared consciousness of one's role and relationships. One's inner and outer selves are inseparable. In this model, one is self-conscious, not in the sense of being able to isolate and objectify one's essential self, but in the sense of being aware of oneself as a locu of observation by others. The locus of self-consciousness is not in the 'I' detached from the 'me', but in the consciousness of the 'me'. This involves an image of self determined by the esteem with which one is regarded in the community, an image of self that is captured in the language of face and shame.

Interestingly, as a consequence of this, there is little talk of individual "rights" in Chinese philosophy. As Bockover says:[77]

In essence, for Confucius, to be a person is to stand in significant relation to others. Thus, the focus of his philosophy is on the interpersonal dimension of human life, which can be sharply contrasted with our highly intrapersonal focus on the individual.

According to Fingarette, Confucius never mentions "rights", "choice", "freedom", "liberty", "autonomy", "individual" or "anxiety" is his writings.[78]

Bockover continues:[79]

Confucius' notion of individuality differs from the traditional Western notion of the isolated and autonomous self, however. According to Confucius, one's unique individuality is socially determined, i.e. the self for Confucius is a complex of social roles that one ideally and distinctively embodies in the course of his or her life. To be a person then, or to cultivate one's self, is to develop an open and responsible stance towards all others in accordance with one's various social roles.

Fingarette says:[80]

Confucius showed that human nature is communal. He then showed that this communal nature is 'ceremonial'. For Confucius, life itself is a sacred ceremony. Utterly absent is the central Western metaphor of the 'inner drama' on the 'inward stage' of the soul.

Rosemont describes well the differences between the Confucian and the Western concept of self. He says that in Confucian philosophy, the "I" is defined first of all within a web of family relationships. If I am a young person, I am primarily a *son* with all its implications in terms of social roles; if I am older and married with children, "I" am primarily a *father*, but also a *son* to my parents, a *husband*, etc.

Rosemont says:[81]

All of this is obvious but note how different it is from focussing on me as an autonomous, freely-choosing individual self. For the early Confucians, there can be no me in isolation to be considered abstractly: I am the totality of roles I live in relation to specific others. It would be misleading to say that I 'perform' or 'play' those roles: for Confucius, I am my *roles. When all the roles have been specified and their interconnections made manifest, then I have been specified fully as a unique person, with few discernible loose threads with which to piece together a free, autonomous, choosing self.*

What distinguishes the Confucian self even more from the Western self is that the community of social and family relations and roles does not end with death; the link with our parents does not end when they die, so that there is a community of the dead and living.

The uniqueness of a Chinese person is immanent and embedded within a ceaseless process of social, cultural and natural changes. Hall and Ames contend that what Confucius means by "self" is *ren* 仁, i.e. "humanity" or "benevolence". This is a crucial difference between the concept of "self" in Western psychology and that in Chinese (Confucian) philosophy.

Ames stresses the social dimension of "self" in Chinese culture:[82]

The centrality of ritual practice in Confucianism is clear when we begin from Confucius's premise that a person is irreducibly social, measurable in terms of the quality of the relationships that one is able to effect. It is ritual practice, taken in its broadest sense, that enables persons to assume roles and, literally, to find their appropriate place in relationship to others. It is a social syntax that enables them to communicate with others and, in so doing, to constitute themselves as a matrix of relationships.

Ames says that "*For Confucius, a human being is not a sort of 'being' at all, but first and foremost a human 'doing' or 'making'.*"[83] Interestingly, the Confucian "self-cultivation" was not so much inner-directed as "outer-directed", i.e. always with ethical consideration in mind. The Confucians were concerned with self-control and self-cultivation so as to minimize friction with the family, the village, the clan and within society at large, and to make it easier to obey the requirements of the state.[84]

It was a self-cultivation, aimed not at individual freedom and development as it was in ancient Greece, but at social harmony and cohesion. Such family and social harmony was ensured also by each individual assuming their proper role and following proper "rites". In China, there was no counterpart to the ancient Greek sense of personal liberty. Individual rights in China were one's "share" of the rights of the community as a whole, not a license to do as one pleases.[85] Social harmony, not individual liberty, was the watchword in ancient (and I would say also in modern) China.

The divergence between the Western and the Chinese concepts of self can be observed right from the beginning, i.e. from the 4th century BC when Confucianism developed and when ancient Greek philosophy flourished. Nisbett says:[86]

[Ancient] *Greeks thought of themselves as individuals with distinctive properties, as units separate from others within society, and in control of their own destinies. Similarly, Greek philosophy started from the individual object – the person, the atom, the house – as the unit of analysis and it dealt with the properties of the object. Chinese social life was interdependent and it was not liberty but harmony that was the watchword – the harmony of humans and Nature for the Daoists and the harmony of humans with other humans for the Confucianists. The Way* [Dao] *and not the discovery of truth was the goal of philosophy. The Chinese philosopher would see a family with inter-related members where the Greeks saw a collection of persons with attributes that were independent of any connections with others.*

The modern Chinese philosopher Hu Shi says: "*In the Confucian human-centered philosophy man cannot exist alone; all action must be in the form of interaction between man and man.*"[87]

In substance, in Confucian philosophy, the self is a center of relationships rather than an isolable individuality. As Tu Wei Ming says:[88]

This is actually another reason why respect of one's parents is so important in Chinese society. The Confucians believe that our sympathetic bonding to our parents is not only biologically natural but morally imperative, for it is the first step in learning to appreciate ourselves not in isolation but in communication. Therefore the ability to show intimacy and respect to those who are intimate is vitally important for allowing the closed private ego to acquire a taste for the open communicating self.

Tan and Yip confirm that the self in Confucian philosophy is a "center of relationships" in the family and society; it is the basis of the cultivating process in which persons exist and cultivate themselves for the purpose of perfecting the self to better serve others.[89] Indeed, Confucius wrote: "*Cultivate oneself, regulate the family, govern the state, and bring peace to the world.*"[90]

Hence the Confucian self is a relational, not an individual self. The Confucians regarded the self as primarily a role-self, expressed in familial and social relationships. Confucius said: "*Let the ruler be ruler; the minister, minister; the father, father; and the son, son.*"[91] Tam and Yip say: "*In this relationship persons are not completely individuals, for they have little individual identity or individuality, and exist only to fulfil dutifully the various roles expected of them.*"[92]

Rosemont says:[93]

For the early Confucians there can be no me in isolation to be considered abstractly: I am the totality of roles I live in relation to specific others ... Taken collectively, they weave for each of us a unique pattern of personal identity, such as if some of my roles change, the others will of necessity change also, literally making me a different person.

Another important difference in the concept of self in East and West is the relationship between mind and body; in China, the dichotomy between mind and matter never existed.

Gernet says:[94]

Not only was the substantial opposition between the soul and the body something quite unknown to the Chinese, but so was the distinction between the sensible and the rational. The Chinese had never believed in the existence of a sovereign and independent faculty of reason. The concept of a soul endowed with reason and capable of acting freely for good or for evil, which is so fundamental to Christianity, was alien to them.

In the classical Chinese world there is no equivalent to the conflict between the heart and the mind associated with self-realization in Western philosophy. Chinese philosophy sees mind and body as a unit, while most of Western philosophy (with exceptions such as Hume and Spinoza) sees the individual, inner-directed mind as totally separate from the body. As we have seen above, the body is a "container" for the mind.

By contrast, in Chinese there are three terms to indicate "body": *shen* 身, *xing* 形, and *ti* 体. Interestingly, the word *shen* does not always simply indicate the body but instead often denotes one's entire psychosomatic person. Ames thinks it is not by chance that *shen* as "body" and *Shen* as "Mind" (of the Heart) are phonetically the same (although denoted by different characters). He thinks it suggestive that a person was seen as having correlative physical and mental aspects denoted by the above instances of *shen*.[95]

That the word *shen* refers to more than just a "body" is also highlighted by the fact that many Chinese expressions containing the word *shen* can be translated into English only by using words such as "person", "self" or "life". The following are some Chinese expressions containing the word *shen* with their English translations (first a literal one, then a contemporary one):[96]

- *an shen*: make one's body peaceful = "settle down in life"
- *chu shen*: put forth one's body = "start one's career"
- *shen fen*: one's body allocation = "personal status"
- *shen shi*: body's world = "one's lifetime experiences"
- *zhong shen*: to body's end = "to the end of one's life"
- *ben shen*: basic body = "oneself"
- *sui shen*: following the body = "on one's person".

EMOTIONS IN NEO-CONFUCIANISM

To the Confucians, emotions are disturbing factors that sway us from the path of *ren* and *li*. Confucianists believed that human nature is "pure" and untainted like a still pond; emotions cloud our human nature, just like stirring up the mud at the bottom of the pond makes it cloudy. Interestingly, some sinologists even think that the word *qing*, normally translated as "emotion" or "feeling", came to mean this only during the Song dynasty under the influence of Neo-Confucian thinking. Before that, *qing* meant "condition", "facts", "genuine" or "essence".[97] This would throw a completely different light on ancient Chinese medicine's classics like the *Yellow Emperor's Classic of Internal Medicine*. As this classic is fragmentary and has been received by us in its Tang dynasty transcription, some ancient passages refer to *qing* as "essence" and passages clearly influenced by Confucianism (the majority) refer to *qing* as emotion.

Hansen says that, in pre-Han literature, *qing* means "essence" or "essence of humanity". He thinks it was what he calls "authoritarian" Confucianism that:[98]

> *... promoted the Buddhist appropriation in sharing with Indo-European systems the negative attitude towards qing. The domination of authoritarian Confucianism when Buddhism first reached China gives us the outline of an explanation why Buddhist translators would have adapted qing to refer to our familiar Western feeling-concepts. Qing threatens the order of rituals for Xun Zi* [a Confucian scholar] *as passions or emotions disturb Reason for Buddhists and Greeks.*

Neo-Confucianists use the image of the mirror to deal with emotions. Bearing in mind that Neo-Confucianism absorbed Daoist ideas, the following statement by Zhuang Zi (a Daoist philosopher) says: "*The stillness of the sage's Mind (Xin) is mirror to the whole world and mirror to the myriad things.*"[99]

The Huai Nan Zi says:[100]

> *The sage is like a mirror: he neither sees things off, nor goes out to meet them. He responds to everything without storing anything up. Thus, he is never injured through the myriad transformations he undergoes.*

The sage has emotions but is without ensnarement. Chuang Zi said:

> *The mind of the perfect man is like a mirror. It does not move with things nor does it anticipate them. It responds to things but does not retain them. Therefore the perfect man is able to deal successfully with things but is not affected by them.*

Wang Pi elaborated on the above, saying:[101]

> *That in which the sage is superior to ordinary people is the spirit. But what the sage has in common with ordinary people is the emotions. The sage has a superior spirit and is therefore able to be in harmony with the universe ... but he has ordinary emotions and therefore cannot respond to things without joy or sorrow. He responds to things, yet he is not ensnared by them.*

The Neo-Confucian method of dealing with the emotions consists essentially in disconnecting them from the self. It could be said that Chinese medicine's view of the emotions as factors which have an *objective* effect on Qi (they make it rise, descend, etc.) is a reflection of the Confucianist attempt to separate the self from the emotions.

!

The Neo-Confucian method of dealing with the emotions consists essentially in disconnecting them from the self. It could be said that Chinese medicine's view of the emotions as factors which have an *objective* effect on Qi (they make it rise, descend, etc.) is a reflection of the Confucianist attempt to separate the self from the emotions.

Cheng Hao says:[102]

The normality of the sage is that his emotions follow the nature of things, yet of himself he has no emotions. Therefore for the superior person, nothing is better than being impersonal and impartial and responding to things spontaneously as they come. The general trouble with man is that he is selfish and rationalistic. Being selfish, he cannot take action as a spontaneous response. Being rationalistic, he cannot take intuition as his natural guide. When the sage is pleased, it is because the thing is there that is rightly the object of pleasure. When the sage is angry, it is because the thing is there that is rightly the object of anger. Therefore the pleasure and anger of the sage are not connected with his mind but with things.

The impersonality, impartiality and spontaneity that Cheng Hao talks about is the same as the vacuity and straightforwardness spoken by Zhou Tun Yi. According to Cheng Hao, it is natural that even the sage should experience pleasure or anger. But since his mind has an impersonal, objective and impartial attitude, when these feelings come, they are simply objective phenomena of the universe and are not especially connected with the self. When he is pleased or angry, it is simply the external things, deserving of either pleasure or anger, that produce corresponding feelings in his mind. His mind is like a mirror on which anything may be reflected. As a result of this attitude, when the object is gone, the emotion that it produced goes with it. In this way, the sage, even though he has emotions, is without ensnarement.

The Neo-Confucianists said of Yen Hui that he "does not transfer his anger". When people are angry, they often transfer their anger to someone who was not the object of their anger. Cheng Yi comments:

We must understand why Yen Hui did not transfer his anger. In a bright mirror, a beautiful object produces a bright reflection while an ugly object produces an ugly reflection. But the mirror itself has no likes or dislikes. There are some people, being offended in their home, discharge their anger in the street. But the anger of the sage operates only according to the nature of things; it is never he himself who possesses the anger. The superior man is the master of things; the small man is their slave.

Thus, according to the Neo-Confucianists, the reason Yen Hui did not transfer his anger is because his emotions were *not connected with the self*. A thing might happen that produces an emotion in his mind, just as an object may appear in a mirror, but his self is not connected with the emotion.

In Neo-Confucian views on emotions, the mind of the sage is responsive to things in accordance with what they are and he or she expresses his or her joy at those things that call for joy, and anger at those that call for anger. His joy and anger are therefore connected with external things not with his or her mind.

The great Neo-Confucianist philosopher Cheng Hao (1032–1085) said:[103]

The constancy of the sage is that his feelings are in accord with the myriad things without having feelings of his own. The sage's joy is determined by the joyous nature of things, and the sage's anger is determined by the hateful nature of things. Therefore, the joy and anger of the sage are not related to his own mind, but to things. In this sense, does not the sage respond to things? Why should it be considered wrong to follow external things and right to seek what is internal? Is there not a great difference between the joy and anger of the selfish and cunning and the correctness of the joy and anger of the sage?

Cheng Hao also said: "*If one compares the pleasure and displeasure of an ordinary person who is selfish, to that of a sage, one will see where the difference lies.*"[104]

This is a very important aspect of Neo-Confucian views on emotions and one that I think is reflected in Chinese medicine. The Chinese medicine view of the emotions as disharmonies of Qi (anger makes Qi rise, fear makes Qi descend, etc.) in my opinion reflects the Neo-Confucian view of emotions as a reaction to *objective* forces and it is a way of "objectivizing" the emotions from the self. Thus, emotions are not psychic forces springing from the self and serving a function in the health of our psyche; they are, instead, objective forces to which our physiology reacts with a disharmony of Qi. If we rectify Qi (make it descend if it rises, make it ascend if it descends), emotions will be dissipated. As we have seen in Chapter 14, emotions are far more than objective disharmonies of Qi.

There are passages as early as in the *Nei Jing* that reflect a Confucianist view of the emotions. Chapter 5 of the *Simple Questions* says:[105]

Anger injures the Liver, sadness counteracts anger ... joy injures the Heart, fear counteracts joy ... pensiveness injures the Spleen, anger counteracts pensiveness ... worry injures the Lungs, joy counteracts worry ... fear injures the Kidneys, pensiveness counteracts fear.

An interesting feature of this passage is that each emotion is said to counteract another along the Controlling Sequence of the Five Elements (see Fig. 9.4). For example, fear pertains to the Kidneys and Water, Water controls Fire (Heart), the emotion related to the Heart is joy, hence fear counteracts joy.

Thus, according to this scheme, emotions counteract each other as follows.

- Anger counteracts pensiveness
- Joy counteracts sadness
- Pensiveness counteracts fear
- Sadness counteracts anger
- Fear counteracts joy

This thinking presents some interesting ideas which are certainly true in practice, e.g. that "anger counteracts pensiveness". However, it would be very strange indeed to try to counteract anger with sadness. Most of all, this rather "mechanical" view of the emotions reflects a view of the emotions as disengaged from the self; emotions are pathologies of Qi that can be "cured" or "rectified" by eliciting an opposite emotion along the Controlling cycle of the Five Elements. This is precisely because Confucianism did not have a concept of a self as an individual, autonomous, inward-directed, psychological center of our being.

Emotions are seen as disturbing factors which cloud our human nature (*Xing*). The Yuan Dao says:[106]

When the intellect comes into contact with things, feelings of attraction and aversion are produced. Where these feelings of attraction and aversion have taken shape, and the intellect has been enticed from the outside, one is unable to return to himself, and the heavenly (Tian) principles in him are destroyed.

Cheng Yi confirms the Confucian view of emotions as psychic factors that cloud human nature:[107]

When a physical form comes into existence and in contact with the external world, he is stimulated within. This stimulation from within arouses the seven emotions, namely pleasure, anger, sorrow, joy, love, hate and desire. As his emotions become agitated and increasingly restless, man's nature is injured. Therefore, the enlightened person controls his emotions, so as to be in accord with the Mean, he rectifies his mind and nourishes his human nature. This is called letting human nature control emotions. The stupid person does not know how to control his emotions, but lets them go to extremes to the extent of impeding and destroying his nature. This is called letting emotions control human nature.

Cheng Yi then clarifies the connection between Heaven (*Tian*), Destiny (*Ming*), Principle (*Li*), Human Nature (*Xing*), Mind (*Xin*) and Emotions (qing):[108]

What is received from Heaven is called Destiny; what is in things is Principle. What is endowed in man is his human nature (Xing); what is in control of the body is the Mind: all these are actually one. The Mind is originally good, but when it expresses itself in thoughts, there is good and not good. And what has been expressed is called emotions (qing) and not Mind.

This passage highlights a clear dualism between the Mind and the emotions which, as we have seen in Chapter 14, does not correspond to reality as emotions are actually an important way in which our Mind works.

A dialogue between Cheng Yi and his disciples clarifies the relation between human nature and emotions:[109]

Do joy, anger, sorrow and pleasure come from human nature? Certainly. As soon as there is life and consciousness, there is human nature. When there is human nature, there are emotions. Without human nature, how could there be emotions? How to explain that joy, anger, sorrow and pleasure come from outside? They do not come from outside. When under the influence from outside, they are stirred from within. Does human nature have joy and anger as water has waves? Yes. It is the nature of water to be clear and still like a mirror. How can waves be the nature of water? In human nature there are the Four Virtues (ren, yi, li and zhi); how can there be evil things in it? But without water, how can there be waves? Without human nature, how can there be emotions?

Zhu Xi developed a tripartite relationship among human nature, Mind and emotions. Human nature is the substance of the Mind while the emotions are the manifestation of the Mind. Human nature (substance of the Mind) consists of humanity (*ren*), righteousness (*yi*), propriety (*li*) and wisdom (*zhi*); emotions (manifestation of the Mind) consist of commiseration, shame, dislike, humility, and right and wrong.[110]

An important Neo-Confucian view of the emotions is that they are psychic factors that cloud our human nature. Zhu Xi distinguished two states of human nature: the first before it is stirred by emotions; the second after it is stirred by emotions. The former he called the original human nature, the Mind of the Dao and the Principle of Heaven. The latter he called the Mind of a human being externally manifested in emotions.[111]

Neo-Confucianists railed against desire as being the root of all emotional suffering. Wang Yang Ming (1472–1529) argued that the sage is able to keep and nourish his original human nature, while the lower man has lost it through his indulging in selfish desire. Selfish desire obscures human nature. Interestingly, according to Chang, the Neo-Confucianists of the Song dynasty changed the term "emotion" into "desire".[112] This is probably also in reaction to the Buddhist emphasis on desire as the root of all suffering and to absorb some of the Buddhist ideas into Confucianism. Hansen concurs that "desire" was assimilated with "emotion" by Neo-Confucianists under a Buddhist influence:[113]

I implicitly accept the possibility that the introduction of Buddhism imported an Indo-European psychological theory and thus introduced new theoretical roles for qing (emotion) and yu (desire).

A passage by Dong Zhong Shu (179–104 BC) highlights how much emotions were considered disturbing factors which had to be "regulated", just as the emperor needs to regulate governance. Dong says:[114]

The natural quality of human beings is called human nature (xing) and this cannot be fulfilled save by moral education and transformation. Human desires are called emotions (qing) and these cannot be regulated except by institution and rules. This is why the human sovereign carefully receives the intention of Heaven from above, so that he may conform with the Mandate. Down below he strives to educate and transform his norms for law and institutions, distinguishing between the upper and the lower orders of society to preclude desire. If he achieves these three aims, the fundamental basis will be established.

This is another clear example of the influence of the Legalist School on Chinese medicine.

The following passage by Li Ao confirms clearly that emotions were considered by the Neo-Confucianists to be factors that cloud our human nature:[115]

How can someone's human nature be corrupted? By the emotions. There are seven emotions: joy, anger, grief, fear, love, disgust and desire. When the emotions are out of control human nature lives in obscurity. It is not that human nature should be blamed. Rather it is the coming and going, by turn, of the seven emotions which prevents human nature from being fully developed. For example, when water is troubled at its source, its stream will be impure; when fire is smoking, its light will not be bright. One cannot say that the water is impure or that the fire is not bright. When there is no sand, the stream will be clear; when there is no smoke, the fire will be bright. When emotions are not aroused, human nature will be fully developed. Yet human nature and emotions cannot be separated from each other. Without human nature, there would be no expression of emotions. The emotions are derived from human nature. Emotions are not self-constituted; they depend upon human nature. Human nature cannot constitute itself: it expresses itself through the emotions. Human nature is ordained by Heaven. Emotions are what is expressed when human nature is in action. When people indulge themselves in the emotions, they are blind to what is fundamental. A sage is not a man who is without emotions. A sage is a man who is master of his emotions and keeps calmness of mind. Though he has emotions, he does not seem to have them. Ordinary people have their human nature too and it is not different from that of the sage. But they can be blinded by their emotions and they do not know what human nature is.

This passage is interesting because, although it reiterates that emotions do cloud human nature, they are an inevitable way in which human nature expresses itself.

One important Confucian influence on the Chinese medicine view of emotions can be observed in the emotion of anger. In my opinion, anger is overemphasized as an emotional cause of disease in Chinese books. I feel that this is very much due to the Confucian influence on Chinese medicine. A very important aspect of Confucianism is the emphasis laid on social harmony which, according to them, begins with family harmony which, in turn, is based on the rigid respect of family hierarchy. For example, the younger brother obeys the older brother, the sister obeys the brother, all the children obey the parents, the wife obeys the husband, etc. When every member of the family and society takes his or her proper place and role in the family and social hierarchy, then familial, social and political harmony reigns.

It is easy to see that the emotion that most threatens the established order is anger because this emotion may lead people to rebel. Given the Confucian influence on Chinese medicine, I believe it is for this reason that anger plays such a predominant role among the emotional causes of disease. Cheng Hao (1032–1085), a great Neo-Confucian philosopher of the Song dynasty, says: "*Of all human emotions, anger is the easiest to arouse but the most difficult to control.*"[116] He also said: "*If one can stop one's anger as soon as it takes form, and coolly appeal to reason to find out what is right and what is wrong, one need not worry about external stimuli. This kind of self-control will take one half way to the Dao!*"[117]

Anger makes Qi "rebel", i.e. go in the wrong direction. It is interesting to note that the Chinese character for "rebellious" Qi is *ni* 逆, which means "rebellious", "contrary", "to counter", "to disobey", "to defy", "to go against"; thus it is easy to see the "social" nature of this pathological movement of Qi. Indeed, the opposite of *ni* is *shun* 顺 which, in Chinese medicine, denotes Qi going the right, proper way; again it is easy to see the social implication of this term which means "to conform", "in the same direction as", "to obey", "to yield to", "to act in submission to".

The deep significance and resonance of these two terms *ni* (rebellion) and *shun* (conforming) with a Confucian viewpoint of *Li* (Principle) is apparent from the *Four Political Treatises of the Yellow Emperor*, a Ma Wang Dui text which says:[118]

All things having laws of their own are called Principle (Li). To abide where Li exists is called compliance (shun). Doing things not according with Dao is called losing Li. To abide where Li is lost is called rebelliousness (ni).

We can therefore see what a deep significance "rebelliousness" (*ni*) has to a Confucian mind as it negates the very Principle (*Li*) that is basis of the universe.

Indeed, it is interesting to note how frequently the word *ni* recurs in the *Four Political Treatises of the Yellow Emperor* to denote a deplorable state of disharmony and social unrest. For example:

When the five kinds of rules are promulgated, there should be five officials to manage according to the correct regulations and thereby be prepared against rebellious (ni) armies.[119]

Those who go against righteousness and disobey (ni) their lord will be punished by death according to the law.[120]

I will let him satisfy his rebellious (ni) ambitions and then kill him and reappoint the six ministers so as to accord with sincerity.[121]

Punishment and reward nourish one another and therefore the distinction between compliance (shun) and rebelliousness (ni) is established.[122]

It must be a person of rectitude who can take righteousness as the measure for rectifying rebelliousness (ni).[123]

It is called waging war for righteousness when a military expedition is carried out to suppress disorders (ni).[124]

!

The terms *ni* and *shun* (meaning "rebellious" and "conforming" Qi, respectively), clearly show a strong social and political connotation.

Yen Hui, a disciple of Confucius, said:[125]

A person comes into contact with the external world and thus becomes stimulated within. With this stimulation, seven kinds of emotions are expressed: joy, anger, sorrow, fear, love, dislike and greed. When the emotions are agitated and become violent, man's nature suffers from a lack of equilibrium. The sages hold their emotions in check. The emotions can thus play no more than their natural part. But those who are ignorant do not know how to control their emotions. Rather, they indulge themselves in violent expressions and this leads them astray. Thus they injure their nature by putting an axe to it, as it were. Emotions get the upper hand of man's nature and he is no longer master of himself.

INFLUENCE OF NEO-CONFUCIANISM ON CHINESE MEDICINE

The influence of Neo-Confucianism on Chinese medicine can be summarized as follows.

The Neo-Confucianists were the first to integrate Daoist and Buddhist elements in a unified system of Chinese medicine. This is an important "systematization" of Chinese medicine which came much earlier

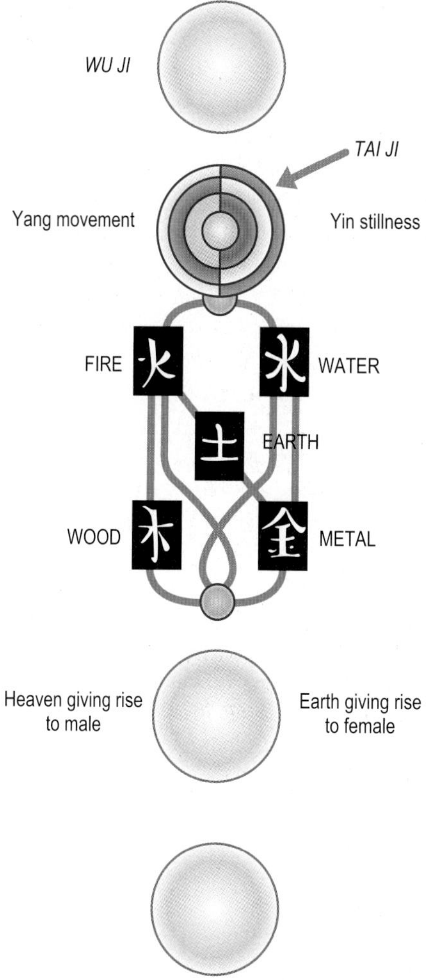

Figure 15.9 Zhou Dun Yi's *Tai Ji* diagram.

than the "systematization" of Chinese medicine carried out by the modern Chinese. Such systematization carried out in China post 1949 is often criticized.

The Neo-Confucianists integrated different ideas from various schools in a unified system: see Zhou Dun Yi's *Tai Ji* diagram (Fig. 15.9). The following is Zhu Xi's commentary on the Supreme Ultimate diagram of Zhou Dun Yi:

The uppermost figure represents that which has no Ultimate and yet is the Supreme Ultimate. It is the original substance of that motion which generates the Yang and of that rest which generates the Yin. It should be regarded neither as a separate form, nor as identical with the Two Forces [of Yin and Yang].

The opening statement of Zhu Xi's commentary is essentially that of a synthetic philosophy uniting in itself the streams of Daoist and Confucian thought, because *Wu Ji* comes from the Dao De Jing and *Tai Ji* comes from the *Yi Jing*. Zhu Xi himself reaffirms the identity, saying that the *Wu Ji* is not something outside or beyond the *Tai Ji*; nor is *Tai Ji* something outside or beyond the world; it constitutes and resides in the myriad things. The Daoist *Wu Ji* is an affirmation that the true and entire Universe depended on no cardinal point, for every part of it took the leadership in turn. The Confucian *Tai Ji*, on the other hand, was a recognition of immanent power informing the wholeness of the Universe, and present everywhere within it.

The Neo-Confucianists were the first to apply systematic correspondences to herbal medicine, i.e. the assignment of tastes following the Five Elements to herbs. The Song dynasty also saw the detailed classification of herbal drugs according to taste, energy and channel entered, a necessary prerequisite for the application of the Yin-Yang and Five-Element theory to herbal medicine.

It would appear that this systematization was partly a reaction by professional physicians to counteract the attempts by Confucian philosophers to ask the educated to acquire sufficient medical knowledge to treat themselves and their families rather than to turn to professional physicians. The famous book of prescriptions *Imperial Grace Formulae for the Assistance of the People from the Tai Ping Era* (*Tai Ping Hui Min He Ji Ju Fang*) arranged the formulae according to disease states (rather than patterns) that were widely known by the educated and could therefore be used without an individualized diagnosis.

Zhu Zhen Heng (1282–1358) wrote a commentary to this book, which was later included in it as an appendix, saying:[126]

These pharmacy formulae are published as a book so that one can design formulae according to signs of disease. This means that, in order to apply drugs, one does not need to visit a doctor and one does not need to prepare anything extra. One buys something and there is instant success. Pills and powders effect the cure of illness and pain in a simple and effective manner. An attitude of love towards the public has reached visible perfection here!

Neo-Confucianist government officials also downgraded the role of physicians by encouraging direct access of patients to pharmacists. It is as a direct result of this policy that pharmacies in China since then often employ physicians called *zuo tang yi*, i.e. "physicians sitting in a pharmacy".[127]

The Confucian, moralistic view of etiology and often of diagnosis began to enter Chinese medicine in the Song dynasty. For example, some old texts say that a good *shen* of the eyes reflects "benevolence" (*ren*), the most important Confucian quality.

The most negative influence of the Confucian approach to education (in my opinion) is the slavish attitude and blind following of the teacher that is characteristic of Chinese medicine. In my opinion, such an unquestioning attitude slowed down the progress of Chinese medicine in subsequent dynasties (and also in modern times).

The rejection of supernatural influences in the etiology of diseases did not start with Marxism but was already a feature of Zhu Xi's Neo-Confucianism. Zhu Xi forged disparate philosophical trends into a unified system in which *Li* constituted the immaterial organizational Principle controlling all genesis, existence and decay, and Qi the material finest influence that brings genesis, existence and decay into fruition. In addition, Zhu Xi combined the doctrines of *Li* and Qi with the cosmogony developed by Zhou Dun Yi, creating an organic model of the universe in which each material phenomenon and each ethical category could be explained.

For Confucians, always "accused" of being interested only in ethics and not in the study of nature, the study of nature was now legal. Moreover, Zhu Xi's construct conferred upon human existence a meaning within a metaphysical system without recourse to deities, spirits and demons of competing doctrines. Zhu Xi demonstrated that the evolution of the Universe in accord with an all-embracing organizational Principle is accompanied at the appropriate time by the genesis of certain conceptions of morality and virtuous conduct; the necessity for some beings beyond space and time, who control the destiny of mankind and watch over his adherence to certain moral values, simply did not exist in this conceptual system.

Neo-Confucianism had an important influence on the suppression of any manifestations of sexuality with many repercussions on Chinese medicine. Under the Neo-Confucian influence, during the Song dynasty there was an increasing prudery and suppression of sexual manifestations. It was during the Song dynasty that the custom of binding women's feet started. One of the explanations of this custom is that it was fostered by the Confucianists because it helped to restrict a woman's movements and kept them within the house, and thus bound feet came to stand as a symbol of womanly modesty and subservience. Interestingly, the Chinese words for many negative characters and traits are based on the radical for "woman" (nu): for example, *wang* (absurdity), *ji* (jealousy), *du* (envy), *lan* (greed), *jian* (lewdness), *mei* (flattery) and *nu* (slavehood), to mention just a few.

During the Tang dynasty there was no taboo on women showing their neck and breasts which started during the Song dynasty; the elegant, Chinese high-collared jacket or dress was introduced during these times. During the Song dynasty the revival of Confucianism started to influence the free association of men and women, and sexual relations began to be restricted by the numerous stringent rules recorded in the Classics. Zhu Xi advocated a strict interpretation of the old Classics. He stressed the inferiority of women and the strict separation of the sexes, and forbade all manifestations of heterosexual love outside the intimacy of the wedded bed.

Confucianists condemned women to a subservient state. Confucius said in the Analects: "*Women and people of lowly station are difficult to deal with. If one is too friendly with them, they become obstreperous, and if one keeps them at a distance they become resentful.*" The Confucianist School states that a woman is absolutely and unconditionally inferior to a man. Her first and foremost duty is to serve and obey her husband and his parents, to look after the household well, and bear healthy male children. Her biological function is emphasized, and her emotional life given secondary consideration. Chastity being a requisite for an orderly family life and undisturbed continuation of the lineage, great stress was laid on women leading a blameless life. To ensure this, the Confucianists advocated the complete separation of the sexes, and carried it through its most absurd consequences, such as that husband and wife should not hang their garments on the same clothes rack. Interestingly, modern Communist China adopted this Confucian repressive attitude towards any manifestations of sexuality.

As indicated above, many passages of the *Simple Questions* and *Spiritual Axis* clearly show the superimposition of Neo-Confucian views on ancient Chinese medicine concepts.

CONCLUSIONS

In conclusion, on the basis of what was discussed in the present chapter and in Chapter 14, I list below my main theses.

- Chinese medicine has been strongly influenced by Confucianism and Neo-Confucianism, probably even more than by Daoism.
- The Confucian influence on Chinese medicine should be recognized in order to evaluate whether some of their ideas are applicable to Western patients.
- Especially in the field of emotions, the Chinese medicine view is strongly influenced by Confucianism and a Confucian concept and practice of Self that is entirely different from that of Western patients. There is no conception of an individual, autonomous, inward-looking Self with an individual psychic life; the Confucian self is identified by its belonging to a family and a society.
- The Chinese medicine view of emotions as derangements of Qi at a physical and an emotional level simultaneously is brilliant and with important practical applications. However, it does also reflect a Confucian attempt to "objectivize" the emotions as something outside our Self: something causes us to be angry, this makes Qi rise, we treat it by subduing Qi. As we have seen in Chapter 14, emotions are value judgments and an essential way in which our mind works.
- From a philosophical point of view, I have also tried to point out some Legalist influences on Chinese medicine that are not usually recognized.

END NOTES

1. Unschuld P 1985 Medicine in China – A History of Ideas. University of California Press, Berkeley, p. 80.
2. Ibid., p. 100.
3. Hall D, Ames R 1998 Thinking from the Han. State University of New York Press, New York, pp. 242–243.
4. Ames RT, Rosemont H 1999 The Analects of Confucius – A Philosophical Translation. Ballantine Books, New York, p. 46.
5. Ibid., pp. 46–47.
6. Ibid., p. 47.
7. Kim Yung Sik 2000 The Natural Philosophy of Chu Hsi. American Philosophical Society, Philadelphia, p. 135.
8. The Analects of Confucius – A Philosophical Translation, p. 48.
9. Ibid., p. 49.
10. Kasulis TP, Ames RT, Dissanayke W 1993 Self as Body in Asian Theory and Practice. State University of New York Press, New York, p. 164.
11. Fingarette H 1972 Confucius – The Secular as Sacred. Waveland Press, Prospect Heights, Illinois, p. 37.
12. Ibid., p. 45.
13. The Analects of Confucius – A Philosophical Translation, p. 312.
14. Huang Siu-chi 1999 Essentials of Neo-Confucianism. Greenwood Press, Westport, Connecticut, p. 93.
15. Gardner DK 2003 Zhu Xi's Reading of the Analects. Columbia University Press, New York, p. 70.
16. The Analects of Confucius – A Philosophical Translation, p. 54.
17. Marks J, Ames RT 1995 Emotions in Asian Thought. State University of New York Press, New York, p. 168.
18. Self as Body in Asian Theory and Practice, p. 152.
19. Confucius – The Secular as Sacred, p. 43.
20. Self as Body in Asian Theory and Practice, p. 115.
21. Chang C 1977 The Development of Neo-Confucian Thought. Greenwood Press, Westport, Connecticut, p. 66.
22. Ibid., p. 67.
23. Needham J 1977 Science and Civilization in China, Vol. 2. Cambridge University Press, Cambridge, pp. 300–301.
24. Medicine in China – A History of Ideas, p. 67.
25. Ibid., p. 63.
26. Tian Dai Hua 2005 Ling Shu Jing 灵枢经 [Spiritual Axis]. People's Health Publishing House, Beijing, p. 73. First published *c.*100 BC.
27. 1981 Huang Di Nei Jing Tai Su 黄帝内经太素 [An Elucidation of the Yellow Emperor's Classic of Internal Medicine]. People's Health Publishing House, Beijing, p. 2. *An Elucidation of the Yellow Emperor's Classic of Internal Medicine* was written by Yang Shang Shan and first published AD 581–618.
28. Graham AC 1999 The Book of Lieh-Tzu – A Classic of Tao. Columbia University Press, New York, p. 9.
29. Ibid., p. 13.
30. Ng On-cho 2001 Cheng-Zhu Confucianism in the Early Qing. State University of New York Press, New York, p. 4.
31. Ibid., p. 4.
32. Ibid., p. 4.
33. Chang LS, Feng Y 1998 The Four Political Treatises of the Yellow Emperor. University of Hawai'i Press, Honolulu, p. 37.
34. Wang Ai He 1999 Cosmology and Political Culture in Early China. Cambridge University Press, Cambridge, p. 193.
35. The Natural Philosophy of Chu Hsi, p. 35.
36. The Development of Neo-Confucian Thought, p. 190.
37. The Natural Philosophy of Chu Hsi, p. 45.
38. Ibid., p. 48.
39. Cosmology and Political Culture in Early China, p. 146.
40. Cheng-Zhu Confucianism in the Early Qing, p. 39.
41. Essentials of Neo-Confucianism, p. 73.
42. Ibid., p. 76.
43. The Development of Neo-Confucian Thought, p. 191.
44. Ibid., p. 104.
45. Ibid., p. 104.
46. Ibid., p. 130.
47. The Natural Philosophy of Chu Hsi, p. 5.
48. Cheng-Zhu Confucianism in the Early Qing, p. 39.
49. Ibid., p. 44.
50. Ibid., p. 72.
51. Ibid., p. 73.
52. Essentials of Neo-Confucianism, p. 131.
53. Ibid., p. 131.
54. Science and Civilization in China, p. 475.
55. Essentials of Neo-Confucianism, p. 133.
56. Ibid., p. 133.
57. Ibid., p. 194.
58. Lau DC, Ames RT 1998 Yuan Dao – Tracing Dao to its Source. Ballantine Books, New York, pp. 47–48.
59. Taylor C 2003 Sources of the Self – The Making of Modern Identity. Cambridge University Press, Cambridge, p. 111
60. Ibid., p. 111.
61. Ibid., p. 111.
62. Ibid., p. 111.
63. Ibid., p. 131.
64. Damasio A 2000 The Feeling of What Happens – Body and Emotion in the Making of Consciousness. Harcourt, San Diego, p. 12.

65. Ibid., p. 16.
66. Ibid., p. 17.
67. Sources of the Self, p. 185.
68. Jones D (ed) 2008 Confucius Now. Open Court, Chicago, pp. 18–19.
69. Ibid., p. 46.
70. Ibid., p. 261.
71. Crabbe J 1999 From Soul to Self. Routledge, London, p. 132.
72. Confucius – The Secular as Sacred, p. 45.
73. Thinking from the Han, p. 32.
74. Yuan Dao – Tracing Dao to its Source, p. 48.
75. Thinking from the Han, p. 47.
76. Ibid., p. 26.
77. Bockover M (ed) 1991 Rules, Ritual and Responsibility – Essays Dedicated to Herbert Fingarette. Open Court, La Salle, Illinois, p. xvii.
78. Ibid., p. xxv.
79. Ibid., p. xviii.
80. Ibid., p. xxvi.
81. Ibid., p. 90.
82. Self as Body in Asian Theory and Practice, p. 152.
83. Ibid., p. 154.
84. Nisbett RE 2003 The Geography of Thought – How Asians and Westerners Think Differently and Why. Free Press, New York, p. 5.
85. Ibid., p. 6.
86. Ibid., p. 19.
87. Ibid., p. 50.
88. Ames RT (ed) 1994 Self as Person in Asian Theory and Practice. State University of New York Press, New York, p. 181.
89. Ames RT, Kasulis TP, Dissanayake W 1998 Self as Image in Asian Theory and Practice. State University of New York Press, New York, p. 200.
90. Ibid., p. 200.
91. Ibid., p. 200.
92. Ibid., p. 200.
93. The Geography of Thought – How Asians and Westerners Think Differently and Why, p. 5.
94. Gernet J 1983 China and the Christian Impact: a Conflict of Cultures. Cambridge University Press, Cambridge, p. 147.
95. Self as Image in Asian Theory and Practice, p. 165.
96. Ibid., pp. 219–220.
97. Emotions in Asian Thought, pp. 182–183.
98. Ibid., p. 203.
99. Thinking from the Han, p. 49.
100. Ibid., p. 49.
101. Emotions in Asian Thought, p. 216.
102. The Four Political Treatises of the Yellow Emperor, p. 90.
103. Essentials of Neo-Confucianism, pp. 90–91.
104. The Development of Neo-Confucian Thought, p. 201.
105. 1979 Huang Di Nei Jing Su Wen 黄帝内经素问 [The Yellow Emperor's Classic of Internal Medicine – Simple Questions]. People's Health Publishing House, Beijing, p. 37. First published c.100 BC.
106. Yuan Dao – Tracing Dao to its Source, p. 51.
107. Essentials of Neo-Confucianism, pp. 108–109.
108. Ibid., p. 112.
109. Ibid., p. 114.
110. Ibid., p. 152.
111. Ibid., p. 153.
112. The Development of Neo-Confucian Thought, p. 106.
113. Emotions in Asian Thought, p. 183.
114. Cosmology and Political Culture in Early China, p. 193.
115. The Development of Neo-Confucian Thought, pp. 105–106.
116. Essentials of Neo-Confucianism, p. 91.
117. The Development of Neo-Confucian Thought, p. 201.
118. The Four Political Treatises of the Yellow Emperor, p. 31.
119. Ibid., pp. 152–153.
120. Ibid., p. 154.
121. Ibid., p. 158.
122. Ibid., p. 161.
123. Ibid., p. 169.
124. Ibid., p. 172.
125. The Development of Neo-Confucian Thought, pp. 225–226.
126. Unschuld P 2000 Medicine in China – Historical Artefacts and Images. Prestel, Munich, p. 28.
127. Unschuld P, personal communication.

郁证

CHAPTER 16

DEPRESSION

DEFINITION AND WESTERN MEDICINE'S VIEW *342*
Major depressive syndrome *343*

PATHOLOGY OF DEPRESSION IN CHINESE MEDICINE *344*
Yu as stagnation *344*
Yu as mental depression *345*
Depression and the relationship between the Mind (*Shen*) and the Ethereal Soul (*Hun*) *345*
The Will-Power (*Zhi*) of the Kidneys in Depression *346*
Distinction between Depression in *Yu* Syndrome and in *Dian* Syndrome *346*
Lilium Syndrome (*Bai He Bing*) *347*
Agitation (*Zang Zao*) *348*
Plum-Stone Syndrome (*Mei He Qi*) *349*
Palpitations and Anxiety (*Xin Ji Zheng Chong*) *350*
Liver-Qi deficiency *351*
"Neurasthenia" and Depression *353*
Elements of the pathology of Depression *353*

ETIOLOGY *354*
Emotional stress *354*
Constitutional traits *355*
Irregular diet *356*
Overwork *356*

PATHOLOGY *356*

IDENTIFICATION OF PATTERNS AND TREATMENT *357*
Liver-Qi stagnation *358*
Heart- and Lung-Qi stagnation *361*
Stagnant Liver-Qi turning into Heat *362*
Phlegm-Heat harassing the Mind *364*
Blood stasis obstructing the Mind *365*
Qi stagnation with Phlegm *367*
Diaphragm Heat *369*
Worry injuring the Mind *370*
Heart and Spleen deficiency *372*
Heart-Yang deficiency *373*
Kidney- and Heart-Yin deficiency, Empty Heat blazing *375*
Kidney-Yang deficiency *376*

ACUPUNCTURE POINTS FOR DEPRESSION *378*

HERBS FOR DEPRESSION *386*

MODERN CHINESE LITERATURE *389*

CLINICAL TRIALS *392*

CASE HISTORIES *399*

PATIENTS' STATISTICS *407*

WESTERN DRUG TREATMENT *407*
Introduction and pharmacology *408*
Clinical use *410*
Types of antidepressants *410*
Combination of Chinese and Western medicine *415*

- Liver-Qi stagnation
- Heart- and Lung-Qi stagnation
- Stagnant Liver-Qi turning into Heat
- Phlegm-Heat harassing the Mind
- Blood stasis obstructing the Mind
- Qi stagnation with Phlegm
- Diaphragm Heat
- Worry injuring the Mind
- Heart and Spleen deficiency
- Heart-Yang deficiency
- Kidney- and Heart-Yin deficiency, Empty Heat blazing
- Kidney-Yang deficiency

DEPRESSION

The complex of symptoms that we call "depression" in the West corresponds not to one but to at least five main categories of mental-emotional disturbances in the classics as follows.

- *Yu Zheng* 郁证 Depression
- *Bai He Bing* 百合病: Lilium Syndrome. This is mentioned in *Essential Prescriptions of the Golden Chest (Jin Gui Yao Lue)*, Chapter 3-1.[1]
- *Mei He Qi* 梅核气: Plum-Stone Syndrome. This is mentioned in the chapter "Pulse, syndromes and treatment of miscellaneous gynecological diseases" of the *Essential Prescriptions of the Golden Chest (Jin Gui Yao Lue*, c.AD 220).
- *Zang Zao* 脏燥: Agitation. This is mentioned in the *Essential Prescriptions of the Golden Chest (Jin Gui Yao Lue)* written by Zhang Zhong Jing, Chapter 22 on women's problems.
- *Xin Ji Zheng Chong* 心悸怔忡: Palpitations and anxiety (see Fig. 16.1).

The discussion of depression will be conducted according to the following topics.

- Definition and Western medicine's view
- Pathology of Depression in Chinese medicine
- Etiology
- Pathology
- Identification of Patterns and Treatment

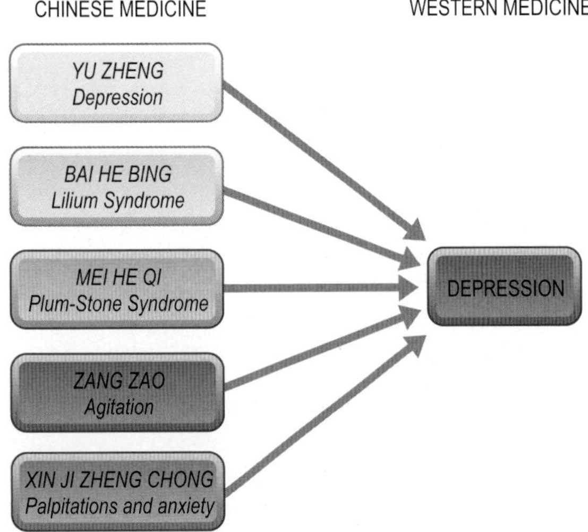

Figure 16.1 Correspondence between Chinese mental-emotional conditions and Depression in Western medicine.

- Acupuncture points for Depression
- Herbs for Depression
- Modern Chinese literature
- Clinical trials
- Case histories
- Patients' statistics
- Western drug treatment

DEFINITION AND WESTERN MEDICINE'S VIEW

A depressive illness is primarily characterized by a change in mood consisting of a feeling of sadness which may vary from mild despondency to the most abject despair. The change in mood is relatively fixed and persists over a period of days, weeks, months or years. Associated with the change in mood are characteristic changes in behavior, attitude, thinking, efficiency and physiological functioning.

In distinguishing the normal reaction from pathological depression, a quantitative judgment has to be made. If the precipitant seems inadequate, the depression too severe and too long lasting, the condition is regarded as abnormal. In addition, the severity and incapacity in depressive illness differ qualitatively as well as quantitatively from depressed feelings which are part of normal experience.

Depression accounts for 35–40% of all psychiatric illnesses. It is twice as common in women as in men. The onset of depression increases towards middle age, with a maximum onset in the 55–60 age group.

Depressive illness that is predominantly determined by genetic–constitutional factors is referred to as endogenous depression. This is characterized by being worse in the morning. Depressive illness that is predominantly a reaction to external influences is referred to as reactive depression.

The main symptoms and signs of depression are:

- painful thoughts
- a feeling of sadness
- anxiety and agitation
- loss of interest
- loss of self-esteem
- derealization and depersonalization
- hypochondriasis
- disorders of perception
- insomnia
- loss of appetite
- diurnal variation (worse in the morning).

The Mayo Clinic gives a detailed description of the clinical manifestations of Depression.[2] This clinic considers two main symptoms to be the hallmarks of depression:

- loss of interest in normal daily activities
- depressed mood, feeling of sadness, helplessness, hopelessness, crying.

The Mayo Clinic also considers the following signs and symptoms (which must be present for at least 2 weeks) as essential to diagnose depression:

- sleep disturbances
- impaired thinking or concentration
- changes in weight
- agitation
- fatigue or slowing of body movements
- low self-esteem
- feelings of guilt
- less interest in sex
- thoughts of death.

The Mayo Clinic distinguishes the following types of depression.

- *Major depression*: This type of mood disturbance lasts more than 2 weeks. Symptoms may include overwhelming feelings of sadness and grief, loss of interest or pleasure in activities you usually enjoy, and feelings of worthlessness or guilt. This type of depression may result in poor sleep, a change in appetite, severe fatigue and difficulty concentrating. Severe depression may increase the risk of suicide.
- *Dysthymia*: Dysthymia is a less severe but more chronic form of depression. Signs and symptoms usually are not disabling, and periods of dysthymia can alternate with short periods of feeling normal.
- *Adjustment disorders*: This is a feeling of depression elicited by external events, mostly to do with loss, e.g. death of a loved one, loss of a job, a diagnosis of cancer. People who cannot adjust to such a loss suffer a feeling of depression which is called "adjustment disorder".
- *Seasonal affective disorder*: Seasonal affective disorder (SAD) is a pattern of depression related to changes in seasons and a lack of exposure to sunlight. It may cause headaches, irritability and a low energy level.

Major depressive syndrome

A "major depressive syndrome" has four main aspects.

1. A particular set of symptoms.
2. It has no organic factor and is not the normal reaction to the death of a family member.
3. There are no delusions or hallucinations in the absence of mood symptoms.
4. It is not superimposed on schizophrenia, delusional disorders or psychotic disorders.

The main symptoms of major depressive syndrome are:

- depressed mood most of the day nearly every day
- markedly diminished interest or pleasure in all, or almost all, activities most of the day, nearly every day
- significant weight loss (or gain), decrease or increase in appetite
- insomnia or sleepiness
- psychomotor agitation or retardation every day
- fatigue nearly every day
- feelings of worthlessness or guilt (which may be delusional) nearly every day (not merely self-reproach or guilt about being ill)
- diminished ability to think or concentrate, indecisiveness nearly every day
- recurrent thoughts of death, recurrent suicidal ideation without a specific plan, or a suicide attempt or a specific plan for committing suicide.

According to Bowlby,[3] depression is a mood that most people experience on occasion and it is an inevitable accompaniment of any state in which behavior becomes disorganized, as it is likely to do after a loss.

So long as there is active interchange between ourselves and the external world, either in thought or in action, our subjective experience is not one of depression: hope, fear, anger, satisfaction, frustration or any combination of these may be experienced. It is when interchange has ceased that depression occurs until such time as new patterns of interchange have become organized towards a new object or goal. It is characteristic of the mentally healthy person that he can bear this phase of depression and disorganization, and emerge from it after not too long a time with behavior, thought and feeling beginning to be reorganized for interactions of a new sort. A person prone to depression will not be able to reorganize new patterns of interaction between himself or herself and the external world.

According to Seligman,[4] depression is characterized by a feeling of helplessness. Principally, the issue about which a person feels helpless is his or her ability to make and to maintain affectional relationships. The feeling of helplessness can be attributed to experiences in the family of origin from childhood to adolescence.

- He or she is likely to have had the bitter experience of never having attained a stable and secure relationship with his or her parents, despite having made repeated efforts to do so. These childhood experiences result in developing a strong bias to interpret any loss he or she may later suffer as yet another of his or her failures to make or maintain a stable affectional relationship.
- He or she may have been told repeatedly how unlovable, inadequate and/or incompetent he or she is. These experiences would result in developing a model of him or herself as unlovable and unwanted, and attachment figures as likely to be unavailable, rejecting or punitive. Whenever such a person suffers adversity, far from expecting others to be helpful, he or she expects them to be hostile and rejecting.
- He or she is more likely than others to have experienced actual loss of a parent during childhood.

Therefore, the particular pattern of depressive illness that a person develops will turn on the particular pattern of childhood experiences he or she has had.

Exposure to such experiences in childhood also explains why, in individuals prone to depression, there is a strong tendency for the sadness, yearning and perhaps anger aroused by a loss to become disconnected from the situation that aroused them.

PATHOLOGY OF DEPRESSION IN CHINESE MEDICINE

The Chinese term for depression is *Yu* 郁. *Yu* has the double meaning of "depression" and "stagnation".

Yu as stagnation

The *Simple Questions* in Chapter 71 discusses the five stagnations of Wood, Fire, Earth, Metal and Water. It says:[5]

When Wood stagnates it extends, when Fire stagnates it rises, when Earth stagnates it seizes, when Metal stagnates it discharges, when Water stagnates it pours.

The *Essential Method of Dan Xi* (*Dan Xi Xin Fa*, 1347) talks about six stagnations, i.e. stagnation of Qi, Blood, Dampness, Phlegm, Heat and Food. It says:[6]

When Qi and Blood are harmonized, no disease arises. If they stagnate diseases arise. Many diseases are due to stagnation ... stagnation makes things accumulate so that they would like to descend but cannot, they would like to transform but cannot ... thus the six stagnations come into being.

Zhu Dan Xi formulated a prescription for these six stagnations called Yue Ju Wan *Gardenia-Chuanxiong Pill* which is an important formula for mental depression deriving from Qi stagnation. Of the six stagnations mentioned above, Qi stagnation is the primary factor.

The *Complete Book of Jing Yue* (*Jing Yue Quan Shu*, 1624) gives an emotional interpretation to stagnation and talks about the six stagnations in a different way from Zhu Dan Xi, i.e. stagnation of anger, pensiveness, worry, sadness, shock and fear. This statement confirms that all emotions can lead to stagnation of Qi, even those (such as sadness) that initially lead to depletion of Qi. Zhang Jing Yue said: "*In the six stagnations, stagnation is the cause of the disease. In emotional stagnation, the disease* [i.e. the emotion] *is the cause of the stagnation.*"[7]

SUMMARY

The six stagnations according to Zhu Dan Xi (1347)

1. Qi
2. Blood
3. Dampness
4. Phlegm
5. Heat
6. Food

SUMMARY

The six stagnations according to Zhang Jing Yue (1624)

1. Anger
2. Pensiveness
3. Worry
4. Sadness
5. Shock
6. Fear

Yu as mental depression

Besides meaning "stagnation, *Yu* also means "mental depression"; some Chinese doctors say that, in a broad sense, *Yu* indicates stagnation and it is the pathological basis for very many diseases; in a narrow sense, *Yu* refers to the disease category of "mental depression".

The connection between "stagnation" and "depression" is not casual because, as we have seen in Chapter 9, emotional stress affects Qi first, usually causing Qi stagnation (which may occur in conjunction with depletion of Qi). However, although Qi stagnation usually characterizes the initial stages of depression, this does not mean that all cases of depression are due purely to Qi stagnation. As we shall see, when the disease progresses, many other pathological factors play a role and they may be characterized by both Full and Empty patterns.

Chinese books ascribe Depression always to Full causes, at least in its beginning stages, with Liver-Qi stagnation being the main, fundamental pathology underlying this disease. Other Full pathologies include Qi stagnation turning into Heat, Phlegm and Blood stasis. A heavy emphasis is put on Liver-Qi stagnation, at least in the beginning stages.

In the later stages, the Fullness can change into a Deficiency, leading to Empty types of mental depression. In fact, Heat can injure Yin and lead to Yin deficiency. On the other hand, Phlegm can impair the function of the Spleen and lead to Spleen deficiency. The main Empty conditions underlying depression are deficiency of Blood of the Spleen and Heart, deficiency of Qi and Yin of the Heart and Lungs, and Liver- and Kidney-Yin deficiency.

Thus, in Chinese medicine, stagnation and mental depression are almost synonymous, implying that all depression is due, at least initially, to stagnation.

When discussing Qi stagnation, it is important to stress that this affects not only the Liver but also, especially in emotional stress, the Heart, Lungs and Spleen. In my opinion, in both ancient and modern China, too much stress is placed on Liver-Qi stagnation as the main cause of mental depression.

!

In Chinese medicine, stagnation (*Yu*) and mental depression (*Yu*) are almost synonymous, implying that all depression is (at least initially) due to stagnation.

SUMMARY

_Yu_ as mental depression

- Besides meaning "stagnation", *Yu* also means "mental depression".
- Emotional stress affects Qi first, usually causing Qi stagnation.
- Not all cases of depression are due purely to Qi stagnation.
- Depression is due to Full causes, at least in its beginning stages.
- In the later stages, the Fullness can change into a Deficiency, leading to Empty types of mental depression.
- In depression, Qi stagnation affects also Heart, Lungs and Spleen.

Depression and the relationship between the Mind (*Shen*) and the Ethereal Soul (*Hun*)

The relationship between Mind (*Shen*) of the Heart and Ethereal Soul (*Hun*) of the Liver has already been discussed in Chapter 3. As we have seen, the Ethereal Soul gives the Mind inspiration, creativity, ideas, plans, life dreams and aspirations; this psychic energy is the result of the "coming and going of the Ethereal Soul" and it is the psychic manifestation of the free flow of Liver-Qi (and, in particular, of the physiological ascending of Liver-Qi).

On the other hand, the Mind needs to control the Ethereal Soul somewhat and to integrate the psychic material deriving from it. It is in the nature of the Ethereal Soul to "come and go", i.e. it is always searching, it has ideas, inspiration, aims, life dreams, etc. It will be remembered that the Ethereal Soul is the *gui* of our human nature and it has its own independent existence.

The Mind needs to integrate the material deriving from the Ethereal Soul in the general psyche. The Ethereal Soul is the source of many ideas simultaneously; the Mind can only deal with one at a time. Therefore "control" and "integration" are the key words describing the function of the Mind in relation to the Ethereal Soul (*see Fig. 3.13*).

When the "coming and going" of the Ethereal Soul is deficient, there is a lack of inspiration, creativity, ideas, plans, life dreams and aspirations; this is an important feature of mental depression. It is important to note that the psychic "coming and going" of the Ethereal Soul may be deficient either because itself is deficient or because the Mind is over-controlling it. The latter is common in individuals with strong, rigid beliefs ("religious" in a broad sense), which lead the Mind to suppress the psychic ideas coming from the Ethereal Soul. This situation may also arise as a consequence of guilt.

In severe depression, there is a disconnection between the Mind (*Shen* of the Heart) and Ethereal Soul (*Hun*): the Ethereal Soul lacks its normal "movement" and the person lacks creativity, ideas, imagination and, most of all, plans, projects, life aims and inspiration, so that depression results.

!

In severe depression, there is a disconnection between the Mind (*Shen* of the Heart) and Ethereal Soul (*Hun*): the Ethereal Soul lacks its normal "movement" and the person lacks creativity, ideas, imagination and, most of all, plans, projects, life aims and inspiration, so that depression results.

SUMMARY

Depression and the relationship between the Mind (*Shen*) and the Ethereal Soul (*Hun*)

- The Ethereal Soul gives the Mind inspiration, creativity, ideas, plans, life dreams and aspirations.
- The Mind needs to control the Ethereal Soul somewhat and to integrate the psychic material deriving from it.
- When the "coming and going" of the Ethereal Soul is deficient, there is a lack of inspiration, creativity, ideas, plans, life dreams and aspirations: this is an important feature of mental depression.

The Will-Power (*Zhi*) of the Kidneys in Depression

The *Zhi* of the Kidneys has several different meanings; for example, it can mean "memory", reflecting the influence of the Kidneys on the Sea of Marrow and the Brain and therefore memory. *Zhi* can also mean "Will-Power" and it is in this context that it plays an important role in depression. "Will-Power" as a translation of *Zhi* includes will-power itself, drive, determination, steadfastness, enthusiasm, and physical and mental power.

CLINICAL NOTE

Will-Power (*Zhi*) of the Kidneys

"Will-Power" as a translation of *Zhi* includes will-power, drive, determination, steadfastness, enthusiasm, and physical and mental power.

In my experience, depression always involves a weakening of "will-power" intended in the broad sense described above, i.e. including drive, determination, steadfastness, enthusiasm, and physical and mental power. These are all qualities that are missing in a depressed person and, for this reason, I therefore always tonify the Kidneys in depression, even if there are no specific symptoms and signs of Kidney deficiency. I do so because the mental-emotional lack of drive and will-power seen in depression is indeed a Kidney-deficiency symptom by itself.

To tonify the will-power and drive deriving from the Kidneys, I generally use BL-23 Shenshu and BL-52 Zhishi.

CLINICAL NOTE

Will-Power (*Zhi*) of the Kidneys

A deficiency of the Kidneys' "Will-Power" (*Zhi*) is nearly always a feature of depression and, for this reason, in depression I tonify the Will-Power with BL-23 Shenshu and BL-52 Zhishi.

Distinction between Depression in *Yu* Syndrome and in *Dian* Syndrome

Many modern Chinese books often discuss Depression Syndrome (*Yu Zheng*) as if it were identical to the depressive phase of Dullness and Mania (*Dian* of *Dian Kuang* 癫狂). Many Chinese books, therefore, when giving the symptoms of "depression", give the symptoms of *Dian*. I personally feel this is unhelpful and not

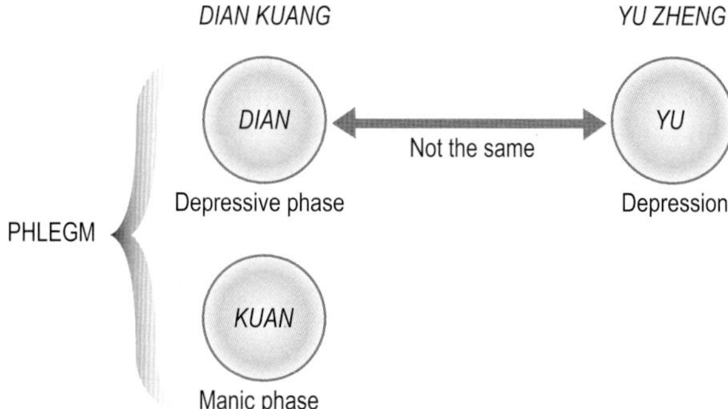

Figure 16.2 Difference between *Dian Kuang* (bipolar disorder) and *Yu Zheng* (depression).

corresponding to clinical practice. The "depression" in clinical depression is quite different from the "depression" in bipolar disorder (Dullness and Mania) from both a Western and a Chinese perspective.

From a Chinese perspective, the depressive and manic phases of Dullness and Mania (*Dian Kuang*) are two poles of a pathological spectrum with the same pathology. Central to the pathology of *Dian Kuang* is Phlegm obstructing the Mind (*Shen*); this accounts for *both* the depressive and the manic phases of the disease. Phlegm obstructs the Mind (*Shen*) but also the Ethereal Soul (*Hun*) so that it interferes with its "coming and going", resulting in depression when it does not "come and go" enough and mania when it "comes and goes" too much (Fig. 16.2).

As Phlegm obstructing the Mind's orifices is central to the pathology of *Dian Kuang*, this disease is always a case of Mind Obstructed; in severe and chronic cases of Depression, the Mind may be obstructed too but it is seldom so. Mind Obstructed has been discussed in Chapter 12.

By contrast, in Depression (*Yu Zheng*) Phlegm is not always present and the "coming and going" of the Ethereal Soul is always impaired (without a manic phase), resulting in a depressed mood, a lack of inspiration, lack of sense of direction in life, lack of life dreams and plans, etc. *Dian Kuang* is discussed in Chapter 19.

If we look at some of the symptoms of *Dian* (being withdrawn, unresponsiveness, incoherent speech, inappropriate laughter or crying, taciturnity), we can see that they do not describe what we call "depression".

SUMMARY

Distinction between Depression in "*Yu*" Syndrome and in "*Dian*" Syndrome

- Many modern Chinese books often discuss Depression Syndrome (*Yu Zheng*) as if it were identical to the depressive phase of Dullness and Mania (*Dian* of *Dian Kuang*).
- The "depression" in clinical depression is quite different from the "depression" in bipolar disorder (Dullness and Mania) from both a Western and a Chinese perspective.
- From a Chinese perspective, the depressive and manic phases of Dullness and Mania (*Dian Kuang*) are two poles of a pathological spectrum with the same pathology.
- Central to the pathology of *Dian Kuang* is Phlegm obstructing the Mind (*Shen*); this accounts for *both* the depressive and the manic phases of the disease.
- In Depression (*Yu Zheng*) Phlegm is not always present and the "coming and going" of the Ethereal Soul is always impaired (without a manic phase), resulting in a depressed mood.

Lilium Syndrome (*Bai He Bing*)

The Lilium Syndrome (*Bai He Bing*) is described in the *Essential Prescriptions of the Golden Chest (Jin Gui Yao Lue*, c.AD 220), Chapter 3-1. This syndrome sounds remarkably like the description of a depressed patient. It says:[8]

The patient wants to eat, but is reluctant to swallow food and unwilling to speak. He or she wants to lie in bed but cannot lie quietly as he or she is restless. He or she wants to walk but is soon tired. Now and then he or she may enjoy eating but cannot tolerate the smell of food. He or she feels cold or hot but without fever or chills, bitter taste or dark urine [i.e. it is not external Wind or internal Heat]. *No drugs are able to cure this syndrome. After taking the medicine the patient may vomit or have diarrhoea. The disease haunts the patient (hu huo)* [*hu* means "fox" and *huo* means "bewildered"] *and, although he or she looks normal, he or she is suffering. The pulse is rapid.*

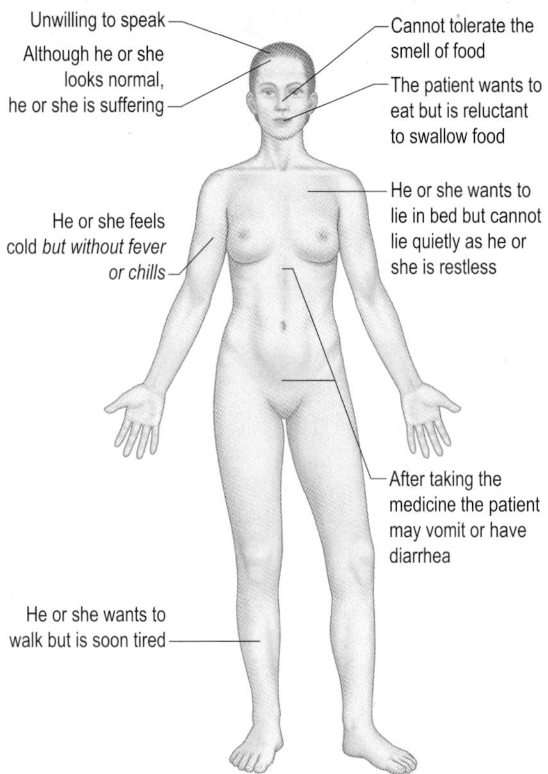

Figure 16.3 Lilium Syndrome.

See Figure 16.3.

Modern books describe the syndrome with the following symptoms: "as if in a trance" or "absent-minded" (*huang hu*), mental restlessness, bitter taste, dark urine, anxiety, depression, red tongue (which may be without coating) and rapid pulse.

The treatment principle recommended by modern doctors is to moisten and nourish the Heart and Lungs, tonify Qi, nourish Yin, clear Heat (or Empty Heat), calm the Mind and strengthen the Will-Power (*Zhi*).

The points suggested by the book *Chinese Acupuncture Therapy* (*Zhong Guo Zhen Jiu Liao Xue*) are as follows.[9]

- HE-7 Shenmen, KI-3 Taixi, LU-9 Taiyuan
- HE-5 Tongli, LU-7 Lieque, KI-4 Dazhong, SP-6 Sanyinjiao
- HE-9 Shaochong, P-9 Zhongchong, KI-7 Fuliu
- BL-15 Xinshu, BL-13 Feishu, BL-23 Shenshu
- LU-7 Lieque, KI-6 Zhaohai, LIV-3 Taichong

With herbal medicine, the formula Bai He Zhi Mu Tang *Lilium-Anemarrhena Decoction* treats this syndrome; the formula is composed only of the two herbs Bai He *Bulbus Lilii* and Zhi Mu *Radix Anemarrhenae*. In fact, I use these two herbs in any situation when a patient is depressed against a background of a Lung and Heart syndrome, but especially Qi and Yin deficiency of these two organs or Heart-Heat. The combination of these two herbs is particularly good to treat sadness and grief. In such cases, I frequently add these two herbs to whatever formula I am using.

CLINICAL NOTE

Bai He (*Bulbus Lilii*) and Zhi Mu (*Radix Anemarrhenae*)

I use the combination of Bai He *Bulbus Lilii* and Zhi Mu *Radix Anemarrhenae* to treat Lilium Syndrome (*Bai He Bing*). In fact, I use these two herbs in any situation when a patient is depressed against a background of a Lung and Heart syndrome, but especially Qi and Yin deficiency of these two organs or Heart-Heat. The combination of these two herbs is particularly good to treat sadness and grief. In such cases, I frequently add these two herbs to whatever formula I am using.

SUMMARY

Lilium Syndrome (*Bai He Bing*)

- The patient wants to eat, but is reluctant to swallow food.
- Unwilling to speak.
- He or she wants to lie in bed but cannot lie quietly as he or she is restless.
- He or she wants to walk but is soon tired.
- Cannot tolerate the smell of food.
- He or she feels cold or hot.
- Rapid pulse.

Agitation (*Zang Zao*)

Zang Zao, literally meaning "visceral restlessness", was first mentioned in the chapter *Pulse, Syndromes and Treatment of Miscellaneous Gynecological Diseases of the Essential Prescriptions of the Golden Chest* (Jin Gui Yao Lue, c.AD 220) specifically in relation to women. This text says:[10]

The patient suffers from Agitation [Zang Zao], feels sad and tends to weep constantly as if she were haunted. She stretches frequently and yawns repeatedly. The decoction

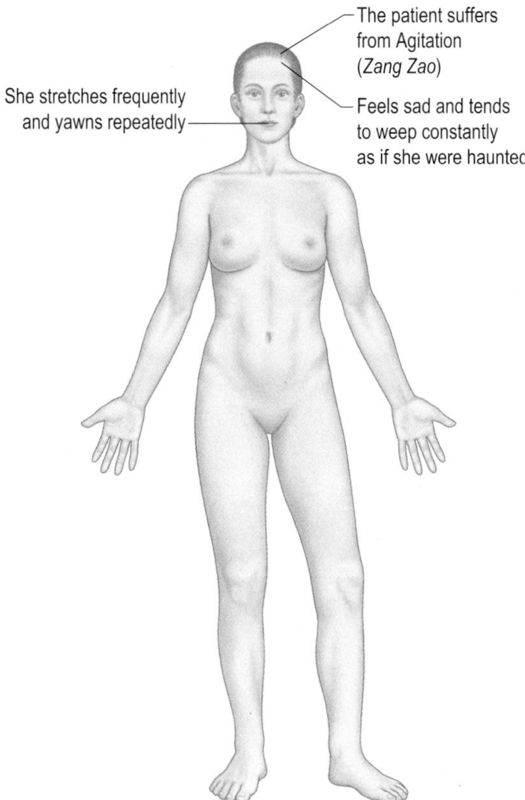

Figure 16.4 Agitation Syndrome.

of Fu Xiao Mai, Zhi Gan Cao and Da Zao can calm the patient.

See Figure 16.4.

The formula for Agitation (*Zang Zao*) is therefore Gan Mai Da Zao Tang *Glycyrrhiza-Triticum-Jujuba Decoction*. Modern Chinese books say that this formula is for Liver-Qi stagnation and that it soothes the Liver by its sweet taste (reverse Controlling cycle of the Five Elements). I tend to disagree with this interpretation that is driven by what I consider an excessive focus on Liver-Qi stagnation.

I personally use this formula not only for Agitation but also for Depression arising against a background of Qi and Blood deficiency. As the formula is composed of only three herbs (all of which are mild in taste and action), I may frequently add this formula to other formulae I am using when I suspect that the problem is of emotional origin and there is Qi and Blood deficiency.

The syndrome described in the *Essential Prescriptions of the Golden Chest* corresponds to that of a patient who is both depressed and anxious. Of course, although mentioned in a chapter on gynecology, both men and women can suffer from this syndrome.

SUMMARY

Agitation (*Zang Zao*)

- *Zang Zao*, literally meaning "visceral restlessness", was first mentioned in the *Essential Prescriptions of the Golden Chest* (*Jin Gui Yao Lue*, c.AD 220).
- The formula for Agitation (*Zang Zao*) is Gan Mai Da Zao Tang *Glycyrrhiza-Triticum-Jujuba Decoction*.
- Modern Chinese books say that this formula is for Liver-Qi stagnation and that it soothes the Liver by its sweet taste.
- I personally use this formula not only for Agitation but also for Depression arising against a background of Qi and Blood deficiency.

Plum-Stone Syndrome (*Mei He Qi*)

Plum-Stone Syndrome was first described in the chapter *Pulse, Syndromes and Treatment of Miscellaneous Gynecological Diseases* of the *Essential Prescriptions of the Golden Chest* (*Jin Gui Yao Lue*, c.AD 220). This text says: *"The patient has a suffocating feeling as if there was a piece of roast meat stuck in the throat. Use Ban Xia Hou Po Tang."*[11] See Figure 16.5.

Therefore, as can be seen from the above statement, originally the symptom of Plum-Stone Syndrome was compared to the feeling of having a piece of meat (rather than a plum stone) in the throat. The etiology of this syndrome is emotional and is due to depression.

Subsequent Chinese books attributed this syndrome to the combination of Qi stagnation and Phlegm obstructing the throat. This type of Phlegm is actually called Qi-Phlegm and it is the most non-substantial type of Phlegm.

Although all modern Chinese books attribute the Plum-Stone Syndrome to stagnation of Liver-Qi, the formula Ban Xia Hou Po Tang *Pinellia-Magnolia Decoction* actually acts on Lung- and Stomach-Qi. I therefore use it primarily for stagnation of Qi of the Heart and Lungs in the chest area deriving from sadness, grief and worry.

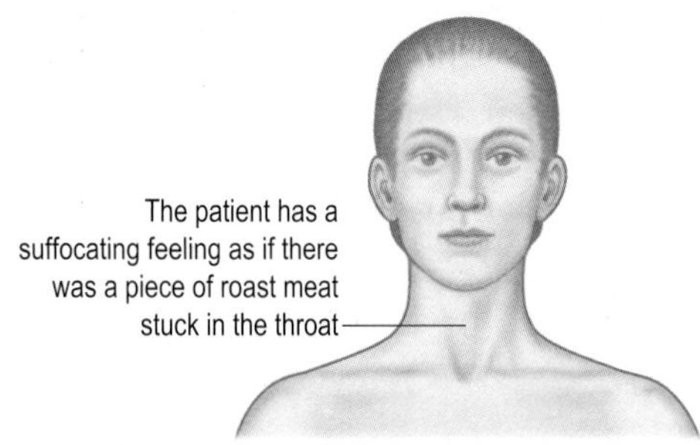

Figure 16.5 Plum-Stone Syndrome.

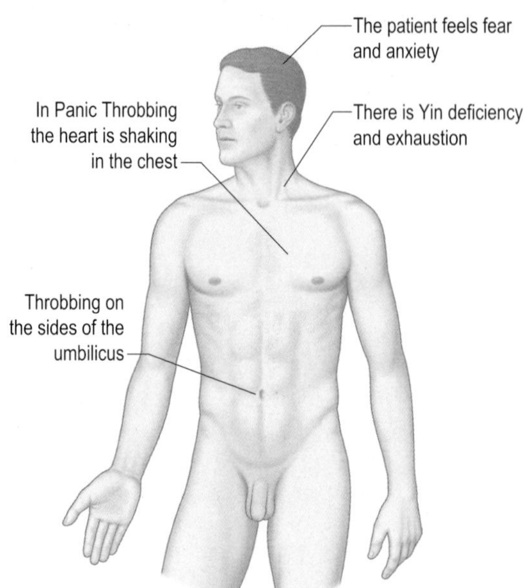

Figure 16.6 Palpitations and anxiety.

CLINICAL NOTE

Plum-Stone Syndrome

Although all modern Chinese books attribute the Plum-Stone Syndrome to stagnation of Liver-Qi, the formula Ban Xia Hou Po Tang actually acts on Lung- and Stomach-Qi. I therefore use it primarily for stagnation of Qi of the Heart and Lungs in the chest area deriving from sadness, grief and worry.

SUMMARY

Plum-Stone Syndrome (*Mei He Qi*)

- Plum-Stone Syndrome was first described in the *Essential Prescriptions of the Golden Chest* (*Jin Gui Yao Lue*, C.AD 220).
- The etiology of this syndrome is emotional and is due to depression.
- Subsequent Chinese books attributed this syndrome to the combination of Qi stagnation and Phlegm obstructing the throat.
- The formula Ban Xia Hou Po Tang *Pinellia-Magnolia Decoction* actually acts on Lung- and Stomach-Qi.

Palpitations and Anxiety (*Xin Ji Zheng Chong*)

What I translate as "palpitations and anxiety" corresponds to two separate conditions in Chinese medicine: the first is *Xin Ji* ("Fear and Palpitations"); the second *Zheng Chong* ("Panic Throbbing"). In modern Chinese medicine, *Xin Ji* is more frequently called *Jing Ji*.

Both these conditions involve a state of fear, worry and anxiety, the first with palpitations and the second with a throbbing sensation in the chest and below the umbilicus. "Fear and Palpitations" is usually caused by external events such as a fright or shock and it comes and goes; it is more frequently of a Full nature. "Panic Throbbing" is not caused by external events and it is continuous; this condition is usually of an Empty nature and is more serious than the first. In chronic cases, "Fear and Palpitations" may turn into "Panic Throbbing". In severe cases, "Panic Throbbing" may correspond to panic attacks. Despite the name "Fear and Palpitations", such states of fear and anxiety may occur without palpitations.

Zhu Dan Xi (1281–1358) says:[12]

In both Fear and Palpitations and Panic Throbbing there is Blood deficiency. Fear and Palpitations come in bouts; Panic Throbbing is constant. Panic Throbbing is due to worry and pensiveness agitating within, causing a deficiency and Phlegm-Heat.

See Figure 16.6.

Zhang Jing Yue says of "Panic Throbbing" in his *Complete Book of Jing Yue* (*Jing Yue Quan Shu*, 1624):[13]

In Panic Throbbing the heart is shaking in the chest, the patient feels fear and anxiety. There is Yin deficiency and exhaustion; there is Yin deficiency below so that the Gathering Qi [Zong Qi] has no root and Qi cannot return to its origin. For this reason, there is shaking [or throbbing] *of the chest above and also throbbing on the sides of the umbilicus.*

Both "Fear and Palpitations" and "Panic Throbbing" may accompany depression and I shall refer to these two conditions collectively as "palpitations and anxiety".

SUMMARY

Palpitations and Anxiety (*Xin Ji Zheng Chong*)

- What I translate as "palpitations and anxiety" corresponds to two separate conditions in Chinese medicine: the first is *Xin Ji* ("Fear and Palpitations"); the second *Zheng Chong* ("Panic Throbbing").
- Both these conditions involve a state of fear, worry and anxiety, the first with palpitations and the second with a throbbing sensation in the chest and below the umbilicus.
- Both "Fear and Palpitations" and "Panic Throbbing" may accompany depression and I shall refer to these two conditions collectively as "anxiety and palpitations".

Liver-Qi deficiency

It is often said that, while Liver-Blood may be deficient, Liver-Qi can never be deficient. This is not quite true, as Liver-Qi may indeed be deficient. In order to understand the pathology of Liver-Qi deficiency, we need to revise the physiological and pathological movements of Liver-Qi. The free flow of Liver-Qi is well known; in physiology, Liver-Qi flows smoothly in all directions, in particular helping Stomach-Qi to descend and Spleen-Qi to ascend. By assisting these two movements, Liver-Qi helps the Stomach to rot and ripen food, and the Spleen to separate the food essences and to transform and transport.

We also know that, in pathology, Liver-Qi frequently ascends too much and this situation leads to "Liver-Yang rising". However, in physiology, Liver-Qi needs to rise to a certain extent and this rising is coordinated with the descending of Lung-Qi.

The Lungs govern Qi and Qi regulates the functions of the Internal Organs. The Lungs have the function of *jie zhi*, which means to govern, control, to check, to moderate. The Lung's function of "restricting", regulating and adjusting the functions of all the Internal Organs is dependent on the descending of Lung-Qi. The descending of Lung-Qi partially depends on the ascending of Liver-Qi.

Liver-Qi normally ascends and this makes the Qi Mechanism work smoothly, so that Qi and Blood are harmonized and flow freely. There is a saying that states: "*The ascending of Qi stems from the Liver.*" Ye Tian Shi said: "*The Liver is on the left and its Qi rises, the Lung is on the right and its Qi descends.*" Obviously, this statement should not be interpreted anatomically (as the liver is on the right side), but energetically. Indeed, if we look at the diagram of the Five Elements with the Earth in the middle, the Liver is on the left and the Lungs on the right.

Ye Tian Shi also said: "*The Qi mechanism of our body is mirrored on heaven and earth in nature, the Liver is on the left and its Qi rises, the Lung is on the right and its Qi descends. When Lung-Qi does not descend, Liver-Qi rebels horizontally.*"

Therefore, the ascending of Liver-Qi and descending of Lung-Qi are essential for the correct functioning of the ascending and descending of Qi in the Qi Mechanism (Fig. 16.7).

Liver-Qi deficiency implies a failure of Liver-Qi to ascend. Where does Liver-Qi ascend to? Besides being coordinated with the descending of Lung-Qi as outlined above, Liver-Qi ascends to the Heart and the movement from Wood to Fire in the Nourishing cycle of the Five Elements is an aspect of the movement of Liver-Qi towards the Heart (Fig. 16.8).

Liver-Qi deficiency usually occurs in conjunction with Liver-Blood deficiency and, for this reason, the clinical manifestations of Liver-Qi deficiency include all those of Liver-Blood deficiency. In addition to these,

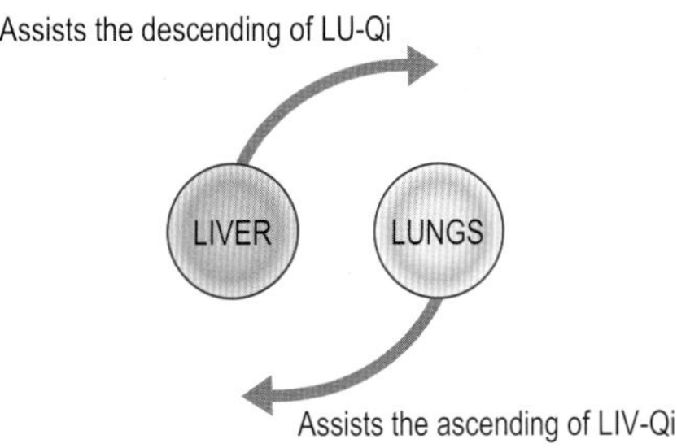

Figure 16.7 Coordination between descending of Lung-Qi and ascending of Liver-Qi.

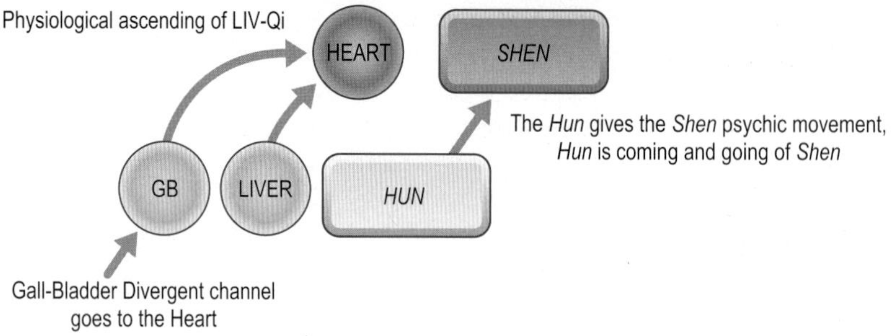

Figure 16.8 Ascending of Liver-Qi to the Heart.

there will be depression. In other words, in the presence of symptoms of Liver-Blood deficiency, mental depression is the characteristic symptom that indicates Liver-Qi deficiency. Of course, this does not mean that all depression is due to Liver-Qi deficiency as Liver-Qi stagnation is a common cause of it. What it does mean is that, in the presence of Empty patterns, depression is often due to Liver-Qi deficiency and to the failure of its Qi to ascend.

A deficiency of Liver-Blood and Liver-Qi leads to an insufficient movement of the Ethereal Soul and therefore to depression, lack of inspiration, lack of life dreams and confusion about a sense of direction in life.

A deficiency of Liver-Qi also implies a deficiency of the Gall-Bladder, as failure to rise is a deficiency of Yang (as rising is a Yang movement) and the Gall-Bladder is the Yang aspect of the Liver. A deficiency of the Gall-Bladder leads to timidity, depression, lack of resolve and an inability to make decisions (Fig. 16.9).

In the presence of depression occurring against the background of Empty patterns and a deficiency of Liver-Qi, I tonify the latter with acupuncture by tonifying the Gall-Bladder and I use in particular the point G.B.-40 Qiuxu. With herbal medicine, most Qi tonics will raise Liver-Qi, e.g. Huang Qi *Radix Astragali* or Ren Shen *Radix Ginseng*.

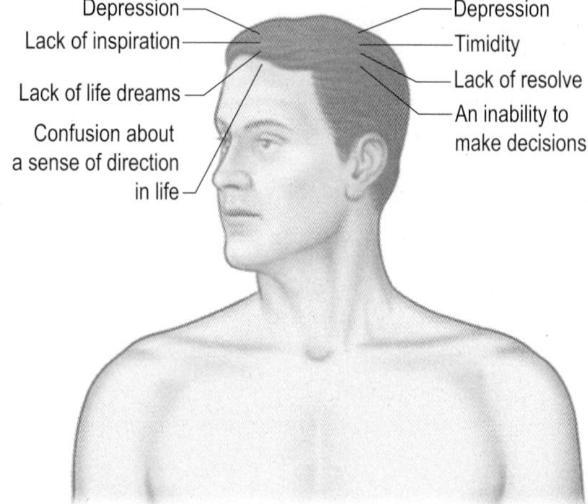

Figure 16.9 Liver-Qi deficiency.

SUMMARY

Liver-Qi deficiency

- Liver-Qi may be deficient.
- In physiology, Liver-Qi rises in coordination with the descending of Lung-Qi.
- The descending of Lung-Qi partially depends on the ascending of Liver-Qi.
- Ye Tian Shi: "*The Liver is on the left and its Qi rises, the Lung is on the right and its Qi descends.*"
- Liver-Qi ascends to the Heart.
- Liver-Qi deficiency usually occurs in conjunction with Liver-Blood deficiency and the clinical manifestations of Liver-Qi deficiency include all those of Liver-Blood deficiency, plus depression.
- A deficiency of Liver-Blood and Liver-Qi leads to an insufficient movement of the Ethereal Soul and therefore to depression, lack of inspiration, lack of life dreams and confusion about a sense of direction in life.
- A deficiency of Liver-Qi also implies a deficiency of the Gall-Bladder, leading to timidity, depression, lack of resolve and an inability to make decisions.

"Neurasthenia" and Depression

The term "neurasthenia" was used frequently in conventional medicine in the 19th century. This term has fallen out of use and "neurasthenia" is no longer a diagnosis in Western medicine. However, some Chinese books still use this term to indicate a state of emotional, mental and physical decline; the Chinese term is *Jing Shen Shuai Ruo* 精神衰弱 which literally means "nervous feebleness". Some aspects of neurasthenia, especially those seen in Empty conditions, correspond to a state of mild depression (Fig. 16.10).

"Neurasthenia" was a Western category of disease and Chinese books say that it may correspond to various Chinese disease entities, e.g. "Depression" (*Yu Zheng*), "Headaches", "Insomnia", "Palpitations and Anxiety" (*Jing Ji*), "Poor Memory" or "Exhaustion" (*Xu Lao*).

Modern Chinese books list the following patterns causing neurasthenia.

- Deficiency of Heart and Spleen
- Heart and Kidneys not harmonized
- Deficiency of Heart and Gall-Bladder
- Liver- and Kidney-Yin deficiency with rising of Liver-Yang
- Deficiency of Kidney-Essence
- Yin deficiency with Empty Heat
- Phlegm-Heat harassing upwards
- Liver-Qi stagnation
- Qi stagnation giving rise to Heat
- Heart-Fire
- Blood stasis
- Stomach-Qi not harmonized

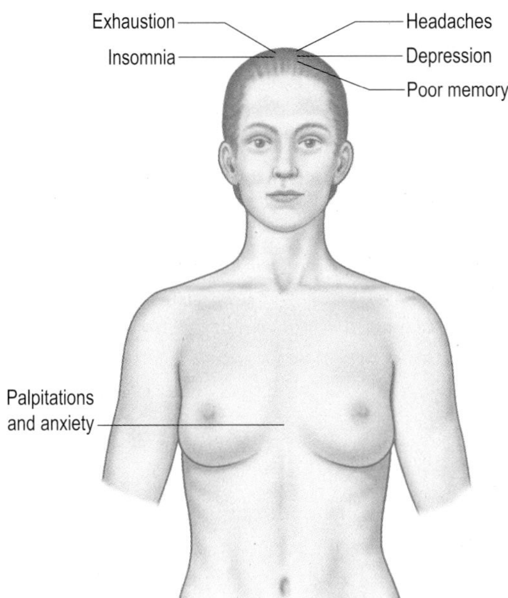

Figure 16.10 Neurasthenia and depression.

As we can see from the above list, many of the patterns occurring in neurasthenia are the same as those occurring in depression. Indeed, I feel that, in modern China, the term "neurasthenia" is used as a diagnosis that avoids the use of the word "depression"; this is because, in China, there is still a certain social stigma associated with depression.

However, although the term "neurasthenia" is somewhat meaningless, it does correspond to situations in the clinic when the patient suffers from a deficiency which affects him or her at both a physical and a mental-emotional level. This occurs in patients whose mental-emotional low state is below the level of what we could call "depression".

Elements of the pathology of Depression

In conclusion, the pathology of Depression has many facets. These are summarized as follows, with the acupuncture points suggested for each aspect.

Will-Power (*Zhi*)

The Will-Power (*Zhi*) is impaired, there is lack of will-power, drive, initiative, enthusiasm and momentum to break out of depression: BL-23 Shenshu, BL-52 Zhishi, KI-3 Taixi.

Ethereal Soul (*Hun*)

The Ethereal Soul does not come and go enough (which may be from stagnation or deficiency), there is a lack of plans, ideas, life dreams, hope, inspiration and a sense of direction: G.B.-40 Xiuxu, BL-47 Hunmen.

Mind (*Shen*)

The Mind (and Spirit in general) is affected with angst, anxiety, despair and sadness: Du-24 Shenting, Ren-15 Jiuwei, HE-7 Shenmen.

Corporeal Soul (*Po*)

The constriction of the Corporeal Soul gives rise to morbid thoughts of death: Du-24 Shenting, BL-13 Feishu ("suicidal"), Du-12 Shenzhu ("desire to kill people"), BL-42 Pohu ("three corpses flowing").

Intellect (*Yi*)

The Intellect is affected by overthinking, giving rise to obsessive thinking, pensiveness and brooding: G.B.-15 Toulinqi, BL-49 Yishe.

Gall-Bladder's "courage"

Deficiency of the Gall-Bladder's "courage" leads to indecisiveness and timidity: G.B.-40 Qiuxu, Du-20 Baihui.

Pericardium and Triple Burner

Affliction of the Pericardium and Triple Burner leads to problems in forming or maintaining relationships: T.B.-5 Waiguan, P-7 Daling, P-6 Neiguan, Ren-17 Shanzhong.

The above are not alternative pathologies of depression but aspects of its pathology; although not all of them need to be present, most of them usually are.

SUMMARY

Elements of the pathology of Depression

Will-Power (Zhi)

BL-23 Shenshu, BL-52 Zhishi, KI-3 Taixi.

Ethereal Soul (Hun)

G.B.-40 Xiuxu, BL-47 Hunmen.

Mind (Shen)

Du-24 Shenting, Ren-15 Jiuwei, HE-7 Shenmen.

Corporeal Soul (Po)

Du-24 Shenting, BL-13 Feishu, Du-12 Shenzhu, BL-42 Pohu.

Intellect (Yi)

G.B.-15 Toulinqi, BL-49 Yishe.

Gall-bladder's "courage"

G.B.-40 Qiuxu, Du-20 Baihui.

vii. Pericardium and triple burner

T.B.-5 Waiguan, P-7 Daling, P-6 Neiguan, Ren-17 Shanzhong.

SUMMARY

Pathology of Depression in Chinese medicine

- *Yu* as stagnation.
- *Yu* as mental depression.
- Depression and the relationship between the Mind (*Shen*) and the Ethereal Soul (*Hun*).
- The Will-Power (*Zhi*) of the Kidneys in depression.
- Distinction between depression in *Yu* Syndrome and in *Dian* Syndrome.
- Lilium Syndrome (*Bai He Bing*).
- Agitation (*Zang Zao*).
- Plum-Stone Syndrome (*Mei He Qi*).
- Palpitations and Anxiety (*Xin Ji Zheng Zhong*).
- "Neurasthenia" and depression.
- Elements of the pathology of depression.

ETIOLOGY

The etiology of depression includes the following factors.

- Emotional stress
- Constitutional traits
- Irregular diet
- Overwork

Emotional stress

Emotional stress is the main etiological factor in depression. The main emotions that may give rise to depression are anger, sadness, grief, worry and guilt.

Anger

Anger (intended in a broad sense to include frustration, resentment and hatred) causes either Liver-Qi stagnation or Liver-Yang rising. When it is suppressed, it is more likely to cause Liver-Qi stagnation and depression. Liver-Qi stagnation is a frequent cause of mental depression, especially in its beginning stages.

Liver-Qi stagnation causes depression by restraining the "coming and going" of the Ethereal Soul, resulting in a lack of ideas, projects, aims, life dreams, inspiration and a general lack of sense of direction in life.

One of the most significant and important signs of Liver-Qi stagnation is a Wiry pulse. If the pulse is generally Wiry in all positions, it is often a sign that the mental depression is due to Liver-Qi stagnation and, usually, to anger. Often the pulse picture contradicts the first appearance of the patient. In fact, the patient may appear depressed, slow in movement, pale with a weak voice – all signs pointing to a Deficiency as the cause of the problem – but the pulse is Full and Wiry in every position; this is a sure sign that the depression is due to Qi stagnation and to anger. Indeed, in some cases (and in my experience, especially in men), the person may seek treatment for tiredness as his or her main complaint, but if the pulse is Full and Wiry in every position, it almost certainly indicates that the person is depressed with Liver-Qi stagnation as the main cause of it.

I would go so far as saying that if the pulse is not Wiry, then anger is not the cause of the depression.

Sadness and grief

Sadness and grief initially deplete Qi and therefore lead to Qi deficiency of the Spleen, Heart and Lungs. However, after some time, the very deficiency of Qi impairs its circulation and leads also to some Qi stagnation; this is a Qi stagnation that affects not the Liver but the Heart and Lungs.

The Heart- and/or Lung-Qi stagnation also affect the Ethereal Soul and restrain its "coming and going", resulting in a lack of ideas, projects, aims, life dreams, inspiration and a general lack of sense of direction in life.

Sadness and grief are frequent causes of depression from loss of a family member or partner from death or separation; this is called reactive depression in Western psychiatry.

When sadness and grief are the cause of the depression, the pulse is Weak in general and especially so on the Lung position.

Worry

Worry "knots" Qi, which means it causes Qi stagnation. Worry causes stagnation of Qi of the Spleen, Lungs and Heart; in my experience, worry also affects the Liver and may cause either Liver-Qi stagnation or Liver-Yang rising.

The Heart- and/or Lung-Qi stagnation also affect the Ethereal Soul and restrain its "coming and going", resulting in a lack of ideas, projects, aims, life dreams, inspiration and a general lack of sense of direction in life.

When worry is the cause of the depression, the pulse is Tight on the Lung position.

Guilt

Guilt is, in my experience, a common cause of Qi stagnation and of depression; it affects primarily the Heart and Kidneys.

The Heart-Qi stagnation also affects the Ethereal Soul and restrains its "coming and going", resulting in a lack of ideas, projects, aims, life dreams, inspiration and a general lack of sense of direction in life.

As guilt also affects the Kidneys, it weakens the Will-Power (*Zhi*), the weakness of which is an important feature of depression.

CLINICAL NOTE

Emotions and Qi stagnation

- All emotions lead to some Qi stagnation initially (also those that deplete Qi such as sadness and grief).
- Not all Qi stagnation is related to the Liver.
- In emotional problems, other organs suffer from Qi stagnation, notably the Lungs and Heart.
- Note that Liver-Qi stagnation may also derive from emotions other than "anger", e.g. worry and guilt.

Constitutional traits

In my experience, constitutional traits play an important role in the etiology of depression. For example, a constitutional deficiency of the Kidneys, with its resulting weakness of the Will-Power (*Zhi*) is a frequent underlying background for the development of depression.

A constitutional tendency to Heart patterns is also an important contributory factor to the development of depression. The most important and reliable sign of a tendency to emotional problems is a midline Heart crack on the tongue (*see Fig. 11.6 and Plate 11.2*).

Irregular diet

Diet plays a secondary role in the etiology of depression; in my experience, it contributes to the development of depression in the presence of emotional stress.

Excessive consumption of dairy foods, sweets, sugar and bread may lead to the formation of Phlegm. Phlegm may become a contributory pathological element of depression as, first of all, it impairs Qi and would therefore aggravate any deficiency and stagnation of Qi. It is also obstructive and heavy and therefore would cloud the Mind, leading to mental confusion; this condition would aggravate a condition of restraint of the Ethereal Soul so that its movement is impaired.

In my experience, a dietary factor that contributes to the development of depression is a diet lacking in nourishment. This occurs when patients follow strict slimming diets or when they apply a vegetarian diet inappropriately. This leads to deficiency of Qi and Blood, which are the conditions underlying Deficiency types of depression.

Overwork

Overwork in the sense of working long hours without adequate rest for several years leads to Kidney-Yin deficiency, and this often forms the background for depression in older people.

SUMMARY

Etiology and pathology

- Emotional stress
  - Anger
  - Sadness and grief
  - Worry
  - Guilt
- Constitutional traits
- Irregular diet
- Overwork

PATHOLOGY

The pathology of depression usually starts either with Qi stagnation or with a combination of Qi stagnation with Qi deficiency. As discussed in Chapters 9 and 10, emotional stress usually upsets the Qi Mechanism first and causes either Qi stagnation or Qi deficiency, or both. Anger, worry and guilt will cause Qi stagnation initially, while sadness and grief cause a combination of Qi deficiency and Qi stagnation.

It is important to remember that Qi stagnation affects not only the Liver but, especially in depression, may affect also the Lungs and/or Heart. The patterns of Lung- and Heart-Qi stagnation have been described in Chapter 12. Qi stagnation impairs the movement of the Ethereal Soul and this leads to depression, as explained in Chapter 3.

As indicated above, although the term *Yu* means both "stagnation" and "depression", this does not mean that there is always Qi stagnation in depression as, initially, there may be only Qi deficiency. Furthermore, in late stages, many other patterns appear.

When Qi stagnation persists, it leads to Heat. This manifests with a slight redness on the sides of the tongue if the Heat is in the Liver, on the sides (chest area) if in the Lungs, and on the tip if in the Heart. Heat agitates the Mind and the Ethereal Soul and it may lead to anxiety, which very often accompanies depression.

Phlegm is a very common pathogenic factor in depression. Please remember that Phlegm is formed not only when there is a deficiency of Qi (of the Lungs, Spleen or Kidneys) but it may also derive from Qi stagnation. Dr Ma Pei Zhi of the Qing dynasty thinks that Phlegm in depression may derive from three possible conditions: a deficiency of Heart and Spleen with stagnation in the Stomach and Liver, a condition of deficient Spleen-Qi not rising and disharmony of Spleen and Liver.[14]

Long-term Qi stagnation may lead to Blood stasis, in which case the tongue will be Purple. Again, Blood stasis affects not only the Liver but also the Lungs and/or Heart. Blood stasis is more likely to occur when the emotional stress is connected to guilt. Blood stasis always aggravates the feeling of depression and it causes a very "dark" feeling of depression and despair.

When Heat persists for a long time, it may injure Yin and lead to Yin deficiency of any of these organs: Heart, Lungs, Stomach/Spleen, Liver and Kidneys. When there is Yin deficiency, the tongue lacks a coating. Please remember that Yin deficiency is not contradictory with Phlegm, as the former is a deficiency of physiological fluids, while the latter is an accumulation of pathological fluids. Indeed, the combination of Phlegm

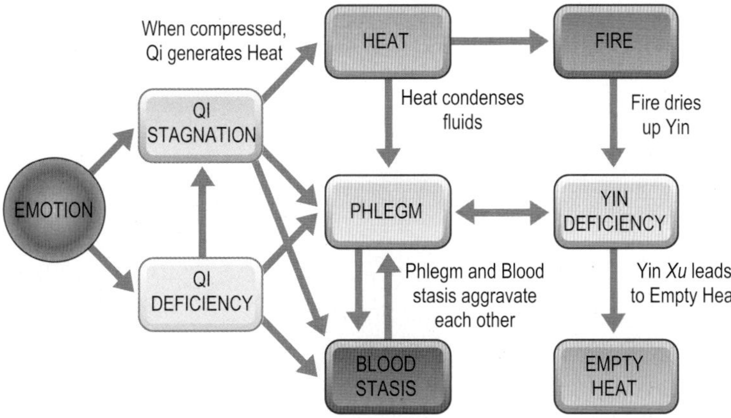

Figure 16.11 Pathology of depression.

and Yin deficiency is relatively common in the elderly in whom the tongue will be Swollen (indicating Phlegm) and lacking in coating (indicating Yin deficiency).

When Yin deficiency goes on for a protracted time, Empty Heat is generated and, in this case, the tongue will be Red and without coating. Empty Heat agitates the Mind and the Ethereal Soul (in the same way as Heat does) and it may cause anxiety and insomnia.

Figure 16.11 illustrates the pathology of depression.

SUMMARY

Pathology

- The pathology of depression usually starts either with Qi stagnation or with a combination of Qi stagnation with Qi deficiency.
- Qi stagnation affects not only the Liver but, especially in depression, it may affect also the Lungs and/or Heart.
- Although the term *Yu* means both "stagnation" and "depression", that does not mean that there is always Qi stagnation in depression as, initially, there may be only Qi deficiency.
- When Qi stagnation persists, it leads to Heat and this manifests with a slight redness on the sides of the tongue if the Heat is in the Liver, on the sides (chest area) if in the Lungs, and on the tip if in the Heart.
- Phlegm is a very common pathogenic factor in depression. Phlegm is formed not only when there is a deficiency of Qi (of the Lungs, Spleen or Kidneys) but it may also derive from Qi stagnation.
- Long-term Qi stagnation may lead to Blood stasis, in which case the tongue will be Purple.
- When Heat persists for a long time, it may injure Yin and lead to Yin deficiency of Heart, Lungs, Stomach/Spleen, Liver or Kidneys.
- When Yin deficiency goes on for a protracted time, Empty Heat is generated and, in this case, the tongue will be Red and without coating.

IDENTIFICATION OF PATTERNS AND TREATMENT

The patterns discussed will be:

- Liver-Qi stagnation
- Heart- and Lung-Qi stagnation
- Stagnant Liver-Qi turning into Heat
- Phlegm-Heat harassing the Mind
- Blood stasis obstructing the Mind
- Qi stagnation with Phlegm
- Diaphragm Heat
- Worry injuring the Mind
- Heart and Spleen deficiency
- Heart-Yang deficiency
- Kidney- and Heart-Yin deficiency, Empty Heat blazing
- Kidney-Yang deficiency

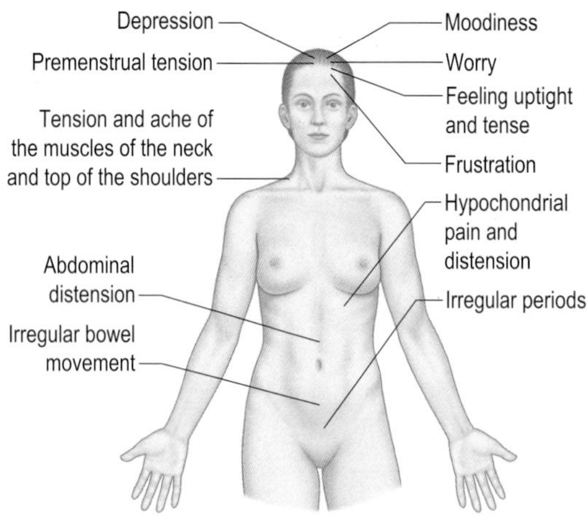

Figure 16.12 Liver-Qi stagnation.

Liver-Qi stagnation

Clinical manifestations

Depression, moodiness, worry, frustration, feeling uptight and tense, hypochondrial pain and distension, tension and ache of the muscles of the neck and top of the shoulders, abdominal distension, irregular bowel movement, irregular periods, premenstrual tension (Fig. 16.12).

Tongue: the tongue-body color may be normal or slightly red on the sides.

Pulse: Wiry.

Pathology and mental-emotional pattern

Depression is characterized by the insufficient "coming and going" of the Ethereal Soul, resulting in a lack of life dreams, aspirations, plans, ideas and inspiration. Liver-Qi stagnation is one of the most common causes of constraint of the movement of the Ethereal Soul.

Liver-Qi stagnation may derive from anger intended in a broad sense (including frustration and resentment); anger is even more prone to cause Liver-Qi stagnation when it is repressed. However, in my experience, Liver-Qi stagnation may also derive from worry and guilt.

The patient who is depressed against a background of Liver-Qi stagnation will not only be depressed but also moody and prone to outbursts of anger. He or she will also suffer from irritability and an intense feeling of frustration.

An important sign of Liver-Qi stagnation as the cause of depression is a Wiry pulse.

Patient's profile

Liver-Qi stagnation is a common cause of depression in young people, roughly from teenage years to about 35. Although Liver-Qi stagnation is obviously seen in depression in older persons, by then other patterns are also likely to be present. Liver-Qi stagnation is usually due to repressed anger, frustration or resentment, or to worry.

Treatment principle

Soothe the Liver, move Qi, eliminate stagnation.

Acupuncture

Points

P-6 Neiguan, LIV-3 Taichong, G.B.-34 Yanglingquan, T.B.-3 Zhongzhu, G.B.-13 Benshen, BL-47 Hunmen, Du-20 Baihui. Reducing or even method on all points except on Du-20, which should be reinforced.

Explanation

- P-6 is an important point for depression from Liver-Qi stagnation. It moves Liver-Qi by virtue of the association between the Pericardium and Liver channels within the Terminal Yin (*Jue Yin*). This point acts on the Liver and has a "centrifugal" movement; it therefore stimulates the "coming and going" of the Ethereal Soul in depression from Liver-Qi stagnation. As it lies on the Pericardium channel, P-6 also acts on the Heart, lifting mood. It is frequently used for this purpose in modern China.
- LIV-3 and G.B.-34 move Liver-Qi and therefore stimulate the "coming and going" of the Ethereal Soul to relieve depression. LIV-3 also has a calming effect and is good when the patient also suffers from anxiety.
- T.B.-3 lifts mood and stimulates the "coming and going" of the Ethereal Soul to relieve depression.
- G.B.-13 lifts mood, calms the Mind and stimulates the "coming and going" of the Ethereal Soul.

- BL-47 regulates the "coming and going" of the Ethereal Soul; it can either stimulate it when it is deficient or calm it when it is excessive.
- Du-20 lifts mood and depression.

> **CLINICAL NOTE**
>
> **P-6 Neiguan**
>
> P-6 is an important point for depression from Liver-Qi stagnation. It combines the function of moving Liver-Qi by virtue of the association between the Pericardium and Liver channels within the Terminal Yin (*Jue Yin*) with that of nourishing the Heart and moving Heart-Qi, because of the close connection between the Heart and Pericardium. This point acts on the Liver and has a "centrifugal" movement; it therefore stimulates the "coming and going" of the Ethereal Soul in depression from Liver-Qi stagnation. As it lies on the Pericardium channel, P-6 also acts on the Heart, lifting mood.

Herbal therapy

Prescription

YUE JU WAN
Gardenia-Chuanxiong Pill

Explanation

Yue Ju Wan is *the* formula for mental depression deriving from Liver-Qi stagnation. It was formulated by Zhu Dan Xi for the six stagnations of Qi, Blood, Food, Dampness, Phlegm and Heat. It contains five herbs for six stagnations because Cang Zhu treats stagnation both from Dampness and from Phlegm. Although this formula is for the six stagnations, it is primarily for Qi stagnation and therefore Xiang Fu is its emperor herb.

This is an intriguing formula as, when considered individually, none of its ingredients has a particularly strong mental effect (indeed, one of them, Shen Qu, is a digestive herb), but together they form a prescription that has an undoubted mental effect in relieving depression.

When this formula is used as an individualized prescription (as opposed to a remedy), the ingredients' dosage can be modified to take into account the presenting pattern. For example, if Phlegm is predominant, then the dosage of Cang Zhu is increased; if Blood stasis is present, then Chuan Xiong is increased, etc.

An important sign for the use of this formula is a Wiry pulse.

> **CLINICAL NOTE**
>
> **Yue Ju Wan**
>
> I find the formula Yue Ju Wan excellent to treat depression from Liver-Qi stagnation. If the pulse is Full and Wiry in every position in a depressed person, this is the first formula I consider.

Prescription

CHAI HU SHU GAN TANG Variation
Bupleurum Soothing the Liver Decoction Variation

Explanation

This is a well-known and much-used formula for Liver-Qi stagnation. It acts primarily on the Lower Burner and it would therefore be suitable if the patient somatizes his or her feelings in the lower abdomen with digestive problems such as abdominal distension and pain and bowel irregularity.

Qing Pi strengthens the moving-Qi effect and it directs it to the upper part of the body and the head; Yu Jin moves Qi and invigorates Blood and opens the Mind's orifices. It has a specific effect on mental depression from Qi stagnation.

Prescription

XIAO YAO SAN
Free and Easy Wanderer Powder

This formula is selected when the stagnation of Liver-Qi occurs against a background of Liver-Blood deficiency, which is more likely to occur in women. The tongue could therefore be Pale and the pulse is not Wiry on all positions (as for Yue Ju Wan), but only slightly Wiry on the left and Fine in general (indicating Blood deficiency). This situation is more common in women and this formula is therefore particularly suited to women.

Explanation

This formula is selected when Liver-Qi stagnation derives from or occurs against a background of Liver-Blood deficiency and Spleen-Qi deficiency.

Table 16.1 Differences between Xiao Yao San and Yue Ju Wan

	XIAO YAO SAN	YUE JU WAN
Patterns	Liver-Qi stagnation, Liver-Blood deficiency, Spleen-Qi deficiency	Liver-Qi stagnation
Etiology	Emotional stress combined with overwork and irregular diet	Emotional stress
Pulse	Fine and slightly Wiry; Weak in general and slightly Wiry on the left	Full and Wiry on all positions
Tongue	Body color may be normal or Pale	Slightly red sides
Emotional symptoms	Depression, sadness, crying	Depression, repressed anger

In my experience, this formula is probably overused to treat mental depression from Liver-Qi stagnation; it is specifically for Liver-Qi stagnation deriving from or occurring against a background of Liver-Blood deficiency. In "pure" Liver-Qi stagnation with a Full and Wiry pulse on all positions, one should use Yue Ju Wan rather than Xiao Yao San.

Table 16.1 illustrates the differences between Yue Ju Wan and Xiao Yao San.

Prescription

WU GE KUAN ZHONG SAN
Five Diaphragms Relaxing the Center Powder

Explanation

This formula is specific for mental depression from Qi stagnation. It has a wider range of effect than the previous formulae and it is particularly indicated when the Qi stagnation manifests in the Middle Burner.

It is called *Five Diaphragms Relaxing the Center Powder* because it treats five different pathological conditions of the diaphragm, all of them with an underlying Qi stagnation. The five conditions are:

- Worry diaphragm
- Anger diaphragm
- Qi diaphragm
- Cold diaphragm
- Heat diaphragm.

The symptoms of each of these five conditions are as follows.

Worry diaphragm
Stagnation of Qi in the chest, fluids not being transformed, food does not go down, shortness of breath.

Anger diaphragm
Fullness under the heart, food not digested, difficulty in urination and defecation.

Qi diaphragm
Fullness in chest and hypochondrium, choking sensation.

Cold diaphragm
Distension and fullness of abdomen and heart region, cough, wheezing, feeling of cold in the abdomen, flatulence, umbilical pain, inability to digest fats.

Heat diaphragm
Five-palm heat, mouth ulcers, burning and heaviness of the limbs, dry lips and mouth, feeling of heat of the body, lower backache, chest pain radiating to the upper back, inability to eat much.

Table 16.2 compares Yue Ju Wan, Chai Hu Shu Gan Tang, Xiao Yao San and Wu Ge Kuan Zhong San.

SUMMARY

Liver-Qi stagnation

Points

P-6 Neiguan, LIV-3 Taichong, G.B.-34 Yanglingquan, T.B.-3 Zhongzhu, G.B.-13 Benshen, BL-47 Hunmen, Du-20 Baihui. Reducing or even method on all points except on Du-20, which should be reinforced.

Herbal therapy

Prescriptions

YUE JU WAN
Gardenia-Chuanxiong Pill

Table 16.2 Comparison of Yue Ju Wan, Chai Hu Shu Gan Tang, Xiao Yao San and Wu Ge Kuan Zhong San

	PATTERNS	PULSE	TONGUE	EMOTIONAL SYMPTOMS
Yue Ju Wan	Liver-Qi stagnation	Full and Wiry on all positions	Slightly red sides	Depression, repressed anger
Chai Hu Shu Gan Tang	Liver-Qi stagnation in Lower Burner	Wiry, may be Wiry only on left	Slightly red sides	Depression, anger
Xiao Yao San	Liver-Qi stagnation, Liver-Blood deficiency, Spleen-Qi deficiency	Fine and slightly Wiry; Weak in general and slightly Wiry on the left	Body color may be normal or Pale	Depression, sadness, crying
Wu Ge Kuan Zhong San	Liver-Qi stagnation in Middle and Upper Burner	Wiry on Stomach and Lung positions	Slightly red sides	Depression, worry

CHAI HU SHU GAN TANG Variation
Bupleurum Soothing the Liver Decoction Variation
XIAO YAO SAN
Free and Easy Wanderer Powder
WU GE KUAN ZHONG SAN
Five Diaphragms Relaxing the Center Powder

Heart- and Lung-Qi stagnation

Clinical manifestations

Depression, sadness, slight anxiety, palpitations, a feeling of distension or oppression of the chest, a slight feeling of lump in the throat, slight shortness of breath, sighing, poor appetite, chest and upper epigastric distension, dislike of lying down, weak and cold limbs, pale complexion (Fig. 16.13).

Tongue: slightly Red on the sides in the chest areas.

Pulse: Empty but very slightly Overflowing on the left Front position and very slightly Tight on the right Front position.

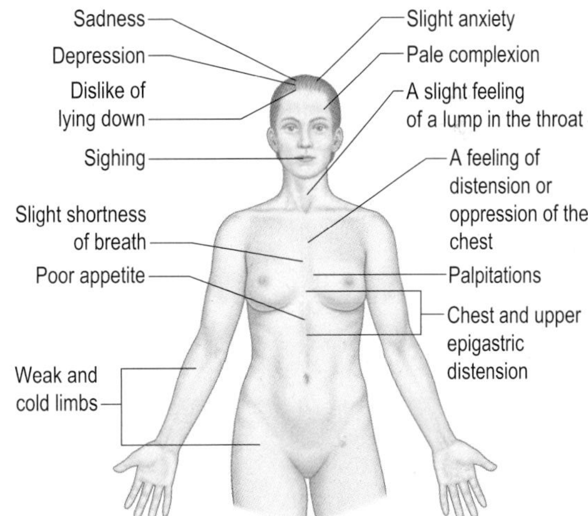

Figure 16.13 Heart- and Lung-Qi stagnation.

!

Remember: Qi stagnation occurs not only in the Liver but, especially in emotional problems, also in the Lungs and Heart.

Pathology and mental-emotional pattern

Sadness, grief and worry affect the Heart and Lungs; whilst sadness and grief initially deplete Qi and worry knots Qi, all three emotions, after some time, lead to Qi stagnation in the chest area. The Lungs are particularly affected by the sadness and grief deriving from separation and loss; this is a very frequent cause of depression.

The Qi stagnation deriving from the above emotions affects the circulation of Heart-Qi and Lung-Qi in the chest and constricts the Corporeal Soul; on a physical level, this causes a feeling of distension or tightness of the chest and sighing. On a mental-emotional level, the person is sad, depressed and tends to weep a lot.

Patient's profile

Heart- and Lung-Qi stagnation are common in young people (up to about 35). They nearly always derive from sadness and grief due to loss.

Treatment principle

Move Heart- and Lung-Qi, calm the Mind, lift mood, settle the Corporeal Soul.

Acupuncture

Points

HE-5 Tongli, HE-7 Shenmen, P-6 Neiguan, Ren-15 Jiuwei, Ren-17 Shanzhong, LU-7 Lieque, ST-40 Fenglong, L.I.-4 Hegu. All with even method.

Explanation

- HE-5, HE-7 and P-6 move Heart-Qi, lift the mood and calm the Mind.
- Ren-15 calms the Mind and nourishes the Heart.
- Ren-17 and LU-7 move Lung-Qi.
- ST-40 and L.I.-4 regulate the ascending and descending of Qi. ST-40 is used here not for Phlegm but to restore the descending of Qi and open the chest.

Herbal therapy

Prescription

MU XIANG LIU QI YIN
Aucklandia Flowing Qi Decoction

Explanation

This formula moves Qi in the Heart and Lungs, subdues rebellious Qi in the chest and tonifies Qi and Yin.

Prescription

BAN XIA HOU PO TANG
Pinellia-Magnolia Decoction

Explanation

This formula moves Qi in the Heart and Lungs and relieves depression. It is used when the physical symptoms are centered in the chest area, with a feeling of oppression and distension of the chest and sighing.

SUMMARY

Heart- and Lung-Qi stagnation

Points

HE-5 Tongli, HE-7 Shenmen, P-6 Neiguan, Ren-15 Jiuwei, Ren-17 Shanzhong, LU-7 Lieque, ST-40 Fenglong, L.I.-4 Hegu. All with even method.

Herbal therapy

Prescriptions

MU XIANG LIU QI YIN
Aucklandia Flowing Qi Decoction
BAN XIA HOU PO TANG
Pinellia-Magnolia Decoction

Stagnant Liver-Qi turning into Heat

Clinical manifestations

Depression, moodiness, worry, frustration, feeling uptight and tense, anxiety, agitation, short temper, dry mouth, bitter taste, constipation, headache, red face and eyes, hypochondrial pain and distension, tension and ache of the muscles of the neck and top of shoulders, abdominal distension, irregular bowel movement, irregular periods, premenstrual tension (Fig. 16.14).

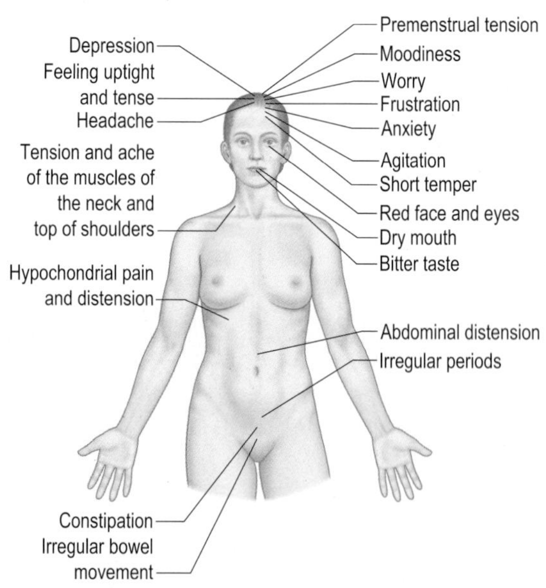

Figure 16.14 Stagnant Liver-Qi turning into Heat.

Tongue: Red body color with redder sides or normal body color with red sides.
Pulse: Wiry-Rapid.

Pathology and mental-emotional pattern

In Liver-Qi stagnation, the clinical manifestations are centered primarily in the hypochondrium and abdomen, while in Stagnant Liver-Qi turning into Heat, there are also manifestations in the head, such as headache, dry mouth, red eyes and face and bitter taste.

Liver-Qi stagnation impairs the "coming and going" of the Ethereal Soul, leading to depression in the same way as that described above under the pattern of "Liver-Qi stagnation". The Heat deriving from the long-term Qi stagnation, on the other hand, agitates the Mind and leads to anxiety.

Patient's profile

Stagnant Liver-Qi turning into Heat tends to be more common in people over 35. The etiology of this pattern is usually repressed anger combined with overwork and excessive consumption of alcohol.

Treatment principle

Soothe the Liver, move Qi, eliminate stagnation, clear Liver-Heat.

Acupuncture

Points

P-6 Neiguan, LIV-3 Taichong, LIV-2 Xingjian, G.B.-34 Yanglingquan, T.B.-3 Zhongzhu, G.B.-43 Xiaxi, G.B.-13 Benshen, Taiyang, BL-47 Hunmen, Du-20 Baihui. Reducing or even method on all points except on Du-20, which should be reinforced.

Explanation

- P-6, LIV-3, G.B.-34, T.B.-3, G.B.-13, BL-47 and Du-20 have all been explained above under the pattern of Liver-Qi stagnation. As the Heat here derives from Qi stagnation, it must be cleared primarily by moving Qi and eliminating stagnation.
- LIV-2 clears Liver-Heat.
- G.B.-43 clears Liver-Heat and treats headaches. It clears Heat from the head region. It is added to the point combination because the Heat in the Liver (as opposed to purely Liver-Qi stagnation) causes some symptoms to appear in the head (headache, dry mouth, bitter taste, red face and eyes).
- Taiyang calms the Mind.

Herbal therapy

Prescription

DAN ZHI XIAO YAO SAN
Moutan-Gardenia Free and Easy Wanderer Powder

Explanation

This is the representative formula to clear Liver-Heat deriving from Liver-Qi stagnation. It is based on Xiao Yao San to move Liver-Qi and eliminate stagnation, with the addition of Mu Dan Pi and Shan Zhi Zi to clear Liver-Heat.

Prescription

XIAO YAO SAN plus **ZUO JIN WAN**
Free and Easy Wanderer Powder plus *Left Metal Pill*

Explanation

When Heat derives from Qi stagnation, the primary treatment principle is to move Qi and eliminate stagnation; when this is eliminated, Heat is also automatically cleared. However, some herbs to clear Heat are also added, hence the addition of Zuo Jin Wan (that clears Liver-Heat) to Xiao Yao San (that moves Liver-Qi).

> **CLINICAL NOTE**
> When Heat derives from Qi stagnation, the primary herbal therapy principle must be to move Qi and eliminate stagnation.

Prescription

JIE YU QING XIN TANG
Eliminating Stagnation and Clearing the Heart Decoction

Explanation

This formula moves Liver-Qi, clears Heart-Heat and calms the Spirit. It is used when stagnant Liver-Qi has given rise to Heart-Heat.

> **SUMMARY**
>
> **Stagnant Liver-Qi turning into heat**
>
> *Points*
>
> P-6 Neiguan, LIV-3 Taichong, LIV-2 Xingjian, G.B.-34 Yanglingquan, T.B.-3 Zhongzhu, G.B.-43 Xiaxi, G.B.-13 Benshen, Taiyang, BL-47 Hunmen, Du-20 Baihui. Reducing or even method on all points except on Du-20, which should be reinforced.
>
> *Herbal therapy*
>
> *Prescriptions*
>
> **DAN ZHI XIAO YAO SAN**
> *Moutan-Gardenia Free and Easy Wanderer Powder*
> **XIAO YAO SAN** plus **ZUO JIN WAN**
> *Free and Easy Wanderer Powder* plus *Left Metal Pill*
> **JIE YU QING XIN TANG**
> *Eliminating Stagnation and Clearing the Heart Decoction*

Phlegm-Heat harassing the Mind

Clinical manifestations

Depression, mental restlessness, anxiety, agitation, restless sleep, excessive dreaming, insomnia, palpitations, a feeling of heaviness of the head, dizziness, a feeling of oppression of the chest, expectoration of phlegm, nausea, bitter taste, sticky taste (Fig. 16.15).

Tongue: Red, Swollen, sticky tongue coating, possibly Heart crack.

Pulse: Slippery-Rapid.

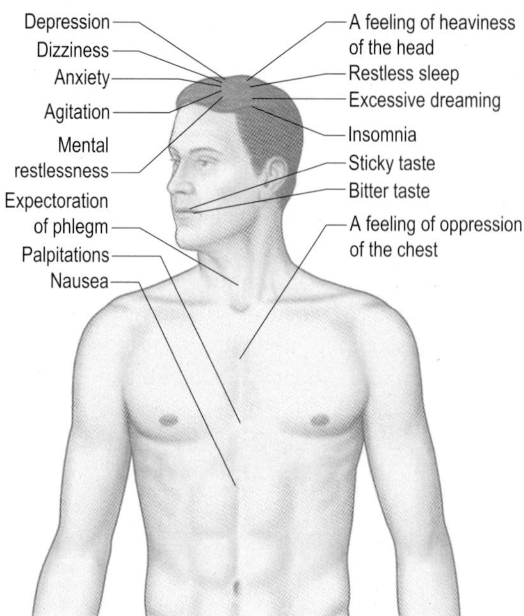

Figure 16.15 Phlegm-Heat harassing the Mind.

Pathology and mental-emotional pattern

Phlegm obstructs the Mind, while Heat agitates it. Phlegm obstructing the Mind causes mental confusion and, in severe cases, a certain loss of insight; Heat makes the person agitated, restless and anxious. In some cases, the person may alternate between periods of depression and confusion (due to Phlegm obstructing the Mind and also impairing the "coming and going" of the Ethereal Soul) and periods of abnormal elation, agitation and manic behavior (due to Fire). In severe cases this leads to manic-depression.

> **CLINICAL NOTE**
>
> Phlegm obstructs the Mind (causing a certain loss of insight) and Heat agitates it (causing anxiety and mental restlessness).

Patient's profile

The pattern of Phlegm-Heat harassing the Mind is more common in people over 45 and with a tendency to obesity. The etiology is usually long-standing emotional stress (particularly worry, guilt and anger), together with irregular diet and the excessive consumption of greasy foods and alcohol.

Treatment principle

Resolve Phlegm, clear Heat, open the Mind's orifices.

Acupuncture

Points

Ren-12 Zhongwan, BL-20 Pishu, ST-40 Fenglong, SP-9 Yinlingquan, SP-6 Sanyinjiao, P-5 Jianshi, P-7 Daling, ST-8 Touwei, Du-24 Shenting, G.B.-13 Benshen, G.B.-17 Zhengying, G.B.-18 Chengling, Du-20 Baihui. All points with reducing or even method except for Ren-12 and BL-20, which should be reinforced.

Explanation

- Ren-12, BL-20, ST-40, SP-9 and SP-6 resolve Phlegm. In particular, ST-40 resolves Phlegm and calms the Mind and SP-6 calms the Mind.
- P-5 and P-7 calm the Mind and open the Mind's orifices.
- ST-8 resolves Phlegm from the head.
- Du-24 and G.B.-13 calm the Mind and lift mood.
- G.B.-17 and G.B.-18 open the Mind's orifices.
- Du-20 lifts mood.

Herbal therapy

Prescription

WEN DAN TANG
Warming the Gall-Bladder Decoction

Explanation

This interesting formula has two main interpretations. Originally it was used for a Gall-Bladder deficiency following a severe acute disease, the Gall-Bladder deficiency manifesting with timidity, jumpiness, insomnia (waking up early in the morning) and mental restlessness. In more recent times, it is more frequently used for Phlegm-Heat affecting the Stomach, Heart or Lungs. The main manifestations for which it is used in this context are mental restlessness, jumpiness, insomnia, a bitter and sticky taste, a flustered feeling in the heart region, a feeling of oppression of the chest, nausea, vomiting, palpitations, dizziness, a Swollen tongue with a sticky-yellow coating and a Wiry or Slippery pulse.

A characteristic tongue configuration strongly indicates the use of this formula. It is a tongue that is Swollen and has a combination of Heart and Stomach crack with a rough, brush-like yellow coating inside the Stomach crack. A combined Heart and Stomach crack extends all the way to the tip, as a Heart crack would do, but it is wide and shallow in the center, as a Stomach crack would be (*see Fig. 11.6*).

Wen Dan Tang is an excellent formula for the pattern of Phlegm-Heat agitating and obstructing the Mind and causing depression; I generally modify it with the addition of Yuan Zhi *Radix Polygalae* and Suan Zao Ren *Semen Ziziphi spinosae.*

SUMMARY

Phlegm-Heat harassing the Mind

Points

Ren-12 Zhongwan, BL-20 Pishu, ST-40 Fenglong, SP-9 Yinlingquan, SP-6 Sanyinjiao, P-5 Jianshi, P-7 Daling, ST-8 Touwei, Du-24 Shenting, G.B.-13 Benshen, G.B.-17 Zhengying, G.B.-18 Chengling, Du-20 Baihui. All points with reducing or even method except for Ren-12 and BL-20, which should be reinforced.

Herbal therapy

Prescription

WEN DAN TANG
Warming the Gall-Bladder Decoction

Blood stasis obstructing the Mind

Clinical manifestations

Depression, mental restlessness, agitation at night, short temper, restless sleep, dreaming a lot, pain in the chest (Fig. 16.16).

Tongue: Purple.

Pulse: Wiry.

Pathology and mental-emotional pattern

Blood is the "residence" of the Mind (*Shen*) and of the Ethereal Soul, and a deficiency of Blood frequently affects both the Mind and the Ethereal Soul, depriving them of their "residence". However, it is important to note that Blood stasis also affects the Mind and the Ethereal Soul. In particular, Blood stasis tends to obstruct the Mind in a similar way that Phlegm does and, in serious cases, it can lead to a certain loss of insight.

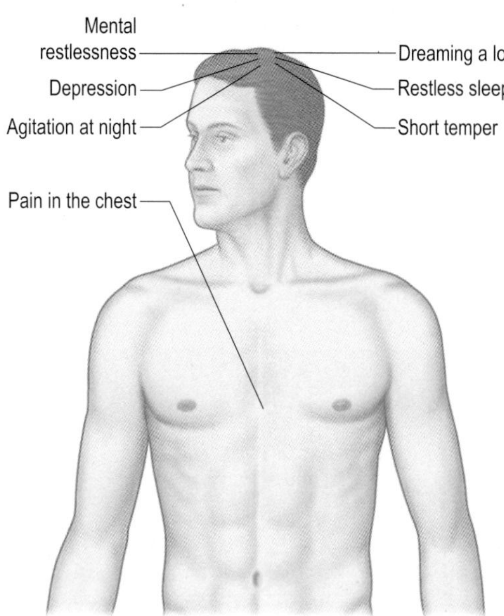

Figure 16.16 Blood stasis obstructing the Mind.

The patient is depressed but also anxious and agitated and may dream a lot, as Blood stasis frequently causes an aggravation of symptoms at night.

> **!**
>
> Remember: not only Blood deficiency but also Blood stasis affects the Mind (*Shen*) and the Ethereal Soul (*Hun*).

Patient's profile

The pattern of Blood stasis obstructing the Mind is more common in people over 40 and in women. It is usually due to long-standing repressed anger, worry or guilt.

Treatment principle

Invigorate Blood, calm the Mind, eliminate stasis.

Acupuncture

Points

P-6 Neiguan, BL-17 Geshu, SP-10 Xuehai, Ren-14 Juque, HE-5 Tongli, SP-6 Sanyinjiao, LIV-3 Taichong, G.B.-15 Toulinqi, Du-20 Baihui. All with reducing or even method except for Du-20, which should be reinforced.

Explanation

- P-6 invigorates Blood and affects the Upper Burner and therefore the head. It also calms the Mind and regulates the "coming and going" of the Ethereal Soul.
- BL-17 and SP-10 invigorate Blood. Both these points invigorate Blood and they are often used together, as the former invigorates Blood in the Upper Burner and the latter in the Lower Burner.
- Ren-14 and HE-5 invigorate Blood in the Heart and therefore calm the Mind when this is agitated by Blood stasis. HE-5 invigorates Blood by virtue of its being the Connecting point.
- SP-6 and LIV-3 calm the Mind and invigorate Blood.
- G.B.-15 has a deep effect on the emotional life and is particularly indicated to balance the moods when the person oscillates between periods of low spirits and periods of elation.[15] In my experience, this point is effective to stop obsessive thoughts and pensiveness.
- Du-20 lifts mood.

Herbal therapy

Prescription

XUE FU ZHU YU TANG
Blood Mansion Eliminating Stasis Decoction

Explanation

This formula is very widely used for stasis of Blood in the Upper Burner causing chest pain. Since Blood is the residence of the Mind, any Blood pathology can affect the Mind. Blood stasis agitates and obstructs the Mind. It agitates the Mind because Qi and Blood cannot flow smoothly and this is reflected on the mental-emotional level. It obstructs the Mind because the impeded flow of Blood retards the circulation of Blood to the Mind and thus obfuscates its orifices.

Anger, frustration, resentment, shock and guilt can all lead to Heart-Blood stasis. This usually occurs only after a long period of time, going through the stage of Qi stagnation first.

When stagnant Blood in the Heart affects the Mind, it may cause depression, palpitations, insomnia, a suffocating sensation in the chest, irritability, mood swings and, in severe cases, psychosis. Sleep is very disturbed, the patient waking up frequently at night, tossing and turning and with nightmares.

Shi Chang Pu *Rhizoma Acori graminei* and Yu Jin *Radix Curcumae* should be added to open the Mind's orifices and invigorate Blood.

SUMMARY

Blood stasis obstructing the Mind

Points

P-6 Neiguan, BL-17 Geshu, SP-10 Xuehai, Ren-14 Juque, HE-5 Tongli, SP-6 Sanyinjiao, LIV-3 Taichong, G.B.-15 Toulinqi, Du-20 Baihui. All with reducing or even method except for Du-20, which should be reinforced.

Herbal therapy

Prescription

XUE FU ZHU YU TANG

Blood Mansion Eliminating Stasis Decoction

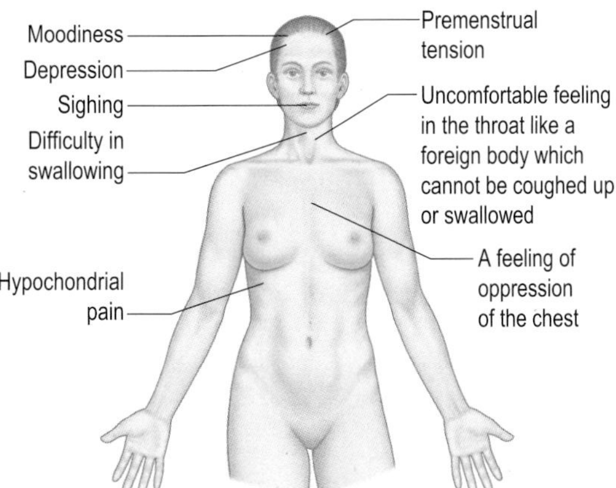

Figure 16.17 Qi stagnation with Phlegm.

Qi stagnation with Phlegm

Clinical manifestations

Depression, moodiness, uncomfortable feeling in the throat like a foreign body which cannot be coughed up or swallowed, difficulty in swallowing, sighing, a feeling of oppression of the chest, hypochondrial pain, premenstrual tension (Fig. 16.17).

Tongue: Swollen body, possibly red sides, sticky coating.

Pulse: Wiry or Slippery.

Pathology and mental-emotional pattern

The Ethereal Soul, residing in the Liver, is responsible for ideas, projects, life dreams, aims, creativity, etc. The Ethereal Soul provides this "movement" on a mental and psychic level to the Mind (*Shen*) and, for this reason, the Ethereal Soul is said to be the "coming and going of the Mind".

When the Ethereal Soul does not "come and go" enough, the person lacks life dreams, aims, projects, inspiration and creativity, he or she lacks a sense of direction and feels frustrated. These people are often at crossroads (which may have to do with relationships or work) in life and lack a sense of direction; in short, the person is depressed.

When Qi stagnates over a long period of time, the free flow of Qi in the Triple Burner is impaired and this leads to impairment of the metabolism of fluids; after time, this may result in the formation of Phlegm.

The "coming and going" of the Ethereal Soul may be restrained both by Qi stagnation and by Phlegm, hence the patient is depressed and lacks a sense of direction in life.

When, in addition to Qi stagnation, there is Phlegm, this clouds the Mind's orifices and it leads to a certain loss of insight. The person feels confused and bewildered, without being able to pinpoint what the trouble is.

On a physical level, the clinical manifestations are centered around the throat and chest, with a feeling of obstruction of the throat (that comes and goes) and a feeling of tightness of the chest.

Patient's profile

The pattern of Qi stagnation with Phlegm is more common in patients between 35 and 45. It is usually due to sadness, grief, worry or shame.

Treatment principle

Resolve Phlegm, move Qi, eliminate stagnation.

Acupuncture

Points

ST-40 Fenglong, Ren-12 Zhongwan, BL-20 Pishu, SP-9 Yinlingquan, SP-6 Sanyinjiao, P-5 Jianshi, T.B.-6 Zhigou, P-6 Neiguan, LIV-3 Taichong, Ren-17 Shanzhong, Ren-15 Jiuwei, Du-21 Qianding, Du-20 Baihui. All with reducing or even method except for Ren-12 and BL-20, which should be reinforced to tonify the Spleen.

Explanation

- ST-40, Ren-12, BL-20, SP-9 and SP-6 resolve Phlegm. In particular, ST-40 resolves Phlegm and calms the Mind and SP-6 calms the Mind.
- P-5 resolves Phlegm from the Mind and opens the Mind's orifices.
- T.B.-6, P-6, LIV-3 and Ren-17 move Qi and calm the Mind. T.B.-6 is particularly indicated if there is hypochondrial pain.
- Ren-15 and Du-21 open the Mind's orifices and calm the Mind.
- Du-20 lifts mood.

Herbal therapy

Prescription

BAN XIA HOU PO TANG
Pinellia-Magnolia Decoction

Explanation

This formula, from the *Discussion of Cold-Induced Diseases*, is normally used for the plum-stone pattern characterized by a feeling of obstruction in the throat, mental depression and irritability. In modern times, this pattern is related to stagnation of Liver-Qi, for which this formula is used. An analysis of the formula, however, reveals that it contains no herbs that move Liver-Qi or even enter the Liver. The main emphasis of the formula is to move stagnant Heart- and Lung-Qi.

Stagnation of Heart- and Lung-Qi derives from sadness and grief over a long period of time. These emotions first deplete Heart-Qi and Lung-Qi and depress the Mind and Corporeal Soul. The depletion of Lung-Qi from sadness and grief leads to shallow breathing and poor circulation of Qi in the chest and, eventually, to stagnation of Lung-Qi in the chest. The simultaneous weakness and stagnation of Lung-Qi may also lead to Phlegm. The Lung channel influences the throat and its stagnation can cause a feeling of obstruction in the throat.

The person becomes depressed, anxious as well as sad, sighs frequently and has the typical feeling of obstruction in the throat and chest. This is caused by the constriction of the Corporeal Soul in the throat and chest. The chronic stagnation of Heart-Qi obstructs the Mind and causes severe confusion.

Modifications

- Similarly as for stagnation of Liver-Qi, Shi Chang Pu *Rhizoma Acori tatarinowii* and Yuan Zhi *Radix Polygalae* should be added to open the Mind's orifices and He Huan Pi *Cortex Albiziae* to treat depression.
- If there is a pronounced feeling of oppression of the chest from Qi stagnation (slightly Wiry pulse), add Qing Pi *Pericarpium Citri reticulatae viride* and Mu Xiang *Radix Aucklandiae*.
- If there is a feeling of heaviness under the heart, add Zhi Shi *Fructus Aurantii immaturus*.
- If mental restlessness and irritability are pronounced, add Suan Zao Ren *Semen Ziziphi spinosae*.

Prescription

SHI WEI WEN DAN TANG Variation
Ten-Ingredient Warming the Gall-Bladder Decoction Variation

Explanation

This formula is a variation of Wen Dan Tang *Warming the Gall-Bladder Decoction*. Of the original prescription, it preserves the element of resolving Phlegm, but, contrary to it, it does not clear Heat. It moves Qi, eliminates stagnation, opens the Mind's orifices, calms the Mind and relieves depression.

Prescription

SHUN QI DAO TAN TANG Variation
Rectifying Qi and Eliminating Phlegm Decoction Variation

Explanation

This formula resolves Phlegm, moves Qi and subdues rebellious Qi; it resolves Phlegm not only by using herbs that dry up Phlegm but also by using herbs that make Qi flow in the right direction. Shi Chang Pu *Rhizoma Acori tatarinowii* and Yuan Zhi *Radix Polygalae* are added to open the Mind's orifices.

Prescription

YI SHEN NING
Benefiting the Tranquillity of the Spirit Formula

Explanation

This formula moves Liver-Qi, resolves Phlegm, clears Heat and calms the Spirit. According to its modern author Dr Hu Xi Ming, it is specific for menopausal depression.[16]

> **SUMMARY**
>
> **Qi stagnation with Phlegm**
>
> *Points*
>
> ST-40 Fenglong, Ren-12 Zhongwan, BL-20 Pishu, SP-9 Yinlingquan, SP-6 Sanyinjiao, P-5 Jianshi, T.B.-6 Zhigou, P-6 Neiguan, LIV-3 Taichong, Ren-17 Shanzhong, Ren-15 Jiuwei, Du-21 Qianding, Du-20 Baihui. All with reducing or even method except for Du-20, which should be reinforced.
>
> *Herbal therapy*
>
> *Prescriptions*
>
> **BAN XIA HOU PO TANG**
> *Pinellia-Magnolia Decoction*
> **SHI WEI WEN DAN TANG** Variation
> *Ten-Ingredient Warming the Gall-Bladder Decoction* Variation
> **SHUN QI DAO TAN TANG** Variation
> *Rectifying Qi and Eliminating Phlegm Decoction* Variation
> **YI SHEN NING**
> *Benefiting the Tranquillity of the Spirit Formula*

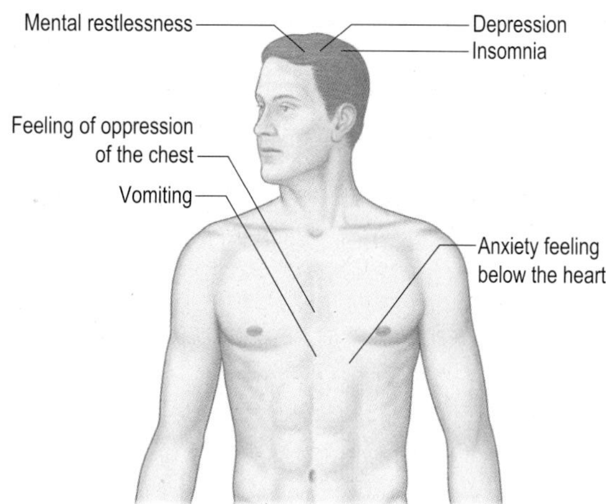

Figure 16.18 Diaphragm Heat.

Diaphragm Heat

Clinical manifestations

Depression, mental restlessness, anxiety feeling below the heart, insomnia, feeling of oppression of the chest, vomiting (Fig. 16.18).

Tongue: yellow coating.

Pulse: Rapid and slightly Wiry.

Pathology and mental-emotional pattern

This pattern occurs in the aftermath of an invasion of exterior Wind-Heat; the exterior Wind-Heat moves into the Interior and changes into Heat. If the patient does not take care, it may give rise to residual Heat in the diaphragm, resulting in depression and the other physical symptoms listed above.

Heat agitates the Mind and the person suffers also from anxiety and insomnia. This pattern occurs only after an invasion of external Wind and it is usually a short-lasting condition. However, if the residual Heat is not cleared, it may also lead to long-term consequences and the patient may suffer from depression for years. This chronic pattern of depression is seen in patients suffering from post-viral fatigue syndrome. Interestingly, Chinese medicine's view of this type of depression (as deriving from external Heat lodged in the diaphragm) cuts through the Western medicine conundrum as to whether chronic fatigue syndrome is "all in the mind" or not.

CLINICAL NOTE

Depression deriving from Diaphragm Heat has a fairly acute onset and is more common in young people and teenagers. It is relatively easy to treat by clearing residual Heat, calming the Mind and lifting mood.

Patient's profile

The pattern of Diaphragm Heat as a cause of depression is more common in teenagers and young people. It is due to residual Heat after a febrile disease but occurring against a pre-existing background of emotional stress and particularly repressed anger or guilt.

Treatment principle

Clear the diaphragm, clear Lung-Heat, calm the Mind.

Acupuncture

Points

T.B.-5 Waiguan, L.I.-11 Quchi, Ren-15 Jiuwei, BL-17 Geshu, Du-9 Zhiyang, P-6 Neiguan, LU-5 Chize. All points with reducing method except P-6 and LU-5, which should be needled with even method.

Explanation

- T.B.-5 and L.I.-11 clear residual Heat.
- Ren-15, BL-17 and Du-9 clear Heat from the diaphragm.
- P-6 lifts mood and clears the diaphragm.
- LU-5 clears Lung-Heat.

Prescription

ZHI ZI CHI TANG
Gardenia-Soja Decoction

Explanation

This is the standard formula to eliminate residual Heat after an invasion of Wind-Heat. It is often modified with the addition of Zhi Shi *Fructus Aurantii immaturus*.

Modifications

- To treat depression, the formula should be modified with the addition of Yuan Zhi *Radix Polygalae* and He Huan Pi *Cortex Albiziae*.

SUMMARY

Diaphragm Heat

Points

T.B.-5 Waiguan, L.I.-11 Quchi, Ren-15 Jiuwei, BL-17 Geshu, Du-9 Zhiyang, P-6 Neiguan, LU-5 Chize. All points with reducing method except P-6 and LU-5, which should be needled with even method.

Herbal therapy

Prescription

ZHI ZI CHI TANG
Gardenia-Soja Decoction

Worry injuring the Mind

Clinical manifestations

Depression, mental confusion, feeling absent, anxiety, no desire to do anything, insomnia, sadness, worry, crying, stretching and yawning (Fig. 16.19).

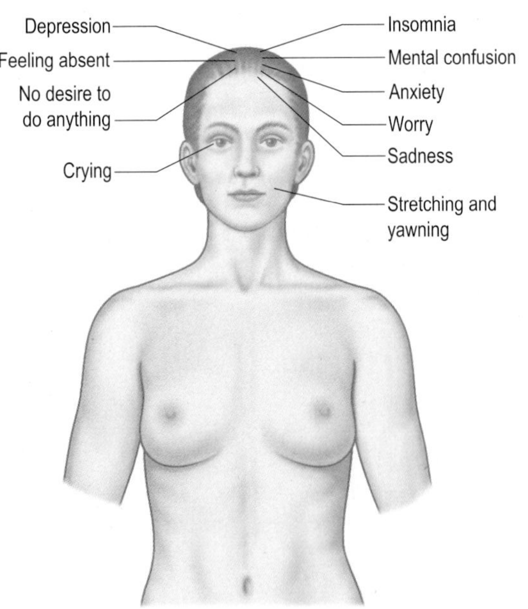

Figure 16.19 Worry injuring the Mind.

Tongue: Pale, sticky-white coating.
Pulse: Fine and very slightly Wiry.

Pathology and mental-emotional pattern

The pattern of "Worry injuring the Mind" is an Empty pattern giving rise to depression. It is caused primarily by worry which knots Qi but also, in the long run, leads to depletion of Qi and Blood. Heart-Blood is the residence of the Mind and, when it is deficient, the Mind is deprived of its residence, resulting in depression, anxiety and insomnia.

The patient presents with characteristic manifestations of Deficiency, i.e. pallor, slow walking, slow speech, sad expression, Weak pulse, etc. The Deficiency makes the patient lacking in drive so that he or she feels unwilling or incapable of doing things.

Patient's profile

The pattern of Worry injuring the Mind is more common in young women.

Treatment principle

Nourish the Heart, calm the Mind.

Acupuncture

Points

LU-9 Taiyuan, LU-3 Tianfu, BL-13 Feishu, Du-12 Shenzhu, Ren-6 Qihai, HE-5 Tongli, ST-36 Zusanli, BL-20 Pishu, BL-49 Yishe, BL-47 Hunmen, Du-20 Baihui.

- Crying: Du-20 and Du-26 (ancient formula).
- Mental dullness due to worry, thinking, shock, fear: Ren-12 Zhongwan, 50 moxa cones (ancient formula).

  All points with reinforcing method.

Explanation

- LU-9, LU-3, BL-13 and Du-12 tonify Lung-Qi and lift mood. LU-3 is a Window of Heaven point.
- Ren-6 tonifies Qi in general.
- HE-5 tonifies Heart-Qi.
- ST-36 and BL-20 tonify Spleen Qi.
- BL-49 tonifies the Intellect (*Yi*) that resides in the Spleen. It is used to brighten the Mind.
- BL-47 stimulates the "coming and going" of the Ethereal Soul.
- Du-20 lifts mood.

Herbal therapy

Prescription

GAN MAI DA ZAO TANG
Glycyrrhiza-Triticum-Jujuba Decoction

Explanation

This ancient formula from the *Essential Prescriptions of the Golden Chest* is specific for mental depression and confusion occurring against a background of Qi deficiency. It is an intriguing formula as it has a profound mental effect and yet it is composed of only three apparently mild herbs, two of which are items of food as well as herbs, i.e. wheat husks (Fu Xiao Mai) and black dates (Da Zao).

Modern Chinese books, which always tend to emphasize Liver-Qi stagnation in mental-emotional problems, say that this formula tonifies Spleen-Qi, nourishes the Heart, calms the Mind and pacifies the Liver through its sweet taste. The explanation is that the sweet taste (taste of the Earth Element) pacifies the Liver (Wood Element). I find this explanation unconvincing and think that this formula is not for Qi stagnation but primarily for Qi and Blood deficiency.

I find this formula excellent when the patient is not only depressed but also mentally confused and kind of "absent". Often, this can be the result of heavy cannabis use in the past. I use this formula when these mental-emotional symptoms occur against a background of deficiency of Qi of the Spleen, Heart and Lungs and of Heart-Blood deficiency.

This formula may also be effective in the treatment of attention deficit disorder and hyperactivity in children.

Modifications

- To treat depression, this formula should be modified with the addition of Yuan Zhi *Radix Polygalae* and He Huan Pi *Cortex Albiziae*.

SUMMARY

Worry injuring the Mind

Points

LU-9 Taiyuan, LU-3 Tianfu, BL-13 Feishu, Du-12 Shenzhu, Ren-6 Qihai, HE-5 Tongli, ST-36 Zusanli, BL-20 Pishu, BL-49 Yishe, BL-47 Hunmen, Du-20 Baihui. All points with reinforcing method.

Herbal therapy

Prescription

GAN MAI DA ZAO TANG

Glycyrrhiza-Triticum-Jujuba Decoction

Heart and Spleen deficiency

Clinical manifestations

Depression, brooding, always thinking, palpitations, timidity, difficulty in falling asleep, pale face, dizziness, poor appetite (Fig. 16.20).

Tongue: Pale.

Pulse: Weak or Choppy.

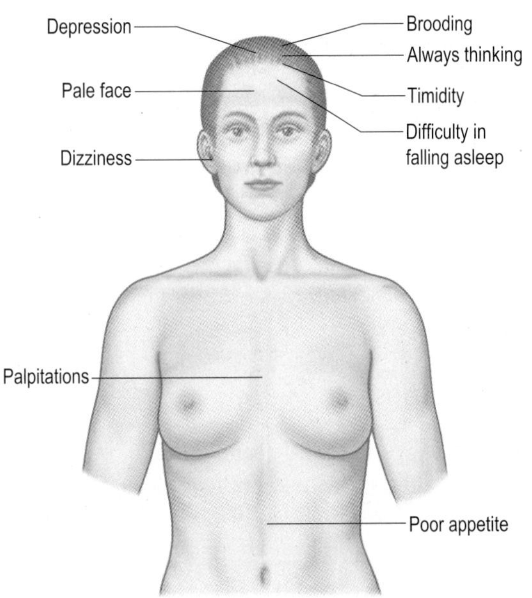

Figure 16.20 Heart and Spleen deficiency.

Pathology and mental-emotional pattern

Heart-Blood is the residence of the Mind and, when it is deficient, the Mind is deprived of its residence, resulting in depression, anxiety and insomnia.

This pattern is characterized by Qi and Blood deficiency, the latter affecting three organs, i.e. the Heart, Spleen and Liver. Heart-Blood houses the Mind and its deficiency causes depression, anxiety and insomnia; Liver-Blood houses the Ethereal Soul and its deficiency causes insomnia and dream-disturbed sleep.

Patient's profile

The pattern of Heart and Spleen deficiency is more common in young women. It is usually caused by sadness and grief.

Treatment principle

Tonify Spleen-Qi, nourish Heart-Blood, calm the Mind.

Acupuncture

Points

ST-36 Zusanli, SP-6 Sanyinjiao, BL-20 Pishu, BL-21 Weishu, Ren-15 Jiuwei, P-6 Neiguan, BL-15 Xinshu, HE-7 Shenmen, Du-14 Dazhui with moxa cones, Du-20 Baihui. All points with reinforcing method.

Explanation

- ST-36, SP-6, BL-20 and BL-21 tonify the Stomach and Spleen and Qi and Blood in general.
- Ren-15, P-6, BL-15 and HE-7 nourish Heart-Blood, calm the Mind and lift mood.
- Du-14 tonifies Heart-Yang (with direct moxa cones).
- Du-20 lifts mood.

Herbal therapy

Prescription

GUI PI TANG

Tonifying the Spleen Decoction

Explanation

This is a widely-used formula that tonifies Spleen-Qi, nourishes Heart-Blood and calms the Mind. As it is a tonic, it also lifts mood and can be used when the patient is depressed and anxious. The tongue is Pale and the pulse is Choppy or Fine.

Prescription

YANG XIN TANG (I)
Nourishing the Heart Decoction

Explanation

This formula is similar to Gui Pi Tang but it differs from it in that it also tonifies Yang (as it contains Rou Gui).

Prescription

BU XIN DAN Variation
Tonifying the Heart Pill Variation

Explanation

The original formula tonifies Qi, nourishes Blood and Yin and calms the Mind. It differs from the previous two in that it also nourishes Yin. Shi Chang Pu *Rhizoma Acori tatarinowii* and He Huan Pi *Cortex Albiziae* open the Mind's orifices and lift mood. The tongue lacks a coating (totally or partially), indicating Yin deficiency.

Table 16.3 compares Gui Pi Tang, Yang Xin Tang and Bu Xin Dan.

SUMMARY

Heart and Spleen deficiency

Points

ST-36 Zusanli, SP-6 Sanyinjiao, BL-20 Pishu, BL-21 Weishu, Ren-15 Jiuwei, P-6 Neiguan, BL-15 Xinshu, HE-7 Shenmen, Du-14 Dazhui with moxa cones, Du-20 Baihui. All points with reinforcing method.

Herbal therapy

Prescriptions

GUI PI TANG
Tonifying the Spleen Decoction
YANG XIN TANG (I)
Nourishing the Heart Decoction
BU XIN DAN Variation
Tonifying the Heart Pill Variation

Heart-Yang deficiency

Clinical manifestations

Depression, feeling cold with desire to curl up, not wanting to do anything, palpitations, tiredness, easily startled (Fig. 16.21).

Tongue: Pale.

Pulse: Weak or Knotted.

Pathology and mental-emotional pattern

The Heart houses the Mind and a deficiency of Yang of the Heart affects the Mind, causing depression. As

Table 16.3 Comparison of Gui Pi Tang, Yang Xin Tang and Bu Xin Dan

	GUI PI TANG	YANG XIN TANG	BU XIN DAN
Patterns	Qi and Blood deficiency of Spleen, Liver and Heart	Qi, Blood and Yang deficiency of Spleen and Heart	Blood and Yin deficiency of Liver and Heart
Emotional symptoms	Depression, insomnia	Depression	Depression, anxiety, insomnia, mental restlessness
Tongue	Pale, teethmarks	Pale	Pale or normal-colored without coating
Pulse	Choppy or Fine	Choppy, Fine, Deep, Slow	Fine

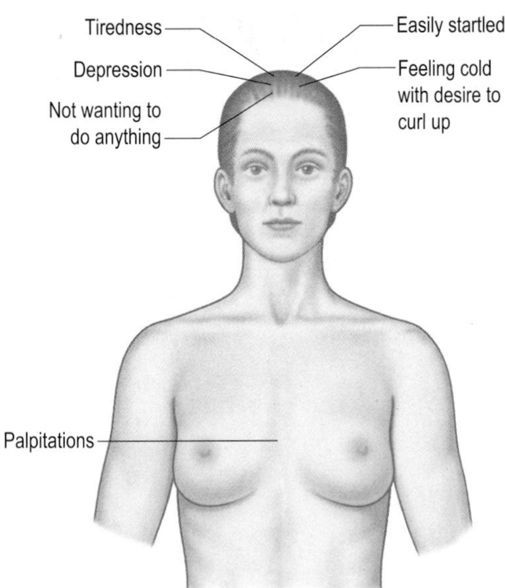

Figure 16.21 Heart-Yang deficiency.

there is Yang deficiency, there is in particular a lack of activity and of drive, so that the patient does not wish to do anything and finds everything a struggle.

Note that, as there is Yang rather than Blood deficiency of the Heart, there is no anxiety or insomnia but a propensity to be startled.

Patient's profile

The pattern of Heart-Yang deficiency is more common in middle-aged or elderly patients.

Treatment principle

Warm and tonify the Heart, calm the Mind, lift mood.

Acupuncture

Points

HE-5 Tongli, Du-14 Dazhui with moxa cones, BL-15 Xinshu, Ren-6 Qihai, ST-36 Zusanli, SP-6 Sanyinjiao, Du-20 Baihui. All points with reinforcing method, moxa should be used.

Explanation

- HE-5, Du-14 and BL-15 tonify Heart-Qi and Heart-Yang.
- Ren-6 tonifies Qi and Yang in general.
- ST-36 and SP-6 tonify Spleen-Qi.
- Du-20 lifts mood.

Herbal therapy

Prescription

ROU FU BAO YUAN TANG
Cinnamomum-Aconitum Preserving the Source Decoction

Explanation

This formula strongly tonifies and warms Heart-Yang; compared to the previous formula, it has a stronger action in tonifying and warming Heart-Yang and a weaker action in calming the Mind. The tongue is very Pale and wet and the pulse is Weak, Deep and Slow.

Prescription

GUI ZHI GAN CAO LONG GU MU LI TANG
Cinnamomum-Glycyrrhiza-Mastodi Ossis fossilia-Concha Ostreae Decoction

Explanation

This formula tonifies Heart-Yang and strongly calms the Mind.

SUMMARY

Heart-Yang deficiency

Points

HE-5 Tongli, Du-14 Dazhui with moxa cones, BL-15 Xinshu, Ren-6 Qihai, ST-36 Zusanli, SP-6 Sanyinjiao, Du-20 Baihui. All points with reinforcing method, moxa should be used.

Herbal therapy

Prescriptions

ROU FU BAO YUAN TANG
Cinnamomum-Aconitum Preserving the Source Decoction.

GUI ZHI GAN CAO LONG GU MU LI TANG
Cinnamomum-Glycyrrhiza-Mastodi Ossis fossilia-Concha Ostreae Decoction

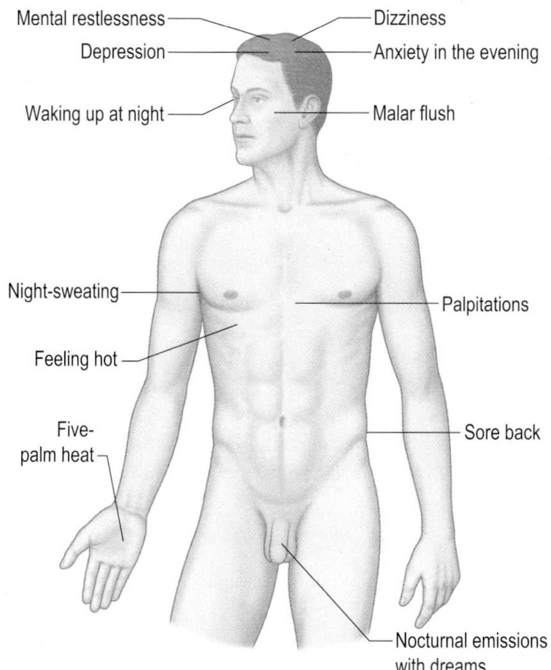

Figure 16.22 Kidney- and Heart-Yin deficiency, Empty Heat blazing.

Kidney- and Heart-Yin deficiency, Empty Heat blazing

Clinical manifestations

Depression, anxiety in the evening, feeling hot, malar flush, dizziness, palpitations, waking up at night, five-palm heat, night-sweating, mental restlessness, nocturnal emissions with dreams, sore back (Fig. 16.22).

Tongue: Red without coating.

Pulse: Floating-Empty or Fine and very slightly Wiry.

Pathology and mental-emotional pattern

This pattern is characterized by deficiency of Yin of the Kidneys and Heart and by Empty Heat of the Heart. The deficiency of Yin of the Kidneys leads to Empty Heat, which blazes upwards to affect the Heart.

This combination of patterns is more common in the middle-aged or elderly. The deficiency of Yin itself causes the patient to become depressed, while the Empty Heat harasses the Mind and the Ethereal Soul, causing the person to become anxious and restless.

An important sign for this combination of patterns is a Red tongue without coating.

!

Remember: it is the lack of coating (and not its redness) on the tongue that indicates Yin deficiency. A tongue without coating indicates Yin deficiency; a Red tongue without coating indicates Yin deficiency with Empty Heat.

Patient's profile

The pattern of Heart- and Kidney-Yin deficiency with Heart Empty Heat is more common in middle-aged or elderly patients. It is usually due to worry, fear, sadness, guilt or grief.

Treatment principle

Nourish Kidney- and Heart-Yin, clear Heart Empty Heat, calm the Mind, lift mood.

Acupuncture

Points

KI-3 Taixi, KI-6 Zhaohai, SP-6 Sanyinjiao, KI-2 Rangu, KI-9 Zhubin, BL-52 Zhishi, HE-6 Yinxi, P-7 Daling, Du-24 Shenting, Du-19 Houding, Ren-15 Jiuwei. Reinforcing method on all points except KI-2, HE-6 and P-7, which should be needled with even method.

Explanation

- KI-3, KI-6 and SP-6 nourish Kidney-Yin.
- KI-2 clears Empty Heat.
- KI-9 nourishes Kidney-Yin and calms the Mind.
- HE-6 and P-7 clear Heart Empty Heat.
- Du-24, Du-19 and Ren-15 calm the Mind.

Herbal therapy

Prescription

ZI SHUI QING GAN YIN
Nourishing Water and Clearing the Liver Decoction

Explanation

This formula nourishes Kidney-Yin and clears Liver-Heat. It is indicated for patients suffering from depression and irritability.

Prescription

TIAN WANG BU XIN DAN
Heavenly Emperor Tonifying the Heart Pill

Explanation

This prescription nourishes Kidney- and Heart-Yin, clears Heart Empty Heat and calms the Mind. The tongue is Red without coating.

Prescription

JIE FAN YI XIN TANG
Calming Mental Restlessness and Benefiting the Heart Decoction

Explanation

This prescription nourishes Yin and calms the Mind but it also tonifies Qi.

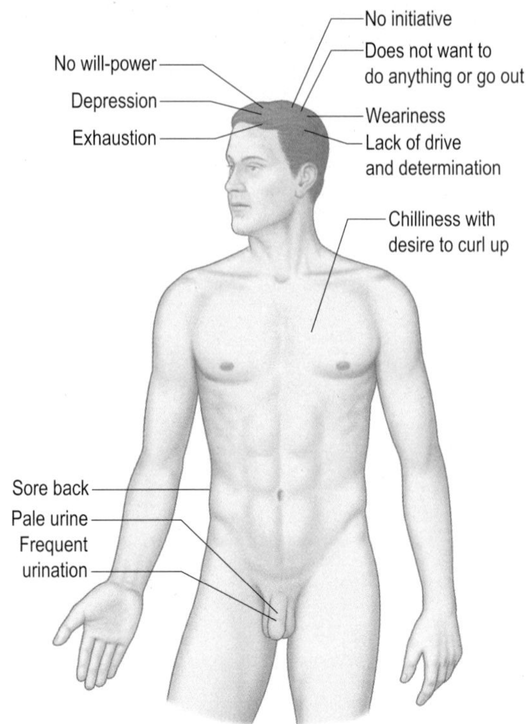

Figure 16.23 Kidney-Yang deficiency.

SUMMARY

Kidney- and Heart-Yin deficiency, Empty Heat blazing

Points

KI-3 Taixi, KI-6 Zhaohai, SP-6 Sanyinjiao, KI-2 Rangu, KI-9 Zhubin, BL-52 Zhishi, HE-6 Yinxi, P-7 Daling, Du-24 Shenting, Du-19 Houding, Ren-15 Jiuwei. Reinforcing method on all points except KI-2, HE-6 and P-7, which should be needled with even method.

Herbal therapy

Prescriptions

ZI SHUI QING GAN YIN
Nourishing Water and Clearing the Liver Decoction
TIAN WANG BU XIN DAN
Heavenly Emperor Tonifying the Heart Pill
JIE FAN YI XIN TANG
Calming Mental Restlessness and Benefiting the Heart Decoction

Kidney-Yang deficiency

Clinical manifestations

Depression, exhaustion, does not want to do anything or go out, weariness, chilliness with desire to curl up, sore back, frequent urination, pale urine, no will-power, no initiative, lack of drive and determination (Fig. 16.23).

Tongue: very Pale, wet.

Pulse: Weak-Deep-Slow.

Pathology and mental-emotional pattern

The Kidneys house the Will-Power (*Zhi*). "Will-power", as a translation of *Zhi*, includes will-power itself, drive, determination, steadfastness and physical and mental power. As Yang implies activity and movements towards the outside, in this pattern of Kidney-Yang deficiency there is a lack of drive, determination and initiative. The person is deeply depressed, lacks enthusiasm and is unable to find the drive to do anything.

> **CLINICAL NOTE**
>
> Depression occurring against a background of Kidney-Yang deficiency is particularly characterized by a weakness of the Kidney's Will-Power (*Zhi*) and therefore lack of drive and initiative.

Patient's profile

The pattern of Kidney-Yang deficiency is more common in middle-aged patients. It is due to worry, sadness, grief or fear.

Treatment principle

Tonify and warm the Kidneys.

Acupuncture

Points

KI-7 Fuliu, KI-3 Taixi, Ren-4 Guanyuan with moxa cones, Du-4 Mingmen, BL-23 Shenshu, BL-52 Zhishi, BL-47 Hunmen, Du-20 Baihui. All points with reinforcing method. Moxa should be used.

Explanation

- KI-7 tonifies Kidney-Yang.
- KI-3, Source point, tonifies the Kidneys.
- Ren-4, with moxa cones, tonifies Kidney-Yang and the Original Qi.
- Du-4 tonifies Kidney-Yang and warms the Fire of the Gate of Life.
- BL-23 tonifies Kidney-Yang.
- BL-52 and BL-47 in combination, strengthen drive, determination and will-power and stimulate the "coming and going" of the Ethereal Soul.
- Du-20 lifts mood.

Herbal therapy

Prescription

YOU GUI WAN
Restoring the Right [Kidney] *Pill*

Explanation

This formula from Zhang Jing Yue (1624) tonifies Kidney-Yang. This is my preferred formula to tonify Kidney-Yang because it is balanced by the presence of Kidney-Yin tonics (Gou Qi Zi *Fructus Lycii chinensis* and Shan Zhu Yu *Fructus Corni*).

Prescription

JIN GUI SHEN QI WAN
Golden Chest Kidney-Qi Pill

Explanation

This well-known formula from Zhang Zhong Jing (*c.*AD 200) tonifies Kidney-Yang.

Prescription

NAN GENG TANG
Male Menopause Decoction

Explanation

This formula tonifies Kidney-Yang, nourishes the Kidney-Essence and clears Empty Heat. It can be modified to enhance its Yang or Yin tonifying effect. It is reported by the modern book *Great Treatise of Secret Formulae in Chinese Medicine* as a specific formula for depression in elderly men.[17]

Modifications

- To treat Liver-Qi stagnation, add Xiang Fu *Rhizoma Cyperi* and Chai Hu *Radix Bupleuri*.
- To enhance the tonification of Kidney-Yang, add Lu Jiao *Cornu Cervi*.
- To enhance the tonification of Kidney-Yin, add Gou Qi Zi *Fructus Lycii chinensis*.
- To treat insomnia, add Suan Zao Ren *Semen Ziziphi spinosae* and Ye Jiao Teng *Caulis Polygoni multiflori*.

> **SUMMARY**
>
> **Kidney-Yang deficiency**
>
> *Points*
>
> KI-7 Fuliu, KI-3 Taixi, Ren-4 Guanyuan with moxa cones, Du-4 Mingmen, BL-23 Shenshu, BL-52

Zhishi, BL-47 Hunmen, Du-20 Baihui. All points with reinforcing method. Moxa should be used.

Herbal therapy

Prescriptions

YOU GUI WAN
Restoring the Right [Kidney] *Pill*
JIN GUI SHEN QI WAN
Golden Chest Kidney-Qi Pill
NAN GENG TANG
Male Menopause Decoction

ACUPUNCTURE POINTS FOR DEPRESSION

I am going to discuss various acupuncture points that I may use for depression without categorizing them according to a pattern as we do for herbs or formulae. There are important differences between the mode of action of acupuncture and that of herbal medicine. For example, to treat depression deriving from Liver-Qi stagnation, one naturally uses a formula from the category of formulae for Qi stagnation; to treat depression from Spleen- and Heart-Blood deficiency, one naturally uses a formula from the category of formulae for Blood deficiency.

Although this approach may be followed also for acupuncture points and point prescriptions, acupuncture works in a different way from herbal medicine. Acupuncture points are not as closely related to patterns as herbs are. For example, a herb from the moving-Qi category (e.g. Xiang Fu *Rhizoma Cyperi*) cannot nourish Blood. By contrast, an acupuncture point such as LIV-3 Taichong can be used to move Liver-Qi but it can also be used to nourish Liver-Blood (as it is the Source point).

As for Qi stagnation, it is indeed my opinion that *every* acupuncture point moves Qi; by the very nature of Qi and of the channels, one cannot insert a needle in a channel *without* moving Qi (and Blood). This is a very useful characteristic of acupuncture compared to herbal medicine. In fact, with herbal medicine, if we use a formula to nourish Blood, this contains herbs that are "sticky" in nature and that may have the tendency to give rise to some Qi stagnation; for this reason, it may be a good idea to add one or two herbs to move Qi (that is why Gui Pi Tang *Tonifying the Spleen Decoction* has Mu Xiang *Radix Aucklandiae*). By contrast, when we use acupuncture to nourish Blood with points such as ST-36 Zusanli, SP-6 Sanyinjiao and LIV-8 Ququan, there is no danger of these points giving rise to Qi stagnation because they automatically also move Qi.

Finally, as explained in Chapter 8, I use acupuncture points to "nourish the Mind" in general; in this case, I use the term "nourishing the Mind" in a general sense and not as a specific treatment technique. In other words, the Mind may be "nourished" whether Heart-Blood is deficient (an Empty condition) or if there is Heart-Fire (a Full condition). Nourishing the Mind is necessary because the Mind plays a unifying, controlling and integrating function towards the other "four *shen*", i.e. the Ethereal Soul, Corporeal Soul, Intellect and Will-Power.

Lung channel

LU-3 Tianfu

The actions and indications of this point are closely related to its being a Window of Heaven point. One of the characteristics of these points is that they regulate the ascending and descending of Qi from the body to and from the head; they do so in the crucial neck area (the gateway between the body and the head). Therefore, they can both subdue rebellious Qi and promote the ascending of clear Qi to the head (Fig. 16.24).

On a psychic level, this point's action in regulating the ascending and descending of Qi to and from the head has a mental-emotional effect. For example, insomnia is due to Qi ascending too much to the head (or not descending from it), while somnolence and forgetfulness are due to clear Qi not ascending to the head.

The *Explanation of the Acupuncture Points* says that LU-3 can make Qi rise to treat forgetfulness, sadness and weeping due to Qi not rising to the head.[18] Forgetfulness is an important indication for this point: this is forgetfulness due to clear Qi not rising to the head. According to the *Explanation of the Acupuncture Points*, this point treats forgetfulness by stimulating the ascending of Qi of both the Lungs and Heart.[19]

Finally, "talking to ghosts" features heavily in this point's indications. Generally speaking, when ancient books mention such symptoms as talking or seeing ghosts among the indications of a point, it means that the point is indicated for relatively serious mental-emotional problems and, in particular, when the Mind

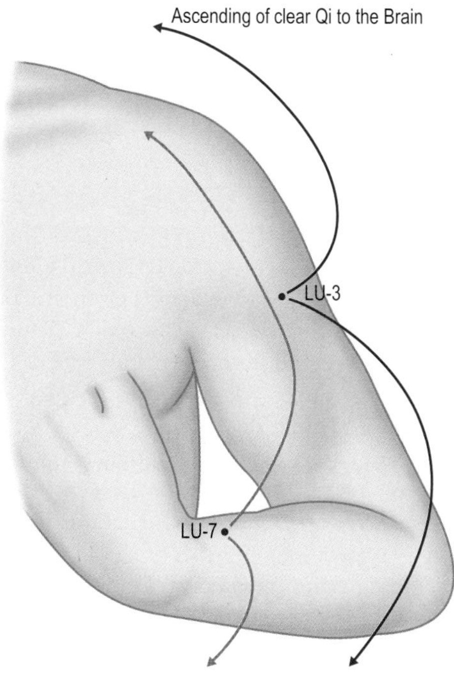

Figure 16.24 Effect of LU-7 Lieque and LU-3 Tianfu.

is obstructed. Obstruction of the Mind can potentially cause serious mental problems such as manic-depression or psychosis.

Again, this point can open the Mind's orifices, i.e. de-obstruct the Mind by regulating the ascending and descending of Qi to and from the head; it opens the Mind's orifices by promoting the descending of turbid Qi from the head and the ascending of clear Qi to the head.

LU-7 Lieque

LU-7 brings clear Qi up to the head and promotes the descending of turbid Qi from the head (Fig. 16.24). On a physical level, this means that LU-7 can treat problems of the nose and sinuses. On a psychic level, it clears the Mind and lifts mood. I use it for most types of depression, whatever the pattern involved, but especially when there is stagnation of Lung-Qi.

Large Intestine channel

L.I.-4 Hegu

In my experience, L.I.-4 has a strong influence on the Mind and can be used to soothe the Mind and allay anxiety, particularly if combined with LIV-3 Taichong and with Du-24 Shenting and G.B.-13 Benshen. I use this combination in depression accompanied by anxiety.

Stomach channel

ST-36 Zusanli

ST-36 has a powerful tonic action and, on the psychic level, it lifts mood in patients who are depressed against a background of Qi and Blood deficiency.

ST-40 Fenglong

ST-40 has a long history of use for mental-emotional conditions; it is especially indicated to open the Mind's orifices in persons tending to manic behavior.

This point has a profound "calming the Mind" action and I use it frequently in patients who are depressed and anxious.

The Phlegm-resolving of this point should not be overemphasized, overlooking its other functions. Apart from its use to resolve Phlegm, ST-40 can also be used to subdue rebellious Qi of the Stomach and Lungs when the person is very anxious, and the anxiety reflects on the Stomach function, with such symptoms as tightness of the epigastrium, a feeling of a knot in the Stomach or, as some people say, a feeling of "butterflies in the stomach" (Fig. 16.25).

Apart from the epigastrium, ST-40 also has an action on the chest; it relaxes and "opens" the chest, both from a physical point of view when it is obstructed by Phlegm, and from a psychic point of view when Qi stagnates in the chest from emotional problems.

CLINICAL NOTE

ST-40 Fenglong

The Phlegm-resolving effect of ST-40 should not be overemphasized. This point has many other actions:

- it calms the Mind
- it opens the Mind's orifices
- it treats all Full conditions of the Stomach
- it subdues rebellious Stomach-Qi
- it treats the epigastrium
- it opens the chest and makes Lung-Qi descend when the chest is obstructed by Phlegm
- it relaxes and opens the chest when Qi stagnates here from emotional problems.

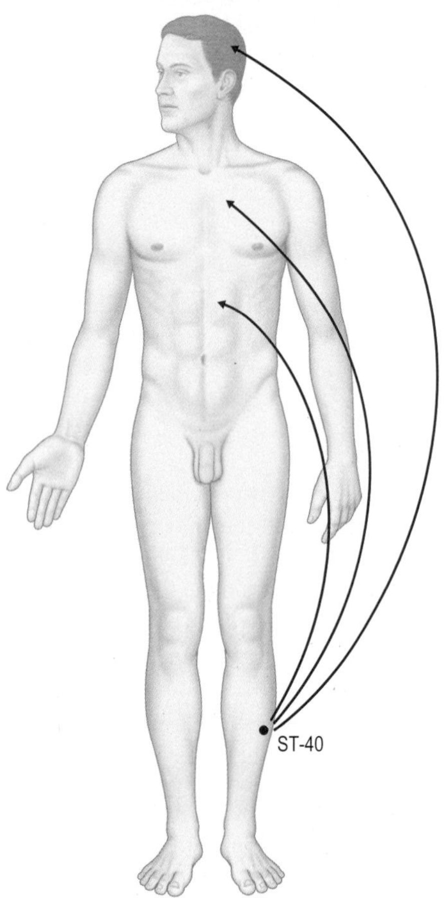

Figure 16.25 Effect of ST-40 Fenglong.

Spleen channel

SP-6 Sanyinjiao

From the emotional point of view, it helps to smooth Liver-Qi to calm the Mind and allay irritability. It can therefore be used in depression occurring against a background of Liver-Qi stagnation.

However, from the mental-emotional point of view, SP-6 has a wide range of actions. It can calm the Mind and is often used for insomnia, particularly if from Blood or Yin deficiency. In particular, it is used for Spleen- and Heart-Blood deficiency, when the Spleen is not making enough Blood, the Heart is not supplied with enough Blood and the Mind lacks residence and floats at night, so that insomnia ensues.

SP-6 is the point to use in this case as it will simultaneously tonify the Spleen, nourish Blood and calm the Mind. If such a comparison could be made, this action is comparable to that of the formula Gui Pi Tang *Tonifying the Spleen Decoction.*

Heart channel

HE-5 Tongli

I use HE-5 as the main point to tonify Heart-Qi and Heart-Blood and it is therefore my point of choice for depression occurring against a background of Qi and Blood deficiency. Its indications include sadness, mental restlessness, anger, fright, depression, agitation, palpitations and weak Heart-Qi.

My use of HE-5 in depression is also connected to this point's nature of Connecting (*Luo*) point. As a Connecting point, it moves Qi and removes obstructions in the channel; on a psychic level, this means that it can lift mood and stimulate the "coming and going" of the Ethereal Soul.

HE-7 Shenmen

I use HE-7 as a point to both lift mood in depression and calm the Mind in anxiety. Its indications include insomnia, poor memory, manic-depression, inappropriate laughter, shouting at people, sadness, fear, mental restlessness, agitation and palpitations.

HE-7 primarily nourishes Heart-Blood and is the point of choice for Heart-Blood deficiency causing the Mind to be deprived of its "residence", resulting in anxiety, insomnia, poor memory, palpitations and a Pale tongue. Again, this action could be compared to that of Gui Pi Tang *Tonifying the Spleen Decoction*. Indeed, the combination of the two points SP-6 mentioned above and HE-7 closely resembles the action of Gui Pi Tang.

I use HE-7 frequently to "nourish" the Mind in the general sense outlined above, irrespective of patterns (e.g. Heart-Blood deficiency, Heart-Heat).

Bladder channel

BL-15 Xinshu

Indications for this point include anxiety, weeping, fright, insomnia, excessive dreaming, manic-depression, disorientation, delayed speech development, poor memory, poor concentration and mental confusion.

I use BL-15 to tonify Heart-Qi and Heart-Blood in depression occurring against a background of Qi and Blood deficiency.

BL-42 Pohu

The indications of this point include sadness, grief, feeling of oppression of the chest, depression, suicidal thoughts and "three corpses flowing".

On a psychological level, BL-42 is related to the Corporeal Soul (*Po*), which is the mental-spiritual aspect residing in the Lungs. It strengthens and roots the Corporeal Soul in the Lungs. It frees breathing when the Corporeal Soul is constricted by worry, sadness or grief.

It is therefore used for emotional problems related to the Lungs, particularly sadness, grief and worry. It has a very soothing effect on the spirit and it nourishes Qi when this is dispersed by a prolonged period of depression, sadness or grief.

The *Explanation of the Acupuncture Points* reports the interesting indication "three corpses flowing" for this point.[20] The association with corpses and death should be interpreted in the way that this point is indicated for suicidal thought.

Because of the connection between the Corporeal Soul and death, points associated with the Corporeal Soul (such as BL-13 Feishu and BL-42 Pohu) are indicated for suicidal thoughts.

BL-44 Shentang

Indications for this point include depression, insomnia, anxiety, mental restlessness, sadness, grief and worry.

BL-44 is mostly used for emotional and psychological problems related to the Heart. It is best used in conjunction with BL-15 Xinshu for anxiety, insomnia and depression. BL-44 strengthens and calms the Mind. It stimulates the Mind's clarity and intelligence.

BL-47 Hunmen

Indications for this point include fear, depression, insomnia, excessive dreaming, lack of sense of direction in life and "possession by corpse".[21]

BL-47 is used for emotional problems related to the Liver, such as depression, frustration and resentment over a long period of time. This point settles and roots the Ethereal Soul in the Liver. It strengthens the Ethereal Soul's capacity of planning, sense of aim in life, life dreams and projects. It is a "door", so this point regulates the "coming and going" of the Ethereal Soul and Mind, i.e. relationships with other people and the world in general. It has an outward movement that could be compared and contrasted with the inward movement of BL-42 Pohu.

The *Explanation of Acupuncture Points* (1654) confirms that, due to this point's nature of "window", "gate" or "door", the Ethereal Soul goes in and out through it. This confirms the dynamic nature of this point in stimulating the movement of the Ethereal Soul and Mind; however, it can also work the other way, i.e. to calm down the excessive movement of the Ethereal Soul.

In my experience, when used in conjunction with BL-18 Ganshu, it has a profound influence on a person's capacity of planning his or her life by rooting and steadying the Ethereal Soul. It can help a person find a sense of direction and purpose in life. This point will also help to lift mental depression associated with such difficulties.

BL-52 Zhishi

Indications for this point include depression, lack of motivation, lack of drive and lack of will-power.

This point strengthens will-power and determination, which are the mental-spiritual phenomena pertaining to the Kidneys. It is a very useful point in the treatment of certain types of depression, when the person lacks motivation and drive and lacks the will-power and mental strength to make an effort to get out of the spiral of depression. Needling this point with reinforcing method, especially if combined with BL-23, will stimulate the will-power and lift the spirit.

BL-52 strengthens will-power, drive, determination, the capacity of pursuing one's goals with single-mindedness, spirit of initiative and steadfastness. I often use this point if there is a Kidney deficiency, in combination with one of the other four points affecting the Spiritual Aspects of the Yin organs, i.e. BL-42 Pohu, BL-44 Shentang, BL-47 Hunmen and BL-49 Yishe, as a solid mental-emotional foundation for the other aspects of the psyche.

In particular, for depression I use the following combination:

- BL-23 Shenshu, BL-52 Zhishi and BL-47 Hunmen to strengthen will-power and drive, and to instill a sense of direction and aim in one's life. This combination is excellent to treat the mental exhaustion, lack of drive and aimlessness and confusion that are typical of chronic depression.

If we analyze the names of the above five points we get the following pattern.

- BL-42 Pohu (*hu* means "window") = "Window of Po"
- BL-44 Shentang (*tang* means "hall") = "Hall of Shen"
- BL-47 Hunmen (*men* means "door") = "Door of Hun"
- BL-49 Yishe (*she* means "abode") = "Abode of Yi"
- BL-52 Zhishi (*shi* means "room") = "Room of Zhi" (*see Fig. 13.9*)

We can detect a pattern as the points correspond to a house – an image for the psyche – with the Mind (*Shen*), Will-Power (*Zhi*) and Intellect (*Yi*) corresponding to "hall", "room" and "abode", respectively, and the Ethereal Soul (*Hun*) and Corporeal Soul (*Po*) corresponding to a "door" and "window", respectively.

The images of door and window fit well the nature of the Ethereal Soul and Corporeal Soul which provide movement to the psyche, the former providing the "coming and going of the Mind" and the latter the "entering and exiting of the Essence". For this reason, BL-47 Hunmen is particularly important in the treatment of depression.

Kidney channel

KI-3 Taixi

KI-3 is the Source (*Yuan*) point of the Kidney channel and it is the best point to tonify the Kidneys. I use this point in depression from a Kidney deficiency to strengthen the will-power, drive and initiative.

KI-9 Zhubin

Indications for this point include anxiety, insomnia, palpitations and manic behavior. KI-9 is an excellent point to calm the Mind in cases of deep anxiety and mental restlessness deriving from Kidney-Yin deficiency.

It also relaxes any tension or feeling of oppression felt in the chest, often with palpitations. Because it tonifies Kidney-Yin, calms the Mind and treats palpitations, this point is particularly indicated in the pattern of "Heart and Kidneys not harmonized".

It is the starting point of the Yin Linking Vessel (*Yin Wei Mai*) and its mental-emotional effect is largely due to this. The Yin Linking Vessel nourishes Heart-Blood and calms the Mind.

Pericardium channel

P-6 Neiguan

P-6 is an extremely important point for depression. It is always used in modern China for mental depression.

P-6 helps depression in different ways which are related to its different connections. First, P-6 affects the Mind and therefore the Heart. The Heart is more Yin, it governs Blood which houses the Mind. The Pericardium is more Yang, and it controls movement of Qi on a mental-emotional level. This effect on Qi is due also to its relationship with the Liver within the Terminal Yin (*Jue Yin*).

P-6 treats especially depression deriving from Liver-Qi stagnation in two ways. First, it moves Liver-Qi due to its connection with the Liver channel within the Terminal Yin (*Jue Yin*) channels. Being connected to the Liver and moving Qi, P-6 is an important point to stimulate the movement of the Ethereal Soul. Second, it treats the Mind (*Shen*) due to its close connection with the Heart. Finally, P-6 has a synergistic effect on acupuncture point prescriptions. The addition of P-6 to any prescription increases the therapeutic effect.

Indications for this point include insomnia, manic behavior, poor memory, anxiety, fright, sadness and depression.

Triple Burner channel

T.B.-3 Zhongzhu

In my experience, T.B.-3 moves Qi and eliminates stagnation. Due to its relationship with the Gall-Bladder (within the Lesser Yang), and between this latter organ and the Liver, T.B.-3 indirectly affects the Liver, so that it can be used to eliminate stagnation of Liver-Qi manifesting with hypochondrial pain, depression and mood swings.

On a psychological level, it moves Qi and lifts depression deriving from stagnation of Liver-Qi, particularly in combination with Du-20 Baihui. It is extremely effective in lifting the Mind when a person is depressed.

Gall-Bladder channel

G.B.-13 Benshen

G.B.-13 is a very important point for mental and emotional problems. Combined with HE-5 Tongli and G.B.-38 Yangfu, it is used in China in psychiatric practice for schizophrenia and split personality.[22] It is also indicated when the person has persistent and unreasonable feelings of jealousy and suspicion.

Apart from these mental traits, it has a powerful effect in calming the Mind and relieving anxiety deriving from constant worry and fixed thoughts. Its effect is enhanced if it is combined with Du-24 Shenting.

However, apart from anxiety, G.B.-13 can also be used for depression. In fact, its deep mental and emotional effect is due to its action of "gathering" Essence to the head. The Kidney-Essence is the root of our Pre-Heaven Qi and is the foundation for our mental and emotional life. A strong Essence is the fundamental prerequisite for a clear Mind (*Shen*) and a balanced emotional life. This is the meaning of this point's name "Root of the Mind", i.e. this point gathers the Essence which is the root of the Mind (*Shen*). The Kidney-Essence is the source of Marrow which fills up the Brain (called Sea of Marrow); G.B.-13 is a point where Essence and Marrow "gather".

The *Great Dictionary of Acupuncture* says that this point "*makes the Mind [Shen] return to its root*";[23] the "root" of the Mind is the Essence, hence this point "gathers" the Essence to the Brain and affects the Mind. As it connects the Mind and the Essence, it also treats both the Heart and the Kidneys and therefore the Mind (*Shen*) and Will-Power (*Zhi*); for this reason, it is an important point in the treatment of depression.

When combined with other points to nourish Essence (such as Ren-4 Guanyuan), G.B.-13 attracts Essence towards the head, with the effect of calming the Mind and strengthening clarity of mind, memory and willpower. The connection between G.B.-13 and the Essence is confirmed by the text *An Enquiry into Chinese Acupuncture*, which has among the indications of this point: "*excessive menstrual bleeding, impotence and seminal emissions*".[24]

Liver channel

LIV-3 Taichong

LIV-3 is a major point for depression deriving from stagnation of Liver-Qi. It moves Liver-Qi, stimulates the "coming and going" of the Ethereal Soul in depression and also calms the Mind.

It has a particularly calming effect when it is combined with L.I.-4 Hegu.

Governing Vessel

Du-4 Mingmen

Du-4 tonifies the Fire of the Gate of Life (*Ming Men*) and Kidney-Yang. As this is the sea of Will-Power (*Zhi*), this point strongly tonifies the will-power, drive and determination in patients who suffer from depression. However, please note that this point should be used only in the presence of Kidney-Yang deficiency.

Du-11 Shendao

Indications for this point include sadness, anxiety, poor memory, palpitations, disorientation and timidity.

Du-11 is on the same level as BL-15 Xinshu, the Back-Transporting point of the Heart, and its action mostly extends to the Heart. It nourishes the Heart and calms the Mind, and therefore treats depression, sadness and anxiety.

Du-12 Shenzhu

Indications for this point include agitation, mad walking, delirious raving, seeing ghosts and rage with desire to kill people.

This point is indicated for manic behavior and morbid thoughts of death, for conditions in which the Ethereal Soul comes and goes too much. It settles the Corporeal Soul. This point should be seen in conjunction with BL-13 Feishu and BL-42 Pohu.

Please note that the *shen* in this point's name means "body" and not the *shen* that means "Mind" as in the previous point Du-11 Shendao.

Du-14 Dazhui

This point strengthens the Heart, tonifies Yang, strengthens the Will-Power (*Zhi*) and tonifies Heart-

and Kidney-Yang. It is very effective for depression, lack of will-power and drive, with the Ethereal Soul not coming and going enough.

Du-16 Fengfu

Indications for this point include manic behavior, incessant talking, mad walking, desire to commit suicide, sadness and fear.

I use this point for depression and anxiety with morbid thoughts of death.

Du-19 Houding

Indications for this point include mad walking and insomnia. This point calms the Mind and nourishes the Heart and is good for sadness and depression. It is good combined with Ren-15 Jiuwei.

Du-20 Baihui

I use Du-20 in many cases of depression deriving from various patterns, whether Full or Empty, to lift Qi; on a psychic level, lifting Qi has the effect of lifting mood.

This point's lifting action on Yang has a mental effect in that it promotes the rise of clear Yang to the Brain and the Mind. In my experience, Du-20 has a powerful effect in lifting depression and clearing the mind.

The only situation when the use of Du-20 might be contraindicated is when there is Heat (whether Full or Empty) blazing upwards.

Du-24 Shenting

An important feature of this point which makes it particularly useful in mental-emotional problems is that it can both calm and lift the Mind; therefore it is used not only for anxiety and insomnia but also for depression and sadness. It is also used in psychiatric practice for schizophrenia and split thoughts.[25]

The name of this point refers to its strong influence on the Mind and Spirit. The courtyard was traditionally considered to be a very important part of the house as it was the one that gave the first impression to visitors; it is the entrance. Thus, this point could be said to be the "entrance" to the Mind and Spirit, and its being a courtyard highlights its importance.

Indications for this point include manic-depression, depression, anxiety, poor memory and insomnia.

Directing Vessel

Ren-4 Guanyuan

I use Ren-4 frequently to tonify the Kidneys and the Will-Power in patients suffering from depression. In Kidney deficiency, I tend to use Ren-4 more than Du-4 as the former has a more balanced effect. In fact, it can tonify Kidney-Yang with direct moxa cones, but, with needling, it also nourishes Blood and tonifies the Original (*Yuan*) Qi.

Ren-4 can calm the Mind (*Shen*) and settle the Ethereal Soul (*Hun*) by nourishing Blood and Yin. It can strengthen the Lower Burner in persons who are very anxious, especially if such anxiety derives from Yin deficiency. This point tonifies the Qi of the Lower Burner, thus rooting Qi downwards and subduing the rising of Qi to the head, which happens in severe anxiety. In this way it has a powerful calming effect.

Ren-4 can root the Ethereal Soul and can be used for a vague feeling of fear at night which is said to be due to the floating of the Ethereal Soul.

Ren-15 Jiuwei

I use Ren-15 very frequently to nourish the Heart, calm the Mind and lift mood. I prefer this point to Ren-14 Juque. This point nourishes all Yin organs and it calms the Mind, particularly in Deficiency of Yin and/or Blood. It has a very powerful calming action in severe anxiety, worry, emotional upsets, fears or obsessions. Although its indications show that it can be used to open the Mind's orifices in serious mental conditions from a Full condition, I personally use this point in mental-emotional states occurring against a background of deficiency of Blood or Yin.

Indications for this point include manic-depression, palpitations, anxiety and insomnia.

SUMMARY

Acupuncture points for depression

LU-3 Tianfu

Regulates the ascending and descending of Qi to and from the head (forgetfulness, sadness and weeping due to Qi not rising to head, "talking to ghosts"), opens the Mind's orifices.

LU-7 Lieque

Brings clear Qi up to the head and promotes the descending of turbid Qi from the head.

L.I.-4 Hegu

Soothes the Mind and allays anxiety.

ST-36 Zusanli

ST-36 lifts mood in patients who are depressed against a background of Qi and Blood deficiency.

ST-40 Fenglong

Opens the Mind's orifices, calms the Mind, resolves Phlegm, restores the descending of Qi, opens the chest.

SP-6 Sanyinjiao

Smoothes Liver-Qi to calm the Mind and allay irritability, nourishes Blood and Yin to treat insomnia.

HE-5 Tongli

Tonifies Heart-Qi and Heart-Blood and lifts depression, stimulates the movement of the Ethereal Soul.

HE-7 Shenmen

Nourishes Heart-Blood and calms the Mind.

BL-15 Xinshu

Tonifies Heart-Qi and Heart-Blood in depression occurring against a background of Qi and Blood deficiency.

BL-42 Pohu

Strengthens and roots the Corporeal Soul in the Lungs. It frees breathing when the Corporeal Soul is constricted by worry, sadness or grief.

BL-44 Shentang

BL-44 is used for emotional and psychological problems related to the Heart. It is best used in conjunction with BL-15 Xinshu for anxiety, insomnia and depression. BL-44 strengthens and calms the Mind. It stimulates the Mind's clarity and intelligence.

BL-47 Hunmen

BL-47 is used for emotional problems related to the Liver, such as depression, frustration and resentment over a long period of time. This point settles and roots the Ethereal Soul in the Liver. It strengthens the Ethereal Soul's capacity of planning, sense of aim in life, life dreams and projects. It is a "door", so this point regulates the "coming and going" of the Ethereal Soul and Mind.

BL-52 Zhishi

Strengthens will-power and determination in depression.

KI-3 Taixi

KI-3 tonifies the Kidneys to strengthen will-power, drive and initiative.

KI-9 Zhubin

Tonifies Kidney-Yin, calms the Mind and treats palpitations.

P-6 Neiguan

Moves Liver-Qi, stimulates the movement of the Ethereal Soul.

T.B.-3 Zhongzhu

Moves Qi and eliminates stagnation.

G.B.-13 Benshen

For mental and emotional problems related to a Liver disharmony. Calms the Mind and settles the Ethereal Soul, gathers Essence to the Brain and Mind, connects Heart and Kidneys.

LIV-3 Taichong

Moves Liver-Qi, stimulates the "coming and going" of the Ethereal Soul in depression and calms the Mind.

Du-4 Mingmen

Du-4 tonifies the Fire of the Gate of Life (*Ming Men*) and Kidney-Yang and strengthens will-power in depression.

Du-11 Shendao

Nourishes the Heart and calms the Mind, and therefore treats depression, sadness and anxiety.

Du-12 Shenzhu

For manic behavior and morbid thoughts of death, for conditions in which the Ethereal Soul comes and goes too much. It settles the Corporeal Soul.

Du-14 Dazhui

Strengthens the Heart, tonifies Yang, strengthens the Will-Power (*Zhi*), tonifies Heart- and Kidney-Yang. It is very effective for depression, lack of will-power and drive, with the Ethereal Soul not coming and going enough.

Du-16 Fengfu

For depression and anxiety with morbid thoughts of death.

Du-19 Houding

Calms the Mind and nourishes the Heart and it is good for sadness and depression.

Du-20 Baihui

Tonifies and raises Qi and Yang, lifts depression, clears the Mind.

Du-24 Shenting

Calms and lifts the Mind; therefore it is used not only for anxiety and insomnia but also for depression and sadness.

Ren-4 Guanyuan

Tonifies the Kidneys and the Will-Power in patients suffering from depression, calms the Mind (*Shen*) and settles the Ethereal Soul (*Hun*) by nourishing Blood and Yin.

Ren-15 Jiuwei

Nourishes the Heart, calms the Mind and lifts mood.

HERBS FOR DEPRESSION

XIANG YUAN *Fructus Citri medicae*

Category: moving Qi.
Channels entered: Liver, Spleen, Lungs.
Taste and energy: pungent, slightly bitter, sour, warm.

Xiang Yuan moves Qi, eliminates stagnation, relieves depression, resolves Phlegm and benefits the diaphragm.

It is a very important herb for mental depression deriving from Liver-Qi stagnation as it eliminates stagnation and specifically relieves depression. It is especially useful as it also resolves Phlegm that frequently accompanies Qi stagnation. It combines well with Fo Shou *Fructus Citri sarcodactylis*.

FO SHOU *Fructus Citri sarcodactylis*

Category: moving Qi.
Channels entered: Liver, Lungs, Stomach, Spleen.
Taste and energy: pungent, bitter, warm.

Fo Shou is a very important herb for depression from Liver-Qi stagnation. In fact, I frequently use one or two herbs to move Qi in a prescription, even in conditions not involving Liver-Qi stagnation. I do so because the Qi-moving action of these herbs stimulates the "coming and going" of the Ethereal Soul, which is always deficient in depression.

Fo Shou moves Qi, harmonizes the Stomach and Spleen and resolves Phlegm. As for Xiang Yuan, the latter action is useful as Phlegm often accompanies Qi stagnation (because stagnant Qi fails to move correctly in the Triple Burner's Water passages, resulting in the formation of Phlegm).

Finally, within the Qi-moving herbs, Fo Shou has a particularly strong mental effect in relieving depression and I frequently add it to a formula to stimulate the "coming and going" of the Ethereal Soul.

QING PI *Pericarpium Citri reticulatae viride*

Category: moving Qi.
Channels entered: Gall-Bladder, Liver, Stomach.
Taste and energy: pungent, bitter, warm.

Qing Pi has a strong Qi-moving action and it primarily enters the Upper Burner. For this reason, it goes to the chest and head and this makes it particularly suitable to treat depression. Qing Pi has a stronger action than other Qi-moving herbs and this is another reason why I often use it in formulae to treat mental depression as it strongly stimulates the "coming and going" of the Ethereal Soul.

MEI GUI HUA *Flos Rosae rugosae*

Category: moving Qi.
Channels entered: Liver, Spleen.
Taste and energy: sweet, slightly bitter, warm.

Mei Gui Hua is frequently used for mental depression occurring against a background of Liver-Qi stagnation. I personally use this herb frequently in depression from Qi stagnation. Compared to the Qi-moving herbs, especially Qing Pi (mentioned above), it has a gentle Qi-moving effect due to its sweet rather than pungent taste.

Another characteristic that makes it suitable to treat mental depression is that it is a flower; as such, it is light and therefore affects the upper part of the body and the head. Although it is not pungent, it is highly aromatic and that is another feature that makes it suitable to treat mental depression.

HE HUAN HUA *Flos Albiziae*

Category: calming the Mind.
Channels entered: Liver, Stomach.
Taste and energy: sweet, neutral.

Although He Huan Hua is placed in the category of herbs that calm the Mind, it also moves Qi and eliminates stagnation. These two actions make it very useful to treat mental depression accompanied by anxiety and insomnia.

As for Mei Gui Hua, another characteristic that makes He Huan Hua suitable to treat mental depression is that it is a flower; as such, it is light and therefore affects the upper part of the body and the head. Although it is not pungent, it is highly aromatic and that is another feature that makes it suitable to treat mental depression.

HE HUAN PI *Cortex Albiziae*

Category: calming the Mind.
Channels entered: Heart, Liver.
Taste and energy: sweet, neutral.

He Huan Pi is an important herb for the treatment of mental depression. It combines the two actions of moving Qi and eliminating stagnation with that of calming the Mind (in fact, it enters the Liver and Heart).

It has an ancient history of use for mental depression and its indications include depression, bad temper, insomnia and irritability. The *Treasury of Words on the Materia Medica* says: "*He Huan Pi allows the five spirits [Shen, Hun, Po, Yi and Zhi] to open and reach outwards, eliminating extremes of the five emotions.*"[26]

YUAN ZHI *Radix Polygalae*

Category: calming the Mind.
Channels entered: Heart, Lungs.
Taste and energy: bitter, pungent, slightly warm.

Yuan Zhi calms the Mind, opens the Mind's orifices and resolves Phlegm. "Calming the Mind" in the category of herbs that calm the Mind should not be interpreted literally. The category of herbs that "calm the Mind" include herbs that are pungent in taste and "stimulate" the Mind and open the Mind's orifices.

The category of herbs that "calm the Mind" comprises two subcategories of herbs: one subcategory of herbs that are "heavy" and therefore anchor, "sink" and calm the Mind (many of these are minerals) and another subcategory of herbs that "nourish the Heart and calm the Mind".

Within this subcategory, there are two quite distinct group of herbs: some sweet and sour that specifically calm the Mind (such as Suan Zao Ren *Semen Ziziphi spinosae* and Bai Zi Ren *Semen Platycladi*), and others pungent that open the Mind's orifices, such as Yuan Zhi *Radix Polygalae*, or that move Qi, such as He Huan Pi *Cortex Albiziae* (Fig. 16.26).

Yuan Zhi pertains to the latter group and it is a very important herb to open the Mind's orifices and to stimulate the "coming and going" of the Ethereal Soul with its pungent and bitter taste. It is an extremely important herb for depression.

Yuan Zhi is often combined with Suan Zao Ren as these two herbs complement each other very well; one pungent, the other sour, they regulate the coming and going of the Ethereal Soul (as the pungent taste stimulates its coming and going and the sour taste restrains it).

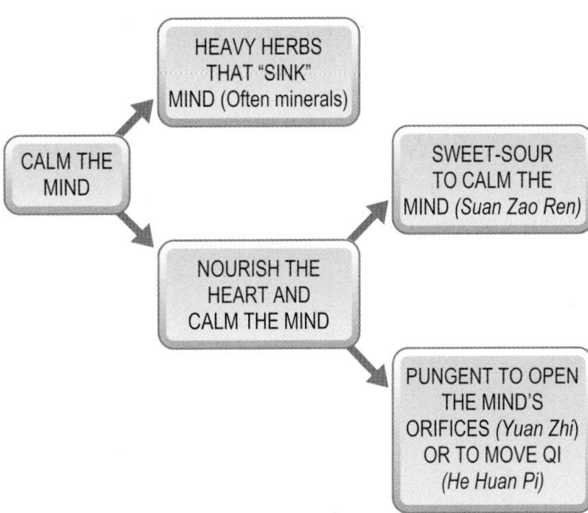

Figure 16.26 Categories of herbs that "calm the Mind".

YU JIN *Radix Curcumae*

Category: invigorating Blood.
Channels entered: Heart, Lungs, Liver.
Taste and energy: pungent, bitter, cold.

Yu Jin moves Qi, invigorates Blood, cools Blood, opens the Mind's orifices and resolves Phlegm. It combines several functions that affect the Mind and the Ethereal Soul. By moving Qi and invigorating Blood, it stimulates the "coming and going" of the Ethereal Soul when this is restrained by stagnation of Qi and/or Blood. By cooling Blood, it calms the Mind when this is affected by Heat. By resolving Phlegm and opening the Mind's orifices, it clears the Mind when this is clouded by Phlegm and it also stimulates the "coming and going" of the Ethereal Soul when this is restrained by Phlegm.

I use this herb very frequently in depression in combination with Yuan Zhi *Radix Polygalae*.

SHI CHANG PU *Rhizoma Acori tatarinowii*

Category: opening the orifices.
Channels entered: Heart, Stomach.
Taste and energy: pungent, bitter, warm, aromatic.

Shi Chang Pu opens the orifices and the Mind's orifices; it resolves Phlegm and calms the Mind. I use this herb very frequently in combination with Yuan Zhi *Radix Polygalae* to open the Mind's orifices and stimulate the "coming and going" of the Ethereal Soul when this is restrained by Phlegm. Shi Chang Pu enters the Heart and is pungent, bitter and aromatic; it is these properties that make it so valuable to open the Mind's orifices and move Qi when the person is depressed.

SUMMARY

Herbs for depression

XIANG YUAN Fructus Citri medicae

Category: moving Qi.
Channels entered: Liver, Spleen, Lungs.
Taste and energy: pungent, slightly bitter, sour, warm.

Xiang Yuan moves Qi, eliminates stagnation, relieves depression, resolves Phlegm and benefits the diaphragm.

FO SHOU Fructus Citri sarcodactylis

Category: moving Qi.
Channels entered: Liver, Lungs, Stomach, Spleen.
Taste and energy: pungent, bitter, warm.

Fo Shou is a very important herb for depression from Liver-Qi stagnation.

QING PI Pericarpium Citri reticulatae viride

Category: moving Qi.
Channels entered: Gall-Bladder, Liver, Stomach.
Taste and energy: pungent, bitter, warm.

Qing Pi has a strong Qi-moving action and it primarily enters the Upper Burner. For this reason, it goes to the chest and head, and this makes it particularly suitable to treat depression.

MEI GUI HUA Flos Rosae rugosae

Category: moving Qi.
Channels entered: Liver, Spleen.
Taste and energy: sweet, slightly bitter, warm.

Mei Gui Hua is frequently used for mental depression occurring against a background of Liver-Qi stagnation.

HE HUAN HUA Flos Albiziae

Category: calming the Mind.
Channels entered: Liver, Stomach.
Taste and energy: sweet, neutral.

He Huan Hua calms the Mind, moves Qi and eliminates stagnation.

HE HUAN PI Cortex Albiziae

Category: calming the Mind.
Channels entered: Heart, Liver.
Taste and energy: sweet, neutral.

He Huan Pi is an important herb for the treatment of mental depression. It combines the two actions of moving Qi and eliminating stagnation with that of calming the Mind (in fact, it enters the Liver and Heart).

YUAN ZHI Radix Polygalae

Category: calming the Mind.
Channels entered: Heart, Lungs.
Taste and energy: bitter, pungent, slightly warm.

Yuan Zhi calms the Mind, opens the Mind's orifices and resolves Phlegm.

YU JIN Radix Curcumae

Category: invigorating Blood.
Channels entered: Heart, Lungs, Liver.
Taste and energy: pungent, bitter, cold.

Yu Jin moves Qi, invigorates Blood, cools Blood, opens the Mind's orifices and resolves Phlegm.

SHI CHANG PU Rhizoma Acori tatarinowii

Category: opening the orifices.
Channels entered: Heart, Stomach.
Taste and energy: pungent, bitter, warm, aromatic.

Shi Chang Pu opens the orifices and the Mind's orifices, it resolves Phlegm and calms the Mind.

MODERN CHINESE LITERATURE

Journal of Chinese Medicine

(*Zhong Yi Za Zhi* 中医杂志), Vol. 32, No. 5, 1991, p. 36.

Liu Guang Zhi et al., "Clinical observations on the treatment of depression in the elderly with electroacupuncture"

Thirty elderly patients suffering from depression were treated with electroacupuncture. The patients ranged in age from 50 to 74, 16 men and 14 women (average age 57.4). The average duration of the disease was 5.5 years.

The points used were Du-20 Baihui and extra point Yintang. Electroacupuncture was applied to the points with dense-sparse wave, ranging from 6 V to 1.5 V, 8–9 mA, Hz 8 × 100. The treatment was given once a day for 6 days a week for a total of 30 sessions.

There were no therapeutic results in five patients. Thirteen patients were completely cured and the rest experienced various degrees of improvement.

Journal of Chinese Medicine

(*Zhong Yi Za Zhi*), Vol. 24, No. 12, 1983, p. 55.

Jiang Ke Ming, "A brief discussion of herbal prescriptions for depression (*Yu Zheng*)"

Dr Jiang emphasizes the dual nature of *Yu Zheng* as "mental depression" and "stagnation". In fact, following the statement from Zhang Jing Yue quoted at the beginning of this chapter, Dr Jiang says that "stagnation may cause depression; conversely, depression may cause stagnation".

Like most Chinese doctors, Dr Jiang says that most cases of mental depression start with Liver-Qi stagnation and the prescriptions he favors are as follows.

- Xiao Yao San *Free and Easy Wanderer Powder*
- Chai Hu Shu Gan Tang *Bupleurum Soothing the Liver Decoction*
- Xuan Fu Dai Zhe Tang *Inula-Hematitum Decoction*
- Ban Xia Hou Po Tang *Pinellia-Magnolia Decoction*
- Su He Xiang Wan *Styrax Pill*
- Yue Ju Wan *Gardenia-Chuanxiong Pill*

As for pathology, Dr Jiang states that, in the beginning, the pathology starts with Liver-Qi stagnation which may later lead to Liver-Blood stasis. The Liver may invade the Stomach and cause Stomach-Qi to rebel upwards. The dysfunction of the Stomach may give rise to Dampness or Phlegm.

In late stages, the Spleen becomes deficient and there may be Blood stasis which affects menstruation in women.

Journal of Chinese Medicine

(*Zhong Yi Za Zhi*), Vol. 24, No. 4, 1983, p. 58.

Tan Jia Ming, "A brief account on the treatment of depression"

Dr Tan states that depression starts with Qi stagnation which may lead to Blood stasis, Phlegm accumulation, Food accumulation, Heat accumulation and, in late stages, Heart and Spleen deficiency and Liver- and Kidney-Yin deficiency.

Dr Tan therefore summarizes the pathology of depression as follows.

- Qi stagnation
- Blood (stasis)
- Dampness
- Phlegm
- Heat
- Food (accumulation)

As for the etiology of depression, Dr Tan thinks that three emotions are the most important ones, i.e. pensiveness, worry and anger. Dr Tan's contribution is interesting as, unlike most other Chinese doctors, he does not place anger at the top of the list as an emotional cause of depression, but he considers pensiveness and worry as main causes. Given my experience with Western patients, I would thoroughly agree with him and would add sadness, grief and guilt to the list.

As for the pathology, Dr Tan says this starts with Liver-Qi stagnation; stagnant Qi may turn into Heat or long-term Qi stagnation may give rise to Blood stasis. Then, either Liver-Qi invades the Spleen or this is directly affected by pensiveness and worry so that Spleen-Qi deficiency develops.

The Spleen-Qi deficiency may give rise to Dampness and Phlegm and Food accumulation. Dampness and Phlegm may combine with Heat. The long-term depression injures Heart-Qi and Heart-Blood, which fails to properly house the Mind; this leads to insomnia and anxiety.

Therefore in chronic cases of depression there is a deficiency of Spleen and Heart; if there is Heat, this may injure Yin and lead to Yin deficiency.

Dr Tan suggests some herbal prescriptions for Full and Empty conditions as follows.

FULL

Qi stagnation
- Chai Hu Shu Gan Tang *Bupleurum Soothing the Liver Decoction*
- Yue Ju Wan *Gardenia-Chuanxiong Pill*

Heat
- Dan Zhi Xiao Yao San *Moutan-Gardenia Free and Easy Wanderer Powder*

Phlegm
- Ban Xia Hou Po Tang *Pinellia-Magnolia Decoction*
- Tan Yu Tang *Phlegm Stagnation Decoction*

Dampness
- Shi Yu Tang *Dampness Stagnation Decoction*

Blood (stasis)
- Xue Yu Tang *Blood Stagnation Decoction*

Food (accumulation)
- Shi Yu Tang *Food Stagnation Decoction*

EMPTY

Worry injuring the Mind
- Gan Mai Da Zao Tang *Glycyrrhiza-Triticum-Jujuba Decoction*

Heart and Spleen deficiency
- Gui Pi Tang *Tonifying the Spleen Decoction*

Yin deficiency with Empty Heat
- Zi Shui Qing Gan Yin *Nourishing Water and Clearing the Liver Decoction*

Journal of Chinese Medicine

(*Zhong Yi Za Zhi*), Vol. 41, No. 11, 2000, p. 654.

Zhang Peng, "The experience of Zhang Tai Kang in the treatment of depression"

Dr Zhang says that, in the beginning stages, depression is characterized by Qi stagnation and Phlegm and it usually occurs against a background of Full conditions; in the late stages, it is characterized by Blood and Yin deficiency and it usually occurs against a background of Empty conditions.

Dr Zhang distinguishes only two major types of pathology: the first is characterized by Liver-Qi stagnation, disharmony of Liver and Spleen, Phlegm and "obstruction of the Brain"; the second by Qi and Blood deficiency, deficiency of Marrow, and deficiency of the Brain.

Liver-Qi stagnation, disharmony of Liver and Spleen, Phlegm and obstruction of the Brain

Pensiveness, sadness, depressed mood, hypochondrial distension, Wiry pulse.

Dr Zhang used the prescription Kai Yu Yue Shen Tang *Opening Stagnation and Cheering the Mind Decoction.*

Qi and Blood deficiency, deficiency of Marrow, deficiency of the Brain

Depression, sadness, decreased mental power, poor memory, decreased capacity in working and studying. This condition is more frequent in the elderly.

Dr Zhang distinguishes two conditions: the first characterized by Heart and Spleen deficiency, for which he uses Yang Xin Jian Pi Tang *Nourishing the Heart and Strengthening the Spleen Decoction*; the other characterized by Liver and Kidney deficiency for which he uses Bu Sui Rong Nao Tang *Tonifying Marrow and Nourishing the Brain Decoction.*

Dr Zhang's work is interesting in that he narrows the pathology of depression to two major categories, one Full, the other Empty. He correlated the first to what he calls "obstruction of the Brain" and the other to "deficiency of the Brain."

Journal of Chinese Medicine

(*Zhong Yi Za Zhi*), Vol. 30, No. 2, 1989. pp. 10–12.

Xu Jing Fan, "Academic thoughts on Ye Tian Shi's diagnosis and treatment of depression"

Dr Xu Jing Fang confirms the two views of the syndrome *Yu* mentioned at the beginning of this chapter. Dr Xu says that in a broad sense, *Yu* indicates "stagnation" and it includes many different conditions; in a narrow sense, *Yu* denotes "mental depression."

When discussing the pathology of Depression, Dr Xu concords with many other Chinese doctors in that, in the beginning, the disease affects the Liver first and is at the Qi level, i.e. Liver-Qi stagnation. He says that the stagnation of Liver-Qi also affects the Gall-Bladder, giving rise to physical symptoms related to this organ and also to the timidity and lack of initiative that is related to a disharmony of the Gall-Bladder.

According to Dr Xu, Ye Tian Shi says: "*Long-term stagnation causes stagnation of the Heart and Spleen.*" This statement is interesting as it confirms that, especially in emotional problems, Qi stagnation does affect the Heart (and also other organs such as the Spleen). The Spleen is also affected directly by the Qi stagnation in the Liver.

Dr Xu therefore says that, in Depression, Qi stagnation affects the Liver and Heart and that the Qi stagnation in this latter organ affects the Mind (*Shen*) as this is deprived of its normal "residence". This is another interesting concept, according to which the Mind is deprived of its residence not only when Heart-Blood is deficient but also when Heart-Qi is stagnant.

Two pathological consequences derive from Qi stagnation: first, the stagnant Qi may give rise to Heat; second, the Qi stagnation in the passages of the Triple Burner impairs the transformation, transportation and excretion of the Body Fluids which therefore accumulate into Phlegm.

Ye Tian Shi says that when pathological Heat is formed, the "Lesser Fire changes into Exuberant Fire". "Lesser Fire" (*Shao Huo*) is another name for the physiological Heat of the Minister Fire and "Exuberant Fire" (*Zhuang Huo*) is a pathological Heat that is formed under the influence of emotional stress.

Ye Tian Shi says that in the elderly, Depression frequently occurs against a background of Yin deficiency, while in young people it occurs against a background of Qi stagnation and Heat.

The pathology of Depression deriving from Qi stagnation becomes complicated due to the several pathological consequences of Qi stagnation. First, Phlegm may be formed as indicated above; second, the Qi stagnation may give rise to Blood stasis and this interacts with Phlegm, the two aggravating each other.

So the pathology of Depression in later stages may be summarized in the three terms of Qi, Phlegm and Stasis (of Blood). In chronic cases, these three pathogenic factors usually give rise to a deficiency which may be of Qi, Yang, Blood or Yin.

As Qi stagnation, Phlegm and Blood stasis may all obstruct the orifices, in treatment Ye Tian Shi placed the emphasis on brightening the orifices (which include the orifices of the Mind). He also placed the emphasis on treatment methods that move, clear obstructions and drain.

The key words Ye Tian Shi used to indicate the treatment methods in Depression are as follows.

- *Da* 达 = "to extend", "to relax".
- *Xuan* 宣 = "to diffuse", "to drain".
- *Chang* 畅 = "to free".
- *Tong* 通 = "to remove obstructions".

In particular, in Qi stagnation, one should move, free and relax; in Blood stasis, one should remove obstructions from the Blood Connecting (*Luo*) channels; in Heat (that derives from Qi stagnation) one should cool with bitter and cool herbs and remove obstructions with Qi-moving herbs.

When the above pathogenic factors are combined with a deficiency, one should combine tonification with moving and removing obstructions.

Journal of Chinese Medicine

(*Zhong Yi Za Zhi*), Vol. 42, No. 9, 2001, p. 566.

Li Bao Ling, "Development of herbal medicine research in depression"

The pathology and treatment discussed by Dr Li are a little different from those discussed by other Chinese doctors. Dr Li discusses five main pathological conditions in Depression.

1. Liver-Qi stagnation giving rise to Heat: this is characterized by depression and irritability. Dr Li suggests using Xiao Chai Hu Tang *Small Bupleurum Decoction* or Xiao Yao San *Free and Easy Wanderer Powder*.

2. Heart not housing the Mind: this is characterized by depression, insomnia, excessive dreaming and mental restlessness. Dr Li suggests using Gan Mai Da Zao Tang *Glycyrrhiza-Triticum-Jujuba Decoction.*
3. Gall-Bladder deficiency: this is characterized by depression, timidity, lack of initiative, difficulty in taking decisions, waking up early in the morning. Dr Li suggests using Yi Lu Kang Jiao Nang *Relieving Depression and Worry Capsule.*
4. Heart- and Lung-Yin deficiency: this is characterized by depression, mental confusion, dislike to speak. Dr Li suggests using Bai He Di Huang Tang *Lilium-Rehmannia Decoction.*
5. Stomach and Spleen deficiency: this is characterized by depression, tiredness, desire to lie down, reluctance in going out and digestive problems. Dr Li suggests using a variation of Er Chen Tang *Two Old Decoction.*

Dr Li suggests various formulae for depression classified according to the organ involved which may be the Liver, Heart, Heart and Lungs, and Spleen as follows.

Liver

- Xiao Chai Hu Tang *Small Bupleurum Decoction*
- Xiao Yao San *Free and Easy Wanderer Powder*
- Gan Mai Da Zao Tang *Glycyrrhiza-Triticum-Jujuba Decoction*
- Yi Lu Kang Jiao Nang *Relieving Depression and Worry Capsule*
- Ping Xin Wang You Tang *Settling the Heart and Forgetting Worry Decoction*

Heart

- Bao Nao Ning Jiao Nang *Preserving the Brain's Tranquillity Capsule*
- Huang Lian Wen Dan Tang *Coptis Warming the Gall-Bladder Decoction*

Heart and Lungs

- Bai He Di Huang Tang *Lilium-Rehmannia Decoction*

Spleen

- Er Chen Tang *Two Old Decoction* Variation

Dr Li also suggests the following acupuncture points for depression: HE-7 Shenmen, P-7 Daling, LIV-3 Taichong, ST-40 Fenglong, ST-36 Zusanli, SP-6 Sanyinjiao, P-5 Jianshi, BL-15 Xinshu and BL-18 Ganshu.

Journal of Chinese Medicine

(*Zhong Yi Za Zhi*), Vol. 46, No. 1, 2005, p. 47.

Chen Ze Qi et al., "Research into the criteria for commonly-seen patterns in depression"

This article confirms what is, in my opinion, an excessive stress by Chinese doctors on Liver-Qi stagnation as the main pattern in Depression.

The authors carried out a multicenter investigation and classification of the main patterns diagnosed in depression. Out of 1731 cases, the following were the five main patterns diagnosed.

- *Liver-Qi stagnation*: 588 (34%)
- *Liver-Qi stagnation with Spleen deficiency*: 487 (28%)
- *Liver-Qi stagnation with Phlegm*: 264 (15%)
- *Heart and Spleen deficiency*: 254 (15%)
- *Liver- and Kidney-Yin deficiency*: 138 (8%).

Therefore, out of a total of 1731 cases, Liver-Qi stagnation in all its variations constituted 77% of cases.

The article reports an interesting correlation between the most common symptoms and patterns (Table 16.4).

CLINICAL TRIALS

Acupuncture

Clinical observation on treatment of depression by electroacupuncture combined with paroxetine

Zhong Guo Zhong Xi Yi Jie He Za Zhi 中国中西医结合杂志 [Chinese Journal of Integrative Medicine] 2007 September, Vol. 13, Issue 3, pp. 228–230.

Zhang GJ, Shi ZY, Liu S, Gong SH, Liu JQ, Liu JS

Objective

To observe the clinical efficacy and adverse reactions of paroxetine combined with electroacupuncture (EA) in treating depression.

Method

Forty-two patients with depression were randomly assigned to an observation group and a control group.

Table 16.4 Correlation between symptoms and patterns in depression

SYMPTOM	LIVER-QI STAGNATION (%)	LIVER-QI STAGNATION AND SPLEEN-QI DEFICIENCY (%)	LIVER-QI STAGNATION WITH PHLEGM (%)	HEART AND SPLEEN DEFICIENCY (%)	LIVER- AND KIDNEY-YIN DEFICIENCY (%)
Depressed mood	99.7	99.6	99.6	99.6	96.4
Sadness and pessimistic mood	89.1	88.5	91.7	88.6	92.0
Affective disorder	95.6	97.1	96.6	98.8	91.3
Tiredness	90.6	95.7	97.7	94.6	98.6
Anxiety	92.3	88.9	87.5	92.5	93.5
Mental restlessness	90.6	83.9	84.5	85.8	91.3
Worry	81.5	91.8	84.8	85.8	86.2
Dejection	81.6	86.5	92.8	90.2	88.4
Listlessness	81.3	94.0	89.8	91.7	88.4
Insomnia	84.3	93.2	89.0	96.9	94.2
Excessive dreaming	81.0	85.2	86.0	88.6	97.1

Twenty-two patients in the observation group were treated with EA combined with paroxetine, and 20 patients comprising the control group were treated with paroxetine alone. The therapeutic course for both groups was 6 weeks. The therapeutic efficacy and adverse reactions were evaluated by the Hamilton Depression Rating Scale (HAMD) and Treatment Emergent Symptoms Scale (TESS) scores, respectively.

Results

HAMD scores determined at the end of the first, second, fourth and sixth week of the treatment course were significantly lower in the observation group than those in the control group ($P<0.05$). The significant improvement rate evaluated at the end of the 6-week treatment was remarkably higher in the observation group than that in the control group (72.7% vs 40%). No significant difference of TESS scores was found between the two groups.

Conclusion

EA combined with paroxetine has better clinical efficacy than that of paroxetine alone, with milder adverse reactions and quicker initiation of effect.

Effects of electroacupuncture and fluoxetine on the density of GTP-binding-proteins in platelet membrane in patients with major depressive disorder

Journal of Affective Disorders 2007 March, Vol. 98, Issue 3, pp. 253–257.
Song Y, Zhou D, Fan J, Luo H, Halbreich U

Background and objective

Electroacupuncture (EA) has been used to treat major depressive disorder (MDD). However, its efficacy is inconclusive and the mechanism is still unclear. Thus, the objective of this study was to investigate the therapeutic effect of EA on GTP-binding-protein (G protein) in platelet membrane using fluoxetine as a comparison.

Method

A randomized controlled trial (RCT) was performed on 90 MDD patients, who were divided into three groups and treated with fluoxetine, EA and sham EA, respectively. Antibodies were utilized to quantify the levels of G protein alpha subtypes in the platelet membrane before and after the 6-week antidepressive treatment. Thirty age- and sex-matched normal individuals were used as controls.

Results

All the treatments had the same therapeutic effects in treating moderate depression. Both levels of $G\alpha i$ and $G\alpha q$ in depression patients were significantly higher than those in controls and were not reduced by treatments, although the severity of the depression was considerably relieved.

Limitations

The duration of treatment was limited to 6 weeks only.

Conclusion

EA might serve as an alternative treatment for moderate depression and it was further demonstrated that the abnormal levels of $G\alpha$ protein in platelet membrane might be a potential risk factor for MDD.

Clinical study on the therapeutic effect of acupuncture in the treatment of post-stroke depression

Acupuncture Research 2007 February, Vol. 32, Issue 1, pp. 58–61.

He J, Shen PF

Objective

To observe the therapeutic effect of Xingnao Kaiqiao Zhenfa (Acupuncture Technique for Restoring Consciousness) in the treatment of post-stroke depression.

Method

A total of 256 stroke patients were divided into the acupuncture group (n = 180: male 138, female 42) and medication group (n = 76: male 57, female 19) according to their visiting sequence to the hospital. Points needled were P-6 Neiguan, Du-26 Renzhong, Du-20 Baihui, Yintang and SP-6 Sanyinjiao on the affected side. The needles were retained for 20 minutes every time. Patients in the medication group were asked to take amitriptyline (50 mg per day at first, then 200 mg per day). Acupuncture treatment was conducted twice daily, and after 1 month's treatment the therapeutic effect was evaluated. Self-Rating Depression Scale (SDS) and Hamilton Rating Scale for Depression (HAMD) were used to assess the patients' state of depression at baseline and after 1 month.

Results

After the treatment, of the 180 and 76 cases in the acupuncture and medication groups, 31 (17.2%) and 13 (17.1%) were cured, 73 (40.6%) and 18 (23.7%) had a marked improvement in their depression state, 27 (15.0%) and 12 (15.8%) had an improvement, 49 (27.2%) and 33 (43.4%) failed, with the effective rates being 72.8% and 56.6%, respectively. The markedly effective rate and the total effective rate of the acupuncture group were significantly higher than those of the medication group ($P < 0.05$). After the treatment, the total scores of SDS and HAMD and the severity index of the two groups greatly decreased in comparison with baseline scores. The therapeutic effects of the acupuncture group were significantly better than those of the medication group in reducing SDS, HAMD and severity index ($P < 0$ .05). In addition, the decreased values of depression, pessimistic mood and irritability of the acupuncture group were all larger than those of the medication group ($P < 0.05$). No significant difference was found between the two groups in the decreased value of insomnia ($P > 0.05$).

Conclusion

The Acupuncture Technique for Restoring Consciousness can effectively improve patients' depression symptoms and the therapeutic effect of acupuncture is markedly superior to that of medication for post-stroke patients.

A systematic review of randomized controlled trials of acupuncture in the treatment of depression

Journal of Affective Disorders 2007 January, Vol. 97, Issue 1–3, pp. 13–22.
Leo RJ, Ligot JS Jnr

Background

Acupuncture has become a popular complementary and alternative treatment approach. This review examined the randomized controlled trials (RCTs) examining the effects of acupuncture treatment of depression.

Methods

RCTs of the treatment of depression with acupuncture were located using MEDLINE, Allied and Complementary Medicine and the Cochrane Central Register of Controlled Trials. The methodology of RCTs was assessed using the Jadad criteria, and elements of research design (randomization, blinding, assessment of attrition rates) were quantified for systematic comparisons among studies.

Results

Among the nine RCTs examined, five were deemed to be of low quality based upon Jadad criteria. The odds ratios derived from comparing acupuncture with control conditions within the RCTs suggests some evidence for the utility of acupuncture in depression. General trends suggest that acupuncture modalities were as effective as antidepressants employed for treatment of depression in the limited studies available for comparison. However, placebo acupuncture treatment was often no different from intended true acupuncture.

Limitations

The RCTs extracted were limited by small sample sizes, imprecise enrollment criteria, problems with randomization and blinding, brief duration of study and lack of longitudinal follow-up.

Conclusion

Despite the findings that the odds ratios of existing literature suggest a role for acupuncture in the treatment of depression, the evidence thus far is inconclusive. However, efforts are being made to standardize complementary approaches to treat depression, and further systematized research into their use is warranted.

Tiaoshenshugan acupuncture versus routine acupuncture for intervention of depression and anxiety

Chinese Journal of Clinical Rehabilitation 2005, Vol. 9, Issue 28, pp. 11–13.
Hou Q, Yan L, Fu L, Du Y-H

Objective

To explore the intervention effects of tiaoshenshugan acupuncture on the depressive and anxious condition of patients with depression.

Method

Seventy-two patients with depression, who were treated in the Department of Acupuncture and outpatient clinic, First Affiliated Hospital, Tianjin University of Traditional Chinese Medicine, were selected between March 2001 and September 2002 with the agreement of the patients or their guardian. According to the order of hospitalization, they were randomly divided into two groups: the observation acupuncture group (40 cases) needled with tiaoshenshugan acupuncture and the control acupuncture group (32 cases). The patients in the tiaoshenshugan acupuncture group were treated with: P-6 Neiguan, Du-26 Renzhong, SP-6 Sanyinjiao, Du-20 Baihui, LIV-3 Taichong and Yintang. All with reinforcing method apart from Du-26, which was manipulated until the eyes watered. Points needled in the control group were LIV-14 Qimen, G.B.-34 Yanglingquan, HE-7 Shenmen and P-5 Jianshi. Reinforcing, reducing or uniform reinforcing reducing method were conducted according to differentiation of symptoms and signs. At baseline and 1 month after treatment, the patients filled out the self-rating depressive scale and the Zung self-rating anxiety scale.

Results

All 72 patients completed the trial. The comparison of baseline versus after-treatment scores in the self-rating depressive scale marks and the anxiety standard marks decreased in both groups, but more significantly in the observation group ($P < 0.05$).

Conclusion

Acupuncture can improve the depressive and anxious condition in patients with depression, while the intervention effect of tiaoshenshugan acupuncture therapy is more effective than routine acupuncture therapy.

Acupuncture: a promising treatment for depression during pregnancy

Journal of Affective Disorders 2004 November, Vol. 83, Issue 1, pp. 89–95.
Manber R, Schnyer RN, Allen J, Rush AJ, Blasey CM

Objective

The aim of this randomized controlled pilot study was to determine whether acupuncture holds promise as a treatment for depression during pregnancy, as there are few medically acceptable treatments in existence.

Method

Sixty-one pregnant women with major depressive disorder and a 17-item Hamilton Rating Scale for Depression (HAMD17) score ≥14 were randomly assigned to one of three treatments, delivered over 8 weeks: active acupuncture ($n = 20$), active control acupuncture ($n = 21$) and massage ($n = 20$). Acupuncture treatments were standardized, but individually tailored, and were provided in a double-blind fashion. Responders to acute phase treatment (HRSD17 score <14 and ≥50% reduction from baseline) continued the treatment until 10 weeks postpartum.

Results

Response rates at the end of the acute phase were statistically significantly higher for the active acupuncture group (69%) than for the massage group (32%), with an intermediate response rate in the active control acupuncture group (47%). The active acupuncture group also exhibited a significantly higher average rate of reduction in Beck Depression Inventory (BDI) scores from baseline to the end of the first month of treatment than the massage group. Responders to the acute phase of all treatments combined had significantly lower depression scores at 10 weeks postpartum than non-responders.

Conclusion

Acupuncture holds promise for the treatment of depression during pregnancy.

Clinical study on electroacupuncture treatment for 30 cases of mental depression

Zhong Yi Za Zhi [Journal of Chinese Medicine] 2004 September, Vol. 24, Issue 3, pp. 172–176.
Han C, Li X, Luo H, Zhao X, Li X

Objective

To compare the effect of electroacupuncture and maprotiline in treating mental depression.

Method

Thirty patients were treated by electroacupuncture on Du-20 Baihui, EX-3 (Yintang extra point) as the main points and other points according to the pattern. The other points were as follows.

- G.B.-34 Yanglingquan and SP-6 Sanyinjiao in cases of disharmony between Liver and Spleen.
- P-6 Neiguan and SP-6 Sanyinjiao in cases of Heart and Spleen deficiency.
- KI-3 Taixi and SP-6 Sanyinjiao in cases of Liver- and Kidney-Yin deficiency.

Maprotiline, which is a medication that strongly inhibits the uptake of noradrenaline (norepinephrine) in the brain and peripheral tissues, was used in the control group of 31 cases. The therapeutic effect and side-effects were evaluated by measurement of the Hamilton Depression Rating Scale (HAMD) and the Asberg Rating Scale.

Results

After the treatment, the scores in HAMD for both groups had decreased ($P < 0.01$) but without significant differences between each group ($P > 0.05$). The total effective rate in the treatment group was 96.7%, and that of the control group was 90.3%, showing no significant differences between the groups ($P > 0.05$). Both groups showed a decrease in Traditional Chinese Medicine (TCM) symptomatic integrals ($P < 0.01$), but the treatment group showed a far greater decrease ($P < 0.05$). The Asberg score decreases, testing the side-effect of antidepressants of the treatment group, were superior to those in the control group. After the treatment, the cortisol (CORT) content and the endothelin-1 (ET-1) content of the two groups were decreased ($P < 0.01$) and registered near normal, without significant differences between the groups ($P > 0.05$).

Conclusion

Electroacupuncture therapy can produce the same clinical therapeutic effect as that produced by the tetracyclic drug maprotiline, giving fewer side-effects and better symptomatic improvement.

Does acupuncture influence the cardiac autonomic nervous system in patients with minor depression or anxiety disorders?

Fortschritte der Neurologie-Psychiatrie [Advances in Neuro-Psychiatry] 2003 March, Vol. 71, Issue 3, pp. 141–149.

Agelink MW, Sanner D, Eich H, Pach J, Bertling R, Lemmer W, Klieser E, Lehmann E

Objective

To evaluate the effects of acupuncture on the cardiac autonomic nervous system (ANS) function in patients with minor depression or anxiety disorder.

Method

Patients ($n = 36$) were randomly distributed into a true acupuncture (TA) group (needles were applied at classic acupuncture points HE-7 Shenmen, P-6 Neiguan, Du-20 Baihui, BL-62 Shenmai, and Ex-6 Yuyao extra point) or a placebo (PL) group (needles were applied only epidermally at non-acupuncture points). Both groups underwent standardized measurements of the 5-minute resting heart rate variability (HRV), which were performed before the first and after the ninth acupuncture session of the acupuncture series, and also three times (before the start, then 5 and 15 minutes after needle application) during the third acupuncture session. Demographic data between the TA and PL group did not differ.

Results

Before the start of the acupuncture there were also no significant differences in HRV data between these groups. Compared to PL, the TA group showed a significant decrease of the mean resting heart rate, both 5 and 15 minutes after needle application, combined with a trend towards an increase of the high frequency (HF; 0.15–0.4 Hz) and a decrease of the low frequency (LF; 0.04–0.15 Hz) spectral power. The latter effects resulted in an overall significant decrease of the mean LF/HF ratio in TA compared to PL treated patients.

Conclusion

This pattern of findings suggests that in patients with minor depression or anxiety only true acupuncture leads to a relative increase of cardiovagal modulation of heart rate, and facilitates the physiological regulatory ANS function in response to alterations of the external or internal environment.

Six-month depression relapse rates among women treated with acupuncture

Complementary Therapies in Medicine 2001 December, Vol. 9, Issue 4, pp. 216–218.

Gallagher SM, Allen JJ, Hitt SK, Schnyer RN, Manber R

Objective

To ascertain the efficacy of acupuncture in treating major depression in women.

Method

Thirty-eight women were randomized to one of three treatment conditions in a double-blind randomized controlled trial of acupuncture in depression. All participants received 8 weeks of acupuncture treatment specifically for depression.

Results

From among the 33 women who completed treatment, 26 (79%) were interviewed after 6 months. Relapse rates were comparable to those of established treatments, with 4 of the 17 women (24%) who achieved full remission at the conclusion of treatment experiencing a relapse 6 months later.

Conclusion

Compared to other empirically validated treatments, acupuncture designed specifically to treat major depression produces results that are comparable in terms of rates of response and of relapse or recurrence.

The benefits of whole body acupuncture in major depression

Journal of Affective Disorders 2000 January–March, Vol. 57, Issue 1–3, pp. 73–81.
Roschke J, Wolf C, Muller MJ, Wagner P, Mann K, Grozinger M, Bech S

Objective

To investigate the efficacy of acupuncture applied in addition to mianserin drug treatment for major depression using a single-blind, placebo-controlled study.

Method

Seventy inpatients with a major depressive episode were randomly included in three different treatment groups: true acupuncture, placebo acupuncture and a control group. All three groups were pharmacologically treated with the antidepressant mianserin. The true group received acupuncture at specific points considered effective in the treatment of depression. The placebo group was treated with acupuncture at non-specific locations and the control group received pharmacological treatment plus clinical management. Acupuncture was applied three times a week over a period of 4 weeks. Psychopathology was rated by judges blind to true/placebo conditions twice a week over 8 weeks.

Results

Patients who experienced acupuncture improved slightly more than patients treated with mianserin alone.

Conclusion

Additionally applied acupuncture improved the course of depression more than pharmacological treatment with mianserin alone. However, no differences were detected between placebo and true acupuncture.

152nd Annual Meeting of the American Psychiatric Association, Washington DC, 15–20 May 1999

Allen JJ, Manber R, Schnyer RN, Hitt SK

Objective

To ascertain the efficacy of acupuncture in the treatment of major depression in women.

Method

Thirty-three women with major depression were randomly assigned to one of three treatment groups. Those in the specific treatment group received acupuncture treatments individually tailored to their symptoms of depression; those in the non-specific group first received acupuncture treatments tailored to address symptoms that were not clearly part of the depressive episode (e.g., back pain), and later received the acupuncture treatments specifically tailored to their symptoms of depression; those in the wait-list group waited without treatment for 8 weeks before receiving the acupuncture treatments tailored for their symptoms of depression.

Results

Following treatments specifically designed to address symptoms of depression, 64% of women experienced remission. Comparing the immediate effect of these three 8-week treatment conditions, subjects receiving specific acupuncture treatments demonstrated greater improvement than those receiving non-specific acupuncture treatments and showed marginally more improvement than wait-list controls.

Conclusion

Based on this outpatient sample of women with major depression, it appears that acupuncture can provide significant symptom relief at rates comparable to standard treatments such as psychotherapy or pharmacotherapy. Acupuncture may hold sufficient promise to warrant a larger-scale clinical trial.

Herbal medicine

Changes in serum tumor necrosis factor (TNF-alpha) with kami shoyo san (Jia Wei Xiao Yao San *Augmented Free and Easy Wanderer Powder*) administration in depressed climacteric patients

American Journal of Chinese Medicine 2004, Vol. 32, Issue 4, pp. 621–629.
Ushiroyama T, Ikeda A, Sakuma K, Ueki M

Objective

To investigate the changes in serum tumor necrosis factor (TNF)-α) in depressed climacteric patients after administration of kami shoyo san (Jia Wei Xiao Yao San TJ-24).

Method

This study included 113 depressed menopausal patients who visited the gynecological and psychosomatic medicine outpatient clinic of the Osaka Medical College Hospital in Japan. Serum TNF-α levels were compared in two treated groups, with and without concurrent use of herbal medicine: 58 patients were administered kami shoyo san and 55 patients were administered antidepressants. Hamilton Rating Scale for depression (HAM-D) scores were determined at baseline and 12 weeks after starting treatment. TNF-α concentrations were analyzed before and after 12 weeks of treatment.

Results

Kami shoyo san significantly increased plasma concentrations of TNF-α after 12 weeks of treatment, to 17.22 ± 6.13 pg/ml from a baseline level of 14.16 ± 6.27 pg/ml (p = 0.048). The percentage change in plasma concentration of TNF-α differed significantly between the kami shoyo san therapy group and the antidepressant therapy group at 4 weeks (12.0 ± 7.8% and −1.22 ± 0.25%, respectively, $p < 0.01$), 8 weeks (19.7 ± 3.4% and −2.45 ± 0.86%, respectively, $p < 0.01$), and 12 weeks (21.3 ± 5.4% and −6.81 ± 2.2%, respectively, $p < 0.001$).

Conclusion

This study found that kami shoyo san increased plasma TNF-α levels in depressed menopausal patients. Cytokines may play various roles in mood and emotional status via the central nervous system and may be regulated by herbal medicines, although the interactions are very complex.

CASE HISTORIES

Case history

A 43-year-old woman had been suffering from depression for several years. This was very apparent as soon as she started talking. She looked very distressed and in mental anguish and frequently burst into tears. She had suffered from the break-up of a relationship and she felt very depressed. She also felt confused about her life aims, both in her work and in relationships. It was very obvious that she had very low self-esteem and harbored suicidal thoughts.

During the first interview she mentioned only her depression and the shock following the break-up of her relationship. A week after the first interview, I got an email from her. In it, she described how she was sexually abused by her teacher when she was 10 years old for 9 months. To keep her quiet, he told her that she was evil, that she had made him do that to her and that she would never amount to anything except a prostitute or similar. He also told her she was stupid. He coerced her not to say anything, threatening that, if she did, people would know what she was, i.e. an evil, twisted, stupid slut who deserved to be abused.

On her 16th birthday she was still a virgin and wanted to remain so. She was raped by her boyfriend.

She had been struggling with this for the past 32 years. She went to university to prove to herself that she was not stupid but she said that she was still now struggling with feeling worthy. She puts herself down all the time and blames herself constantly. Her boyfriend of 11 years left her for a younger woman, telling her there was no-one else and that it was all her fault.

Four and half years later she was still trying to come to terms with this. Her boyfriend's words took her right back to the abuse; it was as if he triggered the same feelings of shame as she had felt when she was abused. She said it also made her feel like a child, totally unable to cope. Then being made redundant 18 months previous to the consultation made her feel really useless and unwanted.

Her letter was very eloquent and bared the roots of her emotional problems very clearly. Her eyes had an anguished look about them, looking like a cry for help. Her periods were regular but she bled for 9 days and suffered from premenstrual tension right from soon after her ovulation.

Her tongue was Red, redder on the sides and with a sticky-yellow coating. Her pulse was Wiry all over in every position.

Diagnosis Obviously the sexual abuse suffered when she was 10 wounded her emotionally in a very deep way. It caused her to have deep feelings of worthlessness and shame. The cruel behavior of her boyfriend resonated with those feelings from the time when she was 10 and triggered her depression.

The emotional stress had caused Qi stagnation; this is evidenced by the tongue and pulse, both of which play a very important role in the diagnosis. Judging from the tongue and pulse, this patient's was definitely a Full condition. The redder color of the sides of the tongue, the Wiry pulse and the premenstrual tension indicate Liver-Qi stagnation as the main pathology.

However, the redness of the tongue clearly indicates that the stagnant Qi has given rise to Heat.

As for the emotional etiology, I feel it would be wrong to attribute it to "anger" simply because there is Liver-Qi stagnation. I personally feel that the Liver is affected by other emotions too; in her case, shame, frustration and feeling of worthlessness.

The stagnation of Liver-Qi restrains the "coming and going" of the Ethereal Soul and this results in her depression and confusion about her life's aims.

Treatment I started off by prescribing a variation of Yue Ju Wan *Gardenia-Chuanxiong Pill*, primarily on the basis of the pulse. In patients who are depressed from Liver-Qi stagnation and have a Wiry pulse, I nearly always use Yue Ju Wan, Zhu Dan Xi's formula for the "six stagnations". After that, my treatment oscillated between using this formula and Dan Zhi Xiao Yao San *Moutan-Gardenia Free and Easy Wanderer Powder*.

My variation of Yue Ju Wan (in the form of concentrated powder) was as follows.

- **Xiang Fu** *Rhizoma Cyperi* 15 g
- **Shen Qu** *Massa medicata fermentata* 10 g
- **Chuan Xiong** *Rhizoma Chuanxiong* 8 g
- **Cang Zhu** *Rhizoma Atractylodis* 10 g
- **Shan Zhi Zi** *Fructus Gardeniae* 10 g
- **Mu Dan Pi** *Cortex Moutan* 10 g
- **Suan Zao Ren** *Semen Ziziphi spinosae* 10 g
- **Yuan Zhi** *Radix Polygalae* 15 g
- **Zhi Gan Cao** *Radix Glycyrrhizae preparata* 10 g
- **Fu Xiao Mai** *Fructus Tritici levis* 10 g
- **Da Zao** *Fructus Jujubae* 10 g

Explanation

The above dosages are for a concentrated powder mixture to be taken one teaspoonful three times a day.

The first five herbs constitute the root formula Yue Ju Wan *Gardenia-Chuanxiong Powder*.

- Mu Dan Pi was added to clear Heat as the tongue is Red and the sides redder.
- Suan Zao Ren and Yuan Zhi work in combination to regulate the "coming and going" of the Ethereal Soul and treat depression. The former is sour and astringent and therefore "absorbs" the Ethereal Soul into the Liver, while the latter is pungent and stimulates the movement of the Ethereal Soul.
- Zhi Gan Cao, Fu Xiao Mai and Da Zao constitute the formula Gan Mai Da Zao Tang *Glycyrrhiza-Triticum-Jujuba Decoction*. Although I normally use this formula for Empty conditions of depression, I do sometimes add it to other

formulae when the patient is very distressed and anguished simply to nourish the Heart, the Mind and the Ethereal Soul.

After two courses of this formula she felt somewhat better and her tongue was considerably less Red but her premenstrual tension was quite bad, with pronounced distension and pain of the breasts. I therefore decided to use Dan Zhi Xiao Yao San *Moutan-Gardenia Free and Easy Wanderer Powder*. I gave her the following variation of it.

- **Bo He** *Herba Menthae* 5 g
- **Chai Hu** *Radix Bupleuri* 6 g
- **Dang Gui** *Radix Angelicae sinensis* 10 g
- **Bai Shao** *Radix Paeoniae alba* 10 g
- **Bai Zhu** *Rhizoma Atractylodis macrocephalae* 10 g
- **Fu Ling** *Poria* 10 g
- **Gan Cao** *Radix Glycyrrhizae* 5 g
- **Mu Dan Pi** *Cortex Moutan* 10 g
- **Shan Zhi Zi** *Fructus Gardeniae* 10 g
- **Yuan Zhi** *Radix Polygalae* 10 g
- **Suan Zao Ren** *Semen Ziziphi spinosae* 10 g
- **Mei Gui Hua** *Flos Rosae rugosae* 10 g
- **He Huan Pi** *Cortex Albiziae* 10 g

Explanation

The first nine herbs constitute the root formula.

- The rationale of Yuan Zhi and Suan Zao Ren has already been explained above.
- Mei Gui Hua was added to move Liver-Qi and lift mood.
- He Huan Pi nourishes the Heart and lifts mood.

I gave her two courses of this formula and then reverted again to the variation of Yue Ju Wan because her pulse was beginning to feel more Wiry. She took five courses of this formula and, after that, she felt very much better, she found a job, she was much more confident, she was not crying so much and was much more optimistic about the future. Her tongue was now of a normal color and the pulse much less Wiry. Her eyes lost the anguished look.

Case history

A 38-year-old woman had been suffering from depression for several years. According to her, this did not seem to have any obvious cause as she was, in her words, happily married and had no financial or work problems.

She initially did not come to me complaining of depression but she sought treatment for chilblains, very cold hands, blue lips and tiredness. She felt very cold all the time. On interrogation, it transpired that she also suffered from dizziness, lower backache, frequent urination and nocturia.

Her tongue was Pale and Swollen in the front part (Lung area); her pulse was Weak in general and especially on both Rear positions but very slightly Wiry on the left.

Diagnosis Judging by her pulse, her condition is clearly primarily Empty. There is a clear deficiency of Kidney-Yang as evidenced by the feeling of cold, cold limbs, tiredness, dizziness, backache, frequent urination, nocturia, Pale tongue and pulse Weak on both Rear positions.

However, there are two Full conditions of which she has no symptoms. First, there is some Phlegm; this is shown by the swelling on the front of the tongue; second, there is some Qi stagnation, shown by the slight Wiry quality of the pulse on the left side.

Therefore, the feeling of depression in her case has two causes, one Empty, the other Full, with a predominance of the first. The deficiency of Kidney-Yang fails to stimulate the "coming and going" of the Ethereal Soul, resulting in depression. On the other hand, this deficiency also implies a weakness of the Kidney's Will-Power and therefore of drive, determination and initiative; this contributes to her feeling of depression.

Treatment In my treatment, I concentrated on treating the Deficiency with a formula to tonify Kidney-Yang, i.e. You Gui Wan *Restoring the Right* [Kidney] *Pill*. This is the variation I used (modified to treat Qi stagnation and Phlegm).

- **Rou Gui** *Cortex Cinnamomi* 5 g
- **Du Zhong** *Cortex Eucommiae ulmoidis* 10 g
- **Shan Zhu Yu** *Fructus Corni* 10 g
- **Tu Si Zi** *Semen Cuscutae* 10 g
- **Lu Jiao Jiao** *Gelatinum Cornu Cervi* 10 g
- **Shu Di Huang** *Radix Rehmanniae preparata* 10 g
- **Shan Yao** *Rhizoma Dioscoreae* 10 g
- **Gou Qi Zi** *Fructus Lycii chinensis* 10 g
- **Dang Gui** *Radix Angelicae sinensis* 5 g
- **Xu Duan** *Radix Dipsaci* 10 g

- **Gui Zhi** *Ramulus Cinnamomi cassiae* 10 g
- **Yuan Zhi** *Radix Polygalae* 10 g
- **Xiang Fu** *Rhizoma Cyperi* 10 g
- **Ban Xia** *Rhizoma Pinelliae preparatum* 10 g

Explanation

The first nine herbs constitute the root formula minus Fu Zi which I do not use.

- Xu Duan was added to tonify Kidney-Yang.
- Gui Zhi was added to tonify Yang and stimulate the circulation of Yang in the limbs.
- Yuan Zhi was added to stimulate the "coming and going" of the Ethereal Soul and lift mood.
- Xiang Fu was added to move Liver-Qi.
- Ban Xia was added to resolve Phlegm.

I gave her one course of the above formula as a concentrated powder, one teaspoonful twice a day. For the second course, I made some changes to strengthen the Phlegm-resolving action, as follows.

- **Rou Gui** *Cortex Cinnamomi* 5 g
- **Du Zhong** *Cortex Eucommiae ulmoidis* 10 g
- **Shan Zhu Yu** *Fructus Corni* 10 g
- **Tu Si Zi** *Semen Cuscutae* 10 g
- **Lu Jiao Jiao** *Gelatinum Cornu Cervi* 10 g
- **Shu Di Huang** *Radix Rehmanniae preparata* 10 g
- **Shan Yao** *Rhizoma Dioscoreae* 10 g
- **Gou Qi Zi** *Fructus Lycii chinensis* 10 g
- **Dang Gui** *Radix Angelicae sinensis* 5 g
- **Gui Zhi** *Ramulus Cinnamomi cassiae* 10 g
- **Yuan Zhi** *Radix Polygalae* 10 g
- **Xiang Fu** *Rhizoma Cyperi* 10 g
- **Ban Xia** *Rhizoma Pinelliae preparatum* 10 g
- **Chen Pi** *Pericarpium Citri reticulatae* 10 g
- **Fu Ling** *Poria* 10 g

After this second course, she said that not only were her limbs much less cold and without chilblains (she was being treated in wintertime), but that her depression had completely and totally lifted. She went out to buy herself new clothes and she said she felt as if she "were on antidepressants".

Case history

A 48-year-old man had been suffering from depression for over 10 years. He was successful in his profession but, in the last 10 years, he felt increasingly dissatisfied and questioned the meaning of life. He was happily married and had no financial problems.

His depression manifested with a low mood, a sense of frustration and irritability, a lack of drive and a feeling of pessimism. From the physical point of view, he had few problems but he did suffer from lower backache and low libido.

His pulse was Wiry but Empty at the deep level. His tongue was Reddish-Purple on the sides and had a deep Heart crack.

After seeing the deep Heart crack on his tongue, I asked him some more questions about his depression and personal history. A deep Heart crack on the tongue always indicates that the person has either been subject to severe emotional stress for many years or that he or she has a family history of mental-emotional problems.

When I asked this patient about his family and personal history he said that his father had suffered from depression for many years when he was a child and a teenager. His memories of his father were of a man who was in the grip of a major depressive disorder and hardly ever left his bedroom. This had affected him deeply (although he himself did not realize this). Therefore the deep Heart crack reflected this situation. The clinical significance of a deep Heart crack concerns also prognosis; in fact, such a crack always indicates that results will be slower to come.

Diagnosis The Wiry pulse and the sense of frustration and irritability indicate Liver-Qi stagnation. As the sides of the tongue are Purple, this indicates that the Qi stagnation has given rise to Blood stasis. The stagnation of Liver-Qi and Liver-Blood contribute to the depression as they restrain the "coming and going" of the Ethereal Soul.

The emptiness of the pulse at the deep level, lower backache and low libido indicate a Kidney deficiency. The Kidney deficiency induces a weakness of Will-Power (*Zhi*) and therefore a lack of drive and enthusiasm that contributes to the feeling of depression.

Treatment The treatment adopted was to move Qi, soothe the Liver, invigorate Blood and tonify the Kidneys. I used primarily acupuncture and some *Three Treasures* remedies.

With acupuncture, I chose the points primarily from the following.

- BL-23 Shenshu, Ren-4 Guanyuan and BL-52 Zhizhi to tonify the Kidneys and strengthen the Will-Power.
- LIV-3 Taichong and BL-47 Hunmen to move Liver-Qi and invigorate Liver-Blood and stimulate the "coming and going" of the Ethereal Soul.
- HE-7 Shenmen, HE-5 Tongli and Ren-15 Jiuwei to nourish the Heart.
- Du-20 Baihui and Du-24 Shenting to lift mood.

The *Three Treasures* remedy used was *Release Constraint* which is based on Zhu Dan Xi's Yue Ju Wan *Gardenia-Chuanxiong Pill* for the six stagnations. This remedy was very well indicated as the patient suffered from Liver-Qi and Liver-Blood stagnation.

I treated this patient with acupuncture only once a month because he lived a long way away. He started to improve after 3 months of treatment with acupuncture and the herbal remedy. After 18 months, he felt a lot better in himself, he was not feeling so frustrated and dejected, and felt much more enthusiastic about life, so much so that he found the mental drive to make a radical change in his career. A deep Heart crack such as the one he had cannot completely disappear but it did get less deep.

Case history

A 51-year-old woman had been suffering from depression for 3 years. This had coincided with the onset of the menopause. She felt very low, dissatisfied with life, sad and was prone to crying. She also felt vulnerable and burst into tears at the slightest negative comment that a member of her family might make. She also lacked drive and enthusiasm.

On interrogation, it transpired that she suffered from lower backache and frequent urination; she felt always cold. Occasionally, she experienced some phlegm in the throat that she needed to expectorate.

Her pulse was Wiry and Slippery and Weak on both Rear positions. Her tongue was Pale, Swollen, with teethmarks and had a sticky coating.

Diagnosis The Wiry pulse indicates that there is Liver-Qi stagnation and this restrains the "coming and going" of the Ethereal Soul, leading to depression. The Weak pulse on both Rear positions, backache and frequent urination indicate a Kidney deficiency, which accounts for the lack of drive and enthusiasm.

There is also some Phlegm as evidenced by the Slippery quality of the pulse, the swelling of the tongue and the occasional expectoration of Phlegm. The Phlegm also restrains the "coming and going" of the Ethereal Soul, contributing to the feeling of depression.

Treatment As she lived far away, I treated her only with herbal medicine and prescribed the *Three Treasures* remedy *Release Constraint* for the stagnation of Liver-Qi and depression. Besides moving Qi, this remedy also resolves Phlegm from which this patient also suffered.

I combined this remedy with the formula Gan Mai Da Zao Tang *Glycyrrhiza-Triticum-Jujuba Decoction* in a powdered form. I prescribed this formula to nourish the Heart and lift mood. I was drawn to using this formula by her emotional symptoms, characterized by vulnerability, sadness and crying. In such cases, I feel the Mind (*Shen*) needs to be nourished and I find the formula Gan Mai Da Zao Tang ideal for this.

After 2 years of treatment, she felt completely different and her depression was completely relieved.

Case history

A 48-year-old woman had been suffering from depression for 12 years. Besides feeling depressed, low and sad, she also felt anxious and slept badly. As she described it, her mind was in constant "turmoil".

She also experienced a feeling of oppression of the chest and palpitations. Her tongue was slightly Red on the sides, Swollen, with a Stomach–Heart crack and a sticky coating. Her pulse was Slippery, Weak on both Rear positions and slightly Overflowing on both Front positions.

Diagnosis The tongue and pulse are absolutely crucial to diagnose this case. The redness of the tongue indicates Heat, while the swelling and sticky coating indicate Phlegm; this is confirmed by the feeling of oppression of the chest. The Stomach–Heart crack is a midline crack that is long and narrow like a Heart crack but also broader in the center, in the Stomach area. The swelling, redness and the crack all indicate the presence of Phlegm-Heat in the Heart and Lungs. This is confirmed by the slightly Overflowing quality on both Front positions (Heart and Lungs) of the pulse. Such an overflowing quality is often related to emotional stress affecting those two organs. Finally, the weakness of the pulse on both Rear positions indicates that there is also a Kidney deficiency.

Treatment I treated this patient only with herbal medicine as she lived a long way away. I actually used three prescriptions in a powdered form.

- Wen Dan Tang *Warming the Gall-Bladder Decoction* to resolve Phlegm and clear Heat from the Heart and Lungs and calm the Mind.
- Bai He Zhi Mu Tang *Lilium-Anemarrhena Decoction* to nourish Heart- and Lung-Yin and nourish the Mind.
- Gan Mai Da Zao Tang *Glycyrrhiza-Triticum-Jujuba Decoction* to nourish the Heart and lift mood.

I added the following herbs to the above prescriptions.

- Yuan Zhi *Radix Polygalae* and Shi Chang Pu *Rhizoma Acori tatarinowii* to stimulate the "coming and going" of the Ethereal Soul and open the Mind's orifices.
- Tu Si Zi *Semen Cuscutae* and Gou Qi Zi *Fructus Lycii chinensis* to tonify the Kidneys.

She took this prescription for over a year and her tongue became gradually less Red and less Swollen; her pulse became stronger on the Rear positions. After 18 months she felt much better in herself, much less depressed and sad but still rather anxious.

Case history

A 73-year-old man had been suffering from depression for many years. He complained of feeling depressed, irritable and frustrated. He conceded that a certain family situation was causing him great frustration and resentment but he did not show any willingness to elaborate on that or to want to discuss it.

Physically, he was in remarkably good health, complaining only of some constipation and abdominal pain. He was not on any medication.

His tongue was quite normal except for being Red on the sides. His pulse was Wiry in all positions.

Diagnosis This is a very clear example of depression occurring against a background of Liver-Qi stagnation and deriving from repressed anger, frustration and resentment. The redness on the sides of the tongue reflects Heat deriving from Liver-Qi stagnation, while the Wiry quality of the pulse in all positions is a clear indication of Liver-Qi stagnation.

The stagnation of Liver-Qi restrains the "coming and going" of the Ethereal Soul and causes him to feel depressed.

Treatment I treated him only with a *Three Treasures* remedy called *Release Constraint* because his condition corresponded very well to that treated by Yue Ju Wan *Gardenia-Chuanxiong Pill* of which *Release Constraint* is a variation.

He felt no change for the first 2 months (taking 2 tablets twice a day), but started feeling an improvement into the third month. He got gradually better and less depressed and, most importantly, he recognized the repressed anger as a cause of his depression and started undergoing psychotherapy.

After 18 months, he felt very much better in himself and his depression lifted completely.

Case history

A 35-year-old woman had been suffering from depression for 7 years. She felt very depressed all the time, sad and cried frequently. The problem started after the break-up of a relationship 8 years previously. She had found this break-up very painful and she had an intense feeling of rejection and loss. She had never recovered from this break-up and had not been in another relationship since then.

She was pale and had a sad expression; she spoke with a very low voice. She sometimes experienced a dry mouth, palpitations and a slight breathlessness.

Her tongue was Pale and the coating was missing in patches. Her pulse was very Weak on the right Front position and Floating-Empty on the left side.

Diagnosis Her symptoms, pulse and tongue all clearly point to a deficiency of Lung-Qi and Lung-Yin. The symptoms indicating deficiency of the Lungs are crying, pale face, sadness, weak voice and a slight breathlessness. The lack of coating in patches on the tongue indicates Yin deficiency.

There is also a deficiency of the Heart as evidenced by the palpitations. In summary, there is therefore a deficiency of Qi and Yin of both Heart and Lungs.

Treatment I treated this patient with herbal medicine. I used the formula Gui Pi Tang *Tonifying the Spleen Decoction* to nourish Heart-Blood and Heart-Yin and lift mood, together with the formula Bai He Zhi Mu Tang *Lilium-Anemarrhena Decoction* (which contains only two herbs) to nourish Heart-Yin and Lung-Yin.

I used these two formulae in concentrated powder form, one teaspoonful twice a day. The patient started improving after taking the prescription for only 1 week. After 6 months, she felt very much better and, significantly, she embarked on a new relationship.

Case history

A 37-year-old woman had been suffering from depression for 2 years after the birth of their fourth child. She had had four children close together. She felt depressed and lacked any drive; she felt confused about her life aims and was torn between the desire to go back to work or to spend all the time at home to look after her children. She felt exhausted all the time with a desire to lie down.

Her periods were regular and not painful but she suffered from premenstrual tension, manifesting with a pronounced irritability and an aggravation of her depression.

Her tongue was slightly Red on the sides but Pale in general. Her pulse was Weak and Choppy.

Diagnosis Again, the tongue and pulse are crucial to the diagnosis. The Choppy quality of the pulse and the Pale color of the tongue indicate Blood deficiency. The redness on the sides of the tongue indicates Liver-Qi stagnation. There is also a Spleen deficiency as evidenced by the tiredness and desire to lie down.

Treatment I treated this patient only with two *Three Treasures* remedies. I gave her *Freeing the Moon* to be taken only for 10 days prior to the period and *Breaking Clouds* to be taken every day. The former remedy is a variation of Xiao Yao San *Free and Easy Wanderer Powder* that nourishes Liver-Blood and moves Liver-Qi; the latter is a variation of Bu Zhong Yi Qi Tang *Tonifying the Center and Benefiting Qi Decoction* that tonifies and lifts Spleen-Qi. This latter formula has been modified to lift mood and treat depression.

After taking these two remedies for 2 months she felt a lot more energetic and positive; after 12 months she felt completely better and her pulse was much stronger.

Case history

A 48-year-old woman had been suffering from depression for over 10 years. Her life had been very difficult in this time, going through the loss of a child and a divorce. She felt depressed, extremely tired, sad and was prone to crying.

She was pale and spoke with a weak voice. She also suffered from backache; on interrogation, it transpired that she felt easily hot and experienced a dry mouth at night. She felt a feeling of constriction of the chest.

Her tongue was Pale but had a red tip; the coating was rootless. Her pulse was Weak on the right Front position and generally empty at the deep level.

Diagnosis There are symptoms of Lung-Qi deficiency: pale face, weak voice, tendency to crying, Weak pulse on the right Front position. The feeling of constriction of the chest indicates some stagnation of Lung-Qi; in emotional problems, this frequently accompanies a Lung-Qi deficiency.

Other symptoms indicate a Kidney-Yin deficiency: lower backache, dry mouth at night, pulse empty at the deep level, rootless tongue coating.

The sadness and grief deriving from her loss and separation injured Lung-Qi and Kidney-Yin, resulting in depression and a restraint of the "coming and going" of the Ethereal Soul. The Kidney deficiency involves a deficiency of the Will-Power (*Zhi*) and this caused her to lack drive and enthusiasm.

Treatment I treated this patient with both acupuncture and herbs. I gave her the *Three Treasures* remedy *Nourish the Root* which is a variation of Zuo Gui Wan *Restoring the Left* [Kidney] *Pill* to nourish Kidney-Yin (in the evening) and *Breaking Clouds* which is a variation of Bu Zhong Yi Qi Tang *Tonifying the Center and Benefiting Qi Decoction* to tonify Lung-Qi and lift mood (in the morning).

With acupuncture, I used points from the following group.

- LU-9 Taiyuan, LU-3 Tianfu, BL-13 Feishu and BL-42 Pohu to tonify the Lungs, soothe the Corporeal Soul and lift mood.
- Ren-4 Guanyuan, SP-6 Sanyinjiao, KI-3 Taixi to nourish Kidney-Yin.
- BL-23 Shenshu and BL-52 Zhishi to strengthen the Will-Power.
- Du-20 Baihui to lift mood.

The combination of acupuncture and herbal medicine produced excellent results in a relatively short time. After 15 months of treatment she felt very much more positive, did not cry and looked forward to the future.

Case history

A 48-year-old woman had been suffering from depression and lack of motivation for some years. Two years previously, she had embarked on a radical change of career, starting to train in Jungian psychotherapy. She founds the course fascinating but also very stressful; as part of the course, she was under therapy herself.

On a physical level, she suffered from lower backache, slight tinnitus, slight night-sweating, tiredness and a dry mouth. Her tongue was fairly normal but with a red tip; her pulse was very Weak on both Rear positions and the left Middle position (Liver) was relatively Full and slightly Wiry.

Diagnosis My main diagnosis was a deficiency of Kidney-Yang and Liver-Qi stagnation. The Kidney deficiency involved a weakness of the Will-Power (*Zhi*), which accounted for depression and lack of motivation. The stagnation of Liver-Qi contributed to the feeling of depression by restraining the movement of the Ethereal Soul.

Treatment I treated this patient only with herbal medicine and I started the treatment by tonifying the Kidneys with a variation of You Gui Wan *Restoring the Right* [Kidney] *Pill*.

- **Shu Di Huang** *Radix Rehmanniae preparata*
- **Shan Yao** *Rhizoma Dioscoreae*
- **Shan Zhu Yu** *Fructus Corni*
- **Tu Si Zi** *Semen Cuscutae*
- **Gou Qi Zi** *Fructus Lycii chinensis*
- **Dang Gui** *Radix Angelicae sinensis*
- **Yuan Zhi** *Radix Polygalae*

I treated her with variations of the above formula (in concentrated powder form) for several months. She improved in general but, at a point where her course was particularly stressful, she lacked motivation and confidence. At that time, I changed the formula to a variation of Gan Mai Da Zao Tang *Glycyrrhiza-Triticum-Jujuba Decoction*.

- **Zhi Gan Cao** *Radix Glycyrrhizae uralensis preparata*
- **Fu Xiao Mai** *Fructus Tritici levis*
- **Da Zao** *Fructus Jujubae*
- **Bai He** *Bulbus Lilii*
- **Zhi Mu** *Radix Anemarrhaenae*
- **Yuan Zhi** *Radix Polygalae*
- **Lian Zi Xin** *Plumula Nelumbinis*
- **Du Zhong** *Cortex Eucommiae ulmoidis*

I use the formula Gan Mai Da Zao Tang in depression occurring against a background of Qi and Blood deficiency. I frequently combine this formula with Bai He and Zhi Mu to soothe Lungs and allay sadness. Yuan Zhi is used to raise Liver-Qi with its pungent taste; Lian Zi Xin was used to calm the Mind and clear Heart-Heat; Du Zhong was used to tonify the Kidneys and strengthen Will-Power and motivation.

I used variations of this formula for several months. In total, she was treated for over 2 years, after which she reported a great improvement in her mental and emotional state and she was able to successfully complete her course.

PATIENTS' STATISTICS

I have compiled a statistic of 68 patients with depression from my practice. There were 47 women (69%) and 21 men (31%); this is almost exactly in line with the overall percentage of women in my practice (67%). The age distribution was as follows.

- 21 to 30: 1 (1%)
- 31 to 40: 4 (6%)
- 41 to 50: 28 (41%)
- 51 to 60: 13 (19%)
- 61 to 70: 10 (15%)
- 71 to 80: 8 (12%)
- 81 to 90: 3 (4%)
- 91 to 100: 1 (1%)

Therefore, the highest incidence of depression is in the 41–50 age bracket and the second highest in the 51–60 age bracket. If we take these two bands together, they account for 60% of cases of depression. This finding is in line with the etiology of depression and its incidence in mid-life. During the mid-life years, the ego-building of the earlier years does not satisfy the individual any longer and the demands of the Soul are being felt. From a Jungian perspective, depression in mid-life is a way for the Soul to make its demands on the individual felt.

In terms of patterns, 33% of patients displayed a purely Full condition, 40% a purely Empty condition and 27% a mixed Full-Empty one. The figure of 33% for a purely Full condition is interesting as it shows that a substantial proportion of patients with depression suffer from a purely Full condition; from the manifestations of depression (slow movement, weak voice, sadness, etc.) it would be easy to conclude wrongly that it is always caused by an Empty condition.

Quite a high percentage of patients (30%) suffered from either Liver-Qi stagnation or Liver-Blood stasis, showing that stagnation is an important feature of the pathology of depression.

In terms of Internal Organs involved, these were as follows.

- *Liver*: 29 (42.6%)
- *Kidneys*: 26 (38.2%)
- *Spleen*: 17 (25%)
- *Heart*: 13 (19.1%)
- *Lungs*: 9 (13.2%)

Please note that the total of the above numbers do not add up to 68 (the total number of patients) and the percentages do not add up to 100 because many patients suffer from patterns from more than one organ, e.g. Liver-Qi stagnation with Kidney deficiency.

The Liver patterns were overwhelmingly of the Full type and the breakdown is as follows.

- *Liver total*: 29 (42%)
- *Liver Blood* Xu: 6 (21%)
- *Liver Blood stasis*: 8 (27%)
- *Liver Fire*: 5 (17%)
- *Liver Wind*: 2 (7%)
- *Liver-Qi stagnation*: 12 (41%)
- *Liver Yang rising*: 1 (3%)
- *Liver Yin* Xu: 1 (3%)

Please note that the numbers on the left do not add up to 29 or the percentages to 100 because one patient may have more than one pattern (e.g. Liver-Qi stagnation with Liver-Blood deficiency); in other words, some patients may appear in more than one box.

In terms of pathogenic factors, the main ones were those related to the Liver and especially Liver-Qi stagnation, Liver-Blood stasis and Liver-Fire. The other important pathogenic factor was Phlegm, accounting for 26 patients (39%); this correlates with the incidence of Swollen tongue, i.e. 24 cases (36%).

As for the tongue, many more tongues were Red than Pale, i.e. 42 (63%) against 14 (21%), respectively. This shows how common Heat is in depression; this is obviously due to the Qi stagnation from emotional stress giving rise to Heat.

Quite a high percentage of tongues were Purple (17 or 25%), showing that Blood stasis is a common pathogenic factor in depression. An interesting finding is the percentage of patients with a Heart crack. These were 9 or 13%; this percentage is above the norm, which for all patients is 7%.

WESTERN DRUG TREATMENT

I shall describe below the Western medicine approach to the treatment of depression and the main classes of antidepressants. I shall also discuss the integration of Chinese with Western medicine in the treatment of depression.

The discussion will be conducted according to the following topics.

- Introduction and pharmacology
- Clinical use
- Types of antidepressants
- Combination of Western and Chinese medicine

Introduction and pharmacology

The treatment of depression in Western psychiatry has been dominated by pharmacological treatment with antidepressants since the 1960s. The first class of antidepressants used was the tricyclic ones (see below) and, since the 1980s, selective serotonin reuptake inhibitors (SSRIs) have been mostly used.

In order to understand how these antidepressants work, we should look briefly at nerve conduction in neurons and the role of neurotransmitters. Neurons communicate through electrical impulses but these cannot cross gaps (synapses) among neurons. The gap is bridged by neurotransmitters. Figure 16.27 illustrates the anatomy of a neuron.

Neurons release neurotransmitters to communicate with other neurons across synapses. Neurotransmitters transmit signals across a gap (synapse) between the nerve cells. Neurons send a signal and then reabsorb the neurotransmitters after they have communicated with another neuron. The process of reabsorption is called reuptake (Figs 16.28 and 16.29).

In depression, there is a lack of certain neurotransmitters. Neurotransmitters associated with depression are serotonin, noradrenaline (norepinephrine) and possibly dopamine. Research suggests that people with depression have lower levels of one or more of these neurotransmitters.

Antidepressants interfere with the reuptake of neurotransmitters across the synapse; this results in higher levels of a particular neurotransmitter in the synapse (Fig. 16.30). This can change the activity of certain nerve cells and influence brain activity. Maintaining a higher level of neurotransmitters improves neurotransmission which, in turn, improves mood.

Tricyclic and tetracyclic antidepressants work by preventing neurotransmitters from binding with certain nerve cell receptors. This indirectly increases the levels of noradrenaline (norepinephrine) and serotonin in the brain. The net result is the same as that taking place when selective serotonin reuptake inhibitors are used, i.e. increased levels of a particular neurotransmitter.

Monoamine oxidase inhibitors (MAOIs) work by inhibiting the action of monoamine oxidase. This com-

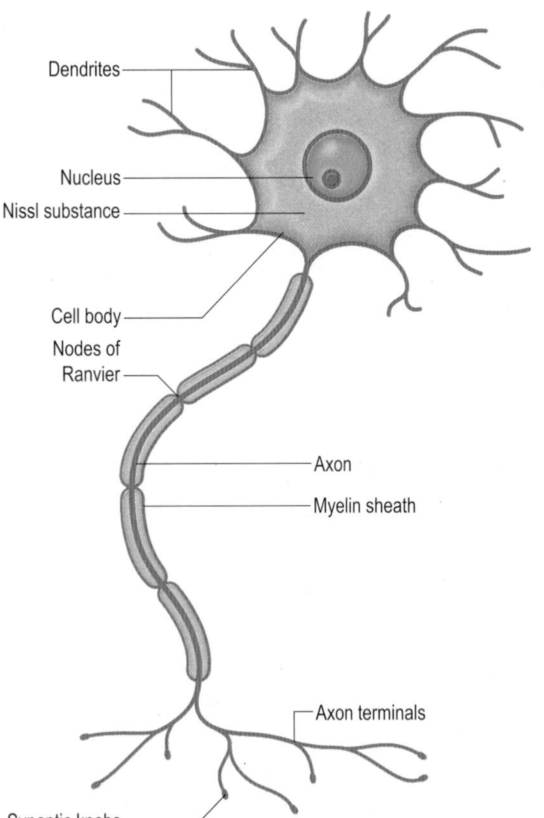

Figure 16.27 Anatomy of a neuron.

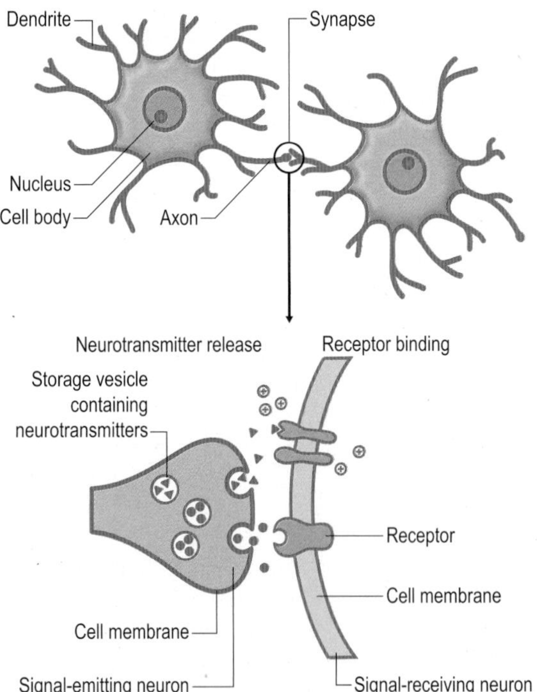

Figure 16.28 Reuptake of neurotransmitters.

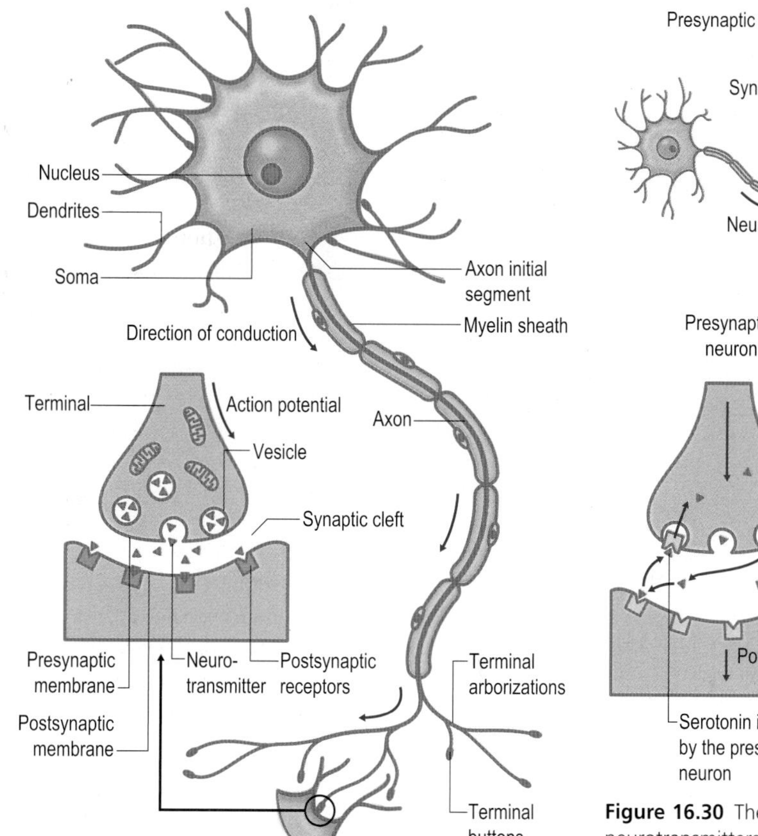

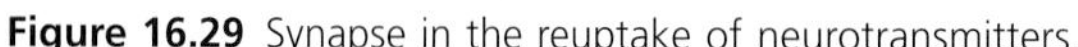

Figure 16.29 Synapse in the reuptake of neurotransmitters.

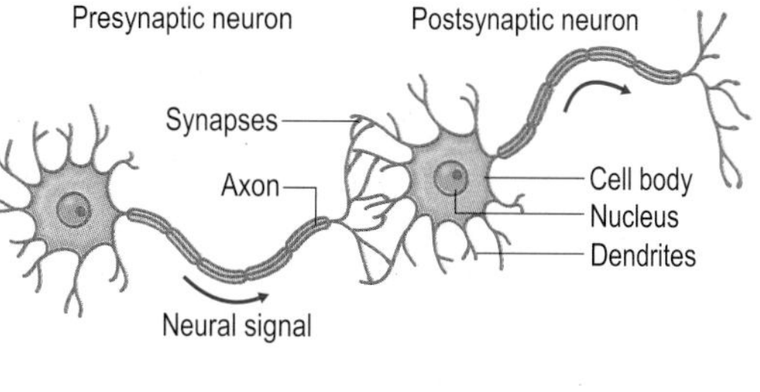

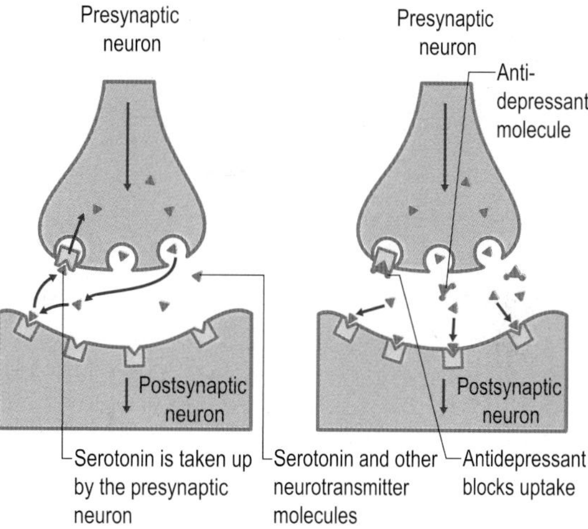

Figure 16.30 The effect of antidepressants upon reuptake of neurotransmitters.

pound metabolizes (and therefore reduces levels of) neurotransmitters such as serotonin and dopamine. MAOIs are not used as much as the SSRIs due to their side-effects and restrictions placed on diet when taking them. However, there is a new generation of selective MAOIs that do not require such restrictions placed on diet. In contrast to the non-selective inhibitors, used in the years 1957–1970, the selective inhibitors bind to and block only one of the two isoenzymes, MAO-A or MAO-B. The MAO-A inhibitors and part of the MAO-B inhibitors differ also from the classic drugs by their reversibility.

The inhibition of MAO-A causes the rise of noradrenaline (norepinephrine), dopamine and serotonin in the synaptic cleft; the inhibition of MAO-B only of dopamine. The new inhibitors diminish also to some extent the reuptake of monoamines. The selective block of one of the isoenzymes does not stop the metabolism of tyramine (from cheese, red wine); this means that the patient does not need to restrict consumption of such foods.

The different modes of action of the three main classes of antidepressants are summarized as follows.

- Monoamine oxidase inhibitors (MAOIs) reduce the metabolism of (and therefore lead to increased levels of) serotonin and noradrenaline (norepinephrine) by inhibiting monoamine oxidase.
- Tricyclic antidepressants inhibit the reuptake of serotonin and noradrenaline (norepinephrine) across the synapses; as these neurotransmitters are not recycled back into the neurons, there are increased levels of them in the synapses. Tricyclic antidepressants also alter the sensitivity of some serotonin and noradrenaline (norepinephrine) receptors.
- Selective serotonin reuptake inhibitors (SSRIs) block the reuptake pumps for serotonin so that this cannot be reshuffled back into the neuron.

Clinical use

After 3 months of treatment, the proportions of people with depression who will be much improved are 50–65% if given an antidepressant compared with 25–30% if given an inactive placebo.[27]

Antidepressants are generally not addictive; they do not often cause the addictions that one gets with tranquillizers, alcohol or nicotine. However, there is a debate about this. In spite of not having the symptoms of addiction described above, up to a third of people who stop SSRIs and serotonin and noradrenaline reuptake inhibitors (SNRIs) do have withdrawal symptoms. These may include:[28]

- stomach upsets
- flu-like symptoms
- anxiety
- dizziness
- vivid dreams at night
- sensations in the body that feel like electric shocks.

In most people these withdrawal effects are mild, but for a small number of people they can be quite severe. They seem to be most likely to happen with paroxetine (Seroxat) and venlafaxine (Efexor). It is generally best to taper off the dose of an antidepressant rather than to stop it suddenly.

The Committee of Safety of Medicines in the UK reviewed the evidence in 2004 and concluded:[29]

There is no clear evidence that the SSRIs and related antidepressants have a significant dependence liability or show development of a dependence syndrome according to internationally accepted criteria.

All antidepressants may cause a complication called "serotonin syndrome". This is a rare but potentially life-threatening side-effect of SSRIs. This condition, characterized by dangerously high levels of serotonin in the brain, can occur when an SSRI interacts with MAOIs. Serotonin syndrome can also occur when SSRIs are taken with other medications or supplements that affect serotonin levels, such as Hypericum (St John's Wort). Serotonin syndrome requires immediate medical treatment.

Signs and symptoms of serotonin syndrome include:[30]

- confusion
- restlessness
- hallucinations
- extreme agitation
- fluctuations in blood pressure
- increased heart rate
- nausea and vomiting
- fever
- seizures
- coma.

Types of antidepressants

I discuss below the seven main classes of antidepressants as follows.

- Selective serotonin reuptake inhibitors (SSRIs)
- Noradrenaline (norepinephrine) and dopamine reuptake inhibitors (NDRIs)
- Serotonin and noradrenaline (norepinephrine) reuptake inhibitors (SNRIs)
- Tricyclic antidepressants (TCAs)
- Tetracyclic antidepressants
- Combined reuptake inhibitors and receptor blockers
- Monoamine oxidase inhibitors (MAOIs)

These antidepressants are listed according to their generic name, followed by the brand name in brackets. The brand names are followed by the designations [US] or [UK] according to whether they are marketed under that name in the USA or the UK; if no country designation is indicated, it means that they have the same brand name in the USA and the UK.

Selective serotonin reuptake inhibitors (SSRIs)

As explained above, SSRI antidepressants work by inhibiting the reuptake of serotonin across the synapses, resulting in higher levels of this neurotransmitter. The main SSRI antidepressants, with generic name and brand names in brackets, are as follows.

- Citalopram (Celexa [US], Cipramil [UK])
- Escitalopram (Lexapro [US], Cipralex [UK])
- Fluoxetine (Prozac)
- Paroxetine (Paxil, Pexeva [US], Seroxat [UK])
- Sertraline (Zoloft [US], Lustral [UK])

Side-effects of SSRIs

SSRIs are generally considered safer than other classes of antidepressants. They are less likely to have adverse interactions with other medications and are less dangerous if taken as an overdose.[31] Individual SSRIs have some different pharmacological characteristics and therefore patients may react differently with one antidepressant compared to another.

The side-effects of SSRIs include:[32]

- nausea
- sexual dysfunction, including reduced desire or orgasm difficulties
- headache
- diarrhea
- nervousness
- rash
- agitation
- restlessness
- increased sweating
- weight gain
- drowsiness
- insomnia.

SUMMARY

Selective serotonin reuptake inhibitors (SSRIs)

- Citalopram (Celexa [US], Cipramil [UK])
- Escitalopram (Lexapro [US], Cipralex [UK])
- Fluoxetine (Prozac)
- Paroxetine (Paxil, Pexeva [US], Seroxat [UK])
- Sertraline (Zoloft [US], Lustral [UK])

Side-effects of SSRIs

- Nausea
- Sexual dysfunction, including reduced desire or orgasm difficulties
- Headache
- Diarrhea
- Nervousness
- Rash
- Agitation
- Restlessness
- Increased sweating
- Weight gain
- Drowsiness
- Insomnia

Noradrenaline (norepinephrine) and dopamine reuptake inhibitors (NDRIs)

Noradrenaline (norepinephrine) and dopamine reuptake inhibitors (NDRIs) are a type of antidepressant medication that increases the levels of both noradrenaline (norepinephrine) and dopamine by inhibiting their reabsorption into cells.

The main NDRI is bupropion (Wellbutrin [US], Zyban [UK]). Zyban is an NDRI antidepressants but it is used mostly as an anti-smoking medication.

Side-effects of NDRIs

Side-effects of NDRIs include:[33]

- loss of appetite
- weight loss
- headache
- dry mouth
- skin rash
- sweating
- ringing in the ears
- shakiness and nervousness
- stomach pain
- agitation
- constipation
- anxiety
- dizziness
- trouble sleeping
- muscle pain
- nausea and vomiting
- fast heartbeat
- sore throat
- more frequent urination.

Safety concerns with NDRIs

Bupropion can increase blood pressure in some people, so regular monitoring is important. The risk of developing high blood pressure may increase if one also uses nicotine replacement therapy, such as a nicotine patch, to stop smoking.

There is a small chance that taking bupropion can cause a seizure if there is a history of previous seizures, a head injury or a nervous system tumor, or if there is a history of bulimia or anorexia.

SUMMARY

Noradrenaline (norepinephrine) and dopamine reuptake inhibitors (NDRIs)

- Bupropion (Wellbutrin [US], Zyban [UK])

Side-effects of NDRIs

- Loss of appetite
- Weight loss
- Headache

- Dry mouth
- Skin rash
- Sweating
- Ringing in the ears
- Shakiness and nervousness
- Stomach pain
- Agitation
- Constipation
- Anxiety
- Dizziness
- Trouble sleeping
- Muscle pain
- Nausea and vomiting
- Fast heartbeat
- Sore throat
- More frequent urination

Serotonin and noradrenaline (norepinephrine) reuptake inhibitors (SNRIs)

Serotonin and noradrenaline (norepinephrine) reuptake inhibitors (SNRIs) are a type of antidepressant medication that increases the levels of both serotonin and noradrenaline (norepinephrine) by inhibiting their reabsorption into cells in the brain. Medications in this group of antidepressants are sometimes known as dual reuptake inhibitors.

The main SNRIs are as follows.

- Duloxetine (Cymbalta [US], Yentreve [UK])
- Venlafaxine (Efexor)

Side-effects of SNRIs

Side-effects of SNRIs include:[34]

- nausea
- vomiting
- dizziness
- insomnia
- sleepiness
- trouble sleeping
- abnormal dreams
- constipation
- sweating
- dry mouth
- yawning
- tremor
- gas
- anxiety
- agitation
- abnormal vision, such as blurred vision or double vision
- headache
- sexual dysfunction.

SUMMARY

Serotonin and noradrenaline (norepinephrine) reuptake inhibitors (SNRIs)

- Duloxetine (Cymbalta [US], Yentreve [UK])
- Venlafaxine (Efexor)

Side-effects of SNRIs

- Nausea
- Vomiting
- Dizziness
- Insomnia
- Sleepiness
- Trouble sleeping
- Abnormal dreams
- Constipation
- Sweating
- Dry mouth
- Yawning
- Tremor
- Gas
- Anxiety
- Agitation
- Abnormal vision, such as blurred vision or double vision
- Headache
- Sexual dysfunction

Tricyclic antidepressants (TCAs)

TCAs inhibit the reabsorption (reuptake) of serotonin and noradrenaline (norepinephrine). As explained above, tricyclic and tetracyclic antidepressants work by preventing neurotransmitters from binding with certain nerve cell receptors. To a lesser extent, TCAs also inhibit reabsorption of dopamine. These antidepressants also block other cell receptors, which accounts for this class of antidepressants causing more side-effects than others. TCAs were among the earliest antidepressants, having been introduced in the 1960s, and they remained the first line of treatment for depression through the 1980s, before newer antidepressants arrived.

The main tricyclic antidepressants are as follows.

- Amitriptyline (Elavil [US], Tryptizol [UK])
- Amoxapine (Asendin [US], Asendis [UK])
- Clomipramine (Anafranil [UK])
- Desipramine (Norpramin)
- Dosulepin (Prothiaden [UK])
- Doxepin (Sinequan [US])
- Imipramine (Tofranil [US])
- Lofepramine (Gamanil [US])
- Nortriptyline (Aventyl, Pamelor [US], Allegron [UK])
- Protriptyline (Vivactil [US])
- Trazodone (Molipaxin [UK])
- Trimipramine (Surmontil)

Side-effects of TCAs

Because TCAs are less selective about which cells they affect, they typically have more side-effects than other antidepressants.

Side-effects of TCAs include:[35]

- drowsiness
- dry mouth
- blurred vision
- constipation
- urinary retention
- dizziness
- impaired sexual functioning
- increased heart rate
- disorientation or confusion
- headache
- low blood pressure
- sensitivity to sunlight
- increased appetite
- weight gain
- nausea
- weakness.

SUMMARY

Tricyclic antidepressants (TCAs)

- Amitriptyline (Elavil [US], Tryptizol [UK])
- Amoxapine (Asendin [US], Asendis [UK])
- Clomipramine (Anafranil [UK])
- Desipramine (Norpramin)
- Dosulepin (Prothiaden [UK])
- Doxepin (Sinequan [US])
- Imipramine (Tofranil [US])
- Lofepramine (Gamanil [US])
- Nortriptyline (Aventyl, Pamelor [US], Allegron [UK])
- Protriptyline (Vivactil [US])
- Trazodone (Molipaxin [UK])
- Trimipramine (Surmontil)

Side-effects of TCAs

- Drowsiness
- Dry mouth
- Blurred vision
- Constipation
- Urinary retention
- Dizziness
- Impaired sexual functioning
- Increased heart rate
- Disorientation or confusion
- Headache
- Low blood pressure
- Sensitivity to sunlight
- Increased appetite
- Weight gain
- Nausea
- Weakness

Tetracyclic antidepressants

Instead of inhibiting the reabsorption of certain neurotransmitters as other antidepressants do, tetracyclic antidepressants prevent neurotransmitters from binding with nerve cell receptors called alpha-2 receptors. This indirectly increases the levels of noradrenaline (norepinephrine) and serotonin in the brain.

The main tetracyclic antidepressant is mirtazapine (Remeron [US], Zispin [UK]).

Side-effects of tetracyclic antidepressants

Side-effects of tetracyclic antidepressants include:[36]

- drowsiness
- weight gain
- dry mouth
- dizziness
- lightheadedness
- thirst

- muscle or joint aches
- constipation
- increased appetite
- increased cholesterol.

SUMMARY

Tetracyclic antidepressants
- Mirtazapine (Remeron [US], Zispin [UK])

Side-effects of tetracyclic antidepressants
- Drowsiness
- Weight gain
- Dry mouth
- Dizziness
- Lightheadedness
- Thirst
- Muscle or joint aches
- Constipation
- Increased appetite
- Increased cholesterol

Combined reuptake inhibitors and receptor blockers

Combined reuptake inhibitors and receptor blockers are dual-action antidepressants. That is, they act both by inhibiting the reabsorption (reuptake) of neurotransmitters into nerve cells (as SSRIs do) and by blocking nerve cell receptors (as tetracyclic antidepressants do).

The main combined reuptake inhibitors and receptor blocker antidepressants are as follows.

- Trazodone (Desyrel [US])
- Nefazodone (Serzone)
- Maprotiline (Ludiomil [UK])
- Mirtazapine (Remeron [US])

Side-effects of combined reuptake inhibitors and receptor blockers

Side-effects of combined inhibitors and blockers include:[37]

- dry mouth
- dizziness
- drowsiness
- lightheadedness
- nervousness
- nausea
- constipation
- weakness
- vision problems
- confusion
- headache.

SUMMARY

Combined reuptake inhibitors and receptor blockers
- Trazodone (Desyrel [US])
- Nefazodone (Serzone [US])
- Maprotiline (Ludiomil [UK])
- Mirtazapine (Remeron [US])

Side-effects of combined reuptake inhibitors and receptor blockers
- Dry mouth
- Dizziness
- Drowsiness
- Lightheadedness
- Nervousness
- Nausea
- Constipation
- Weakness
- Vision problems
- Confusion
- Headache

Monoamine oxidase inhibitors (MAOIs)

MAOIs relieve depression by preventing the enzyme monoamine oxidase from metabolizing the neurotransmitters noradrenaline (norepinephrine), serotonin and dopamine in the brain.

The main MAOIs are as follows.

- Moclobemide (Manerix [UK])
- Phenelzine (Nardil)
- Tranylcypromine (Parnate)
- Isocarboxazid (Marplan)
- Selegiline (Emsam [US], Eldepryl [UK])

Side-effects of MAOIs

Because they can cause serious side-effects, MAOIs are usually reserved for people whose depression does not improve with other antidepressant medications.

Side-effects of MAOIs include:[38]

- drowsiness
- constipation
- nausea
- diarrhea
- stomach upset
- fatigue
- dry mouth
- dizziness
- low blood pressure
- lightheadedness, especially when getting up from a lying or sitting position
- decreased urine output
- decreased sexual function
- sleep disturbances
- muscle twitching
- weight gain
- blurred vision
- headache
- increased appetite
- restlessness
- shakiness
- trembling
- weakness
- increased sweating.

SUMMARY

Monoamine oxidase inhibitors (MAOIs)

- Moclobemide (Manerix [UK])
- Phenelzine (Nardil [US])
- Tranylcypromine (Parnate [US])
- Isocarboxazid (Marplan [US])
- Selegiline (Emsam [US])

Side-effects of MAOIs

- Drowsiness
- Constipation
- Nausea
- Diarrhea
- Stomach upset
- Fatigue
- Dry mouth
- Dizziness
- Low blood pressure
- Lightheadedness, especially when getting up from a lying or sitting position
- Decreased urine output
- Decreased sexual function
- Sleep disturbances
- Muscle twitching
- Weight gain
- Blurred vision
- Headache
- Increased appetite
- Restlessness
- Shakiness
- Trembling
- Weakness
- Increased sweating

Combination of Chinese and Western medicine

First of all, I find that antidepressants do not change the clinical manifestations substantially. Most antidepressants do affect the pulse, giving it a quality that defies description according to the traditional pulse qualities. I describe it as "stagnant" and "reluctant". The pulse feels like it does not flow properly and it lacks a "wave". However, it does not lack a wave in the same way as the "Sad" pulse: this pulse is rather weak and Choppy. The pulse from antidepressants is not weak.

As for interactions, I have never in my practice observed any negative interactions between antidepressants and acupuncture or Chinese herbs. Acupuncture especially certainly does not have any negative interaction with antidepressants.

If a patient is taking antidepressants, I do not ask them to come off them before starting the treatment. This is very important, especially in the case of patients who are extremely depressed. I usually start the treatment (with acupuncture and herbs) and maintain the same level of medication for about 2 months, after which I ask them to try to reduce the dosage. Of course, this must be done with the knowledge of the doctor or psychiatrist who prescribed the medication.

END NOTES

1. 1981 Jin Gui Yao Lue Fang Xin Jie 金匮要略方新解[A New Explanation of the Essential Prescriptions of the Golden Chest]. Zhejiang Scientific Publishing House, Zhejiang, pp. 24–26. The *Essential Prescriptions of the Golden Chest* was written by Zhang Zhong Jing and first published *c.*AD 220.
2. Mayo Clinic website: http://www.mayoclinic.com/health/depression/DS00175. [Accessed 2008].
3. Bowlby J 1980 Loss, Sadness and Depression. Hogarth Press, London, p. 246.

4. Seligman MEP 1975 Helplessness. W.H. Freeman, San Francisco, pp. 21–40.
5. 1979 Huang Di Nei Jing Su Wen 黄帝内经素问[The Yellow Emperor's Classic of Internal Medicine – Simple Questions]. People's Health Publishing House, Beijing, pp. 501–502. First published c.100 BC.
6. Cited in Zhang Bo Yu 1986 Zhong Yi Nei Ke Xue 中医内科学 [Chinese Internal Medicine]. Shanghai Science Publishing House, Shanghai, p. 121.
7. Ibid., p. 121.
8. A New Explanation of the Essential Prescriptions of the Golden Chest, p. 26.
9. Chen You Bang 1990 Zhong Guo Zhen Jiu Zhi Liao Xue 中国针灸治疗学 [Chinese Acupuncture Therapy]. China Science Publishing House, Shanghai, pp. 511–512.
10. A New Explanation of the Essential Prescriptions of the Golden Chest, p. 185.
11. Ibid., p. 185.
12. Cited in Wang Yong Yan 2004 Zhong Yi Nei Ke Xue 中医内科学 [Chinese Internal Medicine]. People's Health Publishing House, Beijing, p. 265.
13. Cited in Zhang Bo Yu 1986 Chinese Internal Medicine, p. 107.
14. Qin Bo Wei 1991 Qing Dai Ming Yi Yi An Jing Hua 清代名医医案精华 [The Essence of Medical Records of Famous Doctors of the Qing Dynasty]. Shanghai Science and Technology Press, Shanghai, p. 233.
15. Dr Zhang Ming Jiu, personal communication, Nanjing 1982.
16. Hu Xi Ming 1989 Zhong Guo Zhong Yi Mi Fang Da Quan 中国中医秘方大全 [Great Treatise of Secret Formulae in Chinese Medicine]. Literary Publishing House, Shanghai, p. 773.
17. Ibid., p. 772.
18. Shan Chang Hua 1990 Jing Xue Jie 经穴解 [An Explanation of the Acupuncture Points]. People's Health Publishing House, Beijing, pp. 26–27. *An Explanation of the Acupuncture Points was written by* Yue Han Zhen and first published in 1654.
19. Ibid., p. 27.
20. Ibid., p. 207.
21. Ibid., p. 211.
22. Dr Zhang Ming Jiu, personal communication, Nanjing 1982.
23. Cheng Bao Shu 1988 Zhen Jiu Da Ci Dian 针灸大辞典 [Great Dictionary of Acupuncture]. Beijing Science Publishing House, Beijing, p. 11.
24. Jiao Shun Fa 1987 Zhong Guo Zhen Jiu Xue Qiu Zhen 中国针学求诊 [An Enquiry into Chinese Acupuncture]. Shanxi Science Publishing House, Shanxi, p. 52.
25. Dr Zhang Ming Jiu, personal communication, Nanjing 1982.
26. Cited in Bensky D, Clavey S, Stöger E 2004 Materia Medica, 3rd edn. Eastland Press, Seattle, p. 936.
27. Royal College of Psychiatrists website: http://www.rcpsych.ac.uk/mentalhealthinformation/mentalhealthproblems/depression/antidepressants.aspx. [Accessed 2008].
28. Ibid.
29. Ibid.
30. Mayo Clinic website: http://www.mayoclinic.com/health/antidepressants/HQ01069 [Accessed 2008].
31. Ibid.
32. Ibid.
33. Ibid.
34. Ibid.
35. Ibid.
36. Ibid.
37. Ibid.
38. Ibid.

惊悸
怔忡

CHAPTER 17

ANXIETY

ANXIETY IN WESTERN MEDICINE *417*

ANXIETY IN CHINESE MEDICINE *418*
Chinese disease entities corresponding to anxiety *419*
Rebellious Qi of the Penetrating Vessel (*Chong Mai*) *419*
Palpitations in Chinese diagnosis *422*
Difference between Mind Unsettled and Mind Obstructed in anxiety *422*

ETIOLOGY *422*
Emotional stress *422*
Constitution *423*
Irregular diet *423*
Loss of blood *423*
Overwork *423*

PATHOLOGY AND TREATMENT PRINCIPLES *423*
Heart *424*
Lungs *425*
Kidneys *426*
Spleen *427*
Liver *427*

ACUPUNCTURE TREATMENT OF ANXIETY *427*
Distal points according to channel *427*
Head points *428*

IDENTIFICATION OF PATTERNS AND TREATMENT *430*
Heart and Gall-Bladder deficiency *430*
Heart-Blood deficiency *431*
Kidney- and Heart-Yin deficiency with Empty Heat *432*
Heart-Yang deficiency *433*
Lung- and Heart-Qi deficiency *434*
Lung- and Heart-Qi stagnation *435*
Lung- and Heart-Yin deficiency *435*
Heart-Blood stasis *436*
Phlegm-Heat harassing the Heart *437*

MODERN CHINESE LITERATURE *438*

CLINICAL TRIALS *439*

CASE HISTORIES *443*

- Heart and Gall-Bladder deficiency
- Heart-Blood deficiency
- Kidney- and Heart-Yin deficiency with Empty Heat
- Heart-Yang deficiency
- Lung- and Heart-Qi deficiency
- Lung- and Heart-Qi stagnation
- Lung- and Heart-Yin deficiency
- Heart-Blood stasis
- Phlegm-Heat harassing the Heart

ANXIETY

Anxiety is a normal reaction to stress. In general, it helps one to cope. But when anxiety becomes an excessive, irrational dread of everyday situations, it has become a disabling disorder.

The discussion of anxiety will be conducted according to the following topics.

- Anxiety in Western medicine
- Anxiety in Chinese medicine
- Etiology
- Pathology and treatment principles
- Acupuncture treatment of anxiety
- Identification of patterns and treatment
- Modern Chinese literature
- Clinical trials
- Case histories

ANXIETY IN WESTERN MEDICINE

The anxiety disorders discussed in Western medicine are:

- generalized anxiety disorder
- panic disorder

- obsessive-compulsive disorder
- post-traumatic stress disorder (PTSD)
- social phobia (or social anxiety disorder)
- specific phobias.

Each anxiety disorder has its own distinct features, but they are all bound together by the common theme of excessive, irrational fear, worry and dread.

A chronic state of anxiety is usually called generalized anxiety disorder. The essential characteristic of generalized anxiety disorder (GAD) is an excessive uncontrollable worry about everyday things. This constant worry affects daily functioning and can cause physical symptoms.

GAD can occur with other anxiety disorders, depressive disorders or substance abuse. GAD is often difficult to diagnose because it lacks some of the dramatic symptoms such as unprovoked panic attacks that are seen with other anxiety disorders; for a diagnosis to be made, worry must be present more days than not for at least 6 months.

Physical symptoms may include:

- muscle tension
- sweating
- nausea
- cold, clammy hands
- difficulty in swallowing
- jumpiness
- gastrointestinal discomfort or diarrhea
- irritability, feeling on edge
- tiredness
- insomnia.

A panic attack is defined as the abrupt onset of an episode of intense fear or discomfort, which peaks in approximately 10 minutes, and includes at least four of the following symptoms:

- a feeling of imminent danger or doom
- the need to escape
- palpitations
- sweating
- trembling
- shortness of breath or a smothering feeling
- a feeling of choking
- chest pain or discomfort
- nausea or abdominal discomfort
- dizziness or lightheadedness
- a sense of things being unreal, depersonalization
- a fear of losing control
- a fear of dying
- tingling sensations
- chills or hot flushes.

Panic disorder is diagnosed when an individual suffers at least two unexpected panic attacks, followed by at least 1 month of concern over having another attack. Sufferers are also prone to situationally predisposed attacks. The frequency and severity of the attacks varies from person to person: an individual might suffer from repeated attacks for weeks, while another will have short bursts of very severe attacks.

Panic disorder affects about 2.4 million adult Americans,[1] and is twice as common in women as in men.[2] Interestingly, human phobias are more resistant to extinction, and more irrational, than conditioned fear in animals.

Arne Öhman, a leader in the study of human fear and anxiety, has recently argued that:[3]

When comparing the physiological responses seen in phobics exposed to their feared objects with those seen in PTSD patients exposed to relevant traumatic scenes for the disorder, and with physiological responses during panic attacks, one is much more struck by the similarities than by the differences.

He goes on to argue that panic, phobic fear and PTSD reflect the activation of one and the same underlying anxiety response.

SUMMARY

Anxiety in Western medicine

The anxiety disorders discussed in Western medicine are:

- generalized anxiety disorder
- panic disorder
- obsessive-compulsive disorder
- post-traumatic stress disorder
- social phobia (or social anxiety disorder)
- specific phobias.

All anxiety disorders involve excessive, irrational fear, worry and dread.

ANXIETY IN CHINESE MEDICINE

"Anxiety" is a modern term that does not have an exact equivalent in Chinese medicine. Chinese medicine assigns quite a prominent role to "fear" among the emotions. However, there are differences between fear and anxiety. Some differentiate fear from anxiety according to the stimulus: fear is "post-stimulus", i.e. a stimulus generates a feeling of fear; anxiety is "pre-stimulus", i.e. the person feels anxious without a stimulus.

Others differentiate fear and anxiety in a different way. Epstein argues that fear is related to coping behavior, particularly escape and avoidance. When coping attempts fail (because the situation is uncontrollable), fear is turned into anxiety.[4] Anxiety can be defined as unresolved fear. According to LeDoux, anxiety and fear are closely related in so far as they are both reactions to harmful or potentially harmful situations. Anxiety is usually distinguished from fear by the lack of an external stimulus that elicits the reaction: anxiety comes from within us, fear from the outside world.[5]

I shall discuss the view of anxiety in Chinese medicine according to the following topics.

- Chinese disease entities corresponding to anxiety
- Rebellious Qi of the Penetrating Vessel (*Chong Mai*)
- Palpitations in Chinese diagnosis
- Difference between Mind Unsettled and Mind Obstructed in anxiety

Chinese disease entities corresponding to anxiety

There is no Chinese medicine term that corresponds exactly to what we call "anxiety" but several ancient Chinese disease entities closely resemble anxiety. The three main disease entities that correspond to anxiety are as follows.

- "Fear and Palpitations" (*Jing Ji*)
- "Panic Throbbing" (*Zheng Chong*)
- "Agitation" (*Zang Zao*)

The first two conditions involve a state of fear, worry and anxiety, the first with palpitations and the second with a throbbing sensation in the chest and below the umbilicus. "Fear and Palpitations" is usually caused by external events such as a fright or shock and it comes and goes; it is more frequently of a Full nature.

"Panic Throbbing" is not caused by external events and is continuous; this condition is usually of an Empty nature and is more serious than the first. In chronic cases, "Fear and Palpitations" may turn into "Panic Throbbing". In severe cases, "Panic Throbbing" may correspond to panic attacks. Despite the name "Fear and Palpitations", such states of fear and anxiety may occur without palpitations.

Zhu Dan Xi (1281–1358) says:[6]

In both Fear and Palpitations and Panic Throbbing there is Blood deficiency. Fear and Palpitations come in bouts; Panic Throbbing is constant. Panic Throbbing is due to worry and pensiveness agitating within, causing a deficiency and Phlegm-Heat.

Zhang Jing Yue says of "Panic Throbbing" in his *Complete Book of Jing Yue* (*Jing Yue Quan Shu*, 1624):[7]

In Panic Throbbing the heart is shaking in the chest, the patient feels fear and anxiety. There is Yin deficiency and exhaustion; there is Yin deficiency below so that the Gathering Qi [Zong Qi] has no root and Qi cannot return to its origin. For this reason, there is shaking [or throbbing] *of the chest above and also throbbing on the sides of the umbilicus.*

"Agitation" (*Zang Zao*) was discussed first in Chapter 22 of the *Essential Prescriptions of the Golden Chest* (*Jin Gui Yao Lue*, AD 220) by Zhang Zhong Jing. Although in this book Agitation is discussed in the chapter entitled *Miscellaneous Gynecological Diseases*, it applies also to men. The original text says of agitation: "*The woman is sad and cries a lot, she looks haunted* [literally: she looks like a lost soul], *she stretches and yawns repeatedly; use Gan Mai Da Zao Tang.*"[8]

SUMMARY

Chinese disease entities corresponding to "anxiety"

- "Fear and Palpitations" (*Jing Ji*)
- "Panic Throbbing" (*Zheng Chong*)
- "Agitation" (*Zang Zao*)
- Rebellious Qi of the Penetrating Vessel (*Li Ji*)

Rebellious Qi of the Penetrating Vessel (*Chong Mai*)

There is a third Chinese condition that may correspond to anxiety and especially to panic attacks and that is the condition of Rebellious Qi of the Penetrating Vessel

(*Chong Mai*) causing the symptom of "internal urgency" (*Li Ji*).

One of the most common pathologies of the Penetrating Vessel is rebellious Qi and "internal urgency" (*Li Ji*); this has been recognized since the times of the *Classic of Difficulties* (*Nan Jing*). Chapter 29 of the *Classic of Difficulties* says: "*The pathology of the Penetrating Vessel is rebellious Qi with internal urgency* [*Li Ji*]."[9]

"Internal urgency" indicates a feeling of anxiety and restlessness; in severe cases, there may be panic attacks with palpitations. On a physical level, it may also be interpreted as an uncomfortable, tight sensation from the lower abdomen radiating upwards towards the heart.

Palpitations are frequently associated with the anxiety or panic attacks deriving from rebellious Qi of the Penetrating Vessel because this vessel flows through the heart. This type of anxiety or panic attack may also be accompanied by a throbbing abdominal sensation which is also due to rebellious Qi of the Penetrating Vessel in the abdomen. From this point of view, Rebellious Qi of the Penetrating Vessel could be considered as a form of "Panic Throbbing" (*Zheng Chong*).

Li Shi Zhen said: "*When Qi rebels upwards, there is internal urgency* [*Li Ji*] *and a feeling of heat; this is rebellious Qi of the Penetrating Vessel.*"[10]

Rebellious Qi of the Penetrating Vessel causes various symptoms at different levels of the abdomen and chest. It causes primarily fullness, distension or pain in these areas. By plotting the pathway of the Penetrating Vessel, we can list the possible symptoms of rebellious Qi of the Penetrating Vessel starting from the bottom (Fig. 17.1):

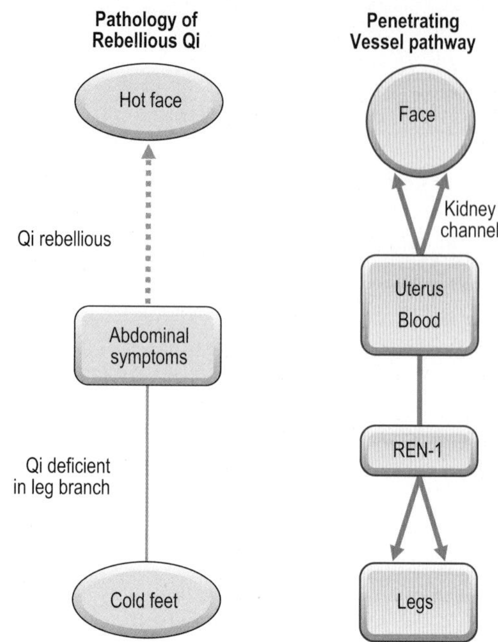

Figure 17.1 Rebellious Qi of the Penetrating Vessel.

- cold feet
- fullness/distension/pain of the lower abdomen
- hypogastric fullness/distension/pain
- painful periods, irregular periods
- fullness/distension/pain of the umbilical area
- fullness/distension/pain of the epigastrium
- feeling of tightness below the xiphoid process
- feeling of tightness of the chest
- palpitations
- feeling of distension of the breasts in women
- slight breathlessness
- sighing
- feeling of lump in the throat
- feeling of heat of the face
- headache
- anxiety, mental restlessness, "internal urgency" (*Li Ji*). See Figure 17.2.

Obviously, not all these symptoms need occur simultaneously to diagnose rebellious Qi of the Penetrating Vessel, but it is necessary to have at least three or four symptoms at different levels, e.g. lower abdomen, epigastrium, chest, throat. For example, if someone had fullness, distension or pain of the lower abdomen, that would not be enough to diagnose the condition of rebellious Qi of the Penetrating Vessel. A feeling of energy rising from the lower abdomen up towards the throat would be a strong indication of rebellious Qi of the Penetrating Vessel.

What makes the Qi of the Penetrating Vessel rebel upwards? In my experience, this may happen for two reasons manifesting with two conditions, one Full, the other mixed Full/Empty. First, the Qi of the Penetrating Vessel can rebel upwards by itself from emotional stress that makes Qi rise or stagnate, e.g. anger, repressed anger, worry, frustration, resentment, etc. In this case, Qi rebels upwards by itself and the condition is Full; I call this "primary" rebellious Qi of the Penetrating Vessel.

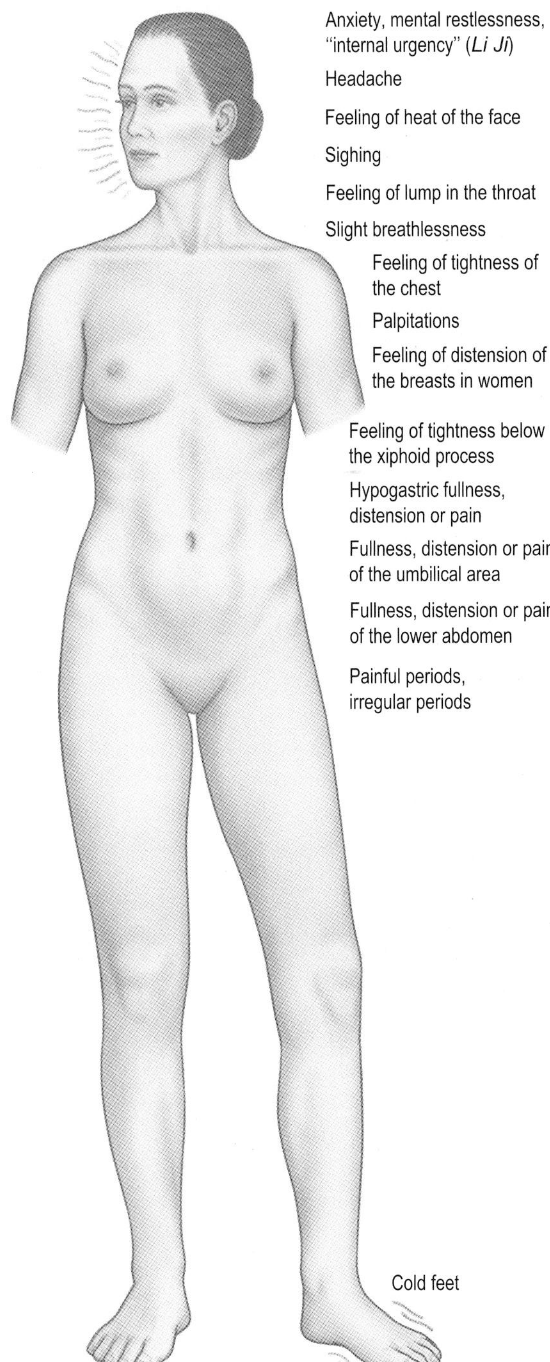

Figure 17.2 Symptoms of Rebellious Qi of the Penetrating Vessel.

Qi of the Penetrating Vessel may rebel upwards also as a consequence of a Deficiency in this vessel in the lower abdomen. In such cases, Qi of the lower *Dan Tian* is weak and the Qi of the Penetrating Vessel "escapes" upwards; this is therefore a mixed Full/Empty condition and I call this "secondary" rebellious Qi of the Penetrating Vessel. The Empty condition is deficiency of Blood and/or deficiency of the Kidneys (which may be Yin or Yang). This second condition is more common in women.

Li Shi Zhen mentions the possibility of this pattern when he says: "*When there is Blood deficiency leading to internal urgency, use Dang Gui.*"[11] The *Classic of Categories* also hints to Blood deficiency as a background for rebellious Qi of the Penetrating Vessel:[12]

The Qi of the Penetrating Vessel rises up to the chest, Qi is not regulated and therefore it rebels in the diaphragm, Blood is deficient and therefore there is internal urgency in the abdomen and chest.

CLINICAL NOTE

- *"Primary" rebellious Qi of the Penetrating Vessel*: the Qi of the Penetrating Vessel rebels upwards by itself from emotional stress that makes Qi rise or stagnate. Full condition.
- *"Secondary" rebellious Qi of the Penetrating Vessel*: Qi of the Penetrating Vessel rebels upwards as a consequence of a Deficiency (of Blood and Kidneys) in this vessel in the lower abdomen. Full/Empty condition.

A particular feature of the syndrome of rebellious Qi of the Penetrating Vessel is that it is characterized by a feeling of heat in the face and cold feet simultaneously. This is due to Qi rebelling upwards towards the face causing a feeling of heat there; on the other hand, as it rebels upwards, there is proportionately less Qi in the descending branch of the Penetrating Vessel which causes cold feet. In fact, as we have seen above, the old texts specifically say that the descending branch of the Penetrating Vessel warms the feet.

This feeling of heat in the face, therefore, is neither Full nor Empty Heat but just the result of a disharmony of Qi in the Penetrating Vessel, i.e. Qi rebelling upwards in its abdominal and head branches and being deficient in the descending branch in the legs.

CLINICAL NOTE

The feeling of heat in the face caused by Rebellious Qi of the Penetrating Vessel is neither Full Heat nor Empty Heat; it is simply an imbalance within the Penetrating Vessel. It is accompanied by cold feet because the Qi of the Penetrating Vessel escapes upwards and not enough flows into its descending branch. This apparent contradictory picture of hot feeling of the face and cold feet is particularly common in women.

SUMMARY

Rebellious Qi of the Penetrating Vessel

- Cold feet
- Fullness/distension/pain of the lower abdomen
- Hypogastric fullness/distension/pain
- Painful periods, irregular periods
- Fullness/distension/pain of the umbilical area
- Fullness/distension/pain of the epigastrium
- Feeling of tightness below the xiphoid process
- Feeling of tightness of the chest
- Palpitations
- Feeling of distension of the breasts in women
- Slight breathlessness
- Sighing
- Feeling of lump in the throat
- Feeling of heat of the face
- Headache
- Anxiety, mental restlessness, "internal urgency" (*Li Ji*)

Palpitations in Chinese diagnosis

On the subject of "palpitations", it is worth explaining what this term indicates. If we ask most Western patients whether they have "palpitations", most of them will reply in the negative because they think that by "palpitations" we mean "tachycardia", i.e. a rapid beat of the heart.

In reality, "palpitations" denotes simply an uncomfortable, subjective sensation of the heart beating in the chest; it has nothing to do with the speed or rate of the heart. Therefore, when I want to ask a Western patient about this symptom, I do not ask "*Do you get palpitations?*" but ask instead "*Are you sometimes aware of your heart beating in an uncomfortable way?*" If we ask in this manner, we will see that palpitations are a more common symptom than we think.

CLINICAL NOTE

"Palpitations" denotes simply an uncomfortable, subjective sensation of the heart beating in the chest; it has nothing to do with the speed or rate of the heart. Therefore, when I want to ask a Western patient about this symptom, I do not ask "*Do you get palpitations?*" but ask instead "*Are you sometimes aware of your heart beating in an uncomfortable way?*"

Difference between Mind Unsettled and Mind Obstructed in anxiety

The difference between anxiety and panic attacks is a good illustration of the difference between Mind Unsettled and Mind Obstructed. In anxiety, the person's Mind is unsettled either by a Full condition (such as Heart-Heat) or by an Empty condition (such as Heart-Blood deficiency). The person is anxious and restless but the Mind is unobstructed and insight is not affected. In obsessive compulsive disorder and in some cases of panic attacks, the Mind is also obstructed.

When the Mind is obstructed there is a certain loss of insight and rationality as may happen in severe panic attacks when the person may have an irrational fear of death. The main pathogenic factors that obstruct the Mind are Phlegm and Blood stasis; severe Qi stagnation may also lead to mild obstruction of the Mind.

We can therefore say that in "Fear and Palpitations" (*Jing Ji*) the Mind is unsettled, while in severe panic attacks, which are more likely to correspond to "Panic Throbbing" (*Zheng Chong*), the Mind is unsettled but also mildly obstructed.

ETIOLOGY

The main etiological factor in anxiety is obviously emotional stress. However, other factors play a role too, and constitution and diet are important etiological factors.

Emotional stress

"Anxiety" is a general term that indicates a chronic state of fear and uneasiness. However, that does not

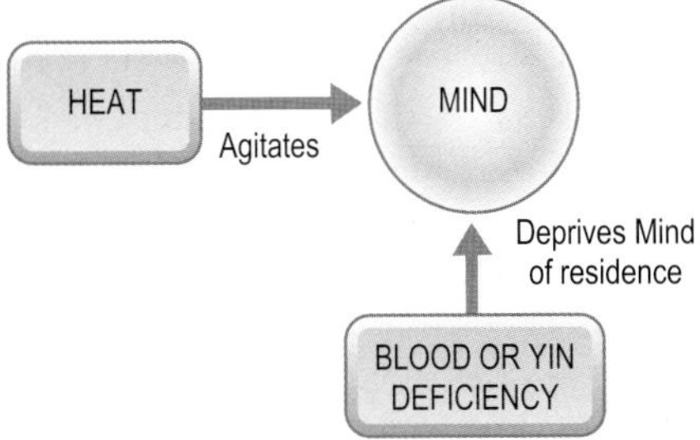

Figure 17.3 Consequences of emotional stress.

mean that, among the emotions, only fear leads to anxiety. A chronic state of anxiety may derive from many emotions, and particularly worry, fear, excess joy, shock, guilt, shame or pensiveness.

Any of the above emotions may lead to some Qi stagnation initially. After some time, stagnant Qi generates Heat and, with time, this injures Blood and Yin leading to Blood and/or Yin deficiency. Therefore Heat may agitate the Mind causing anxiety; on the other hand, Blood and Yin deficiency deprive the Mind of its residence and also lead to anxiety (Fig. 17.3).

The Qi stagnation and Qi deficiency deriving from emotional stress may also lead to the formation of Phlegm, which may obstruct the Mind and lead to more serious anxiety or panic attacks.

Chapter 39 of the *Simple Questions* says: "*When shock affects the Heart, it deprives it of its residence, the Mind has no place to return to, thoughts come ceaselessly* [i.e. anxiety] *and Qi becomes chaotic.*"[13]

Constitution

In my experience, a constitutional tendency is an important and frequent etiological factor in chronic anxiety. There are many people who simply have a constitutional tendency to worry and anxiety for no apparent external reasons. When I have treated various members and even generations of one family, I have also noticed that there is often a familial incidence.

An important sign indicating a constitutional tendency to emotional stress and anxiety is a Heart crack on the tongue (*see Fig. 11.6*).

According to the National Institute of Mental Health, the risk of developing panic disorder appears to be inherited.[14] This confirms the importance of constitution in the etiology of chronic anxiety and panic disorders.

Irregular diet

Irregular eating causes deficiency of Qi and Yin of the Stomach; in the long run, this may affect the Heart and lead to Heart-Yin deficiency and anxiety.

Irregular eating and the excessive consumption of Damp-producing foods lead to the formation of Phlegm. This may obstruct the Mind and aggravate anxiety and panic disorders.

Loss of blood

A heavy loss of blood, such as that which may happen during childbirth, leads to Blood deficiency. The Heart governs Blood and this may therefore lead to Heart-Blood deficiency and anxiety.

Overwork

Overwork in the sense of working long hours without adequate rest for many years seriously depletes Kidney-Yin. A deficiency of Kidney-Yin eventually affects the Heart and may cause chronic anxiety. A deficiency of Kidney-Yin may also cause chronic anxiety by itself, without affecting the Heart.

SUMMARY

Etiology
- Emotional stress
- Constitution
- Irregular diet
- Loss of blood
- Overwork

PATHOLOGY AND TREATMENT PRINCIPLES

In Chinese books, the pathology of "Fear and Palpitations" (*Jing Ji*) and of "Panic Throbbing" (*Zheng Chong*) is always related primarily to the Heart and secondarily to the Liver and Kidneys. These two conditions are related primarily to the Heart because they are closely linked to the symptom of "palpitations". Indeed, all modern Chinese books include the disease entities of "Fear and Palpitations" and "Panic Throbbing" under the disease entity of "Palpitations" (*Xin Ji*).

Strangely, although the essential feature of anxiety is worry, Chinese books do not report Lung patterns in relation to the above two diseases. I have therefore added Lung patterns according to my clinical experience.

Chinese books attribute the pathology of anxiety primarily to Heart patterns, which may include any of the Deficiency patterns (Qi, Yang, Blood and Yin) as well as Full patterns such as Heart-Heat or Heart-Blood stasis.

In my experience, apart from the Heart, the Lungs and Kidneys are also very much involved in the pathology of anxiety, the Lungs because they are affected by worry and the Kidneys because they are affected by fear.

Zhu Dan Xi recommends resolving Phlegm in "Fear and Palpitations" and transforming Water in "Panic Throbbing".

Zhang Jing Yue says in the *Complete Book of Jing Yue (Jing Yue Quan Shu*, 1624):[15]

In Fear and Palpitations, the Heart, Spleen, Liver and Kidneys are involved. Yang is connected to Yin and the Heart to the Kidneys. [In this disease] *the upper part of the body is restless because it cannot link with the lower part; Heart-Qi is deficient and cannot connect with the Essence* [of the Kidneys]. *In Fear and Palpitations the main treatment principles are to nourish the Heart and the Mind* [*Shen*], *supplement the Liver and Gall-Bladder and tonify the Original Qi.*

The above statement from Zhang Jing Yue is interesting because it confirms my clinical experience, according to which fear often makes Qi rise (rather than descend). In fact, in the statement above, Zhang Jing Yue says that in "Fear and Palpitations" there is restlessness above and a disconnection between the Heart and Kidneys with Qi rising.

Fright makes Qi rise and it is therefore necessary to make Qi sink with sinking substances such as Long Gu *Mastodi Ossis fossilia* or Zhen Zhu Mu *Concha Margaritifera usta*. As Fire dries up Blood, it is also necessary to nourish Yin, clear Heart-Heat and nourish Blood. Fright also deprives the Mind of its residence in the Heart, fluids change into Phlegm and they enter the space left vacant so that the Mind cannot return to it; therefore one must resolve Phlegm with formulae such as Shi Wei Wen Dan Tang *Ten-Ingredient Warming the Gall-Bladder Decoction*.[16]

Wang Qing Ren (late Qing dynasty) thought that the main cause of anxiety is Blood stasis. He thought that nourishing Blood and calming the Mind does not yield good results in anxiety and he advocated using his own Xue Fu Zhu Yu Tang *Blood Mansion Eliminating Stasis Decoction* to invigorate Blood and eliminate stasis.[17]

Lin Pei Qin (late Qing dynasty) thought that in Fear and Palpitations caused by fright, the Mind is chaotic and one should tonify and nourish it with a formula like Da Bu Yin Wan *Great Tonifying Yin Qi Decoction*: if there is Yin deficiency he advocates using Zuo Gui Yin *Restoring the Left* [Kidney] *Decoction*; if Yang deficiency, use You Gui Yin *Restoring the Right* [Kidney] *Decoction*.[18]

In my experience, independently of the patterns involved, in chronic anxiety there is always a disconnection between the Heart and Kidneys. In physiology, Heart- and Kidney-Qi communicate with each other, with Heart-Qi descending towards the Kidneys and Kidney-Qi ascending towards the Heart. Chronic anxiety makes Qi rise towards the Heart and "cramps" it. Heart-Qi cannot descend to the Kidneys and the Kidneys cannot root it (Fig. 17.4).

Apart from the patterns with which anxiety may present, it is useful to differentiate the pathology and symptoms of anxiety from the point of view of Internal Organs; this approach is also more relevant to the acupuncture treatment of anxiety.

In my experience, the main organs involved in anxiety are therefore the Heart, Lungs, Liver and Kidneys. The symptoms and characteristics of anxiety for each organ are indicated below.

Heart

The cardinal symptom of a Heart pattern is palpitations (see above); if there are palpitations, there is a Heart pattern.

The patient suffering from anxiety from a Heart disharmony will suffer from palpitations and the anxiety will be experienced in the chest. This may be a feeling of tightness, discomfort or oppression of the chest. In Full conditions, there may be a tight feeling of the chest, while in Empty conditions a feeling of the heart being "suspended".

The person suffering from anxiety with a Heart disharmony will appear flustered and somewhat "haunted". They will be restless and fidgety and they will tend to move in rapid movements (Fig. 17.5).

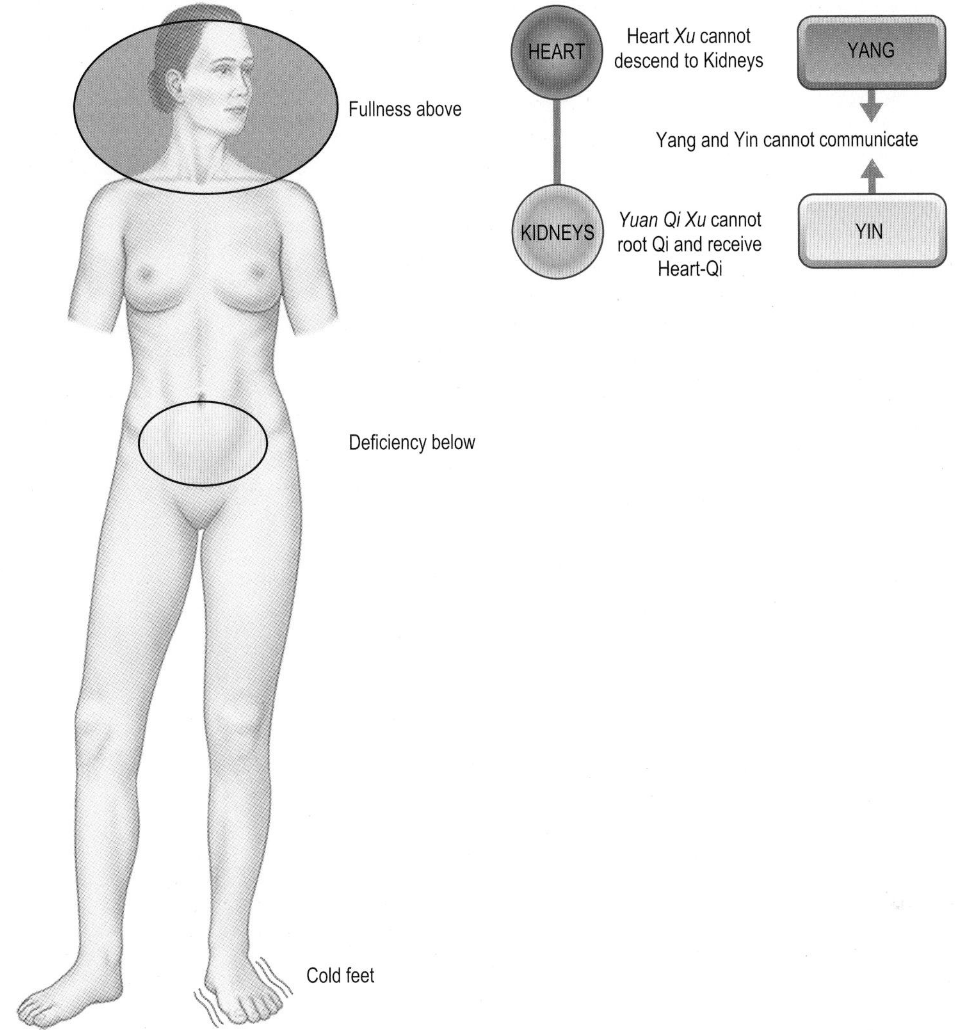

Figure 17.4 Disconnection between Heart and Kidneys in chronic anxiety.

There will be insomnia, and other symptoms will depend on whether it is a Full or an Empty condition of the Heart. Deficiency of Heart-Blood is more common in women who, besides being anxious, will tend to feel sad and cry.

Lungs

The Lungs are affected by sadness and grief, usually deriving from loss. The patient will therefore be sad and prone to crying. Sighing is also a characteristic symptom of mental-emotional patterns of the Lungs. The person will also tend to be pale and speak with a weak voice (Fig. 17.6).

Sadness and grief deplete Qi and therefore lead to Qi deficiency, especially of the Lungs and Heart. This makes the pulse Weak or Empty. However, after some time, the Qi deficiency in the chest may also give rise to some Qi stagnation in this area, affecting the Heart and Lungs. This may make the Lung pulse very slightly Tight. When the Lungs are affected by Qi stagnation, a mild anxiety may follow the initial sadness (Fig. 17.7).

The anxiety of the Lungs is often about spiritual matters, the meaning of life and existential suffering.

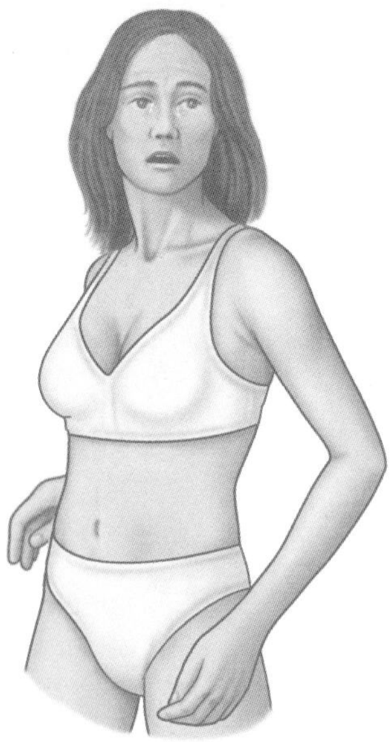

Figure 17.5 Heart-type anxiety.

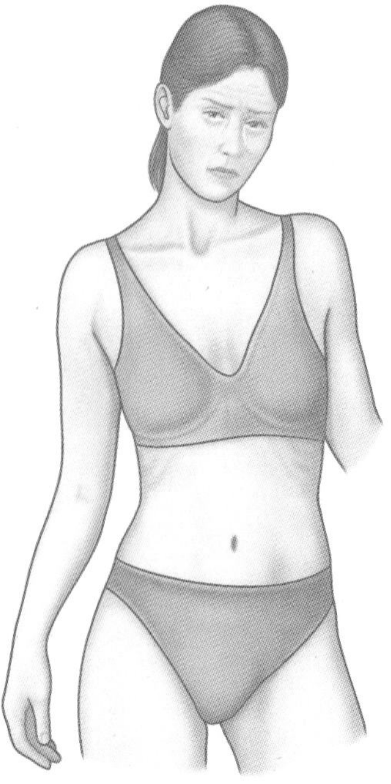

Figure 17.6 Lung-type anxiety.

Kidneys

The emotion of the Kidneys is fear; this emotion, together with worry, is the one that is most closely linked to anxiety. The patient will appear gaunt and scared, with almost a look of panic in the eyes. He

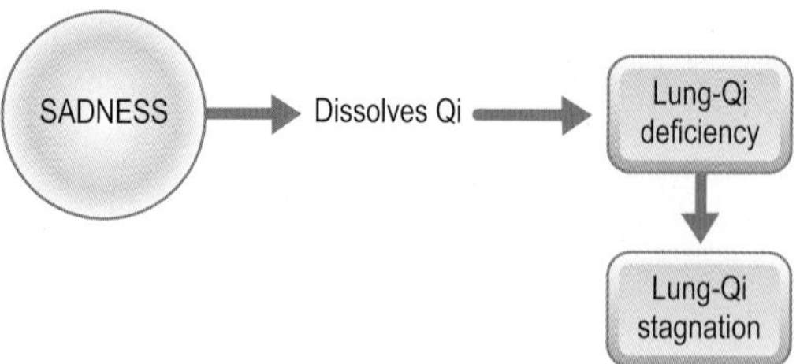

Figure 17.7 Lung-Qi deficiency and Lung-Qi stagnation.

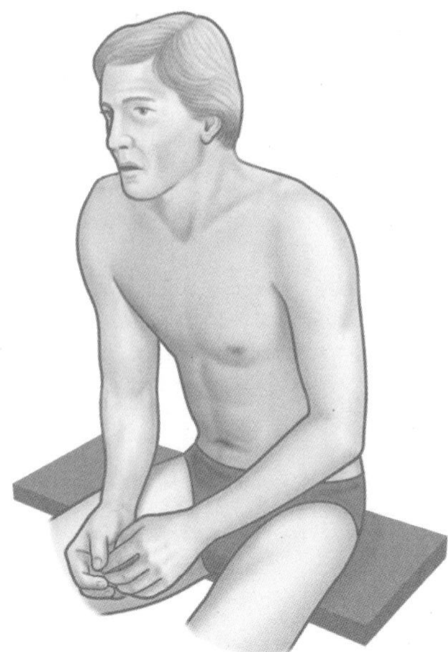

Figure 17.8 Kidney-type anxiety.

or she may have a dark complexion. The person will always fear the worst in any situation (Fig. 17.8).

The fear of the Kidneys has a "dark" quality about it and is different from the anxiety related to other organs. The anxiety of the Kidneys is usually about life situations; the person is deeply pessimistic and the anxiety derives from such pessimism. The Kidney-related anxiety is often due to guilt.

Although it is said that fear makes Qi descend, in my experience, chronic fear and anxiety of the Kidney makes Qi rise to the head, so that the person feels hot in the face, slightly dizzy and anxious.

In my experience, the Kidneys are also affected by guilt, which may cause sinking or stagnation of Kidney-Qi. In both cases, the person may become anxious, being constantly haunted by the feeling of guilt.

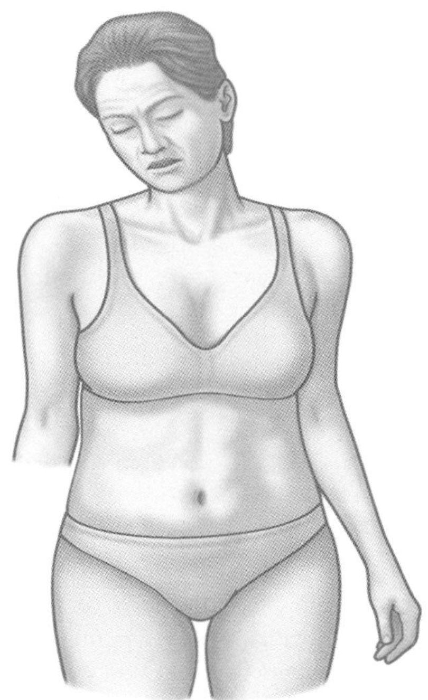

Figure 17.9 Spleen-type anxiety.

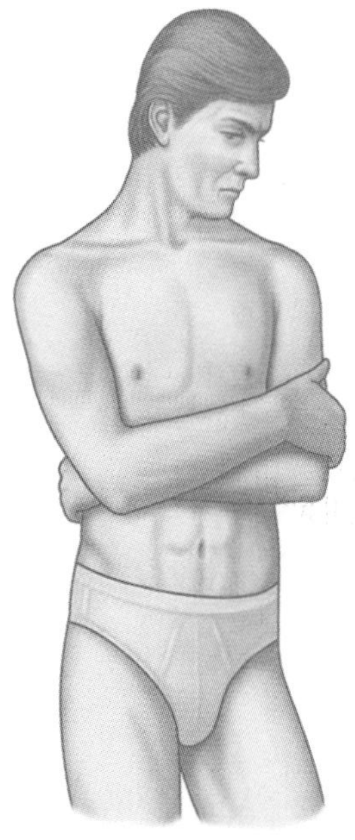

Figure 17.10 Liver-type anxiety.

Spleen

The emotion related to the Spleen is pensiveness; this is akin to worry. Pensiveness is encountered in people whose thoughts go "round in circles" or have "mental arguments"; in severe cases, pensiveness may become obsessive. In chronic cases, pensiveness may cause anxiety as the person is constantly anxious about his or her own mental arguments (Fig. 17.9).

The Spleen anxiety may also be related to nurturing Earth issues, such as being overprotective towards one's children, ignoring one's own needs and putting the needs of others first, or suffering from a lack of mothering.

Liver

The anxiety related to the Liver is akin to worry. People of the Wood type tend to worry easily, they are often tense and sometimes perfectionists. Their anxiety derives from the high standards they set themselves and it is therefore related to a feeling of not achieving what one has set out to achieve (Fig. 17.10).

The Liver houses the Ethereal Soul, which is responsible for our ideas, plans, projects, life dreams and vision. The Liver anxiety is therefore also related to a dissatisfaction with one's achievements.

SUMMARY

Pathology and treatment principles

The pathology of "Fear and Palpitations" (*Jing Ji*) and of "Panic Throbbing" (*Zheng Chong*) are related primarily to the Heart and secondarily to the Liver, Lungs and Kidneys.

ACUPUNCTURE TREATMENT OF ANXIETY

Distal points according to channel

I shall discuss the distal points according to channels, starting with the Yin Organs.

Heart

HE-7 Shenmen

HE-7 is the main point on the Heart channel to calm the Mind and relieve anxiety. It is effective in both Full and Empty conditions, but I personally use it more for Empty conditions when anxiety derives from Heart-Blood or Heart-Yin deficiency.

HE-7 combines well with Ren-15 Jiuwei.

HE-8 Shaofu

I use HE-8 to calm the Mind and relieve anxiety primarily in Full conditions such as Heart-Fire.

Liver

LIV-3 Taichong

LIV-3 is the main point on the Liver channel to calm the Mind and settle the Ethereal Soul. It combines well with L.I.-4 Hegu to calm the Mind.

It also combines well with G.B.-13 Benshen to calm the Mind and settle the Ethereal Soul.

Spleen

SP-6 Sanyinjiao

SP-6 is the main point on the Spleen channel to calm the Mind. It is particularly indicated when the person is affected by worry and pensiveness. It also promotes sleep and it combines well with HE-7 Shenmen.

Lungs

LU-7 Lieque

I use LU-7 to calm the Mind, especially when the person is affected by worry, sadness or grief. LU-7 has a "centrifugal" movement so it promotes the surfacing of emotions that may have been repressed or not acknowledged.

Kidneys

KI-4 Dazhong

I use KI-4 to nourish the Kidneys and relieve anxiety deriving from a Kidney disharmony.

KI-9 Zhubin

I use KI-9 to calm the Mind and relieve anxiety, especially in women suffering from a deficiency of the Kidneys and of Blood. I often combine this point with the opening points of the Yin Linking Vessel (*Yin Wei Mai*), i.e. P-6 Neiguan and SP-4 Gongsun.

Pericardium

P-6 Neiguan

P-6 calms the Mind and relieves anxiety. I use it particularly when there is anxiety against a background of Qi stagnation (which may be of the Liver, Heart or Lungs) or Heart-Blood deficiency.

P-7 Daling

I use P-7 to calm the Mind, settle the Ethereal Soul and relieve anxiety more in Full conditions such as Heart-Fire or Liver-Fire.

Large Intestine

L.I.-4 Hegu

L.I.-4 has a strong calming action with or without LIV-3 Taichong. It regulates the ascending and descending of Qi to and from the head, and it therefore subdues Qi in the head when the person is anxious.

Stomach

ST-40 Fenglong

ST-40 has a strong action in calming the Mind and relieving anxiety. It has a particular action on the chest and it is therefore particularly indicated for anxiety that is related to the Heart and/or Lungs with a feeling of tightness or oppression in the chest.

Head points

In order to calm the Mind and relieve anxiety, it is important to combine distal points with points on the head. The following are the main head points I use for anxiety.

Du-24 Shenting

Du-24's traditional indications include manic-depression, depression, anxiety, poor memory and insomnia.

The most important aspect of Du-24's energetic action is its downward movement; it makes Qi descend and subdues rebellious Yang. This is a very important and powerful point to calm the Mind. It is frequently combined with G.B.-13 Benshen for severe anxiety and fears against the background of Liver patterns.

To calm the Mind and nourish the Heart in mental-emotional problems occurring against a background of Deficiency, I frequently combine Du-24 with Ren-15 Jiuwei.

An important feature of Du-24 that makes it particularly useful is that it can both calm and lift the Mind; therefore it is used not only for anxiety and insomnia but also for depression and sadness. It is also used in psychiatric practice for schizophrenia and split personality.[19]

The name of this point refers to its strong influence on the Mind and Spirit. The courtyard was traditionally considered to be very important as it was the part that gave visitors their first impression of the house; it is the entrance. Thus, this point could be said to be the "entrance" to the Mind and Spirit, and it being called a courtyard highlights its importance.

G.B.-13 Benshen

G.B.-13 calms the Mind (*Shen*) and subdues Liver-Yang. It also extinguishes Wind, resolves Phlegm, gathers Essence (*Jing*) to the head and clears the brain. Its classic indications include manic behavior and fright.

G.B.-13 is a very important point for mental and emotional problems and for anxiety, especially those occurring against a background of Liver patterns. It is very much used in psychiatric practice for schizophrenia and split personality combined with HE-5 Tongli and G.B.-38 Yangfu.[20] It is also indicated when the person has persistent and unreasonable feelings of jealousy and suspicion.

Apart from these mental traits, it has a powerful effect in calming the Mind and relieving anxiety deriving from constant worry and fixed thoughts. Its effect is enhanced if it is combined with Du-24 Shenting.

Its deep mental and emotional effect is also due to its action of "gathering" Essence to the head. The Kidney-Essence is the root of our Pre-Heaven Qi and is the foundation for our mental and emotional life. A strong Essence is the fundamental prerequisite for a clear Mind (*Shen*) and a balanced emotional life. This is the meaning of this point's name "Root of the Mind", i.e. this point gathers the Essence which is the root of the Mind (*Shen*).

The Kidney-Essence is the source of Marrow which fills up the Brain (called Sea of Marrow); G.B.-13 is a point where Essence and Marrow "gather". The *Great Dictionary of Acupuncture* says that this point "*makes the Mind [Shen] return to its root*".[21] The "root" of the Mind is the Essence, hence this point "gathers" the Essence to the Brain, calms the Mind and relieves anxiety.

When combined with other points to nourish Essence (such as Ren-4 Guanyuan), G.B.-13 attracts Essence towards the head with the effect of calming the Mind and strengthening clarity of mind, memory and willpower. The connection between G.B.-13 and the Essence is confirmed by the text *An Enquiry into Chinese Acupuncture*, which has among the indications of this point "*excessive menstrual bleeding, impotence and seminal emissions*".[22]

Finally, G.B.-13 resolves Phlegm in the context of mental-emotional disorders or epilepsy, i.e. it opens the Mind's orifices when these are clouded by Phlegm. The *Explanation of the Acupuncture Points* says: "*The indications of G.B.-13 show that it eliminates the three pathogenic factors of Wind, Fire and Phlegm from the Lesser Yang, in which cases this point should be reduced.*"[23]

Du-19 Houding

Du-19 calms the Mind and opens the Mind's orifices. Its classic indications include manic behavior, anxiety, mental restlessness and insomnia.

Du-19 has a powerful calming effect on the Mind and is very often used in severe anxiety, especially in combination with Ren-15 Jiuwei.

SUMMARY

Acupuncture treatment of anxiety

Distal points according to channel

Heart
- HE-7 Shenmen
- HE-8 Shaofu

Liver
- LIV-3 Taichong

Spleen
- SP-6 Sanyinjiao

Lungs
- LU-7 Lieque

Kidneys
- KI-4 Dazhong
- KI-9 Zhubin

Pericardium
- P-6 Neiguan
- P-7 Daling

Large Intestine
- L.I.-4 Hegu

Stomach
- ST-40 Fenglong

Head points
- Du-24 Shenting
- G.B.-13 Benshen
- Du-19 Houding

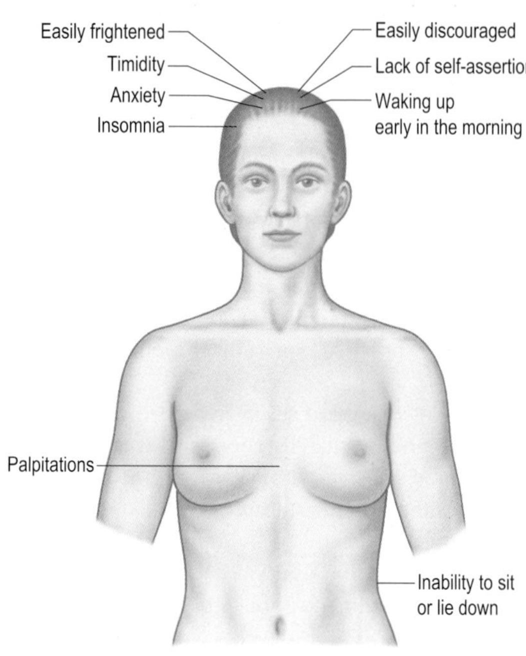

Figure 17.11 Heart and Gall-Bladder deficiency.

IDENTIFICATION OF PATTERNS AND TREATMENT

Heart and Gall-Bladder deficiency

Clinical manifestations

Palpitations, anxiety, timidity, easily frightened, lack of self-assertion, easily discouraged, cannot sit or lie down, insomnia, waking up early in the morning (Fig. 17.11).

Tongue: Pale.

Pulse: Weak.

Mental-emotional profile

This person is timid, shy and lacking in drive. He or she is easily discouraged and finds it difficult to make decisions. The anxiety is mild.

Treatment principle

Tonify the Heart and Gall-Bladder, calm the Mind.

Acupuncture

Points

HE-7 Shenmen, HE-5 Tongli, BL-15 Xinshu, Ren-14 Juque, G.B.-40 Qiuxu, ST-36 Zusanli. All with reinforcing method. Moxa is applicable if the tongue is Pale.

Explanation

- HE-7, HE-5, BL-15 and Ren-14 tonify the Heart and calm the Mind.
- G.B.-40 tonifies the Gall-Bladder. I use this point in particular to stimulate the psychic aspect of the Gall-Bladder, i.e. courage and assertiveness.
- ST-36 is used to tonify the Heart.

Herbal therapy

Prescription

AN SHEN DING ZHI WAN Variation
Calming the Mind and settling the Spirit Pill Variation

Explanation

The original formula tonifies the Heart and calms the Mind. It has been modified with the addition of sinking substances that calm the Spirit. Please note that the use of minerals in herbal prescriptions is not allowed in the UK.

Prescription

PING BU ZHEN XIN DAN Variation
Calming and Tonifying the Heart Pill Variation

Explanation

This formula differs from the previous one in that it provides a more general tonification of the Heart as it tonifies Qi and nourishes Blood.

Prescription

WU WEI ZI TANG Variation
Schisandra Decoction Variation.

Explanation

This formula tonifies the Heart and calms the Mind, emphasizing nourishing the Yin.

SUMMARY

Heart and Gall-Bladder deficiency

Points

HE-7 Shenmen, HE-5 Tongli, BL-15 Xinshu, Ren-14 Juque, G.B.-40 Qiuxu, ST-36 Zusanli. All with reinforcing method. Moxa is applicable if the tongue is Pale.

Herbal therapy

Prescription

AN SHEN DING ZHI WAN Variation
Calming the Mind and settling the Spirit Pill Variation

Prescription

PING BU ZHEN XIN DAN Variation
Calming and Tonifying the Heart Pill Variation

Prescription

WU WEI ZI TANG Variation
Schisandra Decoction Variation

Heart-Blood deficiency

Clinical manifestations

Palpitations, anxiety, dizziness, pale face, insomnia, poor memory, tiredness (Fig. 17.12).

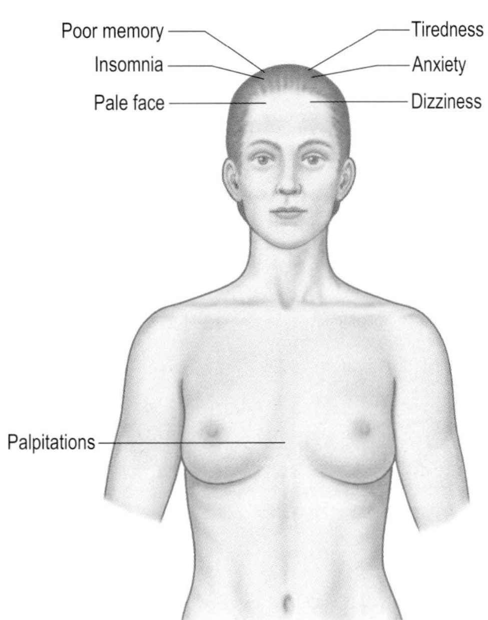

Figure 17.12 Heart-Blood deficiency.

Tongue: Pale and Thin.
Pulse: Choppy or Fine.

Mental-emotional profile

This person is more likely to be a woman, pale, depressed and anxious. The anxiety is mild and may be worse in the evening; it may also be worse after the period.

Treatment principle

Nourish Heart-Blood, calm the Mind.

Acupuncture

Points

HE-7 Shenmen, Ren-14 Juque, ST-36 Zusanli, SP-6 Sanyinjiao. All with reinforcing method. Moxa may be used.

Explanation

- HE-7 and Ren-14 nourish Heart-Blood and calm the Mind.

- ST-36 and SP-6 are used to nourish Blood in general.

Herbal therapy

Prescription

GUI PI TANG Variation
Tonifying the Spleen Decoction Variation

Explanation

The original formula nourishes Qi and Blood of Heart, Spleen and Liver and calms the Mind. It has been modified only slightly by removing Mu Xiang *Radix Aucklandiae* and adding Bai Zi Ren *Semen Platycladi*.

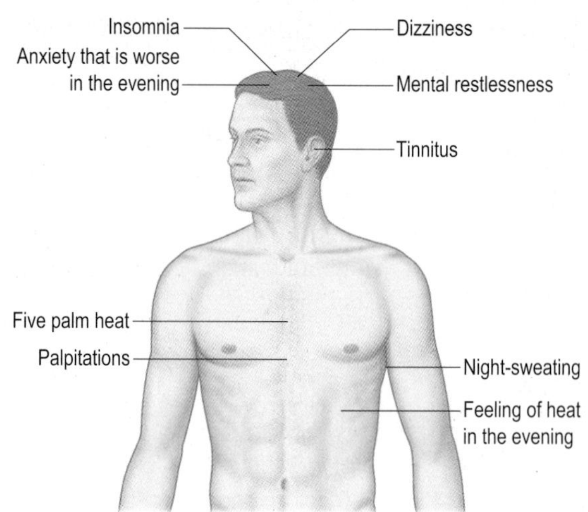

Figure 17.13 Kidney- and Heart-Yin deficiency.

SUMMARY

Heart-Blood deficiency

Points

HE-7 Shenmen, Ren-14 Juque, ST-36 Zusanli, SP-6 Sanyinjiao. All with reinforcing method. Moxa may be used.

Herbal therapy

Prescription

GUI PI TANG Variation
Tonifying the Spleen Decoction Variation

Kidney- and Heart-Yin deficiency with Empty Heat

Clinical manifestations

Palpitations, anxiety that is worse in the evening, mental restlessness, insomnia, night-sweating, feeling of heat in the evening, five-palm heat, dizziness, tinnitus (Fig. 17.13).

Tongue: Red without coating.

Pulse: Floating-Empty and Rapid.

Mental-emotional profile

This person is more likely to be middle-aged. The anxiety is marked and is experienced more in the evenings. In women, this type of anxiety is markedly aggravated with the onset of the menopause. There is a characteristic restlessness and fidgetiness.

Treatment principle

Nourish Heart- and Kidney-Yin, clear Empty Heat, calm the Mind.

Acupuncture

Points

HE-7 Shenmen, Ren-14 Juque, KI-3 Taixi, Ren-4 Guanyuan, SP-6 Sanyinjiao, HE-6 Yinxi, KI-7 Fuliu. Reinforcing method.

Explanation

- HE-7 and Ren-14 nourish Heart-Yin.
- KI-3, Ren-4 and SP-6 nourish Kidney-Yin.
- HE-6 clears Heart Empty Heat; together with KI-7 it treats night-sweating.

Herbal therapy

Prescription

TIAN WANG BU XIN DAN
Heavenly Emperor Tonifying the Heart Pill

Explanation

This formula nourishes Heart- and Kidney-Yin, clears Empty Heat and calms the Mind.

SUMMARY

Kidney- and Heart-Yin deficiency with Empty Heat

Points

HE-7 Shenmen, Ren-14 Juque, KI-3 Taixi, Ren-4 Guanyuan, SP-6 Sanyinjiao, HE-6 Yinxi, KI-7 Fuliu. Reinforcing method.

Herbal therapy

Prescription

TIAN WANG BU XIN DAN
Heavenly Emperor Tonifying the Heart Pill

Heart-Yang deficiency

Clinical manifestations

Palpitations, anxiety, pale face, feeling cold, cold hands, slight breathlessness, discomfort in the chest (Fig. 17.14).

Tongue: Pale, wet.
Pulse: Deep-Weak.

Mental-emotional profile

This person is anxious but also depressed and listless. Everything is an effort and they speak with difficulty.

Treatment principle

Tonify Heart-Yang, calm the Mind.

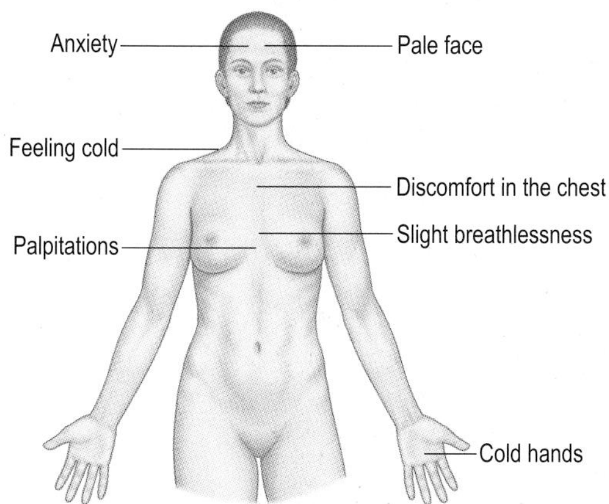

Figure 17.14 Heart-Yang deficiency.

Acupuncture

Points

HE-5 Tongli, BL-15 Xinshu, Du-14 Dazhui, Ren-6 Qihai, ST-36 Zusanli. Reinforcing method; moxa is applicable.

Explanation

- HE-5, BL-15 and Du-14 tonify Heart-Yang and calm the Mind.
- Ren-6 and ST-36 with moxa tonify Yang in general.

Herbal therapy

Prescription

GUI ZHI GAN CAO LONG GU MU LI TANG Variation
Cinnamomum-Glycyrrhiza-Mastodi Ossis fossilia-Concha Ostreae Decoction Variation

Explanation

This formula tonifies Heart-Yang and calms the Mind. It also stops sweating from Heart-Yang deficiency.

Prescription

YANG XIN TANG (I) or **(II)**
Nourishing the Heart Decoction

Explanation

This formula tonifies Heart-Qi and calms the Mind. Its calming the Mind effect is stronger than that of the previous formula. Either (I) or (II) may be used; however, if Yang deficiency is pronounced, use (I).

SUMMARY

Heart-Yang deficiency

Points

HE-5 Tongli, BL-15 Xinshu, Du-14 Dazhui, Ren-6 Qihai, ST-36 Zusanli. Reinforcing method; moxa is applicable.

Herbal therapy

Prescription

GUI ZHI GAN CAO LONG MU MU LI TANG Variation

Cinnamomum-Glycyrrhiza-Mastodi Ossis fossilia-Concha Ostreae Decoction Variation

Prescription

YANG XIN TANG (I) or **(II)**

Nourishing the Heart Decoction

Lung- and Heart-Qi deficiency

Clinical manifestations

Palpitations, anxiety, timidity, easily frightened, sadness, tendency to crying, weak voice, slight breathlessness, propensity to catching colds (Fig. 17.15).

Tongue: Pale.

Pulse: Weak on both Front positions.

Mental-emotional profile

This person is anxious but also sad. They are often affected by grief following a loss. They will tend to be pale and speak with a weak voice. The anxiety is experienced in the chest.

Treatment principle

Tonify Heart- and Lung-Qi, calm the Mind.

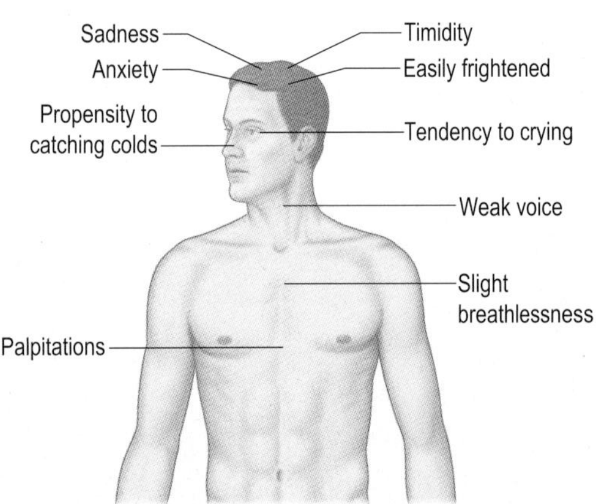

Figure 17.15 Lung- and Heart-Qi deficiency.

Acupuncture

Points

HE-5 Tongli, HE-7 Shenmen, BL-15 Xinshu, Ren-14 Juque, LU-9 Taiyuan, LU-7 Lieque, BL-13 Feishu, Du-12 Shenzhu, Ren-12 Zhongwan, Ren-6 Qihai, ST-36 Zusanli. Reinforcing method.

Explanation

- HE-5, HE-7, BL-15 and Ren-14 tonify the Heart and calm the Mind.
- LU-9, LU-7, BL-13 and Du-12 tonify Lung-Qi.
- Ren-12, Ren-6 and ST-36 tonify Qi in general.

Herbal therapy

Prescription

YANG XIN TANG (I)
Nourishing the Heart Decoction

Explanation

This formula tonifies Heart- and Lung-Qi and calms the Mind.

Prescription

BU FEI TANG Variation
Tonifying the Lungs Decoction Variation

SUMMARY

Lung- and Heart-Qi deficiency

Points

HE-5 Tongli, HE-7 Shenmen, BL-15 Xinshu, Ren-14 Juque, LU-9 Taiyuan, LU-7 Lieque, BL-13 Feishu, Du-12 Shenzhu, Ren-12 Zhongwan, Ren-6 Qihai, ST-36 Zusanli. Reinforcing method.

Herbal therapy

Prescription

YANG XIN TANG (I)
Nourishing the Heart Decoction

Prescription

BU FEI TANG Variation
Tonifying the Lungs Decoction Variation

Lung- and Heart-Qi stagnation

Clinical manifestations

Palpitations, anxiety, a feeling of distension or oppression of the chest, depression, a slight feeling of a lump in the throat, slight shortness of breath, sighing, sadness, chest and upper epigastric distension, slightly purple lips, pale complexion (Fig. 17.16).

Tongue: slightly Pale-Purple on the sides in the chest area.

Pulse: Empty but very slightly Overflowing on both Front positions.

Mental-emotional profile

This person is anxious but also worried and sad. They will tend to be pale and speak with a weak voice. The anxiety is experienced in the chest.

Treatment principle

Move Qi in the Heart and Lung, relax the chest, calm the Mind.

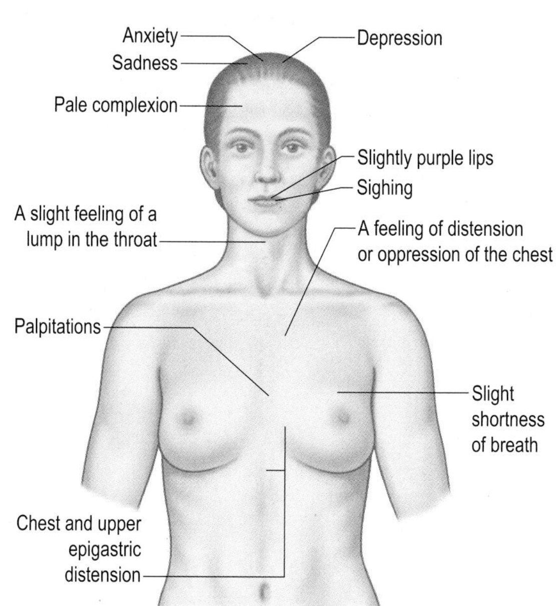

Figure 17.16 Lung- and Heart-Qi stagnation.

Acupuncture

Points

HE-5 Tongli, HE-7 Shenmen, P-6 Neiguan, Ren-15 Jiuwei, Ren-17 Shanzhong, LU-7 Lieque, ST-40 Fenglong. Even method.

Explanation

- HE-5, HE-7 and P-6 move Heart-Qi and calm the Mind.
- Ren-15 and Ren-17 relax the chest and calm the Mind.
- LU-7 moves Lung-Qi.
- ST-40, in combination with LU-7 and P-6, relaxes the chest and calms the Mind.

Herbal therapy

Prescription

BAN XIA HOU PO TANG
Pinellia-Magnolia Decoction

> **SUMMARY**
>
> **Lung- and Heart-Qi stagnation**
>
> *Points*
>
> HE-5 Tongli, HE-7 Shenmen, P-6 Neiguan, Ren-15 Jiuwei, Ren-17 Shanzhong, LU-7 Lieque, ST-40 Fenglong. Even method.
>
> *Herbal therapy*
>
> *Prescription*
>
> **BAN XIA HOU PO TANG**
> *Pinellia-Magnolia Decoction*

Lung- and Heart-Yin deficiency

Clinical manifestations

Anxiety, cough which is dry or with scanty-sticky sputum, weak and hoarse voice, dry mouth and throat, tickly throat, palpitations, insomnia, dream-disturbed sleep, poor memory, propensity to be startled, mental restlessness, uneasiness, dry mouth and throat in the afternoon or evening, tiredness, a dislike of speaking, thin body or thin chest, night-sweating (Fig. 17.17).

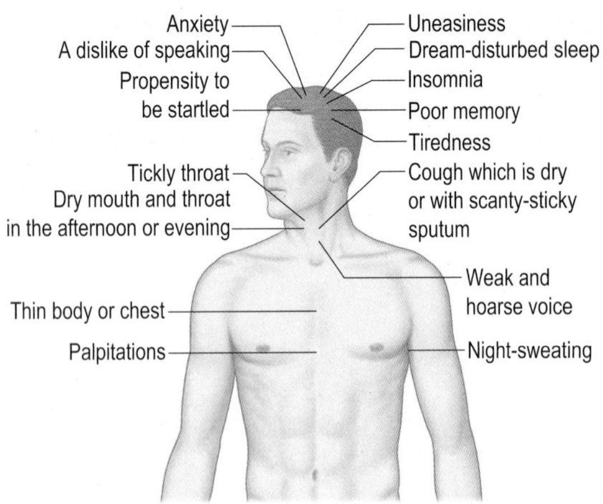

Figure 17.17 Lung- and Heart-Yin deficiency.

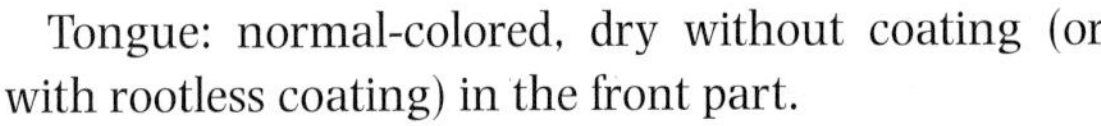

Tongue: normal-colored, dry without coating (or with rootless coating) in the front part.

Pulse: Floating-Empty.

Treatment principle

Nourish Lung- and Heart-Yin and calm the Mind.

Acupuncture

Points

LU-9 Taiyuan, Ren-17 Shanzhong, BL-43 Gaohuangshu, BL-13 Feishu, Ren-4 Guanyuan, Ren-12 Zhongwan, SP-6 Sanyinjiao, HE-7 Shenmen, Ren-14 Juque, Ren-15 Jiuwei. Reinforcing method.

Explanation

- LU-9, Ren-17, BL-43 and BL-13 nourish Lung-Yin.
- Ren-4, Ren-12 and SP-6 nourish Yin in general.
- HE-7, Ren-14 and Ren-15 nourish Heart-Yin and calm the Mind.

Herbal therapy

Prescription

BAI HE GU JIN TANG Variation
Lilium Consolidating Metal Decoction Variation

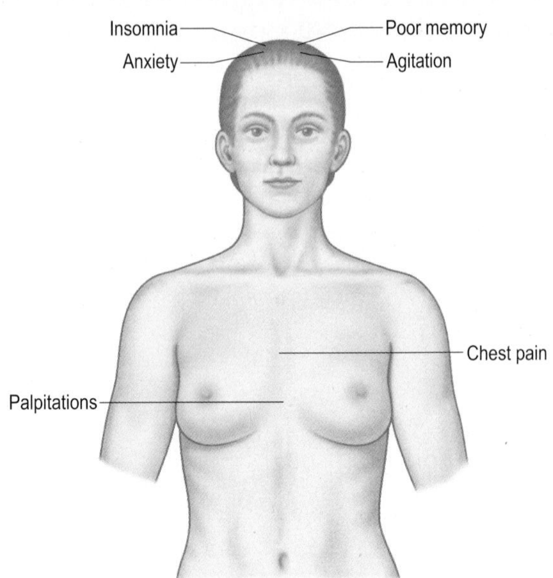

Figure 17.18 Heart-Blood stasis.

Explanation

This formula variation nourishes Lung- and Heart-Yin and calms the Mind.

> **SUMMARY**
>
> **Lung- and Heart-Yin deficiency**
>
> *Points*
>
> LU-9 Taiyuan, Ren-17 Shanzhong, BL-43 Gaohuangshu, BL-13 Feishu, Ren-4 Guanyuan, Ren-12 Zhongwan, SP-6 Sanyinjiao, HE-7 Shenmen, Ren-14 Juque, Ren-15 Jiuwei. Reinforcing method.
>
> *Herbal therapy*
>
> *Prescription*
>
> **BAI HE GU JIN TANG** Variation
> *Lilium Consolidating Metal Decoction* Variation

Heart-Blood stasis

Clinical manifestations

Palpitations, anxiety, insomnia, agitation, poor memory, chest pain (Fig. 17.18).

Tongue: Purple on the sides (chest area).

Pulse: Wiry, Choppy or Firm.

Mental-emotional profile

This person will tend to be middle-aged. The anxiety is experienced more in the evening and often also in the middle of the night, when they might wake up with a panicky feeling.

Treatment principle

Invigorate Heart-Blood, eliminate stasis, calm the Mind.

Acupuncture

Points

HE-5 Tongli, P-6 Neiguan, Ren-14 Juque, Ren-15 Jiuwei, LIV-3 Taichong, SP-6 Sanyinjiao. Even method.

Explanation

- HE-5, P-6, Ren-14 and Ren-15 invigorate Heart-Blood and calm the Mind.
- LIV-3 invigorates Blood in general.
- SP-6 invigorates Blood and calms the Mind.

Herbal therapy

Prescription

TAO REN HONG HUA JIAN
Persica-Carthamus Decoction

Explanation

This formula invigorates Heart-Blood and calms the Mind.

SUMMARY

Heart-Blood stasis

Points

HE-5 Tongli, P-6 Neiguan, Ren-14 Juque, Ren-15 Jiuwei, LIV-3 Taichong, SP-6 Sanyinjiao. Even method.

Herbal therapy

Prescription

TAO REN HONG HUA JIAN
Persica-Carthamus Decoction

Phlegm-Heat harassing the Heart

Clinical manifestations

Palpitations, anxiety, insomnia, dreaming a lot, feeling of oppression of the chest, sputum in the throat, slightly "manic" behavior (Fig. 17.19).

Tongue: Red, Swollen with sticky-yellow coating.

Pulse: Slippery-Rapid.

Mental-emotional profile

In this case, the anxiety is marked, to the point of agitation. The person may be hyperactive and slightly chaotic because, besides being unsettled, the Mind is also obstructed.

Treatment principle

Resolve Phlegm, clear Heart-Heat, calm the Mind, open the Mind's orifices.

Acupuncture

Points

P-5 Jianshi, HE-8 Shaofu, Ren-12 Zhongwan, ST-40 Fenglong, ST-8 Touwei, G.B.-13 Benshen, Ren-15 Jiuwei, Du-24 Shenting. Even method on all points except Ren-12, which should be needled with reinforcing method.

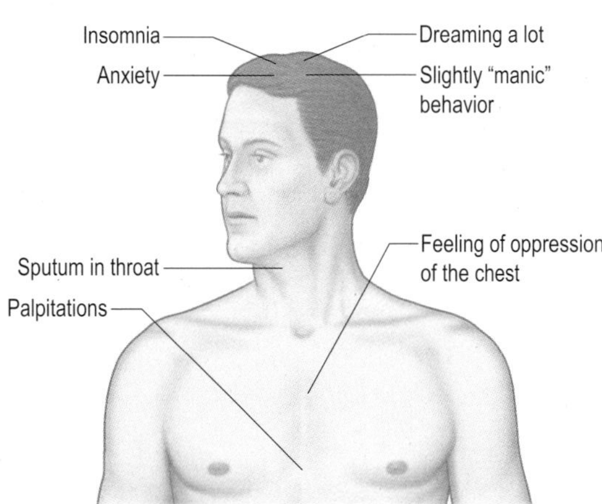

Figure 17.19 Phlegm-Heat harassing the Heart.

Explanation

- P-5 and HE-8 clear Heart-Heat and resolve Phlegm from the Heart.
- Ren-12 and ST-40 resolve Phlegm.
- ST-8 resolves Phlegm from the Brain.
- G.B.-13, Ren-15 and Du-24 calm the Mind and resolve Phlegm from the head.

Herbal therapy

Prescription

WEN DAN TANG
Warming the Gall-Bladder Decoction

Explanation

This formula clears Heart-Heat, resolves Phlegm and calms the Mind.

Prescription

GUI SHEN TANG
Restoring the Mind Decoction

Explanation

This formula opens the Mind's orifices, tonifies the Heart, resolves Phlegm and calms the Mind. Its clearing-Heat effect is not strong.

Please note that the original formula contains Zi He Che *Placenta hominis* and Zhu Sha *Cinnabaris*, which should be omitted as the use of these two substances is not allowed.

SUMMARY

Phlegm-Heat harassing the Heart

Points

P-5 Jianshi, HE-8 Shaofu, Ren-12 Zhongwan, ST-40 Fenglong, ST-8 Touwei, G.B.-13 Benshen, Ren-15 Jiuwei, Du-24 Shenting. Even method on all points except Ren-12, which should be needled with reinforcing method.

Herbal therapy

Prescription

WEN DAN TANG
Warming the Gall-Bladder Decoction

Prescription

GUI SHEN TANG
Restoring the Mind Decoction

MODERN CHINESE LITERATURE

Journal of Chinese Medicine

(*Zhong Yi Za Zhi* 中医杂志), Vol. 41, No. 2, 2000, p. 95.

Sun Song, "The treatment of generalized anxiety disorder with a variation of Chai Hu Long Gu Mu Li Tang *Bupleurum-Mastodi Ossis fossilia-Concha Ostreae* decoction"

Seventy-two cases of generalized anxiety disorder were treated with a variation of the formula Chai Hu Long Gu Mu Li Tang *Bupleurum-Mastodi Ossis fossilia-Concha Ostreae* decoction.

The age distribution of the patients was as follows.

- 16–20: 2 cases
- 21–40: 38 cases
- 41–60: 24 cases
- over 60: 8

There were 29 men and 43 women. The formula used was as follows:

- **Chai Hu** *Radix Bupleuri* 10 g
- **Huang Qin** *Radix Scutellariae* 10 g
- **Ban Xia** *Rhizoma Pinelliae preparatum* 10 g
- **Gui Zhi** *Ramulus Cinnamomi cassiae* 10 g
- **Da Huang** *Radix et Rhizoma Rhei* 10 g
- **Long Gu** *Mastodi Ossis fossilia* 30 g
- **Mu Li** *Concha Ostreae* 30 g
- **Zhen Zhu Mu** *Concha Margaritifera usta* 30 g
- **Fu Xiao Mai** *Fructus Tritici levis* 30 g
- **Da Zao** *Fructus Jujubae* 5 pieces
- **Zhi Gan Cao** *Radix Glycyrrhizae uralensis preparata* 10 g
- **Shu Di Huang** *Radix Rehmanniae preparata* 10 g.

Modifications

- In case of Phlegm, add Dan Nan Xing *Rhizoma Arisaematis preparatum* and Zhu Ru *Caulis Bambusae in Taeniam*.
- In case of Liver-Fire, add Long Dan Cao *Radix Gentianae* and Shan Zhi Zi *Fructus Gardeniae*.
- In case of Empty Heat from Yin deficiency, remove Gui Zhi *Ramulus Cinnamomi cassiae* and add Zhi Mu *Radix Anemarrhenae* and Huang Bo *Cortex Phellodendri*.

- In case of Stomach- and Liver-Yin deficiency, remove Gui Zhi *Ramulus Cinnamomi cassiae* and add Bei Sha Shen *Radix Glehniae* and Mai Men Dong *Radix Ophiopogonis*.

The results were as follows.

- *Complete cure*: 48 cases (68.6%)
- *Significant improvement*: 13 cases (18.05%)
- *Moderate improvement*: 7 cases (9.72%)
- *No results*: 3 cases (4.17%).

CLINICAL TRIALS

Acupuncture

Effect of Jin-3-needling therapy on plasma corticosteroid, adrenocorticotropic hormone and platelet 5-HT levels in patients with generalized anxiety disorder

Zhong Guo Zhong Xi Yi Jie He Za Zhi 中国中西医结合杂志 [Chinese Journal of Integrative Medicine] 2007 December, Vol. 13, Issue 4, pp. 264–268.
Yuan Q, Li JN, Liu B, Wu ZF, Jin R

Objective

To observe the therapeutic efficacy of Jin-3-needling therapy (J3N) on generalized anxiety disorder (GAD) using the clinical global impression scale (CGI), and to measure the plasma levels of corticosteroid (CS), adrenocorticotropic hormone (ACTH) and platelet 5-hydroxytryptamine (5-HT) before and after treatment.

Method

Eighty-six GAD patients with the diagnosis matching the inclusion criteria were assigned, according to the sequence of visiting time, to three groups. The 29 patients in the Western medicine group were treated mainly with fluoxetine or paroxetine; however, alprazolam was additionally administered in severe conditions; the 29 patients in the needling group received J3N therapy using the points Sishencong (the four acupuncture points 1.5 *cun* anterior, posterior, right and left from Du-20), Dingshenzhen (three extra points around Yintang and G.B.-14 Yangbai), P-6 Neiguan, HE-7 Shenmen and SP-6 Sanyinjiao; and the 28 patients in the combined treatment group were treated with both drugs and needling in the same way as applied in the above two groups. The therapeutic course for all was 6 weeks. Conditions of patients were evaluated before and after treatment with CGI, and levels of CS, ACTH as well as 5-HT were measured by high performance liquid chromatography-electrochemistry.

Results

The CGI severity index and the general index scores were not significantly different in the three groups; however, the efficacy index proved to be the highest in the needling group, the second in the combined treatment group and the lowest in the drug group. Plasma levels of ACTH and platelet content of 5-HT were lowered in all three groups after treatment, showing statistical significance ($P < 0.05$), but no significant change was found in CS level ($P > 0.05$).

Conclusion

The efficacy index results of J3N treatment for GAD is significantly higher than that of conventional treatment. Moreover, when combined with drugs, needling might effectively prevent the side-effects of the routinely used Western drugs. The regulatory action of needling on platelet 5-HT and plasma ACTH is probably one of the acting pathways for J3N treatment on GAD.

Acupuncture for mild to moderate emotional complaints in pregnancy – a prospective, quasi-randomized, controlled study

Acupuncture in Medicine 2007 September, Vol. 25, Issue 3, pp. 65–71.
Bosco Guerreiro da Silva J

Objective

The aim of this study was to describe the effects of acupuncture under real life conditions, in the treatment of emotional complaints during pregnancy.

Method

Fifty-one conventionally treated pregnant women (with counseling by their physicians and nurses) were randomly allocated into an acupuncture study group and a control group receiving no treatment. Both groups (28 in the study group and 23 in the control group) presented emotional complaints such as anxiety, depression and irritability. They reported the severity of symptoms using a numerical rating scale (NRS) from 0 to 10, and they rated how much the symptoms disturbed five aspects of their lives: mood, sleep, relationships, social activities and sexual life. Traditional acupuncture was used. A set pattern of points was used in order to facilitate protocols; however, additionally up to four points were permitted as optional points.

Results

Three women from the acupuncture group and four from the control group dropped out of the study. Over the study period, the NRS scores of intensity of emotional distress decreased for at least half of the patients in the study group: 15/25 (60%) and in 5/19 (26%) of those in the control group ($p = 0.013$). The impact of the distress on three out of the five aspects of life was significantly less in the acupuncture group when compared with the control group ($P < 0.05$).

Conclusion

Emotional complaints are very common in pregnancy and medication is always a risk. In this study, acupuncture seems to be an efficacious means of reducing symptoms and improving the quality of life of women with emotional complaints during pregnancy. Large randomized studies are recommended to confirm these results.

Acupuncture for post-traumatic stress disorder: a randomized controlled pilot trial

Journal of Nervous and Mental Disease 2007 June, Vol. 195, Issue 6, pp. 504–513.

Hollifield M, Sinclair-Lian N, Warner TD, Hammerschlag R

Objective

The purpose of the study was to evaluate the potential efficacy and acceptability of acupuncture for post-traumatic stress disorder (PTSD).

Method

People diagnosed with PTSD were randomized to an empirically developed acupuncture treatment (ACU), a group cognitive-behavioral therapy (CBT) or a wait-list control (WLC). The primary outcome measure was self-reported PTSD symptoms at baseline, end treatment and 3-month follow-up. Repeated measures (multivariate analysis of variance) were used to detect predicted Group × Time effects in both intent-to-treat (ITT) and treatment completion models.

Results

Compared with the WLC condition in the ITT model, acupuncture provided large treatment effects for PTSD ($F [1, 46] = 12.60$; $p < 0.01$; Cohen's d (statistical effect size model = 1.29), similar in magnitude to group CBT ($F [1, 47] = 12.45$; $p < 0.01$; $d = 1.42$) (ACU vs. CBT, $d = 0.29$). Symptom reductions at end treatment were maintained at 3-month follow-up for both interventions.

Conclusion

Acupuncture may be an efficacious and acceptable non-invasive treatment option for PTSD. Larger trials with additional controls and methods are warranted to replicate and extend these findings.

Acupuncture for anxiety and anxiety disorders – a systematic literature review

Acupuncture in Medicine 2007 June, Vol. 25, Issue 1–2, pp. 1–10.

Pilkington K, Kirkwood G, Rampes H, Cummings M, Richardson J

Background

The aim of this study was to evaluate the evidence for the efficacy of acupuncture in the treatment of anxiety and anxiety disorders by systematic review of the relevant research.

Method

Searches of the major biomedical databases (MEDLINE, EMBASE, CINAHL, PsycINFO, Cochrane Library) were conducted between February and July 2004. Specialist complementary medicine databases were also searched and efforts made to identify unpublished research. No language restrictions were imposed and translations were obtained where necessary. Study methodology was appraised and clinical commentaries obtained for studies reporting clinical outcomes.

Results

Twelve controlled trials were located, of which 10 were randomized controlled trials (RCTs). Four RCTs focused on acupuncture in generalized anxiety disorder or anxiety neurosis, while six focused on anxiety in the perioperative period. No studies were located on the use of acupuncture specifically for panic disorder, phobias or obsessive-compulsive disorder. In generalized anxiety disorder or anxiety neurosis, it is difficult to interpret the findings of the studies of acupuncture because of the range of interventions against which acupuncture was compared. All trials reported positive findings but the reports lacked many basic methodological details. Reporting of the studies of perioperative anxiety was generally better and the initial indications are that acupuncture, specifically auricular acupuncture, is more effective than acupuncture at sham points and may be as effective as drug therapy in this situation. The results were, however, based on subjective measures and blinding could not be guaranteed.

Conclusion

Positive findings are reported for acupuncture in the treatment of generalized anxiety disorder or anxiety neurosis but there is currently insufficient research evidence for firm conclusions to be drawn. No trials of acupuncture for other anxiety disorders were located. There is some limited evidence in favor of auricular acupuncture in perioperative anxiety. Overall, the promising findings indicate that further research is warranted in the form of well-designed, adequately powered studies.

Effects of acupuncture as a treatment for hyperventilation syndrome: a pilot, randomized crossover trial

Journal of Alternative and Complementary Medicine 2007 January–February, Vol. 13, Issue 1, pp. 39–46.

Gibson D, Bruton A, Lewith GT, Mullee M

Background

Sustained and subtle hyperventilation can result in a wide variety of symptoms, leading to a chronic condition that has been termed hyperventilation syndrome (HVS). Treatment options include physiotherapy, in the form of breathing retraining (BR), but additional approaches aim to reduce the anxiety that is recognized as being a frequent component of this condition.

Objective

The aim of this study was to evaluate whether acupuncture is an appropriate treatment for HVS to reduce anxiety, and whether a crossover trial is an appropriate study design to evaluate acupuncture in this condition.

Method

A single-blind crossover trial was carried out comparing the effects of 4 weeks (30 minutes twice weekly) of acupuncture and BR on patients with HVS. Ten patients diagnosed with HVS were recruited to the trial and randomized into two groups. Both groups received acupuncture and BR with a washout period of 1 week. The primary outcome measure used was the Hospital Anxiety and Depression (HAD) Scale. Other outcome measures used were the Nijmegen questionnaire and Medical Research Council Dyspnoea Scale.

Results

The results showed statistically significant treatment differences between acupuncture and breathing retraining, in favor of acupuncture. Reductions were found in the HAD A (anxiety) ($p = 0.02$) and Nijmegen (symptoms) ($p = 0.03$) scores. There was no statistical evidence of any carryover effects. However, when graphically examining individual anxiety scores, in those who received acupuncture first, there was a reduction in anxiety levels which persisted through the washout period, suggesting that there may have been some carryover effect from this treatment.

Conclusion

This study suggests that acupuncture may be beneficial in the management of HVS in terms of reducing anxiety levels and symptom severity. However, there may be some carryover effect after acupuncture treatment, which went undetected because of the small sample size. This preliminary study provides the basis for a larger, sufficiently powered and methodologically sound trial.

Effect of acupuncture treatment on the immune function impairment found in anxious women

American Journal of Chinese Medicine 2007, Vol. 35, Issue 1, pp. 35–51.
Arranz L, Guayerbas N, Siboni L, De La Fuente M

Objective

It is presently accepted that emotional disturbances lead to immune system impairment, and that therefore their treatment could restore the immune response. Thus, the aim of the present work was to study the effect of an acupuncture treatment, designed specifically to relieve the emotional symptoms stemming from anxiety, on several functions (adherence, chemotaxis, phagocytosis, basal and stimulated superoxide anion levels, lymphocyte proliferation in response to phytohemagglutinin A (PHA) and natural killer (NK) activity) of leukocytes (neutrophils and lymphocytes) from anxious women.

Method

The acupuncture protocol consisted of manual needle stimulation of 19 acupuncture points, with each session lasting 30 minutes. It was performed on 34 female 30–60-year-old patients, suffering from anxiety, as determined by the Beck Anxiety Inventory (BAI). Before and 72 hours after receiving the first acupuncture session, peripheral blood samples were drawn. In 12 patients, samples were also collected immediately after the first single acupuncture session and 1 month after the end of the whole acupuncture treatment, which consisted of 10 sessions during a year, until the complete remission of anxiety. Twenty healthy non-anxious women in the same age range were used as controls.

Results

The results showed that the most favorable effects of acupuncture on the immune functions appear 72 hours after the single session and persist 1 month after the end of the complete treatment. Impaired immune functions in anxious women (chemotaxis, phagocytosis, lymphoproliferation and NK activity) were significantly improved by acupuncture, and augmented immune parameters (superoxide anion levels and lymphoproliferation of the patient subgroup whose values had been too high) were significantly diminished.

Conclusion

Acupuncture brought the above-mentioned parameters to values closer to those of healthy controls, exerting a modulatory effect on the immune system.

Acupuncture in patients with minor depression or generalized anxiety disorders – results of a randomized study

Fortschritte der Neurologie Psychiatrie [Advances in Neuro-Psychiatry] 2000, Vol. 68, Issue 3, pp. 137–144.
Eich H, Agelink MW, Lehmann E, Lemmer W, Klieser E

Objective

To ascertain the affects of acupuncture upon patients with minor depression and generalized anxiety disorder.

Method

In a placebo-controlled, randomized, modified double-blind study the effects were investigated of body acupuncture ($n = 10$) in 43 patients with minor depression (ICD-10 F32.0, F32.1) and 13 patients with generalized anxiety disorders (ICD-10 F41.1). Points needled were Du-20 Baihui, Sishencong, HE-7 Shenmen, P-6 Neiguan and BL-62 Shenmai. The severity of the disease was assessed by the Clinical Global Impression Scale (CGI). Treatment response was defined as a significant improvement in CGI. An intent-to-treat analysis was performed to compare treatment responses between true and placebo acupuncture.

Results

After completing a total of 10 acupuncture sessions, the true acupuncture group ($n = 28$) showed a significantly larger clinical improvement compared to the placebo group (Mann-Whitney test, $p < 0.05$). There were significantly more responders in the true compared to the placebo group (60.7% vs. 21.4%; chi-square test, $p < 0.01$). In contrast, no differences in the response rates were evident after just five acupuncture sessions. A multivariate analysis with the independent factor acupuncture (true vs. placebo) and the results of the additional rating scales (total score of HAMA, HAMD, Bf-S, BL) as dependent variables (ANOVA, 1;54 D.F.) revealed a clear trend towards lower HAMA scores in the true group after completing 10 acupuncture sessions (F3.29, $p = 0.075$). This corresponds well to the high response rate of 85.7% in patients with generalized anxiety disorders, in whom true acupuncture was applied.

Conclusion

The results indicate that acupuncture leads to a significant clinical improvement, as well as to a remarkable reduction in anxiety symptoms in patients with minor depression or with generalized anxiety disorders. The total sum of acupuncture sessions and the specific location of acupuncture needle insertions might be important factors for bringing about therapeutic success.

CASE HISTORIES

Case history

A 40-year-old woman had been suffering from severe anxiety for many years. She was constantly anxious with a panicky feeling that she experienced in the chest. She had a frightened and restless look in her eyes. Her severe anxiety caused her great distress.

Although she did have some problems with her work and finances, these were not serious enough to warrant that level of anxiety. On interrogation, it transpired that she had always been a "worrier" ever since she was a teenager.

She also suffered from dizziness, occasional tinnitus and night-sweating. When she was anxious, she also suffered from palpitations and sweating. Her face was red and her tongue was Red, with a deep Heart crack and almost totally without coating. Her pulse was Fine and Rapid.

Diagnosis Her tongue and pulse indicate a clear condition of Yin deficiency (tongue without coating) with Empty Heat (tongue Red). The Heart crack, palpitations and anxiety indicate that the Yin deficiency is affecting the Heart; the dizziness, tinnitus and night-sweating indicate that the Kidneys are also affected.

In her case, therefore, the anxiety is due not only to the Heart but also the Kidneys (fear). My feeling was that her anxiety was largely of constitutional origin, the deep Heart crack leading me to this conclusion. Such patients are very difficult to treat as the anxiety is ingrained in their mental-emotional constitution. The look in her eyes also led me to believe that her anxiety might also be due to a feeling of guilt, but she did not show any willingness to discuss this.

Treatment I chose the formula Tian Wang Bu Xin Dan *Heavenly Emperor Tonifying the Heart Pill* as it was perfectly suited to her configuration of patterns, i.e. Heart- and Kidney-Yin deficiency with Heart Empty Heat.

I used the following variation of this formula:

- **Sheng Di Huang** *Radix Rehmanniae* 6 g
- **Mai Men Dong** *Radix Ophiopogonis* 6 g
- **Tian Men Dong** *Radix Asparagi* 6 g
- **Ren Shen** *Radix Ginseng* 6 g
- **Fu Ling** *Poria* 9 g
- **Wu Wei Zi** *Fructus Schisandrae* 4 g
- **Dang Gui** *Radix Angelicae sinensis* 6 g
- **Dan Shen** *Radix Salviae miltiorrhizae* 6 g
- **Suan Zao Ren** *Semen Ziziphi spinosae* 6 g
- **Bai Zi Ren** *Semen Platycladi* 6 g
- **Yuan Zhi** *Radix Polygalae* 6 g
- **Lian Zi Xin** *Plumula Nelumbinis* 6 g
- **Jie Geng** *Radix Platycodi* 3 g.

I also treated this patient with acupuncture and selected points from the following pool of points: HE-7 Shenmen, P-7 Daling, Du-24 Shenting, Ren-15 Jiuwei, ST-36 Zusanli, SP-6 Sanyinjiao, Ren-4 Guanyuan, KI-3 Taixi.

I treated this patient for over a year with both acupuncture and herbal medicine. She made a remarkable improvement with a marked reduction in her levels of anxiety. However, she could never be free of it completely. This is probably due to the fact that it was constitutional. I therefore stopped the treatment but advised her to come back for a few treatments every 3–4 months, which she did.

Case history

A 42-year-old woman had been suffering from anxiety ever since the birth of her second child 5 years previously. Her anxiety was mild but constant and disabling. She had a vague feeling of anxiety without being able to pin-point the cause or the object of it. She also slept badly.

Her health was otherwise good apart from complaining of palpitations, blurred vision and tingling of the limbs. Her tongue was Pale and her pulse Choppy.

Diagnosis This is a very clear example of anxiety deriving from Heart-Blood deficiency as evidenced by the anxiety, insomnia and palpitations. There was some Liver-Blood deficiency as evidenced by the blurred vision and tingling. Her tongue and pulse confirm the Blood deficiency.

In her case, the Blood deficiency arose after the birth of her second child. This is a common cause of Blood deficiency in women and one that may also give rise to postnatal depression.

Treatment I treated this patient primarily with acupuncture and with a herbal remedy. The points I used were selected from the following.

- Ren-4 Guanyuan, ST-36 Zusanli, LIV-8 Ququan and SP-6 Sanyinjiao to nourish Liver-Blood.
- HE-7 Shenmen to nourish Heart-Blood.
- Du-24 Shenting and Ren-15 Jiuwei to calm the Mind.

In addition to acupuncture, I used the *Three Treasures* remedy *Calm the Shen*, which nourishes Liver- and Heart-Blood and calms the Mind.

I treated her for 9 months, after which her anxiety was completely relieved.

Case history

A 50-year-old woman had been suffering with anxiety for a long time. She experienced her anxiety more in the daytime and her sleep was good. She worried very easily about the smallest things.

She was rather overweight and felt cold easily. She suffered from lower backache and dizziness, and her urination was frequent and her urine pale.

I enquired about her working life and she had been overworking for many years, leaving home early in the morning and returning in the evening. Her tongue was Pale and her pulse was Weak and Deep, particularly on both Rear positions.

Diagnosis In this case, the anxiety derives clearly from a deficiency of the Kidneys and specifically Kidney-Yang. Fear is the emotion pertaining to the Kidneys.

Treatment I treated this patient with a combination of acupuncture and a herbal remedy. The acupuncture points I used were selected from the following.

- Ren-4 Guanyuan with moxa, BL-23 Shenshu, KI-7 Fuliu and KI-3 Taixi to tonify Kidney-Yang.
- Du-24 Shenting and Ren-15 Jiuwei to calm the Mind.

I also used the *Three Treasures* remedy *Strengthen the Root*, which is a variation of You Gui Wan *Restoring the Right* [Kidney] *Pill* to tonify Kidney-Yang.

Case history

A 59-year-old woman complained of palpitations. It is not often that a Western patient presents with "palpitations" as their main problem. Besides the palpitations, she also suffered from anxiety and insomnia (difficulty in both falling asleep and staying asleep). She also complained of feeling cold and having cold hands, and suffering from catarrh.

From a Western medicine perspective, she had been diagnosed as suffering from Hashimoto thyroiditis and had been put on thyroxine 7 years before.

Her tongue was slightly Pale, with Pale sides, Swollen in general and had a Heart crack. Her pulse was Slippery and a little Slow; it was Weak on the right Middle position (Stomach and Spleen).

Diagnosis I thought this patient suffered from a complex combination of patterns. There was, first of all, a deficiency of Yang of the Spleen (tiredness, feeling cold, Pale tongue with Pale sides and Weak

Stomach/Spleen pulse). This had obviously given rise to Phlegm (Swollen tongue, catarrh, Slippery pulse). The deficiency of Yang of the Spleen had affected Heart-Yang too, and caused the palpitations and cold feeling of the hands. The palpitations are also caused by the retention of Phlegm in the chest.

Therefore, the condition is characterized by Emptiness (deficiency of Yang of the Spleen and Heart) and Fullness (Phlegm and Cold).

Treatment As I often do in chronic Full-Empty conditions, I decided to start by resolving Phlegm and expelling Cold. I used a variation of Wen Dan Tang *Warming the Gall-Bladder Decoction*.

- **Zhu Ru** *Caulis Bambusae in Taeniam*
- **Zhi Shi** *Fructus Aurantii immaturus*
- **Ban Xia** *Rhizoma Pinelliae preparatum*
- **Fu Ling** *Poria*
- **Chen Pi** *Pericarpium Citri reticulatae*
- **Gui Zhi** *Ramulus Cinnamomi cassiae*
- **Yuan Zhi** *Radix Polygalae*
- **Suan Zao Ren** *Semen Ziziphi spinosae*
- **Bai Zi Ren** *Semen Platycladi*
- **Bai Zhu** *Rhizoma Atractylodis macrocephalae*

Explanation

The main formula resolves Phlegm from the Lungs, Heart and chest. I modified it with the addition of Gui Zhi to make it warmer and herbs to calm the Mind to treat the insomnia and anxiety. I added Bai Zhu to tonify the Spleen.

I treated her with variations of this formula for 6 months, during which her palpitations disappeared and her sleep got gradually better although it was still a problem. After 6 months, I continued giving her variations of the above formula, but I modified it with the addition of more Spleen tonics as follows.

- **Zhu Ru** *Caulis Bambusae in Taeniam*
- **Zhi Shi** *Fructus Aurantii immaturus*
- **Ban Xia** *Rhizoma Pinelliae preparatum*
- **Fu Ling** *Poria*
- **Chen Pi** *Pericarpium Citri reticulatae*
- **Gui Zhi** *Ramulus Cinnamomi cassiae*
- **Yuan Zhi** *Radix Polygalae*
- **Suan Zao Ren** *Semen Ziziphi spinosae*
- **Bai Zi Ren** *Semen Platycladi*
- **Bai Zhu** *Rhizoma Atractylodis macrocephalae*
- **Huang Qi** *Radix Astragali*
- **Dang Gui** *Radix Angelicae sinensis*

After another 4 months of treatment with the above formula, her sleep improved further and I therefore decided to turn my attention to treating the Root (Ben), i.e. tonify Spleen-Yang with the following formula.

- **Ren Shen** *Radix Ginseng*
- **Huang Qi** *Radix Astragali*
- **Bai Zhu** *Rhizoma Atractylodis macrocephalae*
- **Chen Pi** *Pericarpium Citri reticulatae*
- **Fu Ling** *Poria*
- **Ban Xia** *Rhizoma Pinelliae preparatum*
- **Gui Zhi** *Ramulus Cinnamomi cassiae*
- **Gan Jiang** *Rhizoma Zingiberis*
- **Dang Gui** *Radix Angelicae sinensis*
- **Bai Zi Ren** *Semen Platycladi*

Although the main impact of this formula was to tonify Spleen-Yang, it still contains herbs to resolve Phlegm. The patient continued to improve with this formula and she is still under treatment at the time of writing.

END NOTES

1. National Institute of Mental Health website: www.nimh.nih.gov. [Accessed 2008].
2. Robins LN, Regier DA (eds) 1991 Psychiatric Disorders in America: the Epidemiologic Catchment Area Study. Free Press, New York.
3. LeDoux J 1996 The Emotional Brain. Simon and Schuster, New York, pp. 229–230.
4. Cited in Lewis M, Haviland-Jones JM (eds) 2004 Handbook of Emotions. Guilford Press, New York, p. 574.
5. The Emotional Brain, p. 228.
6. Cited in Wang Yong Yan 2004 Zhong Yi Nei Ke Xue 中医内科学 [Chinese Internal Medicine]. People's Health Publishing House, Beijing, p. 265.
7. Cited in Zhang Bo Yu 1986 Zhong Yi Nei Ke Xue 中医内科学 [Chinese Internal Medicine]. Shanghai Science Publishing House, Shanghai, p. 107.
8. He Ren 2005 Jin Gui Yao Lue 金匮要略通俗讲话[Essential Prescriptions of the Golden Chest]. People's Health Publishing House, Beijing, p. 83. The *Essential Prescriptions of the Golden Chest* was written by Zhang Zhong Jing and first published *c.*AD 220.
9. Nanjing College of Traditional Chinese Medicine 1979 Nan Jing Jiao Shi 难经校释 [A Revised Explanation of the Classic of Difficulties]. People's Health Publishing House, Beijing, pp. 73–74. First published *c.*AD 100.
10. Wang Luo Zhen 1985 Qi Jing Ba Mai Kao Jiao Zhu 奇经八脉考校注 [A Compilation of the Study of the Eight Extraordinary Vessels]. Shanghai Science Publishing House, Shanghai, p. 60. The *Study of the Eight Extraordinary Vessels* was written by Li Shi Zhen and first published in 1578.
11. Ibid., p. 61.
12. 1982 Lei Jing 类经 [Classic of Categories]. People's Health Publishing House, Beijing, p. 281. The *Classic of Categories* was written by Zhang Jie Bin and first published in 1624.
13. 1979 Huang Di Nei Jing Su Wen 黄帝内经素问[The Yellow Emperor's Classic of Internal Medicine-Simple Questions]. People's Health Publishing House, Beijing, p. 222. First published *c.*100 BC.

14. The NIMH Genetics Workgroup 1998 Genetics and mental disorders. National Institute of Mental Health, Rockville, MD. NIH Publication No. 98: 4268.
15. Cited in Zhang Bo Yu 1986 Chinese Internal Medicine, p. 270.
16. Ibid., p. 270.
17. Ibid., p. 270.
18. Ibid., p. 270.
19. Dr Zhang Ming Jiu, personal communication, Nanjing 1982.
20. Dr Zhang Ming Jiu, personal communication, Nanjing 1982.
21. Cheng Bao Shu 1988 Zhen Jiu Da Ci Dian 诊灸大辞典 [Great Dictionary of Acupuncture]. Beijing Science Publishing House, Beijing, p. 11.
22. Jiao Shun Fa 1987 Zhong Guo Zhen Jiu Qiu Zhen 中国针灸求诊 [An Enquiry into Chinese Acupuncture]. Shanxi Science Publishing House, Shanxi, p. 52.
23. Shan Chang Hua 1990 Jing Xue Jie 经穴解 [An Explanation of the Acupuncture Points]. People's Health Publishing House, Beijing, p. 334. *An Explanation of the Acupuncture Points* was written by Yue Han Zhen and first published in 1654.

失眠

CHAPTER 18

INSOMNIA (EXCESSIVE DREAMING, SOMNOLENCE, POOR MEMORY)

ETIOLOGY *450*

Emotional stress *450*
Overwork *450*
"Gall-Bladder timid" *450*
Irregular diet *450*
Childbirth *451*
Residual Heat *451*
Excessive sexual activity *451*

PATHOLOGY *451*

DIAGNOSIS *454*

Sleep *454*
Dreams *454*
Sleeping positions *455*
Snoring *455*

IDENTIFICATION OF PATTERNS AND TREATMENT *456*

Liver-Fire blazing *456*
Heart-Fire blazing *457*
Phlegm-Heat harassing the Mind *459*
Heart-Qi stagnation *460*
Heart-Blood stasis *461*
Residual Heat in the diaphragm *462*
Retention of Food *464*
Liver-Qi stagnation *465*
Heart- and Spleen-Blood deficiency *466*
Heart-Yin deficiency *468*
Heart and Kidneys not harmonized *468*
Heart and Gall-Bladder deficiency *470*
Liver-Yin deficiency *471*
Liver- and Kidney-Yin deficiency *473*

MODERN CHINESE LITERATURE *475*

CLINICAL TRIALS *478*

PATIENTS' STATISTICS *484*

APPENDIX 1 EXCESSIVE DREAMING *484*

IDENTIFICATION OF PATTERNS AND TREATMENT *486*

Phlegm-Heat *486*
Liver-Fire *486*
Deficiency of Qi of Heart and Gall-Bladder *487*
Heart- and Lung-Qi deficiency *487*
Deficiency of Heart and Spleen *488*
Heart and Kidneys not harmonized *489*

APPENDIX 2 SOMNOLENCE *489*

IDENTIFICATION OF PATTERNS AND TREATMENT *489*

Dampness obstructing the Brain *489*
Phlegm misting the Brain *490*
Spleen deficiency *491*
Kidney-Yang deficiency (Deficiency of Sea of Marrow) *492*

APPENDIX 3 POOR MEMORY *493*

ETIOLOGY *493*

Worry and pensiveness *493*
Overwork and excessive sexual activity *493*
Childbirth *493*
Sadness *493*
"Recreational" drugs *493*

IDENTIFICATION OF PATTERNS AND TREATMENT *494*

Spleen deficiency *494*
Kidney-Essence deficiency *494*
Heart deficiency *495*

INSOMNIA

Full
- Liver-Fire blazing
- Heart-Fire blazing
- Phlegm-Heat harassing the Mind
- Heart-Qi stagnation
- Heart-Blood stasis
- Residual Heat in the diaphragm
- Retention of Food
- Liver-Qi stagnation

Empty
- Heart- and Spleen-Blood deficiency
- Heart-Yin deficiency
- Heart and Kidneys not harmonized
- Heart and Gall-Bladder deficiency
- Liver-Yin deficiency
- Liver- and Kidney-Yin deficiency

EXCESSIVE DREAMING
- Phlegm-Heat
- Liver-Fire
- Deficiency of Qi of Heart and Gall-Bladder
- Heart- and Lung-Qi Deficiency
- Deficiency of Heart and Spleen
- Heart and Kidneys not harmonized

SOMNOLENCE
- Dampness obstructing the Brain
- Phlegm misting the Brain
- Spleen deficiency
- Kidney-Yang deficiency (Deficiency of Sea of Marrow)

POOR MEMORY
- Spleen deficiency
- Kidney-Essence deficiency
- Heart deficiency

INSOMNIA (EXCESSIVE DREAMING, SOMNOLENCE, POOR MEMORY)

The term "insomnia" covers a number of different problems such as inability to fall asleep easily, waking up during the night, sleeping restlessly, waking up early in the morning and dream-disturbed sleep.

The amount and quality of sleep depend of course on the state of the Mind (*Shen*). The Mind is rooted in the Heart and specifically in Heart-Blood and Heart-Yin. If the Heart is healthy and the Blood abundant, the Mind is properly rooted and sleep will be sound. If the Heart is deficient or if it is agitated by pathogenic factors such as Fire, the Mind is not properly rooted and sleep will be affected (Fig. 18.1).

As always in Chinese medicine, there is an interrelationship between body and Mind. On the one hand, a deficiency of Blood or a pathogenic factor such as Fire may affect the Mind; on the other hand, emotional stress affecting the Mind may cause a disharmony of the Internal Organs.

If the disharmony of the Internal Organs, whether it is due to a Deficiency or an Excess, affects Blood and Essence, this affects the Mind. Since the Essence and Qi are the root of the Mind (the "Three Treasures"), the Mind then has no residence and insomnia may result. The *Simple Questions* in Chapter 46 says:[1]

> *When a person lies down and cannot sleep,* [it means] *the Yin organs are injured* [so that] *the Essence has no residence and is not quiet and the person cannot sleep.*

See Figure 18.2.

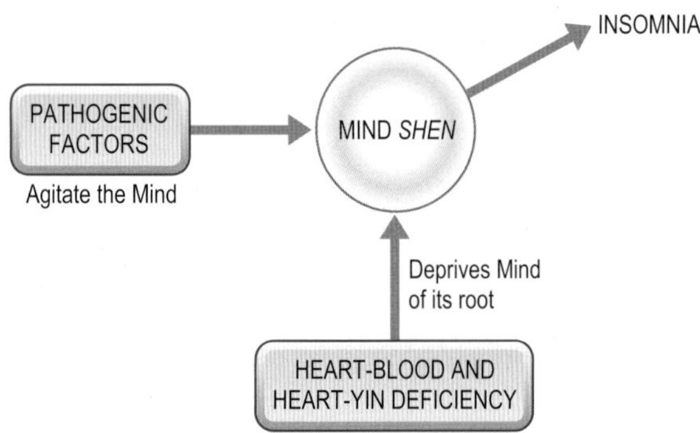

Figure 18.1 Pathology of insomnia.

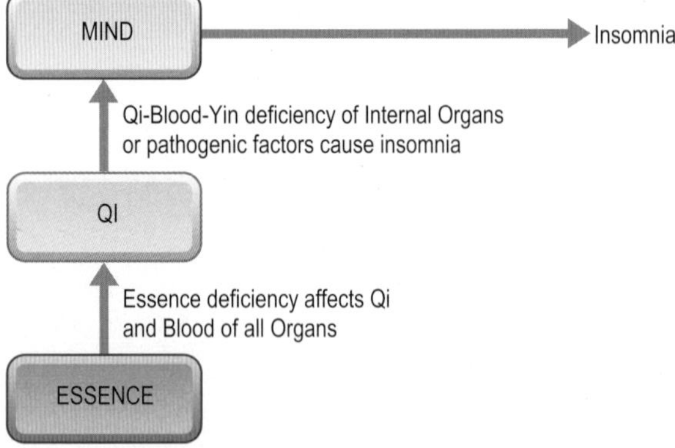

Figure 18.2 The *Three Treasures* (*Jing-Qi-Shen*) and sleep.

As far as sleep is concerned, the Mind is not the only mental-spiritual faculty involved. The Ethereal Soul (*Hun*) also plays an important role in the physiology and pathology of sleep and the length and quality of sleep are related to its state (*see Chapter 3*). In particular, the Ethereal Soul controls dreaming and therefore dream-disturbed sleep is often due to a disharmony of the Ethereal Soul.

If the Ethereal Soul is well rooted in the Liver (Liver-Blood or Liver-Yin), sleep is normal, sound and without too many dreams. If Liver-Blood or Liver-Yin is deficient, the Ethereal Soul is deprived of its residence and wanders off at night, causing a restless sleep with many tiring dreams. Tang Zong Hai says: "*At night during sleep the Ethereal Soul returns to the Liver; if the Ethereal Soul is not peaceful, there are a lot of dreams.*"[2]

The Ethereal Soul is affected not only by a deficiency of the Liver but also by any pathogenic factor (such as Fire or Wind) agitating the Liver. The *Complete Book of Jing Yue* (1624) by Zhang Jing Yue says: "*Overexertion, worrying and excessive thinking injure Blood and fluids so that the Mind and Ethereal Soul are deprived of residence and insomnia results.*"[3] It also says: "*Worrying and excessive thinking injure the Spleen so that it cannot make Blood and insomnia results.*"[4]

Another organ and mental-spiritual aspect influencing sleep are the Kidneys and the Will-Power (*Zhi*). I translate *Zhi* as "Will-Power" but *Zhi* encompasses also other aspects of the psyche. The *Zhi* is the root of the Mind (*Shen*) and it controls memory and sleep. Thus, when the Kidneys and the *Zhi* are deficient, the person may sleep badly; in particular, he or she may wake up frequently during the night.

CLINICAL NOTE

Sleep depends on the following.

- Heart and Mind (*Shen*): BL-44 Shentang
- Liver and Ethereal Soul (*Hun*): BL-47 Hunmen
- Kidneys and Will-Power (*Zhi*): BL-52 Zhishi

When a patient complains of poor sleep we must ascertain that the condition is true insomnia and not an inability to sleep well due to other external or temporary causes. For example, a sudden change in weather, jetlag, a bedroom that is too hot or too cold, drinking a lot of tea or coffee, an emotional upset or worrying about something specific may all cause a person to sleep badly but cannot be defined as "insomnia". In fact, once the above causes are removed, the person sleeps well. Also, one cannot diagnose insomnia when sleep is disturbed by other medical conditions such as asthma, a pain (e.g. shoulder, hip or back pain) or itching from a skin disease; in such cases, sleep is restored once the relevant disease is treated successfully.

It should be remembered that because in old people there is a physiological decline of Qi and Blood, they normally need less sleep than younger people. Chapter 18 of the *Spiritual Axis* says:[5]

Young people have abundant Qi and Blood ... [so that] *they are energetic in the daytime and sleep well at night. Old people have declining Qi and Blood* ... [so that] *they are less active in daytime and cannot sleep at night.*

Of course, normal sleep time depends on age, and the book *Chinese Medicine Psychology* defines normal sleep hours according to age as follows.[6]

- *From birth to 6 months*: 16 hours
- *From 6 months to 2 years*: 13 hours
- *From 2 to 12 years*: 10–12 hours
- *From 12 to 18 years*: 9–10 hours
- *Young adult*: 7–8 hours
- *Over 60 years*: 5–7 hours

Finally, according to traditional Chinese views, the best sleeping position is lying on the right side, with the legs slightly bent, the right arm bent and resting in front of the pillow, and the left arm resting on the left thigh. According to these views, with this position the heart is in a high position so that Blood can circulate freely; the liver is in a low position so that Blood can collect there and root the Ethereal Soul to promote sleep; and the stomach and duodenum are in such a position that facilitates the downward movement of food.

Insomnia will be discussed according to the following topics.

- Etiology
- Pathology
- Diagnosis
- Identification of patterns and treatment
- Modern Chinese literature
- Clinical trials
- Patients' statistics

ETIOLOGY

Emotional stress

Worry and pensiveness

Worry and pensiveness injure the Spleen, Lungs and Heart. When the Spleen is deficient, it cannot produce enough Blood; this deficiency affects the Heart and the Mind is deprived of its residence.

Worry may also injure Heart-Blood directly and this also leads to the Mind's being deprived of its residence and therefore to insomnia. In some cases, worry may lead to Heart-Heat (through Heart-Qi stagnation); this harasses the Mind and may lead to insomnia.

Worry leads to Heart-Qi stagnation and, with time, this may lead to Heart-Blood stasis. Stagnant Heart-Blood harasses the Mind and may lead to insomnia (Fig. 18.3).

Anger

Anger, intended in a broad sense including frustration, resentment and irritation, leads to either Liver-Yang rising or Liver-Fire. Liver-Yang or Liver-Fire agitates the Ethereal Soul so that this is not rooted in the Liver at night. This causes insomnia and dream-disturbed sleep.

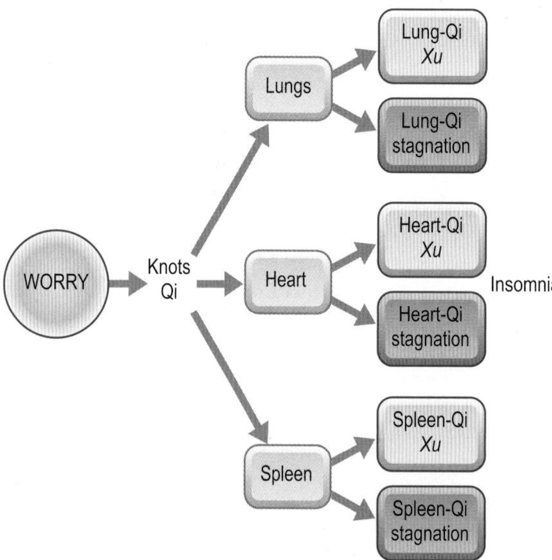

Figure 18.3 Worry and insomnia.

Guilt

Guilt causes stagnation of Qi and it frequently affects the Kidneys (as well as the Heart). By affecting the Kidneys, it injures the *Zhi* and the Essence so that the Mind cannot be rooted in the Kidneys and this causes insomnia.

Overwork

Working long hours without adequate rest, working under conditions of severe stress combined with irregular diet, all weaken Kidney-Yin. When Kidney-Yin is deficient over a long period of time, it fails to nourish Heart-Yin so that Heart Empty Heat develops. This especially happens when the person worries a lot.

The same pattern may be the result of the reverse process. Severe emotional strain over a long period of time may lead to the formation of Heart-Fire, which flares upwards and fails to communicate downwards with the Kidneys. On the other hand, Fire injures the Yin and may lead to Kidney-Yin deficiency. The end result is a similar condition: Heart and Kidneys are not harmonized. This is a common cause of insomnia in the elderly.

"Gall-Bladder timid"

A constitutional weakness of both Heart and Gall-Bladder may give rise to a timid character. The Gall-Bladder is the mother of the Heart and a person whose Gall-Bladder is weak will be timid, fearful and indecisive, and will lack self-assertiveness. Chinese language bears out this connection between the Gall-Bladder and timidity: "big gall-bladder" means "courageous"; "small gall-bladder" means "timid" or "cowardly".

This constitutional deficiency of Heart and Gall-Bladder causes insomnia, especially waking up early.

Irregular diet

Irregular diet, overeating or eating too much greasy and hot food may lead to the formation of Phlegm in the Stomach; this harasses the Mind, leading to insomnia.

Overeating leads to Retention of Food in the Stomach; this disturbs the Heart and the Mind and leads to insomnia. This is a frequent cause of poor sleep in children.

The excessive consumption of hot foods (red meat, spices and alcohol) are conducive to the formation of Heat, which harasses the Heart and Liver, and therefore the Mind and the Ethereal Soul, leading to insomnia.

Childbirth

A large loss of blood during childbirth may induce a deficiency of Blood of the Liver. This may also happen not because the loss of blood is substantial but because of a pre-existing condition of deficiency of Blood. In either case, it causes a fairly sudden and severe deficiency of Liver-Blood. Deprived of its residence, the Ethereal Soul floats at night, causing insomnia and excessive dreaming.

On the other hand, as the Liver is the Mother of the Heart, a deficiency of Liver-Blood may induce a deficiency of Heart-Blood; the Mind is deprived of its residence and it floats at night, causing insomnia.

Residual Heat

During an invasion of Wind-Heat, the pathogenic factor may progress into the Interior and give rise to interior Heat. If this is not cleared properly, the person may make an apparent recovery but residual Heat is left in the body. This is said to lodge in the diaphragm where it harasses the Heart and may lead to insomnia.

This residual Heat in the diaphragm is often the cause of insomnia and mental restlessness in patients suffering from chronic fatigue syndrome.

Excessive sexual activity

Excessive sexual activity applies more to men than women. Sperm (a form of *Tian Gui* in men) is a direct manifestation of the Kidney-Essence. If sexual activity is so frequent that it does not allow the Kidney-Essence to replenish sperm fast enough, this is defined as "excessive" sexual activity. This leads to a deficiency of the Kidneys (which may be Yang or Yin) and to a deficiency of the Will-Power (*Zhi*); *Zhi* fails to root the Mind and insomnia may result.

Excessive sexual activity is seldom a cause of disease in women as, in women, *Tian Gui* (a manifestation of Essence) is menstrual blood and ova, and these are not lost during sexual activity in the same way as sperm is lost in men.

SUMMARY

Etiology

- Emotional stress
  - Worry
  - Anger
  - Guilt
- Overwork
- "Gall-Bladder timid"
- Irregular diet
- Childbirth
- Residual Heat
- Excessive sexual activity

PATHOLOGY

The pathology of insomnia (as that of many other diseases) revolves around Fullness and Emptiness. Empty conditions of insomnia usually involve a deficiency of either Blood or Yin, which deprives the Mind and/or Ethereal Soul of their residence; Full conditions involve a pathogenic factor (usually Heat/Fire or Blood stasis) agitating the Mind and/or the Ethereal Soul. In other words, the Mind and the Ethereal Soul may be restless, either because they are not rooted in Heart- and Liver-Blood/Yin, respectively, or because a pathogenic factor is agitating them. The various etiological factors and pathologies may be summarized in a diagram (Fig. 18.4).

As can be seen from the diagram, the Deficiency conditions causing insomnia occur mostly in the Heart, Spleen, Liver and Kidneys, whilst the Excess conditions occur in the Liver or Stomach.

Worry and pensiveness may weaken Heart-Blood so that the Mind is deprived of its residence and the person cannot sleep. In some people, worry, anxiety and pensiveness lead not to Heart-Blood deficiency, but to Heart-Fire. This is also due to a constitutional tendency to Yang Excess. Heart-Fire flares upwards to agitate the Mind, and insomnia results.

Worry, pensiveness, sadness, grief and guilt may lead to Heart-Qi stagnation; Qi stagnation obstructs the Heart so that this cannot house the Mind and insomnia results. The same emotions in the long term may lead to Heart-Blood stasis; the stagnant Blood in

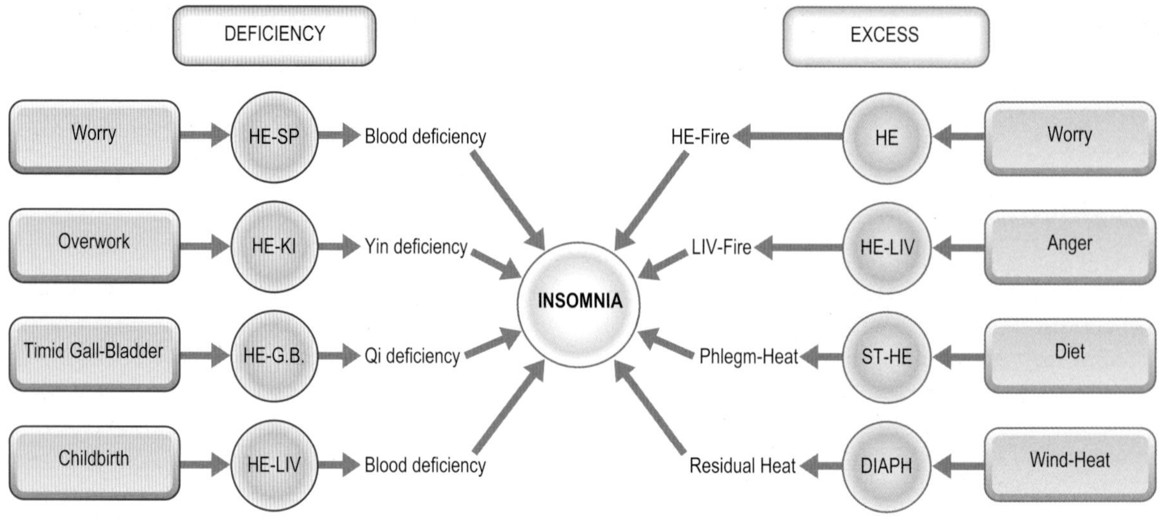

Figure 18.4 Etiology and pathology of insomnia.

the Heart prevents it from housing the Mind and insomnia results.

When Kidney-Yin is deficient over a long period of time, it fails to nourish Heart-Yin so that Heart Empty Heat develops. This especially happens when the person worries a lot. This pattern is also called "Heart and Kidneys not harmonized".

The same pattern may be the result of the reverse process. Severe emotional strain over a long period of time may lead to the formation of Heart-Fire, which flares upwards and fails to communicate downwards with the Kidneys. On the other hand, Fire injures the Yin and may lead to Kidney-Yin deficiency. The end result is a similar condition: Heart and Kidneys are not harmonized. This is a common cause of insomnia in the elderly.

Liver-Yang rising or Liver-Fire may both cause insomnia, especially in young or middle-aged people. A constitutional deficiency of Heart and Gall-Bladder causes insomnia, especially waking up early.

Phlegm-Heat in the Stomach harasses the Mind leading to insomnia. Loss of Blood causes a fairly sudden and severe deficiency of Liver-Blood. Deprived of its residence, the Ethereal Soul floats at night, causing insomnia and excessive dreaming. A deficiency of Liver-Blood often induces a deficiency of Heart-Blood, which also deprives the Mind of its residence and leads to insomnia.

Residual Heat lodges itself in the diaphragm, where it harasses the Heart and may lead to insomnia.

Retention of Food in the Stomach may affect the Heart due to the close relationship between these two organs, and insomnia results. This is a common cause of insomnia, especially in children.

Acupuncture

From the perspective of the channel system, insomnia is due to a breakdown of the interconnection of Yin and Yang. Yang-Qi and Yin-Qi have to be harmonized and flow into one another in a daily cycle. Defensive Qi flows in the Yang during the day and in the Yin during the night. If it remains in the Yang by night as well as by day, the person cannot sleep. The *Spiritual Axis* in Chapter 80 says:[7]

If Defensive Qi does not enter into the Yin at night and remains in the Yang, Yang-Qi becomes Full and the Yang Stepping Vessel (Yang Qiao Mai) in Excess, Yin becomes deficient and the eyes cannot close.

The *Spiritual Axis* in Chapter 21 says:[8]

The Yin and Yang of the Yin and Yang Stepping Vessels interconnect; Yang enters Yin and Yin exits towards

Yang, and the two meet at the corner of the eyes. When Yang-Qi is in Excess the eyes stay open; when Yin-Qi is in Excess, they stay closed.

For this reason, the beginning points of the Yang and Yin Stepping Vessels (*Yang* and *Yin Qiao Mai*), i.e. BL-62 Shenmai and KI-6 Zhaohai, respectively, can be used, together with BL-1 Jingming, for insomnia (see below). See Figure 18.5.

This combination can be used for any type of insomnia in addition to the points appropriate for the relevant pattern.

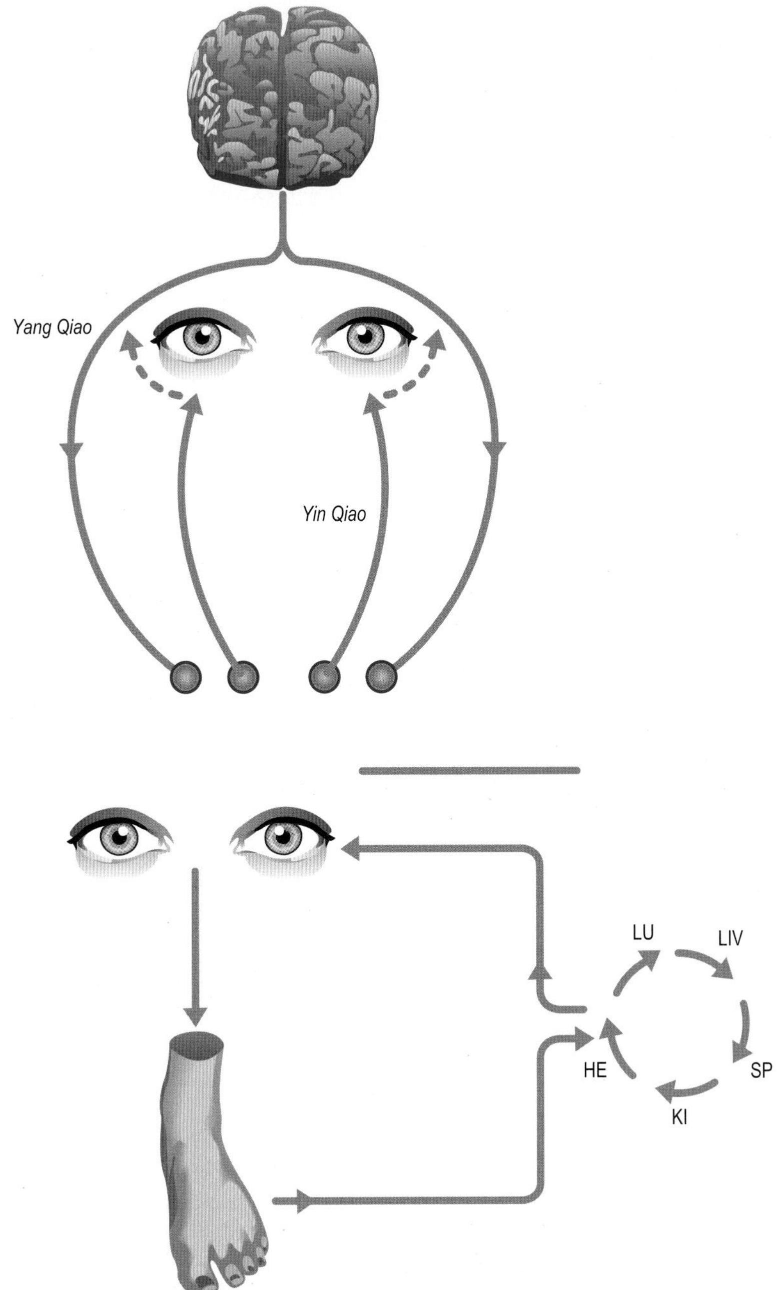

Figure 18.5 Circulation of Defensive Qi.

SUMMARY

Pathology

- The pathology of insomnia (as that of many other diseases) revolves around Fullness and Emptiness.
- Empty conditions involve a deficiency of either Blood or Yin.
- Full conditions involve a pathogenic factor (usually Heat/Fire or Blood stasis).
- Deficiency conditions occur mostly in Heart, Spleen, Liver or Kidneys.
- Excess conditions occur in the Liver or Stomach.
- Heart-Blood deficiency deprives the Mind of its residence and the person cannot sleep.
- Stagnation of Qi or stasis of Blood of the Heart may cause insomnia.
- Heart-Fire agitates the Mind and leads to insomnia.
- Deficient Kidney-Yin fails to nourish Heart-Yin so that Heart Empty Heat develops.
- Liver-Yang rising or Liver-Fire may both cause insomnia, especially in young or middle-aged people.
- A constitutional deficiency of Heart and Gall-Bladder causes insomnia, especially waking up early.
- Phlegm-Heat in the Stomach harasses the Mind leading to insomnia.
- Loss of blood causes a fairly sudden and severe deficiency of Liver-Blood and insomnia.
- Residual Heat lodges itself in the diaphragm, where it harasses the Heart and may lead to insomnia.
- Retention of Food obstructs the Stomach and affects the Heart and Mind, causing insomnia.

DIAGNOSIS

Sleep

When questioning a patient about insomnia, it is important to establish clearly what the main problem is.

Difficulty in falling asleep usually indicates deficiency of Blood, whilst falling asleep easily but waking up frequently during the night often denotes Yin deficiency. This is not, however, an absolute rule. Of course the two conditions may coexist, in which case the person has both difficulty in falling asleep and wakes up during the night.

Waking up early in the morning indicates Heart and Gall-Bladder deficiency. Restless sleep may be due to Heat or Fire agitating the Mind and/or Ethereal Soul. Occasionally, it may be due to Retention of Food.

Dreams

As for dreams, they are due to the wandering of the Mind and/or Ethereal Soul at night. A certain amount of dreaming is therefore normal. Ancient Chinese books do not define what "normal" dreaming is. I personally would say that "excessive dreaming" certainly includes nightmares; I think it also involves anxious dreams or dreams of being angry. Finally, dreaming is excessive also when a person dreams so much all night that he or she wakes up exhausted from it.

Dreaming that does not make the sleep restless, is not frightening, does not disturb the Mind the morning after, and does not leave the person very tired in the morning, can be described as normal and is not a pathological condition.

The old classics described various types of unpleasant dreams such as nightmares, waking up screaming, sleepwalking and talking in one's sleep. They related dreaming to the wandering of the Ethereal Soul at night.

When a person's physical body receives something it is real; when the Mind receives something it produces dreams. When the Mind is slave to objects [i.e. pursues objects] *the Ethereal Soul and the Corporeal Soul become restless, they fly around and, gathering at the eyes, they produce dreams. Grasping* [i.e. excessive craving] *in daytime produces dreaming at night.*

Excessive dreaming may be due to deficiency of Blood or Yin. Frightening dreams that wake one up denote a deficiency of Gall-Bladder and Heart. Restless dreams are often due to Heat affecting Stomach and Heart. The following is a list of dreams from the *Simple Questions* and *Spiritual Axis*.

- *Flying*: Emptiness in the Lower Burner[9]
- *Falling*: Fullness in the Lower Burner[10]
- *Floods and fear*: Excess of Yin[11]
- *Fire*: Excess of Yang[12]
- *Killing and destruction*: Yin and Yang both in Excess[13]

- *Giving away things*: Excess condition[14]
- *Receiving things*: Deficiency condition[15]
- *Being angry*: Liver in Excess[16]
- *Crying, weeping*: Lungs in Excess[17]
- *Crowds*: round worms in the intestines[18]
- *Attack and destruction*: tapeworms in the intestines[19]
- *Fires*: Heart deficiency[20]
- *Volcanic eruptions (if the dream takes place in summertime)*: Heart deficiency[21]
- *Laughing*: Heart in Excess[22]
- *Mountains, fire and smoke*: Heart deficiency[23]
- *Very fragrant mushrooms*: Liver deficiency[24]
- *Lying under a tree being unable to get up (if the dream takes place in springtime)*: Liver deficiency[25]
- *Forests on mountains*: Liver deficiency[26]
- *White objects or bloody killings*: Lung deficiency[27]
- *Battles and war (dream taking place in the autumn)*: Lung deficiency[28]
- *Worry, fear, crying, flying*: Lungs in Excess[29]
- *Flying and seeing strange objects made of gold or iron*: Lung deficiency[30]
- *Being hungry*: Spleen deficiency[31]
- *Building a house (dream taking place in late summer)*: Spleen deficiency[32]
- *Singing and feeling very heavy*: Spleen in Excess[33]
- *Abysses in mountains and marshes*: Spleen deficiency[34]
- *Swimming after a shipwreck*: Kidney deficiency[35]
- *Plunging into water and being scared (dream taking place in wintertime)*: Kidney deficiency[36]
- *Spine being detached from the body*: Kidneys in Excess (i.e. Dampness in Kidneys)[37]
- *Being immersed in water*: Kidney deficiency[38]
- *Having a large meal*: Stomach deficiency[39]
- *Large cities*: Small Intestine deficiency[40]
- *Open fields*: Large Intestine deficiency[41]
- *Fights, trials, suicide*: Gall-Bladder deficiency[42]
- *Voyages*: Bladder deficiency[43]
- *Crossing the sea and being scared*: Excess of Yin[44]

Sleeping positions

If a person is unable to sleep supine (lying on the back), it indicates an Excess condition, often of the Lungs or Heart. The *Simple Questions* in Chapter 46 says:[45]

The Lung is the 'lid' of the other organs; when Lung-Qi is in Excess [i.e. obstructed by a pathogenic factor] *the channels and blood vessels are full and the person cannot lie on the back.*

This often occurs in asthma, for example when the Lungs are obstructed by Phlegm.

If a person can sleep only on the back with the arms outstretched, it indicates a Heat condition. If a person always sleeps in a prone position, it indicates a Deficiency condition, often of the Stomach.

If a person can sleep only on one side it indicates that there is either a deficiency of Qi-Blood on that side of the body or an Excess on the opposite side. This especially applies to Heart or Lungs and can be checked on the pulse. By rolling the finger medially and laterally on the Lung pulse, one can feel the state of Qi in right (laterally) and left (medially) lung. If an imbalance is felt, the patient is only able to sleep on the deficient side.

Snoring

Snoring is usually due to Phlegm affecting the Stomach channel and to rebellious Qi in the three Yang channels of the leg. Chapter 34 of the *Simple Questions* says:[46]

Those who suffer from rebellious Qi cannot sleep well and have noisy breathing [snoring]*; this is due to rebellious Qi in the Bright Yang channels. When the Qi of the three Yang channels of the leg cannot flow down and rebels upwards, it causes insomnia and snoring.*

SUMMARY

Diagnosis

Sleep

- Difficulty in falling asleep usually indicates deficiency of Blood.
- Waking up frequently during the night denotes Yin deficiency.
- Waking up early in the morning indicates Heart and Gall-Bladder deficiency.

Dreams

- Dreams are due to the wandering of the Mind and/or Ethereal Soul at night.
- Excessive dreaming may be due to Liver-Blood/Yin deficiency, or to Liver-Fire or Heart-Fire.
- Frightening dreams which wake one up denote a deficiency of Gall-Bladder and Heart.
- Restless dreams are often due to Phlegm Heat affecting Stomach and Heart.

Sleeping positions

- *Inability to sleep supine (lying on the back)*: Excess condition.
- *Sleeping on the back with the arms outstretched*: Heat condition.
- *Sleeping in a prone position*: Deficiency condition, often of the Stomach.
- *Can sleep only on one side*: either a deficiency of Qi-Blood on that side of the body or an Excess on the opposite side.

Snoring

- Snoring is usually due to Phlegm affecting the Stomach channel and to rebellious Qi in the three Yang channels of the leg.

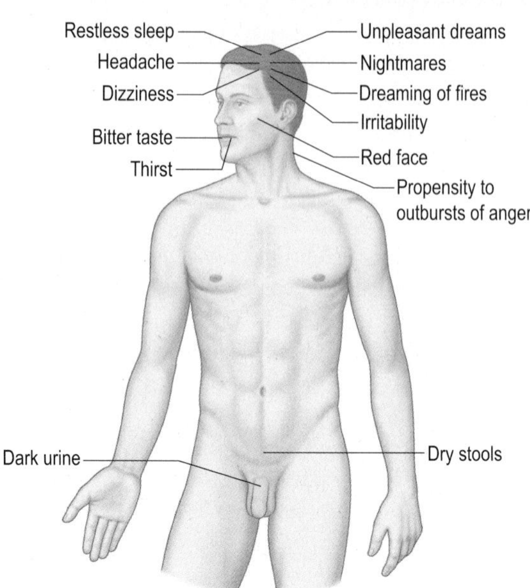

Figure 18.6 Liver-Fire blazing.

IDENTIFICATION OF PATTERNS AND TREATMENT

The most important distinction is that between Full and Empty types of insomnia. The main patterns are as follows.

Full
- Liver-Fire blazing
- Heart-Fire blazing
- Phlegm-Heat harassing the Mind
- Heart-Qi stagnation
- Heart-Blood stasis
- Residual Heat in the diaphragm
- Retention of Food
- Liver-Qi stagnation

Empty
- Heart- and Spleen-Blood deficiency
- Heart-Yin deficiency
- Heart and Kidneys not harmonized
- Heart and Gall-Bladder deficiency
- Liver-Yin deficiency
- Liver- and Kidney-Yin deficiency

Liver-Fire blazing

Clinical manifestations

Restless sleep, unpleasant dreams, nightmares, dreaming of fires, irritability, propensity to outbursts of anger, bitter taste, headache, dizziness, red face, thirst, dark urine and dry stools (Fig. 18.6).

Tongue: Red, redder on the sides with a dry-yellow coating.

Pulse: Wiry and Rapid.

Treatment principle

Drain Liver-Fire, calm the Mind and settle the Ethereal Soul.

Acupuncture

Points

LIV-2 Xingjian, LIV-3 Taichong, G.B.-44 Qiaoyin, G.B.-12 Wangu, G.B.-20 Fengchi, SP-6 Sanyinjiao, BL-18 Ganshu, Du-24 Shenting, G.B.-13 Benshen, G.B.-15 Toulinqi, BL-47 Hunmen, BL-62 Shenmai (reduced), BL-1 Jingming (even), KI-6 Zhaohai (reinforced). Reducing method, no moxa.

Explanation

- LIV-2 is the main point to drain Liver-Fire.
- LIV-3 is added because it has a better Mind-calming effect than LIV-2.

- G.B.-44 clears Liver and Gall-Bladder Heat and is specific for dream-disturbed sleep.
- G.B.-12 and G.B.-20 subdue rebellious Liver-Qi and promote sleep.
- SP-6 cools Blood and calms the Mind.
- BL-18 regulates the Liver and drains Liver-Fire.
- Du-24 and G.B.-13 in combination have a strong effect in calming the Mind and settling the Ethereal Soul in Liver patterns.
- G.B.-15 is used instead of G.B.-13 if the Mind is very overactive and the person cannot stop thinking obsessively.
- BL-47 roots the Ethereal Soul into Liver-Yin at night, thus promoting sleep.
- BL-62 (reduced), BL-1 (even) and KI-6 (in combination) harmonize the flow of the Yin and Yang Stepping Vessels (*Yin* and *Yang Qiao Mai*) to the eyes and promote sleep. The Yin Stepping Vessel carries Yin-Qi, and the Yang Stepping Vessel Yang-Qi, to the eyes. If Yang is in Excess, Yang-Qi cannot flow back into the Yin at night, the eyes stay open at night and insomnia results. The opposite would cause somnolence. The *Spiritual Axis* in Chapter 21 says:[47]

The Yin and Yang of the Yin and Yang Stepping Vessels interconnect; Yang enters Yin and Yin exits towards Yang and the two meet at the corner of the eyes. When Yang-Qi is in Excess the eyes stay open; when Yin-Qi is in Excess, they stay closed.

These points may be used for any of the other Full types of insomnia.

Herbal therapy

Prescription

LONG DAN XIE GAN TANG Variation
Gentiana Draining the Liver Decoction Variation

Modifications

- If the symptoms and signs of Fire are not too evident (no thirst, no bitter taste, urine not dark, stools not dry), omit Huang Qin and Shan Zhi Zi.
- If there are symptoms of Liver-Yang rising (frequent headaches, dizziness, tinnitus), add Tian Ma *Rhizoma Gastrodiae*.

Prescription

XIE QING WAN Variation
Draining the Green Pill Variation

Explanation

This formula drains Liver-Fire by moving downwards; it is therefore particularly applicable if there is constipation or if the stools are dry.

SUMMARY

Liver-Fire blazing

Points

LIV-2 Xingjian, LIV-3 Taichong, G.B.-44 Qiaoyin, G.B.-12 Wangu, G.B.-20 Fengchi, SP-6 Sanyinjiao, BL-18 Ganshu, Du-24 Shenting, G.B.-13 Benshen, G.B.-15 Toulinqi, BL-47 Hunmen, BL-62 Shenmai (reduced), BL-1 Jingming (even), KI-6 Zhaohai (reinforced). Reducing method, no moxa.

Herbal therapy

Prescription

LONG DAN XIE GAN TANG Variation
Gentiana Draining the Liver Decoction Variation

Prescription

XIE QING WAN Variation
Draining the Green Pill Variation

Heart-Fire blazing

Clinical manifestations

Waking up during the night, nightmares, dreams of flying, mental restlessness, bitter taste, thirst, tongue ulcers and palpitations (Fig. 18.7).

Tongue: Red, redder tip with red points, yellow coating.

Pulse: Rapid and Overflowing on the left Front position.

Treatment principle

Drain Heart-Fire, calm the Mind.

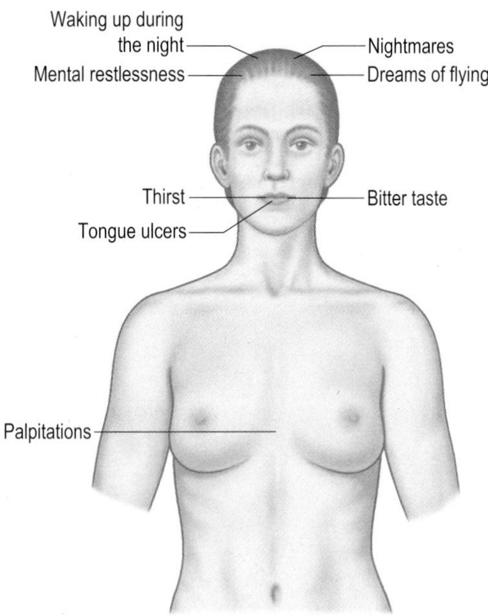

Figure 18.7 Heart-Fire blazing.

Acupuncture

Points

HE-8 Shaofu, HE-7 Shenmen, SP-6 Sanyinjiao, L.I.-11 Quchi, Ren-15 Jiuwei, Du-19 Houding, BL-15 Xinshu, BL-44 Shentang. Reducing method, no moxa.

Explanation

- HE-8 drains Heart-Fire.
- HE-7 calms the Mind and promotes sleep.
- SP-6 cools Blood and calms the Mind.
- L.I.-11 is used if there are pronounced general signs of Fire.
- Ren-15 clears the Heart, calms the Mind and promotes sleep.
- Du-19 in combination with Ren-15 calms the Mind and promotes sleep.
- BL-15 drains Heart-Fire.
- BL-44 calms the Mind and promotes sleep.

Herbal therapy

Prescription

XIE XIN TANG
Draining the Heart Decoction

Explanation

This formula drains Heart-Fire by moving downwards. It is applicable only if there is Full Fire without any signs of Yin deficiency. An important condition for the use of this formula is that the tongue should have a thick, dry and yellow coating.

Prescription

DAO CHI SAN
Eliminating Redness Powder

Explanation

This formula differs from the previous one in so far as, in addition to draining Heart-Fire, it also cools Blood and nourishes Yin (because of the inclusion of Sheng Di Huang). It is therefore suitable for cases when Fire has begun to injure the Yin. The tongue would therefore be Red with a yellow coating, though this coating might be rootless or missing in places.

Modifications

- Other versions of this formula include Deng Xin Cao *Medulla Junci* to clear Heart-Heat and calm the Mind.
- To enhance the sleep-promoting effect of both this formula and the previous one, add Ye Jiao Teng *Caulis Polygoni multiflori*, Fu Shen *Sclerotium Poriae pararadicis* and Yuan Zhi *Radix Polygalae*.

SUMMARY

Heart-Fire blazing

Points

HE-8 Shaofu, HE-7 Shenmen, SP-6 Sanyinjiao, L.I.-11 Quchi, Ren-15 Jiuwei, Du-19 Houding, BL-15 Xinshu, BL-44 Shentang. Reducing method, no moxa.

Herbal therapy

Prescription

XIE XIN TANG
Draining the Heart Decoction

Prescription

DAO CHI SAN
Eliminating Redness Powder

Phlegm-Heat harassing the Mind

Clinical manifestations

Restless sleep, tossing and turning, unpleasant dreams, nightmares, snoring, a feeling of heaviness, dizziness, a feeling of oppression of the chest, nausea, no appetite, palpitations, feeling of heat, sputum in the throat, mental restlessness and a sticky taste (Fig. 18.8).

Tongue: Red with a sticky-yellow coating. Heart crack (or Stomach–Heart crack) with sticky-rough yellow coating inside it.

Pulse: Slippery and Rapid.

This pattern is due to Phlegm-Heat in the Stomach and Heart, with Stomach-Qi rebelling upwards. When Phlegm is present, Stomach-Qi rebelling upwards will carry Phlegm and Heat to the Upper Burner to harass the Heart and Mind, thus causing insomnia. In severe cases this causes mental illness. The *Simple Questions* in Chapter 34 says: "*The Stomach is the Sea of the five Yin and six Yang organs; its Qi must go downwards; when Stomach-Qi rebels upwards ... one cannot sleep.*"[48]

Treatment principle

Clear Heat, resolve Phlegm and calm the Mind.

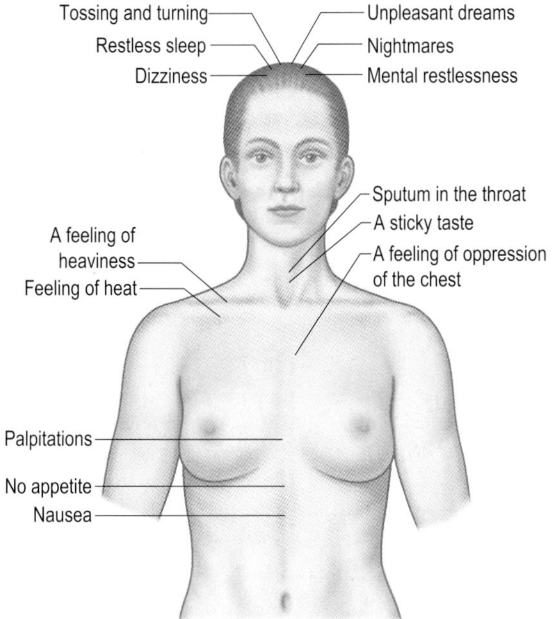

Figure 18.8 Phlegm-Heat harassing the Mind.

Acupuncture

Points

ST-40 Fenglong, Ren-12 Zhongwan, Ren-9 Shuifen, SP-9 Yinlingquan, BL-20 Pishu, L.I.-11 Quchi, ST-8 Touwei, G.B.-12 Wangu, SP-6 Sanyinjiao, ST-45 Lidui, SP-1 Yinbai. Reducing method except for Ren-12 and BL-20, which should be reinforced. No moxa, except for ST-45 (see below).

Explanation

- ST-40 resolves Phlegm and calms the Mind.
- Ren-12, Ren-9 and BL-20 tonify the Spleen to resolve Phlegm.
- SP-9 and SP-6 resolve Dampness which helps to resolve Phlegm. SP-6 also calms the Mind.
- L.I.-11 resolves Phlegm and clears Heat.
- ST-8 is the main local point to resolve Phlegm from the head and it promotes sleep.
- G.B.-12 promotes sleep.
- ST-45 relieves retention of food, calms the Mind and promotes sleep. Very small moxa cones can be used after needling to conduct Fire downwards. This is one of the few cases when moxa is used to counteract Heat.
- SP-1, often combined with ST-44, clears Heat in the Stomach and Spleen, calms the Mind and promotes sleep. The points ST-44 and SP-1 are also specific for excessive and unpleasant dreaming.

Herbal therapy

Prescription

SHI WEI WEN DAN TANG
Ten-Ingredient Warming the Gall-Bladder Decoction

Explanation

This prescription is used if there is Phlegm-Heat in the Stomach and Heart together with some deficiency of Qi and Blood, which is a very common situation.

Prescription

HUANG LIAN WEN DAN TANG
Coptis Warming the Gall-Bladder Decoction

Explanation

This formula is used in preference to the previous one if symptoms and signs of Heat are more pronounced and the tongue is definitely Red with a thick-yellow coating.

Modifications

These formulae have a powerful effect in calming the Mind and promoting sleep, and may need little variation or addition.

- To enhance the sleep-promoting effect, add Ye Jiao Teng *Caulis Polygoni multiflori* and Yuan Zhi *Radix Polygalae.*
- If there are symptoms of retention of food, add Shen Qu *Massa medicata fermentata* and Lai Fu Zi *Semen Raphani.*
- If there are more symptoms of retention of food rather than those of Phlegm-Heat, use Bao He Wan *Preserving and Harmonizing Pill* instead.
- If there is constipation, add Da Huang *Radix et Rhizoma Rhei.*

SUMMARY

Phlegm-Heat harassing the Mind

Points

ST-40 Fenglong, Ren-12 Zhongwan, Ren-9 Shuifen, SP-9 Yinlingquan, BL-20 Pishu, L.I.-11 Quchi, ST-8 Touwei, G.B.-12 Wangu, SP-6 Sanyinjiao, ST-45 Lidui, SP-1 Yinbai. Reducing method except for Ren-12 and BL-20, which should be reinforced. No moxa, except for ST-45.

Herbal therapy

Prescription

SHI WEI WEN DAN TANG
Ten-Ingredient Warming the Gall-Bladder Decoction

Prescription

HUANG LIAN WEN DAN TANG
Coptis Warming the Gall-Bladder Decoction

Heart-Qi stagnation

Clinical manifestations

Insomnia, palpitations, a feeling of distension or oppression of the chest, depression, a slight feeling of lump in the throat, slight shortness of breath, sighing, poor appetite, weak and cold limbs, slightly purple lips, pale complexion (Fig. 18.9).

Tongue: slightly Pale-Purple on the sides in the chest area.

Pulse: Empty but very slightly Overflowing on the left Front position.

Treatment principle

Move Heart-Qi, open the chest, calm the Mind.

Acupuncture

Points

P-6 Neiguan, HE-5 Tongli, HE-7 Shenmen, Ren-15 Jiuwei, Ren-17 Shanzhong, LU-7 Lieque, ST-40 Fenglong, L.I.-4 Hegu. Reducing or even method on all points.

Explanation

- P-6 opens the chest, moves Qi and calms the Mind.
- HE-5 and HE-7 move Heart-Qi and calm the Mind.

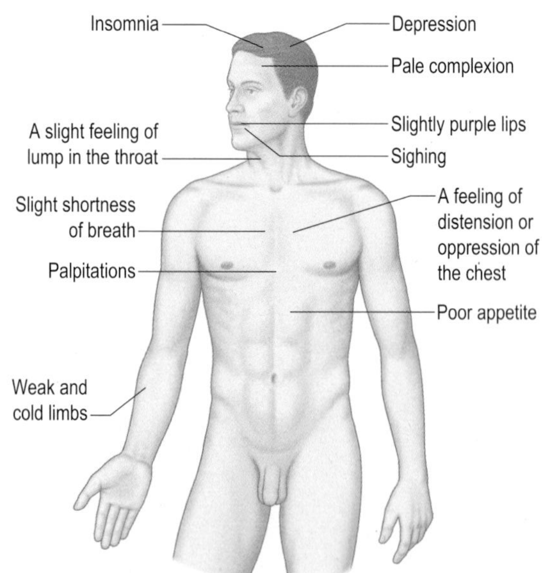

Figure 18.9 Heart-Qi stagnation.

- Ren-15 opens the chest and calms the Mind.
- Ren-17 moves Qi in the chest.
- LU-7 moves Qi in the chest.
- ST-40 is used here not to resolve Phlegm but to open the chest and move Qi in the chest.
- L.I.-4 regulates the ascending and descending of Qi and therefore moves Qi.

Herbal therapy

Prescription

MU XIANG LIU QI YIN
Aucklandia Flowing Qi Decoction

Explanation

This formula moves Heart-Qi.

Prescription

BAN XIA HOU PO TANG
Pinellia-Magnolia Decoction

Explanation

This formula moves Qi of the Heart and Lungs and frees the throat and chest.

Prescription

YUE JU WAN plus **SI NI SAN**
Gardenia-Chuanxiong Pill plus *Four Rebellious Powder*

Explanation

These two formulae move Liver- and Heart-Qi, relieve depression, calm the Mind and settle the Ethereal Soul. These two formulae should be selected when stagnation of Heart-Qi is accompanied by that of Liver-Qi.

Modifications

- These formulae should be modified with the addition of herbs to promote sleep such as Ye Jiao Teng *Caulis Polygoni multiflori* and Suan Zao Ren *Semen Ziziphi spinosae*.

> **SUMMARY**
>
> **Heart-Qi stagnation**
>
> *Points*
>
> P-6 Neiguan, HE-5 Tongli, HE-7 Shenmen, Ren-15 Jiuwei, Ren-17 Shanzhong, LU-7 Lieque, ST-40 Fenglong, L.I.-4 Hegu. Reducing or even method on all points.
>
> *Herbal therapy*
>
> *Prescription*
>
> **MU XIANG LIU QI YIN**
> *Aucklandia Flowing Qi Decoction*
>
> *Prescription*
>
> **BAN XIA HOU PO TANG**
> *Pinellia-Magnolia Decoction*
>
> *Prescription*
>
> **YUE JU WAN** plus **SI NI SAN**
> *Gardenia-Chuanxiong Pill* plus *Four Rebellious Powder*

Heart-Blood stasis

Clinical manifestations

Insomnia, dream-disturbed sleep, tossing and turning in bed during the night, palpitations, chest ache, mental restlessness, anxiety (Fig. 18.10).

Tongue: Purple (it may be Purple only in the chest area). See Figure 18.11.

Pulse: Choppy or Firm.

Treatment principle

Invigorate Blood, calm the Mind.

Acupuncture

Points

HE-7 Shenmen, HE-5 Tongli, P-6 Neiguan, Ren-15 Jiuwei, Ren-17 Shanzhong, BL-17 Geshu, BL-44 Shentang. Even method on all points.

Explanation

- HE-7, HE-5, P-6 and Ren-15 invigorate Heart-Blood and calm the Mind.

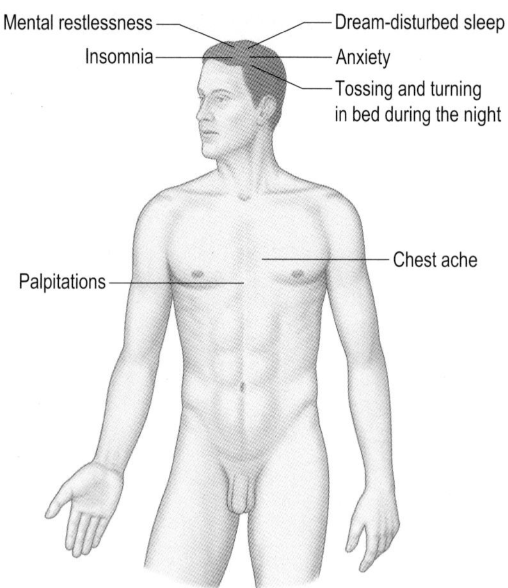

Figure 18.10 Heart-Blood stasis.

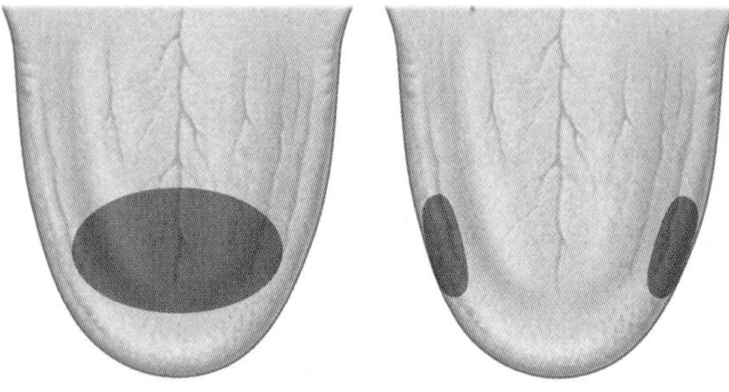

Figure 18.11 Chest area on tongue.

- Ren-17 invigorates Heart-Blood and opens the chest.
- BL-17 invigorates Blood in the Upper Burner.
- BL-44 calms the Mind.

Herbal therapy

Prescription

XUE FU ZHU YU TANG Variation
Blood Mansion Eliminating Stasis Decoction Variation

Explanation

The original formula Xue Fu Zhu Yu Tang invigorates Blood in the Upper Burner. It has been modified with the addition of herbs that calm the Mind (Ye Jiao Teng *Caulis Polygoni multiflori* and Suan Zao Ren *Semen Ziziphi spinosae*).

Prescription

TONG QIAO HUO XUE TANG
Opening the Orifices and Invigorating Blood Decoction

Explanation

This formula is specific to eliminate Blood stasis from the head. Replace She Xiang *Moschus* with Shi Chang Pu *Rhizoma Acori tatarinowii.*

SUMMARY

Heart-Blood stasis

Points

HE-7 Shenmen, HE-5 Tongli, P-6 Neiguan, Ren-15 Jiuwei, Ren-17 Shanzhong, BL-17 Geshu, BL-44 Shentang. Even method on all points.

Herbal therapy

Prescription

XUE FU ZHU YU TANG Variation
Blood Mansion Eliminating Stasis Decoction Variation

Prescription

TONG QIAO HUO XUE TANG
Opening the Orifices and Invigorating Blood Decoction

Residual Heat in the diaphragm

Clinical manifestations

Restless sleep, waking up during the night, mental restlessness, cannot lie down or sit, a feeling of stuffiness of the chest, epigastric discomfort and sour regurgitation (Fig. 18.12).

Tongue: Red in the front part or red points around the center.

Pulse: Deep and slightly Rapid.

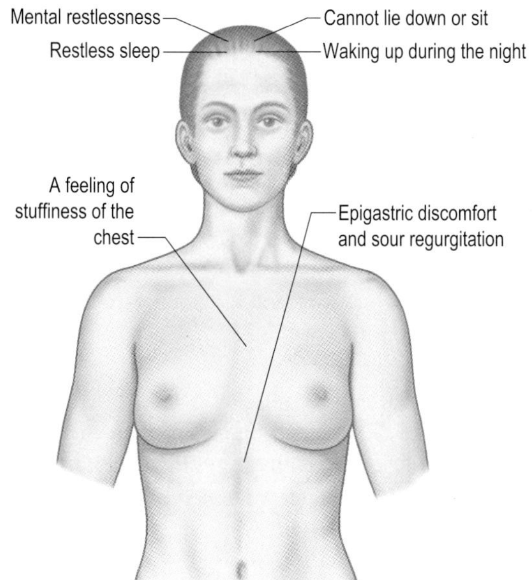

Figure 18.12 Residual Heat in the diaphragm.

This condition arises after an invasion of Wind-Heat which has turned into Interior Heat and has not been cleared properly, often through the inappropriate use of antibiotics; some residual Heat remains in the body and settles in the diaphragm area. From here it rebels upwards to disturb the Heart and Mind.

Treatment principle

Clear residual Heat, calm irritability and calm the Mind.

Acupuncture

Points

LU-10 Yuji, HE-8 Shaofu, BL-17 Geshu, ST-40 Fenglong, L.I.-11 Quchi, SP-6 Sanyinjiao, Ren-15 Jiuwei. Reducing method, no moxa.

Explanation

- LU-10 and HE-8 clear Lung-Heat and Heart-Heat respectively. They are chosen because, from the point of view of channels, residual Heat in the diaphragm is located in Lungs and Heart. Besides this, HE-8 also calms the Mind.
- BL-17 relaxes the diaphragm.
- ST-40 relaxes the diaphragm, subdues rebellious Qi and calms the Mind.
- L.I.-11 clears Heat.
- SP-6 calms the Mind and protects Yin from injury from Heat.
- Ren-15 relaxes the diaphragm, clears the Heart and calms the Mind.

Herbal therapy

Prescription

ZHU YE SHI GAO TANG
Phyllostachys Gipsum Decoction

Explanation

This is one of the formulae for clearing residual Heat, especially from the diaphragm area.

Prescription

ZHI ZI CHI TANG
Gardenia-Soja Decoction

Explanation

This formula lightly clears Heat and is often used to clear residual Heat.

- To enhance the sleep-promoting effect, add Fu Shen *Sclerotium Poriae pararadicis*, Deng Xin Cao *Medulla Junci* and Ye Jiao Teng *Caulis Polygoni multiflori*.

SUMMARY

Residual Heat in the diaphragm

Points

LU-10 Yuji, HE-8 Shaofu, BL-17 Geshu, ST-40 Fenglong, L.I.-11 Quchi, SP-6 Sanyinjiao, Ren-15 Jiuwei. Reducing method, no moxa.

Herbal therapy

Prescription

ZHU YE SHI GAO TANG
Phyllostachys Gipsum Decoction

Prescription

ZHI ZI CHI TANG
Gardenia-Soja Decoction

Retention of Food

Clinical manifestations

Insomnia, restless sleep, excessive dreaming, fullness, pain and distension of the epigastrium which is relieved by vomiting, nausea, vomiting of sour fluids, foul breath, sour regurgitation, belching, loose stools or constipation, poor appetite (Fig. 18.13).

Tongue: thick coating (which could be white or yellow).

Pulse: Full-Slippery.

Treatment principle

Resolve retention of food, stimulate the descending of Stomach-Qi, calm the Mind.

Acupuncture

Points

Du-24 Shenting, Ren-15 Jiuwei, Ren-13 Shangwan, Ren-10 Xiawan, ST-21 Liangmen, ST-44 Neiting, ST-45 Lidui, SP-4 Gongsun, P-6 Neiguan, ST-40 Fenglong, ST-19 Burong, KI-21 Youmen, Ren-12 Zhongwan. Reducing or even method.

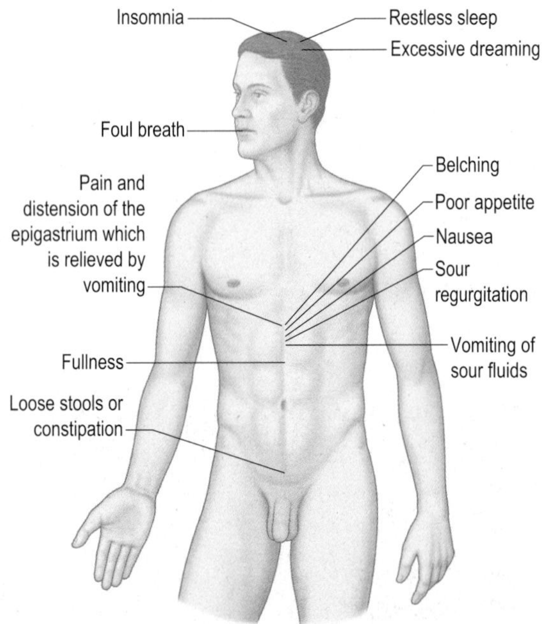

Figure 18.13 Retention of Food.

Explanation

- Du-24 and Ren-15 calm the Mind.
- Ren-13 subdues rebellious Stomach-Qi.
- Ren-10 stimulates the descending of Stomach-Qi.
- ST-21 stimulates the descending of Stomach-Qi and resolves stagnant food.
- ST-44 resolves stagnant food and clears Heat.
- ST-45 resolves stagnant food and calms the Mind (if there is insomnia).
- SP-4 resolves stagnant food.
- P-6 stimulates the descending of Stomach-Qi.
- ST-40 restores the descending of Stomach-Qi.
- ST-19 and KI-21 Youmen restore the descending of Stomach-Qi. ST-19 is specific to resolve Retention of Food.
- Ren-12 resolves Retention of Food.

Herbal therapy

Prescription

BAN XIA SHU MI TANG
Pinellia-Sorghum Decoction

Explanation

This formula resolves Retention of Food. It should be modified with the addition of Ye Jiao Teng *Caulis Polygoni multiflori* to promote sleep.

Prescription

ZHI SHI DAO ZHI WAN
Aurantium Eliminating Stagnation Pill

Explanation

This formula relieves Retention of Food and promotes the descending of Stomach-Qi. It is indicated when Retention of Food is accompanied by Heat or Damp-Heat.

Modifications

Both these formulae should be modified with the addition of herbs that promote sleep such as Ye Jiao Teng *Caulis Polygoni multiflori* and Suan Zao Ren *Semen Ziziphi spinosae*.

SUMMARY

Retention of Food

Points

Du-24 Shenting, Ren-15 Jiuwei, Ren-13 Shangwan, Ren-10 Xiawan, ST-21 Liangmen, ST-44 Neiting, ST-45 Lidui, SP-4 Gongsun, P-6 Neiguan, ST-40 Fenglong, ST-19 Burong, KI-21 Youmen, Ren-12 Zhongwan. Reducing or even method.

Herbal therapy

Prescription

BAN XIA SHU MI TANG
Pinellia-Sorghum Decoction

Prescription

ZHI SHI DAO ZHI WAN
Aurantium Eliminating Stagnation Pill

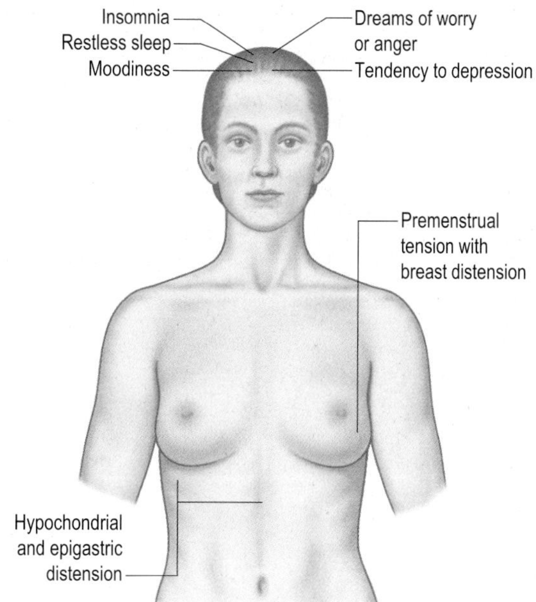

Figure 18.14 Liver-Qi stagnation.

Liver-Qi stagnation

Clinical manifestations

Insomnia, restless sleep, dreams of worry or anger, hypochondrial and epigastric distension, moodiness, tendency to depression, premenstrual tension with breast distension (Fig. 18.14).

Tongue: normal or with slightly red sides.

Pulse: Wiry.

Treatment principle

Regulate the Liver, move Qi, eliminate stagnation, regulate the Ethereal Soul, calm the Mind.

Acupuncture

Points

T.B.-6 Zhigou, P-6 Neiguan, LIV-3 Taichong, G.B.-34 Yanglingquan, G.B.-13 Benshen, Du-24 Shenting, BL-47 Hunmen. Reducing or even method.

Explanation

- T.B.-6, P-6, LIV-3 and G.B.-34 regulate the Liver, move Qi and eliminate stagnation.
- G.B.-13 and Du-24 calm the Mind and settle the Ethereal Soul; they are particularly effective in calming the Mind in the presence of Liver patterns.
- BL-47 regulates the coming and going of the Ethereal Soul.

Herbal therapy

Prescription

YUE JU WAN plus **SI NI SAN** Variation
Gardenia-Chuanxiong Pill plus *Four Rebellious Powder* Variation

Explanation

These two formulae regulate the Liver, move Qi, eliminate stagnation, regulate the Ethereal Soul and calm the Mind. They are particularly indicated if the patient is depressed.

SUMMARY

Liver-Qi stagnation

Points

T.B.-6 Zhigou, P-6 Neiguan, LIV-3 Taichong, G.B.-34 Yanglingquan, G.B.-13 Benshen, Du-24 Shenting, BL-47 Hunmen. Reducing or even method.

Herbal therapy

Prescription

YUE JU WAN plus **SI NI SAN** Variation
Gardenia-Chuanxiong Pill plus *Four Rebellious Powder* Variation

Heart- and Spleen-Blood deficiency

Clinical manifestations

Insomnia, difficulty in falling asleep, palpitations, tiredness, poor appetite, slight anxiety, blurred vision, dizziness, poor memory, pale face (Fig. 18.15).

Tongue: Pale.

Pulse: Choppy.

This is a very common type of insomnia, due to deficiency of Blood of the Heart and Spleen. Since Blood is deficient, the person cannot fall asleep easily but, once asleep, because Yin is sufficient, he or she stays asleep. This pattern is more common in women.

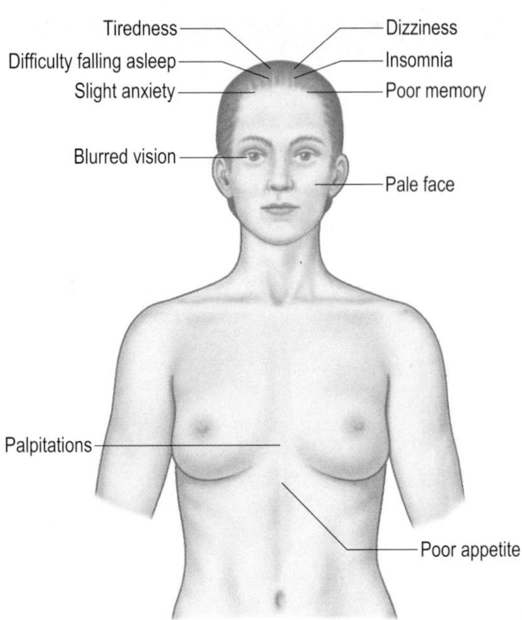

Figure 18.15 Heart- and Spleen-Blood deficiency.

Treatment principle

Tonify the Spleen, nourish Blood, tonify the Heart and calm the Mind.

Acupuncture

Points

ST-36 Zusanli, SP-6 Sanyinjiao, HE-7 Shenmen, Ren-14 Juque, Ren-15 Jiuwei, BL-20 Pishu, BL-15 Xinshu, Yintang, P-6 Neiguan and SP-4 Gongsun in combination together with KI-9 Zhubin. Reinforcing method, moxa may be used.

Explanation

- ST-36, SP-6 and BL-20 tonify the Spleen to produce Blood. SP-6 also calms the Mind.
- HE-7, Ren-14 and Ren-15 nourish Heart-Blood and calm the Mind.
- BL-15 nourishes Heart-Blood and calms the Mind.
- Yintang calms the Mind and promotes sleep, especially in Empty conditions. The patient may also be advised to apply gentle moxibustion to this point with a moxa stick every night.
- P-6 and SP-4 in combination open the Yin Linking Vessel (*Yin Wei Mai*); KI-9 is the starting point of this vessel. I use these three points to nourish Blood and calm the Mind, especially in women.

Herbal therapy

Prescription

GUI PI TANG
Tonifying the Spleen Decoction

Explanation

This formula tonifies Spleen-Qi and Heart-Qi, nourishes Heart-Blood and calms the Mind. This formula is specific for this pattern and it promotes sleep, therefore no modifications are needed.

SUMMARY

Heart- and Spleen-Blood deficiency

Points

ST-36 Zusanli, SP-6 Sanyinjiao, HE-7 Shenmen, Ren-14 Juque, Ren-15 Jiuwei, BL-20 Pishu, BL-15 Xinshu, Yintang, P-6 Neiguan and SP-4 Gongsun in combination together with KI-9 Zhubin. Reinforcing method, moxa may be used.

Herbal therapy

Prescription

GUI PI TANG

Tonifying the Spleen Decoction

Case history

A 42-year-old woman had been suffering from insomnia for some years. The problem became much worse after the birth of twins 8 years previously. She was also very anxious and revealed that she had suffered tremendous emotional strain throughout her life due to her mother's bipolar disorder. She said during the first consultation of her mother's disease: "*It destroyed me.*" She used zopiclone for the insomnia.

She also suffered from recurrent headaches, which also had become worse after the childbirth. The headaches occurred in the forehead and were dull in nature. She also said that she felt "foggy" in her head. She had been prescribed Prozac and she was on it at the time of the consultation.

Her periods were regular but were very heavy, lasting 7–8 days. She also complained of dizziness, palpitations and blurred vision.

Her tongue was Pale and Swollen; her pulse was Weak and Deep and especially weak on both Rear positions (Kidneys).

Diagnosis The insomnia was due to Blood deficiency of the Spleen, Liver and Heart (palpitations, blurred vision, dizziness, Pale tongue). However, there were other factors at play. First, there was a pronounced deficiency of Kidney-Yang (pulse very Weak on both Rear positions); this was evidenced by the aggravation of both insomnia and headaches after childbirth.

The headaches were due partly to Blood deficiency and partly to Phlegm in the head ("foggy" feeling, Swollen tongue).

Treatment This patient was treated only with herbal medicine. To concentrate on treating the insomnia and headaches, I nourished Heart-Blood and calmed the Mind with a variation of Gui Pi Tang *Tonifying the Spleen Decoction*:

- **Bai Zhu** *Rhizoma Atractylodis macrocephalae*
- **Huang Qi** *Radix Astragali*
- **Dang Gui** *Radix Angelicae sinensis*
- **Bai Shao** *Radix Paeoniae alba*
- **Gou Teng** *Ramulus cum Uncis Uncariae*
- **Yuan Zhi** *Radix Polygalae*
- **Suan Zao Ren** *Semen Ziziphi spinosae*
- **Bai Zi Ren** *Semen Platycladi*
- **Long Yan Rou** *Arillus Longan*
- **Ye Jiao Teng** *Caulis Polygoni multiflori*
- **Dan Shen** *Radix Salviae milthiorrizae*
- **Tu Si Zi** *Semen Cuscutae*

After the first course of herbs (in concentrated powder form) she reported feeling very much better in herself. She also reported a breakthrough in her psychotherapy and said she felt like she had "discarded a lot of luggage".

I continued treating her with similar prescriptions for about 8 months, during which all her problems underwent a remarkable improvement (insomnia, headaches, heavy periods). She was also able to stop taking zopiclone and Prozac.

After about 8 months, I turned my attention to tonifying the Kidneys and changed the formula, using a variation of You Gui Wan *Restoring the Right* [Kidney] *Pill*, modified with the addition of herbs to calm the Mind as the sleep was still a problem.

- **Shu Di Huang** *Radix Rehmanniae preparata*
- **Shan Yao** *Rhizoma Dioscoreae*
- **Shan Zhu Yu** *Fructus Corni*
- **Tu Si Zi** *Semen Cuscutae*
- **Gou Qi Zi** *Fructus Lycii chinensis*
- **Dang Gui** *Radix Angelicae sinensis*
- **Dan Shen** *Radix Salviae milthiorrizae*
- **Suan Zao Ren** *Semen Ziziphi spinosae*
- **Bai Zi Ren** *Semen Platycladi*
- **Ye Jiao Teng** *Caulis Polygoni multiflori*
- **Bai Zhu** *Rhizoma Atractylodis macrocephalae*
- **Du Zhong** *Cortex Eucommiae ulmoidis*
- **Sheng Di Huang** *Radix Rehmanniae*
- **Xu Duan** *Radix Dipsaci*

After a further 3 months of treatment with this formula, she reported a total improvement in all her main symptoms, i.e. the insomnia, headaches and heavy periods.

Heart-Yin deficiency

Clinical manifestations

Insomnia, waking up frequently during the night, dry throat, mental restlessness, palpitations, night-sweating, poor memory (Fig. 18.16).

Tongue: without coating, Heart crack, red tip. If there is Empty Heat, Red body.

Pulse: Floating-Empty.

Treatment principle

Nourish Heart-Yin and calm the Mind.

Acupuncture

Points

HE-7 Shenmen, BL-15 Xinshu, Ren-14 Juque, SP-6 Sanyinjiao, ST-36 Zusanli, Ren-4 Guanyuan. Reinforcing method.

Explanation

- HE-7 nourishes the Heart, calms the Mind and promotes sleep.
- BL-15 and Ren-14, Back-Transporting point and Front-Collecting point of the Heart, respectively, nourish the Heart and calm the Mind.
- SP-6 and ST-36 nourish Qi and Yin in general.
- Ren-4 nourishes Yin in general and calms the Mind.

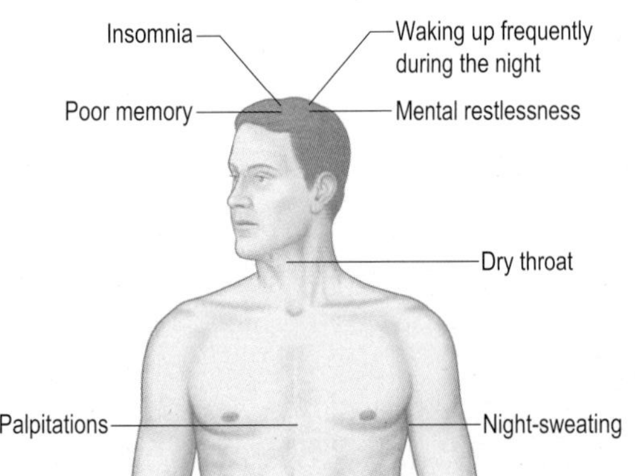

Figure 18.16 Heart-Yin deficiency.

Herbal therapy

Prescription

YANG XIN TANG (II)
Nourishing the Heart Decoction

Explanation

This formula tonifies Heart-Qi, Heart-Blood and Heart-Yin. It shares the same name as another formula (Yang Xin Tang I) which tonifies Heart-Qi and Heart-Blood. When used for Heart-Yin, it can be modified by reducing the dosage of the Qi tonics and increasing that of the Yin tonics.

Modifications

- If the symptoms of Yin deficiency are pronounced, add Tian Men Dong *Radix Asparagi* and Sheng Di Huang *Radix Rehmanniae*.
- If there are pronounced symptoms of Empty Heat, add Qing Hao *Herba Artemisiae annuae* and Mu Li *Concha Ostreae*.

SUMMARY

Heart-Yin deficiency

Points

HE-7 Shenmen, BL-15 Xinshu, Ren-14 Juque, SP-6 Sanyinjiao, ST-36 Zusanli, Ren-4 Guanyuan. Reinforcing method.

Herbal therapy

Prescription

YANG XIN TANG (II)
Nourishing the Heart Decoction.

Heart and Kidneys not harmonized

Clinical manifestations

Insomnia, waking up frequently during the night, difficulty in falling asleep, dry throat, night-sweating, five-palm heat, poor memory, palpitations, dizziness, mental restlessness, tinnitus, backache (Fig. 18.17).

Tongue: Red without coating, tip redder, Heart crack, dry.

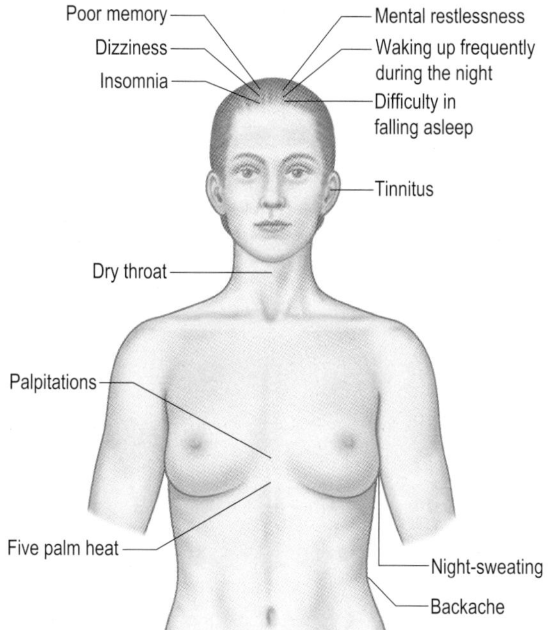

Figure 18.17 Heart and Kidneys not harmonized.

Pulse: Floating-Empty and slightly Rapid.

This pattern consists of deficiency of Kidney-Yin, deficiency of Heart-Yin and Heart Empty Heat.

Treatment principle

Nourish Yin, tonify Kidneys and Heart, clear Empty Heat and calm the Mind.

Acupuncture

Points

HE-7 Shenmen, HE-6 Yinxi, P-7 Daling, Ren-4 Guanyuan, SP-6 Sanyinjiao, KI-3 Taixi, KI-6 Zhaohai, Ren-15 Jiuwei, BL-15 Xinshu, BL-23 Shenshu, BL-44 Shentang, BL-52 Zhishi. Reinforcing method on all points except HE-6, which should be reduced.

Explanation

- HE-7 calms the Mind and promotes sleep.
- HE-6 clears Heart Empty Heat.
- P-7 calms the Mind.
- Ren-4 nourishes Kidney-Yin and calms the Mind.
- SP-6, KI-3 and KI-6 nourish Kidney-Yin.
- Ren-15 nourishes the Heart and calms the Mind.
- BL-15 and BL-23 harmonize Heart and Kidneys.
- BL-44 and BL-52 harmonize the Mind and Will-Power.

Herbal therapy

Prescription

TIAN WANG BU XIN DAN
Heavenly Emperor Tonifying the Heart Pill

Explanation

This prescription nourishes Kidney- and Heart-Yin, clears Empty Heat and calms the Mind.

Prescription

JIAO TAI WAN Variation
Grand Communication Pill Variation

Explanation

This formula is used if there is Heart-Heat above and deficiency of Kidney-Yang below.

Modifications

- To enhance the sleep-promoting effect, add Ye Jiao Teng *Caulis Polygoni multiflori*.
- If there are pronounced symptoms of Empty Heat, add Mu Li *Concha Ostreae* and Qing Hao *Herba Artemisiae annuae*.

SUMMARY

Heart and Kidneys not harmonized

Points

HE-7 Shenmen, HE-6 Yinxi, P-7 Daling, Ren-4 Guanyuan, SP-6 Sanyinjiao, KI-3 Taixi, KI-6 Zhaohai, Ren-15 Jiuwei, BL-15 Xinshu, BL-23 Shenshu, BL-44 Shentang, BL-52 Zhishi. Reinforcing method on all points except HE-6, which should be reduced.

Herbal therapy

Prescription

TIAN WANG BU XIN DAN
Heavenly Emperor Tonifying the Heart Pill

Prescription

JIAO TAI WAN Variation
Grand Communication Pill Variation

Case history

A 58-year-old man had been suffering from insomnia for 2 years. He fell asleep easily but woke up several times during the night with a feeling of dryness of the throat. He had also been suffering from impotence for 3 years.

His tongue was Red, the coating was too thin and it had a Heart crack. His pulse was Empty at the deep level and extremely Weak and Fine on the left Rear and Middle positions.

He was born with one kidney.

Diagnosis The insomnia in this case was due to Kidney-Yin deficiency and Kidney and Heart not harmonized. Although he had comparatively few symptoms, judging from the pulse, the Kidney deficiency was very severe and this obviously also had something to do with his congenital anatomical abnormality.

Treatment principle Nourish Kidney-Yin and Heart-Yin and calm the Mind.

Acupuncture The main points used were as follows.

- S.I.-3 Houxi and BL-62 Shenmai to open the Governing Vessel and strengthen the Kidneys. Although this combination strengthens Kidney-Yang more than Kidney-Yin, it was used to help his impotence which was worrying him more than the insomnia.
- Ren-4 Guanyuan, SP-6 Sanyinjiao and KI-3 Taixi nourish Kidney-Yin.
- BL-23 Shenshu to strengthen the Kidneys.
- HE-7 Shenmen, Ren-15 Jiuwei and Du-19 Houding to calm the Mind.
- G.B.-12 Wangu and Yintang to promote sleep.

Herbal therapy No herbs were prescribed but only the patent remedy Tian Wang Bu Xin Dan *Heavenly Emperor Tonifying the Heart Pill* to nourish Kidney- and Heart-Yin and calm the Mind.

His sleep became normal after 6 months of treatment, while his impotence improved by about 50%.

Heart and Gall-Bladder deficiency

Clinical manifestations

Waking up very early in the morning and being unable to fall asleep again, light sleep, dreaming a lot, propensity to being easily startled, timidity, lack of initiative and assertiveness, palpitations, breathlessness, tiredness, depression (Fig. 18.18).

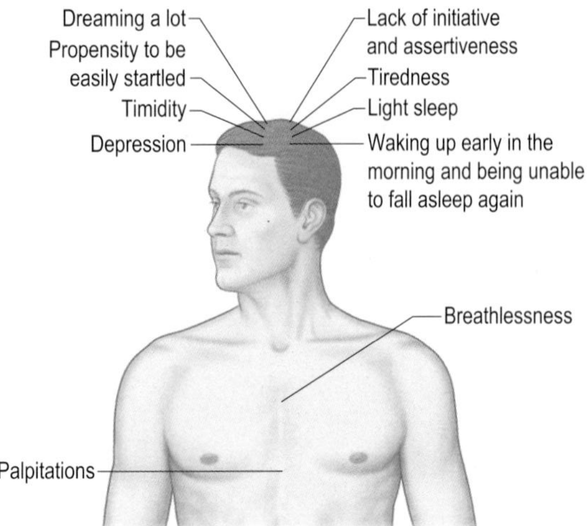

Figure 18.18 Heart and Gall-Bladder deficiency.

Tongue: Pale, Heart crack.

Pulse: Empty.

More than a pattern, this describes a certain character type of a person. Such character may be constitutional or may arise as a consequence of a protracted illness; for example glandular fever (mononucleosis). Originally, the formula Wen Dan Tang *Warming the Gall-Bladder Decoction* was used for this condition, but nowadays this formula is more often used for Phlegm-Heat.

Treatment principle

Tonify Heart and Gall-Bladder, calm the Mind.

Acupuncture

Points

HE-7 Shenmen, G.B.-40 Qiuxu. Reinforcing method.

Explanation

HE-7 and G.B.-40, both Source points, tonify Heart and Gall-Bladder, calm the Mind and stimulate the person's drive and assertiveness.

Herbal therapy

Prescription

AN SHEN DING ZHI WAN
Calming the Mind and Settling the Spirit Pill

Explanation

This formula tonifies Heart-Qi and calms the Mind.

Prescription

DING ZHI WAN Variation
Settling the Spirit Pill Variation

Explanation

This formula tonifies Heart-Qi and Heart-Blood and calms the Mind.

SUMMARY

Heart and Gall-Bladder deficiency

Points

HE-7 Shenmen, G.B.-40 Qiuxu. Reinforcing method.

Herbal therapy

Prescription

AN SHEN DING ZHI WAN
Calming the Mind and Settling the Spirit Pill

Prescription

DING ZHI WAN Variation
Settling the Spirit Pill Variation

Liver-Yin deficiency

Clinical manifestations

Waking up during the night, dreaming a lot, talking in one's sleep, in severe cases sleepwalking, dry throat, irritability, blurred vision, feeling of heat, sore and dry eyes, dry skin and hair, dizziness (Fig. 18.19).

Tongue: without coating.

Pulse: Floating-Empty, especially on the left side.

The deficiency of Liver-Yin causes the Ethereal Soul to be deprived of its root and to "wander" at night during sleep. This causes insomnia and excessive dreaming and, in some cases, even sleep-walking.

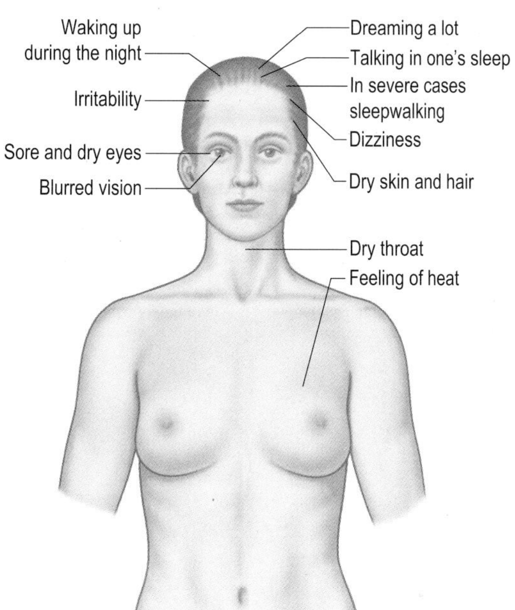

Figure 18.19 Liver-Yin deficiency.

Treatment principle

Nourish Liver-Yin, root the Ethereal Soul and calm the Mind.

Acupuncture

Points

LIV-8 Ququan, Ren-4 Guanyuan, Hunshe extra point, SP-6 Sanyinjiao, P-7 Daling, Du-24 Shenting and G.B.-13 Benshen, BL-47 Hunmen, Anmien. Reinforcing method, no moxa.

Explanation

- LIV-8 nourishes Liver-Blood and Liver-Yin.
- Ren-4 nourishes Liver- and Kidney-Yin and calms the Mind.
- Hunshe (situated level with Ren-8 Shenque and 1 *cun* lateral to it) roots the Ethereal Soul into the Liver.
- SP-6 nourishes Liver-Yin, calms the Mind and settles the Ethereal Soul.
- P-7 harmonizes the Liver (due to the relationship between Pericardium and Liver within the

Terminal Yin), calms the Mind and settles the Ethereal Soul.
- Du-24 and G.B.-13 calm the Mind, especially in Liver patterns.
- BL-47, called the "Door of the Ethereal Soul", settles the Ethereal Soul into the Liver at night. Some old books give sleepwalking as an indication for this point.
- Anmien calms the Ethereal Soul and the Mind and promotes sleep in Liver patterns.

Herbal therapy

Prescription

SUAN ZAO REN TANG
Ziziphus Decoction

Explanation

This is an excellent formula for this condition and is very reliable in its sleep-promoting effect.

Modifications

- If there is Empty Heat arising from Liver-Yin deficiency, add Han Lian Cao *Herba Ecliptae* and Mu Li *Concha Ostreae*.
- If there are symptoms of Liver-Yang rising, add Tian Ma *Rhizoma Gastrodiae* and Gou Teng *Ramulus cum Uncis Uncariae*.

Prescription

YIN MEI TANG
Attracting Sleep Decoction

Explanation

This formula is specific to nourish Liver-Yin and promote sleep by rooting the Ethereal Soul in the Liver. Compared to the previous formula, it is used when the person has many unpleasant dreams.

Modifications

These modifications apply to both above formulae.

- If there is Empty Heat (in which case the tongue is Red and without a coating), add Zhi Mu *Radix Anemarrhaenae* and Mu Dan Pi *Cortex Moutan*.

SUMMARY

Liver-Yin deficiency

Points

LIV-8 Ququan, Ren-4 Guanyuan, Hunshe extra point, SP-6 Sanyinjiao, P-7 Daling, Du-24 Shenting and G.B.-13 Benshen, BL-47 Hunmen, Anmien. Reinforcing method, no moxa.

Herbal therapy

Prescription

SUAN ZAO REN TANG
Ziziphus Decoction

Prescription

YIN MEI TANG
Attracting Sleep Decoction

Case history

A 61-year-old man had been suffering from insomnia ever since his wife died 2 years previously. He found it difficult to fall asleep and also woke up frequently during the night. He was extremely sad about his wife's death and found it very difficult to come to terms with it.

His vision was sometimes blurred and his memory was affected. His tongue was Red, dry and its coating was too thin (Plate 18.1). His pulse was Floating-Empty and very slightly Wiry on the left side.

Diagnosis In this case sadness affected the Liver and Heart rather than the Lungs and Heart. In particular, sadness weakened Liver-Yin so that the Ethereal Soul was deprived of its root. When this happens it wanders at night, causing insomnia.

The Spiritual Axis in Chapter 8 clearly states that sadness can affect the Liver: "*The Liver's sadness and shock injure the Ethereal Soul...*" and:[49]

> *When sadness affects the Liver it injures the Ethereal Soul; this causes mental confusion ... the Yin is damaged, the tendons contract and there is hypochondrial discomfort.*

This quotation clearly indicates that Liver-Yin may be damaged by sadness.

The blurred vision confirms the deficiency of Liver-Yin.

Treatment principle Nourish Liver-Yin, root the Ethereal Soul and calm the Mind.

Acupuncture The points used were:

- LIV-8 Ququan, SP-6 Sanyinjiao and Ren-4 Guanyuan to nourish Liver-Yin.
- HE-7 Shenmen and Ren-15 Jiuwei to calm the Mind.
- Du-24 Shenting and G.B.-13 Benshen to calm the Mind and root the Ethereal Soul.

Herbal therapy No herbs were prescribed but only the patent remedy Suan Zao Ren Tang Pian *Tablet of the Ziziphus Decoction*, which specifically treats insomnia from Liver-Yin deficiency.

This patient's sleep pattern first improved by being able to fall asleep easily although he still woke up during the night. Presumably this is because Liver-Blood (responsible for not falling asleep) was helped before Liver-Yin. After about 6 months of fortnightly treatments he started sleeping through the night.

Case history

A 53-year-old woman had been suffering from insomnia for over 10 years. This started after suffering two shocks in the 2 years preceding its onset. Her problem was not so much falling asleep as waking up during the night. Occasionally she sweated at night.

She has a red rash on the face and neck and her eyes were often dry. Her tongue was slightly Red and without coating, with a shallow Heart crack. Her pulse was Empty at the deep level and very slightly Overflowing on the Liver position.

Diagnosis This is a clear case of Liver-Yin deficiency with some Empty Heat. The Yin deficiency is evidenced by the lack of coating on the tongue, the pulse being Empty at the deep level and night-sweating, and the Liver involvement by the insomnia, dry eyes and red rash.

Treatment I treated this patient with only two *Three Treasures* remedies. The first was *Nourish the Soul*, which is a variation of Suan Zao Ren Tang *Ziziphus Decoction*; this formula nourishes Liver-Yin, clears Empty Heat, calms the Mind and settles the Ethereal Soul. I prescribed three tablets twice a day for this remedy.

The second remedy was *Female Treasure*, which subdues Liver-Yang, clears Empty Heat and nourishes Liver-Yin. I prescribed only two tablets a day to be taken in the evening.

The combination of these two remedies had a very good effect on her sleep and she gradually slept better. The patient is still being treated at the time of writing.

Liver- and Kidney-Yin deficiency

Clinical manifestations

Waking up during the night, dreaming a lot, talking in one's sleep, in severe cases sleepwalking, dry throat, irritability, blurred vision, feeling of heat, sore and dry eyes, dry skin and hair, dizziness, tinnitus, lower backache, night-sweating (Fig. 18.20).

Tongue: without coating.

Pulse: Floating-Empty, especially on the left side.

The deficiency of Liver-Yin causes the Ethereal Soul to be deprived of its root and to "wander" at night during sleep. This causes insomnia and excessive dreaming and, in some cases, even sleepwalking. The deficiency of Kidney-Yin weakens the Will-Power (*Zhi*) and fails to anchor the Mind (*Shen*), leading to insomnia. A deficiency of Kidney-Yin leads to

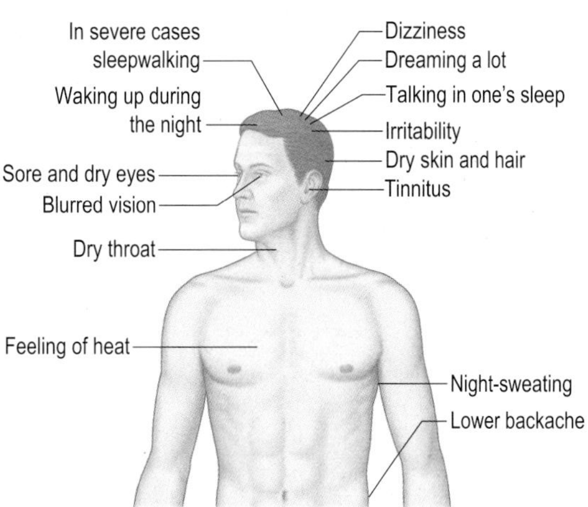

Figure 18.20 Liver- and Kidney-Yin deficiency.

insomnia also because the deficient Kidney-Yin fails to nourish Liver-Yin, which therefore cannot anchor the Ethereal Soul. This type of insomnia is common in the elderly.

Treatment principle

Nourish Liver- and Kidney-Yin, strengthen Will-Power, root the Ethereal Soul and calm the Mind.

Acupuncture

Points

LIV-8 Ququan, Ren-4 Guanyuan, Hunshe extra point, SP-6 Sanyinjiao, P-7 Daling, Du-24 Shenting and G.B.-13 Benshen, BL-47 Hunmen, Anmien, KI-3 Taixi. Reinforcing method, no moxa.

Explanation

- LIV-8 nourishes Liver-Blood and Liver-Yin.
- Ren-4 nourishes Liver- and Kidney-Yin and calms the Mind.
- Hunshe (situated level with Ren-8 Shenque and 1 *cun* lateral to it) roots the Ethereal Soul into the Liver.
- SP-6 nourishes Liver- and Kidney-Yin, calms the Mind and settles the Ethereal Soul.
- P-7 harmonizes the Liver (due to the relationship between Pericardium and Liver within the Terminal Yin), calms the Mind and settles the Ethereal Soul.
- Du-24 and G.B.-13 calm the Mind, especially in Liver patterns.
- BL-47, called the "Door of the Ethereal Soul", settles the Ethereal Soul into the Liver at night. Some old books give sleepwalking as an indication for this point.
- Anmien calms the Ethereal Soul and the Mind and promotes sleep in Liver patterns.
- KI-3 Taixi tonifies the Kidneys and strengthens Will-Power.

Herbal therapy

Prescription

ER ZHI WAN Variation
Two Solstices Pill Variation

Explanation

This formula nourishes Liver- and Kidney-Yin, settles the Ethereal Soul and calms the Mind.

Prescription

ZUO GUI WAN Variation
Restoring the Left [Kidney] *Pill* Variation

Explanation

This formula nourishes Liver- and Kidney-Yin, strengthens the Will-Power, settles the Ethereal Soul and calms the Mind. Compared to the previous formula, it has a more comprehensive action in nourishing Liver- and Kidney-Yin.

Modifications

These modifications apply to both above formulae.

- If there is Empty Heat (in which case the tongue is Red and without a coating), add Zhi Mu *Radix Anemarrhaenae* and Mu Dan Pi *Cortex Moutan*.

SUMMARY

Liver- and Kidney-Yin deficiency

Points

LIV-8 Ququan, Ren-4 Guanyuan, Hunshe extra point, SP-6 Sanyinjiao, P-7 Daling, Du-24 Shenting and G.B.-13 Benshen, BL-47 Hunmen, Anmien, KI-3 Taixi. Reinforcing method, no moxa.

Herbal therapy

Prescription

ER ZHI WAN Variation
Two Solstices Pill Variation

Prescription

ZUO GUI WAN Variation
Restoring the Left [Kidney] *Pill* Variation.

MODERN CHINESE LITERATURE

Journal of Chinese Medicine (Zhong Yi Za Zhi 中医杂志), Vol. 35, No. 3, 1994, p. 180.

Anwei Province Hospital of Chinese Medicine, "What to do when Suan Zao Ren and Ye Jiao Teng fail in the treatment of insomnia"

The authors of this article say that, in insomnia, it is essential to distinguish between a condition with a pathogenic factor (Full) from one without a pathogenic factor (Empty).

Empty conditions without a pathogenic factor are due to worry, pensiveness and overwork injuring the Spleen and Heart, resulting in insomnia, anxiety and palpitations. The formula to use in this case is Shou Pi Jian *Spleen Longevity Decoction.*

- **Dang Shen** *Radix Codonopsis*
- **Bai Zhu** *Rhizoma Atractylodis macrocephalae*
- **Shan Yao** *Rhizoma Dioscoreae*
- **Zhi Gan Cao** *Radix Glycyrrhizae uralensis preparata*
- **Suan Zao Ren** *Semen Ziziphi spinosae*
- **Yuan Zhi** *Radix Polygalae*
- **Gan Jiang** *Rhizoma Zingiberis*
- **Lian Rou** *Fructus Nelumbinis*

If fear injures the Kidneys and the Gall-Bladder, the Mind and Ethereal Soul are deprived of their residence, the Yin and Essence are deficient and insomnia ensues. The formula to use is Da Bu Yuan Jian *Great Tonifying the Original* [Qi] *Decoction.*

- **Shu Di Huang** *Radix Rehmanniae preparata* 15 g
- **Shan Yao** *Rhizoma Dioscoreae* 12 g
- **Shan Zhu Yu** *Fructus Corni* 9 g
- **Gou Qi Zi** *Fructus Lycii chinensis* 12 g
- **Dang Gui** *Radix Angelicae sinensis* 9 g
- **Ren Shen** *Radix Ginseng* 12 g
- **Du Zhong** *Cortex Eucommiae ulmoidis* 9 g
- **Zhi Gan Cao** *Radix Glycyrrhizae uralensis preparata* 6 g

If overwork injures the Heart, Heart-Yin becomes deficient and Empty Heat harasses the Mind. The tongue lacks a coating and is cracked. In this case, use Tian Wang Bu Xin Dan *Heavenly Emperor Tonifying the Heart Pill.*

If Liver-Qi stagnation agitates the Ethereal Soul, Heart and Gall-Bladder become deficient; in such case, use Wen Dan Tang *Warming the Gall-Bladder Decoction.* Please note that the authors are using this formula for the purpose for which it was originally designed, i.e. to "warm the Gall-Bladder" and strengthen resolve and decisiveness, and treat insomnia and anxiety.

As for the Full conditions of insomnia, if the Stomach suffers from Retention of Food, the authors recommend using Da He Zhong Yin *Great Harmonizing the Center Decoction.*

- **Xing Ren** *Semen Armeniacae*
- **Bai Jie Zi** *Semen Sinapis albae*
- **Sheng Jiang** *Rhizoma Zingiberis recens*

If Phlegm is causing insomnia, the authors recommend using Dao Tan Tang *Conducting Phlegm Decoction.* If there is Phlegm with Heat, they recommend using Di Tan Tang *Washing Away Phlegm Decoction.*

The authors conclude by stressing the importance of pattern identification in the treatment of insomnia and not relying simply on the use of Suan Zao Ren and Ye Jiao Teng. The authors say that these herbs are used for insomnia only if deriving from the specific patterns they address, i.e. Liver-Blood deficiency for Suan Zao Ren and Liver-Yin deficiency for Ye Jiao Teng.

Journal of Chinese Medicine (*Zhong Yi Za Zhi*), Vol. 39, No. 11, 1998, p. 658.

Qian Yan Fang, "The treatment of stubborn insomnia based on identification of patterns"

Dr Qian discusses what he considers to be the main patterns causing stubborn insomnia.

Disharmony of the Nutritive and Defensive Qi

The first pattern is disharmony of the Nutritive (*Ying*) and Defensive (*Wei*) Qi. Defensive Qi should enter into the Yin at night; if it does not, and stays in the Yang, it remains on the Exterior of the body and in the eyes, the Yang Stepping Vessel (*Yang Qiao Mai*) is full, the eyes cannot close and insomnia ensues.

The symptoms of this type of insomnia are difficulty in falling asleep or difficulty in staying asleep, inability to close the eyes, excessive dreaming, headache, a sensation rising from the chest to the head, aversion to wind and a Wiry pulse.

The formula Dr Qian suggests is Gui Zhi Jia Long Gu Mu Li Tang *Cinnamomum-Mastodi Ossis fossilia-Concha Ostreae Decoction*. Gui Zhi Tang harmonizes Nutritive and Defensive Qi while Long Gu and Mu Li calm the Mind and settle the Ethereal Soul.

Deficiency of Qi and Yin, disharmony of Heart and Kidneys

The second pattern discussed is deficiency of Qi and Yin and disharmony of Heart and Kidneys. Overwork and pensiveness injure the Spleen and Heart, leading to Blood deficiency, or Heat may injure Yin and lead to Kidney-Yin deficiency. This leads to deficiency of Heart-Yin and Heart Empty Heat.

The formula to use is Sheng Mai San *Generating the Pulse Power*, together with Huang Lian E Jiao Tang *Coptis Colla Corii Asini Decoction*.

Phlegm-Heat

The third pattern is Phlegm-Heat. Dr Qian considers the main symptoms of Phlegm-Heat causing insomnia to be chronic insomnia, palpitations, excessive dreaming, a feeling of heaviness of the head, anxiety, expectoration of sputum, bitter taste, tinnitus, belching, nausea, loose stools, sticky tongue coating and a Slippery-Wiry pulse.

The recommended formula is Huang Lian Wen Dan Tang *Coptis Warming the Gall-Bladder Decoction*.

Heart-Blood stasis

The fourth pattern is Blood stasis of the Heart. The main manifestations are inability to close the eyes at night, startled as soon as the eyes close, headache, blurred vision, poor memory, numbness of limbs, chest pain, Purple tongue, Wiry or Choppy pulse.

The formula recommended is Tong Qiao Huo Xue Tang *Opening the Orifices and Invigorating Blood Decoction*.

Journal of Chinese Medicine (Zhong Yi Za Zhi), Vol. 34, No. 2, 1993, p. 117.

Zhou Jing Ming, "Clinical significance of Zhang Jing Yue's treatment principle of insomnia according to the differentiation between that with and that without pathogenic factors"

The article discusses Zhang Jing Yue (1624) treatment of insomnia: Dr Zhang differentiates clearly insomnia with a pathogenic factor and insomnia without. The author mentions two main patterns with a pathogenic factor: Liver- and Heart-Fire and Phlegm-Heat.

Patterns with pathogenic factors

Liver- and Heart-Fire

For Liver- and Heart-Fire, Dr Zhang uses Qing Huo An Shen Tang *Clearing Fire and Calming the Mind Decoction*.

- **Sheng Di Huang** *Radix Rehmanniae* 12 g
- **Huang Lian** *Rhizoma Coptidis* 3 g
- **Huang Qin** *Radix Scutellariae* 6 g
- **Shan Zhi Zi** *Fructus Gardeniae* 9 g
- **Long Gu** *Mastodi Ossis fossilia* 15 g
- **Mu Li** *Concha Ostreae* 15 g
- **Long Dan Cao** *Radix Gentianae* 3 g
- **Lian Qiao** *Fructus Forsythiae suspensae* 6 g
- **Gan Cao** *Radix Glycyrrhizae uralensis* 3 g

Phlegm-Heat

For insomnia from Phlegm-Heat, Dr Zhang uses He Zhong An Shen Tang *Harmonizing the Center and Calming the Mind Decoction*.

- **Ban Xia** *Rhizoma Pinelliae preparatum* 6 g
- **Fu Ling** *Poria* 9 g
- **Chen Pi** *Pericarpium Citri reticulatae* 6 g
- **Zhi Shi** *Fructus Aurantii immaturus* 9 g
- **Huang Lian** *Rhizoma Coptidis* 3 g
- **Zhu Ru** *Caulis Bambusae in Taeniam* 6 g
- **Bei Shu Mi** *Sorghum* 9 g
- **Gan Cao** *Radix Glycyrrhizae uralensis* 3 g

Patterns without pathogenic factors

The three main patterns without pathogenic factors causing insomnia are Heart and Spleen deficiency, deficiency of Heart and Gall-Bladder, deficiency of Liver- and Kidney-Yin.

Deficiency of Heart and Spleen

For deficiency of Heart and Spleen, Dr Zhang uses Yang Xin An Shen Tang *Nourishing the Heart and Calming the Mind Decoction*.

- **Dang Shen** *Radix Codonopsis* 9 g
- **Bai Zhu** *Rhizoma Atractylodis macrocephalae* 9 g
- **Huang Qi** *Radix Astragali* 12 g

- **Dang Gui** *Radix Angelicae sinensis* 12 g
- **Fu Shen** *Sclerotium Poriae pararadicis* 9 g
- **Yuan Zhi** *Radix Polygalae* 3 g
- **Long Yan Rou** *Arillus Longan* 12 g
- **Suan Zao Ren** *Semen Ziziphi spinosae* 9 g
- **Bai Zi Ren** *Semen Platycladi* 10 g
- **Bai Shao** *Radix Paeoniae alba* 12 g
- **Mu Xiang** *Radix Aucklandiae* 3 g
- **Zhi Gan Cao** *Radix Glycyrrhizae uralensis preparata* 4.5 g

Deficiency of Heart and Gall-Bladder

The second Empty pattern is deficiency of the Heart and Gall-Bladder with the following manifestations: anxiety, Mind (*Shen*) and Ethereal Soul (*Hun*) unsettled, easily sad, excessive dreaming, waking up at night, palpitations, shortness of breath, tiredness.

The formula recommended for this pattern is Ding Zhi An Shen Tang *Settling the Spirit and Calming the Mind Decoction.*

- **Dang Shen** *Radix Codonopsis* 6 g
- **Fu Ling** *Poria* 9 g
- **Yuan Zhi** *Radix Polygalae* 3 g
- **Suan Zao Ren** *Semen Ziziphi spinosae* 9 g
- **Shi Chang Pu** *Rhizoma Acori tatarinowii* 3 g
- **Long Chi** *Fossilia Dentis Mastodi* 15 g
- **Zhen Zhu Mu** *Concha Margaritiferae usta* 15 g
- **Fu Xiao Mai** *Fructus Tritici levis* 15 g
- **Zhi Gan Cao** *Radix Glycyrrhizae uralensis preparata* 3 g

Liver- and Kidney-Yin deficiency

The third Empty pattern in insomnia is deficiency of Liver- and Kidney-Yin, for which Dr Zhang uses Zi Yin An Shen Tang *Nourishing Yin and Calming the Mind Decoction.*

- **Sheng Di Huang** *Radix Rehmanniae* 9 g
- **Shan Zhu Yu** *Fructus Corni* 9 g
- **Shan Yao** *Rhizoma Dioscoreae* 9 g
- **Fu Ling** *Poria* 10 g
- **Huang Lian** *Rhizoma Coptidis* 3 g
- **Mu Dan Pi** *Cortex Moutan* 6 g
- **Bai Shao** *Radix Paeoniae alba* 9 g
- **E Jiao** *Colla Corii Asini* 9 g
- **Ze Xie** *Rhizoma Alismatis* 9 g

Of particular interest in this article is also the small dosage of the herbs, which is contrary to modern Chinese use.

Journal of Chinese Medicine

(*Zhong Yi Za Zhi*), Vol. 45, No. 11, 2004, p. 843.

Hong Yong Bo et al., "Clinical observation on the treatment of 31 cases of insomnia with Jie Yu Wan"

Fifty-three patients suffering from insomnia were randomly divided into a treatment group (31) treated with Jie Yu Wan *Eliminating Stagnation Pill* and a control group (22) treated with trazodone. The patients were assessed before treatment and at the 14th and 28th days of therapy with the Sleeping Questionnaire (SQ), Self-Rating Depression Scale (SDS) and Self-Rating Anxiety Scale (SAS). Adverse effects and efficacy index were evaluated by the method of Clinical Global Impression (CGI).

The marked improvement rate was 54.9% in the treatment group and 59.1% in the control group, with no significant difference between the groups ($P > 0.05$). After treatment, the scores for SQ, SDS and SAS decreased significantly in both groups, with no significant difference between them, although patients reported fewer side-effects in the treatment group.

The formula Jie Yu Wan *Eliminating Stagnation Pill* contained the following (dosages for a batch of pills).

- **Bai Shao** *Radix Paeoniae alba* 270 g
- **Chai Hu** *Radix Bupleuri* 190 g
- **Yu Jin** *Radix Curcumae* 140 g
- **Fu Ling** *Poria* 170 g
- **Bai He** *Bulbus Lilii* 170 g
- **He Huan Pi** *Cortex Albiziae* 170 g
- **Gan Cao** *Radix Glycyrrhizae uralensis* 85 g
- **Fu Xiao Mai** *Fructus Tritici levis* 210 g
- **Da Zao** *Fructus Jujubae* 140 g

This trial is reported here as a typical example of a study that is poorly designed from the point of view of Chinese medicine. First, it treats all patients suffering from insomnia with the same formula, something that we would never do in practice. As the formula's main aim is to move Qi and eliminate stagnation, it assumes that all patients with insomnia suffer from Qi stagnation, something that is clearly not true.

Second, the formula seems aimed more at treating depression than insomnia (see use of Yu Jin and He Huan Pi). As such, there is a basic misunderstanding underlying this trial, as there is a difference between the insomnia that is secondary to depression and insomnia that occurs by itself.

Chinese Acupuncture and Moxibustion (*Zhong Guo Zhen Jiu* 中国针灸), Vol. 20, No. 2, 2000, p. 90.

Ren Jian Jun, "38 cases of insomnia treated with moxibustion on KI-1 Yongquan"

Dr Ren reports on the use of moxibustion on KI-1 Yongquan for the treatment of insomnia. The point was heated with a moxa stick once a day for 15–20 minutes each time. Treatment was given in 7-day courses.

Dr Ren reports 100% success in the treatment of 38 cases of insomnia with this method.

CLINICAL TRIALS

Acupuncture

Randomized and controlled study on effect of acupuncture on sleep quality of primary insomnia patients

Zhong Guo Zhen Jiu [Chinese Acupuncture and Moxibustion] 2007 December, Vol. 27, Issue 12, pp. 886–888.
Xuan YB, Guo J, Wang LP, Wu X

Objective

To observe the effectiveness of acupuncture in improving sleep quality in insomnia patients.

Method

Forty-six cases of primary insomnia were randomly divided into an observation group (n = 24) and a control group (n = 22). The observation group was treated by the needling method for regulating mental activity, with Du-20 Baihui, Du-24 Shenting and HE-7 Shenmen selected as the main points; the control group was treated with an oral administration of estazolam. The therapeutic effects and scores of Pittsburgh Sleep Quality Index Scale before and after treatment were compared between the two groups.

Results

The total effective rate was 83.3% in the observation group and 72.7% in the control group, the observation group being better than the control group ($P < 0.05$). Estazolam was better than acupuncture treatment in prolonging sleeping time, and the acupuncture treatment was better than the control group in the improvement of somnipathy and the increase of daytime functional state ($P < 0.05$).

Conclusion

Acupuncture treatment has advantages of improving somnipathy and increasing daytime functional state.

Clinical observation on the effect of electroacupuncture at Sishencong in treating insomnia

Zhong Guo Zhong Xi Yi Jie He Za Zhi 中国中西医结合杂志 [Chinese Journal of Integrative Medicine] 2007 November, Vol. 27, Issue 11, pp. 1030–1032.
Tang SC, Liu JM, Liu GL

Objective

To evaluate the clinical therapeutic effect of electroacupuncture (EA) at Sishencong on insomnia.

Method

Two hundred and seventy-six patients were randomly assigned to two groups, 138 in each group, the EA group treated with EA at Sishencong, and the control group with oral administration of Tianmeng capsule. The treatment course for both groups was 3 weeks. The quality and related parameters of sleep before and after treatment were evaluated with a multi-channel sleep detector.

Results

After treatment, the quality of sleep was improved in both groups ($P < 0.05$), the difference in related parameters was significant respectively ($P < 0.05$ or $P < 0.01$); however, the improvement in the EA group was superior to that in the control group ($P < 0.01$).

Conclusion

EA at Sishencong has a positive effect on insomnia.

Multiple center clinical studies on the needling method for regulating Wei Qi (Defensive Qi) and strengthening the Brain for treatment of insomnia

Zhong Guo Zhen Jiu [Chinese Acupuncture and Moxibustion] 2007 August, Vol. 27, Issue 8, pp. 623–625.
Gao XY, Wei YL, Shao SJ, Li XR, Zhang HJ, Wang J et al.

Objective

To observe the clinical therapeutic effect of the needling method for regulating Defensive Qi and strengthening the brain in insomnia patients.

Method

Two hundred cases of insomnia were randomly divided into a test group and a control group, 100 cases in each group. The test group was treated with the needling method for regulating Defensive Qi and strengthening the brain – Du-20 Baihui, Du-14 Dazhui, BL-62 Shenmai, KI-6 Zhaohai and ear points Yuanzhong and Shenmen; in the control group, Sishencong, HE-7 Shenmen and SP-6 Sanyinjiao were selected. Acupuncture was given once daily for 15 days. Pittsburgh Sleep Quality Index (PSQI) was used for scoring before and after treatment.

Results

The total effective rate was 89.0% in the test group and 65.0% in the control group, with a very significant difference between the two groups ($P < 0.01$); the difference in PSQI scores before and after was -9.15 ± 5.68 in the test group and -5.64 ± 5.73 in the control group, with a very significant difference before and after treatment in the two groups ($P < 0.01$).

Conclusion

The therapeutic effect of the needling method for regulating Defensive Qi and strengthening the brain in patients with insomnia is better than that of a different selection of acupuncture points.

Auricular acupuncture treatment for insomnia: a systematic review

Journal of Alternative and Complementary Medicine 2007 July–August, Vol. 13, Issue 6, pp. 669–676.
Chen HY, Shi Y, Ng CS, Chan SM, Yung KK, Zhang QL

Objective

To review trials on the efficacy and safety of auricular acupuncture (AA) treatment for insomnia and to identify the most commonly used auricular acupoints for treating insomnia in the studies via a frequency analysis.

Data sources

The international electronic databases searched included: (1) AMED, (2) the Cochrane Library, (3) CINAHL, (4) EMBASE and (5) MEDLINE. Chinese electronic databases searched included: (1) VIP Information, (2) CBMdisc and (3) CNKI. STUDY.

Selection

Any randomized controlled trials using AA as an intervention without using any co-interventions for insomnia were included. Studies using AA versus no treatment, placebo, sham AA or Western medicine were included.

Data extraction

Two independent reviewers were responsible for data extraction and assessment. The efficacy of AA was estimated by the relative risk (RR) using a meta-analysis.

Results

Eight hundred and seventy-eight papers were searched. Six trials (402 treated with AA among 673 participants) that met the inclusion criteria were retrieved. A meta-analysis showed that AA was chosen with a higher priority among the treatment subjects than among the controls ($p < 0.05$). The recovery and improvement rates produced by AA were significantly higher than those of diazepam ($p < 0.05$). The rate of success was higher when AA was used for enhancement of sleeping hours up to 6 hours in treatment subjects ($p < 0.05$). The efficacy of using Semen vaccariae ear seeds was better than that of the controls ($p < 0.01$), while magnetic pearls did not show statistical significance ($p = 0.28$). Six commonly used auricular acupoints were Shenmen (100%), Heart (83.33%), Occiput (66.67%), Subcortex (50%), Brain and Kidney (each 33.33%, respectively).

Conclusion

AA appears to be effective for treating insomnia. Because the trials were low quality, further clinical trials with higher design quality, longer duration of treatment and longer follow-up should be conducted.

Acupuncture for insomnia in pregnancy – a prospective, quasi-randomized, controlled study

Acupuncture in Medicine 2005 June, Vol. 23, Issue 2, pp. 47–51.

Da Silva JB, Nakamura MU, Cordeiro JA, Kulay LJ

Objective

This study was undertaken to test the effects of acupuncture on insomnia in a group of pregnant women under real life conditions, and to compare the results with a group of patients undergoing conventional treatment alone (sleep hygiene).

Method

A total of 30 conventionally treated pregnant women were allocated at random into groups with or without acupuncture: 17 patients formed the study group and 13 the control group. The pregnant women scored the severity of insomnia using a numerical rating scale from 0 to 10. Women were monitored for 8 weeks and interviewed five times, at 2-week intervals.

Results

Eight women dropped out: five in the study group and three in the control group. The study group reported a larger reduction in insomnia rating (5.1) than the control group (0.0), a difference which was statistically significant ($P = 0.0028$). Average insomnia scores decreased by at least 50% over time in nine (75%) patients in the study group and in three (30%) of the control group.

Conclusion

The results of this study suggest that acupuncture alleviates insomnia during pregnancy and further research is justified.

Intradermal acupuncture on HE-7 Shenmen and P-6 Neiguan acupoints in patients with insomnia after stroke

American Journal of Chinese Medicine 2004, Vol. 32, Issue 5, pp. 771–778.

Kim YS, Lee SH, Jung WS, Park SU, Moon SK, Ko CN et al.

Department of Cardiovascular and Neurological Diseases (Stroke Center), College of Oriental Medicine, Kyung-Hee University, Seoul, Korea.

Objective

To analyze the effects of intradermal acupuncture on insomnia after stroke.

Method

Hospitalized stroke patients with insomnia were enrolled and assigned to a real intradermal acupuncture group (RA group) or a sham acupuncture group (SA group) by randomization. The RA group received intradermal acupuncture on HE-7 Shenmen and P-6 Neiguan for 2 days, and the SA group received sham acupuncture on the same points. The effectiveness was measured by the Morning Questionnaire (MQ), Insomnia Severity Index (ISI) and Athens Insomnia Scale (AIS). These scales were examined by an independent, blinded neurologist before, and 1 and 2 days after treatment, repeatedly. Thirty subjects (15 in the RA group and 15 in the SA group) were included in the final analysis.

Results

The RA group showed more improvement in insomnia than the SA group. Repeated measures analysis detected that there were significant between-subject effects in the MQ, the ISI and the AIS.

Conclusion

It is suggested that intradermal acupuncture on HE-7 Shenmen and P-6 Neiguan is a useful treatment for post-stroke-onset insomnia.

Acupuncture increases nocturnal melatonin secretion and reduces insomnia and anxiety: a preliminary report

Journal of Neuropsychiatry and Clinical Neurosciences 2004 Winter, Vol. 16, Issue 1, pp. 19–28.

Spence DW, Kayumov L, Chen A, Lowe A, Jain U, Katzman MA et al.
Center for Addiction and Mental Health, Toronto, Ontario, Canada.

Extract

The response to acupuncture by 18 anxious adult subjects who complained of insomnia was assessed in an open pre-post clinical trial study. Five weeks of acupuncture treatment was associated with a significant ($p = 0.002$) nocturnal increase in endogenous melatonin secretion (as measured in urine) and significant improvements in polysomnographic measures of sleep onset latency ($p = 0.003$), arousal index ($p = 0.001$), total sleep time ($p = 0.001$) and sleep efficiency ($p = 0.002$). Significant reductions in state ($p = 0.049$) and trait ($p = 0.004$) anxiety scores were also found. These objective findings are consistent with clinical reports of acupuncture's relaxant effects. Acupuncture treatment may be of value for some categories of anxious patients with insomnia.

Effects of individualized acupuncture on sleep quality in HIV disease

Journal of Associated Nurses AIDS Care 2001 January–February, Vol. 12, Issue 1, pp. 27–39.

Phillips KD, Skelton WD
Department of Administrative and Clinical Nursing, College of Nursing, University of South Carolina, USA.

Objective

Although it may begin at any point, sleep disturbance often appears early in HIV disease and contributes to decreased quality of life during the course of the illness. The purpose of this study was threefold: to explore the nature of sleep quality in HIV disease, to test the relationship between pain and sleep quality, and to test the effectiveness of acupuncture delivered in a group setting for improving sleep quality in those who are HIV infected.

Method

A pre-test, post-test, pre-experimental design was used to test the effects of acupuncture on sleep quality. Participating in the study were 21 HIV-infected men and women between the ages of 29 and 50 years who reported sleep disturbance three or more times per week and who scored greater than 5 on the Pittsburgh Sleep Quality Index. The Wrist Actigraph was used to measure sleep activity, and the Current Sleep Quality Index was used to measure sleep quality for 2 nights before and after a 5-week acupuncture intervention (10 treatments). Acupuncture was individualized to address insomnia and other symptoms reported by the participants.

Results

Sleep activity and sleep quality significantly improved following 5 weeks of individualized acupuncture delivered in a group setting.

Conclusion

The results suggest that acupuncture may be an effective therapy to address problems of insomnia for HIV sufferers.

Acupuncture and insomnia

Forschende Komplementar Medizin 1999 February, Vol. 6 (Suppl. 1), pp. 29–31.

Montakab H

Objective

To ascertain the effect of acupuncture on insomnia.

Method

Forty patients with primary difficulties in either falling asleep or remaining asleep were diagnosed according to traditional Chinese medicine, allocated to specific diagnostic subgroups and treated individually by a practitioner in his private practice. The patients were randomized into two groups, one group receiving true acupuncture and the other needled at non-acupuncture points for three to five sessions at weekly intervals. The outcome of the therapy was assessed in several ways, first and foremost by an objective measurement of the sleep quality by polysomnography in a specialized sleep laboratory, performed once before and once after termination of the series of treatments. Additional qualitative results were obtained from several questionnaires.

Results

The objective measurement showed a statistically significant effect only in the patients who received the true acupuncture. The subjective, qualitative assessment was better in the proper treatment group than in the control group, but was not calculated statistically for methodological reasons.

Conclusion

Based on the results of this study, it can be concluded that true and individualized acupuncture indeed shows efficacy in primary sleep disorders. However, a direct influence by the therapist cannot be excluded.

Herbal medicine

The involvement of serotonin receptors in Suan Zao Ren Tang-induced sleep alteration

Journal of Biomedical Science 2007 November, Vol. 14, Issue 6, pp. 829–840.
Yi PL, Lin CP, Tsai CH, Lin JG, Chang FC
Department of Medical Technology, Jen-Teh Junior College of Medicine, Nursing and Management, Miaoli, Taiwan.

Background

Sedative-hypnotic medications, including benzodiazepines and non-benzodiazepines, are usually prescribed for insomniac patients; however, the addiction, dependence and adverse effects of those medications have drawn much attention. In contrast, Suan Zao Ren Tang, a traditional Chinese herb remedy, has been used effectively for insomnia relief in China, although its mechanism remains unclear.

Objective

This study was designed to further elucidate the underlying mechanism of Suan Zao Ren Tang on sleep regulation. One ingredient of Suan Zao Ren Tang, *Semen Ziziphi Spinosae*, exhibits binding affinity for serotonin (5-hydroxytryptamine, 5-HT) receptors, 5-HT(1A) and 5-HT(2), and for GABA receptors. Previous results have suggested that GABA(A) receptors, but not GABA(B), mediate Suan Zao Ren Tang-induced sleep alteration. In this current study the involvement of serotonin was further elucidated.

Results

It was found that a high dose of Suan Zao Ren Tang (4 g/kg/2 ml) significantly increased non-rapid eye movement sleep (NREMS) in comparison to a starch placebo, although placebo at a dose of 4 g/kg also enhanced NREMS compared to baseline figures. Rapid eye movement sleep (REMS) was not altered. Administration of either 5-HT(1A) antagonist (NAN-190), 5-HT(2) antagonist (ketanserin) or 5-HT(3) antagonist (3-(4-Allylpiperazin-1-yl)-2-quinoxaline-carbonitrile) blocked Suan Zao Ren Tang-induced NREMS increase.

Conclusion

These results implicate the hypnotic effect of Suan Zao Ren Tang and its effects may be mediated through serotonergic activation.

TCM treatment for 63 cases of senile dyssomnia

Zhong Yi Za Zhi [Journal of Chinese Medicine] 2005 March, Vol. 25, Issue 1, pp. 45–49.
Yang Y, Li H, Zhang S, Li Q, Yang X, Chen X et al.
Beijing University of Chinese Medicine, Beijing, China.

Objective

To ascertain the therapeutic effects of Chinese herbal medicine on senile dyssomnia.

Method

A total of 121 such patients were randomly divided into a treatment group of 63 cases (given the TCM drugs) and a control group of 58 cases (given estazolam). The changes shown in the SDRS and HAMA scores and the other indices were observed in both of the two groups to evaluate the therapeutic effects.

Results

The results showed that the effective rate was 76.3% in the treatment group and 69.1% in the control group, and that the TCM drugs had better effects in improving such symptoms as lethargy, dry mouth and rebound of insomnia.

Conclusion

It can be concluded that the effect of the TCM drugs is better for senile dyssomnia than that of the Western drug estazolam.

The effects of Yoku-kan-san on undifferentiated somatoform disorder with tinnitus

European Psychiatry 2005 January, Vol. 20, Issue 1, pp. 74–75.
Okamoto H, Okami T, Ikeda M, Takeuchi T
Department of Psychiatry, Teikyo University Ichihara Hospital, Ichihara City, Chiba, Japan.

Extract

Up to the present, there have been few strategies that are completely effective in treating undifferentiated somatoform disorder with tinnitus. Yoku-kan-san (TJ-54), one of Japan's traditional herbal medicines, is an effective treatment for tinnitus in undifferentiated somatoform disorder complicated with headache and insomnia. TJ-54 has also been used as an effective treatment for insomnia and irritability in recent centuries and is considered to have some effects on the excitability of nerves. Further studies are needed to confirm the efficacies of Japanese herbal medicines.

Effects of Yoku-kan-san-ka-chimpi-hange on the sleep of healthy adult subjects

Psychiatry and Clinical Neurosciences 2002 June, Vol. 56, Issue 3, pp. 303–304.
Aizawa R, Kanbayashi T, Saito Y, Ogawa Y, Sugiyama T, Kitajima T et al.
Japanese Red Cross Junior College of Akita, Akita City, Japan.

Extract

Yoku-kan-san-ka-chimpi-hange (YKCH) is a drug used for insomnia in Japanese traditional herbal medicine. The present study evaluated the effects of YKCH on sleep by all-night polysomnography using the double-blind method. Yoku-kan-san-ka-chimpi-hange increased the total sleep time significantly, and tended to cause an increase in sleep efficiency and of stage 2 sleep, as well as a decrease of sleep latency and of stage 3 + 4 sleep. There was no apparent influence on rapid eye movement (REM) sleep. In terms of non-REM sleep, the effects of YKCH exhibit a profile similar to those of benzodiazepines.

Clinical trial of Suan Zao Ren Tang in the treatment of insomnia

Clinical Therapeutics 1985, Vol. 7, Issue 3, pp. 334–337.
Chen HC, Hsieh MT

Objective

To ascertain the effect of Suan Zao Ren Tang, an ancient Chinese remedy for insomnia, on patients with sleep disorders.

Method

The hypnotic effect of Suan Zao Ren Tang was studied in 60 patients with sleep disorders. After receiving placebo for 1 week, patients ingested capsules containing 1 g of Suan Zao Ren Tang each night, 30 minutes before bedtime, for 2 weeks. Treatment was followed by another week of placebo administration. Each morning during the study, patients completed questionnaires relating to their sleep the night before and to their ability to function during the previous day.

Results

Analysis of the responses showed statistically significant improvements ($P < 0.001$) in all ratings of sleep quality and well-being during active treatment compared with both placebo periods. Laboratory tests performed before and after treatment with Suan Zao Ren Tang showed no alterations in any test value. No side-effects were noted.

Conclusion

Suan Zao Ren Tang improved the sleep quality of patients with insomnia and the findings warrant further extensive investigation.

PATIENTS' STATISTICS

I have compiled statistics of 73 patients suffering from insomnia in my practice. There were 45 women (62%) and 28 men (38%). The age distribution was as follows.

- 0–10: 3 (4%)
- 11–20: 0 (0%)
- 21–30: 6 (8%)
- 31–40: 20 (27%)
- 41–50: 14 (19%)
- 51–60: 23 (32%)
- 61–70: 7 (10%)

As can be observed, the highest incidence of insomnia is in the 51–60 age group and the overwhelming majority falls in the 31–60 age group.

As for patterns, these were as follows.

- *Purely Empty patterns*: 20 (27%)
- *Purely Full patterns*: 18 (25%)
- *Combined Full-Empty patterns*: 35 (48%)

The breakdown of the main Empty patterns is as follows.

- *Blood deficiency (of Liver and/or Heart)*: 22 (30%)
- *Kidney deficiency*: 33 (45%)
- *Heart deficiency (of Blood, Qi or Yin)*: 9 (12%)

Interestingly, a deficiency of the Kidneys is a more common Empty pattern in insomnia than Blood deficiency.

The breakdown of the main Full patterns is as follows.

- *Phlegm*: 28 (38%)
- *Blood stasis*: 8 (11%)
- *Fire (of Liver and/or Heart)*: 8 (11%)
- *Qi stagnation*: 6 (8%)

Again, it is interesting that Phlegm (rather than Fire) is the most common pathogenic factor in insomnia. Phlegm is a pathogenic factor in insomnia, especially in the elderly.

The most common pulse qualities were as follows.

- *Wiry*: 18 (25%)
- *Slippery*: 24 (34%)
- *Weak*: 25 (35%)
- *Choppy*: 9 (13%)
- *Deep* 12 (17%)
- *Fine*: 12 (17%)

The main types of tongue seen in insomnia were as follows.

- *Pale*: 21 (29%)
- *Red*: 29 (40%)
- *Purple*: 10 (14%)
- *Swollen*: 37 (51%)
- *Peeled*: 13 (18%)
- *Red tip*: 9 (12%)

An interesting feature of the tongues seen in insomnia is the high percentage of tongues with a red tip (12%); in my database of 2786 patients, 1.8% have a red tip.

APPENDIX 1 EXCESSIVE DREAMING

Dr Fang Wen Xian presents a differentiation of excessive dreaming in his book Chinese Internal Medicine which is reported below.[50]

Sleep disturbances linked to excessive dreaming are particularly related to the Ethereal Soul. As it is in the nature of the Ethereal Soul to "wander", at night it wanders, giving rise to dreams. Tang Zong Hai says: *"At night during sleep the Ethereal Soul returns to the Liver; if the Ethereal Soul is not peaceful, there are a lot of dreams."*[51]

The *Secret of the Golden Flower* in Chapter 2 says: *"In the daytime the Ethereal Soul is in the eyes and at night in the Liver. When it is in the eyes we can see; when it is in the Liver we dream."*[52] It also says: *"Dreams constitute the wandering of the Ethereal Soul in the nine Heavens and nine Earths. When one wakes up, one feels obscure and confused* [because] *one is constrained by the Corporeal Soul."*[53]

Quoting an ancient text, *Chinese Medicine Psychology* says:[54]

The Ethereal Soul goes to the eyes and to the Liver at night. When in the eyes, it allows us to see; when in the Liver, it makes us dream. When we dream a lot, the Corporeal Soul is restricting the hun; when we wake up, the Ethereal Soul is victorious over the Corporeal Soul.

As discussed above, few Chinese books explain what is meant by "excessive dreaming". In my experience, dreaming can be defined as excessive either when the sleeper has nightmares or when he or she has unpleasant or anxiety-causing dreams the whole night, waking up exhausted.

"Excessive dreaming" certainly includes nightmares; I think it also involves anxious dreams or dreams of being angry. Dreaming is excessive also when a person dreams so much all night that he or she wakes up exhausted from it.

Dreaming that does not make the sleep restless, is not frightening, does not disturb the Mind the morning after, and does not leave the person very tired in the morning, can be described as normal and is not a pathological condition.

Dr Wang Ke Qin defines "normal" dreaming as that characterized by short, pleasant dreams and not too many of them. According to him, "excessive" dreaming is characterized by nightmares and too many dreams, and by ones that are very long.[55]

Some doctors classify dreams as "chaotic dreams", dreams of fear, dreams of shock, strange dreams, "absurd dreams". They are considered pathological. These are due to the Mind's and the Ethereal Soul's being unsettled and to the "Ethereal Soul leaving the body".

The *Classic of Categories* by Zhang Jie Bin distinguishes six types of dream. These are as follows.

- Normal dreams
- Shock dreams
- Worry dreams
- Sleep dreams
- Pleasure dreams
- Fear dreams

Normal dreaming is not associated with any particular emotion. The second type is "shock" dreams characterized by a feeling of fear. The third type is "worry" dreams characterized by a feeling of worry about the events of the day. The fourth type is "sleep" dreams in which one at the time of waking up is still dreaming. The fifth type is "pleasure" dreams which are pleasurable. The sixth type is "fear" dreams characterized by fear and anxiety dreaming.[56]

Other modern doctors consider excessive dreaming that characterized by fear and anxiety and also sexual dreams and nocturnal emissions.[57]

Considering sexual dreams and nocturnal emissions a pathology is typical of Chinese culture, and we need not take necessarily the same view. Chinese medicine books frequently discuss the symptoms of sexual dreams and nocturnal emissions, and they often present a sophisticated differentiation of nocturnal emissions with or without dreams.

For example, Dr Ren Ying Qiu discusses the pathology and treatment of nocturnal emissions and sleep quality in his article:

In nocturnal emissions [one] *must distinguish with or without dreams in relation to Damp-Heat. In treatment, first calm the Shen and firm the Zhi, second consolidate Jing.*

Dr Ren says that the Essence is stored in the Kidneys but it is directed (governed) by the Heart. In nocturnal emissions, one must distinguish whether there are dreams or not and whether there is Damp-Heat. In general, nocturnal emissions with dreams are light; those without dreams are abundant; nocturnal emissions from Damp-Heat are light.

In treatment, the main method is to calm the Mind (*Shen* of the Heart) and settle the Will-Power (*Zhi* of the Kidneys); consolidate Essence only secondarily.

Nocturnal emissions *with dreams* are due to the Heart and specifically Heart-Blood deficiency or Heart-Fire, both of which agitate the Mind. Dr Ren identifies four subcategories of this type of emissions. The four subcategories and formulae are:

- *Lot of dreams*: Fu Shen Tang *Sclerotiun Poriae pararadicis Decoction*
- *Young person with Heart-Fire*: Qing Xin Wan *Clearing the Heart Pill*
- *Depression, irritability*: Si Qi Tang *Four Seasons Decoction for the Seven Emotions*
- *Anxiety, Heart deficiency*: Yuan Zhi Wan *Polygala Pill.*

Nocturnal emissions *without dreams* are due to the Kidneys. The Kidneys store the Essence; when Kidney-Qi is not firm (*bu gu*), the Essence may leak out. There are four subcategories:

- *Kidney-Yin deficiency with Empty Heat*: use San Cai Feng Sui Dan *Three Abilities Banking Up the Marrow Pill*.
- *Kidney-Qi not Firm, Essence not Consolidated*: use Sang Piao Xiao San *Ootheca Mantidis Pill*.
- *Heart Timid, Heart-Qi deficiency*: use Zhen Zhu Fen Wan *Pearl Pill* (just pearl powder), together with Ding Zhi Wan *Settling the Spirit Pill*.
- *Excessive sexual desire, Original (Yuan) Qi deficiency*: use Jing Gong Sha Xiang San *Palace of Essence Cinnabaris Fragrant Powder*.

Nocturnal emissions from Damp-Heat have two subcategories:

- *Damp-Heat infusing downwards*: dark urine, sweaty genitals, nocturnal emissions with or without dreams; use Er Huang San *Two Yellows Powder*.
- *Damp-Heat severe, swelling of genitals, profuse nocturnal emissions*: use Variation of Cang Bai Er Chen Tang *Gray and White Atractylodes Two Old Decoction*.

IDENTIFICATION OF PATTERNS AND TREATMENT

Phlegm-Heat

Clinical manifestations

Excessive dreaming, dreams of worry, dizziness, palpitations, feeling of oppression of the chest, expectoration of phlegm.

Tongue: Red, Swollen, sticky-yellow coating.

Pulse: Slippery-Rapid.

Treatment principle

Resolve Phlegm, clear Heat, calm the Mind.

Acupuncture

Points

P-5 Jianshi, LU-5 Chize, ST-40 Fenglong, SP-6 Sanyinjiao, Ren-9 Shuifen, L.I.-11 Quchi, HE-7 Shenmen, Du-24 Shenting, Ren-15 Jiuwei. All with reducing or even method.

Explanation

- P-5 resolves Phlegm from the Mind.
- LU-5, ST-40, SP-6 and Ren-9 resolve Phlegm.
- L.I.-11 clears Heat.
- HE-7, Du-24 and Ren-15 calm the Mind.

Herbal therapy

Prescription

HUANG LIAN WEN DAN TANG Variation
Coptis Warming the Gall-Bladder Decoction Variation

Explanation

This formula resolves Phlegm, clears Heat and opens the Mind's orifices.

SUMMARY

Phlegm-Heat

Points

P-5 Jianshi, LU-5 Chize, ST-40 Fenglong, SP-6 Sanyinjiao, Ren-9 Shuifen, L.I.-11 Quchi, HE-7 Shenmen, Du-24 Shenting, Ren-15 Jiuwei. All with reducing or even method.

Herbal therapy

Prescription

HUANG LIAN WEN DAN TANG Variation
Coptis Warming the Gall-Bladder Decoction Variation

Liver-Fire

Clinical manifestations

Excessive dreaming, irritability, headache, red eyes, bitter taste, dizziness, tinnitus.

Tongue: Red, redder sides.

Pulse: Wiry-Rapid.

Treatment principle

Clear Liver and Gall-Bladder, drain Fire, calm the Mind, settle the Ethereal Soul.

Acupuncture

Points

LIV-2 Xingjian, G.B.-44 Zuqiaoyin, L.I.-11 Quchi, P-8 Laogong, HE-8 Shaofu, BL-44 Shentang, BL-47 Hunmen. Reducing or even method.

Explanation

- LIV-2 and G.B.-44 drain Liver- and Gall-Bladder Fire.
- L.I.-11 clears Heat.
- P-8 and HE-8 drain Heart-Fire.
- BL-44 calms the Mind.
- BL-47 regulates the movement of the Ethereal Soul.

Herbal therapy

Prescription

LONG DAN XIE GAN TANG Variation
Gentiana Draining the Liver Decoction Variation

Explanation

This formula drains Liver-Fire, settles the Ethereal Soul and calms the Mind.

SUMMARY

Liver-Fire

Points

LIV-2 Xingjian, G.B.-44 Zuqiaoyin, L.I.-11 Quchi, P-8 Laogong, HE-8 Shaofu, BL-44 Shentang, BL-47 Hunmen. Reducing or even method.

Herbal therapy

Prescription

LONG DAN XIE GAN TANG Variation
Gentiana Draining the Liver Decoction Variation

Deficiency of Qi of Heart and Gall-Bladder

Clinical manifestations

Excessive dreaming, anxiety, easily startled, cannot settle, bewilderment, palpitations, sits down but is restless.

Tongue: Pale.
Pulse. Weak.

Treatment principle

Benefit Qi, calm the Heart, resolve Phlegm, calm the Mind.

Acupuncture

Points

HE-7 Shenmen, HE-5 Tongli, G.B.-40 Qiuxu, ST-36 Zusanli, SP-6 Sanyinjiao. All with reinforcing method.

Explanation

- HE-7 calms the Mind.
- HE-5 tonifies the Heart.
- G.B.-40 tonifies the Gall-Bladder.
- ST-36 and SP-6 tonify Qi in general.

Herbal therapy

Prescription

SHI WEI WEN DAN TANG Variation
Ten-Ingredient Warming the Gall-Bladder Decoction Variation

Explanation

This formula is used for the ancient use of Wen Dan Tang *Warming the Gall-Bladder Decoction*, i.e. literally warming the Gall-Bladder and strengthening the resolve and "courage" associated with this organ.

SUMMARY

Deficiency of Qi of Heart and Gall-Bladder

Points

HE-7 Shenmen, HE-5 Tongli, G.B.-40 Qiuxu, ST-36 Zusanli, SP-6 Sanyinjiao. All with reinforcing method.

Herbal therapy

Prescription

SHI WEI WEN DAN TANG Variation
Ten-Ingredient Warming the Gall-Bladder Decoction Variation

Heart- and Lung-Qi deficiency

Clinical manifestations

Excessive dreaming, palpitations, pale complexion, shortness of breath.

Tongue: Pale.
Pulse: Weak on both Front positions.

Treatment principle

Strengthen Heart and Lungs, calm the Mind.

Acupuncture

Points

HE-7 Shenmen, HE-5 Tongli, BL-15 Xinshu, Ren-15 Jiuwei, LU-9 Taiyuan, LU-3 Tianfu. All with reinforcing method.

Explanation

- HE-7, HE-5, BL-15 and Ren-15 strengthen the Heart and calm the Mind.
- LU-9 tonifies Lung-Qi.
- LU-3 stimulates the ascending of clear Qi to and the descending of turbid Qi from the Mind.

Herbal therapy

Prescription

BU FEI TANG Variation
Tonifying the Lungs Decoction Variation

Explanation

This formula tonifies Heart- and Lung-Qi and calms the Mind.

Deficiency of Heart and Spleen

Clinical manifestations

Excessive dreaming, waking up during the night, insomnia, poor memory, palpitations, poor appetite, tiredness, pale complexion.
Tongue: Pale, paler sides.
Pulse: Weak or Choppy.

Treatment principle

Tonify Qi, nourish Blood, strengthen the Spleen, nourish the Heart.

Acupuncture

Points

HE-7 Shenmen, Du-24 Shenting, Ren-15 Jiuwei, HE-5 Tongli, ST-36 Zusanli, SP-6 Sanyinjiao. All with reinforcing method.

Explanation

- HE-7, Du-24 and Ren-15 calm the Mind.
- HE-5 tonifies the Heart.
- ST-36 and SP-6 tonify the Spleen.

Herbal therapy

Prescription

GUI PI TANG Variation
Tonifying the Spleen Decoction Variation

Explanation

This variation of Gui Pi Tang tonifies Qi and Blood of the Spleen and Heart, calms the Mind and settles the Ethereal Soul.

SUMMARY

Heart- and Lung-Qi Deficiency

Points

HE-7 Shenmen, HE-5 Tongli, BL-15 Xinshu, Ren-15 Jiuwei, LU-9 Taiyuan, LU-3 Tianfu. All with reinforcing method.

Herbal therapy

Prescription

BU FEI TANG Variation
Tonifying the Lungs Decoction Variation

SUMMARY

Deficiency of Heart and Spleen

Points

HE-7 Shenmen, Du-24 Shenting, Ren-15 Jiuwei, HE-5 Tongli, ST-36 Zusanli, SP-6 Sanyinjiao. All with reinforcing method.

Herbal therapy

Prescription

GUI PI TANG Variation
Tonifying the Spleen Decoction Variation

Heart and Kidneys not harmonized

Clinical manifestations

Excessive dreaming, insomnia, anxiety, palpitations, dry mouth, nocturnal emissions with dreams, five-palm heat.

Tongue: Red, redder tip, without coating.

Pulse: Floating-Empty and Rapid.

Treatment principle

Nourish Kidney- and Heart-Yin, clear Heart Empty Heat, harmonize Heart and Kidneys, calm the Mind.

Acupuncture

Points

HE-7 Shenmen, HE-6 Yinxi, P-7 Daling, Ren-4 Guanyuan, SP-6 Sanyinjiao, KI-3 Taixi, KI-6 Zhaohai, Ren-15 Jiuwei, BL-15 Xinshu, BL-23 Shenshu, BL-44 Shentang, BL-52 Zhishi. Reinforcing method on all points except HE-6, which should be reduced.

Explanation

- HE-7 calms the Mind and promotes sleep.
- HE-6 clears Heart Empty Heat.
- P-7 calms the Mind.
- Ren-4 nourishes Kidney-Yin and calms the Mind.
- SP-6, KI-3 and KI-6 nourish Kidney-Yin.
- Ren-15 nourishes the Heart and calms the Mind.
- BL-15 and BL-23 harmonize Heart and Kidneys.
- BL-44 and BL-52 harmonize the Mind and Will-Power.

Herbal therapy

Prescription

HUANG LIAN E JIAO TANG Variation
Coptis-Colla Corii Asini Decoction Variation

Explanation

This formula nourishes Heart- and Kidney-Yin and calms the Mind.

Prescription

TIAN WANG BU XIN DAN
Heavenly Emperor Tonifying the Heart Pill

Explanation

This formula is specific to nourish Kidney- and Heart-Yin, clear Heart Empty Heat and calm the Mind.

SUMMARY

Heart and Kidneys not harmonized

Points

HE-7 Shenmen, HE-6 Yinxi, P-7 Daling, Ren-4 Guanyuan, SP-6 Sanyinjiao, KI-3 Taixi, KI-6 Zhaohai, Ren-15 Jiuwei, BL-15 Xinshu, BL-23 Shenshu, BL-44 Shentang, BL-52 Zhishi. Reinforcing method on all points except HE-6, which should be reduced.

Herbal therapy

Prescription

HUANG LIAN E JIAO TANG Variation
Coptis-Colla Corii Asini Decoction Variation

Prescription

TIAN WANG BU XIN DAN
Heavenly Emperor Tonifying the Heart Pill

APPENDIX 2 SOMNOLENCE

Somnolence indicates the tendency to be always rather sleepy and lethargic. Like insomnia, this is also due either to a pathogenic factor obstructing the Mind or to deficient Qi and Blood not reaching and nourishing the Mind (*Shen*).

IDENTIFICATION OF PATTERNS AND TREATMENT

Dampness obstructing the Brain

Clinical manifestations

Sleepiness after lunch, a feeling of heaviness of the head, a feeling of muzziness of the head as if it were full of cotton-wool, a feeling of fullness of the epigastrium and chest.

Tongue: Thick-sticky coating.

Pulse: Slippery or Soggy.

This pattern is due to Dampness obstructing the head and Brain and preventing the clear Qi from rising upwards to brighten the upper orifices. Another explanation of somnolence deriving from Dampness is that this pathogenic factor obstructs the space between the skin and muscles where the Defensive Qi flows. Because this space is obstructed, the Defensive Qi, Yang in nature, cannot flow there, so it stays in the Yin and the patient feels always sleepy.

Chapter 80 of the *Spiritual Axis*[58] says:

Defensive Qi flows in the Yang during the day and in the Yin at night, when Yang slows down one is sleepy, when Yin slows down one is awake. When Stomach and Intestines are big, Defensive Qi stays there for a long time, the skin is obstructed by Dampness ... Defensive Qi slows down, it stays in the Yin for a long time, Qi is not clear and somnolence results.

Treatment principle

Resolve Dampness and tonify the Spleen.

Acupuncture

Points

Ren-12 Zhongwan, BL-20 Pishu, ST-36 Zusanli, Ren-9 Shuifen, SP-6 Sanyinjiao, BL-22 Sanjiaoshu, LU-7 Lieque, ST-8 Touwei, Du-20 Baihui, Du-24 Shenting. Reinforcing method on Ren-12, BL-20 and ST-36. Reducing method on Ren-9, SP-6 and BL-22. Even method on LU-7, ST-8, Du-20 and Du-24.

Explanation

- Ren-12, BL-20 and ST-36 tonify the Spleen to resolve Dampness.
- Ren-9, SP-6 and BL-22 drain Dampness.
- LU-7 removes obstruction from the channels in the head and favors the ascending of clear Qi to the head.
- ST-8 and Du-20 are local points to expel Dampness from the head and facilitate the rising of clear Yang to the head.
- Du-24 clears the brain and improves memory.

Herbal therapy

Prescription

PING WEI SAN Variation
Balancing the Stomach Powder Variation

Explanation

The first six herbs constitute the Ping Wei San which drains Dampness from the Middle Burner. Huo Xiang *Herba Pogostemonis* and Pei Lan *Herba Eupatorii* resolve Dampness in the head (as they are fragrant and their fragrance reaches upwards). Yi Yi Ren *Semen Coicis* drains Dampness through the Lower Burner.

SUMMARY

Dampness obstructing the Brain

Points

Ren-12 Zhongwan, BL-20 Pishu, ST-36 Zusanli, Ren-9 Shuifen, SP-6 Sanyinjiao, BL-22 Sanjiaoshu, LU-7 Lieque, ST-8 Touwei, Du-20 Baihui, Du-24 Shenting. Reinforcing method on Ren-12, BL-20 and ST-36. Reducing method on Ren-9, SP-6 and BL-22. Even method on LU-7, ST-8, Du-20 and Du-24.

Herbal therapy

Prescription

PING WEI SAN Variation
Balancing the Stomach Powder Variation

Phlegm misting the Brain

Clinical manifestations

Sleepiness after lunch, a feeling of heaviness, a feeling of muzziness of the head as if it were full of cotton-wool, a feeling of oppression of the chest, dizziness, blurred vision, sputum in the throat.

Tongue: Swollen and with a sticky coating.

Pulse: Slippery.

This pattern is due to Phlegm obstructing the head and preventing the clear Qi from rising upwards to brighten the upper orifices. Phlegm is more obstructive than Dampness and this causes the dizziness and blurred vision (as Phlegm obstructs the orifices of the head).

Treatment principle

Resolve Phlegm and tonify the Spleen.

Acupuncture

Points

Ren-12 Zhongwan, BL-20 Pishu, ST-36 Zusanli, Ren-9 Shuifen, SP-6 Sanyinjiao, BL-22 Sanjiaoshu, ST-40 Fenglong, LU-7 Lieque, ST-8 Touwei, Du-20 Baihui, Du-24 Shenting. Reinforcing method on Ren-12, BL-20 and ST-36. Reducing method on Ren-9, SP-6, BL-22 and ST-40. Even method on LU-7, ST-8, Du-20 and Du-24.

Explanation

- Ren-12, BL-20 and ST-36 tonify the Spleen to resolve Phlegm.
- Ren-9, SP-6 and BL-22 resolve Dampness.
- ST-40 resolves Phlegm.
- LU-7 removes obstruction from the channels in the head and favors the ascending of clear Qi to the head.
- ST-8 and Du-20 are local points to expel Phlegm from the head and facilitate the rising of clear Yang to the head.
- Du-24 clears the brain and promotes memory.

Herbal therapy

Prescription

WEN DAN TANG plus **BAN XIA SHU MI TANG**
Warming the Gall-Bladder Decoction plus *Pinellia-Sorghum Decoction*

Explanation

These two formulae together resolve Phlegm from the head. To strengthen their effect, add Shi Chang Pu *Rhizoma Acori tatarinowii* to open the head's orifices.

Modifications

- To relieve the muzzy feeling of the head, add Shi Chang Pu *Rhizoma Acori tatarinowii*.
- If there are signs of Spleen deficiency, add Bai Zhu *Rhizoma Atractylodis macrocephalae* and Huang Qi *Radix Astragali*.

> **SUMMARY**
>
> **Phlegm misting the Brain**
>
> *Points*
>
> Ren-12 Zhongwan, BL-20 Pishu, ST-36 Zusanli, Ren-9 Shuifen, SP-6 Sanyinjiao, BL-22 Sanjiaoshu, ST-40 Fenglong, LU-7 Lieque, ST-8 Touwei, Du-20 Baihui, Du-24 Shenting. Reinforcing method on Ren-12, BL-20 and ST-36. Reducing method on Ren-9, SP-6, BL-22 and ST-40. Even method on LU-7, ST-8, Du-20 and Du-24.
>
> *Herbal therapy*
>
> *Prescription*
>
> **WEN DAN TANG** plus **BAN XIA QIU MI TANG**
> *Warming the Gall-Bladder Decoction* plus *Pinellia-Sorghum Decoction*

Spleen deficiency

Clinical manifestations

Somnolence, lethargy, tiredness, feeling of heaviness, slight abdominal distension and fullness, poor appetite, loose stools.

Tongue: Pale, sticky coating.

Pulse: Weak or Soggy.

Although this pattern is primarily one of deficiency, there is also some Dampness.

Treatment principle

Tonify the Spleen and resolve Dampness.

Acupuncture

Points

ST-36 Zusanli, SP-3 Taibai, Ren-12 Zhongwan, BL-20 Pishu, SP-6 Sanyinjiao, BL-22 Sanyinjiao, ST-8 Touwei, Du-20 Baihui. Reinforcing method on the first four points and even method on the others. Moxa can be used.

Explanation

- ST-36, SP-3, Ren-12 and BL-20 tonify the Spleen.
- SP-6 and BL-22 resolve Dampness.
- ST-8 and Du-20 drain Dampness from the head and facilitate the rising of clear Yang to the head.

Herbal therapy

Prescription

LIU JUN ZI TANG Variation
Six Gentlemen Decoction Variation

Explanation

This formula tonifies the Spleen, resolves Dampness and opens the head's orifices.

Prescription

BU ZHONG YI QI TANG Variation
Tonifying the Center and Benefiting Qi Decoction Variation

Explanation

This formula is used if there is Spleen-Yang deficiency. The original formula tonifies the Spleen and raises Qi.

> **SUMMARY**
>
> **Spleen deficiency**
>
> *Points*
>
> ST-36 Zusanli, SP-3 Taibai, Ren-12 Zhongwan, BL-20 Pishu, SP-6 Sanyinjiao, BL-22 Sanyinjiao, ST-8 Touwei, Du-20 Baihui. Reinforcing method on the first four points and even method on the others. Moxa can be used.
>
> *Herbal therapy*
>
> *Prescription*
>
> **LIU JUN ZI TANG** Variation
> *Six Gentlemen Decoction* Variation
>
> *Prescription*
>
> **BU ZHONG YI QI TANG** Variation
> *Tonifying the Center and Benefiting Qi Decoction* Variation

Kidney-Yang deficiency (Deficiency of Sea of Marrow)

Clinical manifestations

Lethargy, tiredness, apathy, lack of will-power, poor memory, lack of initiative, depression, chilliness, lower backache, dizziness, tinnitus, frequent-pale urination.
Tongue: Pale.
Pulse: Deep and Weak.

Treatment principle

Tonify Kidney-Yang, nourish the Sea of Marrow and stimulate the rising of Qi.

Acupuncture

Points

KI-3 Taixi, BL-23 Shenshu, BL-52 Zhishi, Du-20 Baihui, Du-24 Shenting, Ren-6 Qihai, Du-16 Fengfu. Reinforcing method.

Explanation

- KI-3, BL-23 and BL-52 tonify the Kidneys, strengthen Will-Power, promote memory and nourish Marrow.
- Du-20 and Du-24 facilitate the rising of clear Yang to the head.
- Ren-6 with direct moxa tonifies Yang.
- Du-16, point of the Sea of Marrow, nourishes Marrow.

Herbal therapy

Prescription

SHI BU WAN
Ten Tonifications Pill

Explanation

This formula tonifies the Kidneys and nourishes Marrow.

> **SUMMARY**
>
> **Kidney-Yang deficiency (Deficiency of Sea of Marrow)**
>
> *Points*
>
> KI-3 Taixi, BL-23 Shenshu, BL-52 Zhishi, Du-20 Baihui, Du-24 Shenting, Ren-6 Qihai, Du-16 Fengfu. Reinforcing method.
>
> *Herbal therapy*
>
> *Prescription*
>
> **SHI BU WAN**
> *Ten Tonifications Pill*

APPENDIX 3 POOR MEMORY

In Chinese medicine, memory depends on the state of the Spleen, Kidneys and Heart, and there is a considerable overlap among these three organs' functions.

The Spleen houses Intellect and influences memory in the sense of memorization, studying and concentrating. Its corresponding pathological aspect is excessive thinking and pensiveness.

The Kidneys house Will-Power (*Zhi*) and influence the brain, since the Kidney-Essence produces Marrow which nourishes the brain. As mentioned above, besides meaning "will-power", *Zhi* also means "memory". The Kidneys are responsible for memory in the sense of memorization of both recent and long-past events.

The Heart controls memory because it houses the Mind (*Shen*). There is a considerable overlap between the Kidneys and Heart with regard to memory, but the Heart is responsible more for the memory of recent events (but not exclusively) and also remembering faces, names, etc. The Heart is also responsible for absent-mindedness, forgetting where one has put one's keys, leaving the front door open, etc.

Indeed, memory depends primarily on the *communication* between the Heart and Kidneys. The Heart is above and houses the Mind (*Shen*) and the Kidneys are below and house the Essence (*Jing*) and memory (*Zhi*). One of the functions of the Mind of the Heart is memory and consciousness, and this faculty needs to descend towards the Kidneys. On the other hand, the Kidney-Essence and *Zhi* need to ascend towards the Heart and Brain. When this communication takes place, Essence can generate Qi; Qi, in turn, can generate the Mind and memory is good.

Thus, the Kidneys control memory in two ways: by its *Zhi* reaching the Heart and the Mind, and by its Essence reaching the Brain.

Besides the Heart and Kidneys, memory also relies on the Spleen and its Intellect (*Yi*). The Heart controls the memory of past events, the Kidneys that of everyday events and the Spleen the capacity of memorizing in the course of study.

Chapter 8 of the *Spiritual Axis* clearly refers to the relationship between Heart, Spleen and Kidneys in memory: "*The recollection of the Heart is called Intellect (Yi -Spleen); the storage of memory by the Intellect is called Zhi (of the Kidneys).*"[59] The Yi Xue Ji Cheng says:[60]

With regard to poor memory, in the elderly the Essence dries up; in the young, worry, pensiveness and overwork weaken the Heart. [To strengthen memory] *One must promote the communication between Heart and Kidneys, reinforce the Spleen and harmonize Qi and Blood.*

ETIOLOGY

Worry and pensiveness

Worry and pensiveness affect Lungs, Spleen and Heart, and they influence memory simply because the Spleen and Heart's mental capacity is employed in worrying and obsessive thinking and cannot therefore be used for memorization.

Overwork and excessive sexual activity

Overwork and excessive sexual activity (primarily in men) weaken Kidney-Yin and Kidney-Essence, which decreases mental power and memory.

Childbirth

Excessive bleeding at childbirth weakens Blood and affects the Heart. Deficient Heart-Blood is unable to nourish the brain and the Mind, and poor memory results.

Sadness

Sadness depletes Heart-Qi so that this cannot brighten the Mind and poor memory results.

"Recreational" drugs

Prolonged and continued use of cannabis and other drugs is an important cause of poor memory and concentration. It would appear that the conversion of short-term to long-term memory is impaired by prolonged use of cannabis due to interference by a flow of sensory impressions.[61] Moreover, there have also been reports of loss of brain substance in heavy users of cannabis.[62] I have certainly verified the relationship between heavy, long-term use of cannabis and poor memory in my clinical practice.

SUMMARY

Etiology of poor memory
- Worry and pensiveness
- Overwork and excessive sexual activity
- Childbirth
- Sadness
- "Recreational" drugs

IDENTIFICATION OF PATTERNS AND TREATMENT

Spleen deficiency

Clinical manifestations

Inability to concentrate and study, poor memory, tiredness, poor appetite.

Tongue: Pale.

Pulse: Weak.

Treatment principle

Tonify the Spleen and strengthen the Intellect (*Yi*).

Acupuncture

Points

ST-36 Zusanli, SP-3 Taibai, Du-20 Baihui, BL-15 Xinshu, Du-14 Dazhui with moxa, BL-20 Pishu, BL-49 Yishe. Reinforcing method.

Explanation

- ST-36 and SP-3 tonify the Spleen and strengthen the Intellect.
- Du-20 raises clear Yang to the head to brighten the Mind and Intellect.
- BL-15, Back-Transporting point of the Heart, strengthens the Mind and the Intellect.
- Du-14 with moxa also facilitates the rising of clear Yang to the brain.
- BL-20 and BL-49 tonify the Spleen and strengthen the Intellect and memory.

Herbal therapy

Prescription

GUI PI TANG
Tonifying the Spleen Decoction

Explanation

This formula tonifies Heart-Qi and Heart-Blood and therefore strengthens the Mind and memory.

SUMMARY

Spleen deficiency

Points

ST-36 Zusanli, SP-3 Taibai, Du-20 Baihui, BL-15 Xinshu, Du-14 Dazhui with moxa, BL-20 Pishu, BL-49 Yishe. Reinforcing method.

Herbal therapy

Prescription

GUI PI TANG
Tonifying the Spleen Decoction

Kidney-Essence deficiency

Clinical manifestations

Poor memory of both recent and past events, dizziness, tinnitus, weak knees and back.

Tongue: Pale in case of Kidney-Yang deficiency; without coating in case of Kidney-Yin deficiency.

Pulse: Deep and Weak.

Treatment principle

Tonify the Kidneys, nourish Essence and Marrow and strengthen memory.

Acupuncture

Points

KI-3 Taixi, Ren-4 Guanyuan, BL-23 Shenshu, BL-52 Zhishi, BL-15 Xinshu, Du-20 Baihui. Reinforcing method.

Explanation

- KI-3, Ren-4 and BL-23 tonify the Kidneys.
- BL-52 strengthens the Will-Power and memory.
- BL-15 strengthens the Mind and memory.
- Du-20 facilitates the rising of clear Yang to the head.

Herbal therapy

Prescription

LIU WEI DI HUANG WAN Variation
Six-Ingredient Rehmannia Pill Variation

Explanation

The variation of this formula tonifies the Kidneys, strengthens Marrow and promotes memory.

Modifications

- If there is both Yin and Yang deficiency, add Lu Jiao Jiao *Gelatinum Cornu Cervi*, Ba Ji Tian *Radix Morindae officinalis* and Zi He Che *Placenta hominis*.

SUMMARY

Kidney-Essence deficiency

Points

KI-3 Taixi, Ren-4 Guanyuan, BL-23 Shenshu, BL-52 Zhishi, BL-15 Xinshu, Du-20 Baihui. Reinforcing method.

Herbal therapy

Prescription

LIU WEI DI HUANG WAN Variation
Six-Ingredient Rehmannia Pill Variation

Heart deficiency

Clinical manifestations

Poor memory of both recent and past events, forgetting names, absent-mindedness, palpitations, slight breathlessness on exertion, tiredness.

Tongue: Pale or Red, depending whether there is Yang or Yin deficiency.

Pulse: Weak.

Treatment principle

Tonify the Heart, strengthen the Mind and memory.

Acupuncture

Points

HE-5 Tongli, BL-15 Xinshu, BL-44 Shentang, Ren-6 Qihai, Du-14 Dazhui, with reinforcing method. If Phlegm obstructs the Heart, use ST-40 Fenglong and Ren-14 Juque with reducing method.

Explanation

- HE-5 and BL-15 tonify Heart-Qi and strengthen the Mind.
- BL-44 strengthens the Mind and memory.
- Ren-6 with moxa tonifies Qi in general.
- Du-14 with moxa tonifies the Heart and brightens the Mind. It is coordinated with Ren-6: one is on the Directing Vessel (*Ren Mai*), the other on the Governing Vessel (*Du Mai*), both of which flow through the Heart.
- ST- 40 and Ren-14 resolve Phlegm from the Heart.

Herbal therapy

Prescription

ZHEN ZHONG DAN
Bedside Pill

Explanation

This formula could also be used for poor memory from other Heart patterns such as Heart Empty Heat.

SUMMARY

Heart deficiency

Points

HE-5 Tongli, BL-15 Xinshu, BL-44 Shentang, Ren-6 Qihai, Du-14 Dazhui, with reinforcing method. If Phlegm obstructs the Heart, use ST-40 Fenglong and Ren-14 Juque with reducing method.

Herbal therapy

Prescription

ZHEN ZHONG DAN
Bedside Pill

END NOTES

1. 1979 Huang Di Nei Jing Su Wen 黄帝内经素问 [The Yellow Emperor's Classic of Internal Medicine – Simple Questions]. People's Health Publishing House, Beijing, p. 256. First published c.100 BC.
2. Tang Zong Hai 1892 Zhong Xi Hui Tong Yi Jing Jing Yi [The Essence of the Convergence between Chinese and Western

Medicine], cited in Wang Ke Qin 1988 Zhong Yi Shen Zhu Xue Shuo 中医神主学说 [Theory of the Mind in Chinese Medicine]. Ancient Chinese Medical Texts Publishing House, Beijing, p. 36.
3. 1986 Jing Yue Quan Shu 京岳全书[The Complete Book of Jing Yue]. Shanghai Scientific Publishing House, Shanghai, p. 329. The *Complete Book of Jing Yue* was written by Zhang Jing Yue and first published in 1624.
4. Ibid., p. 329.
5. 1981 Ling Shu Jing 灵书经 [Spiritual Axis]. People's Health Publishing House, Beijing, p. 51. First published c.100 BC.
6. Gu Yu Qi 2005 Zhong Yi Xin Li Xue 中医心理学[Chinese Medicine Psychology]. China Medicine Science and Technology Publishing House, Beijing, p. 46.
7. Spiritual Axis, p. 152.
8. Ibid., p. 56.
9. Simple Questions, p. 102.
10. Ibid., p. 102.
11. Ibid., p. 102.
12. Ibid., p. 102.
13. Ibid., p. 102.
14. Ibid., p. 102.
15. Ibid., p. 102.
16. Ibid., p. 102.
17. Ibid., p. 102.
18. Ibid., p. 102.
19. Ibid., p. 103.
20. Ibid., p. 569.
21. Ibid., p. 569.
22. Spiritual Axis, p. 84.
23. Ibid., p. 84.
24. Simple Questions, p. 569.
25. Ibid., p. 569.
26. Spiritual Axis, p. 85.
27. Simple Questions, p. 569.
28. Ibid., p. 569.
29. Spiritual Axis, p. 85.
30. Ibid., p. 85.
31. Simple Questions, p. 569.
32. Ibid., p. 569.
33. Spiritual Axis, p. 85.
34. Ibid., p. 85.
35. Simple Questions, p. 569.
36. Ibid., p. 569.
37. Spiritual Axis, p. 85.
38. Ibid., p. 85.
39. Ibid., p. 85.
40. Ibid., p. 85.
41. Ibid., p. 85.
42. Ibid., p. 85.
43. Ibid., p. 85.
44. Ibid., p. 85.
45. Simple Questions, p. 256.
46. Ibid., p. 199.
47. Spiritual Axis, p. 56.
48. Simple Questions, p. 199.
49. Spiritual Axis, p. 24.
50. Fang Wen Xian 1989 Zhong Yi Nei Ke Zheng Zhuang Bian Zhi Shou Ce 中医内科证状辨治手册 [A Manual of New Treatment of Internal Medicine Diseases in Chinese Medicine]. Standard China Publishing House, Beijing, p. 75
51. 1979 Xue Zheng Lun 血证论 [Discussion on Blood Patterns]. People's Health Publishing House, Beijing, p. 29. The Discussion on Blood Patterns was written by Tang Zong Hai and first published in 1884.
52. Wilhelm R (translator) 1962 The Secret of the Golden Flower. Harcourt, Brace & World, New York, p. 26.
53. Ibid., p. 26.
54. Chinese Medicine Psychology, p. 35.
55. Theory of the Mind in Chinese Medicine, pp. 94–95.
56. Chinese Medicine Psychology, p. 48.
57. Ibid., p. 51.
58. Spiritual Axis, p. 152.
59. Ibid., p. 23.
60. Cited in Zhou Chao Fan 2000 Li Dai Zhong Yi Zhi Ze Jing Hua 历代中医治则精华 [Essential Chinese Medicine Treatment Principles in Successive Dynasties]. Chinese Herbal Medicine Publishing House, Beijing, p. 456.
61. Laurence DR 1973 Clinical Pharmacology. Churchill Livingstone, Edinburgh, p. 14.29.
62. Ibid., p. 14.30.

癫狂

CHAPTER 19

BIPOLAR DISORDER (MANIC-DEPRESSION) (DULLNESS AND MANIA, *DIAN KUANG*)

BIPOLAR DISORDER IN WESTERN MEDICINE *498*

Symptoms of bipolar disorder *498*

Diagnosis of bipolar disorder *500*

Course of bipolar disorder *501*

Treatment of bipolar disorder *501*

History *502*

BIPOLAR DISORDER IN CHINESE MEDICINE *503*

Historical development of *Dian Kuang* in Chinese medicine *503*

Correspondences and differences between bipolar disorder and *Dian Kuang* *504*

Pathology of *Dian Kuang* *506*

ETIOLOGY OF *DIAN KUANG* *508*

Emotional stress *508*

Diet *508*

Constitution *508*

PATHOLOGY AND TREATMENT PRINCIPLES OF *DIAN KUANG* *509*

Pathology of *Dian Kuang* *509*

Treatment principles for *Dian Kuang* *511*

How to adapt the patterns and treatment of *Dian Kuang* to the treatment of bipolar disorder *513*

ACUPUNCTURE TREATMENT *514*

Points that open the Mind's orifices *514*

Sun Si Miao's 13 ghost points *515*

The Pericardium channel in Manic-Depression *515*

IDENTIFICATION OF PATTERNS AND TREATMENT *516*

Dian *516*

Qi stagnation and Phlegm *516*

Heart and Spleen deficiency with Phlegm *518*

Qi deficiency with Phlegm *519*

Phlegm obstructing the Heart orifices *520*

Kuang *521*

Phlegm-Fire harassing upwards *521*

Fire in Bright Yang *524*

Gall Bladder- and Liver-Fire *524*

Fire injuring Yin with Phlegm *525*

Qi stagnation, Blood stasis, Phlegm *526*

Yin deficiency with Empty Heat *527*

MODERN CHINESE LITERATURE *528*

CLINICAL TRIALS *532*

DIAN

- Qi stagnation and Phlegm
- Heart and Spleen deficiency with Phlegm
- Qi deficiency with Phlegm
- Knotted Heat in the Heart channel
- Phlegm obstructing the Heart orifices

KUANG

- Phlegm-Fire harassing upwards
- Fire in Bright Yang
- Gall Bladder- and Liver-Fire
- Fire injuring Yin with Phlegm
- Qi stagnation, Blood stasis, Phlegm
- Yin deficiency with Empty Heat

BIPOLAR DISORDER (MANIC-DEPRESSION)

Bipolar disorder, also called manic-depression, is a serious mental illness. The discussion of this disease will be conducted according to the following topics.

- Bipolar disorder in Western medicine
- Bipolar disorder in Chinese Medicine
- Etiology of *Dian Kuang*
- Pathology and treatment principles of *Dian Kuang*
- Acupuncture treatment
- Identification of patterns and treatment
- Modern Chinese literature
- Clinical trials

BIPOLAR DISORDER IN WESTERN MEDICINE

Bipolar disorder, also known as manic-depressive illness, is a serious medical illness that causes shifts in a person's mood, energy and ability to function.

More than 2 million American adults, or about 1% of the population age 18 and older in any given year, have bipolar disorder.[1] Bipolar disorder typically develops in late adolescence or early adulthood.

Symptoms of bipolar disorder

Bipolar disorder causes dramatic mood swings – from overly "high" and/or irritable to sad and hopeless, and then back again, often with periods of normal mood in between. Severe changes in energy and behavior go along with these changes in mood. The periods of highs and lows are called episodes of mania and depression, respectively. Previously called manic-depression, this disease is now called bipolar disorder.

Signs and symptoms of *mania* (or a *manic episode*) include:

- elevated and expansive mood (also paranoid or irritable)
- increased energy, activity and restlessness
- excessively "high" euphoric mood
- extreme irritability
- racing thoughts and talking very fast, jumping from one idea to another
- distractibility, inability to concentrate
- extreme impatience
- little sleep needed
- rapid, excitable and intrusive speech
- fast thinking, moving quickly from topic to topic
- unrealistic beliefs in one's abilities and powers
- grandiosity
- chaotic patterns of personal and professional relationships
- impulsive involvement in questionable endeavors
- reckless driving, excessive risk-taking
- certainty of conviction about the correctness and importance of their ideas
- poor judgment
- spending sprees
- a lasting period of behavior that is different from usual
- intense and impulsive romantic or sexual liaisons
- increased sexual drive
- abuse of drugs, particularly cocaine, alcohol and sleeping medications
- provocative, intrusive or aggressive behavior
- denial that anything is wrong
- in its extreme forms, violent agitation, bizarre behavior, delusional thinking, visual and auditory hallucinations.

A manic episode is diagnosed if elevated mood occurs with three or more of the other symptoms most of the day, nearly every day, for 1 week or longer. If the mood is irritable, four additional symptoms must be present.

SUMMARY

Symptoms of mania

- Elevated and expansive mood (also paranoid or irritable)
- Increased energy, activity, and restlessness
- Excessively "high" euphoric mood
- Extreme irritability
- Racing thoughts and talking very fast, jumping from one idea to another
- Distractibility, inability to concentrate
- Extreme impatience
- Little sleep needed
- Rapid, excitable and intrusive speech
- Fast thinking, moving quickly from topic to topic
- Unrealistic beliefs in one's abilities and powers

- Grandiosity
- Chaotic patterns of personal and professional relationships
- Impulsive involvement in questionable endeavors
- Reckless driving, excessive risk-taking
- Certainty of conviction about the correctness and importance of their ideas
- Poor judgment
- Spending sprees
- A lasting period of behavior that is different from usual
- Intense and impulsive romantic or sexual liaisons
- Increased sexual drive
- Abuse of drugs, particularly cocaine, alcohol and sleeping medications
- Provocative, intrusive or aggressive behavior
- Denial that anything is wrong
- In its extreme forms, violent agitation, bizarre behavior, delusional thinking, visual and auditory hallucinations

SUMMARY

Symptoms of depressive phase of bipolar disorder

- Apathy, lethargy
- Lasting sad, anxious or empty mood
- Slowed physical movement
- Feelings of hopelessness or pessimism
- Feelings of guilt, worthlessness or helplessness
- Loss of interest or pleasure in activities once enjoyed, including sex
- Decreased energy, a feeling of fatigue or of being "slowed down"
- Difficulty concentrating, remembering, making decisions
- Restlessness or irritability
- Sleeping too much or insomnia
- Change in appetite and/or unintended weight loss or gain
- Chronic pain or other persistent bodily symptoms that are not caused by physical illness or injury
- Thoughts of death or suicide, or suicide attempts

Signs and symptoms of *depression* (or a *depressive episode*) include:

- apathy, lethargy
- lasting sad, anxious or empty mood
- slowed physical movement
- feelings of hopelessness or pessimism
- feelings of guilt, worthlessness or helplessness
- loss of interest or pleasure in activities once enjoyed, including sex
- decreased energy, a feeling of fatigue or of being "slowed down"
- difficulty concentrating, remembering, making decisions
- restlessness or irritability
- sleeping too much or insomnia
- change in appetite and/or unintended weight loss or gain
- chronic pain or other persistent bodily symptoms that are not caused by physical illness or injury
- thoughts of death or suicide, or suicide attempts.

A depressive episode is diagnosed if five or more of these symptoms last most of the day, nearly every day, for a period of 2 weeks or longer.

A mild to moderate level of mania is called *hypomania*. Hypomania may feel good to the person who experiences it and may even be associated with good functioning and enhanced productivity. Thus, even when family and friends learn to recognize the mood swings as possible bipolar disorder, the person may deny that anything is wrong. Without proper treatment, however, hypomania can become severe mania in some people or can switch into depression.

Occasionally, severe episodes of mania or depression include symptoms of psychosis (or psychotic symptoms). Common psychotic symptoms are hallucinations (auditory or visual) and delusions.

Psychotic symptoms in bipolar disorder tend to reflect the extreme mood state at the time. For example, delusions of grandiosity, such as believing one is Jesus Christ or has special powers or wealth, may occur during mania; delusions of guilt or worthlessness, such as believing that one is ruined and penniless or has committed some terrible crime, may appear during depression. People with bipolar disorder who have these symptoms are sometimes incorrectly diagnosed as having schizophrenia.

Redfield Jamison lists six criteria for the diagnosis of a manic episode, as follows.

A. A distinct period of abnormally and persistently elevated, expansive or irritable mood.
B. At least three of the following symptoms:
   - Inflated self-esteem or grandiosity
   - Decreased need for sleep
   - More talkative than usual
   - Flight of ideas, thoughts racing
   - Distractibility
   - Increase in goal-directed activity (social, work, school, sexual), psychomotor agitation
   - Excessive involvement in pleasurable activities (buying spree, sexual indiscretions, foolish business investments).
C. Mood disturbance (severe).
D. No delusions or hallucinations.
E. Not superimposed on schizophrenia, delusional disorder, psychotic disorder.
F. No organic factor.

(A) plus (B) plus (C) constitutes a manic syndrome, while (A) plus (B) constitutes hypomania.[2]

It may be helpful to think of the various mood states in bipolar disorder as a spectrum or continuous range. In the depressive phase, at one end is severe depression, below which is moderate depression and then mild low mood, which is termed "dysthymia" when it is chronic. In the manic phase, there is normal or balanced mood, above which comes hypomania (mild to moderate mania) and then severe mania (Fig. 19.1).

In some people, however, symptoms of mania and depression may occur together in what is called a mixed bipolar state. Symptoms of a mixed state often include agitation, trouble sleeping, significant change in appetite, psychosis and suicidal thinking. A person may have a very sad, hopeless mood while at the same time feeling extremely energized.

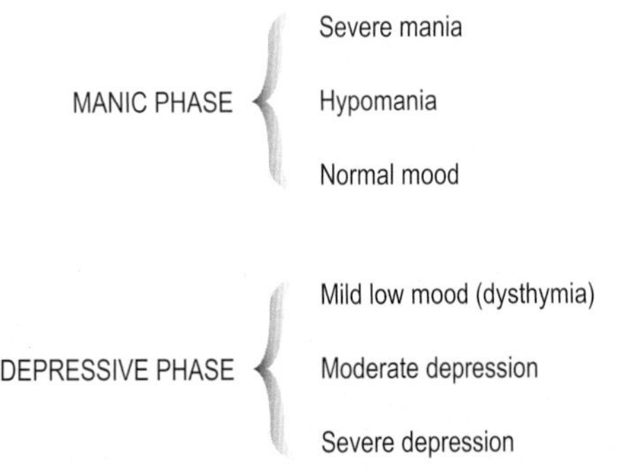

Figure 19.1 Range of mental disturbance between severe mania and severe depression.

Cyclothymia is a milder form of manic-depression, with swings between depression and hypomania. Cyclothymic temperament can be manifested in different ways, i.e. as predominantly depressive, manic, hypomanic or irritable. There are swings between cheerfulness and unhappiness. Not all individuals who have cyclothymia go on to develop the full manic-depressive syndrome, but many do. One out of three persons with cyclothymia goes on to develop full-blown manic-depression.

Redfield Jamison lists five criteria for the diagnosis of cyclothymia, as follows.[3]

A. Numerous hypomanic episodes for 2 years and numerous periods of depressed mood that did not meet the criteria for a major depressive episode.
B. Never without hypomanic or depressive symptoms for 2 years for more than 2 months at a time.
C. No major depressive episode or manic episode.
D. Not superimposed on psychotic disorder.
E. No organic factor.

Diagnosis of bipolar disorder

A diagnosis of bipolar disorder is made on the basis of symptoms, course of illness and, when available, family history. The diagnostic criteria for bipolar disorder are described in the Diagnostic and Statistical Manual for Mental Disorders, 4th edition (DSM-IV).[4]

Descriptions offered by people with bipolar disorder give valuable insights into the various mood states associated with the illness.

Depression

"I doubt completely my ability to do anything well. It seems as though my mind has slowed down and burned out to the point of being virtually useless ... [I am] *haunt*[ed] *... with the total, the desperate hopelessness of it all ... Others say, 'It's only temporary, it will pass, you will get over it,' but of course they haven't any idea of how I feel, although they are certain they do. If I can't feel, move, think or care, then what on earth is the point?"*

Hypomania

"At first when I'm high, it's tremendous ... ideas are fast ... like shooting stars you follow until brighter ones appear ... All shyness disappears, the right words and gestures are suddenly there ... uninteresting people, things become intensely interesting. Sensuality is pervasive, the desire to seduce and be seduced is irresistible. Your marrow is infused

with unbelievable feelings of ease, power, well-being, omnipotence, euphoria ... you can do anything ... but, somewhere this changes."

Mania

"The fast ideas become too fast and there are far too many ... overwhelming confusion replaces clarity ... you stop keeping up with it – memory goes. Infectious humour ceases to amuse. Your friends become frightened ... everything is now against the grain ... you are irritable, angry, frightened, uncontrollable, and trapped."[5]

The following is a description of a manic attack by Redfield Jamison: *"At first, everything seemed so easy. I raced about like a crazed weasel, bubbling with plans and enthusiasm, immersed in sports, staying up all night, night after night, out with friends, reading everything that wasn't nailed down, filling manuscript books with poems, and fragments of plays, and making expansive, completely unrealistic plans for my future."*[6]

The following is a description of a depressive phase: *"Then the bottom became to fall out of my life and mind. My thinking, far from being clearer than a crystal, was tortuous. I would read the same passage over and over again only to realize that I had no memory at all for what I had just read. Each book or poem I picked up was the same way. Incomprehensible, nothing made sense."*[7]

Course of bipolar disorder

Episodes of mania and depression typically recur across the life span. Between episodes, most people with bipolar disorder are free of symptoms, but as many as one-third of people have some residual symptoms. A small percentage of people experience chronic unremitting symptoms despite treatment.

The classic form of the illness, which involves recurrent episodes of mania and depression, is called *bipolar I disorder*. Some people, however, never develop severe mania but instead experience milder episodes of hypomania that alternate with depression; this form of the illness is called *bipolar II disorder*. When four or more episodes of illness occur within a 12-month period, a person is said to have rapid-cycling bipolar disorder. Some people experience multiple episodes within a single week, or even within a single day. Rapid cycling tends to develop later in the course of illness and is more common among women than among men.

People with bipolar disorder can lead healthy and productive lives when the illness is effectively treated. Without treatment, however, the natural course of bipolar disorder tends to worsen. Over time a person may suffer more frequent (more rapid-cycling) and more severe manic and depressive episodes than those experienced when the illness first appeared. In most cases, however, proper treatment can help reduce the frequency and severity of episodes and can help people with bipolar disorder maintain good quality of life.

Treatment of bipolar disorder

Most people with bipolar disorder – even those with the most severe forms – can achieve substantial stabilization of their mood swings and related symptoms with proper treatment. Because bipolar disorder is a recurrent illness, long-term preventative treatment is strongly recommended and almost always indicated. A strategy that combines medication and psychosocial treatment is optimal for managing the disorder over time.

Medication

Medications known as "mood stabilizers" are usually prescribed to help control bipolar disorder. Several different types of mood stabilizer are available. In general, people with bipolar disorder continue treatment with mood stabilizers for extended periods of time (years). Other medications are added when necessary, typically for shorter periods, to treat episodes of mania or depression that break through despite the mood stabilizer. Medications for bipolar disorder include the following.

- *Lithium*, the first mood-stabilizing medication approved by the US Food and Drug Administration (FDA) for treatment of mania, is often very effective in controlling mania and preventing the recurrence of both manic and depressive episodes.
- *Anticonvulsant* medications, such as valproate (Depakote) or carbamazepine (Tegretol), also can have mood-stabilizing effects and may be especially useful for difficult-to-treat bipolar episodes.
- *Newer anticonvulsant* medications, including lamotrigine (Lamictal), gabapentin (Neurontin) and topiramate (Topamax), are being studied to determine how well they work in stabilizing mood cycles.

Generally, children and adolescents with bipolar disorder are treated with lithium, but valproate and carbamazepine also are used. There is some evidence that valproate may lead to adverse hormone changes in teenage girls and polycystic ovary syndrome in women who began taking the medication before age 20.[8] Therefore, young female patients taking valproate should be monitored carefully by a physician.

Research has shown that people with bipolar disorder are at risk of switching into mania or hypomania, or of developing rapid cycling, during treatment with antidepressant medication. Therefore, "mood-stabilizing" medications generally are required, alone or in combination with antidepressants, to protect people with bipolar disorder from this switch. Lithium and valproate are the most commonly used mood-stabilizing drugs today.

Atypical antipsychotic medications, including clozapine (Clozaril), olanzapine (Zyprexa), risperidone (Risperdal), quetiapine (Seroquel) and ziprasidone (Geodon), are being studied as possible treatments for bipolar disorder.

Psychosocial treatments

As an addition to medication, psychosocial treatments – including certain forms of psychotherapy – are helpful in providing support, education and guidance to people with bipolar disorder and their families. Studies have shown that psychosocial interventions can lead to increased mood stability, fewer hospitalizations and improved functioning in several areas.

A licensed psychologist, social worker or counselor typically provides these therapies and often works together with the psychiatrist to monitor a patient's progress. The number, frequency and type of sessions should be based on the treatment needs of each person. Psychosocial interventions commonly used for bipolar disorder are cognitive behavioral therapy, psychoeducation, family therapy and a newer technique, interpersonal and social rhythm therapy.

- *Cognitive behavioral therapy* helps people with bipolar disorder to learn to change inappropriate or negative thought patterns and behaviors associated with the illness.
- *Psychoeducation* involves teaching people with bipolar disorder about the illness and its treatment, and how to recognize signs of relapse so that early intervention can be sought before a full-blown illness episode occurs. Psychoeducation may also be helpful for family members.
- *Family therapy* uses strategies to reduce the level of distress within the family that may either contribute to or result from the ill person's symptoms.
- *Interpersonal and social rhythm therapy* helps people with bipolar disorder both to improve interpersonal relationships and to regularize their daily routines. Regular daily routines and sleep schedules may help protect against manic episodes.

History

Aretaeus of Cappadocia (2nd century AD) was probably the first doctor who correlated melancholia with mania: "*Melancholia is without any doubt the beginning and even part of the disorder called mania.*"[9]

Alexander of Tralles (AD 57) said: "*Mania is nothing else but melancholia in a more intense form.*"[10]

Jason Pratensis (16th century) said: "*Most physicians associate mania and melancholia as one disorder.*"[11] He distinguished mania and melancholia by *degree and manifestation* only.

Dr Thomas Willis (17th century) said:[12]

In the melancholic ... the spirits were sombre and dim; they cast their shadows over the images of things and formed a kind of dark tide; in the manic, on the contrary, the spirits seethed in a perpetual ferment; they were carried by an irregular movement, constantly repeated; a movement that eroded and consumed, and even without fever, sent out its heat. Between mania and melancholia, the affinity is evident; not the affinity of symptoms linked in experience, but the affinity – more powerful and so much more evident in the landscapes of the imagination – that unites in the same fire, both smoke and flame.

Richard Mead (1751) said:[13]

Two kinds of Madness ... the one is attended with audaciousness and fury, the other with sadness and fear; and that they call mania, this melancholy. But these generally differ in degree only. For melancholy very frequently changes, sooner or later, into maniacal madness, and, when the fury is abated, the sadness generally returns heavier than before.

Jean Pierre Falret and Jules Baillarger (mid 19th century) formally posited that mania and depression could represent different manifestations of a single illness.[14]

BIPOLAR DISORDER IN CHINESE MEDICINE

Bipolar disorder follows closely the symptoms of the ancient Chinese disease of *Dian Kuang*, which may be translated as "dullness and raving" or "dullness and mania".

The Chinese characters for *Dian Kuang* are 癫狂.

The character *Dian* is composed of the following parts:

- *Zhen* 真 indicates the Daoist ideal of "gentleman"
- *Ye* 页 is the top of the head through which the soul of the "gentleman" goes out
- *Bing* 疒 is the character for "disease". The "disease" character tells us it is a pathological state, i.e. soul leaving through the top of the head.

The character *Kuang* 狂 indicates the rambling of a mad dog.

Dian indicates a depressive state, indifference, being withdrawn, worry, unresponsiveness, incoherent speech, quiet, inappropriate laughter and taciturnity; *Kuang* indicates agitation, shouting, scolding and hitting people, irritability, aggressive behavior, offensive speech, inappropriate laughter, singing, climbing high places, wild behavior, smashing objects, unusual physical strength, and refusing sleep and food.

Historical development of *Dian Kuang* in Chinese medicine

The earliest mention of the term *Kuang* (mania) is in a non-medical text. The *Rites of Zhou* (1100 BC) says: "*Some people behave strangely in a manic [Kuang] way: this disease is called Mania [Kuang].*"[15]

The conditions of *Dian* and *Kuang* appear as early as in the *Yellow Emperor's Classic of Internal Medicine*. Chapter 74 of the *Simple Questions* says: "*The syndrome of irritable raving [Kuang] is due to Fire.*"[16] Chapter 46 of the *Simple Questions* says: "*Irritable raving is due to* [Excess] *Yang ... and is treated with the formula Sheng Tie Luo Yin.*"[17]

The *Spiritual Axis* says in Chapter 22:[18]

When Dian first appears, there is lack of joy, heavy and painful head, red eyes, eyes looking up. When Kuang first appears, there is little sleep, no hunger, glorification of the self as if one were the most knowledgeable person, shouting at people, no rest in day or night.

Chapter 59 of the *Classic of Difficulties* distinguishes *Dian* from *Kuang*:[19]

Kuang has a sudden onset, the person does not like to lie down or eat, has an inflated opinion of himself or herself, thinks he is wise and from a noble family, is arrogant, laughs and sings inappropriately, is restless and cannot stop. In Dian, the person is unhappy, lies down and stares straight ahead.

The *Classic of Difficulties* says in Chapter 20: "*Excess of Yin causes Dian, Excess of Yang causes Kuang.*"[20]

The *Essential Prescriptions of the Golden Chest* (AD 220) says:[21]

Excessive crying makes the Ethereal Soul and Corporeal Soul restless, Blood and Qi are depleted, when these are depleted the Heart is affected, Heart-Qi becomes deficient, the patient becomes fearful, the eyes close and want to sleep, there are excessive dreams which disperse the Spirit, and the Ethereal Soul and Corporeal Soul are agitated. If there is Yin deficiency, Depression [Dian] develops; if Yang deficiency, Mania [Kuang] develops.

Sun Si Miao describes *Dian Kuang* in his *Thousand Golden Ducats Prescriptions* (AD 652):[22]

In Dullness and Mania [Dian Kuang], the patient may be silent and emit no sound, speak incessantly, sing and cry, chant or laugh, sleep sitting in ditches, eat his or her own feces, discard clothes to be naked, sleep-walk, be angry and shout; these are symptoms of Dullness and Mania [Dian Kuang]. It must be treated with acupuncture and herbs.

A text from the Yuan dynasty attributes the development of *Kuang* to excess Fire and the disconnection between Heart and Kidneys: "*The Kidney Water controls the Will-Power [Zhi] and is in opposition with Fire; when Heart-Fire is exuberant, Kidney Water is depleted with the loss of Will-Power and the development of Mania [Kuang].*"[23] It also says: "*When Heart has Heat, the patient laughs and has Dian; when the Liver has Heat, the patient is angry and there is Kuang.*"[24]

The *Essential Methods of Dan Xi* (*Dan Xi Xin Fa*, 1347) says: "*Dian pertains to Yin and Kuang to Yang ... all cases are due to Phlegm stagnating in the space between the Heart and the chest.*"[25] Zhu Dan Xi was the first doctor who correlated the pathogenesis of *Dian Kuang* with Phlegm. In another passage, he clearly correlates the development of Manic-Depression to stagnation, Phlegm and Fire: "*The Fire of the five spirits* [i.e. Mind, Ethereal Soul, Corporeal Soul, Intellect and Will-Power] *is due to the arousal of the seven emotions and stagnation gives rise to Phlegm.*"[26]

The *Correct Transmission of Medicine* (*Yi Xue Zheng Chuan*) of the Ming dynasty confirms the association of Mania (*Kuang*) with Phlegm and Fire, and says:[27]

Mania [Kuang] is a Full condition due to Phlegm and Fire; Dullness [Dian] is due to Heart deficiency. To treat Mania, use the moving downward method; to treat Dullness calm the Mind and nourish Blood; in both cases eliminate Phlegm-Fire.

The last statement is interesting, as it confirms that Phlegm is central to the pathology of Manic-Depression and is present in both the manic and the depressive phases.

In the ancient literature, the differentiation between *Dian Kuang* and epilepsy is often not clear. Wang Ken Dang of the Ming dynasty was the first to make a clear differentiation between *Dian Kuang* and epilepsy.

The *Complete Book of Jing Yue* (*Jing Yue Quan Shu*, 1624) says: "*In Kuang the patient is always active and angry; in Dian, the patient is quiet and withdrawn as if he or she were unconscious.*"[28] In treatment, Zhang Jing Yue advocates first of all draining Fire as the principal method of treatment; secondarily, one must resolve Phlegm and move Qi.[29]

Wang Qing Ren in his *Corrections of Errors of Medical Circles* (*Yi Lin Gai Cuo*) attributes the pathology of *Dian Kuang* to Blood stasis:[30]

In Dian Kuang the patient cries, laughs, shouts, curses, sings. This is due to Qi and Blood stagnation in the Brain and to stagnation in the Internal Organs.

Correspondences and differences between bipolar disorder and *Dian Kuang*

Although the symptoms of *Dian Kuang* closely resemble those of bipolar disorder, we must always exercise caution when making direct connections between Western and Chinese medicine. As we shall see when we discuss the patterns of *Dian* and of *Kuang*, *Dian* does not exactly correspond to depression and *Kuang* does not exactly correspond to mania. For example, some of the manifestations of *Kuang* would fall under the category of generalized anxiety disorder.

In particular, the symptoms of *Dian* do not necessarily correspond exactly to the depressive phase of bipolar disorder. Moreover, the symptoms of *Dian* do not correspond to what we call "depression" in Western psychiatry. Modern Chinese books equate the symptoms of *Dian* with depression but I find this unhelpful. I maintain that, first, the pathology of depression is quite different from that of the depressive phase of bipolar disorder, and second, the symptoms of *Dian* are not necessarily or always those of the depressive phase of Manic-Depression. Indeed, especially *Dian* may correspond to some cases of schizophrenia.

CLINICAL NOTE

Please note that *Dian Kuang* does not necessarily correspond exactly to bipolar disorder. Indeed, especially *Dian* may correspond to some cases of schizophrenia.

Moreover, when discussing bipolar disorder, some modern books simply merge the patterns of Depression (*Yu Zheng*) with those of *Kuang* to offer a differentiation and treatment for this disease.[31] I personally think this is unhelpful.

It is worth noting that epilepsy (called *Dian Xian* in which "dian" is the same as in *Dian Kuang*) was wrongly classified with mental illnesses in ancient Chinese medicine. One particular modern Chinese doctor actually maintains that the word *Dian* in Chapter 22 of the *Spiritual Axis* refers to epilepsy and not to *Dian Kuang*.[32]

Indeed, the description of the symptoms of *Dian* from Chapter 22 of the *Spiritual Axis* (entitled *Dian Kuang*) sounds a lot more like epilepsy than those of the mental illness *Dian*:[33]

In the initial stages of Dian, the patient is unhappy, there is heaviness and pain of the head, with the eyes looking up ... in later stages, the patient has twitching of the mouth, crying out, panting and palpitations ... then the body is stiff and arched in the wrong direction, and there is pain in the spine.

Further on, the chapter seems to confirm that it is talking about tremors as it distinguishes three types of *Dian*, i.e. Bone *Dian*, Sinews *Dian* and Blood-Vessel *Dian*. Dr Zhang then says that, by contrast, the term *Kuang* in Chapter 22 of the *Spiritual Axis* includes both mental illnesses of *Dian* and *Kuang*.

> **CLINICAL NOTE**
>
> One modern Chinese doctor maintains that the word *Dian* in Chapter 22 of the *Spiritual Axis* refers to epilepsy and not to *Dian Kuang*.

To complicate matters further, the disease category of *Dian Kuang* may even correspond in some cases to schizophrenia in Western medicine. In fact, in a modern Chinese clinical trial, of the 30 patients suffering from *Dian Kuang* that were treated, 16 had a diagnosis of schizophrenia.[34] The modern book *Chinese Internal Medicine* confirms this possibility as, under the chapter of *Dian*, it reports the treatment of four cases of schizophrenia.[35]

People with schizophrenia may hear "voices" or believe that others are reading their minds, controlling their thoughts or plotting to harm them. These experiences are terrifying and can cause fearfulness, withdrawal or extreme agitation. People with schizophrenia may not make sense when they talk, may sit for hours without moving or talking much, or can seem perfectly fine until they talk about what they are really thinking. As can be seen, some of the manifestations may resemble those of *Dian*, e.g. fearfulness, withdrawal, sitting for hours without talking or moving.

The symptoms of schizophrenia fall into three broad categories.

- Positive symptoms are unusual thoughts or perceptions that include hallucinations, delusions and thought disorder.
- Negative symptoms represent a loss or a decrease in the ability to initiate plans, speak, express emotion or find pleasure in everyday life. These symptoms are harder to recognize as part of the disorder and can be mistaken for laziness or depression. Again, these may resemble those of *Dian*.
- Cognitive symptoms (or cognitive deficits) are problems with attention, certain types of memory and the executive functions that allow us to plan and organize.

The term "negative symptoms" refers to reductions in normal emotional and behavioral states, which include:

- flat affect (immobile facial expression, monotonous voice)
- lack of pleasure in everyday life
- diminished ability to initiate and sustain planned activity
- speaking infrequently, even when forced to interact.

As can be seen, the above "negative symptoms" of schizophrenia resemble those of *Dian*. Figure 19.2 summarizes the relationships between *Dian Kuang* and Western psychiatric disorders.

Therefore, although we must be careful in making direct connections between Western and Chinese medical disease entities, the formulae used for the treatment of *Dian Kuang* can be adapted to the treatment of bipolar disorder.

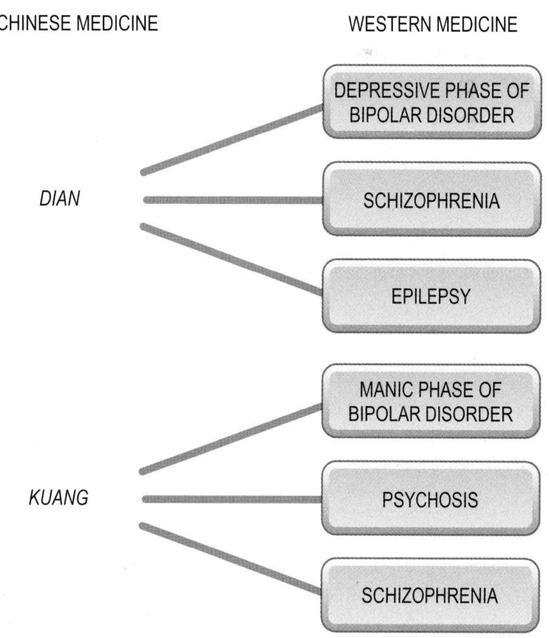

Figure 19.2 Relationships between *Dian Kuang* and Western psychiatric disorders.

SUMMARY

Correspondences and differences between bipolar disorder and *Dian Kuang*

In conclusion, I would summarize the main points regarding the correspondence between *Dian Kuang* and psychiatric diseases as follows.

1. *Dian Kuang* does not necessarily correspond exactly to bipolar disorder.
2. *Dian* is not depression as we intend it in Western psychiatry.
3. *Dian* could correspond to schizophrenia.
4. Epilepsy was often confused with *Dian* of *Dian Kuang* in the past.
5. *Dian Kuang* itself may correspond to schizophrenia.

Pathology of *Dian Kuang*

Disharmony of Yin and Yang

In *Dian Kuang* there is always a disharmony of Yin and Yang. Chapter 3 of the *Simple Questions* says: "*When Yin does not vanquish Yang, the pulse is Overflowing and there is Kuang.*"[36] Chapter 23 of the *Simple Questions* says: "*When pathogenic factors enter Yang, there is Kuang; when they enter Yin, Painful Obstruction syndrome.*"[37]

Chapter 20 of the *Classic of Difficulties* says: "*In Excess of Yang there is Kuang; in Excess of Yin, Dian.*"[38] The *Discussion of the Origin of Symptoms in Diseases* (*Zhu Bing Yuan Hou Lun*) (AD 610) says: "*When Qi merges with Yang, there is Kuang.*"[39]

Thus, as a broad generalization, we can say that in Mania there is an Excess of Yang such as Fire; in this condition, there is an Excess of Yang also in the sense that Yang is rising to the top of the body.

In Dullness, there is broadly speaking an Excess of Yin in the form of Phlegm and Qi stagnation. Of course, that is not to say that there is no Phlegm in Mania as there certainly is, but it is usually combined with Fire.

Phlegm

Central to the pathology of *Dian Kuang* is Phlegm and both the depressive and the manic phases are due to obstruction of the Mind by Phlegm. This is a major difference between the depressive phase of bipolar disorder (or *Dian Kuang*) – Dullness – and "Depression" (*Yu Zheng*, *see Chapter 16*). In Depression (*Yu Zheng*), there are many patterns without Phlegm. Moreover, the depressive and the manic phases of bipolar disorder, although so different from each other in their manifestations, are really two sides of the same coin. I therefore disagree with modern Chinese books which, when describing the symptoms of Depression (*Yu Zheng*), list many of the symptoms of the depressive phase (*Dian*) of *Dian Kuang*.

CLINICAL NOTE

Phlegm is central to the pathology of bipolar disorder (and of *Dian Kuang*) in both its manic and depressive phases.

As there is Phlegm, bipolar disorder is, by definition, a case of Mind Obstructed, while Depression (*Yu Zheng*) is seldom so.

CLINICAL NOTE

The "depression" of the depressive phase of bipolar disorder is different from that of "Depression": in bipolar disorder, the Mind is Obstructed by definition; in Depression, it is only seldom so.

Fire harassing upwards

The constraint of Qi-induced emotional stress usually leads to Heat and Fire. In Manic-Depression, there is nearly always Fire which, together with Phlegm, accounts for the rash behavior during the manic phase. As we have seen above, all the old texts attribute *Kuang* to Fire and Excess of Yang. Fire combines with Phlegm and it harasses upwards to agitate the Mind while the Phlegm obstructs it.

The Fire harassing upwards derives primarily from the Liver and Heart.

Qi stagnation and Blood stasis

The Qi stagnation caused by emotional stress in time leads to Blood stasis; this is a feature of chronic cases of Manic-Depression and one that complicates the conditions of Phlegm and Fire.

Disharmony of the "coming and going" of the Ethereal Soul (*Hun*)

It is also my opinion that, in bipolar disorder (and in *Dian Kuang*), the primary aspect is the manic phase, and the depressive phase is merely a reaction to it.[40] This means that, contrary to what happens in Depression (*Yu Zheng*), in bipolar disorder (and in *Dian Kuang*) the essential pathology is the excessive "coming and going" of the Ethereal Soul, even in its depressive phase (see below).

As described in Chapters 3 and 16, the Ethereal Soul gives the Mind inspiration, creativity, ideas, plans, life dreams and aspirations; this psychic energy is the result of the "coming and going of the Ethereal Soul" and it is the psychic manifestation of the free flow of Liver-Qi (and, in particular, of the physiological ascending of Liver-Qi).

On the other hand, the Mind needs to control the Ethereal Soul somewhat and to integrate the psychic material deriving from it. It is in the nature of the Ethereal Soul to "come and go", i.e. it is always searching, it has ideas, inspiration, aims, etc. The Mind needs to integrate the material deriving from the Ethereal Soul into the general psyche: the Ethereal Soul is the source of many ideas simultaneously; the Mind can only deal with one at a time. Therefore "control" and "integration" are the key words describing the function of the Mind in relation to the Ethereal Soul (*see Fig. 3.15*).

When the "coming and going" of the Ethereal Soul is deficient, there is a lack of inspiration, creativity, ideas, plans, life dreams and aspirations; this is an important feature of mental depression. In severe depression, there is a disconnection between the Mind (*Shen* of the Heart) and Ethereal Soul (*Hun*); the Ethereal Soul lacks its normal "movement" and the person lacks creativity, ideas, imagination and, most of all, plans, projects, life aims and inspiration so that depression results.

When the movement of the Ethereal Soul is excessive by itself, or because the Mind is weak and fails to restrain and control it, this may be too restless and its "movement" excessive; this will only bring confusion and chaos to the Mind, making the person scattered, unsettled and slightly manic. This can be observed in some people who are always full of ideas, dreams and projects, none of which ever comes to fruition because of the chaotic state of the Mind, which is therefore unable to restrain the Ethereal Soul. Figure 3.15 illustrates the two situations when the "coming and going" of the Ethereal Soul is excessive, either by itself (on the left side) or because the Mind does not control it enough (on the right side).

If the movement of the Ethereal Soul is excessive, contents breaking through from the Ethereal Soul cannot be integrated by the Mind. The Mind should integrate the Ethereal Soul so that images, symbols and dreams coming from it can be assimilated. When the "coming and going" of the Ethereal Soul is excessive, there is a steady and excessive stream of ideas, inspiration and plans flooding the Mind; in serious cases, this can lead to mania.

Degrees of "mania"

The important thing to realize is that mania and manic behavior can occur in many degrees of severity, i.e. the border between "mental illness" and "normality" is not a clear-cut separation. There is, however, a broad area of behaviors that, while not normal, do not constitute "mental illness". In other words, in its milder forms, "mania" and "manic behavior" are relatively common; these are states of "mania" that are even below that represented by hypomania. Whenever the "coming and going" of the Ethereal Soul is excessive, there is the possibility of "manic" behavior.

Thus, in mania, there is always an excessive movement of the Ethereal Soul.

CLINICAL NOTE

Mania and manic behavior can occur in many degrees of severity, i.e. the border between "mental illness" and "normality" is not a clear-cut separation between the two. There is, however, a broad area of behaviors that, while not normal, do not constitute "mental illness". In other words, in its milder forms, "mania" and "manic behavior" are relatively common. Whenever the "coming and going" of the Ethereal Soul is excessive, there is the possibility of "manic" behavior.

My own criteria for diagnosing mild "mania" (i.e. in normal people who are not mentally ill and below the level of hypomania) are as follows.

- Mental restlessness, agitation
- Hyperactivity
- Working and being active at night
- Spending a lot

- Having many projects simultaneously, none of which comes to fruition
- Mental confusion
- Obsessive thoughts
- Laughing a lot
- Talking a lot
- Propensity to take risks
- Often artistic

SUMMARY

Symptoms of mild "mania" in normal individuals

- Mental restlessness, agitation
- Hyperactivity
- Working and being active at night
- Spending a lot
- Having many projects simultaneously, none of which comes to fruition
- Mental confusion
- Obsessive thoughts
- Laughing a lot
- Talking a lot
- Propensity to take risks
- Often artistic

It is interesting to note that people suffering from bipolar disorder are often artistic. Or to put it differently, among famous artists there is a disproportionate incidence of bipolar disorder.[41] This is due to the fact that the artistic inspiration derives from the Ethereal Soul; therefore, the same psychic energy of the Ethereal Soul that makes someone artistic, in pathological conditions, may also make them mentally ill.

During manic episodes, the bipolar patient is bristling with ideas, he or she is inspired, feelings intensify, sensations are keener and he or she often writes poetry.[42]

SUMMARY

Pathology of *Dian Kuang*

To summarize, the main elements of the pathology of Manic-Depression are:

- disharmony of Yin and Yang
- Phlegm
- Fire harassing upwards
- Qi stagnation and Blood stasis
- disharmony of the Ethereal Soul.

ETIOLOGY OF *DIAN KUANG*

Emotional stress

Emotional stress is the main etiological factor of bipolar disorder. Anger, worry, excess joy and guilt may all be the initial cause of this disease. The initial Qi stagnation resulting from emotional stress generates Heat, which harasses the Mind. The stagnation of Qi in the Triple Burner leads to the impairment of the transformation of fluids and therefore to Phlegm. This is also aggravated by the condensing action of Heat on fluids.

Anger, shock and fear injure Liver and Kidneys; these become deficient and lose the nourishment of Water, which causes *Dian*. Excess joy and anger injure Heart-Yin; this leads to Heart-Fire and *Kuang*. Pensiveness and worry injure Heart and Spleen, the Heart loses its nourishment, the Spleen cannot transform; this leads to *Dian*.

Worry and pensiveness injure Heart and Spleen; the latter cannot transform and transport, and this gives rise to Phlegm.

The *Complete Book of Jing Yue* (*Jing Yue Quan Shu*) says: "*Kuang is due to Fire deriving from worry, pensiveness and anger.*"[43]

Zhang Jing Yue says:[44]

Kuang is due to Fire deriving from worry and anger; the Qi of Liver and Gall-Bladder rebels upwards, Wood and Fire combine, the condition is Full, pathogenic factors invade the Heart so that the Mind and Ethereal Soul become restless.

Interestingly, Dr Zhang Fa Rong includes shock as an emotional cause of disease for *Dian Kuang*. He says that a big shock injures the Kidneys.[45]

Diet

As Phlegm plays a central role in the pathology of bipolar disorder, irregular diet is an important contributing factor to its etiology. Excessive consumption of dairy foods, fried food, fatty foods, carbohydrates and sugar leads to the formation of Phlegm.

Phlegm may also be formed when the person eats in an irregular and chaotic way, i.e. eating late at night, eating in a hurry, eating while working, etc.

Constitution

A constitutional tendency to mental-emotional problems plays a role in the development of bipolar disorder. Both children and adolescents can develop bipolar disorder. It is more likely to affect the children of parents who have the illness.[46]

Interestingly, as far back as the time when the *Yellow Emperor's Classic of Internal Medicine* was written (approximately 100 BC), Chinese doctors knew that heredity plays a role in the development of Manic-Depression. The *Simple Questions* says in Chapter 47:[47]

The disease of Dian arises in the mother's womb during gestation and it is due to the mother's suffering a big shock so that Qi rises and cannot descend to the residence of Essence [Jing]; this leads to the development of Dian in the fetus.

Because bipolar disorder tends to run in families, researchers have been searching for specific genes passed down through generations that may increase a person's chance of developing the illness. But genes are not the whole story. Studies of identical twins, who share all the same genes, indicate that both genes and other factors play a role in bipolar disorder. If bipolar disorder were caused entirely by genes, then the identical twin of someone with the illness would *always* develop the illness, and research has shown that this is not the case. But if one twin has bipolar disorder, the other twin is more likely to develop the illness than is another sibling.[48]

From the point of view of Chinese medicine, a tongue with a deep Heart crack indicates the tendency to mental-emotional problems (*see Fig. 11.6*).

Figure 19.3 summarizes the etiology of *Dian Kuang*.

SUMMARY

Etiology of *Dian Kuang*
- Emotional stress
- Diet
- Constitution

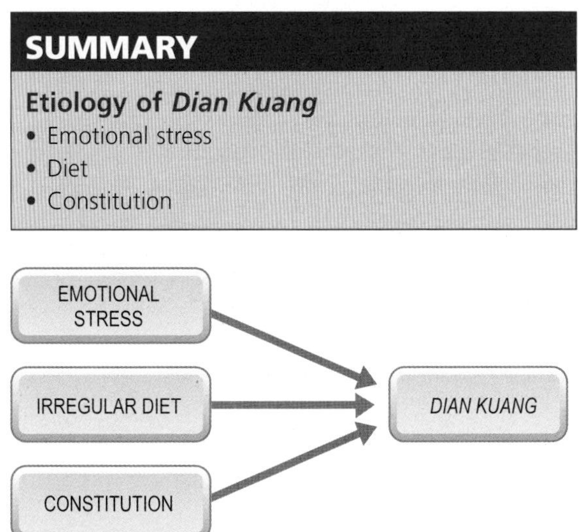

Figure 19.3 Etiology of *Dian Kuang*.

PATHOLOGY AND TREATMENT PRINCIPLES OF *DIAN KUANG*

Pathology of *Dian Kuang*

The pathology of bipolar disorder is complex, especially in chronic conditions. In the beginning stages there is Qi stagnation, Fire and Phlegm, while in later stages, there is also a deficiency (of Qi, Blood or Yin). The manic stage is characterized by more Fullness while the depressive stage is characterized by a mixture of Full and Empty conditions. Four words could summarize the pathology of bipolar disorder: Qi (stagnation), Fire, Phlegm and Stasis (of Blood).

CLINICAL NOTE

Four words could summarize the pathology of bipolar disorder:
- Qi (stagnation)
- Fire
- Phlegm
- Stasis (of Blood).

Central to the pathology of bipolar disorder (and *Dian Kuang*) is Phlegm. Bipolar disorder is a serious mental illness characterized by loss of insight; in Chinese terms, this is due to obstruction of the Mind's orifices. The Mind's orifices can be obstructed by Phlegm or by severe Blood stasis. In bipolar disorder (and *Dian Kuang*), the Mind's orifices are obstructed principally by Phlegm, although, in later stages, Blood stasis may also contribute to the obstruction. Obstruction of the Mind by Phlegm accounts for both the manic and the depressive phases of bipolar disorder.

Please note that Phlegm does not derive only from a Spleen deficiency: Qi stagnation may give rise to Phlegm by obstructing the free flow of Qi in the Three Burners; Fire can also give rise to Phlegm by condensing the body fluids; Blood stasis (which itself derives from Qi stagnation) aggravates Phlegm.

In bipolar disorder, there is usually also Fire, which agitates the Mind and Ethereal Soul and "stokes up" the manic behavior of the person. In chronic cases, Fire injures Yin and the resulting Empty Heat further agitates the Mind.

Furthermore, the Qi stagnation that is usually present in the beginning stages of bipolar disorder may also give rise to Blood stasis; this further clouds the Mind's orifices.

In *Dian*, there is often Phlegm with Qi stagnation and a deficiency of the Heart and Spleen; in *Kuang*, there is often Phlegm-Fire agitating and obstructing the Mind and eventually leading to Yin deficiency. In chronic cases, the Qi stagnation and the Phlegm may also give rise to Blood stasis.

The *Medical Records of the Guide to Clinical Practice* (*Lin Zheng Zhi Nan Yi An*) summarizes the etiology and pathology of *Dian Kuang* as follows:[49]

> *Mania [Kuang] is due to a big shock and big anger; the disease is in the Liver, Gall-Bladder and Stomach channels, the three Yang rise, Fire burns and Phlegm surges, the orifices of the Heart are obstructed. Dullness [Dian] is due to worry, the disease is in the Spleen, Heart and Pericardium channels; the three Yin cannot diffuse, Qi stagnates and Phlegm is formed so that the Mind is confused.*

In conclusion, the pathology of the manic phase of bipolar disorder is characterized by Qi stagnation in its beginning stages; Qi stagnation in the Three Burners leads to the formation of Phlegm that clouds the Mind's orifices. On the other hand, Qi stagnation also leads to Fire, which harasses the Mind and causes mania. In chronic cases, Qi stagnation also leads to Blood stasis, which obstructs the Mind's orifices further. In chronic conditions, Fire injures Yin and leads to Yin deficiency. The main organs involved are Heart, Liver and Spleen.

CLINICAL NOTE

Pathology of manic phase

The pathology of the manic phase of bipolar disorder is characterized by:

- Qi stagnation
- Phlegm that clouds the Mind's orifices
- Fire which harasses the Mind and causes mania
- Blood stasis which obstructs the Mind's orifices further
- Yin deficiency.

The main organs involved are Heart, Liver and Spleen.

Another essential characteristic of the pathology of bipolar disorder in its manic phase is the excessive "coming and going" of the Ethereal Soul, resulting in the flooding of the Mind by ideas, projects, plans, inspiration, etc. in a chaotic way that leads to mania. This has already been discussed above.

The Mind needs to control and integrate the psychic material deriving from the Ethereal Soul; the Mind can deal with only one thing at a time. Flooding of the Mind by the psychic material deriving from the Ethereal Soul results in total immersion of the Mind within the Ethereal Soul and therefore mental illness as in bipolar disorder; this situation is illustrated in Figure 3.21.

The pathology of the depressive phase is characterized by a mixture of Full and Empty conditions. In the beginning stages, there is Qi stagnation and Phlegm which obstructs the Mind's orifices. In chronic cases, there is a deficiency of the Heart and Spleen.

The main organs involved in the pathology of bipolar disorder are therefore the Heart, Liver, Lungs and Spleen. The pathology affecting these organs is summarized in Figure 19.4.

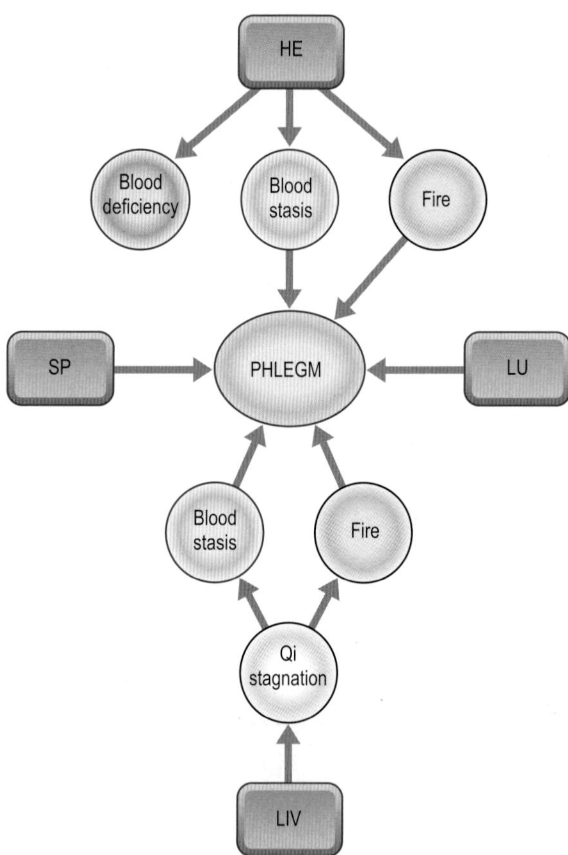

Figure 19.4 Pathology of *Dian Kuang*.

SUMMARY

Pathology of *Dian Kuang*

The pathology of Manic-Depression (*Dian Kuang*) can be summarized as follows.

- Phlegm
- Fire
- Qi stagnation
- Blood stasis
- Deficiency (of Qi, Blood or Yin)

Treatment principles for *Dian Kuang*

In view of the pathology of bipolar disorder, the main treatment principles are as follows.

- Move Qi
- Resolve Phlegm
- Nourish Heart and Spleen
- Drain Fire
- Nourish Blood
- Nourish Yin if necessary
- Invigorate Blood
- Calm the Mind
- Open the Mind's orifices

The veteran Beijing doctor Zhang Li Sheng treated hundreds of cases of *Dian Kuang*. He recommends the following treatment principles.[50]

- *Nourish the Heart and calm the Mind*: Yuan Zhi *Radix Polygalae*, Bai Zi Ren *Semen Platycladi*, Suan Zao Ren *Semen Ziziphi spinosae*, Fu Ling *Poria*, Hu Po *Succinum*.
- *Clear the Heart and open the Mind's orifices*: Shi Chang Pu *Rhizoma Acori tatarinowii*, Yu Jin *Radix Curcumae*, Gou Teng *Ramulus cum Uncis Uncariae*, Lian Zi Xin *Plumula Nelumbinis nuciferae*.
- *Move Liver-Qi*: Xiang Fu *Rhizoma Cyperi*, Hou Po *Cortex Magnoliae officinalis*.
- *Resolve Phlegm*: in case of Phlegm, add Tian Zhu Huang *Concretio Silicea Bambusae* and Dan Nan Xing *Rhizoma Arisaematis preparatum*.

Doctors Shen Quan Yu, Wu Yu Hua and Shen Li Ling advocate the following treatment principles. They say that the condition causing Dullness (*Dian*) is Yin and Empty in character, and that the main pathogenic factors are Phlegm and Qi stagnation. The treatment principle is therefore to resolve Phlegm, move Qi, eliminate stagnation, settle the Heart, calm the Mind, tonify Qi and nourish Blood.

The condition leading to Mania (*Kuang*) is Yang and Full in character; the main pathogenic factors are Fire, Phlegm and Blood stasis. The treatment principle is therefore to drain Fire, resolve Phlegm, invigorate Blood and eliminate stasis; in later stages nourish Yin and clear Empty Heat.

The treatment principle of Dullness in the acute stage must address the Manifestation, resolve Phlegm and open the Mind's orifices. In between attacks, one must tonify the Heart and the Spleen, resolve Phlegm, move Qi and eliminate stagnation (treating the Root).

The treatment principle of Mania in the acute stage must address the Manifestation by resolving Phlegm and opening the Mind's orifices. In between attacks, one must regulate Yin and Yang, nourish Yin and clear Empty Heat (treating the Root). See Table 19.1.

The above doctors recommend the following treatment methods and applicable herbs.

- *Move Qi*: Xiang Fu *Rhizoma Cyperi*, Mu Xiang *Radix Aucklandiae*, Yu Jin *Radix Curcumae*.
- *Resolve Phlegm and open the Mind's orifices*: Dan Nan Xing *Rhizoma Arisaematis preparatum*, Ban Xia *Rhizoma Pinelliae preparatum*, Fu Ling *Poria*, Shi Chang Pu *Rhizoma Acori tatarinowii*, Yu Jin *Radix Curcumae*.
- *Nourish the Heart and calm the Mind*: Dang Gui *Radix Angelicae sinensis*, Bai Zi Ren *Semen Platycladi*, Yuan Zhi *Radix Polygalae*, Suan Zao Ren *Semen Ziziphi spinosae*, Wu Wei Zi *Fructus Schisandrae*.

Table 19.1 Treatment principles for *Dian* and *Kuang*

	ACUTE STAGE (TREAT MANIFESTATION)	IN BETWEEN ATTACKS (TREAT ROOT)
Depression (*Dian*)	Resolve Phlegm, open the Mind's orifices	Tonify Heart and Spleen, resolve Phlegm, move Qi
Mania (*Kuang*)	Resolve Phlegm, open the Mind's orifices	Regulate Yin and Yang, nourish Yin or Blood, clear Empty Heat

- *Strongly resolve Phlegm*: Sheng Tie Luo *Frusta Ferri*, Dai Zhe Shi *Hematitum*, Zhe Bei Mu *Bulbus Fritillariae thunbergii*, Da Huang *Radix et Rhizoma Rhei*, Dan Nan Xing *Rhizoma Arisaematis preparatum*.
- *Drain Fire and resolve Phlegm*: Da Huang *Radix et Rhizoma Rhei*, Long Dan Cao *Radix Gentianae*, Huang Lian *Rhizoma Coptidis*, Shi Gao *Gypsum fibrosum*, Zhi Mu *Radix Anemarrhaenae*.
- *Resolve Phlegm with the attacking method*: Meng Shi *Lapis Chloriti seu Micae*, Ban Xia *Rhizoma Pinelliae* (unprepared), Da Huang *Radix et Rhizoma Rhei*, Huang Qin *Radix Scutellariae*.
- *Draining Fire*: Shi Gao *Gypsum fibrosum*, Zhi Mu *Radix Anemarrhaenae*, Huang Lian *Rhizoma Coptidis*, Da Huang *Radix et Rhizoma Rhei*, Huang Qin *Radix Scutellariae*.
- *Nourish Yin and clear Empty Heat*: Sheng Di Huang *Radix Rehmanniae*, Mai Men Dong *Radix Ophiopogonis*, Xuan Shen *Radix Scrophulariae*, Huang Lian *Rhizoma Coptidis*, Mu Tong *Caulis Akebiae trifoliatae*, Gan Cao *Radix Glycyrrhizae uralensis*.
- *Drain Liver-Fire*: Long Dan Cao *Radix Gentianae*, Lu Hui *Aloe*, Shan Zhi Zi *Fructus Gardeniae*.
- *Invigorate Blood*: Dang Gui *Radix Angelicae sinensis*, Chi Shao *Radix Paeoniae rubra*, Tao Ren *Semen Persicae*, Hong Hua *Flos Carthami tinctorii*, Yu Jin *Radix Curcumae*.
- *Vomiting*: Gua Di *Cucumis melo*, Li Lu *Radix et Rhizoma Veratri*.

Dr Zhang Fa Rong discusses the treatment principles of Manic-Depression in his book *Chinese Internal Medicine*.[51] He advocates the following treatment principles.

- Regulate Yin-Yang
- Calm the Mind
- Settle the Will-Power (*ding Zhi*)
- Resolve Phlegm
- Open the Mind's orifices
- Invigorate Blood

He further distinguishes *Dian* from *Kuang* in identifying the treatment principle. For *Dian*, he advocates moving Qi, resolving Phlegm, opening the Mind's orifices, rectifying Qi; in case of Heart and Spleen deficiency, tonify Heart and Spleen, nourish the Heart and calm the Mind.

For *Kuang*, he advocates resolving Phlegm, draining Fire, sinking Heart-Qi, clearing the Liver. If Fire has injured Yin, nourish Yin, clear Empty Heat and calm the Mind.

Interestingly, Dr Zhang says that until the Yuan dynasty, *Dian Kuang* was often confused with *Dian Xian* (epilepsy) and epilepsy was wrongly classified as a mental illness. Wang Ken Dang of the Ming dynasty was the first to distinguish *Dian Kuang* from *Dian Xian* (epilepsy).

The famous gynecologist of the Qing dynasty, Fu Qing Zhu, wrote a chapter on *Dian Kuang* in both men and women. He went against the prevailing view that mania is always due to Fire and is Yang in nature. He maintained that there are also Cold types of mania due to Spleen-Qi deficiency and Cold Phlegm obstructing the Mind's orifices.[52] He therefore advocates treating the Root (*Ben*) as well as the Manifestation (*Biao*). This means that, in the treatment of *Kuang* due to Cold Phlegm, it is important not only to resolve Phlegm but also to tonify and warm the Spleen, especially with high doses (over 30 g) of Ren Shen *Radix Ginseng* and Bai Zhu *Rhizoma Atractylodis macrocephalae*.

Table 19.2 compares and contrasts Depression (*Dian*) with Mania (*Kuang*).

Table 19.2 Differentiation between *Dian* and *Kuang*

	DIAN	*KUANG*
Pathology	Qi stagnation and Phlegm	Phlegm-Fire harassing the Heart
Mood symptoms	Unhappy, dull thinking	Agitation, mania, anger, anxiety
Speech symptoms	Silent, incoherent speech, stumbling speech	Incessant talking, incoherent speech, shouting abuse, cursing
Movement symptoms	Singing, crying, likes to be alone, sadness, erratic behavior	Mania, anger, ascends to high places and sings, casts off clothes, hitting people, taking risks
Special points	Stillness and depression	A lot of movement and frequent changes
Yin-Yang character	Yin	Yang

SUMMARY

Treatment principles for *Dian Kuang*

The main treatment principles are as follows.

- Move Qi
- Resolve Phlegm
- Nourish Heart and Spleen
- Drain Fire
- Nourish Blood
- Nourish Yin if necessary
- Invigorate Blood
- Calm the Mind
- Open the Mind's orifices

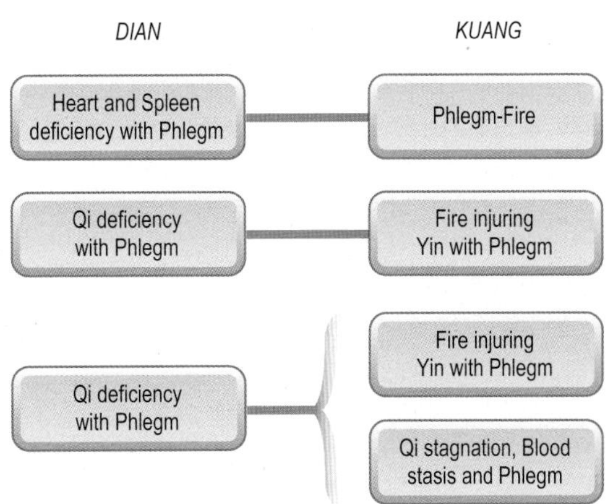

Figure 19.5 Possible combinations of patterns of *Dian* and *Kuang* in bipolar disorder.

How to adapt the patterns and treatment of *Dian Kuang* to the treatment of bipolar disorder

In the ensuing discussion, I follow the Chinese books' discussion of *Dian* and *Kuang* separately as two single disease entities. However, one of the characteristics of bipolar disorder is precisely the alternation, in the same patient, of phases of abnormally elated and abnormally depressed mood.

Therefore, patterns of both *Dian* and *Kuang* may appear in the same patient, and not necessarily in the depressive and the manic phase, respectively. In other words, if, for example, a patient displays the pattern of Heart and Spleen deficiency during the depressive phase, this pattern is not going to disappear during the manic phase, although it may be overshadowed by a Full pattern such as Phlegm-Fire. More often than not, each patient will have a combination of patterns and it is not at all unusual to have a pattern from *Dian* (e.g. Spleen and Heart deficiency) and one from *Kuang* (e.g. Phlegm-Fire harassing upwards).

Figure 19.5 gives three examples of combinations of patterns from *Dian* and *Kuang* in bipolar disorder. Please note that these are only examples and other combinations are possible. The combinations illustrated in Figure 19.5 are:

- Heart and Spleen deficiency with Phlegm (*Dian*) plus Phlegm-Fire (*Kuang*)
- Qi deficiency with Phlegm (*Dian*) plus Fire injuring Yin with Phlegm (*Kuang*)
- Qi deficiency with Phlegm (*Dian*) plus Fire injuring Yin with Phlegm (*Kuang*) plus Qi stagnation, Blood stasis and Phlegm (*Kuang*).

I believe that, in the treatment of bipolar disorder, we need to put the emphasis on the manic rather than the depressive side of the disease. This is because the depressive side is usually a reaction to a manic phase and it is really the other side of the coin of the same disease.

In bipolar disorder there is always Phlegm, and in the manic phase there is bound to be some Fire, usually in the Liver and/or Heart. In chronic conditions, Fire may injure Yin and the clinical picture would become more complex.

Of course, for there to be Phlegm, there must also be a deficiency (and/or a stagnation) of Qi; there is usually a deficiency of the Spleen and/or Lungs giving rise to Phlegm. This deficiency needs to be addressed and we should not concentrate solely on the treatment of Phlegm and Fire.

It is *extremely important* to note that on no account should we advise a patient to discontinue taking lithium or other medication prescribed by a psychiatrist. Any change in the dosage of lithium must be agreed by and discussed with the patient's psychiatrist. Given the possibility of suicide in the depressive phase, this is extremely important.

CLINICAL NOTE

It is *extremely important* to note that on no account should we advise a patient to discontinue taking lithium or other medication prescribed by a psychiatrist. Any change in the dosage of lithium must be agreed by and discussed with the patient's psychiatrist. Given the possibility of suicide in the depressive phase, this is extremely important.

SUMMARY

How to adapt the patterns and treatment of *Dian Kuang* to the treatment of bipolar disorder

- Patterns of both *Dian* and *Kuang* may appear in the same patient and not necessarily in the depressive and the manic phase, respectively.
- For example, if a patient displays the pattern of Heart and Spleen deficiency during the depressive phase, this pattern is not going to disappear during the manic phase, although it may be overshadowed by a Full pattern such as Phlegm-Fire.
- Each patient will have a combination of patterns and it is not at all unusual to have a pattern from *Dian* (e.g. Spleen and Heart deficiency) and one from *Kuang* (e.g. Phlegm-Fire harassing upwards).
- In the treatment of bipolar disorder, put the emphasis on the manic rather than the depressive side of the disease.
- In bipolar disorder there is always Phlegm, and in the manic phase there is bound to be some Fire, usually in the Liver and/or Heart. In chronic conditions, Fire may injure Yin and the clinical picture would become more complex.
- There is also a deficiency (and/or a stagnation) of Qi; there is usually a deficiency of the Spleen and/ or Lungs giving rise to Phlegm.
- It is *extremely important* to note that on no account should we advise a patient to discontinue taking lithium or other medication prescribed by a psychiatrist.

ACUPUNCTURE TREATMENT

Points that open the Mind's orifices

In order to treat bipolar disorder, it is important to use points that open the Mind's orifices. These include the following.

- *LU-3 Tianfu*: somnolence, insomnia, sadness, weeping, forgetfulness and "talking to ghosts".
- *L.I.-5 Yangxi*: manic behavior, propensity to inappropriate laughter, "seeing ghosts" and fright.
- *L.I.-7 Wenliu*: inappropriate laughter, manic behavior and "seeing ghosts".
- *ST-25 Tianshu*: mental restlessness, anxiety, schizophrenia and mania. The Qing dynasty's *An Explanation of the Acupuncture Points* reports Sun Si Miao as saying that ST-25 is the abode of the Corporeal Soul and Ethereal Soul; this would explain the mental effect of this point that is actually not reported by modern books.[53]
- *ST-40 Fenglong*: *Dian Kuang*, inappropriate laughter, inappropriate elation, desire to ascend to high places and sing, undress and run around, mental restlessness and "seeing ghosts".
- *ST-42 Chongyang*: *Dian Kuang*, desire to ascend to high places and sing, discarding clothes and running around.
- *ST-45 Lidui*: excessive dreaming, fright, insomnia, dizziness, *Dian Kuang*, desire to ascend to high places, sing, discard clothes and run around.
- *S.I.-16 Tianchuang*: manic behavior, *Dian Kuang* and "talking with ghosts".
- *BL-10 Tianzhu*: manic behavior, incessant talking and "seeing ghosts".
- *P-5 Jianshi*: palpitations, agitation, feeling of oppression of the chest, manic behavior, fright, mental restlessness, poor memory and "seeing ghosts".
- *G.B.-13 Benshen*: manic behavior and fright.
- *G.B.-17 Zhengying*: obsessive thoughts, pensiveness and manic behavior.
- *G.B.-18 Chengling*: obsessive thoughts and pensiveness, dementia.[54]
- *Du-16 Fengfu*: manic behavior, desire to commit suicide, sadness and fear.
- *Du-19 Houding*: manic behavior, anxiety, mental restlessness and insomnia.
- *Du-20 Baihui*: disorientation, sadness and crying with desire to die, mania.
- *Du-26 Renzhong*: *Dian Kuang*.
- All the Well (*Jing*) points.

The modern *text Chinese Acupuncture Therapy* lists the following points for *Dian* and *Kuang*.[55]

Dian *(two groups of points)*

- BL-15 Xinshu, BL-18 Ganshu, BL-20 Pishu, ST-40 Fenglong, HE-7 Shenmen, LIV-3 Taichong.
- BL-15 Xinshu, Ren-14 Juque, P-6 Neiguan, HE-7 Shenmen, SP-6 Sanyinjiao.

Kuang *(two groups of points)*

- Du-26 Renzhong, Du-16 Fengfu, L.I.-1 Shangyang, P-7 Daling, L.I.-11 Quchi, ST-40 Fenglong, SP-1 Yinbai.

- Du-26 Renzhong, Du-23 Shangxing, Yintang, HE-7 Shenmen, P-6 Neiguan, P-7 Daling, BL-62 Shenmai.

The modern text *A Study of Acupuncture* lists the following points for *Dian* and *Kuang*.[56]

Dian

- HE-7 Shenmen, P-7 Daling, LIV-3 Taichong, ST-40 Fenglong, SP-6 Sanyinjiao, Du-20 Baihui.

Kuang

- Du-26 Renzhong, P-8 Laogong, HE-8 Shaofu, LIV-2 Xiangjian, ST-40 Fenglong.

The modern book *A Collection of Chinese Acupuncture Prescriptions* recommends the following treatment principles and points for *Dian* and *Kuang*.[57]

Dian

- *Treatment principle*: Eliminate stagnation, resolve Phlegm, open the Mind's orifices, regulate Qi.
- *Points*: Du-15 Yamen, HE-4 Lingdao, Du-14 Dazhui, Du-26 Renzhong, HE-7 Shenmen, P-6 Neiguan, BL-15 Xinshu, ST-36 Zusanli.

Kuang

- *Treatment principle*: Move Liver-Qi, resolve Phlegm, drain Fire, calm the Mind, place emphasis on the Governing Vessel's points.
- *Points*: Du-16 Fengfu, Du-14 Dazhui, HE-4 Lingdao, Du-12 Shenzhu, Du-20 Baihui, Du-26 Renzhong, Yintang.

Sun Si Miao's 13 ghost points

Su Si Miao listed 13 points for the treatment of *Dian Kuang*. In the following list, the first name is the most common one and the one next to it is the alternative name. As can be seen, all the alternative names contain the word *gui*, i.e. "ghost". This is due to the fact that some kind of mental illnesses were considered to be due to the invasion of "ghosts".

Du-26 Renzhong	Guigong	"Ghost Palace"
LU-11 Shaoshang	Guixin	"Ghost Message"
SP-1 Yinbai	Guiyan	"Ghost Eye"
P-7 Daling	Guixin	"Ghost Heart"
BL-62 Shenmai	Guilu	"Ghost Road"
Du-16 Fengfu	Guizhen	"Ghost Pillow"
ST-6 Jiache	Guichang	"Ghost Bed"
Ren-24 Chengjiang	Guishi	"Ghost Market"
P-8 Laogong	Guiku	"Ghost Cave"
Du-23 Shangxing	Guitang	"Ghost Hall"
Ren-1 Huiyin	Guicang	"Ghost Hiding"
Yumen	Guicang	"Ghost Hiding"
L.I.-11 Quchi	Guichen	"Ghost Minister"
Haiquan	Guifeng	"Ghost Seal"

Sun Si Miao's instructions

Ren-1 is used in men with moxa cones and Yumen (in the anterior fold of the vagina) is used in women with a moxa stick. Haiquan is a point in the veins under the tongue.

The points were used for insanity from invasion of evil spirits. Use points bilaterally but start on the left for men and the right for women, and withdraw in reverse order.

Modern use

Anxiety, uncontrolled weeping, fear, fright, disorientation, delirium, seizures, depression, hysteria and mania.

The Pericardium channel in Manic-Depression

In the acupuncture treatment of Manic-Depression, it is important to place the emphasis on the Pericardium channel, perhaps even more than on the Heart channel. This is because the Pericardium points have a stronger action in opening the Mind's orifices than the Heart points.

The *Medical Records of the Guide to Clinical Practice* (*Lin Zheng Zhi Nan Yi An*) summarizes the etiology and pathology of *Dian* as follows:[58]

Depression [Dian] is due to worry, the disease is in the Spleen, Heart and Pericardium channels; the three Yin cannot diffuse, Qi stagnates and Phlegm is formed so that the Mind is confused.

According to this statement, therefore, the use of the Pericardium channel is particularly important in the treatment of *Dian*.

The modern doctor Dr Liang Jian Bo stresses the importance of using the Pericardium channel in the treatment of both *Dian* and *Kuang*. Dr Liang thinks that, in *Kuang*, the Liver, Heart, Stomach and Pericardium are affected, with Fire in the Liver, Heart and Stomach. Fire also invades the Pericardium and this causes the Ethereal Soul to become restless.[59]

Dr Liang says that in some cases of *Dian*, although the main manifestations are depression and withdrawn mood, some patients may display some restlessness; this indicates Heat in the Heart, Spleen and Pericardium and that there is some Fullness within the Deficiency.

The main points from the Pericardium channel to open the Mind's orifices are P-7 Daling, P-8 Laogong and P-5 Jianshi: P-7 is selected in case of severe Mania to calm the Mind and settle the Ethereal Soul; P-8 is selected if there is Fire; P-5 resolves Phlegm from the Mind.

SUMMARY

The Pericardium channel in Manic-Depression

- In the acupuncture treatment of Manic-Depression, it is important to place the emphasis on the Pericardium channel to open the Mind's orifices.
- The *Medical Records of the Guide to Clinical Practice* (*Lin Zheng Zhi Nan Yi An*) states: *"Depression [Dian] is due to worry, the disease is in the Spleen, Heart and Pericardium channels."*
- The modern doctor Dr Liang Jian Bo stresses the importance of using the Pericardium channel in the treatment of both *Dian* and *Kuang*.
- The main points from the Pericardium channel to open the Mind's orifices are P-7 Daling, P-8 Laogong and P-5 Jianshi:
  - P-7 is selected in case of severe Mania to calm the Mind and settle the Ethereal Soul
  - P-8 is selected if there is Fire
  - P-5 resolves Phlegm from the Mind.

IDENTIFICATION OF PATTERNS AND TREATMENT

DIAN

Qi stagnation and Phlegm

Clinical manifestations

Depression, apathy, dull thinking, incoherent speech, muttering to oneself, inappropriate laughter, not remembering to eat, emotional dullness, alternation of anger and laughing without reason.

Tongue: Swollen, sticky coating.

Pulse: Wiry and Slippery.

Treatment principle

Move Qi, eliminate stagnation, resolve Phlegm, open the Mind's orifices.

Acupuncture

Points

P-6 Neiguan, LIV-3 Taichong, T.B.-6 Zhigou, P-5 Jianshi, ST-40 Fenglong, Ren-12 Zhongwan, Ren-9 Shuifen, SP-6 Sanyinjiao, Du-20 Baihui. All with reducing or even method.

Explanation

- P-6, LIV-3 and T.B.-6 move Qi and relieve depression.
- P-5 resolves Phlegm from the Heart and the Mind and opens the Mind's orifices.
- ST-40, Ren-12, Ren-9 and SP-6 resolve Phlegm.
- Du-20 lifts mood and opens the Mind's orifices.

Herbal therapy

Prescription

SHUN QI DAO TAN TANG Variation
Rectifying Qi and Eliminating Phlegm Decoction Variation

Explanation

This formula promotes the descending of Qi in the Triple Burner in order to resolve Phlegm. It has been modified with the addition of Huang Lian *Rhizoma Coptidis*, Huang Qin *Radix Scutellariae*, Yuan Zhi *Radix Polygalae*, Shi Chang Pu *Rhizoma Acori tatarinowii* and Chen Xiang *Lignum Aquilariae resinatum*.

Prescription

WEN DAN TANG Variation
Warming the Gall-Bladder Decoction Variation

Explanation

This formula resolves Phlegm-Heat from the Lungs and Heart and calms the Mind. It is used if Phlegm is combined with Heat and the patient is anxious and worried, in addition to being depressed. It is especially indicated if there is a feeling of oppression of the chest.

Prescription

SI QI TANG Variation
Four Seasons Decoction for the Seven Emotions Variation

Explanation

This formula moves Lung- and Heart-Qi in the chest and relieves worry and anxiety. This formula is used if the symptoms of obstruction of the Mind by Phlegm are pronounced (mental dullness, incoherent speech, staring gaze without blinking, very Swollen tongue with very sticky coating).

It has been modified with the addition of herbs to resolve Phlegm and open the Mind's orifices such as Yuan Zhi *Radix Polygalae*, Dan Nan Xing *Rhizoma Arisaematis preparatum*, Yu Jin *Radix Curcumae* and Shi Chang Pu *Rhizoma Acori tatarinowii*.

Prescription

SU HE XIANG WAN plus **SI QI TANG** Variation
Styrax Pill plus *Four Seasons Decoction for the Seven Emotions* Variation

Explanation

This formula is used if Phlegm is very pronounced and the symptoms of obstruction of the Mind are very severe. This formula has a very strong effect in opening the Mind's orifices. Please note that I have removed several banned substances from the formula Su He Xiang Wan.

These two formulae together have the strongest effect in opening the Mind's orifices.

Table 19.3 compares and contrasts the formulae for the pattern of Qi stagnation and Phlegm of *Dian*.

SUMMARY

Qi stagnation and Phlegm

Points

P-6 Neiguan, LIV-3 Taichong, T.B.-6 Zhigou, P-5 Jianshi, ST-40 Fenglong, Ren-12 Zhongwan, Ren-9 Shuifen, SP-6 Sanyinjiao, Du-20 Baihui. All with reducing or even method.

Herbal therapy

Prescription

SHUN QI DAO TAN TANG Variation
Rectifying Qi and Eliminating Phlegm Decoction Variation

Prescription

WEN DAN TANG Variation
Warming the Gall-Bladder Decoction Variation

Prescription

SI QI TANG Variation
Four Seasons Decoction for the Seven Emotions Variation

Prescription

SU HE XIANG WAN plus **SI QI TANG** Variation
Styrax Pill plus *Four Seasons Decoction for the Seven Emotions* Variation

Table 19.3 Differentiation of formulae for the pattern of Qi stagnation and Phlegm of *Dian*

	ACTION	TONGUE
Shun Qi Dao Tan Tang	Restore the descending of Qi, resolve Phlegm	Swollen, sticky coating
Wen Dan Tang	Resolve Phlegm, clear Heat	Swollen, sticky-yellow coating
Si Qi Tang	Restore the descending of Heart- and Lung-Qi, resolve Phlegm	Swollen, very sticky coating
Su He Xiang Wan plus Si Qi Tang	Resolve Phlegm, open the Mind's orifices	Very Swollen, very sticky coating

Heart and Spleen deficiency with Phlegm

Clinical manifestations

Depression, excessive dreaming, insomnia, mental confusion, easily startled, bewilderment, sadness, crying, shutting windows, muttering to oneself, visual or auditory hallucinations, palpitations, dull-pale complexion, slow movement, dislike to speak, loose stools, tiredness, weak limbs, poor appetite.

Tongue: Pale, Swollen with a sticky coating.

Pulse: Soggy.

Treatment principle

Strengthen the Spleen, nourish Heart, benefit Qi, calm the Mind, resolve Phlegm, open the Mind's orifices.

Acupuncture

Points

HE-7 Shenmen, HE-5 Tongli, P-5 Jianshi, ST-36 Zusanli, Ren-12 Zhongwan, BL-20 Pishu, Du-24 Shenting, Du-20 Baihui, ST-40 Fenglong, Ren-9 Shuifen, SP-6 Sanyinjiao. HE-7, HE-5, ST-36, Ren-12 and BL-20 with reinforcing method; all others with even method.

Explanation

- HE-7 and HE-5 tonify the Heart.
- P-5 opens the Mind's orifices and resolves Phlegm from the Mind.
- ST-36, Ren-12 and BL-20 (with reinforcing method) tonify the Spleen.
- Du-24 and Du-20 lift mood and open the Mind's orifices.
- ST-40, Ren-9 and SP-6 resolve Phlegm.

Herbal therapy

Prescription

YANG XIN TANG (I) or **(II)**
Nourishing the Heart Decoction

Explanation

This formula nourishes Heart-Blood and Spleen-Blood. In order to treat bipolar disorder, it should be modified with the addition of herbs to resolve Phlegm and open the Mind's orifices such as Yuan Zhi *Radix Polygalae*, Ban Xia *Rhizoma Pinelliae preparatum* and Shi Chang Pu *Rhizoma Acori tatarinowii*. Either (I) or (II) may be used; however, if Yang deficiency is pronounced, use (I).

Prescription

GAN MAI DA ZAO TANG
Glycyrrhiza-Triticum-Jujuba Decoction

Explanation

This formula is used if there is sadness, crying a lot, disorientation, bewilderment.

Prescription

JI SHENG SHEN QI TANG Variation
Kidney-Qi Decoction from "Formulae to Aid the Living" Variation

Explanation

This formula is used if there a Spleen deficiency and a constitutional deficiency of the Kidneys with Phlegm (mental dullness, incoherent speech, tiredness, weakness).

Table 19.4 compares and contrasts the three formulae for Heart and Spleen deficiency with Phlegm of *Dian*.

Table 19.4 Differentiation of formulae for the pattern of Heart and Spleen deficiency with Phlegm

	ACTION	SYMPTOMS	TONGUE
Yang Xin Tang	Nourish Heart- and Spleen-Blood	Insomnia	Pale, dry, Thin
Gan Mai Da Zao Tang	Tonify the Spleen, nourish Heart-Blood	Sadness, crying, disorientation	Pale
Ji Sheng Shen Qi Tang	Tonify the Spleen and Kidneys, strengthen Will-Power, resolve Phlegm	Mental dullness, lack of Will-Power	Pale, Swollen, wet

> **SUMMARY**
>
> **Heart and Spleen deficiency with Phlegm**
>
> *Points*
>
> HE-7 Shenmen, HE-5 Tongli, P-5 Jianshi, ST-36 Zusanli, Ren-12 Zhongwan, BL-20 Pishu, Du-24 Shenting, Du-20 Baihui, ST-40 Fenglong, Ren-9 Shuifen, SP-6 Sanyinjiao. HE-7, HE-5, ST-36, Ren-12 and BL-20 with reinforcing method; all others with even method.
>
> *Herbal therapy*
>
> *Prescription*
>
> **YANG XIN TANG (I)** or **(II)**
> *Nourishing the Heart Decoction*
>
> *Prescription*
>
> **GAN MAI DA ZAO TANG**
> *Glycyrrhiza-Triticum-Jujuba Decoction*
>
> *Prescription*
>
> **JI SHENG SHEN QI TANG** Variation
> *Kidney-Qi Decoction from "Formulae to Aid the Living"* Variation

Qi deficiency with Phlegm

Clinical manifestations

Chronic condition, emotional dullness, reluctance to move or speak, staring eyes, inappropriate laughter, muttering to oneself, incoherent thinking, visual and auditory hallucinations, self reproach, feeling of guilt, mental dullness, loose stools, pale complexion, tiredness, shortness of breath, no appetite.

Tongue: Pale.

Pulse: Soggy.

Treatment principle

Tonify Lung-, Stomach- and Spleen-Qi, resolve Phlegm, open the Mind's orifices.

Acupuncture

Points

LU-9 Taiyuan, BL-13 Feishu, Ren-12 Zhongwan, BL-20 Pishu, BL-21 Weishu, ST-36 Zusanli, Ren-9 Shuifen, SP-6 Sanyinjiao, ST-40 Fenglong, P-5 Jianshi, P-6 Neiguan, Du-20 Baihui, Du-26 Renzhong. LU-9, BL-13, Ren-12, BL-20, BL-21 and ST-36 with reinforcing method; all others with even method.

Explanation

- LU-9 and BL-13 tonify Lung-Qi.
- Ren-12, BL-20, BL-21 and ST-36 tonify Stomach- and Spleen-Qi.
- Ren-9, SP-6 and ST-40 resolve Phlegm.
- P-5 and P-6 open the Mind's orifices.
- Du-20 and Du-26 open the Mind's orifices and clear the Brain.

Herbal therapy

Prescription

DI TAN TANG
Washing Away Phlegm Decoction

Explanation

This formula resolves Phlegm and tonifies Qi. It should be modified with the addition of Yuan Zhi *Radix Polygalae* to open the Mind's orifices.

Prescription

SHI WEI WEN DAN TANG Variation
Ten-Ingredient Warming the Gall-Bladder Decoction Variation

Explanation

The variation of this formula resolves Phlegm, tonifies Qi and opens the Mind's orifices.

> **SUMMARY**
>
> **Qi deficiency with Phlegm**
>
> *Points*
>
> LU-9 Taiyuan, BL-13 Feishu, Ren-12 Zhongwan, BL-20 Pishu, BL-21 Weishu, ST-36 Zusanli, Ren-9 Shuifen, SP-6 Sanyinjiao, ST-40 Fenglong, P-5 Jianshi, P-6 Neiguan, Du-20 Baihui, Du-26 Renzhong. LU-9, BL-13, Ren-12, BL-20, BL-21 and ST-36 with reinforcing method; all others with even method.

Herbal therapy

Prescription

DI TAN TANG
Washing Away Phlegm Decoction

Prescription

SHI WEI WEN DAN TANG Variation
Ten-Ingredient Warming the Gall-Bladder Decoction Variation

Knotted Heat in the Heart channel

Clinical manifestations

Depression with sudden onset, flustered feeling in the heart region, laughing without reason, insomnia, feeling of heat in the nose and eyes, thirst, mouth ulcers.

Tongue: Red, redder tip, yellow coating.

Pulse: Overflowing-Rapid.

Treatment principle

Drain Heart-Fire, open the Mind's orifices, calm the Mind.

Acupuncture

Points

HE-8 Shaofu, HE-7 Shenmen, Du-24 Shenting, Ren-15 Jiuwei, BL-44 Shentang, P-8 Laogong, P-5 Jianshi. All with reducing or even method.

Explanation

- HE-8 drains Heart-Fire.
- HE-7, Du-24, Ren-15 and BL-44 clear Heart-Heat and calm the Mind.
- P-8 drains Heart-Fire and opens the Mind's orifices.
- P-5 Jianshi resolves Phlegm from the Mind.

Herbal therapy

Prescription

DAO CHI SAN Variation
Eliminating Redness Powder Variation

Explanation

This formula drains Heart-Fire and calms the Mind.

Modifications

- If there is agitation, add Dan Dou Chi *Semen Sojae preparatum* and Shan Zhi Zi *Fructus Gardeniae*.
- If there is a feeling of heat in eyes and nose, add Long Dan Cao *Radix Gentianae*, Shi Jue Ming *Concha Haliotidis* and Huang Qin *Radix Scutellariae*.
- If there is epistaxis, add Da Ji *Radix Euphorbiae seu Knoxiae*, Xiao Ji *Herba Cirisii*, Mu Dan Pi *Cortex Moutan* and Zi Cao *Herba Lithospermi*.
- If the patient is suffering from insomnia, add Suan Zao Ren *Semen Ziziphi spinosae*, Ye Jiao Teng *Caulis Polygoni multiflori* and Zhen Zhu Mu *Concha Margaritiferae usta*.

SUMMARY

Knotted Heat in the Heart channel

Points

HE-8 Shaofu, HE-7 Shenmen, Du-24 Shenting, Ren-15 Jiuwei, BL-44 Shentang, P-8 Laogong, P-5 Jianshi. All with reducing or even method.

Herbal therapy

Prescription

DAO CHI SAN Variation
Eliminating Redness Powder Variation

Phlegm obstructing the Heart orifices

Clinical manifestations

Depression, mental dullness, backwardness, emotional dullness, muttering to oneself, incoherent speech, staring eyes, absence of blinking.

Tongue: Swollen with sticky coating.

Pulse: Slippery.

Treatment principle

Resolve Phlegm, open the Mind's orifices.

Acupuncture

Points

P-5 Jianshi, Du-20 Baihui, Du-24 Shenting, ST-40 Fenglong, SP-6 Sanyinjiao, Ren-9 Shuifen. All with reducing or even method.

Explanation

- P-5, Du-20 and Du-24 open the Mind's orifices.
- ST-40, SP-6 and Ren-9 resolve Phlegm.

Herbal therapy

Prescription

DI TAN TANG
Washing Away Phlegm Decoction

Explanation

This formula resolves Phlegm and opens the Mind's orifices.

> **SUMMARY**
>
> **Phlegm obstructing the Heart orifices**
>
> *Points*
>
> P-5 Jianshi, Du-20 Baihui, Du-24 Shenting, ST-40 Fenglong, SP-6 Sanyinjiao, Ren-9 Shuifen. All with reducing or even method.
>
> *Herbal therapy*
>
> *Prescription*
>
> **DI TAN TANG**
> *Washing Away Phlegm Decoction*

KUANG

Phlegm-Fire harassing upwards

Clinical manifestations

Manic behavior with sudden onset, emotional upsets, shouting, scolding or hitting people, exceptional physical strength, not eating or sleeping, agitation, an angry look in the eyes, shouting abuse, desire to climb to high places, irritability, inability to rest, breaking things, rash/impulsive behavior, rash movements, constipation, headache, insomnia, red face and eyes, anger.

Tongue: Red, thick-sticky-yellow coating, Stomach–Heart crack with rough-sticky-dry yellow coating inside it.

Pulse: Rapid-Wiry-Overflowing-Slippery.

Treatment principle

Calm the Heart, resolve Phlegm, drain Liver-Fire, drain Heart-Fire, open the Mind's orifices.

Acupuncture

Points

P-7 Daling, P-5 Jianshi, LIV-2 Xingjian, HE-8 Shaofu, P-8 Laogong, Du-19 Houding, G.B.-17 Zhengying, G.B.-18 Chengling, ST-40 Fenglong, Ren-12 Zhongwan, Ren-9 Shuifen, SP-6 Sanyinjiao. All with reducing or even method.

Explanation

- P-7 and P-5 open the Mind's orifices.
- LIV-2 and HE-8 drain Liver- and Heart-Fire, respectively.
- P-8 drains Heart-Fire and opens the Mind's orifices.
- Du-19, G.B.-17 and G.B.-18 calm the Mind and open the Mind's orifices.
- ST-40, Ren-12, Ren-9 and SP-6 resolve Phlegm.

Herbal therapy

Prescription

SHENG TIE LUO YIN
Frusta Ferri Decoction

Explanation

This formula resolves Phlegm, calms the Mind and opens the Mind's orifices. The original formula contains Zhu Sha *Cinnabaris* which should be eliminated due to its toxicity.

The formula obviously contains iron, which is actually its emperor herb; the use of minerals in herbal formulae is not allowed in European Union countries.

Prescription

WEN DAN TANG
Warming the Gall-Bladder Decoction

Explanation

This formula resolves Phlegm-Heat from the Heart and Lungs, calms the Mind and opens the Mind's orifices. The formula should be modified with the addition of herbs to resolve Phlegm and open the Mind's orifices, such as Shi Chang Pu *Rhizoma Acori tatarinowii* and Yuan Zhi *Radix Polygalae*.

Prescription

DANG GUI LONG HUI WAN
Angelica-Gentiana-Aloe Pill

Explanation

This formula drains Liver-Fire and calms the Mind. It contains She Xiang which should be removed from the formula.

The formula should be modified with the addition of herbs to resolve Phlegm and open the Mind's orifices, such as Ban Xia *Rhizoma Pinelliae preparatum*, Shi Chang Pu *Rhizoma Acori tatarinowii* and Yuan Zhi *Radix Polygalae*.

Prescription

WEN DAN TANG plus **ZHU SHA AN SHEN WAN**
Warming the Gall-Bladder Decoction plus *Cinnabar Calming the Mind Pill*

Explanation

These two formulae are used if the symptoms of obstruction of the Mind are pronounced (mental confusion, incoherent speech, loss of insight).

Please note that the use of Zhu Sha is not allowed and it should therefore be omitted from the formula.

Prescription

MENG SHI GUN TAN WAN
Chloritum Chasing-away Phlegm Pill

Explanation

This formula strongly resolves Phlegm by moving downwards. It is used if there is constipation or dry stools.

Prescription

XIE XIN TANG Variation
Draining the Heart Decoction Variation

Explanation

This formula is used if there are pronounced manifestations of Heart-Fire.

Table 19.5 compares and contrasts the formulae for the pattern of Phlegm-Fire harassing upwards in *Kuang*.

Table 19.5 Differentiation of formulae for the pattern of Phlegm-Fire harassing upwards in *Kuang*

	ACTION	SYMPTOM	TONGUE
Sheng Tie Luo Yin	Resolve Phlegm, sink the Mind, open the Mind's orifices	Mental confusion, irritability	Swollen, sticky coating
Wen Dan Tang	Resolve Phlegm, clear Heat, restore the descending of Lung-Qi	Anxiety	Red, Swollen, sticky-yellow coating
Dang Gui Long Hui Wan	Drain Liver-Fire, calm the Mind, move downwards	Constipation, dry stools	Red, redder sides
Wen Dan Tang plus Zhu Sha An Shen Wan	Resolve Phlegm, clear Heat, open the Mind's orifices	Mental confusion	Red tip, Swollen, sticky coating
Meng Shi Gun Tan Wan	Resolve Phlegm, sink the Ming, move downwards	Mental confusion, constipation, dry stools	Swollen
Xie Xin Tang	Drain Heart-Fire, calm the Mind	Insomnia	Red, redder tip

SUMMARY

Phlegm-Fire harassing upwards

Points

P-7 Daling, P-5 Jianshi, LIV-2 Xingjian, HE-8 Shaofu, P-8 Laogong, Du-19 Houding, G.B.-17 Zhengying, G.B.-18 Chengling, ST-40 Fenglong, Ren-12 Zhongwan, Ren-9 Shuifen, SP-6 Sanyinjiao. All with reducing or even method.

Herbal therapy

Prescription

SHENG TIE LUO YIN
Frusta Ferri Decoction

Prescription

WEN DAN TANG
Warming the Gall-Bladder Decoction

Prescription

DANG GUI LONG HUI WAN
Angelica-Gentiana-Aloe Pill

Prescription

WEN DAN TANG plus **ZHU SHA AN SHEN WAN**
Warming the Gall-Bladder Decoction plus *Cinnabar Calming the Mind Pill*

Prescription

MENG SHI GUN TAN WAN
Chloritum Chasing-away Phlegm Pill

Prescription

XIE XIN TANG Variation
Draining the Heart Decoction Variation

Case history

A 52-year-old man had been suffering from manic-depression for at least 20 years. His wife confirmed that it would be difficult to pinpoint when the disease started as it was difficult to distinguish pathological traits from his normally boisterous behavior.

He was short and overweight, talked in a loud voice and his speech was frequently interspersed by bursts of laughter. His complexion was reddish. He talked a lot and frequently went off on a tangent, telling a story about his colorful and interesting life. His family was Italian but they had to leave Italy after the beginning of the persecution of the Jews during the Fascist years. So they sailed to Egypt when my patient was 3 years old. He lived in many different countries and was one of the very few people to take part in all three Israeli–Arab wars. He was a tank commander and a decorated war hero. I was struck by the way he talked about his war experiences as if they had been exciting school-boy adventures.

He had a colorful sexual history, with a string of infidelities to the chagrin of his long-suffering wife. When he spoke, he almost shouted and was difficult to stop.

He had been diagnosed with bipolar disorder after a period of intense, ceaseless activity and insomnia. His periods of high energy were always followed by periods of black depression; however, these did not last long and he had longer periods of mania than of depression.

I asked him about his general health and this was quite good; he had few physical symptoms. However, the ones that were significant from the point of view of Chinese medicine were a feeling of oppression in the chest, palpitations and sputum in the throat.

His tongue was quite typical: it was Red, Swollen, with a deep Heart crack and a sticky-yellow coating; his pulse was Slippery-Wiry-Rapid.

Diagnosis The few symptoms of feeling of oppression in the chest, palpitations and sputum in the throat, together with the tongue and pulse, point unmistakably to Phlegm-Fire in the Heart as the cause of his manic-depression. His excessive weight also confirms Phlegm.

Treatment I treated him primarily with acupuncture and selected points from the following.

- HE-7 Shenmen and P-5 Jianshi to calm the Mind and open the Mind's orifices.
- Du-19 Houding and Ren-15 to calm the Mind and open the Mind's orifices.
- Ren-12 Zhongwan, ST-40 Fenglong, Ren-9 Shuifen, SP-6 Sanyinjiao and KI-7 Fuliu to resolve Phlegm.
- HE-8 Shaofu to clear Heart-Heat.

I treated him weekly for a long time (at least 2 years) and then started spacing out the treatments. He improved dramatically, reporting a reduction in his manic phases, feeling much calmer and sleeping better. Significantly, he also stopped his womanizing. Apart from a progressive improvement in his symptoms, he always felt an immediate benefit during each treatment.

This patient continues to be well at the time of writing (15 years later) and I treat him only four or five times a year.

Fire in Bright Yang

Clinical manifestations

Manic behavior, raving walking, shouting, abusing people, climbing to high places, singing, discarding clothes, unusual physical strength, foul breath, red face, constipation.

Tongue: Red with dark-yellow or black, dry coating.

Pulse: Deep and Wiry.

Treatment principle

Drain Stomach-Fire by moving downwards, calm the Mind, open the Mind's orifices, resolve Phlegm.

Acupuncture

Points

ST-44 Neiting, L.I.-11 Quchi, ST-40 Fenglong, P-8 Laogong, HE-8 Shaofu, ST-25 Tianshu, SP-15 Daheng, P-5 Jianshi. All with reducing or even method.

Explanation

- ST-44 and L.I.-11 drain Stomach-Fire.
- ST-40 helps to drain Stomach-Fire.
- P-8 and HE-8 drain Heart-Fire and calm the Mind.
- ST-25 stabilizes the Ethereal Soul and Corporeal Soul.
- SP-15 moves downwards and promotes the bowel movement.
- P-5 Jianshi resolves Phlegm from the Mind.

Herbal therapy

Prescription

DA CHENG QI TANG Variation
Great Conducting Qi Decoction Variation

Explanation

This formula drains Stomach-Fire by moving downwards, resolves Phlegm and opens the Mind's orifices.

> **SUMMARY**
>
> **Fire in Bright Yang**
>
> *Points*
>
> ST-44 Neiting, L.I.-11 Quchi, ST-40 Fenglong, P-8 Laogong, HE-8 Shaofu, ST-25 Tianshu, SP-15 Daheng, P-5 Jianshi. All with reducing or even method.
>
> *Herbal therapy*
>
> *Prescription*
>
> **DA CHENG QI TANG** Variation
> *Great Conducting Qi Decoction* Variation

Gall Bladder- and Liver-Fire

Clinical manifestations

Manic behavior, irritability, propensity to outbursts of anger, red face and eyes, bitter taste, laughing inappropriately, shouting, hypochondrial and chest pain, palpitations.

Tongue: Red with dark-yellow coating.

Pulse: Rapid-Wiry-Slipper.

Treatment principle

Drain Liver-Fire, resolve Phlegm, calm the Mind.

Acupuncture

Points

LIV-2 Xingjian, G.B.-44 Zuqiaoyin, L.I.-11 Quchi, ST-40 Fenglong, SP-6 Sanyinjiao, Ren-9 Shuifen, HE-7 Shenmen, P-5 Jianshi. All with reducing or even method.

Explanation

- LIV-2 and G.B.-44 drain Liver- and Gall Bladder-Fire.
- L.I.-11 clears Heat and cools Blood in general.
- ST-40, SP-6 and Ren-9 resolve Phlegm.

- HE-7 calms the Mind.
- P-5 Jianshi resolves Phlegm from the Mind.

Herbal therapy

Prescription

LONG DAN XIE GAN TANG Variation
Gentiana Draining the Liver Decoction Variation

Explanation

This variation of Long Dan Xie Gan Tang drains Liver-Fire, resolves Phlegm and calms the Mind.

> **SUMMARY**
>
> **Gall Bladder- and Liver-Fire**
>
> *Points*
>
> LIV-2 Xingjian, G.B.-44, L.I.-11 Quchi, ST-40 Fenglong, SP-6 Sanyinjiao, Ren-9 Shuifen, HE-7 Shenmen, P-5 Jianshi. All with reducing or even method.
>
> *Herbal therapy*
>
> *Prescription*
>
> **LONG DAN XIE GAN TANG** Variation
> *Gentiana Draining the Liver Decoction* Variation

Fire injuring Yin with Phlegm

Clinical manifestations

Chronic *Kuang*, talking a lot, easily startled, mental restlessness, thin body (loss of weight), red face, malar flush, feeling of heat in the evening.

Tongue: Red, Swollen, without coating.

Pulse: Fine-Rapid.

Treatment principle

Nourish Yin, clear Empty-Heat, calm the Mind, resolve Phlegm, open the Mind's orifices.

Acupuncture

Points

HE-7 Shenmen, HE-6 Yinxi, P-7 Daling, KI-3 Taixi, Ren-4 Guanyuan, SP-6 Sanyinjiao, ST-40 Fenglong, Ren-12 Zhongwan, Ren-9 Shuifen, Du-24 Shenting, Du-19 Houding, P-5 Jianshi. KI-3, Ren-4 and SP-6 with reinforcing method; all the others with even method.

Explanation

- HE-7, HE-6 and P-7 calm the Mind and open the Mind's orifices.
- KI-3, Ren-4 and SP-6 nourish Yin.
- ST-40, Ren-12 and Ren-9 resolve Phlegm.
- Du-24 and Du-19 calm the Mind and open the Mind's orifices.
- P-5 resolves Phlegm from the Mind.

Herbal therapy

Prescription

ER YIN JIAN
Two Yin Decoction

Explanation

This formula nourishes Yin and calms the Mind. In order to treat bipolar disorder, it should be modified with the addition of some herbs to resolve Phlegm and open the Mind's orifices, such as Ban Xia *Rhizoma Pinelliae preparatum*, Yuan Zhi *Radix Polygalae* and Shi Chang Pu *Rhizoma Acori tatarinowii*.

Please note that the original formula contains Mu Tong which should be eliminated due to its potential toxicity.

Prescription

ER YIN JIAN Variation
Two Yin Decoction Variation

Explanation

This formula nourishes Yin, settles the Ethereal Soul and calms the Mind.

> **SUMMARY**
>
> **Fire injuring Yin with Phlegm**
>
> *Points*
>
> HE-7 Shenmen, HE-6 Yinxi, P-7 Daling, KI-3 Taixi, Ren-4 Guanyuan, SP-6 Sanyinjiao, ST-40 Fenglong,

Ren-12 Zhongwan, Ren-9 Shuifen, Du-24 Shenting, Du-19 Houding, P-5 Jianshi. KI-3, Ren-4 and SP-6 with reinforcing method; all the others with even method.

Herbal therapy

Prescription

ER YIN JIAN
Two Yin Decoction

Prescription

ER YIN JIAN Variation
Two Yin Decoction Variation

Case history

A 45-year-old woman had been suffering from bipolar disorder for 10 years. Her disease seemed to have started after the birth of her third child. Her symptoms during the manic phases were severe and included grossly increased energy and activity, mental restlessness, excessively "high" euphoric mood, talking a lot and very fast, staying up all night, spending sprees and delusional thinking. Her condition was quite severe as it was bordering on psychosis. For example, she once spent a very long time telling me how the KGB had been shadowing her years before.

She was on medication (lithium) but she had not been consistent taking it and her disease was therefore out of control. She was thin, had a gaunt, haunted look and her complexion was red on the cheekbones.

Her tongue was Red, redder on the sides, Swollen, with a sticky but rootless yellow coating; her pulse was Fine and Rapid.

Diagnosis As she displays clear symptoms of obstruction of the Mind, she must have Phlegm and this is confirmed by the swelling of her tongue and the stickiness of the coating. The thinness of her body, the red cheekbones, the rootless coating and the pulse indicate Yin deficiency. This is therefore a case of Fire having injured the Yin fluids, with Phlegm-Fire obstructing the Heart. Fire was also affecting the Liver as indicated by the redder sides of the tongue.

Treatment I treated her with a variation of Er Yin Jian as follows.

- **Ban Xia** *Rhizoma Pinelliae preparatum* 6 g
- **Zhu Ru** *Caulis Bambusae in Taeniam* 6 g
- **Yuan Zhi** *Radix Polygalae* 6 g
- **Shi Chang Pu** *Rhizoma Acori tatarinowii* 6 g
- **Sheng Di Huang** *Radix Rehmanniae* 10 g
- **Mai Men Dong** *Radix Ophiopogonis* 9 g
- **Suan Zao Ren** *Semen Ziziphi spinosae* 15 g
- **Huang Lian** *Rhizoma Coptidis* 3 g
- **Mu Dan Pi** *Cortex Moutan* 6 g
- **Fu Ling** *Poria* 9 g
- **Deng Xin Cao** *Medulla Junci* 6 g
- **Gan Cao** *Radix Glycyrrhizae uralensis* 3 g

I treated her with variations of this formula as well as with acupuncture, selecting points from the following.

- HE-7 Shenmen and P-5 Jianshi to calm the Mind and open the Mind's orifices.
- G.B.-13 Benshen and G.B.-18 Chengling to open the Mind's orifices.
- Du-19 Houding and Ren-15 to calm the Mind.
- LIV-2 Xiangian and HE-8 Shaofu to drain Liver- and Heart-Fire.
- Ren-12 Zhongwan, Ren-9 Shuifen, ST-40 Fenglong and SP-6 Sanyinjiao to resolve Phlegm.
- Ren-4 Guanyuan, KI-3 Taixi and SP-6 Sanyinjiao to nourish Yin.

The combination of herbal medicine and acupuncture greatly helped to stabilize her moods and work out the proper dosage of lithium. Due to the severity of her condition, she will have to be on lithium continuously and she is still being treated with herbal medicine only.

Qi stagnation, Blood stasis, Phlegm

Clinical manifestations

Chronic *Kuang*, talking a lot, easily startled, mental restlessness, abdominal pain, dark complexion, insomnia, agitation at night.

Tongue: Reddish-Purple, Swollen.

Pulse: Wiry-Slippery.

Treatment principle

Move Qi, invigorate Blood, eliminate stasis, resolve Phlegm, calm the Mind, open the Mind's orifices.

Acupuncture

Points

P-6 Neiguan, HE-7 Shenmen, LIV-3 Taichong, SP-10 Xuehai, BL-17 Geshu, ST-40 Fenglong, Ren-12 Zhongwan, Ren-9 Shuifen, Du-24 Shenting, Du-19 Houding, G.B.-17 Zhengying, G.B.-18 Chengling, P-5 Jianshi. All with reducing or even method.

Explanation

- P-6 and HE-7 calm the Mind and invigorate Blood.
- LIV-3, SP-10 and BL-17 invigorate Blood and eliminate stasis.
- ST-40, Ren-12 and Ren-9 resolve Phlegm.
- Du-24 and Du-19 calm the Mind and open the Mind's orifices.
- G.B.-17 and G.B.-18 open the Mind's orifices.
- P-5 resolves Phlegm from the Mind.

Herbal therapy

Prescription

DIAN KUANG MENG XING TANG
Manic-Depression Regaining Consciousness after a Dream Decoction

Explanation

This formula moves Qi, invigorates Blood, resolves Phlegm and opens the Mind's orifices. It is suitable if there is Blood stasis.

Please note that the original formula contains Mu Tong which should be eliminated due to its potential toxicity.

Prescription

DING KUANG ZHU YU TANG
Calming Mania and Eliminating Stasis Decoction

Explanation

This formula invigorates Blood, calms the Mind and opens the Mind's orifices. It should be modified with the addition of herbs to open the Mind's orifices such as Yuan Zhi *Radix Polygalae* and Ban Xia *Rhizoma Pinelliae preparatum*.

> **SUMMARY**
>
> **Qi stagnation, Blood stasis, Phlegm**
>
> *Points*
>
> P-6 Neiguan, HE-7 Shenmen, LIV-3 Taichong, SP-10 Xuehai, BL-17 Geshu, ST-40 Fenglong, Ren-12 Zhongwan, Ren-9 Shuifen, Du-24 Shenting, Du-19 Houding, G.B.-17 Zhengying, G.B.-18 Chengling, P-5 Jianshi. All with reducing or even method.
>
> *Herbal therapy*
>
> *Prescription*
>
> **DIAN KUANG MENG XING TANG**
> *Manic-Depression Regaining Consciousness after a Dream Decoction*
>
> *Prescription*
>
> **DING KUANG ZHU YU TANG**
> *Calming Mania and Eliminating Stasis Decoction*

Yin deficiency with Empty Heat

Clinical manifestations

Chronic manic behavior, listlessness, incessant talking, easily startled, mental restlessness, insomnia.

Tongue: Red without coating.

Pulse: Fine-Rapid.

Treatment principle

Nourish Yin, clear Empty Heat, calm the Mind.

Acupuncture

Points

KI-3 Taixi, LIV-8 Ququan, SP-6 Sanyinjiao, Ren-4 Guanyuan, HE-7 Shenmen, Ren-15 Jiuwei, HE-6 Yinxi, P-7 Daling, ST-40 Fenglong, Ren-9 Shuifen, P-5 Jianshi. KI-3, LIV-8, SP-6 and Ren-4 with reinforcing method; all others with even method.

Explanation

- KI-3, LIV-8, SP-6 and Ren-4 nourish Liver- and Kidney-Yin.
- HE-7, Ren-15, HE-6 and P-7 calm the Mind and clear Empty Heat.

- ST-40 Fenglong and Ren-9 resolve Phlegm.
- P-5 resolves Phlegm from the Mind.

Herbal therapy

Prescription

ER YIN JIAN Variation
Two Yin Decoction Variation

> **SUMMARY**
>
> **Yin deficiency with Empty Heat**
>
> *Points*
>
> KI-3 Taixi, LIV-8 Ququan, SP-6 Sanyinjiao, Ren-4 Guanyuan, HE-7 Shenmen, Ren-15 Jiuwei, HE-6 Yinxi, P-7 Daling, ST-40 Fenglong, Ren-9 Shuifen, P-5 Jianshi. KI-3, LIV-8, SP-6 and Ren-4 with reinforcing method; all others with even method.
>
> *Herbal therapy*
>
> *Prescription*
>
> **ER YIN JIAN** Variation
> *Two Yin Decoction* Variation

MODERN CHINESE LITERATURE

Journal of Chinese Medicine (*Zhong Yi Za Zhi* 中医杂志), Vol. 25, No. 11, 1984, p. 31.

Chen Chao, "Clinical observations on the use of a variation of Wen Dan Tang to treat 30 cases of *Dian Kuang*"

Thirty patients suffering from *Dian Kuang* were treated, 8 men and 22 women ranging in age from 14 to 49; 16 patients had a diagnosis of schizophrenia. Of the total, 26 patients fell under the category of *Dian* and 4 under that of *Kuang*.

The formula used was a variation of Wen Dan Tang *Warming the Gall-Bladder Decoction* as follows.

- **Zhu Ru** *Caulis Bambusae in Taeniam*
- **Chen Pi** *Pericarpium Citri reticulatae*
- **Ban Xia** *Rhizoma Pinelliae preparatum*
- **Fu Ling** *Poria*
- **Zhi Ke** *Fructus Aurantii*
- **Yuan Zhi** *Radix Polygalae*
- **Shi Chang Pu** *Rhizoma Acori tatarinowii*
- **Suan Zao Ren** *Semen Ziziphi spinosae*
- **Long Gu** *Mastodi Ossis fossilia*
- **Mu Li** *Concha Ostreae*
- **Zhen Zhu Mu** *Concha Margaritiferae usta*
- **Mai Men Dong** *Radix Ophiopogonis*

The authors report that 13 patients (43%) were cured; 5 (17%) improved; 8 (27%) somewhat improved; no results, 4 patients (13%).

Chen Jin Guang 1992 Complete Textbook of Chinese Patterns in Contemporary Chinese Medicine

(Xian Dai Zhong Yi Lin Zheng Quan Shu 先代中医临证全书). Beijing Publishing House, Beijing, p. 109.

Dr Wang Ning Ni treated 310 patients with Mania (*Kuang*) with Meng Xia Cheng Qi Tang *Chlorite-Pinellia Conducting Qi Decoction*.

The patients ranged in age from 15 to 59. There were 216 men and 94 women. The results were as follows.

- *Cured*: 165
- *Improved*: 129
- *No results*: 16

The formula used was as follows.

- **Meng Shi** *Lapis Chloriti seu Micae* 20 g
- **Huang Qin** *Radix Scutellariae* 20 g
- **Ban Xia** *Rhizoma Pinelliae preparatum* 10 g
- **Zhi Shi** *Fructus Aurantii immaturus* 10 g
- **Shi Chang Pu** *Rhizoma Acori tatarinowii* 10 g
- **Lian Qiao** *Fructus Forsythiae* 10 g
- **Yu Jin** *Radix Curcumae* 15 g
- **Hou Po** *Cortex Magnoliae officinalis* 12 g
- **Da Huang** *Radix et Rhizoma Rhei* 10 g
- **Mang Xiao** *Natrii Sulfas* 10 g

Modifications

- *Heart-Fire*: Huang Lian *Rhizoma Coptidis*, Zhu Ye *Folium Phyllostachys nigrae*.
- *Liver-Fire*: Long Dan Cao *Radix Gentianae*, Xia Ku Cao *Spica Prunellae*.
- *Stomach-Heat*: Shi Gao *Gypsum fibrosum*, Zhi Mu *Radix Anemarrhaenae*.

Dr Ma Ming Lei treated 75 patients suffering from Manic-Depression. The formula used was a variation of Di Tan Tang *Washing Away Phlegm Decoction*:

- **Long Chi** *Fossilia Dentis Mastodi* 30 g
- **Shi Gao** *Gypsum fibrosum* 15 g
- **Dan Nan Xing** *Rhizoma Arisaematis preparatum* 10 g
- **Shi Chang Pu** *Rhizoma Acori tatarinowii* 10 g
- **Zhi Shi** *Fructus Aurantii immaturus* 10 g
- **Fu Ling** *Poria* 10 g
- **Chen Pi** *Pericarpium Citri reticulatae* 10 g
- **Ban Xia** *Rhizoma Pinelliae preparatum* 10 g
- **Gan Cao** *Radix Glycyrrhizae uralensis* 10 g
- **Dang Shen** *Radix Codonopsis* 10 g
- **Zhu Ru** *Caulis Bambusae in Taeniam* 6 g
- **Wu Gong** *Scolopendra* 2 pieces
- **Sheng Jiang** *Rhizoma Zingiberis recens* 3 slices
- **Da Zao** *Fructus Jujubae* 7 dates.

Liang Jian Bo, "To treat *Dian,* settle the Heart, eliminate Stagnation, calm the Mind and resolve Phlegm; to treat *Kuang,* clear the Stomach, drain Fire and resolve Phlegm"

In: Shi Yu Guang 1992 Dang Dai Ming Yi Lin Zheng Jing Hua 当代名医临证精华 [Essential Clinical Experience of Famous Contemporary Doctors – Manic-Depression and Epilepsy]. Ancient Chinese Medicine Texts Publishing House, Beijing, pp. 14–18.

Dr Liang says that in *Dian* there is a deficiency of the Heart, Liver and Spleen so that the Mind is harassed and Liver-Qi is chaotic.

He thinks *Kuang* is due to sadness, anger, indignation and vexation, which cause the Liver to develop Fire; this invades the Stomach and harasses the Heart, the Heart orifices are obfuscated and Heart-Qi rebels upwards. In *Kuang*, the Liver, Heart, Stomach and Pericardium are affected, with Fire in the Liver, Heart and Stomach. Fire also invades the Pericardium and this causes the Ethereal Soul to become restless. As a broad generalization, Dr Liang says that in *Dian* there is a deficiency of the Yin Organs, while in *Kuang*, an Excess of the Yang Organs.

Interestingly, Dr Liang describes the pulse qualities associated with *Dian* and *Kuang*. He says that in the former the pulse is Deep and Fire, while in the latter it is Overflowing and Full. He says that in *Kuang* the pulse feels Floating, Big, Slippery, Rapid and Long; in *Dian* the pulse feels Empty, soft, Soggy and Weak.

Dr Liang then makes the interesting observation that if in *Dian* the pulse feels Floating from the Rear to the Front in a straight line, it indicates the presence of Phlegm.

For *Dian*, Dr Liang recommends regulating Heart-Qi, eliminating stagnation, calming the Mind and resolving Phlegm. He uses the following variation of the formula Dao Tan Tang *Conducting Phlegm Decoction*.

- **Ban Xia** *Rhizoma Pinelliae preparatum*
- **Chen Pi** *Pericarpium Citri reticulatae*
- **Fu Ling** *Poria*
- **Gan Cao** *Radix Glycyrrhizae uralensis*
- **Dan Nan Xing** *Rhizoma Arisaematis preparatum*
- **Zhi Shi** *Fructus Aurantii immaturus*
- **Mu Xiang** *Radix Aucklandiae*
- **Shi Chang Pu** *Rhizoma Acori tatarinowii*
- **Fu Zi** *Radix Aconiti lateralis preparata*
- **Sheng Jiang** *Rhizoma Zingiberis recens*
- **Da Zao** *Fructus Jujubae*

If in *Dian* there is a complicated condition of Heart-Qi stagnation, Phlegm in the Interior and Liver-Fire with Phlegm, Dr Liang recommends using the above formula Dao Tan Tang *Conducting Phlegm Decoction* plus:

- **Huang Lian** *Rhizoma Coptidis*
- **Huang Qin** *Radix Scutellariae*
- **Yuan Zhi** *Radix Polygalae*
- **Zhu Sha** *Cinnabaris* (we are not allowed to use this)
- **Chen Xiang** *Lignum Aquilariae resinatum.*

Dr Liang says that in some cases of *Dian*, although the main manifestations are depression and withdrawn mood, some patients may display some restlessness; this indicates Heat in the Heart, Spleen and Pericardium and that there is some Fullness within the Deficiency.

In these cases, Dr Liang uses first Di Tan Tang *Washing Away Phlegm Decoction*, then Niu Huang Qing Xin Wan *Calculus Bovis Clearing the Heart Pill.* Afterwards, he nourishes the Heart with Gui Pi Tang *Tonifying the Spleen Decoction* with the addition of:

- **Long Gu** *Mastodi Ossis fossilia*
- **Mu Li** *Concha Ostreae*
- **Shi Chang Pu** *Rhizoma Acori tatarinowii*
- **Wu Wei Zi** *Fructus Schisandrae.*

Alternatively, one can use Shen Zhong Dan *Pillow Pill.*

In chronic *Dian*, there is Heart and deficiency which deprives the Mind of its residence. There is therefore

Heart deficiency, the Mind is scattered and the Original Qi is weakened. In such cases, Dr Liang uses Gui Shen Dan *Tonifying the Spirit Pill.*

- **Suan Zao Ren** *Semen Ziziphi spinosae* 9 g
- **Fu Ling** *Poria* 9 g
- **Ren Shen** *Radix Ginseng* 9 g
- **Zhu Sha** *Cinnabaris* 9 g (we are not allowed to use this)
- **Dang Gui** *Radix Angelicae sinensis* 6 g

As for *Kuang*, Dr Liang thinks this is often due to Fire in the Stomach deriving from emotional stress such as anger, sadness and indignation. These cause the development of Fire in the Liver and Pericardium. For treatment, Dr Liang advocates draining Stomach-Fire and resolving Phlegm with the formula Er Yang Jian *Two Yang Decoction.*

- **Huang Lian** *Rhizoma Coptidis*
- **Meng Shi** *Lapis Chloriti seu Micae*
- **Da Huang** *Radix et Rhizoma Rhei*
- **Long Dan Cao** *Radix Gentianae*
- **Shan Zhi Zi** *Fructus Gardeniae*
- **Qing Dai** *Indigo naturalis*
- **Mang Xiao** *Natrii Sulfas*
- **Dan Nan Xing** *Rhizoma Arisaematis preparatum*
- **Di Long** *Pheretima*
- **Shi Chang Pu** *Rhizoma Acori tatarinowii*
- **Yuan Zhi** *Radix Polygalae*
- **Shi Jue Ming** *Concha Haliotidis*

Dr Liang says that he has been using this formula for bipolar disorder (manic phase) for many years with good results.

As for chronic *Kuang*, Dr Liang says that, in addition to Fire and Phlegm (Full conditions), there is also a deficiency of Heart-Blood or of Yin which, in turn, leads to Empty Heat. In severe cases of chronic *Kuang* he also advocates using the vomiting treatment method.

If there is Fire in the Upper Burner, Dr Liang uses Sheng Tie Luo Yin *Frusta Ferri Decoction*; if there is Fire in Bright Yang, he uses Dang Gui Cheng Qi Tang *Angelica Conducting Qi Decoction* (Dang Gui *Radix Angelicae sinensis*, Da Huang *Radix et Rhizoma Rhei*, Mang Xiao *Natrii Sulfas* and Gan Cao *Radix Glycyrrhizae uralensis*).

If there is Fire in the Middle Burner, Dr Liang uses Liang Ge San *Cooling the Diaphragm Powder*. If there is Heart-Yin deficiency, he uses Long Chi Qing Hun San *Fossilia Dentis Mastodi Clearing the Ethereal Soul Powder*, as follows.

- **Long Chi** *Fossilia Dentis Mastodi*
- **Yuan Zhi** *Radix Polygalae*
- **Suan Zao Ren** *Semen Ziziphi spinosae*
- **Shan Yao** *Rhizoma Dioscoreae*
- **Ren Shen** *Radix Ginseng*
- **Sheng Di Huang** *Radix Rehmanniae*
- **Fu Ling** *Poria*
- **Shi Chang Pu** *Rhizoma Acori tatarinowii*
- **Wu Wei Zi** *Fructus Schisandrae*
- **Mai Men Dong** *Radix Ophiopogonis*
- **Gan Cao** *Radix Glycyrrhizae uralensis*

Dr Liang uses this formula to regulate the Ethereal Soul when this is injured by sadness. When the Corporeal Soul is injured by excessive joy, Dr Liang uses Qing Shen Tang *Clearing the Spirit Decoction*, as follows.

- **Huang Lian** *Rhizoma Coptidis*
- **Fu Ling** *Poria*
- **Bai Zi Ren** *Semen Platycladi*
- **Yuan Zhi** *Radix Polygalae*
- **Shi Chang Pu** *Rhizoma Acori tatarinowii*
- **Gan Cao** *Radix Glycyrrhizae uralensis*
- **Suan Zao Ren** *Semen Ziziphi spinosae*
- **Zhu Li** *Succus Bambusae*

If there is Lung deficiency, add Bei Sha Shen *Radix Glehniae*; if Stomach deficiency, Ren Shen *Radix Ginseng*; if Liver deficiency, Ling Yang Jiao *Cornu Saigae tataricae*.

Wang Ji Ru, "The disease [*Dian Kuang*] is due to Phlegm, Fire and Stagnation; treat it by resolving Phlegm and clearing Heat"

In: Shi Yu Guang 1992 Dang Dai Ming Yi Lin Zheng Jing Hua [Essential Clinical Experience of Famous Contemporary Doctors – Manic-Depression and Epilepsy]. Ancient Chinese Medicine Texts Publishing House, Beijing, pp. 20–22.

Dr Wang treats Mania (*Kuang*) with two main formulae which resolve Phlegm and drain Fire. The first is Huo Tan Ding Kuang Tang *Breaking Phlegm and Stopping Mania Decoction*, as follows.

- **Long Chi** *Fossilia Dentis Mastodi* 30 g
- **Mu Li** *Concha Ostreae* 30 g
- **Shi Jue Ming** *Concha Haliotidis* 30 g
- **Zhen Zhu Mu** *Concha Margaritiferae usta* 30 g
- **Long Dan Cao** *Radix Gentianae* 10 g
- **Tian Zhu Huang** *Concretio Silicea Bambusae* 10 g

- **Shi Chang Pu** *Rhizoma Acori tatarinowii* 10 g
- **Yu Jin** *Radix Curcumae* 10 g
- **Xuan Fu Hua** *Flos Inulae* 10 g
- **Dai Zhe Shi** *Hematitum* 10 g
- **Meng Shi** *Lapis Chloriti seu Micae* 30 g
- **Chen Xiang** *Lignum Aquilariae resinatum* 3 g
- **Huang Qin** *Radix Scutellariae* 10 g
- **Da Huang** *Radix et Rhizoma Rhei* 6 g

The emphasis of this formula is very much on sinking Qi to calm the Mind. The other formula that Dr Wang uses for *Kuang* is Jia Wei Wen Dan Tang *Augmented Warming the Gall-Bladder Decoction*:

- **Ban Xia** *Rhizoma Pinelliae preparatum* 10 g
- **Chen Pi** *Pericarpium Citri reticulatae* 10 g
- **Fu Shen** *Sclerotium Poriae pararadicis* 12 g
- **Yuan Zhi** *Radix Polygalae* 10 g
- **Zhu Ru** *Caulis Bambusae in Taeniam* 12 g
- **Zhi Shi** *Fructus Aurantii immaturus* 10 g
- **Shi Chang Pu** *Rhizoma Acori tatarinowii* 10 g
- **Yu Jin** *Radix Curcumae* 10 g
- **Tian Zhu Huang** *Concretio Silicea Bambusae* 10 g
- **Meng Shi** *Lapis Chloriti seu Micae* 30 g
- **Long Chi** *Fossilia Dentis Mastodi* 15 g
- **Mu Li** *Concha Ostreae* 15 g
- **Long Dan Cao** *Radix Gentianae* 10 g
- **Zhu Sha** *Cinnabaris* 1.5 g (we are not allowed to use this).

Ban Xiu Wen, "To treat *Dian Kuang* distinguish Emptiness from Fullness; in Full conditions, drain Liver and Stomach, in Empty conditions, tonify Heart and Spleen"

In: Shi Yu Guang 1992 Dang Dai Ming Yi Lin Zheng Jing Hua [Essential Clinical Experience of Famous Contemporary Doctors – Manic-Depression and Epilepsy]. Ancient Chinese Medicine Texts Publishing House, Beijing, pp. 20–22.

This text provides useful guidelines for differentiating Full from Empty conditions in Manic-Depression. Dr Ban says that when the disease starts with Depression and then progresses into Mania, it is likely to be of a Full nature with Fire in the Liver and Stomach; when it starts with Mania and progresses into Depression, it is likely to be of an Empty nature with deficiency of the Heart and Spleen.

In treatment for Mania from Fire in the Liver and Stomach Dr Ban uses a variation of Tiao Wei Cheng Qi Tang *Regulating the Stomach Conducting Qi Decoction* with the addition of the following herbs:

- **Long Dan Cao** *Radix Gentianae*
- **Shan Zhi Zi** *Fructus Gardeniae*
- **Zhe Bei Mu** *Bulbus Fritillariae thunbergii*
- **Tian Hua Fen** *Radix Trichosanthis*
- **Gua Lou** *Fructus Trichosanthis*
- **Huang Lian** *Rhizoma Coptidis.*

For Depression from deficiency of the Heart and Spleen, Dr Ban uses a variation of Gui Pi Tang *Tonifying the Spleen Decoction*, with the addition of the following herbs:

- **Zhe Bei Mu** *Bulbus Fritillariae thunbergii*
- **Hai Fu Shi** *Pumice*
- **Tian Zhu Huang** *Concretio Silicea Bambusae.*

If the pulse is Fine and the tongue lacks a coating, indicating deficiency of Heart-Yin, Dr Ban uses a variation of Gan Mai Da Zao Tang *Glycyrrhiza-Triticum-Jujuba Decoction* together with Bai He Di Huang Tang *Lilium-Rehmannia Decoction*, with the addition of the following herbs:

- **He Shou Wu** *Radix Polygoni multiflori preparata*
- **He Huan Pi** *Cortex Albiziae*
- **Gou Qi Zi** *Fructus Lycii chinensis*
- **Ye Jiao Teng** *Caulis Polygoni multiflori*
- **Mu Li** *Concha Ostreae*
- **Long Gu** *Mastodi Ossis fossilia.*

Ma Rui Ting, "An outline of patterns and treatment of Manic-Depression (*Dian Kuang*)"

In: Shi Yu Guang 1992 Dang Dai Ming Yi Lin Zheng Jing Hua [Essential Clinical Experience of Famous Contemporary Doctors – Manic-Depression and Epilepsy]. Ancient Chinese Medicine Texts Publishing House, Beijing, pp. 20–22.

Dr Ma Rui Ting has an interesting view of Manic-Depression for two reasons – saying first that, within Depression, there may be aspects of Mania and vice versa; second, Dr Ma treats the Lungs as well, which other doctors do not stress.

For Mania, Dr Ma moves Liver-Qi, restores the descending of Lung-Qi, subdues rebellious Qi and resolves Phlegm. Dr Ma uses the following prescription.

- **Fu Ling** *Poria* 9 g
- **Gan Cao** *Radix Glycyrrhizae uralensis* 6 g
- **Huang Qin** *Radix Scutellariae* 9 g

- **Bai Shao** *Radix Paeoniae alba* 12 g
- **Mu Dan Pi** *Cortex Moutan* 9 g
- **Chen Pi** *Pericarpium Citri reticulatae* 12 g
- **Gua Lou** *Fructus Trichosanthis* 12 g
- **Ban Xia** *Rhizoma Pinelliae preparatum* 9 g
- **Yu Jin** *Radix Curcumae* 9 g
- **Tian Men Dong** *Radix Asparagi* 9 g
- **Shu Qi** *Lacca* 3 g
- **Zhu Sha** *Cinnabaris* 3 g (we are not allowed to use this)

In case of Depression symptoms, Dr Ma adds Long Gu *Mastodi Ossis fossilia* and Mu Li *Concha Ostreae.*

To treat Depression, Dr Ma strengthens the Spleen, harmonizes the Stomach, clears the Lungs and restores the descending of Qi, subdues rebellious Qi, calms the Mind and resolves Phlegm. Dr Ma uses the following empirical prescription.

- **Fu Ling** *Poria* 9 g
- **Gan Cao** *Radix Glycyrrhizae uralensis* 6 g
- **Bai Shao** *Radix Paeoniae alba* 9 g
- **Mu Dan Pi** *Cortex Moutan* 9 g
- **He Shou Wu** *Radix Polygoni multiflori preparata* 9 g
- **Chen Pi** *Pericarpium Citri reticulatae* 9 g
- **Xing Ren** *Semen Armeniacae* 9 g
- **Ban Xia** *Rhizoma Pinelliae preparatum* 9 g
- **Yu Jin** *Radix Curcumae* 9 g
- **Long Gu** *Mastodi Ossis fossilia* 12 g
- **Mu Li** *Concha Ostreae* 15 g
- **Sheng Jiang** *Rhizoma Zingiberis recens* 6 g
- **Cao Guo** *Fructus Tsaoko* 5 g
- **Shi Chang Pu** *Rhizoma Acori tatarinowii* 12 g
- **Zhu Sha** *Cinnabaris* 1.5 g (we are not allowed to use this)

In case of symptoms of Mania, Dr Ma adds Shu Qi *Lacca*.

CLINICAL TRIALS

Herbal medicine

Adjunctive herbal medicine with carbamazepine for bipolar disorders: a double-blind, randomized, placebo-controlled study

Journal of Psychiatric Research 2007 April–June, Vol. 41, Issue 3–4, pp. 360–369.

Zhang ZJ, Kang WH, Tan QR, Li Q, Gao CG, Zhang FG et al.

Objective

Chinese herbal medicines possess the therapeutic potential for mood disorders. This double-blind, randomized, placebo-controlled study was designed to evaluate the efficacy and side-effects of the herbal medicine called Free and Easy Wanderer Plus (FEWP) as an adjunct to carbamazepine (CBZ) in patients with bipolar disorders.

Method

A total of 124 bipolar depressed and 111 manic patients were randomized to treatment with CBZ alone, CBZ plus FEWP, or equivalent placebo for 12 weeks. CBZ was initiated at 300 mg/day and FEWP was given at a fixed dose of 36 g/day. Efficacy measures included the Hamilton Rating Scale for Depression, Montgomery-Asberg Depression Rating Scale, Young Mania Rating Scale, Bech-Rafaelsen Mania Scale, and Clinical Global Impression-Severity (CGI-S).

Results

CBZ monotherapy produced significantly greater improvement on manic measures at week 2 through endpoint and CGI-S of depression at endpoint compared to placebo. CBZ monotherapy also yielded significantly higher clinical response rates than placebo on bipolar depression (63.8% vs. 34.8%, $P = 0.044$) and mania (87.8% vs. 57.1%, $P = 0.012$). Compared to CBZ monotherapy, adjunctive FEWP with CBZ resulted in significantly better outcomes on the three measures of depression at week 4 and week 8, and significantly greater clinical response rate in depressed subjects (84.8% vs. 63.8%, $P = 0.032$), but failed to produce significantly greater improvement on manic measures and the response rate in manic subjects. There was a lesser incidence of dizziness and fatigue in the combination therapy compared to CBZ monotherapy.

Conclusion

These results suggest that adjunctive FEWP has additive beneficial effects in bipolar patients, particularly for those in the depressive phase.

The beneficial effects of the herbal medicine Free and Easy Wanderer Plus (FEWP) for mood disorders: double-blind, placebo-controlled studies

Journal of Psychiatric Research 2007 November, Vol. 41, Issue 10, pp. 828–836.
Zhang ZJ, Kang WH, Li Q, Tan QR

Objective

To ascertain the effect of the herbal medicine Free and Easy Wanderer Plus (FEWP) as adjunctive therapy with carbamazepine (CBZ) in the treatment of bipolar disorders.

Background

A study published in the *Journal of Psychiatric Research* in 2005 conducted by Zhang ZJ, Kang WH, Tan QR, Li Q, Gao CG, Zhang FG et al. showed the beneficial effects of the herbal medicine Free and Easy Wanderer Plus (FEWP) as adjunctive therapy with carbamazepine (CBZ) in the 12-week treatment of bipolar disorders. Here, follow-up data obtained from a continuation of the 2005 study are presented.

Method

Treatment and clinical evaluation of bipolar patients (n = 188) who had randomly received 12-week CBZ plus placebo (n = 92) or CBZ plus FEWP (n = 96) were extended to 26 weeks under double-blind conditions. Patients in the adjunctive FEWP group showed a significantly lower overall discontinuation rate (31%) at endpoint compared to the placebo group (51%, p = 0.009). Of the patients in the adjunctive FEWP group, 15% discontinued treatment due to intolerable side-effects, markedly lower than those in the placebo group (28%, p = 0.019). No difference in discontinuation for lack of efficacy and exacerbation was observed in the two groups.

Results

Patients receiving adjunctive FEWP had significantly fewer adverse side-effects and lower serum levels of CBZ than those on placebo. A separate study was further conducted to evaluate the effectiveness of FEWP as monotherapy in depressed patients.

Method

A total of 87 unipolar and 62 bipolar depressed patients were randomly assigned to treatment with 36 g/day FEWP (n = 86) or placebo (n = 63) for 12 weeks under double-blind conditions. Efficacy was measured using the Hamilton Rating Scale for Depression (HAMD), Montgomery-Asberg Depression Rating Scale (MADRS) and Clinical Global Impression-Severity (CGI-S).

Results

Both unipolar and bipolar patients assigned to FEWP displayed significantly greater improvement on the three efficacy indices and significantly higher clinical response rate (74%) than those treated with placebo (42%, $p < 0.001$) at endpoint.

Conclusion

These results suggest that adjunctive FEWP improves tolerability of CBZ in the long term, which may be associated with the suppression of blood CBZ concentrations via herb–drug interactions. FEWP monotherapy may also be an effective alternative treatment for depression.

END NOTES

1. Regier DA, Narrow WE, Rae DS et al 1993 The de facto mental and addictive disorders service system. Epidemiologic Catchment Area prospective 1-year prevalence rates of disorders and services. Archives of General Psychiatry 50(2): 85–94.
2. Redfield Jamison K 1993 Touched with Fire – Manic-depressive Illness and the Artistic Temperament. Free Press, New York, pp. 262–263.
3. Ibid., p. 263.
4. American Psychiatric Association 1994 Diagnostic and Statistical Manual for Mental Disorders, 4th edn (DSM-IV). American Psychiatric Press, Washington, DC.
5. National Institute of Mental Health website: www.nimh.nih.gov. [Accessed 2008].
6. Redfield Jamison K 1995 An Unquiet Mind. Picador, London, p. 36.
7. Ibid., p. 37.
8. Vainionpaa LK, Rattya J, Knip M et al. 1999 Valproate-induced hyperandrogenism during pubertal maturation in girls with epilepsy. Annals of Neurology 45(4): 444–450.
9. Touched with Fire – Manic-depressive Illness and the Artistic Temperament, p. 34.
10. Ibid., p. 34.
11. Ibid., p. 34.
12. Ibid., p. 35.
13. Ibid., p. 35.
14. Ibid., p. 35.
15. Shen Quan Yu, Wu Yu Hua, Shen Li Ling 1989 Dian Kuang Xian Zheng Zhi 癫狂病证治 [The Treatment of Manic-Depression and

Epilepsy]. Ancient Chinese Medicine Texts Publishing House, Beijing, p. 1.
16. 1979 Huang Di Nei Jing Su Wen 黄帝内经素问[The Yellow Emperor's Classic of Internal Medicine – Simple Questions]. People's Health Publishing House, Beijing, p. 539. First published *c*.100 BC.
17. Ibid., pp. 257–258.
18. 1981 Ling Shu Jing 灵枢经 [Spiritual Axis]. People's Health Publishing House, Beijing, p. 57. First published *c*.100 BC.
19. Nanjing College of Traditional Chinese Medicine 1979 Nan Jing Jiao Shi 难经教释 [A Revised Explanation of the Classic of Difficulties]. People's Health Publishing House, Beijing, p. 132. First published c. AD 100.
20. Ibid., p. 52.
21. He Ren 2005 Jin Gui Yao Lue 金匮要略[Essential Prescriptions of the Golden Chest]. People's Health Publishing House, Beijing, p. 42. The *Essential Prescriptions of the Golden Chest* was written by Zhang Zhong Jing and first published *c*.AD 220.
22. Cited in The Treatment of Manic-Depression and Epilepsy, p. 3.
23. Ibid., p. 3.
24. Ibid., p. 3.
25. Cited in Zhang Bo Yu 1986 Zhong Yi Nei Ke Xue 中医内科学 [Chinese Internal Medicine]. Shanghai Science Publishing House, Shanghai, p. 125.
26. Cited in The Treatment of Manic-Depression and Epilepsy, p. 4.
27. Ibid., p. 4.
28. Zhang Jing Yue 1986 Jing Yue Quan Shu 京岳全书[Complete Book of Jing Yue]. Shanghai Scientific Publishing House, Shanghai, p. 574. First published 1634.
29. Cited in The Treatment of Manic-Depression and Epilepsy, p. 4.
30. Ibid., p. 5.
31. Huang Tai Tang 2001 Nei Ke Yi Nan Bing Zhong Yi Zhi Liao Xue 内科医疑难病中医治疗学 [The Treatment of Difficult Diseases in Chinese Internal Medicine]. Chinese Herbal Medicine Science Publishing House, Beijing, pp. 761–774.
32. Zhang Gang 1986 [Differentiating terminology and reality of *Dian Kuang* in the Yellow Emperor's Classic of Internal Medicine]. Journal of Chinese Medicine (Zhong Yi Za Zhi 中医杂志) 27(5): 56.
33. Spiritual Axis, p. 57.
34. Chen Chao 1984 [Clinical observations on the use of a variation of Wen Dan Tang to treat 30 Cases of *Dian Kuang*]. Journal of Chinese Medicine 25(11): 31.
35. Wang Yong Yan 2004 Zhong Yi Nei Ke Xue 中医内科学[Chinese Internal Medicine]. People's Health Publishing House, Beijing, p. 354.
36. Tian Dai Hua 2005 Huang Di Nei Jing Su Wen 黄帝内经素问 The Yellow Emperor's Classic of Internal Medicine – Simple Questions]. People's Health Publishing House, Beijing, p. 6. First published *c*.100 BC.
37. Ibid., p. 49.
38. Qin Yue Ren 2004 Nan Jing Jiao Shi 难经教释[Classic of Difficulties]. Scientific and Technical Documents Publishing House, Beijing, p. 13. First published *c*.AD 100.
39. Zhang Bo Yu 1986 Chinese Internal Medicine, p. 125.
40. An Unquiet Mind, pp. 92–93 and p. 120.
41. Touched with Fire – Manic-depressive Illness and the Artistic Temperament.
42. Trimble MR 2007 The Soul in the Brain. Johns Hopkins University Press, Baltimore, p. 105.
43. Cited in The Treatment of Manic-Depression and Epilepsy, p. 6.
44. Ibid., p. 6.
45. Zhang Fa Rong 1989 Zhong Yi Nei Ke Xue 中医内科学[Chinese Internal Medicine]. Sichuan Science Publishing House, Chengdu, p. 103.
46. National Institute of Mental Health website: www.nimh.nih.gov. [Accessed 2008].
47. Tian Dai Hua 2005 The Yellow Emperor's Classic of Internal Medicine – Simple Questions, p. 94.
48. The NIMH Genetics Workgroup 1998 Genetics and mental disorders. National Institute of Mental Health, Rockville, MD. NIH Publication No. 98: 4268.
49. Cited in The Treatment of Manic-Depression and Epilepsy, p. 6.
50. Liu Xiu Zhen 1994 [The experience of Dr Zhang Li Sheng in the treatment of *Dian Kuang* and epilepsy]. Journal of Chinese Medicine 35(2): 77.
51. Zhang Fa Rong 1989 Chinese Internal Medicine, pp. 103–105.
52. Yang Tai De et al. 2001 [Fu Shan's views on *Dian Kuang*]. Journal of Chinese Medicine 42(9): 571.
53. Shan Chang Hua 1990 Jing Xue Jie 经穴解 [An Explanation of the Acupuncture Points]. People's Health Publishing House, Beijing, p. 88. An *Explanation of the Acupuncture Points* was written by Yue Han Zhen and first published in 1654.
54. Dr Zhang Ming Jiu, personal communication, Nanjing 1982.
55. Chen You Bang 1990 Zhong Guo Zhen Jiu Zhi Liao Xue 中国针灸治疗学 [Chinese Acupuncture Therapy]. China Science Publishing House, Shanghai, p. 501.
56. Yang Jia San 1989 Zhen Jiu Xue 针灸学[A Study of Acupuncture]. Beijing Science Publishing House, Beijing, p. 632.
57. Wang Li Cao 1997 Zhong Guo Zhen Jiu Chu Fang Da Cheng 中国针灸处方大成 [A Collection of Chinese Acupuncture Prescriptions]. Shanxi Science Publishing House, Taiyuan, p. 446.
58. Cited in The Treatment of Manic-Depression and Epilepsy, p. 6.
59. Liang Jian Bo 1992 To treat *Dian*, settle the Heart, eliminate Stagnation, calm the Mind and resolve Phlegm; to treat *Kuang*, clear the Stomach, drain Fire and resolve Phlegm. In: Shi Yu Guang 1992 Dang Dai Ming Yi Lin Zheng Jing Hua 当代名医临证精华 [Essential Clinical Experience of Famous Contemporary Doctors – Manic-Depression and Epilepsy]. Ancient Chinese Medicine Texts Publishing House, Beijing, pp. 14–18.

夜惊

CHAPTER 20

NIGHT TERRORS

ETIOLOGY *536*

Emotional stress *536*

Overwork *536*

Irregular diet *536*

Loss of blood during childbirth *536*

PATHOLOGY *536*

IDENTIFICATION OF PATTERNS AND TREATMENT *537*

Liver- and Heart-Fire *537*

Phlegm-Heat harassing the Ethereal Soul and the Mind *537*

Liver- and Heart-Blood deficiency *538*

Liver- and Heart-Yin deficiency *539*

Shock displacing the Mind *540*

- Liver- and Heart-Fire
- Phlegm-Heat harassing the Ethereal Soul and the Mind
- Liver- and Heart-Blood deficiency
- Liver- and Heart-Yin deficiency
- Shock displacing the Mind

NIGHT TERRORS

"Night Terrors" describes a condition whereby a person suddenly screams during sleep, their eyes may be open but they are not awake, and they may sit up suddenly gripped by fear or terror. There may be sweating, confusion, rapid heart rate and palpitations. This may last 5–20 minutes. When the person wakes up, they have no recollection of a nightmare.

Night Terrors are not nightmares. Indeed, nightmares occur during the dream phase of sleep known as rapid eye movement (REM) sleep. Most people enter the REM stage of sleep some time after 90 minutes of sleep. The nightmare frightens the sleeper, and they will wake up with a vivid memory of a bad dream. Night Terrors, on the other hand, occur during a phase of deep non-REM sleep, usually within an hour after the subject goes to bed. This is also known as stage 4. Night Terrors are sometimes associated with sleepwalking.

However, although it is important to make the above distinction between nightmares and Night Terrors, that is *not* to say that patients who suffer from Night Terrors (in the non-REM stage of sleep) may not occasionally also have nightmares (in the REM stage of sleep).

Night Terrors correspond to the Chinese disease of "Fright Cry" (*Jing Ti* 惊啼). The *Discussion of the Origin of Symptoms in Diseases* (*Zhu Bing Yuan Hou Lun*) says:[1]

Fright Cry in children occurs during sleep when they suddenly wake up crying and with a feeling of fear. It is due to Wind-Heat invading the Heart; this leads to Heart-Heat, the Spirit is unsettled and restless, and Fright Cry occurs.

Zhang Jing Yue relates Fright Cry to a pathology of the Ethereal Soul (*Hun*) being restless at night; as the Ethereal Soul follows the Mind (*Shen*), the Mind loses consciousness and the Ethereal Soul is swept away.[2]

The discussion of Night Terrors will be conducted according to the following topics.

- Etiology
- Pathology
- Identification of patterns and treatment

ETIOLOGY

Emotional stress

Anger, resentment, frustration, guilt and worry all affect the Liver causing Liver-Qi stagnation, often leading to Liver-Fire. The Ethereal Soul is housed in the Liver and Liver-Fire agitates the Ethereal Soul, so that it becomes restless at night, causing Night Terrors.

Sadness and grief may lead to Qi and Blood deficiency of the Heart and Liver, and therefore the Mind and Ethereal Soul are deprived of their residence. The Mind and Ethereal Soul are not anchored in the Heart and Liver respectively at night so that they are agitated; this leads to Night Terrors.

Shock displaces the Mind from its residence in the Heart. As the Mind is not anchored in the Heart, it becomes restless at night and this may lead to Night Terrors.

In children, the emotional stress leading to Night Terrors is more likely to be fear or insecurity arising from some situation in the family.

Overwork

Overwork (in the sense of working long hours without adequate rest for many years) weakens Liver- and Kidney-Yin. The deficient Liver-Qi fails to anchor the Ethereal Soul at night, Yang floats and this leads to Night Terrors. This is the cause of this problem in the middle-aged and elderly.

Irregular diet

A diet too rich in carbohydrates, fats, sugars, dairy foods and fried foods often leads to the formation of Phlegm. Phlegm often combines with Heat and it affects the Heart, Lungs and Liver. Phlegm obstructs the Mind's orifices, and Heat agitates the Mind and the Ethereal Soul. This may lead to Night Terrors.

Loss of blood during childbirth

A heavy loss of blood during childbirth weakens Liver-Blood; as the Liver is the mother of the Heart, this induces a deficiency of Heart-Blood too. Heart-Blood and Liver-Blood are the residence of the Mind and Ethereal Soul respectively, so that the Mind and Ethereal Soul become restless at night; this may lead to Night Terrors.

SUMMARY

Etiology
- Emotional stress
- Overwork
- Irregular diet
- Loss of blood during childbirth

PATHOLOGY

The pathology of Night Terrors is characterized by either a Full or an Empty condition. In Night Terrors the Mind and the Ethereal Soul are agitated at night and this may occur for two basic reasons: either there is a pathogenic factor agitating them (Full condition) or there is a deficiency that deprives them of their residence at night (Empty condition) (*see Fig. 18.1*).

The most common Full conditions are Fire or Phlegm-Heat; the most common Empty conditions are Blood or Yin deficiency.

Liver- and Heart-Fire agitate the Ethereal Soul and the Mind at night and this leads to Night Terrors. In the middle-aged or elderly, there is often Phlegm and this frequently combines with Heat. Phlegm obstructs the Mind's orifices and Heat agitates the Mind and Ethereal Soul. When Night Terrors are caused by Phlegm-Heat, they are worse than those caused purely by Heat or Fire, because the obstruction of the Mind by Phlegm distorts perception more.

When the Blood or Yin of the Heart and Liver is deficient, the Mind and the Ethereal Soul are deprived of their residence at night; they fail to be anchored in their respective organs and Night Terrors may ensue.

Whatever the pathology, in Night Terrors the Mind and the Ethereal Soul are mainly involved.

SUMMARY

Pathology
- The pathology of Night Terrors is characterized by either a Full or an Empty condition.
- The most common Full conditions are Fire or Phlegm-Heat.
- The most common Empty conditions are Blood or Yin deficiency.

- In the middle-aged or elderly, there is often Phlegm and this frequently combines with Heat.
- Whatever the pathology, in Night Terrors the Mind and the Ethereal Soul are mainly involved.

IDENTIFICATION OF PATTERNS AND TREATMENT

Liver- and Heart-Fire

Clinical manifestations

Night Terrors, crying in the middle of the night, shouting, red face and eyes, thirst, bitter taste, headache (Fig. 20.1).

Tongue: Red, redder sides and tip, thick-dry-yellow coating.

Pulse: Wiry-Overflowing-Rapid.

Treatment principle

Drain Heart- and Liver-Fire, calm the Mind, settle the Ethereal Soul.

Acupuncture

Points

LIV-2 Xingjian, HE-8 Shaofu, P-8 Laogong, L.I.-11 Quchi, Du-24 Shenting, G.B.-13 Benshen, Ren-15 Jiuwei, BL-47 Hunmen. All with reducing method, except the points on the head which should be needled with even method.

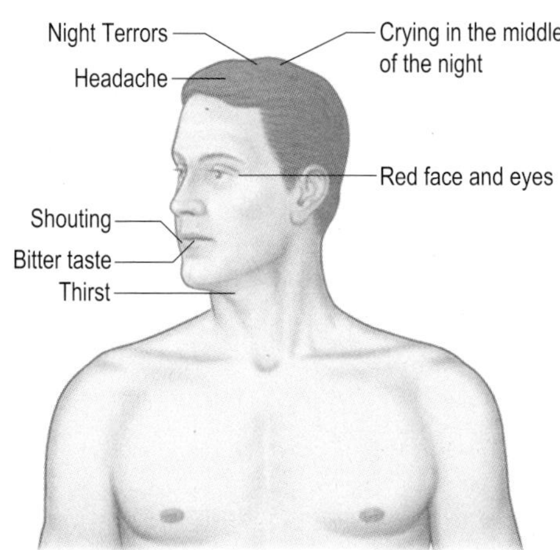

Figure 20.1 Liver- and Heart-Fire.

Explanation

- LIV-2 drains Liver-Fire.
- HE-8 and P-8 drain Heart-Fire.
- L.I.-11 clears Heat.
- Du-24, G.B.-13 and Ren-15 calm the Mind and settle the Ethereal Soul.
- BL-47 regulates the movement of the Ethereal Soul.

Herbal therapy

Prescription

LONG DAN XIE GAN TANG Variation
Gentiana Draining the Liver Decoction Variation

Explanation

This variation of Long Dan Xie Gan Tang drains Liver- and Heart-Fire, settles the Ethereal Soul and calms the Mind.

SUMMARY

Liver- and Heart-Fire

Points

LIV-2 Xingjian, HE-8 Shaofu, P-8 Laogong, L.I.-11 Quchi, Du-24 Shenting, G.B.-13 Benshen, Ren-15 Jiuwei, BL-47 Hunmen. All with reducing method, except the points on the head which should be needled with even method.

Herbal therapy

Prescription

LONG DAN XIE GAN TANG Variation
Gentiana Draining the Liver Decoction Variation

Phlegm-Heat harassing the Ethereal Soul and the Mind

Clinical manifestations

Night Terrors, crying, shouting, nightmares, possibly sleepwalking, a feeling of oppression of the chest, sputum in the throat, mental confusion, irritability (Fig. 20.2).

Tongue: Red with redder sides and tip, Swollen, sticky-yellow coating.

Pulse: Slippery-Rapid.

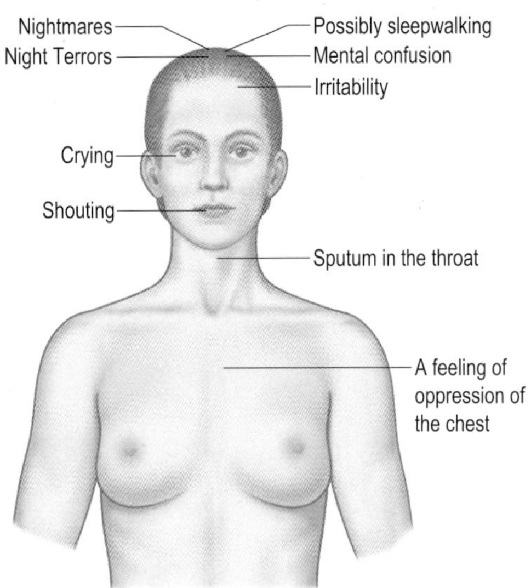

Figure 20.2 Phlegm-Heat harassing the Ethereal Soul and the Mind.

Treatment principle

Clear Heat, resolve Phlegm, open the Mind's orifices, calm the Mind, settle the Ethereal Soul.

Acupuncture

Points

L.I.-11 Quchi, LIV-2 Xiangjian, HE-8 Shaofu, P-8 Laogong, ST-40 Fenglong, Ren-9 Shuifen, SP-6 Sanyinjiao, G.B.-17 Zhengying, Du-24 Shenting, G.B.-13 Benshen, Ren-15 Jiuwei, BL-47 Hunmen. All with reducing method, except the points in the head which should be needled with even method.

Explanation

- L.I.-11 clears Heat.
- LIV-2, HE-8 and P-8 drain Liver- and Heart-Fire.
- ST-40, Ren-9 and SP-6 resolve Phlegm.
- G.B.-17 resolves Phlegm and opens the Mind's orifices. Among its indications are "obsessive thoughts, pensiveness, and manic behavior".
- Du-24, G.B.-13 and Ren-15 calm the Mind and settle the Ethereal Soul.
- BL-47 regulates the movement of the Ethereal Soul.

Herbal therapy

Prescription

WEN DAN TANG Variation
Warming the Gall-Bladder Decoction Variation

Explanation

This formula resolves Phlegm, clears Heat, opens the Mind's orifices, calms the Mind and settles the Ethereal Soul.

SUMMARY

Phlegm-Heat harassing the Ethereal Soul and the Mind

Points

L.I.-11 Quchi, LIV-2 Xiangjian, HE-8 Shaofu, P-8 Laogong, ST-40 Fenglong, Ren-9 Shuifen, SP-6 Sanyinjiao, G.B.-17 Zhengying, Du-24 Shenting, G.B.-13 Benshen, Ren-15 Jiuwei, BL-47 Hunmen. All with reducing method, except the points in the head which should be needled with even method.

Herbal therapy

Prescription

WEN DAN TANG Variation
Warming the Gall-Bladder Decoction Variation

Liver- and Heart-Blood deficiency

Clinical manifestations

Night Terrors, no shouting, waking up with a low-sound cry, difficulty in falling asleep, palpitations, poor memory, dizziness, blurred vision (Fig. 20.3).

Tongue: Pale, slightly dry, possibly Thin.

Pulse: Choppy or Fine.

Treatment principle

Nourish Liver- and Heart-Blood, calm the Mind, settle the Ethereal Soul.

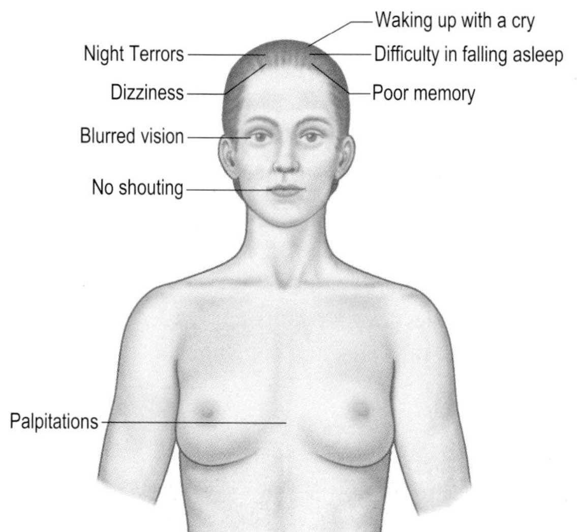

Figure 20.3 Liver- and Heart-Blood deficiency.

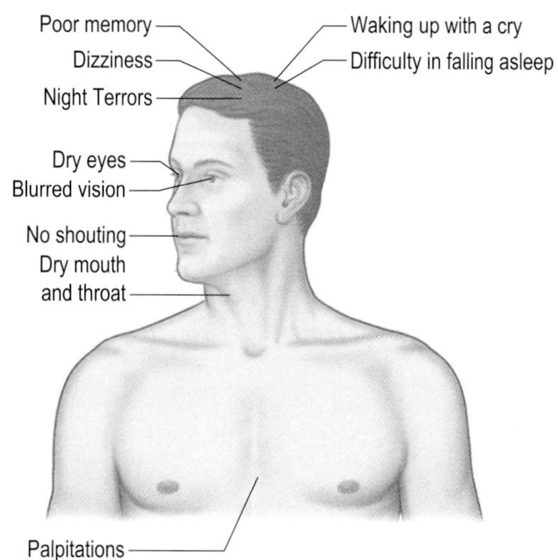

Figure 20.4 Liver- and Heart-Yin deficiency.

Acupuncture

Points

LIV-8 Ququan, SP-6 Sanyinjiao, ST-36 Zusanli, Ren-4 Guanyuan, HE-7 Shenmen, Ren-15 Jiuwei, Du-24 Shenting, BL-47 Hunmen. All with reinforcing method.

Explanation

- LIV-8, SP-6, ST-36 and Ren-4 nourish Liver-Blood.
- HE-7 and Ren-15 nourish Heart-Blood and calm the Mind.
- Du-24 and Ren-15 calm the Mind.
- BL-47 regulates the movement of the Ethereal Soul.

Herbal therapy

Prescription

GUI PI TANG Variation
Tonifying the Spleen Decoction Variation

Explanation

This formula nourishes Liver- and Heart-Blood, calms the Mind and settles the Ethereal Soul.

SUMMARY

Liver- and Heart-Blood deficiency

Points

LIV-8 Ququan, SP-6 Sanyinjiao, ST-36 Zusanli, Ren-4 Guanyuan, HE-7 Shenmen, Ren-15 Jiuwei, Du-24 Shenting, BL-47 Hunmen. All with reinforcing method.

Herbal therapy

Prescription

GUI PI TANG Variation
Tonifying the Spleen Decoction Variation

Liver- and Heart-Yin deficiency

Clinical manifestations

Night Terrors, no shouting, waking up with a low-sound cry, difficulty in falling asleep, palpitations, poor memory, dizziness, blurred vision, dry mouth and throat, dry eyes (Fig. 20.4).

Tongue: normal color, slightly dry, possibly Thin, no coating. If there is Empty Heat, the tongue body is Red.

Pulse: Fine or Floating-Empty.

Treatment principle

Nourish Liver- and Heart-Yin, calm the Mind and settle the Ethereal Soul.

Acupuncture

Points

LIV-8 Ququan, SP-6 Sanyinjiao, ST-36 Zusanli, Ren-4 Guanyuan, HE-7 Shenmen, Ren-15 Jiuwei, Du-24 Shenting, BL-47 Hunmen; if there is Empty Heat, add P-7 Daling and LIV-2 Xingjian. All with reinforcing method except P-7 and LIV-2, which should be needled with even method.

Explanation

- LIV-8, SP-6, ST-36 and Ren-4 nourish Liver-Blood and Liver-Yin.
- HE-7 and Ren-15 nourish Heart-Blood and Heart-Yin and calm the Mind.
- Du-24 and Ren-15 calm the Mind.
- BL-47 regulates the movement of the Ethereal Soul.
- P-7 and LIV-2 clear Empty Heat from the Heart and Liver.

Herbal therapy

Prescription

SUAN ZAO REN TANG Variation
Ziziphus Decoction Variation

Explanation

This formula nourishes Liver-Yin and settles the Ethereal Soul.

Prescription

YIN MEI TANG Variation
Attracting Sleep Decoction Variation

Explanation

This formula is specific to nourish Liver-Yin and promote sleep by rooting the Ethereal Soul in the Liver. Compared to the previous formula, it is used when the person has many unpleasant dreams.

Modifications

These modifications apply to both above formulae.

- If there is Empty Heat (in which case the tongue is Red and without a coating), add Zhi Mu *Radix Anemarrhaenae* and Mu Dan Pi *Cortex Moutan.*
- If there is Liver-Yang rising, add Tian Ma *Rhizoma Gastrodiae* and Gou Teng *Ramulus cum Uncis Uncariae.*

SUMMARY

Liver- and Heart-Yin deficiency

Points

LIV-8 Ququan, SP-6 Sanyinjiao, ST-36 Zusanli, Ren-4 Guanyuan, HE-7 Shenmen, Ren-15 Jiuwei, Du-24 Shenting, BL-47 Hunmen; if there is Empty Heat, add P-7 Daling and LIV-2 Xingjian. All with reinforcing method except P-7 and LIV-2, which should be needled with even method.

Herbal therapy

Prescription

SUAN ZAO REN TANG Variation
Ziziphus Decoction Variation

Prescription

YIN MEI TANG Variation
Attracting Sleep Decoction Variation

Shock displacing the Mind

Clinical manifestations

Night Terrors with sudden onset, cry at night, shouting, a feeling of panic, possibly sleepwalking, pale face, palpitations (Fig. 20.5).

Tongue: Pale or unchanged.

Pulse: Moving-Rapid; Overflowing on the Heart pulse.

Treatment principle

Calm the Mind, nourish the Heart.

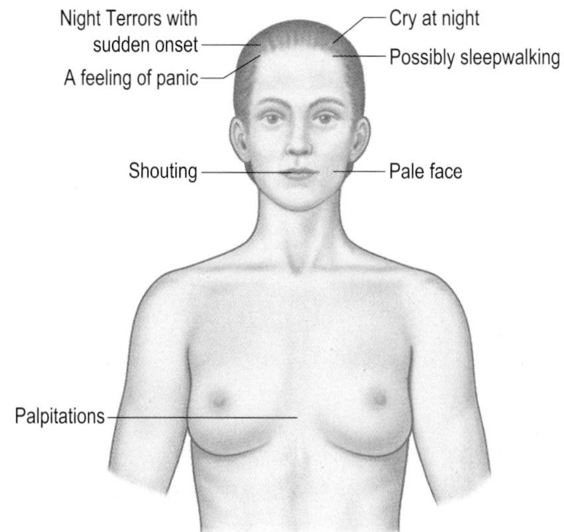

Figure 20.5 Shock displacing the Mind.

Acupuncture

Points

HE-7 Shenmen, Ren-15 Jiuwei, Du-24 Shenting, Ren-4 Guanyuan. All with reinforcing method.

Explanation

- HE-7 and Ren-15 nourish the Heart and calm the Mind.
- Du-24 calms the Mind.
- Ren-4 calms the Mind by rooting Qi in the Lower *Dan Tian*.

Herbal therapy

Prescription

GAN MAI DA ZAO TANG Variation
Glycyrrhiza-Triticum-Jujuba Decoction Variation

Explanation

This formula calms the Mind, nourishes the Heart and tonifies the Spleen. This variation of it strongly sinks the Mind and the Ethereal Soul.

SUMMARY

Shock displacing the Mind

Points

HE-7 Shenmen, Ren-15 Jiuwei, Du-24 Shenting, Ren-4 Guanyuan. All with reinforcing method.

Herbal therapy

Prescription

GAN MAI DA ZAO TANG Variation
Glycyrrhiza-Triticum-Jujuba Decoction Variation

END NOTES

1. Cited in Zeng Shi Zu 1992 Zhi Liao Dian Xian, Yi Bing Xiao Fang An Mo Shi Liao 治疗癫痫癔病效方按摩食疗 [Dietary Treatment, Massage and Herbal Treatment for Epilepsy and Hysteria]. Shanxi Science and Technology Publishing House, Xian, p. 98.
2. Ibid., p. 98.

CHAPTER 21

ATTENTION DEFICIT DISORDER (ADD) AND ATTENTION DEFICIT HYPERACTIVITY DISORDER (ADHD)

ATTENTION DEFICIT DISORDER (ADD) AND ATTENTION DEFICIT HYPERACTIVITY DISORDER (ADHD) *544*

ATTENTION DEFICIT DISORDER IN WESTERN MEDICINE *544*

SYMPTOMS *544*
Hyperactivity–impulsiveness *544*
Inattention *545*

POSSIBLE CAUSES OF ADHD AND ADD *545*
Environmental agents *545*
Brain injury *545*
Food additives and sugar *545*
Genetics *545*

TREATMENT OF ADHD AND ADD *546*

ATTENTION DEFICIT HYPERACTIVITY DISORDER IN ADULTS *547*
Diagnosis *547*
Treatment *547*

ATTENTION DEFICIT DISORDER IN CHINESE MEDICINE *548*

PATHOLOGY *548*
The Mind (*Shen*) *548*
The Ethereal Soul (*Hun*) *548*
The Intellect (*Yi*) *548*
Organ pathology *549*
Phlegm *549*

ETIOLOGY *550*
Heredity *550*
Diet *550*
Emotional stress *550*
Pregnancy and labor *551*

ACUPUNCTURE TREATMENT *551*
Heart *551*
Spleen *551*
Liver *552*
Governing Vessel *552*
Other points *553*
The experience of teachers from the Nanjing University of Traditional Chinese Medicine *554*

IDENTIFICATION OF PATTERNS AND TREATMENT *555*
Deficiency of Heart- and Spleen-Blood *555*
Heart- and Kidney-Yin deficiency *556*
Kidney- and Liver-Yin deficiency with Liver-Yang rising *556*
Heart- and Spleen-Qi deficiency *557*
Liver- and Heart-Fire *558*
Heart and Spleen deficiency with Phlegm *558*

WESTERN MEDICINE CLINICAL TRIALS *559*

CHINESE MEDICINE CLINICAL TRIALS *561*

- Deficiency of Heart- and Spleen-Blood
- Heart- and Kidney-Yin deficiency
- Kidney- and Liver-Yin deficiency with Liver-Yang rising
- Heart- and Spleen-Qi deficiency
- Liver- and Heart-Fire
- Heart and Spleen deficiency with Phlegm

ATTENTION DEFICIT DISORDER (ADD) AND ATTENTION DEFICIT HYPERACTIVITY DISORDER (ADHD)

Attention deficit disorder is characterized by inattention, difficulty in concentrating and impulsiveness. When associated with hyperactivity in children, it is called attention deficit hyperactivity disorder (ADHD). It is the most commonly diagnosed disorder in children. According to the National Institute of Mental Health, between 3 and 5% of all children (in the USA) have ADHD.[1]

Although ADD/ADHD is a behavioral disorder most commonly diagnosed in childhood, symptoms can last into adulthood. In children, ADHD causes poor performance in school, inconsistency in work, emotional immaturity and social difficulties.

Brain maps using quantitative electroencephalographic (QEEG) measurements of brain-wave activity in the various lobes of the brain can demonstrate ADD and ADHD. In the frontal lobe, where focused analytical thinking occurs, ADD/ADHD patients tend to produce an abnormally high amount of alpha and/or theta waves (normally associated with dreamy, closed-eye states) and fewer beta waves (associated with focused analytical thinking).

When given an "eyes-open" challenge involving focused mental calculation or reading, most people will produce fewer alpha (or theta) waves and more beta waves. This state of brain functioning appears to be necessary for optimal focused attention and linear problem solving. When given the same challenge, patients with ADHD appear to be unable to make the appropriate shift into this focused type of brain functioning.

The discussion of ADD and ADHD will be conducted according to the following topics.

- Attention deficit disorder in Western medicine
  - Symptoms
  - Possible causes of ADHD and ADD
  - Treatment of ADHD and ADD
  - Attention deficit hyperactivity disorder in adults
- Attention deficit disorder in Chinese medicine
  - Pathology
  - Etiology
  - Acupuncture treatment
  - Identification of patterns and treatment
- Western medicine clinical trials
- Chinese medicine clinical trials

ATTENTION DEFICIT DISORDER IN WESTERN MEDICINE

SYMPTOMS

The principal characteristics of ADHD are inattention, hyperactivity and impulsiveness. In children, symptoms of ADHD will appear over the course of many months, often with the symptoms of impulsiveness and hyperactivity preceding those of inattention, which may not emerge for a year or more.

When the child's hyperactivity, distractibility, poor concentration or impulsiveness begin to affect performance in school, social relationships with other children or behavior at home, ADHD may be suspected.

According to the most recent version of the Diagnostic and Statistical Manual of Mental Disorders, there are three patterns of behavior that indicate ADHD. These are inattentiveness, hyperactivity and impulsive behaviors.[2] This means that there are three subtypes of ADHD (Table 21.1):

- the predominantly hyperactive–impulsive type (that does not show significant inattention)
- the predominantly inattentive type (that does not show significant hyperactive–impulsive behavior), sometimes called ADD
- the combined type (that displays both inattentive and hyperactive–impulsive symptoms).

Hyperactivity–impulsiveness

Hyperactive children always seem to be "on the go" or constantly in motion. They dash around touching or playing with whatever is in sight, or talk incessantly. They cannot sit still at dinner or during a school lesson

Table 21.1 Types of ADHD

SYMPTOMS	HYPERACTIVE TYPE	INATTENTIVE TYPE
Predominantly hyperactivity	+	–
Predominantly inattentive	–	+
Combined	+	+

or a story. They may run around the room, touch everything or fidget incessantly. Hyperactive teenagers or adults may feel internally restless. They often need to stay busy and they may do several things at once.

Impulsive children will often blurt out inappropriate comments, display their emotions without restraint and act without regard for the later consequences of their conduct. Their impulsiveness may make it hard for them to wait for things they want or to take their turn in games. They may grab a toy from another child or hit them when they are upset.

Inattention

Children who are inattentive find it hard to concentrate on one thing and may get bored with a task after only a few minutes. Focusing and deliberate, conscious attention to organizing and completing a task or learning something new is difficult.

Children diagnosed with the predominantly inattentive type of ADHD are seldom impulsive or hyperactive, yet they have significant problems paying attention. They appear to be daydreaming, easily confused, slow moving and lethargic. They may have difficulty processing information as quickly and accurately as other children.

SUMMARY

ADD in Western medicine – symptoms
- Hyperactivity
- Impulsiveness
- Inattention

POSSIBLE CAUSES OF ADHD AND ADD

Most substantiated causes appear to fall in the realm of neurobiology and genetics. However, environmental factors influence the severity of the disorder, especially the degree of impairment and suffering the child may experience.

Environmental agents

Studies have shown a possible correlation between the use of cigarettes and alcohol during pregnancy and risk for ADHD in the offspring of that pregnancy.

Another environmental agent that may be associated with a higher risk of ADHD is high levels of lead in the bodies of young preschool children. Since lead is no longer allowed in paint and is usually found only in older buildings, exposure to toxic levels is not as prevalent as it once was. Children who live in old buildings in which lead still exists in the plumbing or in lead paint that has been painted over may be at risk.

Brain injury

One early theory maintained that attention disorders were caused by brain injury. Some children who have suffered accidents leading to brain injury may show some signs of behavior similar to that of ADHD, but only a small percentage of children with ADHD have been found to have suffered a traumatic brain injury.

Food additives and sugar

It has been suggested that attention disorders are caused by refined sugar or food additives, or that symptoms of ADHD are exacerbated by sugar or food additives. In 1982, the National Institute of Health held a scientific consensus conference to discuss this issue. It was found that diet restrictions helped about 5% of children with ADHD, mostly young children who had food allergies.[3]

A more recent study on the effect of sugar on children, using sugar one day and a sugar substitute on alternate days, without parents, staff or children knowing which substance was being used, showed no significant effects of the sugar on behavior or learning.[4]

A study by researchers at the University of Southampton has shown evidence of increased levels of hyperactivity in young children consuming mixtures of some artificial food colors and the preservative sodium benzoate.[5]

Genetics

Attention disorders often run in families, so there are likely to be genetic influences. Studies indicate that 25% of the close relatives in the families of ADHD children also have ADHD, whereas the rate is about 5% in the general population.[6] Many studies of twins now show that a strong genetic influence exists in the disorder.[7]

SUMMARY

ADD in Western medicine – possible causes of ADHD and ADD

- Environmental agents
- Brain injury
- Food additives and sugar
- Genetics

TREATMENT OF ADHD AND ADD

The National Institute of Mental Health (NIMH) has funded many studies of treatments for ADHD and has conducted the most intensive study ever undertaken for evaluating the treatment of this disorder. This study is known as the Multimodal Treatment Study of Children with Attention Deficit Hyperactivity Disorder (MTA).[8]

The MTA study included 579 (95–98 at each of six treatment sites) elementary school boys and girls with ADHD, who were randomly assigned to one of four treatment programs: (1) medication management alone; (2) behavioral treatment alone; (3) a combination of both; or (4) routine community care.

The results of the study indicated that long-term combination treatments and the medication management alone were superior to intensive behavioral treatment and routine community treatment. Another advantage of combined treatment was that children could be successfully treated with lower doses of medicine, compared with the medication-only group.

For decades, medications have been used to treat the symptoms of ADHD. The medications that seem to be the most effective are stimulants. Table 21.2 is a list of stimulants (by trade name and generic name) used in the USA. "Approved age" means that the drug has been tested and found safe and effective in children of that age.

The US Food and Drug Administration (FDA) recently approved a medication for ADHD that is not a stimulant. The medication – atomoxetine (Strattera) – works on the neurotransmitter noradrenaline (norepinephrine), whereas the stimulants primarily work on dopamine. Both of these neurotransmitters are believed to play a role in ADHD. The evidence to date indicates that over 70% of children with ADHD given atomoxetine manifest significant improvement in their symptoms.

Table 21.2 Medication for ADHD and ADD

TRADE NAME	GENERIC NAME	APPROVED AGE
Adderall	Amfetamine	3 and older
Concerta	Methylphenidate (long acting)	6 and older
Cylert*	Pemoline	6 and older
Dexedrine	Dexamfetamine	3 and older
Dextrostat	Dexamfetamine	3 and older
Focalin	Dexmethylphenidate	6 and older
Metadate ER	Methylphenidate (extended release)	6 and older
Metadate CD	Methylphenidate (extended release)	6 and older
Ritalin	Methylphenidate	6 and older
Ritalin SR	Methylphenidate (extended release)	6 and older
Ritalin LA	Methylphenidate (long acting)	6 and older

**Because of its potential for serious side-effects affecting the liver, Cylert should not ordinarily be considered as first-line drug therapy for ADHD.*

The stimulant drugs, when used with medical supervision, are usually considered quite safe. Stimulants do not make the child feel "high", although some children say they feel different or funny. To date, there is no evidence that stimulant medications, when used for treatment of ADHD, cause drug abuse or dependence. A review of all long-term studies on stimulant medication and substance abuse, conducted by researchers at Massachusetts General Hospital and Harvard Medical School, found that teenagers with ADHD who remained on their medication during the teen years had a lower likelihood of substance use or abuse than did ADHD adolescents who were not taking medications.[9]

Side-effects of the stimulant medications are minor and are usually related to the dosage. The most common side-effects are decreased appetite, insomnia, increased anxiety and/or irritability. Some children report mild stomach aches or headaches.

Behavioral therapy, emotional counseling and practical support will help ADHD children cope with everyday problems and feel better about themselves.

SUMMARY

ADD in Western medicine – treatment of ADHD and ADD

- Long-term combination treatments and medication management alone are superior to intensive behavioral treatment and routine community treatment.
- The medications that seem to be the most effective are stimulants.
- Atomoxetine (Strattera) is not a stimulant and it works on the neurotransmitter noradrenaline (norepinephrine), whereas the stimulants primarily work on dopamine.
- Side-effects of the stimulant medications include decreased appetite, insomnia, increased anxiety and/or irritability, mild stomach aches or headaches.

ATTENTION DEFICIT HYPERACTIVITY DISORDER IN ADULTS

Several studies done in recent years estimate that between 30 and 70% of children with ADHD continue to exhibit symptoms in the adult years.[10]

Typically, adults with ADHD are unaware that they have this disorder and may attribute their problems to their lack of organization. An adult suffering from ADHD or ADD will find it difficult to perform the simplest everyday tasks of getting up, organizing one's day and being on time.

Diagnosis

Diagnosing an adult with ADHD or ADD is fraught with difficulties. Many adults with ADHD or ADD will seek professional help for depression or anxiety. They may have a history of school failures or problems at work.

To be diagnosed with ADHD, an adult must have childhood-onset, persistent and current symptoms.[11] For an accurate diagnosis, a history of the patient's childhood behavior, together with an interview with his life partner, a parent, close friend or other close associate, will be needed.

Treatment

As with children, if adults take a medication for ADHD or ADD, they often start with a stimulant medication. The stimulant medications affect the regulation of the two neurotransmitters, norepinephrine (noradrenaline) and dopamine. The newest medication approved for ADHD by the FDA, atomoxetine (Strattera), has been tested in controlled studies in both children and adults and has been found to be effective.[12]

Antidepressants are considered a second choice for treatment of adults with ADHD or ADD. The older antidepressants, the tricyclics, are sometimes used because they, like the stimulants, affect noradrenaline (norepinephrine) and dopamine. Venlafaxine (Efexor), a newer antidepressant, is also used for its effect on noradrenaline (norepinephrine). Bupropion (Wellbutrin), an antidepressant with an indirect effect on the neurotransmitter dopamine, has been found useful in clinical trials on the treatment of ADHD in both children and adults.

In prescribing for an adult, special considerations are made. The adult may need less of the medication for his/her weight, as a medication may have a longer "half-life" in an adult.

Caffeine, as found in coffee and other herbal stimulants, has been proposed as an alternative to stimulant drugs in the treatment of ADD/ADHD. The benefit (or its absence) of caffeine stimulation has been addressed in several studies, some of which are reported at the end of this chapter. In general, these studies have demonstrated significant benefits with the administration of caffeine to children with ADD/ADHD. The benefits, however, have not been without side-effects and have failed to match or exceed those derived from the conventional stimulant medication regimens.

SUMMARY

ADD in Western medicine – attention deficit hyperactivity disorder in adults

- Between 30 and 70% of children with ADHD continue to exhibit symptoms in the adult years.
- An adult suffering from ADHD or ADD will find it difficult to perform the simplest everyday tasks of

getting up, organizing one's day and being on time.

Diagnosis

- To be diagnosed with ADHD, an adult must have childhood-onset, persistent and current symptoms.

Treatment

- As with children, if adults take a medication for ADHD or ADD, they often start with a stimulant medication. The stimulant medications affect the regulation of the two neurotransmitters, noradrenaline (norepinephrine) and dopamine.
- Antidepressants are considered a second choice for treatment of adults with ADHD or ADD.
- Caffeine has been proposed as an alternative to stimulant drugs in the treatment of ADD/ADHD.

ATTENTION DEFICIT DISORDER IN CHINESE MEDICINE

The Chinese literature on ADD and ADHD is scanty and the following are ideas derived partly from Chinese text and partly from my own experience. Contrary to what I usually do for other chapters, I will discuss the pathology first and then the etiology.

PATHOLOGY

In my opinion, the pathology of ADD revolves around the Heart, Liver and Spleen and their respective emotional-mental-spiritual faculties, i.e. the Mind (*Shen*), the Ethereal Soul (*Hun*) and the Intellect (*Yi*).

In general, we can say that both ADD and ADHD are characterized by a pathology of both the Intellect (*Yi*) and Ethereal Soul (*Hun*). However, in ADD there is prevalence of a pathology of Intellect (*Yi*), while in ADHD there is more a pathology of Ethereal Soul (*Hun*). The Mind (*Shen*) is involved in both ADD and ADHD (Fig. 21.1).

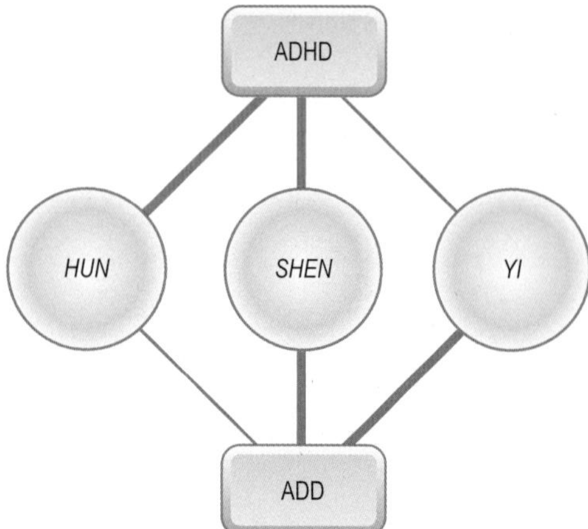

Figure 21.1 Relative involvement of Mind, Ethereal Soul and Intellect in ADHD and ADD.

The Mind (*Shen*)

The Mind is responsible for thinking, memory, emotional life, cognition, intelligence, wisdom and ideas. Therefore, it is obvious that the Mind is involved in the pathology of ADD and ADHD, but especially the former. In this disorder the Mind is weakened, and thinking, memory and concentration are all affected.

The Ethereal Soul (*Hun*)

I believe that the Ethereal Soul plays a pivotal role in the pathology of ADD and ADHD (especially the latter). As we have seen in Chapter 3, the Ethereal Soul is responsible for ideas, plans, projects, inspiration and creativity. The Ethereal Soul is constantly searching and "moving" and I believe that in ADD and ADHD (and especially the latter) there is an excess of such "movement" of the Ethereal Soul. Children and adults suffering from this disorder find it difficult to focus and concentrate on one thing at a time because the Ethereal Soul's movement is excessive.

Crucial to this pathology is the relationship between the Mind and the Ethereal Soul; in ADD and ADHD, the movement of the Ethereal Soul is excessive and the Mind does not perform adequately its function of control and integration (*see Figs 3.13 and 3.15*).

In Chapter 3, we concentrated on manic behavior as a consequence of a pathological, excessive movement of the Ethereal Soul; now we can see another, different pathology of such an excessive movement, i.e. ADHD and ADD. Interestingly, the Ethereal Soul is responsible for artistic inspiration and children suffering from ADHD are often artistic.

The Intellect (*Yi*)

The Intellect of the Spleen is responsible for focusing, concentration and the ability to apply oneself to the job in hand, all qualities that are lacking in those suffering

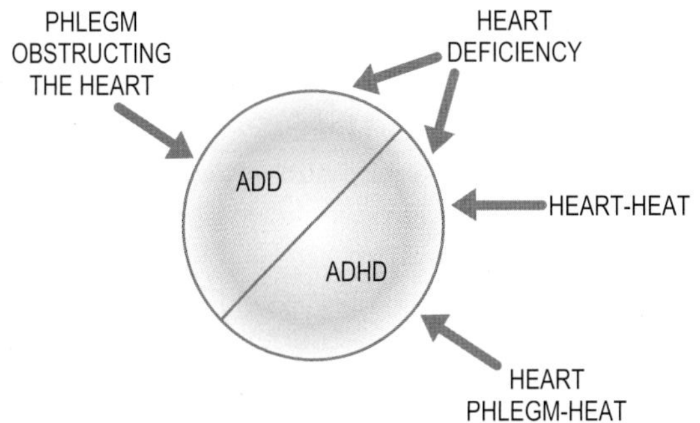

Figure 21.2 Heart pathology in ADD and ADHD.

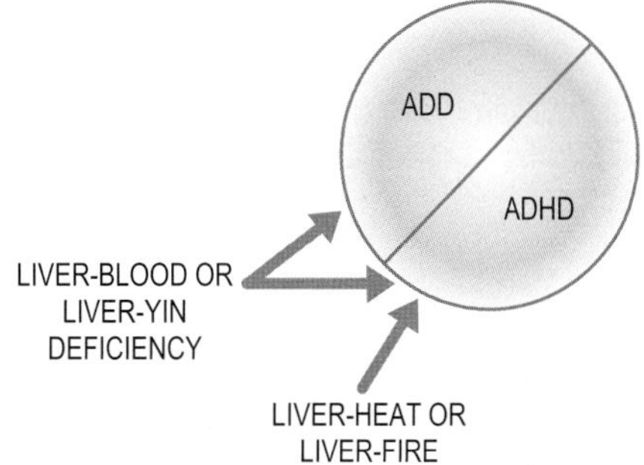

Figure 21.3 Liver pathology in ADD and ADHD.

from ADD or ADHD (especially the former). Thus, a pathology of the Intellect (and therefore of the Spleen) is a definite feature of the pathology of ADD.

Please note that the Intellect is affected not only by a deficiency of the Spleen but also by Full conditions such as Dampness and/or Phlegm obstructing the Spleen (and therefore the Intellect).

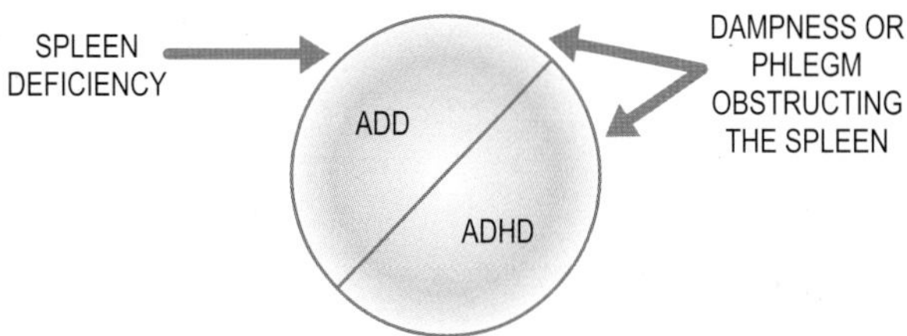

Figure 21.4 Spleen pathology in ADD and ADHD.

Organ pathology

As always in pathology, a disorder may manifest with Full or Empty conditions. I shall list the main conditions according to organ involved, bearing in mind that in practice patterns occur simultaneously.

Heart

A Heart deficiency is nearly always present in ADD and ADHD. Heart-Heat may especially cause ADHD but this is often combined with a deficiency of the Heart. This deficiency may involve Qi, Blood or Yin. Please note that Heart-Heat also stimulates the excessive movement of the Ethereal Soul.

Obstruction of the Heart by Phlegm (with or without Heat) may also be present in ADD; if there is Heat, then this condition is more likely to cause ADHD (Fig. 21.2).

Liver

The movement of the Ethereal Soul may be excessive, either because of a deficiency of Liver-Blood and/or Liver-Yin or because of Heat or Fire in the Liver. In ADHD, there is more likely to be Heat or Fire (Fig. 21.3). The ADHD patient with Liver-Fire is confrontational and particularly difficult.

I present the pattern of combined Liver- and Heart-Fire below and, in practice, this can present with different manifestations according to whether Liver-Fire or Heart-Fire predominates.

Spleen

A deficiency of the Spleen (usually of Qi or Yang) weakens the Intellect and is a feature of ADD. However, the thinking, focusing and concentration of the Intellect may also be impaired by Dampness and/or Phlegm affecting the Spleen (Fig. 21.4).

Phlegm

Phlegm in the Brain is a common factor in ADD and ADHD. Remember that Phlegm may accompany both Full and Empty patterns: for example, Liver- and Heart-Fire with Phlegm or Spleen- and Heart-Blood deficiency with Phlegm.

SUMMARY

ADD in Chinese medicine – pathology

The pathology of ADD revolves around the Heart, Liver and Spleen and their respective emotional-mental-spiritual faculties, i.e. the Mind (*Shen*), the Ethereal Soul (*Hun*) and the Intellect (*Yi*).

The Mind (Shen)

The Mind is responsible for thinking, memory, emotional life, cognition, intelligence, wisdom and ideas. Therefore, it is obvious that the Mind is involved in the pathology of ADD and ADHD, but especially the former.

The Ethereal Soul (Hun)

The Ethereal Soul plays a pivotal role in the pathology of ADD and ADHD (especially the latter). The Ethereal Soul is constantly searching and "moving" and in ADD and ADHD (and especially the latter) there is an excess of such "movement" of the Ethereal Soul. Children and adults suffering from this disorder find it difficult to focus and concentrate on one thing at a time because the Ethereal Soul's movement is excessive.

The Intellect (Yi)

The Intellect of the Spleen is responsible for focusing, concentration and the ability to apply oneself to the job in hand, all qualities that are lacking in those suffering from ADD or ADHD (especially the former). Thus, a pathology of the Intellect (and therefore of the Spleen) is a definite feature of the pathology of ADD.

Organ pathology

- Heart
  - Heart deficiency
  - Heart-Heat
  - Obstruction of the Heart by Phlegm
- Liver
  - Deficiency of Liver-Blood and/or Liver-Yin
  - Liver-Heat or Liver-Fire
- Spleen
  - Deficiency of the Spleen
  - Dampness
  - Phlegm

Phlegm

ETIOLOGY

Heredity

A hereditary weakness of the Heart, Liver and Spleen (and therefore of Mind, Ethereal Soul and Intellect) is a possible cause of ADD and ADHD.

Diet

Obviously ancient Chinese medicine dietary principles are based on an ancient diet that was entirely free of pesticides, colorings, preservatives and flavorings; these are therefore obviously not discussed in Chinese books.

The main way in which diet may affect ADD and ADHD in Western patients is the excessive consumption of foods that lead to Dampness and/or Phlegm, i.e. dairy foods, fats, sugar and excessive consumption of bread. Dampness and Phlegm may obstruct the Heart and Spleen and therefore the Mind and Intellect, leading to ADD.

A study by researchers at the University of Southampton has shown evidence of increased levels of hyperactivity in young children consuming mixtures of some artificial food colors and the preservative sodium benzoate. The research involved studying levels of hyperactivity in 153 3-year-olds and 144 8-year-olds living in the city of Southampton. The children were selected from the general population to represent the full range of behavior, from normal through to hyperactive, and not for any previous behavioral problems or known sensitivities to particular foods.

The children's families were asked to put them on a diet free from the additives used in the study. Over a 6-week period the children were then given a drink each day which contained either one of two mixtures of food colors and benzoate preservative, or just fruit juice – with all the drinks looking and tasting identical.

The results of the Southampton study show that when the children were given the drinks containing the test mixtures, in some cases their behavior was significantly more hyperactive.

The research team used a combination of reports on the children's behavior from teachers and parents, together with recordings of the children's behavior in the classroom made by an observer, and, for the older children, a computer-based test of attention. None of the participants – teachers, parents, the observer or the children – knew which drink each child was taking at any one time.[13]

Emotional stress

Emotional stress in early childhood may cause ADD or ADHD. This is usually due to fear, fright or shock affecting the baby or young child. These emotions weaken the Heart and Spleen and therefore the Mind and Intellect.

In other children, anger plays a role in the etiology of this disorder. In small children, anger may derive from competition with siblings or from anger towards one of the parents (e.g. a parent who is excessively stern and strict or, worse, a parent who physically abuses the child).

Sadness and grief may also play a role in the etiology of ADHD and ADD; these usually derive from lack of affection and tactility from the parents.

Pregnancy and labor

Events affecting the mother's pregnancy and labor may contribute to the development of ADD or ADHD. The consumption of alcohol, smoking and shocks during pregnancy are all events that may adversely affect the brain of the baby in the womb.

A traumatic and prolonged labor may also affect adversely the brain of the newborn.

SUMMARY

ADD in Chinese medicine – etiology

- Heredity
- Diet
- Emotional stress
- Pregnancy and labor

ACUPUNCTURE TREATMENT

Before discussing individual patterns, I shall discuss the general principles of acupuncture treatment of this condition. Although the acupuncture treatment is also given for each pattern, there are some general principles for the acupuncture treatment that apply to all patterns.

As the treatment should focus on the Mind (*Shen*), Intellect (*Yi*) and Ethereal Soul (*Hun*), the acupuncture treatment focuses on the Heart, Spleen and Liver. However, treatment of the Governing Vessels and other head points is also important. I will therefore discuss the points from the Heart, Spleen and Liver channel, then the Governing Vessel points and then points from other channels.

Heart

HE-5 Tongli

I use this as the main point to tonify the Heart and strengthen the Mind in ADD. When I use this point to strengthen the Mind and tonify the Heart, I combine it with general points that tonify Qi such as ST-36 Zusanli and Ren-6 Qihai. I also frequently combine HE-5 with BL-15 Xinshu.

HE-7 Shenmen

I use this point especially to nourish Heart-Blood and calm the Mind. However, besides "calming the Mind", it also stimulates the Mind and memory and, for this reason, it is an important point for ADD. Its indications include poor memory, mental restlessness and agitation.

BL-15 Xinshu

This is an important point to tonify the Heart and strengthen the Mind in ADD. I frequently combine it with HE-5 Tongli. BL-15 nourishes the Heart and stimulates the Brain.

Its indications include anxiety, disorientation, delayed speech development, poor memory, poor concentration, mental confusion and Heart-Qi deficiency in children.

At the same time as calming the Mind, BL-15 also stimulates the brain if used with reinforcing method or with direct moxibustion. In particular, used with direct moxibustion, it has a good effect in stimulating the brain, and is effective for mental confusion and poor concentration in adults and slow development in children.

Spleen

SP-3 Taibai

I use this as the main point from the Spleen channel to stimulate the Intellect (*Yi*) in ADD. Its indications include poor memory, confused thinking, muzziness of the head and difficulty in concentrating.

Another important function of this point is to resolve Dampness, which is a major aspect of its functions. In my experience, SP-3 is particularly useful to resolve

Dampness from the head where it causes a feeling of heaviness and muzziness of the head and poor concentration.

SP-6 Sanyinjiao

SP-6 has a strong calming action on the Mind and it is therefore particularly indicated in the treatment of ADHD, especially if occurring against a background of Blood or Yin deficiency. In particular, SP-6 is used for Spleen- and Heart- Blood deficiency; when the Spleen is not making enough Blood, the Heart is not supplied with enough Blood and the Mind lacks a "residence", so that there is hyperactivity and lack of concentration. SP-6 is the point to use in this case, as it will simultaneously tonify the Spleen, nourish Blood and calm the Mind.

BL-20 Pishu

BL-20 is the Back-Transporting point of the Spleen; it tonifies the Spleen, strengthens the Intellect (*Yi*) and resolves Dampness. In the context of ADD, it stimulates memory and concentration. In order to achieve this, I often combine this point with the point next to it on the outer Bladder line, i.e. BL-49 Yishe.

Liver

BL-47 Hunmen

BL-47 Hunmen regulates the movement of the Ethereal Soul; it can stimulate it or restrain it. In the treatment of ADD and ADHD, I use it to restrain the movement of the Ethereal Soul. The indications of this point include fear, depression, insomnia, excessive dreaming, lack of sense of direction in life and "possession by corpse".[14]

This point settles and roots the Ethereal Soul in the Liver. It is a "door", so this point regulates the "coming and going" of the Ethereal Soul.

The *Explanation of Acupuncture Points* (1654) confirms that, due to this point's nature of "window", "gate" or "door", the Ethereal Soul goes in and out through it. This confirms the dynamic nature of this point in stimulating the movement of the Ethereal Soul and Mind; however, it can also work the other way, i.e. to calm down the excessive movement of the Ethereal Soul.

LIV-3 Taichong

LIV-3 has a profound calming effect on the Mind and the Ethereal Soul, and is effective in calming the hyperactivity of ADHD. Its calming action is enhanced when combined with L.I.-4 Hegu (the "Four Gates").

The indications of this point include propensity to outbursts of anger, irritability, insomnia and worrying.

Governing Vessel

Du-16 Fengfu

Du-16 Fengfu has a deep influence on the Brain and the mental-emotional state due to three of its characteristics: it is a point of the Sea of Marrow, a Window of Heaven point, and one of Sun Si Miao's 13 ghost points. These are its most important characteristics in the context of ADD.

Du-16 nourishes Marrow and benefits the Brain, calms the Mind and opens the Mind's orifices. Among its indications are manic behavior, desire to commit suicide, sadness and fear.

In the context of ADD, Du-16 clears the Mind and stimulates the brain due to its being a point of the Sea of Marrow. Being a Window of Heaven point, it promotes the ascending of clear Qi and descending of turbid Qi to and from the head; this contributes to stimulating memory and concentration.

Du-17 Naohu

The name of Du-17 means "Window of the Brain"; this point nourishes the Brain and stimulates memory and concentration. Among its indications are feeling of heaviness of the head, dizziness and manic behavior. The presence of "feeling of heaviness of the head" and "dizziness" among its indications shows that this point also resolves Phlegm from the Brain.

Du-17 is therefore indicated in the treatment of ADD both to nourish the Brain (in Empty conditions) and to eliminate Phlegm from the Brain (in Full conditions).

Du-19 Houding

Du-19 calms the Mind and opens the Mind's orifices. This point is particularly indicated to calm the Mind in ADHD. Among its indications are manic behavior, anxiety, mental restlessness and insomnia. To calm the

Mind, I frequently combine this point with Ren-15 Jiuwei.

Du-20 Baihui

Du-20 is a point of the Sea of Marrow; it benefits the Brain and the sense organs and clears the Mind. Among its indications are dizziness, "brain noise", tinnitus and poor memory.

Du-20 is a meeting point of many Yang channels which carry clear Yang to the head; it therefore has a powerful effect in stimulating the ascending of Yang. When used with direct moxa, it stimulates the ascending of clear Qi to the head; this point's lifting action on Qi has a mental effect in that it promotes the rise of clear Yang to the Brain and the Mind. For this reason, I frequently use Du-20 to stimulate concentration in ADD.

Du-24 Shenting

Du-24 calms and lifts the Mind and opens the Mind's orifices. Its indications include manic-depression, depression, anxiety, poor memory and insomnia.

This is a very important and powerful point to calm the Mind. It is frequently combined with G.B.-13 Benshen for severe anxiety and fears. An important feature of this point that makes it particularly useful is that it can both calm and lift the Mind; therefore, it is used not only for anxiety and insomnia but also for depression and sadness. This means that this point can be used for both ADD and ADHD.

The name of this point ("Spirit courtyard") refers to its strong influence on the Mind and Spirit. The courtyard was traditionally considered to be a very important part of the house as it was the one that gave the first impression to visitors; it is the entrance. Thus, this point could be said to be the "entrance" to the Mind and Spirit, and its being a courtyard highlights its importance.

Other points

G.B.-13 Benshen

G.B.-13 calms the Mind (*Shen*), resolves Phlegm from the Brain, gathers Essence (*Jing*) to the head and clears the brain. Among its indications are manic behavior, fright and dizziness.

G.B.-13 is a very important point for mental and emotional problems. This point has a powerful effect in calming the Mind and settling the Ethereal Soul when the person is hyperactive. Its effect is enhanced if it is combined with Du-24 Shenting.

Its deep mental and emotional effect is also due to its action of "gathering" Essence to the head. The Kidney-Essence is the root of our Pre-Heaven Qi and is the foundation for our mental and emotional life. A strong Essence is the fundamental prerequisite for a clear Mind (*Shen*) and a balanced emotional life. This is the meaning of this point's name "Root of the Mind", i.e. this point gathers the Essence which is the root of the Mind (*Shen*).

The Kidney-Essence is the source of Marrow which fills up the Brain (called Sea of Marrow); G.B.-13 is a point where Essence and Marrow "gather". The *Great Dictionary of Acupuncture* says that this point "*makes the Mind [Shen] return to its root*":[15] the "root" of the Mind is the Essence, hence this point "gathers" the Essence to the Brain and affects the Mind. As it connects the Mind and the Essence, it also treats both the Heart and the Kidneys and therefore the Mind (*Shen*) and Will-Power (*Zhi*); bearing in mind that the *Zhi* of the Kidneys also involves memory, this point will stimulate memory and concentration by acting on both the Liver and the Kidneys.

When combined with other points to nourish Essence (such as Ren-4 Guanyuan), G.B.-13 attracts Essence towards the head with the effect of calming the Mind and strengthening clarity of mind, memory and concentration. The connection between G.B.-13 and the Essence is confirmed by the text *An Enquiry into Chinese Acupuncture* which has among the indications of this point: "*excessive menstrual bleeding, impotence and seminal emissions*".[16]

Finally, G.B.-13 resolves Phlegm from the Brain. In the context of ADD, it opens the Mind's orifices when these are clouded by Phlegm; this will stimulate memory and concentration.

G.B.-17 Zhengying

G.B.-17 resolves Phlegm and opens the Mind's orifices. Its indications include dizziness, blurred vision from Phlegm, obsessive thoughts, pensiveness and manic behavior.

G.B.-17 has a strong mental-emotional effect in opening the Mind's orifices and resolving Phlegm. In my experience, it is effective to eliminate Phlegm from the head when this obstructs the Mind causing obsessive thoughts, pensiveness and mild manic behavior.

In the context of ADD, I use this point to stimulate memory and concentration when the Brain is obstructed by Phlegm.

G.B.-18 Chengling

G.B.-18 calms the Mind and opens the Mind's orifices. Its indications include dizziness, obsessive thoughts and pensiveness.

G.B.-18 has a deep effect on mental problems such as obsessional thoughts and dementia.[17] I use this point to resolve Phlegm from the Brain and calm the Mind in ADHD.

G.B.-19 Naokong

G.B.-19 calms the Mind. Its indications include dizziness, blurred vision, manic-depression, fright and palpitations.

I use G.B.-19 to calm the Mind in ADHD.

ST-8 Touwei

I use ST-8 primarily to resolve Phlegm from the Brain in ADD.

BL-10 Tianzhu

BL-10 is a Window of Heaven point; its effect on ADD is partly related to this characteristic. It clears the brain and opens the Mind's orifices. Its indications include dizziness, feeling of heaviness of the head, mental confusion, difficulty in concentrating, poor memory, incessant talking, "seeing ghosts" and manic behavior.

Being Yang in nature due to its channel polarity and position, BL-10 treats excess of Yang causing mental problems (incessant talking, "seeing ghosts", manic behavior).

In the context of ADD, being a Window of Heaven point, BL-10 can stimulate the rising of clear Qi to the head and the descending of turbid Qi from the head; this will clear the Brain and stimulate memory and concentration.

BL-23 Shenshu

BL-23 is the Back-Transporting point of the Kidneys. The Kidneys store the Essence which nourishes Marrow and the Brain. Tonifying BL-23 can strengthen the Marrow and nourish the Brain to stimulate memory and concentration in ADD.

The experience of teachers from the Nanjing University of Traditional Chinese Medicine

Professor Wang Ling Ling of the Nanjing University of Traditional Chinese Medicine focuses on the Governing Vessel for the treatment of ADD. She uses a general formula based on the following points: Du-14 Dazhui, L.I.-4 Hegu, LIV-3 Taichong, HE-7 Shenmen and SP-6 Sanyinjiao.

In addition to these points she uses one of the following two sets of points in alternation: (1) Du-20 Baihui, Du-24 Shenting and Yintang, and (2) Sishencong.[18]

Dr Shen Can Rou of the Jiangsu Province Hospital of Traditional Chinese Medicine in Nanjing focuses on tonifying the Spleen and subduing the Liver in the treatment of ADD in children with the following points: G.B.-20 Fengchi, HE-7 Shenmen, ST-36 Zusanli, SP-6 Sanyinjiao, LIV-3 Taichong and Yintang.[19]

Dr Tao Kun lists the following patterns causing ADHD in his experience.

1. Kidney-Yin deficiency, Water failing to nourish Wood.
2. Heart- and Liver-Fire.
3. Heart-Fire with Phlegm.
4. Malnutrition of channels due to Qi stagnation and Blood stasis.
5. Disharmony of Yin and Yang between Liver, Heart, Kidneys and Spleen.

The treatment principle Dr Tao adopts is to treat the underlying pattern and restore normal flow of Qi and Blood, and to adjust *Ren* and *Du Mai* to harmonize Yin and Yang.

Dr Tao selects points from the following list: Du-14 Dazhui, Ren-8 Shenque, Du-20 Baihui, Sishencong, L.I.-4 Hegu, HE-7 Shenmen, KI-3 Taixi and LIV-3 Taichong.[20]

SUMMARY

Attention deficit disorder in Chinese medicine – acupuncture treatment

Heart

- HE-5 Tongli
- HE-7 Shenmen
- BL-15 Xinshu

Spleen

- SP-3 Taibai
- SP-6 Sanyinjiao
- BL-20 Pishu

Liver

- BL-47 Hunmen
- LIV-3 Taichong

Governing Vessel

- Du-16 Fengfu
- Du-17 Naohu
- Du-19 Houding
- Du-20 Baihui
- Du-24 Shenting

Other points

- G.B.-13 Benshen
- G.B.-17 Zhengying
- G.B.-18 Chengling
- G.B.-19 Naokong
- ST-8 Touwei
- BL-10 Tianzhu
- BL-23 Shenshu

The experience of teachers from the Nanjing University of Traditional Chinese Medicine

- *Professor Wang Ling Ling*: Du-14 Dazhui, L.I.-4 Hegu, LIV-3 Taichong, HE-7 Shenmen and SP-6 Sanyinjiao. In addition to these points she uses one of the following two sets of points in alternation: (1) Du-20 Baihui, Du-24 Shenting and Yintang, and (2) Sishencong.
- *Dr Shen Can Rou*: G.B.-20 Fengchi, HE-7 Shenmen, ST-36 Zusanli, SP-6 Sanyinjiao, LIV-3 Taichong and Yintang.
- *Dr Tao Kun*: Du-14 Dazhui, Ren-8 Shenque, Du-20 Baihui, Sishencong, L.I.-4 Hegu, HE-7 Shenmen, KI-3 Taixi and LIV-3 Taichong.

IDENTIFICATION OF PATTERNS AND TREATMENT

The Chinese medicine literature on the treatment of ADHD and ADD is scanty. A review of some of the existing literature is presented at the end of this chapter. As often is the case, Chinese studies are poorly designed but they are reported here to give the reader at least an indication of the treatment strategies adopted in China.

Deficiency of Heart- and Spleen-Blood

Clinical manifestations

Attention deficit disorder, poor memory and concentration, difficulty in sticking to the job in hand, difficulty in keeping time, tendency to daydream, lack of attention, tiredness, insomnia, anxiety, poor appetite, loose stools, palpitations.

Tongue: Pale, Thin.

Pulse: Choppy or Fine.

Treatment principle

Nourish Heart- and Spleen-Blood, strengthen the Mind (*Shen*) and the Intellect (*Yi*).

Acupuncture

Points

HE-7 Shenmen, Ren-15 Jiuwei, Du-24 Shenting, SP-6 Sanyinjiao, Ren-12 Zhongwan, BL-20 Pishu, Du-20 Baihui. All with reinforcing method.

Explanation

- HE-7 and Ren-15 nourish Heart-Blood and strengthen the Mind.
- Du-24 strengthens the Mind and improves memory and concentration.
- SP-6, Ren-12 and BL-20 tonify Spleen-Qi and Spleen-Blood.
- Du-20 improves memory and concentration.

Herbal therapy

Prescription

GUI PI TANG Variation
Tonifying the Spleen Decoction Variation

Explanation

This formula tonifies Qi and Blood of the Heart and Spleen and it stimulates the Brain.

> **SUMMARY**
>
> **Deficiency of Heart- and Spleen-Blood**
>
> *Points*
>
> HE-7 Shenmen, Ren-15 Jiuwei, Du-24 Shenting, SP-6 Sanyinjiao, Ren-12 Zhongwan, BL-20 Pishu, Du-20 Baihui. All with reinforcing method.
>
> *Herbal therapy*
>
> *Prescription*
>
> **GUI PI TANG** Variation
> *Tonifying the Spleen Decoction* Variation

Heart- and Kidney-Yin deficiency

Clinical manifestations

Hyperactive child or adult suffering from ADHD, insomnia, dry mouth, tinnitus, night-sweating, poor memory and concentration.

Tongue: without coating.

Pulse: Floating-Empty.

Treatment principle

Nourish Heart- and Kidney-Yin, strengthen the Mind (*Shen*).

Acupuncture

Points

SP-6 Sanyinjiao, KI-3 Taixi, Ren-4 Guanyuan, HE-7 Shenmen, Du-24 Shenting, Ren-15 Jiuwei. All with reinforcing method.

Explanation

- SP-6, KI-3 and Ren-4 nourish Kidney-Yin.
- HE-7 nourishes Heart-Yin.
- Du-24 and Ren-15 nourish the Heart, strengthen the Mind and stimulate memory and concentration.

Herbal therapy

Prescription

KONG SHENG ZHEN ZHONG DAN
Master Kong's Bedside Pill

Explanation

This formula nourishes Heart- and Kidney-Yin, strengthens the Marrow and Brain and calms the Spirit.

> **SUMMARY**
>
> **Heart-Yin and Kidney-Yin deficiency**
>
> *Points*
>
> SP-6 Sanyinjiao, KI-3 Taixi, Ren-4 Guanyuan, HE-7 Shenmen, Du-24 Shenting, Ren-15 Jiuwei. All with reinforcing method.
>
> *Herbal therapy*
>
> *Prescription*
>
> **KONG SHENG ZHEN ZHONG DAN**
> *Master Kong's Bedside Pill*

Kidney- and Liver-Yin deficiency with Liver-Yang rising

Clinical manifestations

Hyperactive child or adult suffering from ADHD, night-sweating, dry mouth, tinnitus, irritability, propensity to outbursts of anger.

Tongue: without coating, red sides.

Pulse: Floating-Empty and slightly Wiry.

Treatment principle

Nourish Liver- and Kidney-Yin, subdue Liver-Yang.

Acupuncture

Points

SP-6 Sanyinjiao, LIV-8 Ququan, KI-3 Taixi, Ren-4 Guanyuan, HE-7 Shenmen, LIV-3 Taichong, G.B.-13 Benshen, Du-24 Shenting.

Explanation

- SP-6, LIV-8, KI-3 and Ren-4 nourish Liver- and Kidney-Yin.

- HE-7 calms the Mind.
- LIV-3 subdues Liver-Yang.
- G.B.-13 and Du-24 subdue Liver-Yang, calm the Mind and stimulate memory and concentration.

Herbal therapy

Prescription

QI JU DI HUANG WAN Variation
Lycium-Chrysanthemum-Rehmannia Decoction Variation

Explanation

This formula nourishes Liver- and Kidney-Yin, subdues Liver-Yang and calms the Spirit.

> **SUMMARY**
>
> **Kidney- and Liver-Yin deficiency with Liver-Yang rising**
>
> *Points*
>
> SP-6 Sanyinjiao, LIV-8 Ququan, KI-3 Taixi, Ren-4 Guanyuan, HE-7 Shenmen, LIV-3 Taichong, G.B.-13 Benshen, Du-24 Shenting.
>
> *Herbal therapy*
>
> *Prescription*
>
> **QI JU DI HUANG WAN** Variation
> *Lycium-Chrysanthemum-Rehmannia Decoction* Variation

Heart- and Spleen-Qi deficiency

Clinical manifestations

Child or adult with ADD, the child is in his or her own world, lack of concentration, daydreaming, quiet, slow movement, light sleeper, spontaneous sweating, picky eater.

Tongue: Pale.
Pulse: Weak.

Treatment principle

Tonify Heart- and Spleen-Qi, strengthen the Brain.

Acupuncture

Points

HE-5 Tongli, BL-15 Xinshu, Ren-15 Jiuwei, Du-24 Shenting, Du-20 Baihui, Ren-12 Zhongwan, ST-36 Zusanli, BL-20 Pishu, BL-49 Yishe.

Explanation

- HE-5 and BL-15 tonify the Heart.
- Ren-15 and Du-24 calm the Spirit.
- Du-20 stimulates the ascending of clear Qi to the Brain.
- Ren-12, ST-36 and BL-20 tonify the Spleen.
- BL-49 stimulates the Intellect.

Herbal therapy

Prescription

GUI PI TANG plus **GAN MAI DA ZAO TANG**
Tonifying the Spleen Decoction plus *Glycyrrhiza-Triticum-Jujuba Decoction*

Explanation

Gui Pi Tang tonifies Qi and Blood of Spleen, Liver and Heart, while Gan Mai Da Zao Tang tonifies the Heart and calms the Spirit.

> **SUMMARY**
>
> **Heart- and Spleen-Qi deficiency**
>
> *Points*
>
> HE-5 Tongli, BL-15 Xinshu, Ren-15 Jiuwei, Du-24 Shenting, Du-20 Baihui, Ren-12 Zhongwan, ST-36 Zusanli, BL-20 Pishu, BL-49 Yishe.
>
> *Herbal therapy*
>
> *Prescription*
>
> **GUI PI TANG** plus **GAN MAI DA ZAO TANG**
> *Tonifying the Spleen Decoction* plus *Glycyrrhiza-Triticum-Jujuba Decoction*

Liver- and Heart-Fire

Clinical manifestations

Child with ADHD, restless and irritable child, propensity to outbursts of anger, lack of concentration, inability to focus on a task, thirst, dry mouth, insomnia, unpleasant dreams, headaches, bitter taste. Often an artistic child.

Tongue: Red with redder sides, dry-yellow coating.

Pulse: Wiry-Rapid.

Treatment principle

Drain Heart- and Liver-Fire, calm the Mind, settle the Ethereal Soul.

Acupuncture

Points

LIV-2 Xingjian, LIV-3 Taichong, Du-24 Shenting, G.B.-13 Benshen, Ren-15 Jiuwei. All with reducing method.

Explanation

- LIV-2 drains Liver-Fire.
- LIV-3 calms the Spirit and settles the Ethereal Soul.
- Du-24, G.B.-13 and Ren-15 calm the Spirit and settle the Ethereal Soul.

Herbal therapy

Prescription

LONG DAN XIE GAN TANG Variation
Gentiana Draining the Liver Decoction Variation

Explanation

This variation of Long Dan Xie Gan Tang drains Liver- and Heart-Fire, calms the Spirit and settles the Ethereal Soul.

SUMMARY

Liver- and Heart-Fire

Points

LIV-2 Xingjian, LIV-3 Taichong, Du-24 Shenting, G.B.-13 Benshen, Ren-15 Jiuwei. All with reducing method.

Herbal therapy

Prescription

LONG DAN XIE GAN TANG Variation
Gentiana Draining the Liver Decoction Variation

Heart and Spleen deficiency with Phlegm

Clinical manifestations

Child or adult with ADD, the child is in his or her own world, lack of concentration, daydreaming, quiet, slow movement, sleepiness, spontaneous sweating, picky eater, catarrh, feeling of oppression of the chest, expectoration of sputum.

Tongue: Pale and Swollen with a sticky coating.

Pulse: Soggy or Slippery.

Treatment principle

Tonify the Spleen, strengthen the Intellect, resolve Phlegm.

Acupuncture

Points

Ren-12 Zhongwan, Ren-9 Shuifen, SP-6 Sanyinjiao, ST-40 Fenglong, HE-5 Tongli, BL-15 Xinshu, Du-24 Shenting, Ren-15 Jiuwei, ST-36 Zusanli, BL-20 Pishu, BL-49 Yishe. Ren-9, SP-6 and ST-40 with reducing or even method; all others with reinforcing method.

Explanation

- Ren-12, Ren-9, SP-6 and ST-40 resolve Phlegm.
- HE-5 and BL-15 tonify the Heart.
- Du-24 and Ren-15 calm the Spirit.
- ST-36, Ren-12 and BL-20 tonify the Spleen.
- BL-49 stimulates the Intellect.

Herbal therapy

Prescription

GUI PI TANG plus **GAN MAI DA ZAO TANG** Variation
Tonifying the Spleen Decoction plus *Glycyrrhiza-Triticum-Jujuba Decoction* Variation

Explanation

This variation of these two formulae tonifies the Heart and Spleen, calms the Spirit, settles the Ethereal Soul and resolves Phlegm.

SUMMARY

Heart and Spleen deficiency with Phlegm

Points

Ren-12 Zhongwan, Ren-9 Shuifen, SP-6 Sanyinjiao, ST-40 Fenglong, HE-5 Tongli, BL-15 Xinshu, Du-24 Shenting, Ren-15 Jiuwei, ST-36 Zusanli, BL-20 Pishu, BL-49 Yishe. Ren-9, SP-6 and ST-40 with reducing or even method; all others with reinforcing method.

Herbal therapy

Prescription

GUI PI TANG plus **GAN MAI DA ZAO TANG** Variation

Tonifying the Spleen Decoction plus *Glycyrrhiza-Triticum-Jujuba Decoction* Variation

WESTERN MEDICINE CLINICAL TRIALS

High-resolution brain SPECT imaging in ADHD

Annals of Clinical Psychiatry 1997 June, Vol. 9, Issue 2, pp. 81–86.

Amen DG, Carmichael BD
Amen Clinic for Behavioral Medicine, Fairfield, California

Children and adolescents with ADHD were evaluated with high-resolution brain SPECT imaging to determine if there were similarities between reported PET and QEEG findings.

Fifty-four children and adolescents with ADHD by DSM-III-R and Conners' Rating Scale criteria were evaluated. A non-ADHD control group was also studied with SPECT. Two brain SPECT studies were done on each group: a resting study and an intellectual stress study done while participants were doing a concentration task.

Sixty-five percent of the ADHD group revealed decreased perfusion in the prefrontal cortex with intellectual stress, compared to only 5% of the control group. These findings are consistent with PET and QEEG findings. Of the ADHD group who did not show decreased perfusion, two-thirds had markedly decreased activity in the prefrontal cortices at rest.

Sensitivity and specificity of QEEG in children with attention deficit or specific developmental learning disorders

Clinical Electroencephalography 1996 January, Vol. 27, Issue 1, pp. 26–34.

Chabot RJ, Merkin H, Wood LM, Davenport TL, Serfontein G
Department of Psychiatry, New York University School of Medicine, New York

The sensitivity and specificity of QEEG-based discriminant functions were evaluated in populations of children diagnosed with specific developmental learning disorders and those with attention deficit disorders.

Both populations of children could be distinguished from each other, and from the normal population, with high levels of accuracy. Pre-treatment QEEG could be utilized to distinguish ADD/ADHD children who responded to dextroamfetamine [dexamfetamine] from those who responded to methylphenidate, again with high levels of accuracy.

This paper provides a replication of all presented discriminant functions, and should provide the research basis for the generalized utilization of QEEG in the initial evaluation of children with learning and/or attention disorders. As demonstrated in the above study, the effectiveness of stimulant therapy, including indications for specific medication, could be predicted based on QEEG determinations.

Objectively measured hyperactivity – II. Caffeine and amfetamine effects

Journal of Clinical Pharmacology 1985 May–June, Vol. 25, Issue 4, pp. 276–280.

Schechter MD, Timmons GD

Errors of commission and omission, chair movements and reaction times were assessed in 15 previously diagnosed hyperactive children on a Continuous Performance Test after four drug regimens: amfetamine at doses of 1.6 and 5.0 mg twice a day, as well as 300 mg caffeine administered alone, and with 1.6 mg amfetamine twice a day, and produced significant reductions in errors of commission and increased reaction times in those children scoring 24 or more on the Conners' Abbreviated Parent Questionnaire.

In addition, subjective symptoms on this questionnaire were significantly reduced by all drug treatments. The high (600 mg) daily dose of caffeine was observed to significantly control hyperactive symptoms; however, it also produced a number of side-effects as well. It has even been suggested that many ADHD children who go into remission as adults may have learned to self-medicate with regular coffee consumption. In such cases, elimination of caffeine from their diet may actually unmask the underlying ADHD condition.

Will population decreases in caffeine consumption unveil attention deficit disorders in adults?

Medical Hypotheses 1985 October, Vol. 18, Issue 2, pp. 163–167.

Dalby JT

Department of Psychology, Calgary General Hospital, Alberta, Canada

Attention deficit disorders (ADD) represent the commonest behavior disorder observed in children but only recently has the persistence of these disorders into adulthood been acknowledged. As individuals with ADD enter adolescence and then adulthood, some behavioral symptoms appear to cease, others become muted. This change has usually been attributed to physiological maturation.

One environmental factor that may also contribute to the altered clinical picture is the regular ingestion of caffeine beginning in late adolescence. Caffeine has been found to alter the behavior of ADD children in a manner resembling more widely prescribed stimulant medications.

If some adults with ADD have responded positively to caffeine ingestion, then it would be predicted that increases in reports of ADD symptoms will escalate with the rapid decline in caffeine consumption in North America. The following studies comparing caffeine therapy to Ritalin (methylphenidate) showed similar benefits using low-dose caffeine, and even better results when the two stimulants were combined. It may be important to note that the benefits of caffeine were negated using higher doses.

Responses to methylphenidate and varied doses of caffeine in children with attention deficit disorder

Canadian Journal of Psychiatry 1981 October, Vol. 26, Issue 6, pp. 395–401.

Garfinkel BD, Webster CD, Sloman L

Six children with the diagnosis of attention deficit disorder were treated as day hospital patients, using different stimulant medication. They were studied in a double-blind crossover experiment in which they received caffeine in low dose or in a high dose. Methylphenidate (Ritalin) was added to both dosages, as well as administered alone.

Results indicated that caffeine in low dosage when added to methylphenidate was superior to all other treatment conditions. Caffeine in low dosage could not be differentiated from 10 mg of methylphenidate.

High dosage caffeine was no different from placebo or no-drug conditions. This study offers evidence to support a curvilinear pattern of dose–response for caffeine, in attenuating the behavioral manifestations of this syndrome.

Individual responses to methylphenidate and caffeine in children with minimal brain dysfunction

Canadian Medical Association Journal 1975 October, Vol. 113, Issue 8, pp. 729–732.

Garfinkel BD, Webster CD, Sloman L

Eight children with minimal brain dysfunction were studied for their individual responses to two stimulant medications – methylphenidate (Ritalin) hydrochloride and caffeine citrate. Four types of behavioral responses were observed in the double-blind crossover experiment: four children responded favorably to both psychostimulants, one responded to methylphenidate alone and two responded to the placebo. The behavior of one child deteriorated while he was taking methylphenidate and caffeine.

In general, methylphenidate was superior to caffeine in diminishing hyperactive and aggressive behavior. It is apparent that such stimulant medication exerts therapeutic effects and would therefore be useful as one aspect of a complete treatment program for children with this syndrome.

Caffeine versus methylphenidate and D-amfetamine in minimal brain dysfunction: a double-blind comparison

American Journal of Psychiatry 1975 August, Vol. 132, Issue 8, pp. 868–870.
Huestis RD, Arnold LE, Smeltzer DJ

The authors compared the efficacy of caffeine, methylphenidate, and D-amfetamine in children with minimal brain dysfunction using a double-blind crossover design.

The slight improvement with caffeine was not significantly better than placebo. Both prescription drugs resulted in significant improvement and were significantly superior to caffeine.

The authors suggest that the discrepancy between these results and an earlier, more optimistic report may stem from the use in this study of pure caffeine rather than whole coffee.

CHINESE MEDICINE CLINICAL TRIALS

Acupuncture

Effects of electroacupuncture combined with behavior therapy on intelligence and behavior of children with autism

Zhong Guo Zhen Jiu 中国针灸 [Chinese Acupuncture and Moxibustion] 2007 September, Vol. 27, Issue 9, pp. 660–662.
Wang CN, Liu Y, Wei XH, Li LX

Objective

To find out an effective therapy for autism.

Method

Sixty children with autism were randomly divided into an electroacupuncture (EA) plus behavior therapy group and a behavior therapy group, with 30 cases in each group. The patients in the EA plus behavior therapy group were needled at points Du-20 Baihui, Sishencong, Du-24 Shenting, G.B.-13 Benshen, Yintang, Du-17 Naohu, G.B.-19 Naokong, P-6 Neiguan and scalp acupuncture at speech areas I, II and III. The therapeutic effects, Peabody Picture and Vocabulary Test (PPVT) and behavior ability were observed.

Results

The total effective rate was 86.7% in the EA plus behavior therapy group, which was better than the 56.7% in the behavior therapy group. The EA plus behavior therapy group had significant improvement in sensation and ability of self-care ($P < 0.05$) but there was no significant improvement in the PPVT scores in the two groups ($P > 0.05$).

Conclusion

EA combined with behavior therapy can significantly improve clinical symptoms of autism, but does not improve intelligence.

Effect of acupuncture on rehabilitation training for children's autism

Zhong Guo Zhen Jiu [Chinese Acupuncture and Moxibustion] 2007 July, Vol. 27, Issue 7, pp. 503–505.
Yan YF, Wei Y, Chen YH, Chen MM

Objective

To observe the effect of acupuncture on rehabilitation training for children's autism.

Method

Forty autistic children receiving rehabilitation training were divided into a control group and a treatment group, with 20 cases in each group. The control group received rehabilitation training including ABA training, the Conductive Education Approach and the training of sensory integration, with about 90 sessions for each training; the treatment group received acupuncture treatment for 60–90 sessions after the rehabilitation training. Their results were measured by the revised Chinese version of Psycho-Educational Profile for autistic and developmentally disabled children (C-PEP).

Results

The markedly effective rate was 55.0% in the treatment group and 15.0% in the control group, with a very significant difference between the two groups ($P < 0.01$); the differences before and after training in areas such as the total score of development, imitation, oral cognition in the treatment group were very significantly different from those in the control group ($P < 0.01$).

Conclusion

Acupuncture combined with scientific and effective rehabilitation training has a better therapeutic effect than that of simple rehabilitation training for children's autism.

Herbal medicine

Clinical and experimental studies on Tiaoshen Liquor for infantile hyperactive syndrome

(*Zhong Guo Zhong Xi Yi Jie He Za Zhi* 中国中西医结合杂志 [Chinese Journal of Integrative Medicine] 1995 June, Vol. 15, Issue 6, pp. 337–340.

Wang LH, Li CS, Li GZ
Pediatric Department of the Affiliated Hospital of Shandong College of TCM, Jinan

Objective

To ascertain the effect of Tiaoshen Liquor on infantile hyperactive syndrome.

Method

One hundred children with hyperactive syndrome were treated by using Tiaoshen Liquor (TL) consisting of Chinese herbal drugs [the article does not disclose the composition of this remedy].

Results

After the treatment, the behavioral problems grading lowered greatly, attention was improved, and academic records rose. The total effective rate reached 94%.

The results of animal studies showed that TL could reduce spontaneous activities in mice with hyperkinetic behavior elicited by scopolamine; reinforce the learning memory in healthy mice; and improve in different degrees the learning memory of mice with dysmnesia caused by administering scopolamine, sodium nitrite and alcohol, respectively.

Conclusion

This indicates that the therapeutic mechanism of TL for this syndrome was probably related to the improvement of information transfer function of the cholinergic neuron synapses of the central nervous system and to the enhancement of hypoxia tolerance of the cerebral tissues.

Clinical observation and treatment of hyperkinesia in children by Traditional Chinese Medicine

Zhong Yi Za Zhi 中医杂志 [Journal of Chinese Medicine] 1994 June, Vol. 14, Issue 2, p. 105.

Sun Y, Wang Y, Qu X, Wang J, Fang J, Zhang L
Shanxi College of Traditional Chinese Medicine, Xianyang

Extract

Sixty-six children with hyperkinesia were treated with Yizhi syrup, after which their scores on behavioral problems dropped and their school records improved, giving a total effectiveness rate of 84.8%.

After the treatment, examination of the 24-hour urine showed significant increases in its content of norepinephrine (NE), dopamine (DA), 3-4 dihydroxy phenylacetic acid (DOPAC), cyclic adenosine monophosphate (cAMP) and creatinine (Cr).

Preliminary study of Traditional Chinese Medicine treatment of minimal brain dysfunction: analysis of 100 cases

Zhong Guo Zhong Xi Yi Jie He Za Zhi [Chinese Journal of Integrative Medicine] 1990 May, Vol. 10, Issue 5, pp. 260, 278–279.

Zhang H, Huang J
Affiliated Hospital of Guangzhou College of Traditional Chinese Medicine, Zhanjiang, Guangdong

Objective

To ascertain the efficacy of Traditional Chinese Medicine upon minimal brain dysfunction.

Method

One hundred patients with minimal brain dysfunction (MBD) were divided randomly into a Traditional Chinese Medicine [TCM] and a Western medicine [WM] group. The age ranged from 7 to 14.2 years, and the average age was 10.5 years. The TCM group (80 cases) were treated with herbs to subdue Liver-Yang and tonifying the Spleen. The herbs used were as follows.

- **Chai Hu** *Radix Bupleuri*
- **Huang Qin** *Radix Scutellariae*
- **Huang Qi** *Radix Astragali*
- **Dang Shen** *Radix Codonopsis*
- **Nu Zhen Zi** *Fructus Ligustri lucidi*
- **Zhu Ye** *Folium Phyllostachys nigrae*

The WM group (20 cases) were treated with Ritalin [methylphenidate] 5–15 mg twice daily. One course of treatment lasted 1 month, and effects were evaluated after one to three courses of treatment.

Results

In the TCM group, 23 cases were cured (clinical symptoms and signs disappeared, their IQ was increased by 10 points, the electroencephalogram became normal and there was no recurrence during the first 6 months after recovery); 46 cases were improved (clinical symptom and signs markedly improved, their IQ increased by 4 units and electroencephalogram improved); in 11 cases treatment was ineffective. The effective rate was 86.25%.

In the WM group, 6 cases were cured, 12 cases were improved and in 2 cases treatment was ineffective, the clinical effective rate being 90.0%. Therefore, there was no significant difference between the two groups in this study; however, the side-effects of the TCM group were less than the WM group, and the TCM group had more beneficial effects in improving intelligence, enuresis and the dark rings under the eyes.

Conclusion

Traditional Chinese Medicine proved as effective as Western medicine in the treatment of minimal brain dysfunction.

Note: At the time of some of these earlier studies, the terms "Attention Deficit Disorder (ADD)" or "Attention-Deficit/Hyperactivity Disorder (ADHD)" had not been included in the DSM. The term "Minimal Brain Dysfunction" was one of the diagnostic distinctions that we have now come to describe as ADD (DSM-III) or one of the forms of ADHD (DSM-IV)].

END NOTES

1. National Institute of Mental Health website [Accessed 2008]. http://www.nimh.nih.gov/healthinformation/adhdmenu.cfm
2. Diagnostic and Statistical Manual of Mental Disorders, 4th edn. Text revision. American Psychiatric Association, Washington, DC.
3. Consensus Development Panel 1982 Defined Diets and Childhood Hyperactivity. National Institutes of Health Consensus Development Conference Summary, Vol. 4, Number 3, 1982.
4. Wolraich M, Milich R, Stumbo P, Schultz F 1985 The effects of sucrose ingestion on the behavior of hyperactive boys. Pediatrics 106: 657–682.
5. McCann D, Barrett A, Cooper A et al. 2007 Food additives and hyperactive behaviour in 3-year-old and 8/9-year-old children in the community: a randomised, double-blinded, placebo-controlled trial. Lancet 370(9598): 1560–1567.
6. Biederman J, Faraone SV, Keenan K, Knee D, Tsuang MF 1990 Family-genetic and psychosocial risk factors in DSM-III attention deficit disorder. Journal of the American Academy of Child and Adolescent Psychiatry 29(4): 526–533.
7. Faraone SV, Biederman J 1998 Neurobiology of attention-deficit hyperactivity disorder. Biological Psychiatry 44: 951–958.
8. The MTA Cooperative Group 1999 A 14-month randomized clinical trial of treatment strategies for attention-deficit hyperactivity disorder (ADHD). Archives of General Psychiatry 56: 1073–1086.
9. Wilens TE, Faraone SV, Biederman J, Gunawardene S 2003 Does stimulant therapy of attention-deficit/hyperactivity disorder beget later substance abuse? A meta-analytic review of the literature. Pediatrics 111(1): 179–185.
10. Silver LB 2000 Attention-deficit hyperactivity disorder in adult life. Child and Adolescent Psychiatric Clinics of North America 9(3): 511–523.
11. Wilens TE, Biederman J, Spencer TJ 2002 Attention deficit/hyperactivity disorder across the lifespan. Annual Review of Medicine 53:113–131.
12. Attention deficit disorder in adults. Harvard Mental Health Letter 2002; 19(5): 36.
13. McCann D, Barrett A, Cooper A et al. 2007 Food additives and hyperactive behaviour in 3-year-old and 8/9-year-old children in the community: a randomised, double-blinded, placebo-controlled trial. Lancet 370(9598): 1560-1567.
14. Shan Chang Hua 1990 Jing Xue Jie 经穴解 [An Explanation of the Acupuncture Points]. People's Health Publishing House, Beijing, p. 211. An *Explanation of the Acupuncture Points* was written by Yue Han Zhen and first published in 1654.
15. Cheng Bao Shu 1988 Zhen Jiu Da Ci Dian 针灸大辞典 [Great Dictionary of Acupuncture]. Beijing Science Publishing House, Beijing, p. 11.
16. Jiao Shun Fa 1987 Zhong Guo Zhen Jiu Qiu Zhen 中国针灸学求真 [An Enquiry into Chinese Acupuncture]. Shanxi Science Publishing House, p. 52.
17. Dr Zhang Ming Jiu, personal communication, Nanjing 1982.
18. Professor Wang Ling Ling, personal communication, October 2007.
19. Dr Shen Can Ruo, personal communication, October 2007.
20. Dr Tao Kun, personal communication, October 2007.

CHAPTER 22

EPILOGUE: THE ROLE OF CHINESE MEDICINE IN DISORDERS OF THE PSYCHE

I was very young (28) when I started practicing acupuncture and I did not know anything about counseling or psychotherapy. In those early times, colleges of Chinese medicine did not teach "patient skills" as they do now. I was therefore left to wrestle on my own with my patients' mental-emotional problems in the clinic. I soon came to realize that most of my patients had some kind of emotional suffering, whether this was the main cause of their physical problems or not.

As I was left to deal with such emotional suffering on my own, I coped as best as I could with my patients' emotional and mental suffering. For example, if a patient starts to cry a few minutes after the needles have been inserted (something that happened relatively frequently in my clinic and that, incidentally, I have never seen happen in China), what is the practitioner supposed to do? Should I ignore it and pretend it was not happening? Should I comfort the patient? How much physical contact (e.g. stroking their head) would be deemed to be professional? Should I delve into their deep emotional life or not? Was it my role to do so? Having no training in counseling or psychotherapy, was I qualified to do so? And, if the patient did unburden his or her tribulations, how was I supposed to use such information? If a patient is suffering from grief and sadness, should the treatment be changed according to whether the sadness is caused by a loss or by general depression? What if the sadness really hides guilt? How would the treatment differ then?

In the course of studying Chinese medicine, I had read many books on Daoism and Buddhism and also practiced Buddhism and Buddhist meditation. I asked myself, how should I apply these teachings to the treatment of my patients' emotional suffering? I soon found that when a patient is overwhelmed by an emotion, it does not really work trying to convince them that their emotional suffering is all an illusion because there really is no self (*anatta*, Sanskrit for "no self"), this being merely a flux of the five *skandhas*.

Incidentally, some of my patients did find it useful when I discussed the Buddhist view of the mind and emotions, but not when, for example, the husband had left the family home and the patient was right in the middle of a huge emotional upheaval. I had long discussions with interested patients on the subject of Daoism and Buddhism many times.

Another question that often came up is this: if a patient comes to us for a relatively trivial problem such as tenosynovitis of the wrist and, during one of the sessions, it comes to the fore that she suffered sexual abuse in her teenage years, how do we use this information? Should we treat her *Shen*? Is it appropriate to do so anyway or should we do so only if she asks us? Is it invasive to want to treat the *Shen* when a patient comes merely for a superficial tendino-muscular problem? Should we treat the *Shen* without even telling them or should we tell them?

Based on my experience, my answer to the above question now is that, yes, it is always relevant to treat the *Shen* when the patient has a history of deep emotional suffering from the past. My approach would be flexible and depend entirely on the patient's disposition. I always respect the patient's wish; some may want to unburden themselves of their past emotional history and seek treatment for it, some may not want to do so. In this latter case, I would always respect that and not force the issue.

However, that is not to say that I would not keep that into account in my treatment. In the above example, I would obviously treat the presenting problem of tenosynovitis but I would also very gently nourish the *Shen*, perhaps simply with HE-7 Shenmen and Ren-15 Jiuwei. My experience is that nourishing the *Shen* when this is wounded by past emotional suffering *always* helps, whatever problem the patient may present with. Incidentally, HE-7 Shenmen also has an analgesic effect.

So I was left to cope as best as I could with my own home-spun counseling skills. Today, after practicing for 35 years, I still do not have the answer to some of the above questions, although I like to think that I have a lot more experience in knowing how to deal with the emotional crises of my patients. However, such knowledge, I must say, has not derived from Chinese medicine but from my readings about Freud, Jung (especially), psychotherapy and counseling in general, and many other books on the emotions in Western philosophy and in modern neurophysiology.

My new skills, of course, also simply derived from experience and from taking a pragmatic and flexible approach in dealing with patients' emotional upheavals. I soon came to realize that there is no "standard" way of dealing with their crises and we need to adapt our approach according to the patient's personality (and often also sex, as in general women are much better than men at communicating their emotional suffering).

What to do if a patient started telling me about some childhood experiences that were at the root of their suffering? My training in Chinese medicine did not prepare me for that and had nothing to offer me; I think that the situation is the same now, even after much more extensive reading of Chinese books on the subject of mental-emotional problems.

As I have said many times throughout the preceding chapters, in my opinion the Chinese medicine view of emotions is Confucian and the concept of self in Confucianism is completely different from that in the West. As a result, emotions are seen as objective disharmonies of Qi, almost disconnected from the self, that need to be re-balanced purely for the sake of social harmony; emotions are social, ethical issues rather than the intense, personal passions of the Western individual, autonomous, inward-looking self. In Chinese medicine, "rectifying" the disharmonies created by the emotions is an ethical rather than a psychological issue. For this reason, Chinese medicine has nothing to say about how our childhood experiences are the root of our emotions, complexes and projections later on in life.

So what has Chinese medicine got to offer in the treatment of Westerners' emotional suffering? As we all know, a lot. Even though its view of emotions is tainted by Confucianism and the concept of self is completely different from that of the West, Chinese medicine has a deep, healing influence on the mind and the spirit when these are affected by emotional suffering.

Chinese medicine relieves emotional suffering in many ways. The Chinese medicine view of emotions (seen as causes of disease) as disharmonies of Qi that are simultaneously and inextricably physical, emotional and mental is brilliant.

First, by simply moving Qi, it releases the stagnation that is often present in emotional suffering. Second, by moving Qi, Chinese medicine helps the patient to express his or her emotions when these are suppressed. Third, and most importantly, acupuncture and herbs simply "nourish" the *Shen* (intended both as Mind of the Heart and as Spirit); irrespective of the pathology and patterns, acupuncture and herbs simply nurture the *Shen* and so have a deep calming effect on the patient. Fourth, by nourishing the *Shen*, acupuncture and herbs seem to make the patient more sensitive and attuned to his or her emotions.

A question that I have posed myself countless times is the respective role of Chinese medicine and psychotherapy in the treatment of mental-emotional suffering. How far can Chinese medicine go when a patient has a complex history of emotional suffering stretching back many years? What are the boundaries of Chinese medicine, if any? How far should we attempt to counsel the patient if we have no training in psychotherapy?

My ideas on these questions have been taking shape over the years. I definitely think that Chinese medicine does have its limitations when dealing with patients with complex emotional histories, simply because Chinese medicine does not provide a framework for interpreting the emotional suffering of patients with complex emotional histories stretching back to childhood.

Chinese medicine has nothing to say about our childhood emotional upbringing, the question of attachment, bonding and loss, our complexes, projections and defenses developed in childhood. One of the reasons for this is simply, as I have now stated several times, that the Confucian concept of self does not envisage an individual, autonomous, inward-looking center of consciousness formed during our childhood experiences and influencing our adult life.

Therefore, when I treat a patient with a complex and far-stretching emotional history, I first of all gently suggest that they might benefit from seeing a psychotherapist. This has to be done with great tact as, in some countries, this suggestion may almost be offensive. Whenever one of my patients was seeing a psychotherapist concurrently with the Chinese medicine treatment, I always found that a great "relief"; I could get on with my job of interpreting and treating my patient's emotional suffering from a Chinese point of view in the safe knowledge that my patient's deeper emotional issues were being explored with the psychotherapist.

However, that did not mean that I would simply stop talking to the patient about their emotional issues and simply administer my Chinese treatment. When I treat a patient suffering from emotional turmoil, in my mind I tend to wear "two hats": one is the Chinese medicine hat, the other the psychotherapist hat (although, I hasten to add, I am not qualified as a therapist). In particular, I am attracted to Jungian psychology as I personally find it the one that offers the most enlightening explanation of the human psyche. When I say that I wear the "psychotherapist hat", I do not mean that I counsel the patient as a psychotherapist but that I try to interpret their emotional suffering in terms of Jungian psychotherapy to gain an understanding of their situation.

The tricky and interesting question is: can the two be integrated and, if so, how? In other words, if we think (from a Jungian perspective) that a woman patient may be dominated by her negative *animus*, how does that fit in Chinese medicine? Is there a Chinese medicine interpretation (and therefore treatment) of it? I believe there could be, but these questions can only be answered by the accumulated experience of many practitioners over several generations.

I am beginning to formulate my own embryonic ideas and, going back to the above example, I, for example, think that the Ethereal Soul is similar to the *anima* while the *animus* is the Mind (*Shen* of the Heart) and Intellect (*Yi* of the Spleen). Therefore, when a woman is possessed by her negative *animus*, the Ethereal Soul is being hindered and the Mind and Intellect are working in a negative rather than a positive way. Therefore, treating the Liver (for the Ethereal Soul), the Heart (for the Mind) and the Spleen (for the Intellect) might help a woman to overcome her negative *animus* and bring forth the positive qualities of the Mind and Intellect.

This is, I admit, quite speculative, but my experience seems to confirm the above. Is this a replacement of psychotherapy? Most definitely not! We can only truly overcome our mental-emotional suffering by actively engaging our mind in understanding our unconscious drives; it cannot be done for us. Thus, I have never seen Chinese medicine as a replacement for psychotherapy.

Indeed, the combination of Chinese medicine and psychotherapy is an excellent one. The two work in unison with each other and Chinese medicine can shorten the course of psychotherapy. I have noticed this many times in practice. My patients who were undergoing psychotherapy regularly reported that, after receiving Chinese medicine, they had many clear insights that made them progress in their psychotherapeutic journey much faster than would have otherwise been the case.

An interesting passage by Xu Chun Fu (1570) discusses the combination of herbal treatment by a doctor with incantations by a shaman. He said that a pre-existing weakness in the person's Qi made an attack by an evil spirit possible and he advocated combining herbal therapy with incantations by a shaman in a very interesting passage which was quoted in the Preface. His advocating a combination of the methods of the herbalist and shaman is significant; it is tempting to substitute "psychotherapist" for "exorcist" and infer that Xu Chun Fu advocated combining a physical therapy such as herbal medicine with psychotherapy.

This is not to say that every patient should undergo psychotherapy. If the patient is not prepared to undergo psychotherapy, Chinese medicine still helps greatly by alleviating emotional suffering. It also creates a space where Qi is flowing, the Mind (*Shen*) and Ethereal Soul (*Hun*) are more coordinated in their activities, the Corporeal Soul (*Po*) is animating the body better and the Will-Power (*Zhi*) is strong.

For this reason, I have changed my approach to the treatment of mental-emotional suffering somewhat in the past 10 years. Over the years, I have come to think that, although treating according to patterns is essential, simply treating the Mind, Ethereal Soul, Corporeal Soul, Intellect and Will-Power can produce deep psychological changes.

In other words, although I always diagnose the patterns, I also diagnose in the general terms of the pathology of the Mind (*Shen*), Ethereal Soul (*Hun*), Corporeal Soul (*Po*), Intellect (*Yi*) or Will-Power (*Zhi*). I find that when these five *shens* are "nourished" in a broad sense, it brings about deep mental-emotional changes, irrespective of the patterns. This applies especially to acupuncture. I tend to use acupuncture to "nourish" the five *shens* while I tend to use herbal medicine to treat the patterns.

For example, irrespective of the patterns involved, I see depression as a manifestation of an insufficient movement of the Ethereal Soul, which, itself, may be due to an excessive control of the Mind over it. If the movement of the Ethereal Soul is deficient by itself, I then treat the Liver and Gall-Bladder; if the movement of the Ethereal Soul is insufficient due to over-control by the Mind, then I treat the Liver, Gall-Bladder and Heart.

Conversely, if the person is slightly manic, it is due to an excessive movement of the Ethereal Soul, irrespective of the pattern and I therefore treat the Liver. In autism, there is also an insufficient movement of the Ethereal Soul and a wounding of the Mind; I therefore treat Liver and Heart. Conversely, in ADHD, there is an excessive movement of the Ethereal Soul, a lack of control of the Mind and a deficiency of the Intellect; I therefore treat the Liver, Heart and Spleen.

I use the term "nourishing" the *Shen* not necessarily in the specific sense of tonifying (as a treatment method) but simply using acupuncture to affect the Mind, Ethereal Soul, Corporeal Soul, Intellect and Will-Power. For example, in this sense, HE-7 Shenmen will "nourish" the Mind, even though, strictly from a pattern point of view, it may drain Heart-Fire or nourish Heart-Blood. In both patterns, this point will "nourish" the Mind.

As I explained in the Preface, in the last 10 years I have been absorbed by the study of Confucian and Neo-Confucian philosophy to explore its influence on Chinese medicine. My conclusion is that it had a profound influence on Chinese medicine and especially on Chinese medicine's view of the emotions. As I have said in the Preface, the Confucian concept of self is family- and society-determined and is totally different from the Western concept of self. Also, all three philosophies of China, i.e. Daoism, Buddhism and Confucianism, see emotions as factors that cloud our mind.

Interestingly, as Western practitioners, although we have studied Chinese medicine, when faced with a patient in deep emotional turmoil we turn to our Western concept of self and not to a Confucian one. If we have a patient crying his or her heart out, we do not tell them that emotions "obscure our human nature" (Confucianism) and should be avoided, or that emotions distract us from following the *Dao* (Daoism), or that emotions are an illusion because the self really does not exist (Buddhism).

We do not do this but we tell the patient that it is normal to feel such emotions, that it is good to manifest them, that manifesting them may be cathartic, that such emotions are part of our human nature. We therefore instinctively counsel the patient according to our Western, not Confucian, concept of self.

Another important question that always comes up in the treatment of mental-emotional suffering is the integration of our treatment with Western pharmaceutical treatment. Generally speaking, in spite of the great advances in the pharmacological approach to emotional and mental suffering, I personally consider the neurotransmitter approach to treatment essentially very crude.

Indeed, the use of neurotransmitters (e.g. serotonin and noradrenaline) in the treatment of depression is now at least 30 if not 40 years old. It therefore lags behind the exciting advances made in neurophysiology in the last 10–15 years with the use of PET and fMRI imaging.

Neurotransmitters are the symptoms rather than the cause of a mental-emotional imbalance. Modern neurophysiology bears this out and a great many exciting new discoveries are being made every week with the use of PET and fMRI scans of the brain.

As discussed in Chapter 14, the emotional centers of the brain work in a very complex way and interact at every step with the cortical centers. To think that we can influence our mental-emotional life simply by manipulating a neurotransmitter is crude and mechanical.

However, having said that, there are situations when the use of a short course of antidepressants in very severe depression is useful to break the vicious cycle and spiral of depression the patient is in. Incidentally, I have never noticed any negative interaction between Chinese herbs and the use of antidepressants, and the two can definitely be combined – and the same for acupuncture.

In the last 10 years I have pursued three lines of research that have given me a different perspective of Chinese medicine and specifically of how Chinese medicine sees the emotions. These lines of research were the emotions in Western philosophy, the philosophy of Neo-Confucianism and the emotions in modern neurophysiology. I was amazed to discover that practically all Western philosophers tackled the question of emotions from Plato right down to Sartre.

I soon discovered that the ancient Greeks already had a very sophisticated theory of emotions, compared to which the Chinese medicine view of emotions is rather crude. For example, Plato conceived of a three-part soul with a rational soul (*logistikon*), a high-spirited soul (*thumoeides*) and an appetitive soul (*epi-*

thumetikon). This view inspired Freud's concept of the id. The ancient Stoics devised very sophisticated techniques to overcome emotions; these are the forerunners of our modern cognitive behavioral therapy. The Stoics even conceived of music therapy that would affect children from an early age to free them from emotional turmoil later on in life.

My study of emotions in Western philosophy and in modern neurophysiology made me realize that emotions are far more than just the causes of disease envisaged by Chinese medicine. Far from obscuring our human nature, as the Neo-Confucianists tell us, they define our human nature and give meaning to our life.

APPENDIX 1

HERBAL PRESCRIPTIONS

AN SHEN DING ZHI WAN

Calming the Mind and Settling the Spirit Pill
Ren Shen *Radix Ginseng* 9 g
Fu Ling *Poria* 12 g
Fu Shen *Sclerotium Poriae cocos pararadicis* 9 g
Long Chi *Fossilia Dentis Mastodi* 15 g
Yuan Zhi *Radix Polygalae* 6 g
Shi Chang Pu *Rhizoma Acori tatarinowii* 8 g

AN SHEN DING ZHI WAN Variation (Chapter 17, Anxiety, Heart and Gall-Bladder deficiency)

Calming the Mind and Settling the Spirit Pill Variation
Ren Shen *Radix Ginseng* 9 g
Fu Ling *Poria* 12 g
Fu Shen *Sclerotium Poriae cocos pararadicis* 9 g
Long Chi *Fossilia Dentis Mastodi* 15 g
Yuan Zhi *Radix Polygalae* 6 g
Shi Chang Pu *Rhizoma Acori tatarinowii* 8 g
Ci Shi *Magnetitum* 15 g
Ho Po *Succinum* 9 g
Suan Zao Ren *Semen Ziziphi spinosae* 6 g
Bai Zi Ren *Semen Platycladi* 9 g

BAI HE DI HUANG TANG

Lilium-Rehmannia Decoction
Bai He *Semen Platycladi* 9 g
Sheng Di Huang *Radix Rehmanniae* 9 g
Mai Men Dong *Radix Ophiopogonis* 6 g
Wu Wei Zi *Fructus Schisandrae* 6 g
Gan Cao *Radix Glycyrrhizae uralensis* 3 g

BAI HE GU JIN TANG

Lilium Consolidating Metal Decoction
Bai He *Bulbus Lilii* 15 g
Mai Men Dong *Radix Ophiopogonis* 9 g
Xuan Shen *Radix Scrophulariae* 9 g
Sheng Di Huang *Radix Rehmanniae* 9 g
Shu Di Huang *Radix Rehmanniae preparata* 9 g
Dang Gui *Radix Angelicae sinensis* 6 g
Bai Shao *Radix Paeoniae alba* 9 g
Jie Geng *Radix Platycodi* 6 g
Chuan Bei Mu *Bulbus Fritillariae cirrhosae* 6 g
Gan Cao *Radix Glycyrrhizae uralensis* 3 g

BAI HE GU JIN TANG Variation (Chapter 17, Anxiety, Lung- and Heart-Yin deficiency)

Lilium Consolidating Metal Decoction Variation
Bai He *Bulbus Lilii* 15 g
Mai Men Dong *Radix Ophiopogonis* 9 g
Sheng Di Huang *Radix Rehmanniae* 9 g
Dang Gui *Radix Angelicae sinensis* 6 g
Bai Shao *Radix Paeoniae alba* 9 g
Jie Geng *Radix Platycodi* 6 g
Chuan Bei Mu *Bulbus Fritillariae cirrhosae* 6 g
Suan Zao Ren *Semen Ziziphi spinosae* 6 g
Bai Zi Ren *Semen Platycladi* 6 g
Wu Wei Zi *Fructus Schisandrae* 6 g
Zhi Mu *Radix Anemarrhenae* 6 g
Gan Cao *Radix Glycyrrhizae uralensis* 3 g

BAI HE ZHI MU TANG

Lilium-Anemarrhena Decoction
Bai He *Bulbus Lilii* 9 g
Zhi Mu *Rhizoma Anemarrhenae* 6 g

BAI ZI YANG XIN WAN

Platycladum Nourishing the Heart Pill
Bai Zi Ren *Semen Platycladi* 120 g
Fu Shen *Sclerotium Poriae cocos pararadicis* 30 g
Gou Qi Zi *Fructus Lycii chinensis* 90 g

Shu Di Huang *Radix Rehmanniae preparata* 60 g
Dang Gui *Radix Angelicae sinensis* 30 g
Xuan Shen *Radix Scrophulariae* 60 g
Mai Men Dong *Radix Ophiopogonis* 30 g
Shi Chang Pu *Rhizoma Acori tatarinowii* 30 g
Gan Cao *Radix Glycyrrhizae uralensis* 15 g

BAN XIA HOU PO TANG

Pinellia-Magnolia Decoction
Ban Xia *Rhizoma Pinelliae preparatum* 12 g
Hou Po *Cortex Magnoliae officinalis* 9 g
Zi Su Ye *Folium Perillae* 6 g
Fu Ling *Poria* 12 g
Sheng Jiang *Rhizoma Zingiberis recens* 9 g

BAN XIA SHU MI TANG

Pinellia-Sorghum Decoction
Ban Xia *Rhizoma Pinelliae preparatum* 10 g
Fu Ling *Poria* 10 g
Shan Zha *Fructus Crataegi* 6 g
Mai Ya *Fructus Hordei germinatus* 6 g
Shen Qu *Massa medicata fermentata* 6 g
Cang Zhu *Rhizoma Atractylodis* 6 g
Shan Yao *Rhizoma Dioscoreae* 6 g
Shu Mi *Sorghum* husks 5 g

BAO NAO NING JIAO NANG

Preserving the Brain's Tranquillity Capsule
Dan Nan Xing *Rhizoma Arisaematis preparatum* 6 g
Hu Po *Succinum* 6 g
Fu Shen *Sclerotium Poriae cocos pararadicis* 6 g
Shi Chang Pu *Rhizoma Acori tatarinowii* 6 g
Huang Qin *Radix Scutellariae* 6 g
Dang Shen *Radix Codonopsis* 6 g

BU FEI TANG

Tonifying the Lungs Decoction
Ren Shen *Radix Ginseng* 9 g
Huang Qi *Radix Astragali* 12 g
Shu Di Huang *Radix Rehmanniae preparata* 12 g
Wu Wei Zi *Fructus Schisandrae* 6 g
Zi Wan *Radix Asteris* 9 g
Sang Bai Pi *Cortex Mori* 6 g

BU FEI TANG Variation (Chapter 17, Anxiety, Lung- and Heart-Qi deficiency)

Tonifying the Lungs Decoction Variation
Ren Shen *Radix Ginseng* 9 g
Huang Qi *Radix Astragali* 12 g
Shu Di Huang *Radix Rehmanniae preparata* 12 g
Wu Wei Zi *Fructus Schisandrae* 6 g
Sang Bai Pi *Cortex Mori* 6 g
Bai He *Bulbus Lilii* 6 g
Bai Zi Ren *Semen Platycladi* 6 g
Suan Zao Ren *Semen Ziziphi spinosae* 6 g

BU FEI TANG Variation (Chapter 18, Insomnia, Appendix 1 Excessive dreaming, Heart- and Lung-Qi deficiency)

Tonifying the Lungs Decoction Variation
Dang Shen *Radix Codonopsis* 15 g
Huang Qi *Radix Astragali* 15 g
Shu Di Huang *Radix Rehmanniae preparata* 10 g
Wu Wei Zi *Fructus Schisandrae* 10 g
Zi Wan *Radix Asteris* 9 g
Sang Bai Pi *Cortex Mori* 6 g
Fu Shen *Sclerotium Poriae cocos pararadicis* 10 g
Suan Zao Ren *Semen Ziziphi spinosae* 10 g
Long Chi *Fossilia Dentis Mastodi* 10 g
Hu Po *Succinum* 3 g

BU SUI RONG NAO TANG

Tonifying the Marrow and Nourishing the Brain Decoction
Shu Di Huang *Radix Rehmanniae preparata* 9 g
Dang Gui *Radix Angelicae sinensis* 6 g
Bai Shao *Radix Paeoniae alba* 9 g
Nu Zhen Zi *Fructus Ligustri lucidi* 6 g
Gou Qi Zi *Fructus Lycii chinensis* 6 g
Wu Wei Zi *Fructus Schisandrae* 6 g
Sang Shen *Fructus Mori* 6 g

BU XIN DAN

Tonifying the Heart Pill
Sheng Di Huang *Radix Rehmanniae* 6 g
Wu Wei Zi *Fructus Schisandrae* 6 g
Dang Gui *Radix Angelicae sinensis* 6 g
Tian Men Dong *Radix Asparagi* 6 g
Mai Men Dong *Radix Ophiopogonis* 6 g
Bai Zi Ren *Semen Platycladi* 6 g

Suan Zao Ren *Semen Ziziphi spinosae* 6 g
Dang Shen *Radix Codonopsis* 6 g
Xuan Shen *Radix Scrophulariae* 6 g
Dan Shen *Radix Salviae miltiorrhizae* 6 g
Fu Ling *Poria* 6 g
Yuan Zhi *Radix Polygalae* 6 g
Jie Geng *Radix Platycodi* 3 g

BU XIN DAN Variation (Chapter 16, Depression, Heart and Spleen deficiency)

Tonifying the Heart Pill Variation
Sheng Di Huang *Radix Rehmanniae* 6 g
Wu Wei Zi *Fructus Schisandrae* 6 g
Dang Gui *Radix Angelicae sinensis* 6 g
Tian Men Dong *Radix Asparagi* 6 g
Mai Men Dong *Radix Ophiopogonis* 6 g
Bai Zi Ren *Semen Platycladi* 6 g
Suan Zao Ren *Semen Ziziphi spinosae* 6 g
Dang Shen *Radix Codonopsis* 6 g
Xuan Shen *Radix Scrophulariae* 6 g
Dan Shen *Radix Salviae miltiorrhizae* 6 g
Fu Ling *Poria* 6 g
Yuan Zhi *Radix Polygalae* 6 g
Jie Geng *Radix Platycodi* 3 g
Shi Chang Pu *Rhizoma Acori tatarinowii* 6 g
He Huan Pi *Cortex Albiziae* 6 g

BU ZHONG YI QI TANG

Tonifying the Center and Benefiting Qi Decoction
Huang Qi *Radix Astragali* 12 g
Ren Shen *Radix Ginseng* 9 g
Bai Zhu *Rhizoma Atractylodis macrocephalae* 9 g
Dang Gui *Radix Angelicae sinensis* 6 g
Chen Pi *Pericarpium Citri reticulatae* 6 g
Sheng Ma *Rhizoma Cimicifugae* 3 g
Chai Hu *Radix Bupleuri* 3 g

BU ZHONG YI QI TANG Variation (Chapter 18, Insomnia, Appendix 2 Somnolence, Spleen deficiency)

Tonifying the Center and Benefiting Qi Decoction Variation
Huang Qi *Radix Astragali* 12 g
Ren Shen *Radix Ginseng* 9 g
Bai Zhu *Rhizoma Atractylodis macrocephalae* 9 g
Dang Gui *Radix Angelicae sinensis* 6 g
Chen Pi *Pericarpium Citri reticulatae* 6 g
Sheng Ma *Rhizoma Cimicifugae* 3 g
Chai Hu *Radix Bupleuri* 3 g
Zhi Gan Cao *Radix Glycyrrhizae uralensis preparata* 3 g
Gan Jiang *Rhizoma Zingiberis* 3 g

CANG BAI ER CHEN TANG

Gray and White Atractylodes Two Old Decoction
Cang Zhu *Rhizoma Atractylodis* 6 g
Bai Zhu *Rhizoma Atractylodis macrocephalae* 6 g
Chen Pi *Pericarpium Citri reticulatae* 4.5 g
Ban Xia *Rhizoma Pinelliae preparatum* 9 g
Fu Ling *Poria* 6 g
Zhi Gan Cao *Radix Glycyrrhizae uralensis preparata* 3 g
Sheng Jiang *Rhizoma Zingiberis recens* 3 slices

CHAI HU LONG GU MU LI TANG

Bupleurum-Mastodi Ossis fossilia-Concha Ostreae Decoction
Chai Hu *Radix Bupleuri* 12 g
Huang Qin *Radix Scutellariae* 9 g
Ban Xia *Rhizoma Pinelliae preparatum* 9 g
Ren Shen *Radix Ginseng* 6 g
Zhi Gan Cao *Radix Glycyrrhizae uralensis preparata* 5 g
Sheng Jiang *Rhizoma Zingiberis recens* 9 g
Da Zao *Fructus Jujubae* 4 dates
Gui Zhi *Ramulus Cinnamomi cassiae* 4.5 g
Fu Ling *Poria* 4.5 g
Long Gu *Mastodi Ossis fossilia* 4.5 g
Long Gu Long Gu *Concha Ostreae* 4.5 g
Da Huang *Radix et Rhizoma Rhei* 6 g
Qian Dan *Minium* 4.5 g

CHAI HU SHU GAN TANG

Bupleurum Soothing the Liver Decoction
Chai Hu *Radix Bupleuri* 6 g
Bai Shao *Radix Paeoniae alba* 4.5 g
Zhi Ke *Fructus Aurantii* 4.5 g
Zhi Gan Cao *Radix Glycyrrhizae uralensis preparata* 1.5 g
Chen Pi *Pericarpium Citri reticulatae* 6 g
Xiang Fu *Rhizoma Cyperi* 4.5 g
Chuan Xiong *Rhizoma Chuanxiong* 4.5 g

CHAI HU SHU GAN TANG Variation (Chapter 16, Depression, Liver-Qi stagnation)

Bupleurum Soothing the Liver Decoction Variation
Chai Hu *Radix Bupleuri* 6 g
Bai Shao *Radix Paeoniae alba* 4.5 g
Zhi Ke *Fructus Aurantii* 4.5 g
Zhi Gan Cao *Radix Glycyrrhizae uralensis preparata* 1.5 g
Chen Pi *Pericarpium Citri reticulatae* 6 g
Xiang Fu *Rhizoma Cyperi* 4.5 g
Chuan Xiong *Rhizoma Chuanxiong* 4.5 g
Yu Jin *Radix Curcumae* 6 g
Qing Pi *Pericarpium Citri reticulatae viride* 6 g

DA BU YIN WAN

Great Tonifying Yin Pill
Zhi Mu *Radix Anemarrhenae* 9 g
Huang Bo *Cortex Phellodendri* 9 g
Shu Di Huang *Radix Rehmanniae preparata* 12 g
Gui Ban *Plastrum Testudinis* 9 g
Pigs' marrow 20 g

DA BU YUAN JIAN

Great Tonifying the Original [Qi] *Decoction*
Shu Di Huang *Radix Rehmanniae preparata* 15 g
Shan Yao *Rhizoma Dioscoreae* 12 g
Shan Zhu Yu *Fructus Corni* 9 g
Gou Qi Zi *Fructus Lycii chinensis* 12 g
Dang Gui *Radix Angelicae sinensis* 9 g
Ren Shen *Radix Ginseng* 12 g
Du Zhong *Cortex Eucommiae ulmoidis* 9 g
Zhi Gan Cao *Radix Glycyrrhizae uralensis preparata* 6 g

DA CHENG QI TANG

Great Conducting Qi Decoction
Da Huang *Radix et Rhizoma Rhei* 12 g
Mang Xiao *Natrii Sulfas* 9 g
Hou Po *Cortex Magnoliae officinalis* 15 g
Zhi Shi *Fructus Aurantii immaturus* 12 g

DA CHENG QI TANG Variation (Chapter 19, Bipolar Disorder, *Kuang*, Fire in Bright Yang)

Great Conducting Qi Decoction Variation
Da Huang *Radix et Rhizoma Rhei* 15 g
Mang Xiao *Natrii Sulfas* 10 g
Meng Shi *Lapis Chloriti seu Micae* 10 g
Zhi Shi *Fructus Aurantii immaturus* 10 g
Zao Jiao *Spina Gleditsiae sinensis* 3 g
Zhu Dan Ye (pig's bile) 3 g
Vinegar 5 g

DAN ZHI XIAO YAO SAN

Moutan-Gardenia Free and Easy Wanderer Powder
Bo He *Herba Menthae haplocalycis* 3 g
Chai Hu *Radix Bupleuri* 9 g
Dang Gui *Radix Angelicae sinensis* 9 g
Bai Shao *Radix Paeoniae alba* 12 g
Bai Zhu *Rhizoma Atractylodis macrocephalae* 9 g
Fu Ling *Poria* 15 g
Gan Cao *Radix Glycyrrhizae uralensis* 6 g
Sheng Jiang *Rhizoma Zingiberis recens* 3 slices
Mu Dan Pi *Cortex Moutan* 6 g
Shan Zhi Zi *Fructus Gardeniae* 6 g

DANG GUI LONG HUI WAN

Angelica-Gentiana-Aloe Pill
Dang Gui *Radix Angelicae sinensis* 30 g
Long Dan Cao *Radix Gentianae* 15 g
Lu Hui *Aloe* 15 g
Shan Zhi Zi *Fructus Gardeniae* 6 g
Huang Lian *Rhizoma Coptidis* 4 g
Huang Bo *Cortex Phellodendri* 6 g
Huang Qin *Radix Scutellariae* 6 g
Da Huang *Radix et Rhizoma Rhei* 9 g
Mu Xiang *Radix Aucklandiae* 5 g
She Xiang *Moschus* 1.5 g
Qing Dai *Indigo naturalis* 6 g

DAO CHI SAN

Eliminating Redness Powder
Sheng Di Huang *Radix Rehmanniae* 15 g
Mu Tong *Caulis Akebiae trifoliatae* 3 g
Gan Cao *Radix Glycyrrhizae uralensis* 6 g
Zhu Ye *Folium Phyllostachys nigrae* 3 g

DAO CHI SAN Variation (Chapter 19, Bipolar disorder, *Dian*, Knotted Heat in the Heart channel)

Eliminating Redness Powder Variation
Huang Lian *Rhizoma Coptidis* 10 g

Mu Tong *Caulis Akebiae trifoliatae* 10 g
Sheng Di Huang *Radix Rehmanniae* 10 g
Gan Cao *Radix Glycyrrhizae uralensis* 5 g
Da Huang *Radix et Rhizoma Rhei* 10 g
Shi Gao *Gypsum fibrosum* 30 g
Fu Shen *Sclerotium Poriae cocos pararadicis* 10 g
He Huan Pi *Flos Albiziae* 15 g

DAO TAN TANG

Conducting Phlegm Decoction
Ban Xia *Rhizoma Pinelliae preparatum* 6 g
Dan Nan Xing *Rhizoma Arisaematis preparatum* 3 g
Zhi Shi *Fructus Aurantii immaturus* 3 g
Fu Ling *Poria* 3 g
Chen Pi *Pericarpium Citri reticulatae* 3 g
Zhi Gan Cao *Radix Glycyrrhizae uralensis preparata* 2 g
Sheng Jiang *Rhizoma Zingiberis recens* 3 g

DI PO TANG

Earth Corporeal Soul Decoction
Mai Men Dong *Radix Ophiopogonis* 9 g
Bai Shao *Radix Paeoniae alba* 9 g
Wu Wei Zi *Fructus Schisandrae* 3 g
Xuan Shen *Radix Scrophulariae* 9 g
Mu Li *Concha Ostreae* 9 g
Ban Xia *Rhizoma Pinelliae preparatum* 9 g
Gan Cao *Radix Glycyrrhizae uralensis* 3 g

DI TAN TANG

Washing Away Phlegm Decoction
Ban Xia *Rhizoma Pinelliae preparatum* 8 g
Dan Nan Xing *Rhizoma Arisaematis preparatum* 8 g
Zhu Ru *Caulis Bambusae in Taeniam* 2 g
Chen Pi *Pericarpium Citri reticulatae* 6 g
Fu Ling *Poria* 6 g
Zhi Shi *Fructus Aurantii immaturus* 6 g
Shi Chang Pu *Rhizoma Acori tatarinowii* 3 g
Ren Shen (**Dang Shen**) *Radix Ginseng* (*Radix Codonopsis*) 3 g
Zhi Gan Cao *Radix Glycyrrhizae uralensis preparata* 2 g
Sheng Jiang *Rhizoma Zingiberis recens* 3 slices
Da Zao *Fructus Jujubae* 3 dates

DIAN KUANG MENG XING TANG

Manic-Depression Regaining Consciousness after a Dream Decoction
Tao Ren *Semen Persicae* 6 g
Chai Hu *Radix Bupleuri* 6 g
Xiang Fu *Rhizoma Cyperi* 9 g
Mu Tong *Caulis Akebiae trifoliatae* 3 g
Chi Shao *Radix Paeoniae rubra* 6 g
Ban Xia *Rhizoma Pinelliae preparatum* 9 g
Da Fu Pi *Pericarpium Arecae* 6 g
Qing Pi *Pericarpium Citri reticulatae viride* 6 g
Chen Pi *Pericarpium Citri reticulatae* 6 g
Sang Bai Pi *Cortex Mori* 6 g
Su Zi *Fructus Perillae* 6 g
Gan Cao *Radix Glycyrrhizae uralensis* 3 g

DING KUANG ZHU YU TANG

Calming Mania and Eliminating Stasis Decoction
Dan Shen *Radix Salviae milthiorrizae* 9 g
Chi Shao *Radix Paeoniae rubra* 6 g
Tao Ren *Semen Persicae* 6 g
Hong Hua *Flos Carthami tinctorii* 6 g
Chai Hu *Radix Bupleuri* 6 g
Xiang Fu *Rhizoma Cyperi* 6 g
Shi Chang Pu *Rhizoma Acori tatarinowii* 6 g
Yu Jin *Radix Curcumae* 6 g
Hu Po *Succinum* 6 g
Da Huang *Radix et Rhizoma Rhei* 6 g
Zhi Gan Cao *Radix Glycyrrhizae uralensis preparata* 3 g

DING ZHI WAN

Settling the Spirit Pill
Ren Shen *Radix Ginseng* 9 g
Fu Ling *Poria* 6 g
Shi Chang Pu *Rhizoma Acori tatarinowii* 6 g
Yuan Zhi *Radix Polygalae* 6 g

DING ZHI WAN Variation (Chapter 18, Insomnia, Heart and Gall-Bladder deficiency)

Settling the Spirit Pill Variation
Dang Shen *Radix Codonopsis* 10 g
Fu Ling *Poria* 10 g
Fu Shen *Sclerotium Poriae cocos pararadicis* 10 g

Shi Chang Pu *Rhizoma Acori tatarinowii* 9 g
Yuan Zhi *Radix Polygalae* 6 g
Suan Zao Ren *Semen Ziziphi spinosae* 15 g

ER CHEN TANG

Two Old Decoction
Ban Xia *Rhizoma Pinelliae preparatum* 15 g
Chen Pi *Pericarpium Citri reticulatae* 15 g
Fu Ling *Poria* 9 g
Zhi Gan Cao *Radix Glycyrrhizae uralensis preparata* 5 g
Sheng Jiang *Rhizoma Zingiberis recens* 3 g
Wu Mei *Fructus Mume* 1 prune

ER CHEN TANG Variation (Chapter 16, Depression, Experience of Dr Li Bao Ling, Stomach and Spleen deficiency)

Two Old Decoction Variation
Ban Xia *Rhizoma Pinelliae preparatum* 15 g
Chen Pi *Pericarpium Citri reticulatae* 15 g
Fu Ling *Poria* 9 g
Zhi Gan Cao *Radix Glycyrrhizae uralensis preparata* 5 g
Sheng Jiang *Rhizoma Zingiberis recens* 3 g
Wu Mei *Fructus Mume* 1 prune
Zi Su Geng *Caulis Perillae* 4 g
Xiang Fu *Rhizoma Cyperi* 6 g
Huang Qi *Radix Astragali* 6 g
Dang Gui *Radix Angelicae sinensis* 6 g
Bai Zhu *Rhizoma Atractylodis macrocephalae* 6 g
Tian Ma *Rhizoma Gastrodiae* 6 g
Yuan Zhi *Radix Polygalae* 6 g
Shi Chang Pu *Rhizoma Acori tatarinowii* 6 g
Ye Jiao Teng *Caulis Polygoni multiflori* 6 g

ER HUANG SAN

Two Yellows Powder
Huang Bo *Cortex Phellodendri* 9 g
Huang Lian *Rhizoma Coptidis* 6 g

ER YIN JIAN

Two Yin Decoction
Sheng Di Huang *Radix Rehmanniae* 15 g
Mai Men Dong *Radix Ophiopogonis* 12 g
Suan Zao Ren *Semen Ziziphi spinosae* 9 g
Xuan Shen *Radix Scrophulariae* 6 g
Huang Lian *Rhizoma Coptidis* 3 g
Fu Ling *Poria* 9 g
Mu Tong *Caulis Akebiae trifoliatae* 3 g
Deng Xin Cao *Medulla Junci* 6 g
Gan Cao *Radix Glycyrrhizae uralensis* 3 g

ER YIN JIAN Variation (Chapter 19, Bipolar disorder, *Kuang*, Fire injuring Yin with Phlegm)

Two Yin Decoction Variation
Sheng Di Huang *Radix Rehmanniae* 10 g
Mai Men Dong *Radix Ophiopogonis* 10 g
Xuan Shen *Radix Scrophulariae* 15 g
Huang Lian *Rhizoma Coptidis* 6 g
Mu Tong *Caulis Akebiae trifoliatae* 10 g
Fu Shen *Sclerotium Poriae cocos pararadicis* 10 g
Suan Zao Ren *Semen Ziziphi spinosae* 10 g
Gan Cao *Radix Glycyrrhizae uralensis* 5 g

ER YIN JIAN Variation (Chapter 19, Bipolar disorder, *Kuang*, Yin Deficiency with Empty Heat)

Two Yin Decoction Variation
Sheng Di Huang *Radix Rehmanniae* 10 g
Mai Men Dong *Radix Ophiopogonis* 10 g
Suan Zao Ren *Semen Ziziphi spinosae* 10 g
Xuan Shen *Radix Scrophulariae* 10 g
Fu Ling *Poria* 10 g
Huang Lian *Rhizoma Coptidis* 5 g
Mu Tong *Caulis Akebiae trifoliatae* 5 g
Deng Xin Cao *Medulla Junci* 6 g
Zhu Ye *Folium Phyllostachys nigrae* 9 g
Shi Chang Pu *Rhizoma Acori tatarinowii* 9 g
Yuan Zhi *Radix Polygalae* 9 g

ER ZHI WAN

Two Solstices Pill
Nu Zhen Zi *Fructus Ligustri lucidi* 12 g
Han Lian Cao *Herba Ecliptae* 9 g

ER ZHI WAN Variation (Chapter 18, Insomnia, Liver- and Kidney-Yin deficiency)

Two Solstices Pill Variation
Nu Zhen Zi *Fructus Ligustri lucidi* 15 g

Han Lian Cao *Herba Ecliptae* 15 g
Sang Ji Sheng *Herba Taxilli* 15 g

FU SHEN TANG

Sclerotium Poriae Decoction
Fu Shen *Sclerotium Poriae cocos pararadicis* 9 g
Long Gu *Mastodi Ossis fossilia* 15 g
Gan Jiang *Rhizoma Zingiberis* 3 g
Xi Xin *Herba Asari* 1.5 g
Bai Zhu *Rhizoma Atractylodis macrocephalae* 6 g
Ren Shen *Radix Ginseng* 6 g
Yuan Zhi *Radix Polygalae* 9 g
Zhi Gan Cao *Radix Glycyrrhizae uralensis preparata* 3 g
Rou Gui *Cortex Cinnamomi* 3 g
Du Huo *Radix Angelicae pubescentis* 6 g
Suan Zao Ren *Semen Ziziphi spinosae* 9 g
Fang Feng *Radix Saposhnikoviae* 4.5 g

GAN MAI DA ZAO TANG

Glycyrrhiza-Triticum-Jujuba Decoction
Fu Xiao Mai *Fructus Tritici levis* 15 g
Gan Cao *Radix Glycyrrhizae uralensis* 9 g
Da Zao *Fructus Jujubae* 7 dates

GAN MAI DA ZAO TANG Variation (Chapter 20, Night Terrors, Shock displacing the Mind)

Glycyrrhiza-Triticum-Jujuba Decoction Variation
Fu Xiao Mai *Fructus Tritici levis* 30 g
Gan Cao *Radix Glycyrrhizae uralensis* 9 g
Da Zao *Fructus Jujubae* 7 dates
Fu Shen *Sclerotium Poriae cocos pararadicis* 6 g
Long Gu *Mastodi Ossis fossilia* 15 g
Mu Li *Concha Ostreae* 15 g
Gou Teng *Ramulus cum Uncis Uncariae* 6 g

GUI PI TANG

Tonifying the Spleen Decoction
Ren Shen *Radix Ginseng* 6 g
Huang Qi *Radix Astragali* 15 g
Bai Zhu *Rhizoma Atractylodis macrocephalae* 12 g
Dang Gui *Radix Angelicae sinensis* 6 g
Fu Shen *Sclerotium Poriae cocos pararadicis* 9 g
Suan Zao Ren *Semen Ziziphi spinosae* 9 g
Long Yan Rou *Arillus Longan* 12 g
Yuan Zhi *Radix Polygalae* 9 g
Mu Xiang *Radix Aucklandiae* 3 g
Zhi Gan Cao *Radix Glycyrrhizae uralensis preparata* 4 g
Sheng Jiang *Rhizoma Zingiberis recens* 3 slices
Hong Zao *Fructus Jujubae* 5 dates

GUI PI TANG Variation (Chapter 17, Anxiety, Heart-Blood deficiency)

Tonifying the Spleen Decoction Variation
Ren Shen *Radix Ginseng* 6 g
Huang Qi *Radix Astragali* 15 g
Bai Zhu *Rhizoma Atractylodis macrocephalae* 12 g
Dang Gui *Radix Angelicae sinensis* 6 g
Fu Shen *Sclerotium Poriae cocos pararadicis* 9 g
Suan Zao Ren *Semen Ziziphi spinosae* 9 g
Long Yan Rou *Arillus Longan* 12 g
Yuan Zhi *Radix Polygalae* 9 g
Bai Zi Ren *Semen Platycladi* 9 g
Zhi Gan Cao *Radix Glycyrrhizae uralensis preparata* 4 g
Sheng Jiang *Rhizoma Zingiberis recens* 3 slices
Hong Zao *Fructus Jujubae* 5 dates

GUI PI TANG Variation (Chapter 18, Insomnia, Appendix 1 Excessive dreaming, deficiency of Heart and Spleen)

Tonifying the Spleen Decoction Variation
Bai Zhu *Rhizoma Atractylodis macrocephalae* 10 g
Fu Shen *Sclerotium Poriae cocos pararadicis* 10 g
Huang Qi *Radix Astragali* 10 g
Long Yan Rou *Arillus Longan* 10 g
Suan Zao Ren *Semen Ziziphi spinosae* 10 g
Dang Shen *Radix Codonopsis* 10 g
Mu Xiang *Radix Aucklandiae* 5 g
Zhi Gan Cao *Radix Glycyrrhizae uralensis preparata* 6 g
Dang Gui *Radix Angelicae sinensis* 10 g
Yuan Zhi *Radix Polygalae* 6 g
Shi Chang Pu *Rhizoma Acori tatarinowii* 10 g
Hu Po *Succinum* 3 g

GUI PI TANG Variation (Chapter 20, Night Terrors, Liver- and Heart-Blood deficiency)

Tonifying the Spleen Decoction Variation
Bai Zhu *Rhizoma Atractylodis macrocephalae* 10 g
Fu Shen *Sclerotium Poriae cocos pararadicis* 10 g
Huang Qi *Radix Astragali* 10 g
Long Yan Rou *Arillus Longan* 10 g
Suan Zao Ren *Semen Ziziphi spinosae* 10 g
Dang Shen *Radix Codonopsis* 10 g
Mu Xiang *Radix Aucklandiae* 5 g
Zhi Gan Cao *Radix Glycyrrhizae uralensis preparata* 6 g
Dang Gui *Radix Angelicae sinensis* 10 g
Yuan Zhi *Radix Polygalae* 6 g
Long Gu *Mastodi Ossis fossilia* 15 g
Mu Li *Concha Ostreae* 15 g

GUI PI TANG Variation (Chapter 21, Attention Deficit Disorder, Heart- and Spleen-Blood deficiency)

Tonifying the Spleen Decoction Variation
Bai Zhu *Rhizoma Atractylodis macrocephalae* 10 g
Fu Shen *Sclerotium Poriae cocos pararadicis* 10 g
Huang Qi *Radix Astragali* 10 g
Long Yan Rou *Arillus Longan* 10 g
Suan Zao Ren *Semen Ziziphi spinosae* 10 g
Dang Shen *Radix Codonopsis* 10 g
Mu Xiang *Radix Aucklandiae* 5 g
Zhi Gan Cao *Radix Glycyrrhizae uralensis preparata* 6 g
Dang Gui *Radix Angelicae sinensis* 10 g
Yuan Zhi *Radix Polygalae* 6 g
Shi Chang Pu *Rhizoma Acori tatarinowii* 6 g
Bai Zi Ren *Semen Platycladi* 6 g

GUI PI TANG plus **GAN MAI DA ZAO TANG** Variation (Chapter 21, Attention Deficit Disorder, Heart and Spleen deficiency with Phlegm)

Tonifying the Spleen Decoction plus *Glycyrrhiza-Triticum-Jujuba Decoction* Variation
Bai Zhu *Rhizoma Atractylodis macrocephalae* 10 g
Fu Shen *Sclerotium Poriae cocos pararadicis* 10 g
Huang Qi *Radix Astragali* 10 g
Long Yan Rou *Arillus Longan* 10 g
Suan Zao Ren *Semen Ziziphi spinosae* 10 g
Dang Shen *Radix Codonopsis* 10 g
Mu Xiang *Radix Aucklandiae* 5 g
Dang Gui *Radix Angelicae sinensis* 10 g
Yuan Zhi *Radix Polygalae* 6 g
Shi Chang Pu *Rhizoma Acori tatarinowii* 6 g
Bai Zi Ren *Semen Platycladi* 6 g
Zhi Gan Cao *Radix Glycyrrhizae uralensis preparata* 9 g
Da Zao *Fructus Jujubae* 6 g
Fu Xiao Mai *Fructus Tritici levis* 12 g
Ban Xia *Rhizoma Pinelliae preparatum* 6 g
Chen Pi *Pericarpium Citri reticulatae* 3 g
Gua Lou *Fructus Trichosanthis* 6 g
Zhu Ru *Caulis Bambusae in Taeniam* 6 g

GUI SHEN TANG

Restoring the Mind Decoction
Ren Shen *Radix Ginseng* 15 g
Bai Zhu *Rhizoma Atractylodis macrocephalae* 30 g
Ba Ji Tian *Radix Morindae officinalis* 30 g
Fu Shen *Sclerotium Poriae cocos pararadicis* 15 g
Zi He Che *Placenta Hominis* 6 g
Ban Xia *Rhizoma Pinelliae preparatum* 9 g
Chen Pi *Pericarpium Citri reticulatae* 3 g
Bai Jie Zi *Semen Sinapis albae* 9 g
Shi Chang Pu *Rhizoma Acori tatarinowii* 3 g
Zhu Sha *Cinnabaris* 3 g
Mai Men Dong *Radix Ophiopogonis* 6 g
Bai Zi Ren *Semen Platycladi* 6 g
Zhi Gan Cao *Radix Glycyrrhizae uralensis preparata* 3 g

GUI ZHI GAN CAO LONG GU MU LI TANG

Cinnamomum-Glycyrrhiza-Mastodi Ossis fossilia-Concha Ostreae Decoction
Gui Zhi *Ramulus Cinnamomi cassiae* 9 g
Zhi Gan Cao *Radix Glycyrrhizae uralensis preparata* 18 g
Long Gu *Mastodi Ossis fossilia* 30 g
Mu Li *Concha Ostreae* 30 g

GUI ZHI GAN CAO LONG GU MU LI TANG Variation (Chapter 17, Anxiety, Heart-Yang deficiency)

Cinnamomum-Glycyrrhiza-Mastodi Ossis fossilia-Concha Ostreae Decoction Variation
Gui Zhi *Ramulus Cinnamomi cassiae* 9 g
Zhi Gan Cao *Radix Glycyrrhizae uralensis preparata* 18 g

Long Gu *Mastodi Ossis fossilia* 30 g
Mu Li *Concha Ostreae* 30 g
Rou Gui *Cortex Cinnamomi* 3 g
Ren Shen *Radix Ginseng* 9 g
Bai Zi Ren *Semen Platycladi* 6 g

GUI ZHI JIA LONG GU MU LI TANG

Cinnamomum-Mastodi Ossis fossilia-Concha Ostreae Decoction
Gui Zhi *Ramulus Cinnamomi cassiae* 9 g
Bai Shao *Radix Paeoniae alba* 9 g
Sheng Jiang *Rhizoma Zingiberis recens* 9 g
Da Zao *Fructus Jujubae* 3 dates
Zhi Gan Cao *Radix Glycyrrhizae uralensis preparata* 6 g
Long Gu *Mastodi Ossis fossilia* 18 g
Mu Li *Concha Ostreae* 18 g

HE CHE DA ZAO WAN

Placenta Great Fortifying Pill
Zi He Che *Placenta Hominis* 1 placenta
Shu Di Huang *Radix Rehmanniae preparata* 60 g
Sheng Di Huang *Radix Rehmanniae* 45 g
Gou Qi Zi *Fructus Lycii chinensis* 45 g
Tian Men Dong *Radix Asparagi* 20 g
Wu Wei Zi *Fructus Schisandrae* 20 g
Dang Gui *Radix Angelicae sinensis* 20 g
Niu Xi *Radix Achyranthis bidentatae* 20 g
Du Zhong *Cortex Eucommiae ulmoidis* 30 g
Suo Yang *Herba Cynomorii* 20 g
Rou Cong Rong *Herba Cistanches* 20 g
Huang Bo *Cortex Phellodendri* 20 g

HUANG LIAN E JIAO TANG

Coptis-Colla Corii Asini Decoction
Huang Lian *Rhizoma Coptidis* 3 g
Huang Qin *Radix Scutellariae* 9 g
Bai Shao *Radix Paeoniae alba* 9 g
Ji Zi Huang *Egg yolk* 2 yolks
E Jiao *Colla Corii Asini* 9 g

HUANG LIAN E JIAO TANG Variation (Chapter 18, Insomnia, Appendix 1 Excessive dreaming, Heart and Kidneys not harmonized)

Coptis-Colla Corii Asini Decoction Variation
Huang Lian *Rhizoma Coptidis* 6 g
E Jiao *Colla Corii Asini* 6 g
Huang Qin *Radix Scutellariae* 10 g
Bai Shao *Radix Paeoniae alba* 10 g
Ji Zi Huang (egg, 1)
Yuan Zhi *Radix Polygalae* 6 g
Fu Shen *Sclerotium Poriae cocos pararadicis* 10 g
Tian Men Dong *Radix Asparagi* 10 g

HUANG LIAN WEN DAN TANG

Coptis Warming the Gall-Bladder Decoction
Huang Lian *Rhizoma Coptidis* 4.5 g
Ban Xia *Rhizoma Pinelliae preparatum* 6 g
Fu Ling *Poria* 5 g
Chen Pi *Pericarpium Citri reticulatae* 9 g
Zhu Ru *Caulis Bambusae in Taeniam* 6 g
Zhi Shi *Fructus Aurantii immaturus* 6 g
Zhi Gan Cao *Radix Glycyrrhizae uralensis preparata* 3 g
Sheng Jiang *Rhizoma Zingiberis recens* 5 slices
Da Zao *Fructus Jujubae* 1 date

HUANG LIAN WEN DAN TANG Variation (Chapter 18, Insomnia, Appendix 1 Excessive dreaming, Phlegm-Heat)

Coptis Warming the Gall-Bladder Decoction Variation
Huang Lian *Rhizoma Coptidis* 5 g
Huang Qin *Radix Scutellariae* 12 g
Ban Xia *Rhizoma Pinelliae preparatum* 9 g
Zhu Ru *Caulis Bambusae in Taeniam* 6 g
Zhi Shi *Fructus Aurantii immaturus* 6 g
Chen Pi *Pericarpium Citri reticulatae* 10 g
Fu Ling *Poria* 10 g
Dan Nan Xing *Rhizoma Arisaematis preparatum* 6 g
He Huan Pi *Cortex Albiziae* 9 g
Zhi Gan Cao *Radix Glycyrrhizae uralensis preparata* 3 g

JI SHENG SHEN QI TANG

Kidney-Qi Decoction from "Formulae to Aid the Living"
Fu Zi *Radix Aconiti lateralis preparata* 3 g
Gui Zhi *Ramulus Cinnamomi cassiae* 4 g
Gan Jiang *Rhizoma Zingiberis* 4 g
Huang Qi *Radix Astragali* 6 g
Shu Di Huang *Radix Rehmanniae preparata* 6 g

Sha Ren *Fructus Amomi* 3 g
Yin Yang Huo *Herba Epimedii* 6 g
Tu Si Zi *Semen Cuscutae* 6 g
Ze Xie *Rhizoma Alismatis* 6 g

JI SHENG SHEN QI TANG Variation (Chapter 19, Bipolar disorder, *Dian*, Heart and Spleen deficiency with Phlegm)

Kidney-Qi Decoction from "Formulae to Aid the Living" Variation
Yin Yang Huo *Herba Epimedii* 15g
Shi Chang Pu *Rhizoma Acori tatarinowii* 10 g
Yu Jin *Radix Curcumae* 10 g
Shu Di Huang *Radix Rehmanniae preparata* 10 g
Shan Yao *Rhizoma Dioscoreae* 10 g
Shan Zhu Yu *Fructus Corni* 10 g
Mu Dan Pi *Cortex Moutan* 10g
Ze Xie *Rhizoma Alismatis* 10 g
Huai Niu Xi *Radix Achyranthis bidentatae* 10 g
Rou Gui *Cortex Cinnamomi* 3 g

JIAO TAI WAN Variation (Chapter 18, Insomnia, Heart and Kidneys not harmonized)

Grand Communication Pill Variation
Huang Lian *Rhizoma Coptidis* 5 g
Rou Gui *Cortex Cinnamomi* 5 g
Fu Shen *Sclerotium Poriae cocos pararadicis* 10 g
Suan Zao Ren *Semen Ziziphi spinosae* 10 g

JIE FAN YI XIN TANG

Calming Mental Restlessness and Benefiting the Heart Decoction
Ren Shen *Radix Ginseng* 6 g
Huang Lian *Rhizoma Coptidis* 3 g
Suan Zao Ren *Semen Ziziphi spinosae* 9 g
Bai Zhu *Rhizoma Atractylodis macrocephalae* 3 g
Fu Shen *Sclerotium Poriae cocos pararadicis* 6 g
Xuan Shen *Radix Scrophulariae* 15 g
Gan Cao *Radix Glycyrrhizae uralensis* 3 g
Zhi Ke *Fructus Aurantii* 0.5 g
Tian Hua Fen *Radix Trichosanthis* 6 g

JIE YU QING XIN TANG

Eliminating Stagnation and Clearing the Heart Decoction
Chai Hu *Radix Bupleuri* 10 g
Xiang Fu *Rhizoma Cyperi* 10 g
Long Gu *Mastodi Ossis fossilia* 20 g
Mu Li *Concha Ostreae* 20 g
Shi Chang Pu *Rhizoma Acori tatarinowii* 10 g
Yu Jin *Radix Curcumae* 10 g
Sheng Di Huang *Radix Rehmanniae* 15 g
Huang Lian *Rhizoma Coptidis* 5 g
Zhu Ye *Folium Phyllostachys nigrae* 6 g

JIN GUI SHEN QI WAN

Golden Chest Kidney-Qi Pill
Fu Zi *Radix Aconiti lateralis preparata* 3 g
Gui Zhi *Ramulus Cinnamomi cassiae* 3 g
Shu Di Huang *Radix Rehmanniae preparata* 24 g
Shan Zhu Yu *Fructus Corni* 12 g
Shan Yao *Rhizoma Dioscoreae* 12 g
Ze Xie *Rhizoma Alismatis* 9 g
Mu Dan Pi *Cortex Moutan* 9 g
Fu Ling *Poria* 9 g

JIN SUO GU JING WAN

Metal Lock Consolidating the Essence Pill
Sha Yuan Ji Li *Semen Astragali complanati* 60 g
Qian Shi *Semen Euryales ferocis* 60 g
Lian Xu *Stamen Nelumbinis nuciferae* 60 g
Long Gu *Mastodi Ossis fossilia* 30 g
Mu Li *Concha Ostreae* 30 g
Lian Zi *Semen Nelumbinis nuciferae* 120 g

JING GONG SHA XIANG SAN

Palace of Essence Cinnabaris Fragrant Powder
Zhu Sha *Cinnabaris* 1.5 g
Long Gu *Mastodi Ossis fossilia* 12 g
Sha Ren *Fructus Amomi* 4.5 g
Jiu Zi *Semen Allii tuberosi* 6 g

KAI YU YUE SHEN TANG

Opening Stagnation and Cheering the Mind Decoction
Chai Hu *Radix Bupleuri* 6 g
Xiang Fu *Rhizoma Cyperi* 9 g
Qing Pi *Pericarpium Citri reticulatae viride* 6 g
Dan Shen *Radix Salviae miltiorrhizae* 6 g
Chi Shao *Radix Paeoniae rubra* 6 g
Chen Pi *Pericarpium Citri reticulatae* 3 g
Ban Xia *Rhizoma Pinelliae preparatum* 6 g
Shi Chang Pu *Rhizoma Acori tatarinowii* 6 g

Yuan Zhi *Radix Polygalae* 6 g
Huang Qin *Radix Scutellariae* 6 g
Huang Lian *Rhizoma Coptidis* 3 g
Shan Zhi Zi *Fructus Gardeniae* 6 g
Suan Zao Ren *Semen Ziziphi spinosae* 6 g
Fu Ling *Poria* 6 g
He Huan Pi *Cortex Albiziae* 6 g
Zhen Zhu Mu *Concha Margaritiferae usta* 12 g

KONG SHENG ZHEN ZHONG DAN

Master Kong's Bedside Pill
Gui Ban *Plastrum Testudinis* 10 g
Long Gu *Mastodi Ossis fossilia* 10 g
Yuan Zhi *Radix Polygalae* 10 g
Shi Chang Pu *Rhizoma Acori tatarinowii* 10 g
Gou Qi Zi *Fructus Lycii chinensis* 10 g
Mu Li *Concha Ostreae* 15 g
Bai Zi Ren *Semen Platycladi* 9 g
Suan Zao Ren *Semen Ziziphi spinosae* 6 g

LIANG GE SAN[1]

Cooling the Diaphragm Powder
Da Huang *Radix et Rhizoma Rhei* 600 g
Mang Xiao *Mirabilitum* 600 g
Gan Cao *Radix Glycyrrhizae uralensis* 600 g
Huang Qin *Radix Scutellariae* 300 g
Shan Zhi Zi *Fructus Gardeniae* 300 g
Lian Qiao *Fructus Forsythiae* 1200 g
Bo He *Herba Menthae haplocalycis* 300 g

LING JIAO GOU TENG TANG

Cornu Saigae-Uncaria Decoction
Ling Yang Jiao *Cornu Saigae tataricae* 4.5 g
Gou Teng *Ramulus cum Uncis Uncariae* 9 g
Sang Ye *Folium Mori* 6 g
Ju Hua *Flos Chrysanthemi* 9 g
Bai Shao *Radix Paeoniae alba* 9 g
Sheng Di Huang *Radix Rehmanniae* 15 g
Fu Shen *Sclerotium Poriae cocos pararadicis* 9 g
Chuan Bei Mu *Bulbus Fritillariae cirrhosae* 12 g
Zhu Ru *Caulis Bambusae in Taeniam* 15 g
Gan Cao *Radix Glycyrrhizae uralensis* 2.5 g

LIU JUN ZI TANG

Six Gentlemen Decoction
Ren Shen *Radix Ginseng* 10 g
Bai Zhu *Rhizoma Atractylodis macrocephalae* 9 g
Fu Ling *Poria* 9 g
Zhi Gan Cao *Radix Glycyrrhizae uralensis preparata* 6 g
Chen Pi *Pericarpium Citri reticulatae* 9 g
Ban Xia *Rhizoma Pinelliae preparatum* 12 g

LIU JUN ZI TANG Variation (Chapter 18, Insomnia, Appendix 2 Somnolence, Spleen deficiency)

Six Gentlemen Decoction Variation
Ren Shen *Radix Ginseng* 10 g
Bai Zhu *Rhizoma Atractylodis macrocephalae* 9 g
Fu Ling *Sclerotium Poriae cocos* 9 g
Zhi Gan Cao *Radix Glycyrrhizae uralensis preparata* 6 g
Chen Pi *Pericarpium Citri reticulatae* 9 g
Ban Xia *Rhizoma Pinelliae preparatum* 12 g
Mai Ya *Fructus Hordei Vulgaris germinatus* 9 g
Shen Qu *Massa medicata fermentata* 9 g
Shan Zha *Fructus Crataegi* 6 g
Shi Chang Pu *Rhizoma Acori tatarinowii* 6 g

LIU WEI DI HUANG WAN

Six-Ingredient Rehmannia Pill
Shu Di Huang *Radix Rehmanniae preparata* 24 g
Shan Zhu Yu *Fructus Corni* 12 g
Shan Yao *Rhizoma Dioscoreae* 12 g
Ze Xie *Rhizoma Alismatis* 9 g
Mu Dan Pi *Cortex Moutan* 9 g
Fu Ling *Poria* 9 g

LIU WEI DI HUANG WAN Variation (Chapter 12, Patterns in mental-emotional problems, Heart- and Kidney-Yin deficiency with Heart Empty Heat)

Six-Ingredient Rehmannia Pill Variation
Shu Di Huang *Radix Rehmanniae preparata* 24 g
Shan Zhu Yu *Fructus Corni* 12 g
Shan Yao *Rhizoma Dioscoreae* 12 g
Ze Xie *Rhizoma Alismatis* 9 g
Mu Dan Pi *Cortex Moutan* 9 g
Fu Ling *Poria* 9 g
Bai Shao *Radix Paeoniae alba* 15 g
Chai Hu *Radix Bupleuri* 1.5 g
Mai Men Dong *Radix Ophiopogonis* 15 g
Wu Wei Zi *Fructus Schisandrae* 3 g

Suan Zao Ren *Semen Ziziphi spinosae* 15 g
Ju Hua *Flos Chrysanthemi* 9 g

LIU WEI DI HUANG WAN Variation (Chapter 18, Insomnia, Appendix 3 Poor memory, Kidney deficiency)

Six-Ingredient Rehmannia Pill Variation
Shu Di Huang *Radix Rehmanniae preparata* 24 g
Shan Zhu Yu *Fructus Corni* 12 g
Shan Yao *Rhizoma Dioscoreae* 12 g
Ze Xie *Rhizoma Alismatis* 9 g
Mu Dan Pi *Cortex Moutan* 9 g
Fu Ling *Poria* 9 g
Bai Shao *Radix Paeoniae alba* 15 g
Chai Hu *Radix Bupleuri* 1.5 g
Mai Men Dong *Radix Ophiopogonis* 15 g
Wu Wei Zi *Fructus Schisandrae* 3 g
Suan Zao Ren *Semen Ziziphi spinosae* 15 g
Ju Hua *Flos Chrysanthemi* 9 g

LONG DAN XIE GAN TANG

Gentiana Draining the Liver Decoction
Long Dan Cao *Radix Gentianae* 6 g
Huang Qin *Radix Scutellariae* 9 g
Shan Zhi Zi *Fructus Gardeniae* 9 g
Ze Xie *Rhizoma Alismatis* 9 g
Mu Tong *Caulis Akebiae trifoliatae* 9 g
Che Qian Zi *Semen Plantaginis* 9 g
Sheng Di Huang *Radix Rehmanniae* 12 g
Dang Gui *Radix Angelicae sinensis* 9 g
Chai Hu *Radix Bupleuri* 9 g
Gan Cao *Radix Glycyrrhizae uralensis* 3 g

LONG DAN XIE GAN TANG Variation (Chapter 18, Insomnia, Liver-Fire blazing)

Gentiana Draining the Liver Decoction Variation
Long Dan Cao *Radix Gentianae* 6 g
Huang Qin *Radix Scutellariae* 9 g
Shan Zhi Zi *Fructus Gardeniae* 9 g
Ze Xie *Rhizoma Alismatis* 9 g
Mu Tong *Caulis Akebiae trifoliatae* 9 g
Che Qian Zi *Semen Plantaginis* 9 g
Sheng Di Huang *Radix Rehmanniae* 12 g
Dang Gui *Radix Angelicae sinensis* 9 g
Chai Hu *Radix Bupleuri* 9 g
Gan Cao *Radix Glycyrrhizae uralensis* 3 g
Fu Shen *Sclerotium Poriae cocos pararadicis* 6 g
YE Jiao Teng *Caulis Polygoni multiflori* 9 g
Long Chi *Fossilia Dentis Mastodi* 15 g

LONG DAN XIE GAN TANG Variation (Chapter 18, Insomnia, Appendix 1 Excessive dreaming, Liver-Fire)

Gentiana Draining the Liver Decoction Variation
Long Dan Cao *Radix Gentianae* 9 g
Huang Qin *Radix Scutellariae* 9 g
Shan Zhi Zi *Fructus Gardeniae* 9 g
Dang Gui *Radix Angelicae sinensis* 10 g
Sheng Di Huang *Radix Rehmanniae* 10 g
Chai Hu *Radix Bupleuri* 6 g
Bai Shao *Radix Paeoniae alba* 10 g
Chuan Xiong *Rhizoma Chuanxiong* 3 g
Zhi Mu *Radix Anemarrhaenae* 6 g
Gan Cao *Radix Glycyrrhizae uralensis* 6 g

LONG DAN XIE GAN TANG Variation (Chapter 19, Bipolar disorder, *Kuang*, Gall Bladder- and Liver-Fire)

Gentiana Draining the Liver Decoction Variation
Long Dan Cao *Radix Gentianae* 6 g
Huang Qin *Radix Scutellariae* 9 g
Shan Zhi Zi *Fructus Gardeniae* 9 g
Ze Xie *Rhizoma Alismatis* 9 g
Mu Tong *Caulis Akebiae trifoliatae* 9 g
Che Qian Zi *Semen Plantaginis* 9 g
Sheng Di Huang *Radix Rehmanniae* 12 g
Dang Gui *Radix Angelicae sinensis* 9 g
Chai Hu *Radix Bupleuri* 9 g
Gan Cao *Radix Glycyrrhizae uralensis* 3 g
Fu Shen *Sclerotium Poriae cocos pararadicis* 6 g
Zhu Ru *Caulis Bambusae in Taeniam* 10 g
Long Chi *Fossilia Dentis Mastodi* 15 g

LONG DAN XIE GAN TANG Variation (Chapter 20, Night Terrors, Liver- and Heart-Fire)

Gentiana Draining the Liver Decoction Variation
Long Dan Cao *Radix Gentianae* 6 g
Huang Qin *Radix Scutellariae* 6 g
Sheng Di Huang *Radix Rehmanniae* 9 g
Shan Zhi Zi *Fructus Gardeniae* 6 g
Chai Hu *Radix Bupleuri* 4.5 g
Che Qian Zi *Semen Plantaginis* 6 g
Dang Gui *Radix Angelicae sinensis* 6 g
Ze Xie *Rhizoma Alismatis* 6 g

Gou Teng *Ramulus cum Uncis Uncariae* 10 g
Shi Jue Ming *Concha Haliotidis* 12 g
He Huan Pi *Cortex Albiziae* 6 g

LONG DAN XIE GAN TANG Variation (Chapter 21, Attention Deficit Hyperactivity Disorder, Liver- and Heart-Fire)

Gentiana Draining the Liver Decoction Variation
Long Dan Cao *Radix Gentianae* 9 g
Huang Qin *Radix Scutellariae* 9 g
Shan Zhi Zi *Fructus Gardeniae* 9 g
Dang Gui *Radix Angelicae sinensis* 10 g
Sheng Di Huang *Radix Rehmanniae* 10 g
Chai Hu *Radix Bupleuri* 6 g
Bai Shao *Radix Paeoniae alba* 10 g
Chuan Xiong *Rhizoma Chuanxiong* 3 g
Zhi Mu *Radix Anemarrhaenae* 6 g
Gan Cao *Radix Glycyrrhizae uralensis* 6 g
Lian Zi Xin *Plumula Nelumbinis nuciferae* 6 g
Zhu Ye *Folium Phyllostachys nigrae* 6 g

MAI WEI DI HUANG WAN (BA XIAN CHANG SHOU WAN)

Ophiopogon-Schisandra-Rehmannia Pill (Eight Immortals Longevity Pill)
Shu Di Huang *Radix Rehmanniae preparata* 24 g
Shan Zhu Yu *Fructus Corni* 12 g
Shan Yao *Rhizoma Dioscoreae* 12 g
Ze Xie *Rhizoma Alismatis* 9 g
Mu Dan Pi *Cortex Moutan* 9 g
Fu Ling *Poria* 9 g
Mai Men Dong *Radix Ophiopogonis* 6 g
Wu Wei Zi *Fructus Schisandrae* 6 g

MENG SHI GUN TAN WAN

Chloritum Chasing-away Phlegm Pill
Da Huang *Radix et Rhizoma Rhei* 15 g
Mang Xiao *Natrii Sulfas* 3 g
Huang Qin *Radix Scutellariae* 15 g
Chen Xiang *Lignum Aquilariae resinatum* 3 g
Meng Shi *Chloritum* 6 g

MU XIANG LIU QI YIN

Aucklandia Flowing Qi Decoction
Mu Xiang *Radix Aucklandiae* 6 g
Ban Xia *Rhizoma Pinelliae preparatum* 6 g
Chen Pi *Pericarpium Citri reticulatae* 3 g
Hou Po *Cortex Magnoliae officinalis* 4.5 g
Qing Pi *Pericarpium Citri reticulatae viride* 3 g
Gan Cao *Radix Glycyrrhizae uralensis* 3 g
Xiang Fu *Rhizoma Cyperi* 6 g
Zi Su Ye *Folium Perillae* 3 g
Ren Shen *Radix Ginseng* 6 g
Fu Ling *Poria* 6 g
Mu Gua *Fructus Chaenomelis lagenariae* 3 g
Shi Chang Pu *Rhizoma Acori tatarinowii* 3 g
Bai Zhu *Rhizoma Atractylodis macrocephalae* 4.5 g
Bai Zhi *Radix Angelicae dahuricae* 3 g
Mai Men Dong *Radix Ophiopogonis* 6 g
Cao Guo *Fructus Amomi Tsaoko* 3 g
Rou Gui *Cortex Cinnamomi* 1.5 g
E Zhu *Rhizoma Curcumae zedoariae* 3 g
Da Fu Pi *Pericarpium Arecae* catechu 3 g
Ding Xiang *Flos Caryophylli* 3 g
Bing Lang *Semen Arecae catechu* 3 g
Huo Xiang *Herba Pogostemonis* 3 g
Mu Tong *Caulis Akebiae trifoliatae* 1.5 g

NAN GENG TANG

Male Menopause Decoction
Yin Yang Huo *Herba Epimedii* 9 g
Xian Mao *Rhizoma Curculiginis* 9 g
Ba Ji Tian *Radix Morindae officinalis* 9 g
Dang Gui *Radix Angelicae sinensis* 9 g
Zhi Mu *Radix Anemarrhaenae* 9 g
Huang Bo *Cortex Phellodendri* 6 g

NIU HUANG QING XIN WAN

Calculus Bovis Clearing the Heart Pill
Huang Lian *Rhizoma Coptidis* 9 g
Huang Qin *Radix Scutellariae* 6 g
Shan Zhi Zi *Fructus Gardeniae* 6 g
Yu Jin *Radix Curcumae* 6 g
Zhu Sha *Cinnabaris* 4 g
Niu Huang *Calculus Bovis* 1 g

PING BU ZHEN XIN DAN

Calming and Tonifying the Heart Pill
Ren Shen *Radix Ginseng* 9 g
Mai Men Dong *Radix Ophiopogonis* 6 g
Wu Wei Zi *Fructus Schisandrae* 6 g
Shan Yao *Rhizoma Dioscoreae* 6 g
Sheng Di Huang *Radix Rehmanniae* 6 g

Shu Di Huang *Radix Rehmanniae preparata* 9 g
Rou Gui *Cortex Cinnamomi* 3 g
Yuan Zhi *Radix Polygalae* 6 g
Long Chi *Fossilia Dentis Mastodi* 9 g
Suan Zao Ren *Semen Ziziphi spinosae* 6 g
Fu Ling *Poria* 6 g
Fu Shen *Sclerotium Poriae cocos pararadicis* 6 g
Zhu Sha *Cinnabaris* 0.5 g
Che Qian Zi *Semen Plantaginis* 6 g
Tian Men Dong *Radix Asparagi* 6 g
Zhi Gan Cao *Radix Glycyrrhizae uralensis preparata* 3 g

PING BU ZHEN XIN DAN Variation (Chapter 17, Anxiety, Heart and Gall-Bladder deficiency)

Calming and Tonifying the Heart Pill Variation
Ren Shen *Radix Ginseng* 9 g
Mai Men Dong *Radix Ophiopogonis* 6 g
Wu Wei Zi *Fructus Schisandrae* 6 g
Shan Yao *Rhizoma Dioscoreae* 6 g
Sheng Di Huang *Radix Rehmanniae* 6 g
Shu Di Huang *Radix Rehmanniae preparata* 9 g
Rou Gui *Cortex Cinnamomi* 3 g
Yuan Zhi *Radix Polygalae* 6 g
Long Gu *Mastodi Ossis fossilia* 9 g
Mu Li *Concha Ostreae* 9 g
Suan Zao Ren *Semen Ziziphi spinosae* 6 g
Fu Shen *Sclerotium Poriae cocos pararadicis* 6 g
Zhi Gan Cao *Radix Glycyrrhizae uralensis preparata* 3 g

PING WEI SAN

Balancing the Stomach Powder
Cang Zhu *Rhizoma Atractylodis* 9 g
Chen Pi *Pericarpium Citri reticulatae* 6 g
Hou Po *Cortex Magnoliae officinalis* 6 g
Zhi Gan Cao *Radix Glycyrrhizae uralensis preparata* 3 g
Sheng Jiang *Rhizoma Zingiberis recens* 3 g
Da Zao *Fructus Jujubae* 3 dates

PING WEI SAN Variation (Chapter 18, Insomnia, Appendix 2 Somnolence, Dampness obstructing the Brain)

Balancing the Stomach Powder Variation
Cang Zhu *Rhizoma Atractylodis* 9 g
Chen Pi *Pericarpium Citri reticulatae* 6 g
Hou Po *Cortex Magnoliae officinalis* 6 g
Zhi Gan Cao *Radix Glycyrrhizae uralensis preparata* 3 g
Sheng Jiang *Rhizoma Zingiberis recens* 3 g
Da Zao *Fructus Jujubae* 3 dates
Huo Xiang *Herba Pogostemonis* 4.5 g
Pei Lan *Herba Eupatorii fortunei* 4.5 g
Yi Yi Ren *Semen Coicis* 15 g

PING XIN WANG YOU TANG

Settling the Heart and Forgetting Worry Decoction
Ci Shi *Magnetitum* 9 g
Qing Meng Shi *Lapis Chloriti* 9 g
Zhi Shi *Fructus Aurantii immaturus* 6 g
Huang Bo *Cortex Phellodendri* 6 g
Ban Xia *Rhizoma Pinelliae preparatum* 6 g
Hou Po *Cortex Magnoliae officinalis* 6 g
Fu Ling *Poria* 6 g
Shen Qu *Massa medicata fermentata* 6 g
Rou Gui *Cortex Cinnamomi* 3 g
Zi Su Ye *Folium Perillae* 6 g
Shi Chang Pu *Rhizoma Acori tatarinowii* 6 g
Sheng Jiang *Rhizoma Zingiberis recens* 3 slices

QI JU DI HUANG WAN

Lycium-Chrysanthemum-Rehmannia Pill
Gou Qi Zi *Fructus Lycii chinensis* 9 g
Ju Hua *Flos Chrysanthemi* 6 g
Shu Di Huang *Radix Rehmanniae preparata* 24 g
Shan Zhu Yu *Fructus Corni* 12 g
Shan Yao *Rhizoma Dioscoreae* 12 g
Ze Xie *Rhizoma Alismatis* 9 g
Mu Dan Pi *Cortex Moutan* 9 g
Fu Ling *Poria* 9 g

QI JU DI HUANG WAN Variation (Chapter 21, Attention Deficit Disorder, Kidney Deficiency with Liver-Yang rising)

Lycium-Chrysanthemum-Rehmannia Decoction Variation
Gou Qi Zi *Fructus Lycii chinensis* 9 g
Ju Hua *Flos Chrysanthemi* 6 g
Shu Di Huang *Radix Rehmanniae preparata* 24 g
Shan Zhu Yu *Fructus Corni* 12 g
Shan Yao *Rhizoma Dioscoreae* 12 g
Ze Xie *Rhizoma Alismatis* 9 g
Mu Dan Pi *Cortex Moutan* 9 g

Fu Ling *Poria* 9 g
Long Gu *Mastodi Ossis fossilia* 12 g
Mu Li *Concha Ostreae* 12 g

QING XIN TANG

Clearing the Heart Decoction
Fu Shen *Sclerotium Poriae cocos pararadicis* 9 g
Huang Lian *Rhizoma Coptidis* 3 g
Suan Zao Ren *Semen Ziziphi spinosae* 6 g
Shi Chang Pu *Rhizoma Acori tatarinowii* 6 g
Yuan Zhi *Radix Polygalae* 9 g
Bai Zi Ren *Semen Platycladi* 6 g
Gan Cao *Radix Glycyrrhizae uralensis* 3 g

ROU FU BAO YUAN TANG

Cinnamomum-Aconitum Preserving the Source Decoction
Rou Gui *Cortex Cinnamomi* 1.5 g
Fu Zi *Radix Aconiti lateralis preparata* 3 g
Huang Qi *Radix Astragali* 6 g
Ren Shen *Radix Ginseng* 6 g
Zhi Gan Cao *Radix Glycyrrhizae uralensis preparata* 3 g

SAN CAI FENG SUI DAN

Three Abilities Banking Up the Marrow Pill
Tian Men Dong *Radix Asparagi* 6 g
Shu Di Huang *Radix Rehmanniae preparata* 6 g
Ren Shen *Radix Ginseng* 6 g

SANG DAN XIE BAI SAN

Morus-Moutan Draining Whiteness Powder
Sang Ye *Folium Mori* 6 g
Mu Dan Pi *Cortex Moutan* 6 g
Di Gu Pi *Cortex Lycii* 9 g
Sang Bai Pi *Cortex Mori* 9 g
Zhi Gan Cao *Radix Glycyrrhizae uralensis preparata* 3 g
Geng Mi *Semen Oryzae sativae* 6 g

SANG DAN XIE BAI SAN Variation (Chapter 4, Corporeal Soul, contraction of Corporeal Soul)

Morus-Moutan Draining Whiteness Powder Variation
Di Gu Pi *Cortex Lycii* 9 g
Sang Bai Pi *Cortex Mori* 9 g
Zhi Gan Cao *Radix Glycyrrhizae uralensis preparata* 3 g
Geng Mi *Semen Oryzae sativae* 6 g
Sang Ye *Folium Mori* 6 g
Zhu Ru *Caulis Bambusae in Taeniam* 6 g
Chuan Bei Mu *Bulbus Fritillariae cirrhosae* 6 g
Da Zao *Fructus Jujubae* 3 dates
Bai Xian Pi *Cortex Dictamni* 9 g
Zhu Ye *Folium Phyllostachys nigrae* 6 g

SANG PIAO XIAO SAN

Ootheca Mantidis Pill
Sang Piao Xiao *Ootheca Mantidis* 9 g
Long Gu *Mastodi Ossis fossilia* 15 g
Gui Ban *Plastrum Testudinis* 15 g
Dang Gui *Radix Angelicae sinensis* 9 g
Ren Shen *Radix Ginseng* 9 g
Fu Shen *Sclerotium Poriae cocos pararadicis* 6 g
Yuan Zhi *Radix Polygalae* 6 g
Shi Chang Pu *Rhizoma Acori tatarinowii* 6 g

SHEN ZHONG DAN

Pillow Pill
(Zhi) Gui Ban *Plastrum Testudinis* (prepared) 15 g
(Duan) Long Gu *Mastodi Ossis fossilia* (calcined) 15 g
Yuan Zhi *Radix Polygalae* 9 g
Shi Chang Pu *Rhizoma Acori tatarinowii* 6 g

SHENG MAI SAN

Generating the Pulse Powder
Ren Shen *Radix Ginseng* 9 g
Mai Men Dong *Radix Ophiopogonis* 9 g
Wu Wei Zi *Fructus Schisandrae* 3 g

SHENG TIE LUO YIN

Frusta Ferri Decoction
Sheng Tie Luo *Frusta Ferri* 60 g
Dan Nan Xing *Rhizoma Arisaematis preparatum* 9 g
Zhe Bei Mu *Bulbus Fritillariae thunbergii* 9 g
Xuan Shen *Radix Scrophulariae* 9 g
Tian Men Dong *Radix Asparagi* 9 g

Mai Men Dong *Radix Ophiopogonis* 9 g
Lian Qiao *Fructus Forsythiae* 9 g
Dan Shen *Radix Salviae miltiorrhizae* 12 g
Fu Ling *Poria* 12 g
Chen Pi *Pericarpium Citri reticulatae* 6 g
Shi Chang Pu *Rhizoma Acori tatarinowii* 6 g
Yuan Zhi *Radix Polygalae* 6 g
Zhu Sha *Cinnabaris* 1.8 g

SHI BU WAN

Ten Tonifications Pill
Fu Zi *Radix Aconiti lateralis preparata* 3 g
Gui Zhi *Ramulus Cinnamomi cassiae* 3 g
Shu Di Huang *Radix Rehmanniae preparata* 24 g
Shan Zhu Yu *Fructus Corni* officinalis 12 g
Shan Yao *Radix Dioscoreae oppositae* 12 g
Ze Xie *Rhizoma Alismatis* 9 g
Mu Dan Pi *Cortex Moutan* 9 g
Fu Ling *Poria* 9 g
Lu Rong *Cornu Cervi parvum* 6 g
Wu Wei Zi *Fructus Schisandrae* 6 g

SHI WEI WEN DAN TANG

Ten-Ingredient Warming the Gall-Bladder Decoction
Ban Xia *Rhizoma Pinelliae preparatum* 6 g
Chen Pi *Pericarpium Citri reticulatae* 6 g
Fu Ling *Poria* 4.5 g
Zhi Shi *Fructus Aurantii immaturus* 6 g
Ren Shen *Radix Ginseng* 3 g
Shu Di Huang *Radix Rehmanniae preparata* 9 g
Suan Zao Ren *Semen Ziziphi spinosae* 3 g
Yuan Zhi *Radix Polygalae* 3 g
Zhi Gan Cao *Radix Glycyrrhizae uralensis preparata* 1.5 g
Sheng Jiang *Rhizoma Zingiberis recens* 5 slices
Hong Zao *Fructus Jujubae* 1 date

SHI WEI WEN DAN TANG Variation (Chapter 16, Depression, Qi stagnation with Phlegm)

Ten-Ingredient Warming the Gall-Bladder Decoction Variation
Chen Pi *Pericarpium Citri reticulatae* 3 g
Ban Xia *Rhizoma Pinelliae preparatum* 9 g
Fu Ling *Poria* 9 g
Zhi Ke *Fructus Aurantii* 6 g
Qian Hu *Radix Peucedani* 6 g
Zhu Ru *Caulis Bambusae in Taeniam* 6 g
Gan Cao *Radix Glycyrrhizae uralensis* 3 g
Yuan Zhi *Radix Polygalae* 6 g
Shi Chang Pu *Rhizoma Acori tatarinowii* 6 g
Yu Jin *Radix Curcumae* 6 g
Gua Lou *Fructus Trichosanthis* 6 g
Dan Nan Xing *Rhizoma Arisaematis preparatum* 6 g
Shan Zhi Zi *Fructus Gardeniae* 6 g
He Huan Pi *Cortex Albiziae* 6 g

SHI WEI WEN DAN TANG Variation (Chapter 18, Insomnia, Appendix 1 Excessive dreaming, deficiency of Qi of Heart and Gall-Bladder)

Ten-Ingredient Warming the Gall-Bladder Decoction Variation
Ban Xia *Rhizoma Pinelliae preparatum* 10 g
Zhi Shi *Fructus Aurantii immaturus* 6 g
Chen Pi *Pericarpium Citri reticulatae* 6 g
Fu Ling *Poria* 10 g
Suan Zao Ren *Semen Ziziphi spinosae* 15 g
Yuan Zhi *Radix Polygalae* 6 g
Wu Wei Zi *Fructus Schisandrae* 10 g
Shu Di Huang *Radix Rehmanniae preparata* 10 g
Dang Shen *Radix Codonopsis* 10 g
Zhi Gan Cao *Radix Glycyrrhizae uralensis preparata* 6 g
Long Chi *Fossilia Dentis Mastodi* 10 g
Meng Shi *Lapis Chloriti* 10 g

SHI WEI WEN DAN TANG Variation (Chapter 19, Bipolar disorder, *Dian*, Qi deficiency with Phlegm)

Ten-Ingredient Warming the Gall-Bladder Decoction Variation
Ban Xia *Rhizoma Pinelliae preparatum* 9 g
Zhi Shi *Fructus Aurantii immaturus* 10 g
Chen Pi *Pericarpium Citri reticulatae* 9 g
Fu Ling *Poria* 10 g
Ren Shen *Radix Ginseng* 5 g
Shu Di Huang *Radix Rehmanniae preparata* 9 g
Suan Zao Ren *Semen Ziziphi spinosae* 10 g
Yuan Zhi *Radix Polygalae* 9 g
Wu Wei Zi *Fructus Schisandrae* 10 g
Zhi Gan Cao *Radix Glycyrrhizae uralensis preparata* 6 g
Shi Chang Pu *Rhizoma Acori tatarinowii* 10 g
Fu Shen *Sclerotium Poriae cocos pararadicis* 10 g

SHI YU TANG

Dampness Stagnation Decoction
Cang Zhu *Rhizoma Atractylodis* 9 g
Bai Zhu *Rhizoma Atractylodis macrocephalae* 9 g
Xiang Fu *Rhizoma Cyperi* 6 g
Chen Pi *Pericarpium Citri reticulatae* 3 g
Qiang Huo *Rhizoma seu Radix Notopterygii* 3 g
Du Huo *Radix Angelicae pubescentis* 6 g
Chuan Xiong *Rhizoma Chuanxiong* 6 g
Ban Xia *Rhizoma Pinelliae preparatum* 6 g
Hou Po *Cortex Magnoliae officinalis* 6 g
Fu Ling *Poria* 6 g
Sheng Jiang *Rhizoma Zingiberis recens* 3 slices
Gan Cao *Radix Glycyrrhizae uralensis* 3 g

SHI YU TANG

Food Stagnation Decoction
Cang Zhu *Rhizoma Atractylodis* 9 g
Hou Po *Cortex Magnoliae officinalis* 6 g
Chuan Xiong *Rhizoma Chuanxiong* 6 g
Chen Pi *Pericarpium Citri reticulatae* 3 g
Shen Qu *Massa medicata fermentata* 6 g
Shan Zhi Zi *Fructus Gardeniae* 6 g
Zhi Ke *Fructus Aurantii* 6 g
Zhi Gan Cao *Radix Glycyrrhizae uralensis preparata* 3 g
Xiang Fu *Rhizoma Cyperi* 6 g
Shan Ren *Fructus Amomi* 3 g

SHUN QI DAO TAN TANG

Rectifying Qi and Eliminating Phlegm Decoction
Chen Pi *Pericarpium Citri reticulatae* 3 g
Fu Ling *Poria* 3 g
Ban Xia *Rhizoma Pinelliae preparatum* 6 g
Gan Cao *Radix Glycyrrhizae uralensis* 1.5 g
Dan Nan Xing *Rhizoma Arisaematis preparatum* 6 g
Mu Xiang *Radix Aucklandiae* 3 g
Xiang Fu *Rhizoma Cyperi* 6 g
Zhi Shi *Fructus Aurantii immaturus* 6 g

SHUN QI DAO TAN TANG Variation (Chapter 16, Depression, Qi stagnation with Phlegm)

Rectifying Qi and Eliminating Phlegm Decoction Variation
Chen Pi *Pericarpium Citri reticulatae* 3 g
Fu Ling *Poria* 3 g
Ban Xia *Rhizoma Pinelliae preparatum* 6 g
Gan Cao *Radix Glycyrrhizae uralensis* 1.5 g
Dan Nan Xing *Rhizoma Arisaematis preparatum* 6 g
Mu Xiang *Radix Aucklandiae* 3 g
Xiang Fu *Rhizoma Cyperi* 6 g
Zhi Shi *Fructus Aurantii immaturus* 6 g
Shi Chang Pu *Rhizoma Acori tatarinowii* 6 g
Yuan Zhi *Radix Polygalae* 6 g

SHUN QI DAO TAN TANG Variation (Chapter 19, Bipolar disorder, *Dian*, Qi stagnation and Phlegm)

Rectifying Qi and Eliminating Phlegm Decoction Variation
Chen Pi *Pericarpium Citri reticulatae* 3 g
Fu Ling *Poria* 3 g
Ban Xia *Rhizoma Pinelliae preparatum* 6 g
Gan Cao *Radix Glycyrrhizae uralensis* 1.5 g
Dan Nan Xing *Rhizoma Arisaematis preparatum* 6 g
Mu Xiang *Radix Aucklandiae* 3 g
Xiang Fu *Rhizoma Cyperi* 6 g
Zhi Shi *Fructus Aurantii immaturus* 6 g
Huang Lian *Rhizoma Coptidis* 3 g
Huang Qin *Radix Scutellariae* 6 g
Yuan Zhi *Radix Polygalae* 6 g
Shi Chang Pu *Rhizoma Acori tatarinowii* 6 g
Chen Xiang *Lignum Aquilariae resinatum* 6 g

SI NI SAN

Four Rebellious Powder
Chai Hu *Radix Bupleuri* 6 g
Bai Shao *Radix Paeoniae alba* 9 g
Zhi Shi *Fructus Aurantii immaturus* 6 g
Zhi Gan Cao *Radix Glycyrrhizae uralensis preparata* 6 g

SI QI TANG

Four Seasons Decoction for the Seven Emotions
Hou Po *Cortex Magnoliae officinalis* 9 g
Ban Xia *Rhizoma Pinelliae preparatum* 9 g
Fu Ling *Poria* 12 g
Sheng Jiang *Rhizoma Zingiberis recens* 15 g
Zi Su Ye *Folium Perillae* 6 g
Da Zao *Fructus Jujubae* 5 dates

SI QI TANG Variation (Chapter 19, Bipolar disorder, *Dian*, Qi stagnation and Phlegm)

Four Seasons Decoction for the Seven Emotions Variation
Hou Po *Cortex Magnoliae officinalis* 9 g
Ban Xia *Rhizoma Pinelliae preparatum* 9 g
Fu Ling *Poria* 12 g
Sheng Jiang *Rhizoma Zingiberis recens* 15 g
Zi Su Ye *Folium Perillae* 6 g
Da Zao *Fructus Jujubae* 5 dates
Yuan Zhi *Radix Polygalae* 6 g
Dan Nan Xing *Rhizoma Arisaematis preparatum* 6 g
Yu Jin *Radix Curcumae* 6 g
Shi Chang Pu *Rhizoma Acori tatarinowii* 6 g

SU HE XIANG WAN

Styrax Pill
Su He Xiang *Styrax* 30 g
She Xiang *Moschus* 60 g
Bing Pian *Borneolum* 30 g
An Xi Xiang *Benzoinum* 60 g
Mu Xiang *Radix Aucklandiae* 60 g
Tan Xiang *Lignum Santali albi* 60 g
Chen Xiang *Lignum Aquilariae resinatum* 60 g
Ru Xiang *Olibanum* 30 g
Ding Xiang *Flos Caryophylli* 60 g
Xiang Fu *Rhizoma Cyperi* 60 g
Bi Ba *Fructus Piperis longi* 60 g
Shui Niu Jiao *Cornu Bubali* 60 g
Zhu Sha *Cinnabaris* 60 g
Bai Zhu *Rhizoma Atractylodis macrocephalae* 60 g
He Zi *Fructus Chebulae* 60 g

SU HE XIANG WAN plus **SI QI TANG** Variation (Chapter 19, Bipolar disorder, *Dian*, Qi stagnation and Phlegm)

Styrax Pill plus *Four Seasons Decoction for the Seven Emotions* Variation
Su He Xiang *Styrax* 30 g
Bing Pian *Borneolum* 30 g
Mu Xiang *Radix Aucklandiae* 60 g
Tan Xiang *Lignum Santali albi* 60 g
Chen Xiang *Lignum Aquilariae resinatum* 60 g
Ru Xiang *Olibanum* 30 g
Ding Xiang *Flos Caryophylli* 60 g
Xiang Fu *Rhizoma Cyperi* 60 g
Bi Ba *Fructus Piperis longi* 60 g
Bai Zhu *Rhizoma Atractylodis macrocephalae* 60 g
He Zi *Fructus Chebulae* 60 g
Hou Po *Cortex Magnoliae officinalis* 9 g
Ban Xia *Rhizoma Pinelliae preparatum* 9 g
Fu Ling *Poria* 12 g
Sheng Jiang *Rhizoma Zingiberis recens* 15 g
Zi Su Ye *Folium Perillae* 6 g
Da Zao *Fructus Jujubae* 5 dates
Dan Nan Xing *Rhizoma Arisaematis preparatum* 30 g
Yuan Zhi *Radix Polygalae* 30 g
Shi Chang Pu *Rhizoma Acori tatarinowii* 30 g
Yu Jin *Radix Curcumae* 30 g

SUAN ZAO REN TANG

Ziziphus Decoction
Suan Zao Ren *Semen Ziziphi spinosae* 18 g
Chuan Xiong *Rhizoma Chuanxiong* 6 g
Fu Ling *Poria* 12 g
Zhi Mu *Rhizoma Anemarrhenae* 9 g
Gan Cao *Radix Glycyrrhizae uralensis* 3 g

SUAN ZAO REN TANG Variation (Chapter 20, Night Terrors, Liver- and Heart-Yin deficiency)

Ziziphus Decoction Variation
Suan Zao Ren *Semen Ziziphi spinosae* 18 g
Chuan Xiong *Rhizoma Chuanxiong* 6 g
Fu Ling *Poria* 12 g
Zhi Mu *Rhizoma Anemarrhenae* 9 g
Gan Cao *Radix Glycyrrhizae uralensis* 3 g
Long Chi *Fossilia Dentis Mastodi* 15 g
Mu Li *Concha Ostreae* 15 g

TAN YU TANG

Phlegm Stagnation Decoction
Su Zi *Fructus Perillae* 9 g
Ban Xia *Rhizoma Pinelliae preparatum* 9 g
Qian Hu *Radix Peucedani* 6 g
Zhi Gan Cao *Radix Glycyrrhizae uralensis preparata* 3 g
Dang Gui *Radix Angelicae sinensis* 6 g
Chen Pi *Pericarpium Citri reticulatae* 3 g
Chen Xiang *Lignum Aquilariae resinatum* 6 g
Gua Lou *Fructus Trichosanthis* 9 g
Dan Nan Xing *Rhizoma Arisaematis preparatum* 6 g
Zhi Shi *Fructus Aurantii immaturus* 6 g

Xiang Fu *Rhizoma Cyperi* 6 g
Hua Shi *Talcum* 6 g

TAO HE CHENG QI TANG

Persica Conducting Qi Decoction
Tao Ren *Semen Persicae* 12 g
Da Huang *Radix et Rhizoma Rhei* 12 g
Gui Zhi *Ramulus Cinnamomi cassiae* 6 g
Mang Xiao *Natrii Sulfas* 6 g
Zhi Gan Cao *Radix Glycyrrhizae uralensis preparata* 6 g

TAO REN HONG HUA JIAN

Persica-Carthamus Decoction
Tao Ren *Semen Persicae* 6 g
Hong Hua *Flos Carthami tinctorii* 6 g
Chuan Xiong *Rhizoma Chuanxiong* 9 g
Yan Hu Suo *Rhizoma Corydalis* 6 g
Gua Lou *Fructus Trichosanthis* 6 g
Qing Pi *Pericarpium Citri reticulatae viride* 6 g
Tan Xiang *Lignum Santali albi* 3 g
Dang Gui *Radix Angelicae sinensis* 6 g
Long Chi *Fossilia Dentis Mastodi* 9 g
Gui Zhi *Ramulus Cinnamomi cassiae* 6 g

TIAN WANG BU XIN DAN

Heavenly Emperor Tonifying the Heart Pill
Sheng Di Huang *Radix Rehmanniae* 6 g
Xuan Shen *Radix Scrophulariae* 6 g
Mai Men Dong *Radix Ophiopogonis* 6 g
Tian Men Dong *Radix Asparagi* 6 g
Ren Shen *Radix Ginseng* 6 g
Fu Ling *Poria* 9 g
Wu Wei Zi *Fructus Schisandrae* 4 g
Dang Gui *Radix Angelicae sinensis* 6 g
Dan Shen *Radix Salviae miltiorrhizae* 6 g
Suan Zao Ren *Semen Ziziphi spinosae* 6 g
Bai Zi Ren *Semen Platycladi* 6 g
Yuan Zhi *Radix Polygalae* 6 g
Jie Geng *Radix Platycodi* 3 g

TIAO WEI CHENG QI TANG

Regulating the Stomach Conducting Qi Decoction
Da Huang *Radix et Rhizoma Rhei* 12 g
Mang Xiao *Natrii Sulfas* 9 g
Zhi Gan Cao *Radix Glycyrrhizae uralensis preparata* 6 g

TONG QIAO HUO XUE TANG

Opening the Orifices and Invigorating Blood Decoction
Chi Shao *Radix Paeoniae rubra* 3 g
Chuan Xiong *Rhizoma Chuanxiong* 3 g
Tao Ren *Semen Persicae* 9 g
Hong Hua *Flos Carthami tinctorii* 9 g
She Xiang *Moschus* 15 g
Cong Bai *Bulbus Allii fistulosi* 3 g
Hong Zao *Fructus Jujubae* 7 red dates
Sheng Jiang *Rhizoma Zingiberis recens* 3 slices
Rice Wine

WEN DAN TANG

Warming the Gall-Bladder Decoction
Ban Xia *Rhizoma Pinelliae preparatum* 6 g
Fu Ling *Poria* 5 g
Chen Pi *Pericarpium Citri reticulatae* 9 g
Zhu Ru *Caulis Bambusae in Taeniam* 6 g
Zhi Shi *Fructus Aurantii immaturus* 6 g
Zhi Gan Cao *Radix Glycyrrhizae uralensis preparata* 3 g
Sheng Jiang *Rhizoma Zingiberis recens* 5 slices
Da Zao *Fructus Jujubae* 1 date

WEN DAN TANG Variation (Chapter 19, Bipolar disorder, *Dian*, Qi stagnation and Phlegm)

Warming the Gall-Bladder Decoction Variation
Ban Xia *Rhizoma Pinelliae preparatum* 10 g
Chen Pi *Pericarpium Citri reticulatae* 10 g
Zhi Shi *Fructus Aurantii immaturus* 10 g
Zhu Ru *Caulis Bambusae in Taeniam* 6 g
Fu Ling *Poria* 9 g
Huang Lian *Rhizoma Coptidis* 6 g
Dan Nan Xing *Rhizoma Arisaematis preparatum* 6 g
Yu Jin *Radix Curcumae* 10 g
Bai Fan *Alumen* 6 g

WEN DAN TANG Variation (Chapter 20, Night Terrors, Phlegm-Heat harassing the Ethereal Soul and the Mind)

Warming the Gall-Bladder Decoction Variation
Ban Xia *Rhizoma Pinelliae preparatum* 10 g
Chen Pi *Pericarpium Citri reticulatae* 10 g

Zhi Shi *Fructus Aurantii immaturus* 10 g
Fu Ling *Poria* 9 g
Dan Nan Xing *Rhizoma Arisaematis preparatum* 6 g
Shi Chang Pu *Rhizoma Acori tatarinowii* 6 g
Yuan Zhi *Radix Polygalae* 9 g

WU GE KUAN ZHONG SAN

Five Diaphragms Relaxing the Center Powder
Bai Dou Kou *Fructus Amomi rotundus* 1.5 g
Hou Po *Cortex Magnoliae officinalis* 9 g
Sha Ren *Fructus Amomi* 4.5 g
Mu Xiang *Radix Aucklandiae* 3 g
Xiang Fu *Rhizoma Cyperi* 9 g
Qing Pi *Pericarpium Citri reticulatae viride* 4.5 g
Chen Pi *Pericarpium Citri reticulatae* 4.5 g
Ding Xiang *Flos Caryophylli* 3 g
Zhi Gan Cao *Radix Glycyrrhizae uralensis preparata* 6 g
Sheng Jiang *Rhizoma Zingiberis recens* 3 slices

WU WEI ZI TANG

Schisandra Decoction
Wu Wei Zi *Fructus Schisandrae* 9 g
Huang Qi *Radix Astragali* 6 g
Ren Shen *Radix Ginseng* 9 g
Mai Men Dong *Radix Ophiopogonis* 6 g
Zhi Gan Cao *Radix Glycyrrhizae uralensis preparata* 3 g

WU WEI ZI TANG Variation (Chapter 17, Anxiety, Heart and Gall-Bladder deficiency)

Schisandra Decoction Variation
Wu Wei Zi *Fructus Schisandrae* 9 g
Huang Qi *Radix Astragali* 6 g
Ren Shen *Radix Ginseng* 9 g
Mai Men Dong *Radix Ophiopogonis* 6 g
Yu Zhu *Rhizoma Polygonati odorati* 6 g
Bei Sha Shen *Radix Glehniae* 6 g
Suan Zao Ren *Semen Ziziphi spinosae* 6 g
Bai Zi Ren *Semen Platycladi* 6 g
He Huan Pi *Cortex Albiziae* 6 g
Zhi Gan Cao *Radix Glycyrrhizae uralensis preparata* 3 g

XIAO CHAI HU TANG

Small Bupleurum Decoction
Chai Hu *Radix Bupleuri* 12 g
Huang Qin *Radix Scutellariae* 9 g
Ban Xia *Rhizoma Pinelliae preparatum* 9 g
Ren Shen *Radix Ginseng* 6 g
Zhi Gan Cao *Radix Glycyrrhizae uralensis preparata* 5 g
Sheng Jiang *Rhizoma Zingiberis recens* 9 g
Da Zao *Fructus Jujubae* 4 dates

XIAO FENG SAN from Imperial Grace Formulary

Eliminating Wind Powder from Imperial Grace Formulary
Jing Jie *Herba Schizonepetae* 6 g
Bo He *Herba Menthae haplocalycis* 6 g
Qiang Huo *Rhizoma seu Radix Notopterygii* 6 g
Fang Feng *Radix Saposhnikoviae* 6 g
Chuan Xiong *Rhizoma Chuanxiong* 6 g
Chan Tui *Periostracum Cicadae* 6 g
Jiang Can *Bombyx batryticatus* 6 g
Fu Ling *Poria* 6 g
Chen Pi *Pericarpium Citri reticulatae* 3 g
Hou Po *Cortex Magnoliae officinalis* 3 g
Ren Shen *Radix Ginseng* 6 g

XIAO YAO SAN

Free and Easy Wanderer Powder
Bo He *Herba Menthae haplocalycis* 3 g
Chai Hu *Radix Bupleuri* 9 g
Dang Gui *Radix Angelicae sinensis* 9 g
Bai Shao *Radix Paeoniae alba* 12 g
Bai Zhu *Rhizoma Atractylodis macrocephalae* 9 g
Fu Ling *Poria* 15 g
Gan Cao *Radix Glycyrrhizae uralensis* 6 g
Sheng Jiang *Rhizoma Zingiberis recens* 3 slices

XIE GAN AN SHEN WAN

Draining the Liver and Calming the Mind Pill
Long Dan Cao *Radix Gentianae* 9 g
Shan Zhi Zi *Fructus Gardeniae* 6 g
Huang Qin *Radix Scutellariae* 6 g
Bai Ji Li *Fructus Tribuli* 4 g
Shi Jue Ming *Concha Haliotidis* 12 g
Ze Xie *Rhizoma Alismatis* 6 g
Che Qian Zi *Semen Plantaginis* 6 g

Dang Gui *Radix Angelicae sinensis* 6 g
Sheng Di Huang *Radix Rehmanniae* 9 g
Mai Men Dong *Radix Ophiopogonis* 6 g
Zhen Zhu Mu *Concha Margaritiferae usta* 12 g
Long Gu *Mastodi Ossis fossilia* 12 g
Mu Li *Concha Ostreae* 12 g
Fu Shen *Sclerotium Poriae cocos pararadicis* 6 g
Yuan Zhi *Radix Polygalae* 6 g
Bai Zi Ren *Semen Platycladi* 6 g
Suan Zao Ren *Semen Ziziphi spinosae* 6 g
Gan Cao *Radix Glycyrrhizae uralensis* 3 g

XIE QING WAN

Draining the Green Pill
Fang Feng *Radix Saposhnikoviae* 6 g
Qiang Huo *Rhizoma seu Radix Notopterygii* 6 g
Chuan Xiong *Rhizoma Chuanxiong* 6 g
Dang Gui *Radix Angelicae sinensis* 6 g
Long Dan Cao *Radix Gentianae* 9 g
Shan Zhi Zi *Fructus Gardeniae* 6 g
Da Huang *Radix et Rhizoma Rhei* 6 g

XIE QING WAN Variation (Chapter 18, Insomnia, Liver-Fire)

Draining the Green Pill Variation
Dang Gui *Radix Angelicae sinensis* 10 g
Long Dan Cao *Radix Gentianae* 12 g
Chuan Xiong *Rhizoma Chuanxiong* 5 g
Huang Qin *Radix Scutellariae* 10 g
Shan Zhi Zi *Fructus Gardeniae* 9 g
Da Huang *Radix et Rhizoma Rhei* 6 g
Fang Feng *Radix Saposhnikoviae* 3 g
Chai Hu *Radix Bupleuri* 3 g
Gan Cao *Radix Glycyrrhizae uralensis* 6 g

XIE XIN TANG

Draining the Heart Decoction
Da Huang *Radix et Rhizoma Rhei* 9 g
Huang Lian *Rhizoma Coptidis* 6 g
Huang Qin *Radix Scutellariae* 9 g

XIE XIN TANG Variation (Chapter 19, Bipolar disorder, *Kuang*, Phlegm-Fire harassing upwards)

Draining the Heart Decoction Variation
Da Huang *Radix et Rhizoma Rhei* 10 g
Huang Qin *Radix Scutellariae* 10 g
Huang Lian *Rhizoma Coptidis* 10g
Sheng Tie Luo *Frusta Ferri* 9 g
Zhi Mu *Radix Anemarrhaenae* 9 g

XUAN FU DAI ZHE TANG

Inula-Hematitum Decoction
Xuan Fu Hua *Flos Inulae* 9 g
Dai Zhe Shi *Hematitum* 9 g
Ban Xia *Rhizoma Pinelliae preparatum* 9 g
Sheng Jiang *Rhizoma Zingiberis recens* 6 g
Ren Shen *Radix Ginseng* 6 g
Zhi Gan Cao *Radix Glycyrrhizae uralensis preparata* 3 g
Da Zao *Fructus Jujubae* 4 dates

XUE FU ZHU YU TANG

Blood Mansion Eliminating Stasis Decoction
Dang Gui *Radix Angelicae sinensis* 9 g
Sheng Di Huang *Radix Rehmanniae* 9 g
Chi Shao *Radix Paeoniae rubra* 6 g
Chuan Xiong *Rhizoma Chuanxiong* 5 g
Tao Ren *Semen Persicae* 12 g
Hong Hua *Flos Carthami tinctorii* 9 g
Chai Hu *Radix Bupleuri* 3 g
Zhi Ke *Fructus Aurantii* 6 g
Huai Niu Xi *Radix Achyranthis bidentatae* 9 g
Jie Geng *Radix Platycodi* 5 g
Gan Cao *Radix Glycyrrhizae uralensis* 3 g

XUE FU ZHU YU TANG Variation (Chapter 18, Insomnia, Heart-Blood stasis)

Blood Mansion Eliminating Stasis Decoction Variation
Dang Gui *Radix Angelicae sinensis* 9 g
Sheng Di Huang *Radix Rehmanniae* 9 g
Chi Shao *Radix Paeoniae rubra* 6 g
Chuan Xiong *Rhizoma Chuanxiong* 5 g
Tao Ren *Semen Persicae* 12 g
Hong Hua *Flos Carthami tinctorii* 9 g
Chai Hu *Radix Bupleuri* 3 g
Zhi Ke *Fructus Aurantii* 6 g
Niu Xi *Radix Achyranthis bidentatae* 9 g
Jie Geng *Radix Platycodi* 5 g
Ye Jiao Teng *Caulis Polygoni multiflori* 9 g
Suan Zao Ren *Semen Ziziphi spinosae* 6 g
Gan Cao *Radix Glycyrrhizae uralensis* 3 g

XUE YU TANG

Blood Stagnation Decoction
Xiang Fu *Rhizoma Cyperi* 9 g
Mu Dan Pi *Cortex Moutan* 9 g
Su Mu *Lignum Sappan* 6 g
Shan Zha *Fructus Crataegi* 6 g
Tao Ren *Semen Persicae* 6 g
Shen Qu *Massa medicata fermentata* 6 g
Chuan Shan Jia *Squama Manitis Pentadactylae* 6 g
Chen Xiang *Lignum Aquilariae resinatum* 6 g
Tong Cao *Medulla Tetrapanacis* 3 g
Mai Ya *Fructus Hordei germinatus* 6 g

YANG XIN JIAN PI TANG

Nourishing the Heart and Strengthening the Spleen Decoction
Huang Qi *Radix Astragali* 6 g
Suan Zao Ren *Semen Ziziphi spinosae* 6 g
Bai Zi Ren *Semen Platycladi* 6 g
YE Jiao Teng *Caulis Polygoni multiflori* 6 g
He Huan Pi *Cortex Albiziae* 6 g
Wu Wei Zi *Fructus Schisandrae* 6 g
Long Gu *Mastodi Ossis fossilia* 9 g
Mu Li *Concha Ostreae* 9 g
Gui Zhi *Ramulus Cinnamomi cassiae* 4 g
Gan Cao *Radix Glycyrrhizae uralensis* 3 g
Shi Chang Pu *Rhizoma Acori tatarinowii* 6 g
Yuan Zhi *Radix Polygalae* 6 g

YANG XIN TANG (I)

Nourishing the Heart Decoction
Ren Shen *Radix Ginseng* 6 g
Huang Qi *Radix Astragali* 9 g
Fu Ling *Poria* 6 g
Zhi Gan Cao *Radix Glycyrrhizae uralensis preparata* 4.5 g
Dang Gui *Radix Angelicae sinensis* 6 g
Chuan Xiong *Rhizoma Chuanxiong* 4.5 g
Wu Wei Zi *Fructus Schisandrae* 4.5 g
Bai Zi Ren *Semen Platycladi* 6 g
Suan Zao Ren *Semen Ziziphi spinosae* 4.5 g
Yuan Zhi *Radix Polygalae* 6 g
Rou Gui *Cortex Cinnamomi* 1.5 g
Ban Xia *Rhizoma Pinelliae preparatum* 4.5 g

YANG XIN TANG (II)

Nourishing the Heart Decoction
Huang Qi *Radix Astragali* 6 g
Ren Shen *Radix Ginseng* 6 g
Bai Zi Ren *Semen Platycladi* 9 g
Fu Shen *Sclerotium Poriae cocos pararadicis* 6 g
Chuan Xiong *Rhizoma Chuanxiong* 3 g
Yuan Zhi *Radix Polygalae* 6 g
Mai Men Dong *Radix Ophiopogonis* 6 g
Wu Wei Zi *Fructus Schisandrae* 6 g
Zhi Gan Cao *Radix Glycyrrhizae uralensis preparata* 3 g
Sheng Jiang *Rhizoma Zingiberis recens* 1 slice

YI LU KANG JIAO NANG

Relieving Depression and Worry Capsule
Chen Xiang *Lignum Aquilariae resinatum* 6 g
Mu Xiang *Radix Aucklandiae* 6 g
Fo Shou *Fructus Citri sarcodactylis* 6 g
Shan Yao *Rhizoma Dioscoreae* 6 g
Shi Chang Pu *Rhizoma Acori tatarinowii* 6 g
Niu Huang *Calculus Bovis* 3 g
Zhu Sha *Cinnabaris* 2 g
Hu Po *Succinum* 6 g
Yu Jin *Radix Curcumae* 6 g
Chai Hu *Radix Bupleuri* 3 g
Suan Zao Ren *Semen Ziziphi spinosae* 6 g
Yuan Zhi *Radix Polygalae* 6 g

YI SHEN NING

Benefiting the Tranquillity of the Spirit Formula
Chai Hu *Radix Bupleuri* 6 g
Long Gu *Mastodi Ossis fossilia* 30 g
Mu Li *Concha Ostreae* 30 g
Da Huang *Radix et Rhizoma Rhei* 9 g
Huang Qi *Radix Astragali* 9 g
Gui Zhi *Ramulus Cinnamomi cassiae* 9 g
Ban Xia *Rhizoma Pinelliae preparatum* 9 g
Zhi Gan Cao *Radix Glycyrrhizae uralensis preparata* 3 g

YIN MEI TANG

Attracting Sleep Decoction
Bai Shao *Radix Paeoniae alba* 30 g
Dang Gui *Radix Angelicae sinensis* 15 g

Long Chi *Fossilia Dentis Mastodi* 6 g
Tu Si Zi *Semen Cuscutae* 9 g
Mai Men Dong *Radix Ophiopogonis* 15 g
Bai Zi Ren *Semen Platycladi* 6 g
Suan Zao Ren *Semen Ziziphi spinosae* 9 g
Fu Shen *Sclerotium Poriae cocos pararadicis* 9 g

YIN MEI TANG Variation (Chapter 20, Night Terrors, Liver- and Heart-Yin deficiency)

Attracting Sleep Decoction Variation
Bai Shao *Radix Paeoniae alba* 30 g
Dang Gui *Radix Angelicae sinensis* 15 g
Long Chi *Fossilia Dentis Mastodi* 6 g
Tu Si Zi *Semen Cuscutae* 9 g
Mai Men Dong *Radix Ophiopogonis* 15 g
Bai Zi Ren *Semen Platycladi* 6 g
Suan Zao Ren *Semen Ziziphi spinosae* 9 g
Fu Shen *Sclerotium Poriae cocos pararadicis* 9 g
Mu Li *Concha Ostreae* 15 g

YOU GUI WAN

Restoring the Right [Kidney] *Pill*
Fu Zi *Radix Aconiti lateralis preparata* 3 g
Rou Gui *Cortex Cinnamomi* 3 g
Du Zhong *Cortex Eucommiae ulmoidis* 6 g
Shan Zhu Yu *Fructus Corni* 4.5 g
Tu Si Zi *Semen Cuscutae* 6 g
Lu Jiao Jiao *Gelatinum Cornu Cervi* 6 g
Shu Di Huang *Radix Rehmanniae preparata* 12 g
Shan Yao *Rhizoma Dioscoreae* 6 g
Gou Qi Zi *Fructus Lycii chinensis* 6 g
Dang Gui *Radix Angelicae sinensis* 4.5 g

YOU GUI YIN

Restoring the Right [Kidney] *Decoction*
Shu Di Huang *Radix Rehmanniae preparata* 15 g
Shan Zhu Yu *Fructus Corni* 3 g
Shan Yao *Rhizoma Dioscoreae* 6 g
Du Zhong *Cortex Eucommiae ulmoidis* 6 g
Rou Gui *Cortex Cinnamomi* 3 g
Fu Zi *Radix Aconiti lateralis preparata* 3 g
Gou Qi Zi *Fructus Lycii chinensis* 6 g
Zhi Gan Cao *Radix Glycyrrhizae uralensis preparata* 3 g

YUAN ZHI WAN

Polygala Pill
Yuan Zhi *Radix Polygalae* 9 g
Mai Men Dong *Radix Ophiopogonis* 6 g
Chi Shi Zhi *Halloysitum rubrum* 9 g
Shu Di Huang *Radix Rehmanniae preparata* 9 g
Ren Shen *Radix Ginseng* 6 g
Fu Shen *Sclerotium Poriae cocos pararadicis* 6 g
Bai Zhu *Radix Rehmanniae preparata* 6 g
Gan Cao *Radix Glycyrrhizae uralensis* 3 g

YUE JU WAN

Gardenia-Chuanxiong Pill
Cang Zhu *Rhizoma Atractylodis* 6 g
Chuan Xiong *Rhizoma Chuanxiong* 6 g
Xiang Fu *Rhizoma Cyperi* 6 g
Shan Zhi Zi *Fructus Gardeniae* 6 g
Shen Qu *Massa medicata fermentata* 6 g

YUE JU WAN plus SI NI SAN Variation (Chapter 18, Insomnia, Liver-Qi stagnation)

Gardenia-Chuanxiong Pill plus *Four Rebellious Powder* Variation
Xiang Fu *Rhizoma Cyperi* 10 g
Chai Hu *Radix Bupleuri* 9 g
Shen Qu *Massa medicata fermentata* 10 g
Shan Zhi Zi *Fructus Gardeniae* 6 g
Bai Shao *Radix Paeoniae alba* 10 g
Chuan Xiong *Rhizoma Chuanxiong* 6 g
Zhi Ke *Fructus Aurantii* 6 g
Ban Xia *Rhizoma Pinelliae preparatum* 6 g
Gan Cao *Radix Glycyrrhizae uralensis* 6 g

ZHEN ZHONG DAN

Bedside Pill
Gui Ban *Plastrum Testudinis* 10 g
Long Gu *Mastodi Ossis fossilia* 10 g
Yuan Zhi *Radix Polygalae* 10 g
Shi Chang Pu *Rhizoma Acori tatarinowii* 10 g

ZHEN ZHU MU WAN

Concha Margaritiferae Pill
Zhen Zhu Mu *Concha Margaritiferae usta* 30 g
Long Chi *Fossilia Dentis Mastodi* 18 g

Chen Xiang *Lignum Aquilariae resinatum* 3 g
Zhu Sha *Cinnabaris* 1.5 g
Shu Di Huang *Radix Rehmanniae preparata* 12 g
Dang Gui *Radix Angelicae sinensis* 6 g
Ren Shen *Radix Ginseng* 6 g
Suan Zao Ren *Semen Ziziphi spinosae* 6 g
Bai Zi Ren *Semen Platycladi* 6 g
Fu Shen *Sclerotium Poriae cocos pararadicis* 6 g
Shui Niu Jiao *Cornu Bubali* 6 g

ZHI SHI DAO ZHI WAN

Aurantium Eliminating Stagnation Pill
Da Huang *Radix et Rhizoma Rhei* 15 g
Zhi Shi *Fructus Aurantii immaturus* 12 g
Huang Lian *Rhizoma Coptidis* 6 g
Huang Qin *Radix Scutellariae* 6 g
Fu Ling *Poria* 6 g
Ze Xie *Rhizoma Alismatis* 6 g
Bai Zhu *Rhizoma Atractylodis macrocephalae* 6 g
Shen Qu *Massa medicata fermentata* 12 g

ZHI ZI CHI TANG

Gardenia-Soja Decoction
Shan Zhi Zi *Fructus Gardeniae* 9 g
Dan Dou Chi *Semen Sojae preparatum* 9 g

ZHU SHA AN SHEN WAN

Cinnabar Calming the Mind Pill
Huang Lian *Rhizoma Coptidis* 3 g
Sheng Di Huang *Radix Rehmanniae* 12 g
Dang Gui *Radix Angelicae sinensis* 6 g
Fu Ling *Poria* 6 g
Suan Zao Ren *Semen Ziziphi spinosae* 6 g
Zhu Sha *Cinnabaris* 3 g
Yuan Zhi *Radix Polygalae* 6 g
Gan Cao *Radix Glycyrrhizae uralensis* 3 g

ZHU YE SHI GAO TANG

Phyllostachys Gipsum Decoction
Zhu Ye *Folium Phyllostachys nigrae* 15 g
Shi Gao *Gypsum fibrosum* 30 g
Ban Xia *Rhizoma Pinelliae preparatum* 9 g
Mai Men Dong *Radix Ophiopogonis* 15 g
Ren Shen *Radix Ginseng* 5 g
Gan Cao *Radix Glycyrrhizae uralensis* 3 g
Geng Mi *Semen Oryzae sativae* 15 g

ZI SHUI QING GAN YIN

Nourishing Water and Clearing the Liver Decoction
Sheng Di Huang *Radix Rehmanniae* 6 g
Shan Zhu Yu *Fructus Corni* 6 g
Shan Yao *Rhizoma Dioscoreae* 6 g
Fu Ling *Poria* 6 g
Mu Dan Pi *Cortex Moutan* 6 g
Ze Xie *Rhizoma Alismatis* 6 g
Dang Gui *Radix Angelicae sinensis* 6 g
Bai Shao *Radix Paeoniae alba* 6 g
Chai Hu *Radix Bupleuri* 6 g
Shan Zhi Zi *Fructus Gardeniae* 6 g
Suan Zao Ren *Semen Ziziphi spinosae* 6 g

ZUO GUI WAN

Restoring the Left [Kidney] *Pill*
Shu Di Huang *Radix Rehmanniae preparata* 15 g
Shan Yao *Rhizoma Dioscoreae* 9 g
Shan Zhu Yu *Fructus Corni* 9 g
Gou Qi Zi *Fructus Lycii chinensis* 9 g
Chuan Niu Xi *Radix Cyathulae* 6 g
Tu Si Zi *Semen Cuscutae* 9 g
Lu Jiao *Cornu Cervi* 9 g
Gui Ban Jiao *Colla Plastri Testudinis* 9 g

ZUO GUI WAN Variation (Chapter 18, Insomnia, Liver- and Kidney-Yin deficiency)

Restoring the Left [Kidney] *Pill* Variation
Shu Di Huang *Radix Rehmanniae preparata* 15 g
Shan Yao *Rhizoma Dioscoreae* 9 g
Shan Zhu Yu *Fructus Corni* 9 g
Gou Qi Zi *Fructus Lycii chinensis* 9 g
Chuan Niu Xi *Radix Cyathulae* 6 g
Tu Si Zi *Semen Cuscutae* 9 g
Lu Jiao *Cornu Cervi* 9 g
Gui Ban Jiao *Colla Plastri Testudinis* 9 g
Ye Jiao Teng *Caulis Polygoni multiflori* 9 g
Suan Zao Ren *Semen Ziziphi spinosae* 9 g

ZUO GUI YIN

Restore the Left [Kidney] *Decoction*
Shu Di Huang *Radix Rehmanniae preparata* 12 g
Shan Zhu Yu *Fructus Corni* 6 g

Gou Qi Zi *Fructus Lycii chinensis* 6 g
Shan Yao *Rhizoma Dioscoreae* 6 g
Fu Ling *Poria* 6 g
Zhi Gan Cao *Radix Glycyrrhizae uralensis preparata* 3 g

ZUO JIN WAN

Left Metal Pill
Huang Lian *Rhizoma Coptidis* 15 g
Wu Zhu Yu *Fructus Evodiae* 2 g

EMPIRICAL PRESCRIPTIONS

EMPIRICAL PRESCRIPTION by Dr Chen Jia Xu (Chapter 3, The Ethereal Soul)

Huang Qi *Radix Astragali* 6 g
Dang Shen *Radix Codonopsis* 6 g
Bai Zhu *Rhizoma Atractylodis macrocephalae* 6 g
Dang Gui *Radix Angelicae sinensis* 9 g
Chai Hu *Radix Bupleuri* 3 g
Gui Zhi *Ramulus Cinnamomi cassiae* 4 g
Fu Ling *Sclerotium Poriae cocos* 6 g
Bai Shao *Radix Paeoniae alba* 9 g
Wu Wei Zi *Fructus Schisandrae* 3 g
Bai Zi Ren *Semen Platycladi* 6 g
Zhi Gan Cao *Radix Glycyrrhizae uralensis preparata* 3 g

END NOTE

1. Please note that the dosages indicated are to make a batch of pills.

APPENDIX 2

SUGGESTED SUBSTITUTIONS OF CHINESE HERBS

The following is a partial list of suggested substitutions for Chinese herbs that are forbidden to use in Western countries. This may be because they are animal or mineral substances, because they are toxic or because they come from protected species.

Please note that some herbs may be banned in certain countries and not in others. Please note also that certain Chinese herbs are wrongly thought to be toxic and their inclusion in this list does not signify my agreement with such a view. Indeed, in some cases, some herbs (e.g. Fang Ji Radix *Stephaniae tetrandrae*) are banned not because they are toxic but because of the possibility of wrong identification of the herb. In fact, (Han) Fang Ji Radix *Stephaniae tetrandrae* is not toxic but, because when ordering it may be substituted with (Guang) Fang Ji *Radix Aristolochiae Fangchi* which is potentially toxic, (Han) Fang Ji is also banned.

Many Chinese herbs have of course more than one action and it is therefore impossible to recommend a single substitution in such cases. For example, Chuan Shan Jia *Squama Manitis Pentadactylae* may be used to invigorate Blood or to soften masses. In some cases, a herb cannot be substituted by a single herb and it needs two herbs to replicate the action of the herb being substituted.

Toxicity issues

- **Fang Ji** *Radix Stephaniae tetrandrae* (see above)
- **Fu Zi** *Radix Aconiti lateralis preparata*
- **Huang Yao Zi** *Radix Dioscoreae bulbiferae*
- **Mu Tong** *Caulis Akebiae trifoliatae*

Animal products

- **Bie Jia** *Carapax Trionycis*
- **Chuan Shan Jia** *Squama Manitis Pentadactylae*
- **Gui Ban** *Plastrum Testudinis*
- **Long Chi** *Fossilia Dentis Mastodi*
- **Long Gu** *Mastodi Ossis fossilia*
- **She Xiang** *Moschus*
- **Xi Jiao** *Cornu Rhinoceri*

Mineral products

- **Ci Shi** *Magnetitum*
- **Mu Li** *Concha Ostreae*
- **Shi Jue Ming** *Concha Haliotidis*
- **Zhen Zhu Mu** *Concha Margaritifera usta*

Protected species issues

- **Bai Ji** *Rhizoma Bletillae*
- **Gou Ji** *Rhizoma Cibotii*
- **Shi Hu** *Herba Dendrobii*
- **Tian Ma** *Rhizoma Gastrodiae*

Table App. 2.1 lists the above herbs and their substitutions in the same order as above.

Table App 2.1 Herbal substitutions

HERB	SUBSTITUTION ACTION 1	SUBSTITUTION ACTION 2
FANG JI *Radix Stephaniae tetrandrae*	Fu Ling *Poria* with Huang Bo *Cortex Phellodendri* (to resolve Damp Heat in the Lower Burner)	Yi Yi Ren *Semen Coicis* with Cang Zhu *Rhizoma Atractylodis* (to resolve Dampness and remove obstructions from the channels in Painful Obstruction (*Bi*) Syndrome)
FU ZI *Radix Aconiti lateralis preparata*	Rou Gui *Cortex Cinnamomi* (to tonify Yang and the Fire of the Gate of Life)	Gui Zhi *Ramulus Cinnamomi cassiae* (to warm the channels in Painful Obstruction Syndrome)
HUANG YAO ZI *Radix Dioscoreae bulbiferae*	Ban Xia *Rhizoma Pinelliae preparatum* with Bai Hua She She Cao *Herba Hedyotidis diffusae*	
MU TONG *Caulis Akebiae trifoliatae*	Tong Cao *Medulla Tetrapanacis* (to remove obstructions from the Connecting channels)	Fu Ling *Poria* with Huang Bo *Cortex Phellodendri* (to resolve Damp Heat)
BIE JIA *Carapax Trionycis*	Huang Jing *Rhizoma Polygonati* with Gou Qi Zi *Fructus Lycii chinensis* (to nourish Yin)	Yi Yi Ren *Semen Coicis* (to soften masses)
CHUAN SHAN JIA *Squama Manitis Pentadactylae*	Wang Bu Liu Xing *Semen Vaccariae* (to invigorate Blood)	Yi Yi Ren *Semen Coicis* (to soften masses)
GUI BAN *Plastrum Testudinis*	Huang Jing *Rhizoma Polygonati* with Gou Qi Zi *Fructus Lycii chinensis*	
LONG CHI *Fossilia Dentis Mastodi*	Suan Zao Ren *Semen Ziziphi spinosae*	
LONG GU *Mastodi Ossis fossilia*	Suan Zao Ren *Semen Ziziphi spinosae* (to calm the Mind)	Yi Yi Ren *Semen Coicis* (to soften masses)
SHE XIANG *Moschus*	Shi Chang Pu *Rhizoma Acori tatarinowii*	
XI JIAO *Cornu Rhinoceri*	Shui Niu Jiao *Cornu Bubali*	
CI SHI *Magnetitum*	Suan Zao Ren *Semen Ziziphi spinosae*	
MU LI *Concha Ostreae*	Suan Zao Ren *Semen Ziziphi spinosae* (to calm the Mind)	Yi Yi Ren *Semen Coicis* (to soften masses)
SHI JUE MING *Concha Haliotidis*	Gou Teng *Ramulus cum Uncis Uncariae*	
ZHEN ZHU MU *Concha Margaritifera usta*	Gou Teng *Ramulus cum Uncis Uncariae* (to subdue Liver-Yang)	Suan Zao Ren *Semen Ziziphi spinosae* (to calm the Mind)
BAI JI *Rhizoma Bletillae*	Xian He Cao *Herba Agrimoniae*	
GOU JI *Rhizoma Cibotii*	Du Zhong *Cortex Eucommiae ulmoidis*	
SHI HU *Herba Dendrobii*	Yu Zhu *Rhizoma Polygonati odorati*	
TIAN MA *Rhizoma Gastrodiae*	Gou Teng *Ramulus cum Uncis Uncariae*	

APPENDIX 3

THE CLASSICS OF CHINESE MEDICINE

The following is a brief description of the classics of Chinese medicine that I mention most frequently. As I mention some of the classics extensively, it might help the reader to see these in their historical context. This is not a comprehensive list of the classics of Chinese medicine (which would have to be much longer), but simply of those that I mention most frequently. For each classic, I also give the reasons why I mention them frequently and what they add to our clinical practice in the 21st century.

The Yellow Emperor's Classic of Internal Medicine (between 300 and 100 BC, Warring States period, Qin and Han dynasties)

Huang Di Nei Jing

The authorship and date of the *Yellow Emperor's Classic of Internal Medicine* is the subject of intense conjecture. The best source for a discussion of the authorship and date of this classic is Unschuld's *Huang Di Nei Jing Su Wen: Nature, Knowledge, Imagery in an Ancient Chinese Medical Text.*[1]

What is certain is that the *Yellow Emperor's Classic of Internal Medicine* was written between 300 and 100 BC and that it was changed by many different authors over the centuries. My Chinese teachers in Nanjing thought that this classic could not be older than the times of Zou Yan (*c.*350–270 BC), who was the formulator of the main theory of the Five Elements.

That this classic received contributions and changes by many different authors is obvious from the variety of subjects treated and, most of all, by the apparent lack of coordination among subjects. What is also generally accepted is that the bulk of the text we use nowadays was compiled by Wang Bing during the Tang dynasty (AD 762).

The *Yellow Emperor's Classic of Internal Medicine* consists of two parts, each of 81 chapters: the *Simple Questions* (*Su Wen*) and the *Spiritual Axis* (*Ling Shu*). Generally speaking, the *Simple Questions* deals more with the general theory of Chinese medicine, while the *Spiritual Axis* is mostly about acupuncture.

The importance of the *Yellow Emperor's Classic of Internal Medicine* in the history of Chinese medicine cannot be overemphasized. It is the earliest source of physiology, pathology, diagnosis and treatment in Chinese medicine. Besides medicine, this classic also contains theories of meteorology, astrology and calendar. The following is a partial list of the main topics of significance of the *Yellow Emperor's Classic of Internal Medicine*.

1. It established a systematic theory of the channels.
2. It deals in depth with the theories of Yin-Yang and the Five Elements.
3. It discusses the nature and origin of different types of Qi.
4. It describes the physiology and pathology of the Internal Organs.
5. It determines the location of 160 acupuncture points and their names.
6. It describes the various types of needles and their use.
7. It defines the function of the acupuncture points and their contraindications.
8. It discusses many needling techniques, including the reinforcing and reducing methods.
9. It describes the diagnosis, identification of patterns and treatment of many diseases.

From a philosophical point of view, it is clear that the *Yellow Emperor's Classic of Internal Medicine* was influenced by several different philosophical trends that arose during the Warring States period (475–221 BC). In particular, this classic shows the influence of the Confucian, Daoist, Legalist and Naturalist schools of thought. The influence of these schools of thought has been described in Chapter 15.

The influence of the Naturalist School (called "School of Yin-Yang") is manifested throughout this classic because the theory of Yin-Yang and the Five Elements pervades the whole book.

The influence of the Daoist school of thought is evident in the frequent discussion of the ways or "nourishing life" (*yang sheng*), i.e. advice on breathing, exercises, diet and lifestyle to prolong life and avoid disease.

The influence of the Confucian school is manifested by the conception of the Internal Organs as ministers of a government, and has been discussed at length in Chapter 15. The political views of Confucianism are very much reflected in Chinese medicine where the Internal Organs are compared to government officials with an emperor in the form of the Heart. Each internal organ is compared to a minister and health depends on good "governance" by the Internal Organs. Ill health is not so much a medical problem as an ethical problem stemming from not abiding by the rules of behavior.

Finally, the *Yellow Emperor's Classic of Internal Medicine* bears the imprint also of the Legalist School. The Legalist School was called the School of Law in ancient China. This school of thought flourished during the Warring States period and it prevailed during the Qin dynasty (221–206 BC), a brief dynasty started by the first emperor Qin Shi Huang Di who enthusiastically adopted the principles of government advocated by the Legalist School.

The state of Qin in Western China was the first to adopt Legalist doctrines. The Qin were so successful that by 221 BC they had conquered the other Chinese states and unified the empire after centuries of war. Legalist ideas on human nature, society and government could not be further from those of Confucius; the Legalists thought that human nature is essentially unruly, and that order in society can be kept only by strict laws and harsh punishments, not through ethical behavior as the Confucianists thought.

What is interesting about the Legalist school from the Chinese medicine point of view is the fact that the Qin dynasty (which adopted Legalist ideas) was the first to unify China. They established irrigation, unified weights, coins, Chinese script, measures and other things such as the gauge of wheel axles throughout China. The first Qin emperor also initiated a huge program of road building and canal digging. Another important innovation of the Qin dynasty was the fostering of trade among various regions of China on a huge scale.

The Qin dynasty therefore provided the first model of a unified state with an emperor, a central government, a unified economy, local officials and a state-wide irrigation system. This provided the first metaphor of Chinese medicine in which the Heart is the emperor, the other Internal Organs are the officials and the acupuncture channels are the irrigation canals.

One can see an influence of the Legalist school also in the therapeutic approach of the *Yellow Emperor's Classic of Internal Medicine*, i.e. just as human nature cannot be relied upon and must be "straightened" with strict laws and harsh punishments, the body's Qi must be regulated by attacking pathogenic factors decisively and by making sure that the "ruler" and officials do their jobs properly.

The Classic of Difficulties (*c.*100 BC, Han dynasty)

Nan Jing

The *Nan Jing* was written in approximately 100 BC by Qin Yue Ren who used as a pseudonym the name of an ancient, mythical doctor called Bian Que. However, like the *Nei Jing*, the date of compilation of the *Nan Jing* is a subject of controversy. Its date is put by some authors as late as AD 600. The best discussion of the origin of the *Nan Jing* is in Unschuld's *Nan-ching – The Classic of Difficult Issues*.[2]

The *Nan Jing* is a gem of a book; in its Chinese edition, a very thin and small book full of clinical insights. The attraction of the book for me is that, unlike the *Nei Jing*, it clearly seems to have been written by one author because there is quite a logical progression among chapters.

The *Nan Jing* consists of 81 short chapters. The importance of the *Nan Jing* in the history of Chinese medicine cannot be overestimated. For example, the *Nan Jing* was the first text to advocate taking the pulse at the radial artery; previously the pulse was taken in nine different positions of the body on the arms, legs and neck. This classic was also the first to develop the theory of the Original Qi (*Yuan Qi*) and the role of the Triple Burner in relation to it.

The following is a partial list of the reasons for the importance of the *Nan Jing*.

1. It added to the knowledge of the eight extraordinary vessels compared to that of the *Nei Jing*.
2. It developed the theory of the five Transporting (*Shu*) points further than what is discussed in the *Nei Jing*.
3. It put forward for the first time the technique of reinforcing and reducing points according to the Mother–Child relationships within the Five-Element theory (e.g. that the Wood point tonifies the Heart channel because it pertains to Wood, the Heart pertains to Fire and Wood is the Mother of Fire).
4. It established the practice of feeling the pulse at the radial artery.
5. It developed the theory of the Original Qi (*Yuan Qi*) and Gate of Life (*Ming Men*).

Essential Prescriptions of the Golden Chest (AD 220, Han dynasty)

Jin Gui Yao Lue

Written by Zhang Zhong Jing, this is a classic I also quote frequently. In the field of mental-emotional problems, it is the source of three important formulae: Ban Xia Hou Po Tang *Pinellia-Magnolia Decoction*, Gan Mai Da Zao Tang *Glycyrrhiza-Triticum-Jujuba Decoction* and Bai He Tang *Lilium Decoction*.

The Pulse Classic (AD 280, Three Kingdoms period)

Mai Jing

Written by Wang Shu He, *The Pulse Classic* is very important in the development of pulse diagnosis. This classic consolidated and further developed the assignment of the three pulse positions to organs, first done by the *Nan Jing*. *The Pulse Classic* describes 24 pulse qualities and their clinical significance systematically.

Discussion of the Origin of Symptoms in Diseases (AD 610, Sui dynasty)

Zhu Bing Yuan Hou Lun

Written by Chao Yuan Fang, this book is one of the first books describing the symptoms, patterns and treatment of diseases systematically. I consult this book when researching the pathology and treatment of a particular condition.

Thousand Golden Ducats Prescriptions (AD 652, Tang dynasty)

Qian Jin Yao Fang

Written by Sun Si Miao, this book is one of the few to bear a Buddhist influence. Sun Si Miao was an expert on diet and sexuality. He was one of the first doctors to describe goitre and correctly attribute it to living in mountainous regions (with water deprived of iodine); he correctly prescribed the use of seaweeds to treat this condition.

In my mind, Sun Si Miao is forever linked to the formulation of the prescription Wen Dan Tang *Warming the Gall-Bladder Decoction* which I use extensively in the treatment of mental-emotional conditions.

Discussion on Stomach and Spleen (1249, Song dynasty)

Pi Wei Lun

Written by Li Dong Yuan, the *Discussion on Stomach and Spleen* is a very important classic in the history of Chinese medicine. Li Dong Yuan is the founder of the School of Stomach and Spleen which attributes a central importance to the Stomach and Spleen in pathology and treatment.

In my mind, the importance of this classic lies especially in the formulation of the prescription Bu Zhong Yi Qi Tang *Tonifying the Center and Benefiting Qi Decoction*. This is a very important prescription for many different conditions and, in mental-emotional problems, I use it for depression.

Li Dong Yuan was the first to formulate the theory of "Yin Fire", a condition characterized by Heat above deriving from a deficiency of the Stomach and Spleen and of the Original Qi (*Yuan Qi*). In my opinion, Yin Fire is a common pathology in many modern Western diseases such as chronic fatigue syndrome.

Qi Jing Ba Mai Kao (1578, Ming dynasty)

A Study of the Eight Extraordinary Vessels

Written by Li Shi Zhen, the importance of this book cannot be overemphasized. For anyone who uses the eight extraordinary vessels, this book is a must; it is the first book that describes the pathways of the extraordinary vessels in detail, point by point. It also describes the pathology of rebellious Qi of the Penetrating Vessel (*Chong Mai*) which is so common in practice.

I have consulted and quoted this book extensively when writing the *Channels of Acupuncture*.

A Study of the Pulse by the Pin Hu Lake Master (1578, Ming dynasty)

Pin Hu Mai Xue

Written by Li Shi Zhen, this is another must to understand pulse diagnosis. Li Shi Zhen gives the best description of the pulse qualities and their clinical significance.

Compendium of Acupuncture (1601, Ming dynasty)

Zhen Jiu Da Cheng

Written by Yang Ji Zhou, this book is a must for acupuncturists. It occupies a fundamental place in the acupuncture literature for several reasons.

1. It summarized the acupuncture experience of previous centuries.
2. It describes numerous different needling techniques, many of which are used today.
3. It dealt with internal medicine, gynecology and pediatrics.
4. It has many case histories with point prescriptions.
5. It uses the identification of patterns with point prescriptions.
6. It introduced massage therapy for children.

I have used this book extensively when writing the *Channels of Acupuncture*.

Classic of Categories (1624, Ming dynasty)

Lei Jing

Written by Zhang Jing Yue (also called Zhang Jie Bin), this is a very important book in the history of Chinese medicine. Its importance lies in its discussion of theories from the *Nei Jing* arranged according to topics. It therefore joins together scattered passages from the *Nei Jing* according to topics and diseases.

Jing Yue Quan Shu (1624, Ming dynasty)

Complete Book of Jing Yue

Written by Zhang Jing Yue (also called Zhang Jie Bin), this book discusses the diagnosis, pathology and treatment of many different conditions. Zhang Jing Yue formulated the prescriptions Zuo Gui Wan *Restoring the Left* [Kidney] *Pill* and You Gui Wan *Restoring the Right* [Kidney] *Pill*, which tonify Kidney-Yin and Kidney-Yang, respectively. I personally use these two formulae to tonify the Kidneys much more often than Liu Wei Di Huang Wan *Six Ingredients Rehmannia Pill* and Jin Gui Shen Qi Wan *Golden Chest Kidney-Qi Pill*.

An Explanation of the Acupuncture Points (1654, Qing dynasty)

Jing Xue Jie

Written by Yue Han Zhen, this is not a famous classic but it is a gem of a book that I use extensively to consult the actions and functions of acupuncture points. The book explains the meaning of the points' names and it discusses the actions and functions of points according to the channels affected, which is very useful. I find the book also interesting because it gives the action of the points (e.g. Spleen-12 moves Qi), which many people think is a modern adaptation of Chinese acupuncture.

Yi Zong Jin Jian (1742, Qing dynasty)

Golden Mirror of Medicine

Written by Wu Qian, this book discusses the diagnosis, pathology and treatment of many different diseases in the field of internal medicine, gynecology and pediatrics. It is a mine of information and a book that I consult frequently when writing my books.

Discussion on Blood Patterns (1884, Qing dynasty)

Xue Zheng Lun

Written by Tang Zong Hai, this is an important book for the treatment of bleeding disorders. It formulates the four-pronged approach to the treatment of bleeding.

END NOTES

1. Unschuld P 2003 Huang Di Nei Jing Su Wen: Nature, Knowledge, Imagery in an Ancient Chinese Medical Text. University of California Press, Berkeley.
2. Unschuld P 1986 Nan-ching – The Classic of Difficult Issues. University of California Press, Berkeley.

APPENDIX 4

TERMINOLOGY OF TREATMENT PRINCIPLES

In this Appendix, I will explain the terminology of some of the less usual treatment methods in the field of emotional and mental disturbances. I will not explain the treatment methods that are self-evident, e.g. "Tonify Spleen-Qi" or "nourish Blood". However, I shall also point out some terminology issues with the common treatment methods as well.

Calm the Mind

I use the term "calm the Mind" in a different sense from the traditional one. "Calming the Mind" usually means using formulae from the "Calming the Mind" category. "Calming the Mind" here is a general term that includes the treatment principle of calming the Mind by sinking Qi (such as Chai Hu Long Gu Mu Li Tang *Bupleurum-Mastodi Ossis fossilia-Concha Ostreae Decoction*) or by nourishing the Mind (such as Gui Pi Tang *Tonifying the Spleen Decoction*).

I use the term "calm the Mind" in the more specific sense of allaying anxiety.

Clear Heat

I use the term "clear Heat" for the Chinese term *xie re* 泄热. This specifically consists of the use of formulae with a pungent-cold taste that expels the Heat outward. Heat is energetically more superficial than Fire and it can be expelled outwards with the pungent-cold taste (see "Drain Fire" below).

An example of a formula that clears Heat is Bai Hu Tang *White Tiger Decoction*.

Drain Fire

I use the term "Drain Fire" for the Chinese term *xie huo* 泻火. This specifically consists of the use of formulae with a bitter-cold taste to drain Fire downwards (usually also stimulating the bowel movement). Fire is energetically deeper than Heat and it cannot be expelled outwards with pungent-cold herbs; it can only be drained downwards with bitter-cold herbs.

An example of a formula that drains Fire is Long Dan Xie Gan Tang *Gentiana Draining the Liver Decoction*.

Eliminate stagnation

I use the term "eliminate stagnation" for Qi stagnation (for Blood stasis I use "eliminate stasis").

Invigorate Blood

I use the term "invigorate Blood" in the sense of "moving Blood" (*huo xue* 活血), which literally means "to enliven Blood". I use the term "invigorate Blood" as the treatment principle adopted for Blood stasis.

Lift mood

"Lift mood" is not a traditional treatment method terminology. By "lifting mood" I mean using points that lift mood such as Du-20 Baihui. "Lifting mood" is of course used in depression and I contrast it with the term "calming the Mind' used for anxiety.

Move Qi

"Moving Qi" refers specifically to the use of formulae from the moving Qi category. Every acupuncture point moves Qi.

Nourish Blood

I use the term "nourish Blood" specifically in relation to formulae or points that nourish Blood. This is contrasted with the term "tonify Qi" where I use the term "tonify" for Qi.

Nourish the Heart

I use this term in relation to the treatment method of nourishing Heart-Blood.

Open the chest

I use this term to denote the action of acupuncture points that have an effect on the chest, moving Qi and Blood in this area. This term also implies that it is used when emotional stress is somatized in the chest. Examples of points that open the chest are LU-7 Lieque, P-6 Neiguan, ST-40 Fenglong and KI-9 Zhubin.

Open the Mind's orifices

This term refers to the treatment method of eliminating either Phlegm or Blood stasis from the Mind, thus opening the Heart's orifices. I use the term "open the Mind's orifices" in a specific sense in all cases of Mind Obstructed (see Chapter 12).

Settle the Corporeal Soul

This is not a traditional term for a treatment method. By "settling the Corporeal Soul", I mean using formulae or points that soothe the Lungs and treat emotions that are Lung related, such as grief, sadness and worry. I use this treatment method in Lung patterns accompanied by sadness, grief or worry; for example, LU-7 Lieque and LU-3 Tianfu, or the formula Ban Xia Hou Po Tang *Pinellia-Magnolia Decoction*, settle the Corporeal Soul.

Settle the Ethereal Soul

This is not a traditional treatment principle term. By "settling the Ethereal Soul", I mean using formulae or points that calm the Spirit and make Qi go down, with the effect of restraining the movement of the Ethereal Soul. One example of a formula that settles the Ethereal Soul would be Suan Zao Ren Tang *Ziziphus Decoction*. Examples of points that settle the Ethereal Soul would be LIV-3 Taichong and G.B.-13 Benshen.

Soothe the Liver, move Qi

This basically means to move Liver-Qi and stimulate its free going. In herbal medicine, this means using formulae from the "Moving Qi" category.

Strengthen Will-Power

This is not a traditional treatment principle term. By "strengthening Will-Power", I mean tonifying the Kidneys to strengthen the *Zhi*. Examples of points that strengthen the Will-Power are BL-23 Shenshu and BL-62 Zhishi.

ENGLISH–PINYIN GLOSSARY OF CHINESE TERMS

GENERAL

Ancestral Muscle	***Zong Jin*** 宗筋
Area below the xiphoid process	***Xin xia*** 心下
Cavities and Texture (also space between the skin and muscles)	***Cou Li*** 腠理
Central-lower abdominal area	***Xiao Fu*** 小腹
Center of the Thorax	***Shan Zhong*** 膻中
Conforming Qi	***Shun Qi*** 顺气
Contralateral needling	***Miu Ci*** 缪刺
Cun (acupuncture unit of measurement)	***Cun*** 寸
Deep layer of skin	***Ge*** 革
Diffusing (of Lung-Qi)	***Xuan Fa*** 宣发
Eight Ramparts	***Ba Kuo*** 八廓
Emotion	***Qing*** 情
Eye System	***Mu Xi*** 目系
Exuberant Fire	***Zhuang Huo*** 状火
Fat and Muscles	***Fen Rou*** 分肉
Fat Tissue	***Gao*** 膏
Field of Elixir	***Dan Tian*** 丹田
Five Wheels	***Wu Lun*** 五轮
Great Connecting channel of the Stomach (manifesting in apical pulse)	***Xu Li*** 虚里
Heaven (or Heavenly)	***Tian*** 天
Hypochondrium	***Xie Lei*** 胁肋
Identification of the disease	***Bian Bing*** 辨病
Identification of patterns	***Bian Zheng*** 辨证
Image	***Xiang*** 象
Lateral-lower abdominal area	***Shao Fu*** 少腹
Lesser Fire	***Shao Huo*** 少火
Manifestation	***Biao*** 标
Membranes	***Huang*** 肓
Muscles or flesh	***Rou*** 肉
Opposite needling	***Ju Ci*** 巨刺
Palace of Sperm (or Palace of Essence)	***Jing Gong*** 精宫
Pathogenic factor	***Xie*** 邪
Pathogenic factor	***Xie Qi*** 邪气
Pathways of Qi	***Qi Jie*** 气街
Penis	***Yin Jing*** 阴茎
Pores (including sebaceous glands)	***Xuan Fu*** 玄府
Qi Mechanism	***Qi Ji*** 气机
Rebellious Qi	***Ni Qi*** 逆气
Room of Sperm (or Essence)	***Jing Shi*** 精室
Root	***Ben*** 本
Sinews	***Jin*** 筋
Six Climates	***Liu Qi*** 六气
Six Evils (external pathogenic factors)	***Liu Xie*** 六邪
Six Excesses (excessive climates)	***Liu Yin*** 六淫
Sperm Gate	***Jing Guan*** 精关
"Streets", "avenues", "crossroads" (symbols for channels of the abdomen controlled by the Penetrating Vessel)	***Jie*** 街

Subcutaneous muscles	***Ji*** 肌
Superficial layer of skin	***Fu*** 膚
Transformation and transportation (of the Spleen)	***Yun Hua*** 运化
Uterus	***Zi Bao* (sometimes also called "*Bao*")** 子包
Uterus channel	***Bao Luo*** 胞络
Uterus Vessel	***Bao Mai*** 胞脉

SYMPTOMS AND SIGNS

Accumulation (or nodules)	***Jie*** 结
Alopecia	***Tou Fa Tuo Luo*** 头发脱落
Alternation of chills and fever	***Han Re Wang Lai*** 寒热往来
Anxiety (in the context of rebellious Qi of the Penetrating Vessel)	***Li Ji*** 里急
Aversion to cold	***Wu Han*** 恶寒
Aversion to cold and fever, simultaneous	***Wu Han Fa Re*** 恶寒发热
Aversion to food	***Yan Shi*** 厌食
Aversion to wind	***Wu Feng*** 恶风
Blood masses	***Ji*** 积
Blood masses	***Zheng*** 症
Bluish-greenish (color)	***Qing*** 青
Blurred vision and floaters	***Mu Hua*** 目花
Blurred vision	***Mu Yun*** 目晕
Brain noise	***Nao Ming*** 脑鸣
Breakdown	***Jue*** 厥
Breathlessness	***Chuan*** 喘
Clouded vision	***Mu Hun*** 目昏
Collapse	***Tuo*** 脱
Contraction of the fingers	***Shou Zhi Luan*** 手指挛
Cough	***Ke Sou*** 咳嗽
Deficiency	***Xu*** 虚
Depression	***Yu Zheng*** 郁症
Deviation of eye and mouth	***Kou Yan Wai Xie*** 口眼歪斜
Diarrhea	***Xie Xie*** 泄泻
Difficulty in defecation	***Li Ji Hou Zhong*** 里急后重
Discharge from the eyes	***Yan Chi*** 眼眵
Distension, feeling of	***Zhang*** 胀
Dizziness	***Tou Yun*** 头晕
Dizziness	***Xuan Yun*** 眩晕
Drooping head	***Tou Qing*** 头倾
Eczema	***Shi Zhen*** 湿疹
Edema	***Shui Zhong*** 水肿
Emission of heat, fever	***Fa Re*** 发热
Empty	***Xu*** 虚
Emptiness	***Xu*** 虚
Excess	***Shi*** 实
Fear and palpitations	***Jing Ji*** 惊悸
Fear of cold (in exterior invasions of Wind)	***Wei Han*** 畏寒
Feeling of distension	***Zhang*** 胀
Feeling of fullness	***Man*** 满
Feeling of heaviness	***Zhong*** 重
Feeling of heaviness of the body	***Shen Zhong*** 身重
Feeling of heaviness of the head	***Tou Zhong*** 头重
Feeling of oppression	***Men*** 闷
Feeling of stuffiness	***Pi*** 痞
Five Flaccidities	***Wu Ruan*** 五软
Five Retardations	***Wu Chi*** 五迟
Five-palm heat	***Wu Xin Fa Re*** 五心发热
Floaters	***Mu Hua*** 目花
Fetus' Qi rebelling upwards	***Tai Qi Shang Ni*** 胎气上逆
Four Rebellious	***Si Ni*** 四逆
Full	***Shi*** 实
Full, Fullness, Excess	***Shi*** 实
Fullness, feeling of	***Man*** 满
Gnawing hunger	***Cao Za*** 嘈杂
Graying of the hair	***Tou Fa Bian Bai*** 头发变白
Heart feeling vexed	***Xin Zhong Ao Nong*** 心中懊
Heaviness, feeling of	***Zhong*** 重
Heaviness of the head, feeling of	***Tou Zhong*** 头重
Hemiplegia	***Ban Shen Bu Sui*** 半身不遂
Hemp rash (measles)	***Ma Zhen*** 麻疹
Hiccup	***E Ni*** 呃逆

Hypochondrial pain	***Xie Tong*** 胁痛
Incontinence of urine	***Yi Niao*** 遗尿
Internal urgency	***Li Ji*** 里急
Leg Qi	***Jiao Qi*** 脚气
Long retching with loud sound	***Yue*** 哕
Macule (in tongue diagnosis, red spots)	***Ban*** 斑
Manifestation	***Biao*** 标
Mental restlessness	***Xin Fan*** 心烦
Mental restlessness and agitation (restlessness of limbs)	***Fan Zao*** 烦燥
Milky moth (swollen tonsils)	***Ru E*** 乳蛾
Mouth ulcers	***Kou Chuang*** 口疮
Nausea	***E Xin*** 恶心
Night-sweating	***Dao Han*** 盗汗
"Nose pool" (sinusitis)	***Bi Yuan*** 鼻渊
Numbness and/or tingling	***Ma Mu*** 麻木
Oppression, feeling of	***Men*** 闷
Palpitations	***Xin Ji*** 心悸
Panic throbbing	***Zheng Chong*** 怔忡
Papule	***Qiu Zhen*** 丘疹
Phlegm-Fluids (or Phlegm-Fluids in Stomach and Intestines)	***Tan Yin*** 痰饮
Phlegm-Fluids above the diaphragm	***Zhi Yin*** 支饮
Phlegm-Fluids in the hypochondrium	***Xuan Yin*** 玄饮
Phlegm-Fluids in the limbs	***Yi Yin*** 溢饮
Phlegm Nodules	***Tan He*** 痰核
Pustule	***Nong Pao*** 脓泡
Qi masses	***Jia*** 瘕
Qi masses	***Ju*** 聚
Qi edema	***Qi Zhong*** 气肿
Quivering eyeball	***Mu Chan*** 目颤
Rash	***Zhen*** 疹
Rebellious-Qi breathing	***Shang Qi*** 上气
Regurgitation of food	***Fan Wei*** 反胃
Reverse period	***Ni Jing*** 逆经
Robbing of Qi (very feeble voice with interrupted speech)	***Duo Qi*** 夺气
Seminal emissions	***Yi Jing*** 遗精
Shivers	***Han Zhan*** 寒战
Shiver sweating	***Zhan Han*** 颤汗
Short retching with low sound	***Gan Ou*** 干呕
Shortness of breath	***Duan Qi*** 短气
Stone moth (swollen tonsils)	***Shi E*** 石蛾
Streaming eyes	***Liu Lei*** 流泪
Stuffiness, feeling of	***Pi*** 痞
Sweating from Breakdown	***Jue Han*** 厥汗
Tidal fever	***Hu Re*** 湖热
Toxic Heat	***Re Du*** 热毒
Tremor of the feet	***Zu Chan*** 足颤
Tremor of the hands	***Shou Chan*** 手颤
Vesicle	***Pao*** 泡
Vesicle	***Shui Pao*** 水泡
Vomiting (with sound)	***Ou*** 呕
Vomiting (without sound)	***Tu*** 吐
Vomiting	***Ou Tu*** 呕吐
Water pox (chickenpox)	***Shui Dou*** 水痘
Weak breathing	***Qi Shao*** 气少
Wheal	***Feng Tuan*** 风团
Wheezing	***Xiao*** 哮
Wind hidden rash (urticaria)	***Feng Yin Zhen*** 风阴疹
Wind rash (German measles)	***Feng Zhen*** 风疹

DISEASE-SYMPTOMS

Abdominal masses	***Ji Ju*** 积聚
Abdominal masses (in women)	***Zheng Jia*** 症瘕
Accumulation Disorder (in children)	***Ji Dai*** 积滞
Agitation	***Zang Zao*** 脏躁
Atrophy Syndrome	***Wei Zheng*** 痿症
Bleeding between periods	***Jing Jian Qi Chu Xue*** 经间期出血
Blood Urinary Syndrome	***Xue Lin*** 血淋
Brain Discharge	***Nao Lou*** 脑漏
Breakdown Heart Pain	***Jue Xin Tong*** 厥心痛
Breakdown Syndrome	***Jue Zheng*** 厥症
Breast lumps	***Ru Pi*** 乳癖
Chickenpox	***Shui Dou*** 水痘
Childhood nutritional impairment	***Gan*** 疳
Cough	***Ke Sou*** 咳嗽
Cretinism	***Chi Dai*** 痴呆
Convulsions	***Jing Bing*** 痉病
Depression	***Yu Zheng*** 郁症

Diarrhea	***Xie Xie*** 泄泻
Dizziness of Pregnancy	***Zi Yun*** 子晕
Dullness and Mania	***Dian Kuang*** 癫狂
Dysentery	***Li Ji*** 痢疾
Dysphagia and Blockage	***Ye Ge*** 噎膈
Early periods	***Yue Jing Xian Qi*** 月经先其
Eczema (dermatitis)	***Shi Zhen*** 湿疹
Edema	***Shui Zhong*** 水肿
Edema of Pregnancy	***Zi Zhong*** 子肿
Epilepsy	***Dian Xian*** 癫痫
Erectile dysfunction	***Yang Wei*** 阳痿
Essence Turbidity	***Jing Zhuo*** 精浊
Exhaustion	***Xu Lao*** 虚劳
Exhaustion	***Xu Sun*** 虚损
Facial paralysis	***Mian Tan*** 面瘫
Fatigue Urinary Syndrome	***Lao Lin*** 劳淋
Fear and palpitations	***Jing Ji*** 惊悸
Five Flaccidities	***Wu Ruan*** 五软
Five Retardations	***Wu Chi*** 五迟
Flooding and Trickling	***Beng Lou*** 崩漏
Fright Cry	***Jing Ti*** 惊啼
German measles	***Feng Zhen*** 风疹
Gnawing hunger	***Cao Za*** 嘈杂
Goitre	***Ying*** 瘿
Heat Urinary Syndrome	***Re Lin*** 热淋
Heart Pain	***Xin Tong*** 心痛
Heavy periods	***Yue Jing Guo Duo*** 月经过多
Hernial and Genitourinary disorders	***Shan*** 疝
Hiccup	***E Ni*** 呃逆
Hypochondrial pain	***Xie Tong*** 胁痛
Hysteria	***Yi*** 癔
Impotence (erectile dysfunction)	***Yang Wei*** 阳痿
Incontinence of urine	***Yi Niao*** 遗尿
Irregular periods	***Yue Jing Xian Hou Wu Ding Qi*** 月经先后无定期
Late periods	***Yue Jing Hou Qi*** 月经后期
Lilium Syndrome	***Bai He Bing*** 百合病
Lung-Exhaustion	***Fei Xu Lao*** 肺虚劳
Malaria	***Nue Ji*** 疟疾

Measles	***Ma Zhen*** 麻疹
Multiple joints (Wind)	***Li Jie (Feng)*** 历节(风)
No periods	***Bi Jing*** 闭经
"Nose pool" (sinusitis)	***Bi Yuan*** 鼻渊
Painful Obstruction Syndrome	***Bi Zheng*** 痹症
Palpitations	***Xin Ji*** 心悸
Palpitations and anxiety	***Xin Ji Zheng Chong*** 心悸怔
Panic throbbing	***Zheng Chong*** 怔忡
Paralysis	***Tan Huan*** 瘫缓
Phlegm Nodules	***Tan He*** 痰核
Pi masses	***Pi Kuai*** 痞块
Plum-Stone Syndrome	***Mei He Qi*** 梅核气
Qi edema	***Qi Zhong*** 气肿
Qi Urinary Syndrome	***Qi Lin*** 气淋
Red Turbidity	***Chi Zhuo*** 赤浊
Regurgitation of food	***Fan Wei*** 反胃
Running Piglet Syndrome	***Ben Tun*** 奔豚
Scanty periods	***Yue Jing Guo Shao*** 月经过少
Scrofula	***Luo Li*** 瘰疬
Seminal emissions	***Yi Jing*** 遗精
Silent Scrofula	***Yin Luo*** 阴瘰
Sour regurgitation	***Tun Suan*** 吞酸
Sour vomiting	***Tu Suan*** 吐酸
Spermatorrhea	***Bai Yin*** 白淫
Sticky Urinary Syndrome	***Gao Lin*** 膏淋
Stone Urinary Syndrome	***Shi Lin*** 石淋
Stubborn Painful Obstruction Syndrome	***Wan Bi*** 顽痹
Stuffy Nose	***Bi Qiu*** 鼻鼽
Stuffy Nose and Sneezing	***Qiu Ti*** 鼽嚏
Tremors	***Chan Zheng*** 颤证
True Heart Pain	***Zhen Xin Tong*** 真心痛
Turbidity	***Zhuo*** 浊
Urinary Retention	***Long Bi*** 癃闭
Urinary Syndrome	***Lin Zheng*** 淋症
Urinary Syndrome of Pregnancy	***Zi Lin*** 子淋
Warm disease	***Wen Bing*** 温病
Warm epidemic pathogenic factor	***Wen Yi*** 温疫
White Turbidity	***Bai Zhuo*** 白浊
Wind-stroke	***Zhong Feng*** 中风

VITAL SUBSTANCES

Central Qi	***Zhong Qi*** 中气
Channel Qi	***Jing Qi*** 经气
Corporeal Soul	***Po*** 魄
Defensive Qi	***Wei Qi*** 卫气
Emperor Fire	***Jun Huo*** 君火
Essence	***Jing*** 精
Ethereal Soul	***Hun*** 魂
Exuberant Fire (pathological)	***Zhuang Huo*** 壮火
Fire of the Gate of Life	***Ming Men Huo*** 命门火
Gate of Life	***Ming Men*** 命门
Gathering Qi (of the chest)	***Zong Qi*** 宗气
Ghost, spirit, soul of dead person	***Gui*** 鬼
Heavenly Gui	***Tian Gui*** 天癸
Intellect	***Yi*** 意
Marrow	***Sui*** 髓
Mind (the Shen of the Heart)	***Shen*** 神
Minister Fire	***Xiang Huo*** 相火
Nutritive Qi	***Ying Qi*** 营气
Original Qi	***Yuan Qi*** 原气
Physiological Fire of the body	***Shao Huo*** 少火
Postnatal Qi	***Hou Tian Zhi Qi*** 后天之气
Prenatal Qi	***Xian Tian Zhi Qi*** 先天之气
Saliva	***Xian*** 涎
Spirit (the complex of Heart-Shen, Corporeal Soul, Ethereal Soul, Intellect and Will-Power)	***Shen*** 神
Spittle	***Tuo*** 唾
True Qi	***Zhen Qi*** 真气
Upright Qi	***Zheng Qi*** 正气
Will-Power	***Zhi*** 志

EMOTIONS

Anger	***Nu*** 怒
Craving	***Yu*** 愈
Fear, fright	***Kong*** 恐
Joy	***Xi*** 喜
Love	***Ai*** 爱 (or ***Hao*** 好)
Pensiveness	***Si*** 思
Reflection	***Lü*** 虑
Sadness	***Bei*** 悲
Shock	***Jing*** 惊
Worry	***You*** 忧

CHANNELS AND POINTS

Accumulation point	***Xi Xue*** 郗穴
Ah Shi Point	***Ah Shi Xue*** 阿是穴
Ancestral Vessel	***Zong Mai*** 宗脉
Back-Transporting points	***(Bei) Shu Xue*** 背俞穴
Bright Yang	***Yang Ming*** 阳明
Cavities and Texture	***Cou Li*** 腠理
Connecting channel	***Luo Mai*** 络脉
Connecting point	***Luo Xue*** 络穴
Contralateral needling	***Miu Ci*** 缪刺
Directing Vessel	***Ren Mai*** 任脉
Divergent channel	***Jing Bie*** 经别
Five Transporting points	***Wu Shu Xue*** 五输穴
Front-Collecting points	***Mu Xue*** 募穴
Gathering point	***Hui Xue*** 会穴
Girdle Vessel	***Dai Mai*** 带脉
Governing Vessel	***Du Mai*** 督脉
Greater Yang	***Tai Yang*** 太阳
Greater Yin	***Tai Yin*** 太阴
Lesser Yang	***Shao Yang*** 少阳
Lesser Yin	***Shao Yin*** 少阴
Main channel	***Jing Mai*** 经脉
Minute Connecting channel	***Sun Luo*** 孙络
Muscle channel	***Jing Jin*** 经筋
Opposite needling	***Ju Ci*** 巨刺
Origin and Concentration (of channels)	***Gen Jie*** 根结
Pathways of Qi	***Qi Jie*** 气街
Penetrating Vessel	***Chong Mai*** 冲脉
River point	***Jing Xue*** 经穴
Root and Branch (of channels)	***Ben Biao*** 本标
Sea point	***He Xue*** 合穴
Source point	***Yuan Xue*** 原穴
Space between skin and muscles	***Cou Li*** 腠里
Spring point	***Ying Xue*** 荥穴
Stream point	***Shu Xue*** 输穴

Superficial Connecting channel	***Fu Luo*** 浮络
Terminal Yin	***Jue Yin*** 厥阴
Uterus channel	***Bao Luo*** 胞络
Uterus Vessel	***Bao Mai*** 胞脉
Well point	***Jing Xue*** 井穴
Yang Linking Vessel	***Yang Wei Mai*** 阳维脉
Yang Stepping Vessel	***Yang Qiao Mai*** 阳跷脉
Yin Linking Vessel	***Yin Wei Mai*** 阴维脉
Yin Stepping Vessel	***Yin Qiao Mai*** 阴跷脉

PULSE POSITIONS

Front (pulse position)	***Cun*** 寸
Middle (pulse position)	***Guan*** 关
Rear (pulse position)	***Chi*** 尺

PULSE QUALITIES

Big	***Da*** 大
Choppy	***Se*** 涩
Deep	***Chen*** 沉
Empty	***Xu*** 虚
Fine	***Xi*** 细
Firm	***Lao*** 牢
Floating	***Fu*** 浮
Full	***Shi*** 实
Hasty	***Cu*** 促
Hidden	***Fu*** 伏
Hollow	***Kou*** 芤
Hurried	***Ji*** 急
Irregular or Intermittent	***Dai*** 代
Knotted	***Jie*** 结
Leather	***Ge*** 革
Long	***Chang*** 长
Minute	***Wei*** 微
Moving	***Dong*** 动
Overflowing	***Hong*** 洪
Rapid	***Shu*** 数
Scattered	***San*** 散
Short	***Duan*** 短
Slippery	***Hua*** 滑
Slow	***Chi*** 迟
Slowed-Down	***Huan*** 缓
Soggy	***Ru*** 濡
Soggy	***Ruan*** 软
Tight	***Jin*** 紧
Weak	***Ruo*** 弱
Wiry	***Xian*** 弦

TONGUE DIAGNOSIS

Cracked	***Lie Wen*** 裂纹
Deviated	***Bian Wai*** 偏歪
Mouldy	***Fu*** 腐
Moving	***Nong*** 弄
Pale	***Dan Bai*** 淡白
Purple	***Zi*** 紫
Quivering	***Zhan*** 颤
Red	***Hong*** 红
Red points (on the tongue)	***Dian*** 点
Slippery (tongue coating)	***Hua*** 滑
Spots	***Ban*** 斑
Sticky (tongue coating)	***Ni*** 腻
Stiff	***Qiang Geng*** 强硬
Swollen	***Zhong*** 肿
Teethmarks	***Chi Gen*** 齿痕
Tongue body	***She Zhi*** 舌质
Tongue body shape	***She Ti*** 舌体
Tongue coating	***She Tai*** 舌苔

METHODS OF TREATMENT

Benefit the throat	***Li Hou*** 利喉
Break-up Blood	***Po Xue*** 破血
Brighten the eyes	***Li Mu*** 利目
Calm the Fetus	***An Tai*** 安胎
Calm the Liver	***Ping Gan*** 平肝
Circulate Defensive Qi	***Liu Wei*** 疏卫
Clear Heat	***Qing Re*** 清热
Clear (Heat)	***Xie*** 泄
Consolidate	***Gu*** 固
Consolidate Collapse	***Gu Tuo*** 固脱
Consolidate the Exterior	***Gu Biao*** 固表

Dispel stasis (of Blood)	***Gong Yu*** 功瘀
Dissipate accumulation	***San Jie*** 散结
Dissipate nodules	***San Jie*** 散结
Drain (method of treatment as opposed to *Bu* 补, tonify)	***Xie*** 泻
Drain (Fire)	***Xie*** 泻
Eliminate stagnation (of Qi)	***Jie Yu*** 解郁
Eliminate stasis (of Blood)	***Hua Yu*** 化瘀
Eliminate stasis (of Blood)	***Qu Yu*** 去瘀
Expel Cold	***San Han*** 散寒
Expel (external) Wind	***Qu Feng*** 去风
Extinguish Wind (internal)	***Xi Feng*** 熄风
Harmonize Nutritive and Defensive Qi	***Tiao He Ying Wei*** 调和营卫
Invigorate Blood	***Huo Xue*** 活血
Moderate urgency	***Huan Ji*** 缓急
Move downwards	***Xie Xia*** 泻下
Move downwards	***Gong Xia*** 功下
Move Qi	***Li Qi*** 理气
Nourish (Blood)	***Yang (Xue)*** 养血
Obtaining needling sensation	***De Qi*** 得气
Open (the chest)	***Tong Yang*** 通畅(胸)
Open the nose	***Xuan Tong Bi*** 宣通鼻窍
Open the orifices	***Kai Qiao*** 开窍
Open the orifices	***Tong Qiao*** 通窍
Open the Water passages by promoting diuresis	***Tong Li*** 通利
Pacify (the Liver)	***Shu (Gan)*** 疏肝
Penetrate the Yang Organs	***Tong Fu*** 通腑
Promote healing of tissues	***Sheng Xin*** 生新
Promote resuscitation	***Xing Zhi*** 醒志
Promote Water transformation	***Li Shui*** 利水
Rectify Qi	***Shun Qi*** 顺气
Reduce (as a needle technique)	***Xie*** 泻
Regulate the period	***Tiao Jing*** 调经
Regulate the Water passages	***Li Shui Dao*** 理水道
Reinforce (as a needle technique)	***Bu*** 补
Relax the sinews	***Shu Jin*** 舒筋
Release the Exterior	***Jie Biao*** 解表
Remove obstructions from the breasts' Connecting channels	***Tong Ru Luo*** 通乳络
Remove obstructions from the Connecting channels	***Tong Luo*** 通络
Remove obstructions by moving downwards	***Tong Xia*** 通下
Remove obstructions by restoring the correct direction of Qi flow	***Tong Shun*** 通顺
Resolve Dampness	***Hua Shi*** 化湿
Resolve Dampness	***Li Shi*** 利湿
Resolve Phlegm	***Hua Tan*** 化痰
Restore the diffusing of Lung-Qi	***Xuan Fei*** 宣肺
Scatter Cold	***San Han*** 散寒
Tonify (or reinforce as a needle technique)	***Bu*** 补
Use pungent herbs to open and bitter ones to make Qi descend	***Xin Kai Ku Jiang*** 辛开苦降
Warm the menses	***Wen Jing*** 温经

PATHOGENIC FACTORS

Cold	***Han*** 寒
Dampness	***Shi*** 湿
Dryness	***Zao*** 燥
Fire	***Huo*** 火
Heat	***Re*** 热
Pathogenic factor	***Xie*** 邪
Pathogenic factor	***Xie Qi*** 邪气
Phlegm	***Tan*** 痰
Phlegm-Fluids in general and also Phlegm-Fluids in the Stomach	***Tan Yin*** 痰饮
Phlegm-Fluids in the diaphragm	***Zhi Yin*** 支饮
Phlegm-Fluids in the hypochondrium	***Xuan Yin*** 悬饮
Phlegm-Fluids in the limbs	***Yi Yin*** 溢饮
Summer-Heat	***Shu*** 暑
Toxic Heat	***Re Du*** 热毒
Warm epidemic pathogenic factor	***Wen Yi*** 温疫
Wind-Cold	***Feng Han*** 风寒
Wind-Heat	***Feng Re*** 风热

PINYIN–ENGLISH GLOSSARY OF CHINESE TERMS

GENERAL

Ba Kuo 八廓	Eight Ramparts
Bao 胞	Uterus in women and Room of Sperm in men
Bao Luo 胞络	Uterus channel
Bao Mai 胞脉	Uterus Vessel
Ben 本	Root
Bian Bing 辨病	Identification of the disease
Bian Zheng 辨证	Identification of patterns
Biao 标	Manifestation
Cou Li 腠理	Cavities and Texture (also space between the skin and muscles)
Cun 寸	Cun (acupuncture unit of measurement)
Dan Tian 丹田	Field of Elixir
Fen Rou 分肉	Fat and Muscles
Fu 膚	Superficial layer of skin
Gao 膏	Fat Tissue
Ge 革	Deep layer of skin
Huang 肓	Membranes
Ji 肌	Subcutaneous muscles
Jie 街	"Streets", "avenues", "crossroads" (symbols for channels of the abdomen controlled by the Penetrating Vessel)
Jin 筋	Sinews
Jing Gong 精宫	Palace of Sperm (or Palace of Essence)
Jing Guan 精关	Sperm Gate
Jing Shi 精室	Room of Sperm (or Essence)
Ju Ci 巨刺	Opposite needling
Liu Qi 六气	Six Climates
Liu Xie 六邪	Six Evils (external pathogenic factors)
Liu Yin 六淫	Six Excesses (excessive climates)
Miu Ci 缪刺	Contralateral needling
Mu Xi 目系	Eye System
Ni (Qi) 逆气	Rebellious Qi
Qi Ji 气机	Qi Mechanism
Qi Jie 气街	Pathways of Qi
Qing 情	Emotion
Rou 肉	Muscles or flesh
Shan Zhong 膻中	Center of the Thorax
Shao Fu 少腹	Lateral-lower abdominal area
Shao Huo 少火	Lesser Fire
Shun (Qi) 顺气	Conforming Qi
Tian 天	Heaven (or Heavenly)
Wu Lun 五轮	Five Wheels
Xiang 象	Image
Xiao Fu 小腹	Central-lower abdominal area
Xie 邪	Pathogenic factor
Xie Lei 胁肋	Hypochondrium
Xie Qi 邪气	Pathogenic factor
Xin xia 心下	Area below the xiphoid process
Xu Li 虚里	Great Connecting channel of the Stomach (manifesting in apical pulse)
Xuan Fa 宣发	Diffusing (of Lung-Qi)
Xuan Fu 玄府	Pores (including sebaceous glands)
Yin Jing 阴茎	Penis
Yun Hua 运化	Transformation and transportation (of the Spleen)
Zhuang Huo 状火	Exuberant Fire
***Zi Bao* (sometimes also called *"Bao"*)** 子包	Uterus
Zong Jin 宗筋	Ancestral Muscle

SYMPTOMS AND SIGNS

Ban 斑	Macule (in tongue diagnosis, red spots)
Ban Shen Bu Sui 半身不遂	Hemiplegia
Bi Yuan 鼻渊	"Nose pool" (sinusitis)
Biao 标	Manifestation
Cao Za 嘈杂	Gnawing hunger
Chuan 喘	Breathlessness
Dao Han 盗汗	Night-sweating
Duan Qi 短气	Shortness of breath
Duo Qi 夺气	Robbing of Qi (very feeble voice with interrupted speech)
E Ni 呃逆	Hiccup
E Xin 恶心	Nausea
Fa Re 发热	Emission of heat, fever
Fan Wei 反胃	Regurgitation of food
Fan Zao 烦燥	Mental restlessness and agitation (restlessness of limbs)
Feng Tuan 风团	Wheal
Feng Yin Zhen 风阴疹	Wind hidden rash (urticaria)
Feng Zhen 风疹	Wind rash (German measles)
Gan Ou 干呕	Short retching with low sound
Han Re Wang Lai 寒热往来	Alternation of chills and fever
Han Zhan 寒战	Shivers
Hu Re 湖热	Tidal fever
Ji 积	Blood masses
Jia 瘕	Qi masses
Jiao Qi 脚气	Leg Qi
Jie 结	Accumulation (or nodules)
Jing Ji 惊悸	Fear and palpitations
Ju 聚	Qi masses
Jue 厥	Breakdown
Jue Han 厥汗	Sweating from Breakdown
Ke Sou 咳嗽	Cough
Kou Chuang 口疮	Mouth ulcers
Kou Yan Wai Xie 口眼歪斜	Deviation of eye and mouth
Li Ji 里急	Anxiety, internal urgency (in the context of rebellious Qi of the Penetrating Vessel)
Li Ji Hou Zhong 里急后重	Difficulty in defecation
Liu Lei 流泪	Streaming eyes
Ma Mu 麻木	Numbness and/or tingling
Ma Zhen 麻疹	Hemp rash (measles)
Man 满	Feeling of fullness
Men 闷	Feeling of oppression
Mu Chan 目颤	Quivering eyeball
Mu Hua 目花	Blurred vision and floaters
Mu Hun 目昏	Clouded vision
Mu Yun 目晕	Blurred vision
Nao Ming 脑鸣	Brain noise
Ni Jing 逆经	Reverse period
Nong Pao 脓泡	Pustule
Ou 呕	Vomiting (with sound)
Ou Tu 呕吐	Vomiting
Pao 泡	Vesicle
Pi 痞	Feeling of stuffiness
Qi Shao 气少	Weak breathing
Qi Zhong 气肿	Qi edema
Qing 青	Bluish-greenish (color)
Qiu Zhen 丘疹	Papule
Re Du 热毒	Toxic Heat
Ru E 乳蛾	Milky moth (swollen tonsils)
Shang Qi 上气	Rebellious-Qi breathing
Shen Zhong 身重	Feeling of heaviness of the body
Shi 实	Full, Fullness, Excess
Shi E 石蛾	Stone moth (swollen tonsils)
Shi Zhen 湿疹	Eczema
Shou Chan 手颤	Tremor of the hands
Shou Zhi Luan 手指挛	Contraction of the fingers
Shui Dou 水痘	Water pox (chickenpox)
Shui Pao 水泡	Vesicle
Shui Zhong 水肿	Edema
Si Ni 四逆	Four Rebellious
Tai Qi Shang Ni 胎气上逆	Fetus' Qi rebelling upwards
Tan He 痰核	Phlegm Nodules
Tan Yin 痰饮	Phlegm-Fluids (or Phlegm-Fluids in Stomach and Intestines)
Tou Fa Bian Bai 头发变白	Graying of the hair
Tou Fa Tuo Luo 头发脱落	Alopecia

Tou Qing 头倾	Drooping head
Tou Yun 头晕	Dizziness
Tou Zhong 头重	Feeling of heaviness of the head
Tu 吐	Vomiting (without sound)
Tuo 脱	Collapse
Wei Han 畏寒	Fear of cold (in exterior invasions of Wind)
Wu Chi 五迟	Five Retardations
Wu Feng 恶风	Aversion to wind
Wu Han 恶寒	Aversion to cold
Wu Han Fa Re 恶寒发热	Aversion to cold and fever, simultaneous
Wu Ruan 五软	Five Flaccidities
Wu Xin Fa Re 五心发热	Five-palm heat
Xiao 哮	Wheezing
Xie Tong 胁痛	Hypochondrial pain
Xie Xie 泄泻	Diarrhea
Xin Fan 心烦	Mental restlessness
Xin Ji 心悸	Palpitations
Xin Zhong Ao Nong 心中懊	Heart feeling vexed
Xu 虚	Empty, Emptiness, Deficiency
Xuan Yin 玄饮	Phlegm-Fluids in the hypochondrium
Xuan Yun 眩晕	Dizziness
Yan Chi 眼眵	Discharge from the eyes
Yan Shi 厌食	Aversion to food
Yi Jing 遗精	Seminal emissions
Yi Niao 遗尿	Incontinence of urine
Yi Yin 溢饮	Phlegm-Fluids in the limbs
Yu Zheng 郁症	Depression
Yue 哕	Long retching with loud sound
Zhan Han 颤汗	Shiver sweating
Zhang 胀	Feeling of distension
Zhen 疹	Rash
Zheng 症	Blood masses
Zheng Chong 怔忡	Panic throbbing
Zhi Yin 支饮	Phlegm-Fluids above the diaphragm
Zhong 重	Feeling of heaviness
Zhong 重	Heaviness, feeling of
Zu Chan 足颤	Tremor of the feet

DISEASE-SYMPTOMS

Bai He Bing 百合病	Lilium Syndrome
Bai Yin 白淫	Spermatorrhea
Bai Zhuo 白浊	White Turbidity
Ben Tun 奔豚	Running Piglet Syndrome
Beng Lou 崩漏	Flooding and Trickling
Bi Jing 闭经	No periods
Bi Qiu 鼻鼽	Stuffy Nose
Bi Yuan 鼻渊	"Nose pool" (sinusitis)
Bi Zheng 痹症	Painful Obstruction Syndrome
Cao Za 嘈杂	Gnawing hunger
Chan Zheng 颤证	Tremors
Chi Dai 痴呆	Cretinism
Chi Zhuo 赤浊	Red Turbidity
Dian Kuang 癫狂	Dullness and Mania
Dian Xian 癫痫	Epilepsy
E Ni 呃逆	Hiccup
Fan Wei 反胃	Regurgitation of food
Fei Xu Lao 肺虚劳	Lung-Exhaustion
Feng Zhen 风疹	German measles
Gan 疳	Childhood nutritional impairment
Gao Lin 膏淋	Sticky Urinary Syndrome
Ji Dai 积滞	Accumulation Disorder (in children)
Ji Ju 积聚	Abdominal masses
Jing Bing 痉病	Convulsions
Jing Ji 惊悸	Fear and palpitations
Jing Jian Qi Chu Xue 经间期出血	Bleeding between periods
Jing Ti 惊啼	Fright Cry
Jing Zhuo 精浊	Essence Turbidity
Jue Xin Tong 厥心痛	Breakdown Heart Pain
Jue Zheng 厥症	Breakdown Syndrome
Ke Sou 咳嗽	Cough
Lao Lin 劳淋	Fatigue Urinary Syndrome
Li Ji 痢疾	Dysentery
Li Jie (Feng) 历节(风)	Multiple joints (Wind)
Lin Zheng 淋症	Urinary Syndrome
Long Bi 癃闭	Urinary Retention
Luo Li 瘰疬	Scrofula
Ma Zhen 麻疹	Measles

Mei He Qi 梅核气	Plum-Stone Syndrome
Mian Tan 面瘫	Facial paralysis
Nao Lou 脑漏	Brain Discharge
Nue Ji 疟疾	Malaria
Pi Kuai 痞块	Pi masses
Qi Lin 气淋	Qi Urinary Syndrome
Qi Zhong 气肿	Qi edema
Qiu Ti 鼽嚏	Stuffy Nose and Sneezing
Re Lin 热淋	Heat Urinary Syndrome
Ru Pi 乳癖	Breast lumps
Shan 疝	Hernial and Genitourinary disorders
Shi Lin 石淋	Stone Urinary Syndrome
Shi Zhen 湿疹	Eczema (dermatitis)
Shui Dou 水痘	Chickenpox
Shui Zhong 水肿	Edema
Tan He 痰核	Phlegm Nodules
Tan Huan 瘫缓	Paralysis
Tu Suan 吐酸	Sour vomiting
Tun Suan 吞酸	Sour regurgitation
Wan Bi 顽痹	Stubborn Painful Obstruction Syndrome
Wei Zheng 痿症	Atrophy Syndrome
Wen Bing 温病	Warm disease
Wen Yi 温疫	Warm epidemic pathogenic factor
Wu Chi 五迟	Five Retardations
Wu Ruan 五软	Five Flaccidities
Xie Tong 胁痛	Hypochondrial pain
Xie Xie 泄泻	Diarrhea
Xin Ji 心悸	Palpitations
Xin Ji Zheng Chong 心悸怔	Palpitations and anxiety
Xin Tong 心痛	Heart Pain
Xu Lao 虚劳	Exhaustion
Xu Sun 虚损	Exhaustion
Xue Lin 血淋	Blood Urinary Syndrome
Yang Wei 阳痿	Erectile dysfunction
Yang Wei 阳痿	Impotence (erectile dysfunction)
Ye Ge 噎膈	Dysphagia and Blockage
Yi 癔	Hysteria
Yi Jing 遗精	Seminal emissions
Yi Niao 遗尿	Incontinence of urine
Yin Luo 阴瘰	Silent Scrofula
Ying 瘿	Goitre
Yu Zheng 郁症	Depression
Yue Jing Guo Duo 月经过多	Heavy periods
Yue Jing Guo Shao 月经过少	Scanty periods
Yue Jing Hou Qi 月经后期	Late periods
Yue Jing Xian Hou Wu Ding Qi 月经先后无定期	Irregular periods
Yue Jing Xian Qi 月经先其	Early periods
Zang Zao 脏躁	Agitation
Zhen Xin Tong 真心痛	True Heart Pain
Zheng Chong 怔忡	Panic throbbing
Zheng Jia 症瘕	Abdominal masses (in women)
Zhong Feng 中风	Wind-stroke
Zhuo 浊	Turbidity
Zi Lin 子淋	Urinary Syndrome of Pregnancy
Zi Yun 子晕	Dizziness of Pregnancy
Zi Zhong 子肿	Edema of Pregnancy

VITAL SUBSTANCES

Gui 鬼	Ghost, spirit, soul of dead person
Hou Tian Zhi Qi 后天之气	Postnatal Qi
Hun 魂	Ethereal Soul
Jing 精	Essence
Jing Qi 经气	Channel Qi
Jun Huo 君火	Emperor Fire
Ming Men 命门	Gate of Life
Ming Men Huo 命门火	Fire of the Gate of Life
Po 魄	Corporeal Soul
Shao Huo 少火	Physiological Fire of the body
Shen 神	Mind (the Shen of the Heart) or Spirit (the complex of Heart-Shen, Corporeal Soul, Ethereal Soul, Intellect and Will-Power)
Sui 髓	Marrow
Tian Gui 天癸	Heavenly Gui

Tuo 唾	Spittle
Wei Qi 卫气	Defensive Qi
Xian 涎	Saliva
Xian Tian Zhi Qi 先天之气	Prenatal Qi
Xiang Huo 相火	Minister Fire
Yi 意	Intellect
Ying Qi 营气	Nutritive Qi
Yuan Qi 原气	Original Qi
Zhen Qi 真气	True Qi
Zheng Qi 正气	Upright Qi
Zhi 志	Will-Power
Zhong Qi 中气	Central Qi
Zhuang Huo 壮火	Exuberant Fire (pathological)
Zong Qi 宗气	Gathering Qi (of the chest)

EMOTIONS

Ai 爱 (or ***Hao*** 好)	Love
Bei 悲	Sadness
Jing 惊	Shock
Kong 恐	Fear, fright
Lü 虑	Reflection
Nu 怒	Anger
Si 思	Pensiveness
Xi 喜	Joy
You 忧	Worry
Yu 愈	Craving

CHANNELS AND POINTS

Ah Shi Xue 阿是穴	Ah Shi Point
Bao Luo 胞络	Uterus channel
Bao Mai 胞脉	Uterus Vessel
Ben Biao 本标	Root and Branch (of channels)
Chong Mai 冲脉	Penetrating Vessel
Cou Li 腠理	Space between skin and muscles (also Cavities and Texture)
Dai Mai 带脉	Girdle Vessel
Du Mai 督脉	Governing Vessel
Fu Luo 浮络	Superficial Connecting channel
Gen Jie 根结	Origin and Concentration (of channels)
He Xue 合穴	Sea point
Hui Xue 会穴	Gathering point
Jing Bie 经别	Divergent channel
Jing Jin 经筋	Muscle channel
Jing Mai 经脉	Main channel
Jing Xue 井穴	Well point
Jing Xue 经穴	River point
Ju Ci 巨刺	Opposite needling
Jue Yin 厥阴	Terminal Yin
Luo Mai 络脉	Connecting channel
Luo Xue 络穴	Connecting point
Miu Ci 缪刺	Contralateral needling
Mu Xue 募穴	Front-Collecting points
Qi Jie 气街	Pathways of Qi
Ren Mai 任脉	Directing Vessel
Shao Yang 少阳	Lesser Yang
Shao Yin 少阴	Lesser Yin
Shu Xue 输穴	Stream point
(Bei) Shu Xue 背俞穴	Back-Transporting points
Sun Luo 孙络	Minute Connecting channel
Tai Yang 太阳	Greater Yang
Tai Yin 太阴	Greater Yin
Wu Shu Xue 五输穴	Five Transporting points
Xi Xue 郄穴	Accumulation point
Yang Ming 阳明	Bright Yang
Yang Qiao Mai 阳跷脉	Yang Stepping Vessel
Yang Wei Mai 阳维脉	Yang Linking Vessel
Yin Qiao Mai 阴跷脉	Yin Stepping Vessel
Yin Wei Mai 阴维脉	Yin Linking Vessel
Ying Xue 荥穴	Spring point
Yuan Xue 原穴	Source point
Zong Mai 宗脉	Ancestral Vessel

PULSE POSITIONS

Chi 尺	Rear (pulse position)
Cun 寸	Front (pulse position)
Guan 关	Middle (pulse position)

PULSE QUALITIES

Chang 长	Long
Chen 沉	Deep
Chi 迟	Slow
Cu 促	Hasty
Da 大	Big
Dai 代	Irregular or Intermittent
Dong 动	Moving
Duan 短	Short
Fu 浮	Floating
Fu 伏	Hidden
Ge 革	Leather
Hong 洪	Overflowing
Hua 滑	Slippery
Huan 缓	Slowed-Down
Ji 急	Hurried
Jie 结	Knotted
Jin 紧	Tight
Kou 芤	Hollow
Lao 牢	Firm
Ru 濡	Soggy
Ruan 软	Soggy
Ruo 弱	Weak
San 散	Scattered
Se 涩	Choppy
Shi 实	Full
Shu 数	Rapid
Wei 微	Minute
Xi 细	Fine
Xian 弦	Wiry
Xu 虚	Empty

TONGUE DIAGNOSIS

Ban 斑	Spots
Bian Wai 偏歪	Deviated
Chi Gen 齿痕	Teethmarks
Dan Bai 淡白	Pale
Dian 点	Red points (on the tongue)
Fu 腐	Mouldy
Hong 红	Red
Hua 滑	Slippery (tongue coating)
Lie Wen 裂纹	Cracked
Ni 腻	Sticky (tongue coating)
Nong 弄	Moving
Qiang Geng 强硬	Stiff
She Tai 舌苔	Tongue coating
She Ti 舌体	Tongue body shape
She Zhi 舌质	Tongue body
Zhan 颤	Quivering
Zhong 肿	Swollen
Zi 紫	Purple

METHODS OF TREATMENT

An Tai 安胎	Calm the Fetus
Bu 补	Tonify (or reinforce as a needle technique)
De Qi 得气	Obtaining needling sensation
Gong Xia 功下	Move downwards
Gong Yu 功瘀	Dispel stasis (of Blood)
Gu 固	Consolidate
Gu Biao 固表	Consolidate the Exterior
Gu Tuo 固脱	Consolidate Collapse
Hua Shi 化湿	Resolve Dampness
Hua Tan 化痰	Resolve Phlegm
Hua Yu 化瘀	Eliminate stasis (of Blood)
Huan Ji 缓急	Moderate urgency
Huo Xue 活血	Invigorate Blood
Jie Biao 解表	Release the Exterior
Jie Yu 解郁	Eliminate stagnation (of Qi)
Kai Qiao 开窍	Open the orifices
Li Hou 利喉	Benefit the throat
Li Mu 利目	Brighten the eyes
Li Qi 理气	Move Qi
Li Shi 利湿	Resolve Dampness
Li Shui 利水	Promote Water transformation
Li Shui Dao 理水道	Regulate the Water passages
Liu Wei 疏卫	Circulate Defensive Qi
Ping Gan 平肝	Calm the Liver
Po Xue 破血	Break-up Blood
Qing Re 清热	Clear Heat
Qu Feng 去风	Expel (external) Wind

Qu Yu 去瘀	Eliminate stasis (of Blood)
San Han 散寒	Expel (or scatter) Cold
San Jie 散结	Dissipate accumulation or dissipate nodules
Sheng Xin 生新	Promote healing of tissues
Shu (Gan) 疏肝	Pacify (the Liver)
Shu Jin 舒筋	Relax the sinews
Shun Qi 顺气	Rectify Qi
Tiao He Ying Wei 调和营卫	Harmonize Nutritive and Defensive Qi
Tiao Jing 调经	Regulate the period
Tong Fu 通腑	Penetrate the Yang Organs
Tong Li 通利	Open the Water passages by promoting diuresis
Tong Luo 通络	Remove obstructions from the Connecting channels
Tong Qiao 通窍	Open the orifices
Tong Ru Luo 通乳络	Remove obstructions from the breasts' Connecting channels
Tong Shun 通顺	Remove obstructions by restoring the correct direction of Qi flow
Tong Xia 通下	Remove obstructions by moving downwards
Tong Yang 通畅(胸)	Open (the chest)
Wen Jing 温经	Warm the menses
Xi Feng 熄风	Extinguish Wind (internal)
Xie 泻	Reduce (as a needle technique)
Xie 泄	Clear (Heat)
Xie 泻	Drain (Fire)
Xie 泻	Drain (method of treatment as opposed to *Bu* 补, tonify)
Xie Xia 泻下	Move downwards
Xin Kai Ku Jiang 辛开苦降	Use pungent herbs to open and bitter ones to make Qi descend
Xing Zhi 醒志	Promote resuscitation
Xuan Fei 宣肺	Restore the diffusing of Lung-Qi
Xuan Tong Bi 宣通鼻窍	Open the nose
Yang (Xue) 养血	Nourish (Blood)

PATHOGENIC FACTORS

Feng Han 风寒	Wind-Cold
Feng Re 风热	Wind-Heat
Han 寒	Cold
Huo 火	Fire
Re 热	Heat
Re Du 热毒	Toxic Heat
Shi 湿	Dampness
Shu 署	Summer-Heat
Tan 痰	Phlegm
Tan Yin 痰饮	Phlegm-Fluids in general and also Phlegm-Fluids in the Stomach
Wen Yi 温疫	Warm epidemic pathogenic factor
Xie 邪	Pathogenic factor
Xie Qi 邪气	Pathogenic factor
Xuan Yin 悬饮	Phlegm-Fluids in the hypochondrium
Yi Yin 溢饮	Phlegm-Fluids in the limbs
Zao 燥	Dryness
Zhi Yin 支饮	Phlegm-Fluids in the diaphragm

CHRONOLOGY OF CHINESE DYNASTIES

Xia: 21st to 16th century BC
Shang: 16th to 11th century BC
Zhou: 11th century to 771 BC
Spring and Autumn period: 770–476 BC
Warring States period: 475–221 BC
Qin: 221–207 BC
Han: 206 BC–AD 220
Three Kingdoms period: AD 220–280
Jin: 265–420
Northern and Southern dynasties: 420–581
Sui: 581–618
Tang: 618–907
Five Dynasties: 907–960
Song: 960–1279
Liao: 906–1125
Jin: 1115–1234
Yuan: 1271–1368
Ming: 1368–1644
Qing: 1644–1911
Republic of China: 1912–1949
People's Republic of China: 1949–present

COMPARATIVE TIMELINE OF WESTERN AND CHINESE PHILOSOPHERS AND DOCTORS

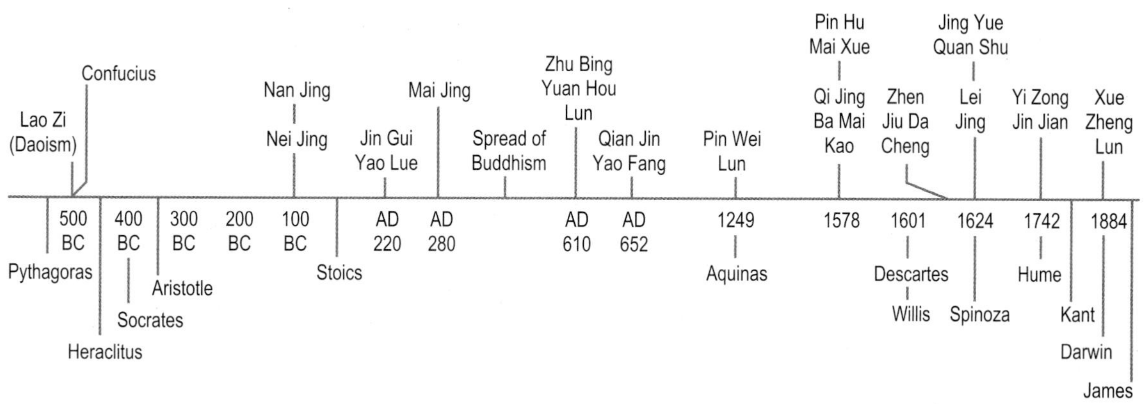

BIBLIOGRAPHY

ANCIENT CLASSICS (listed in chronological order)

1. 1979 Huang Di Nei Jing Su Wen 黄帝内经素问[The Yellow Emperor's Classic of Internal Medicine – Simple Questions]. People's Health Publishing House, Beijing. First published *c.*100 BC.
2. Tian Dai Hua 2005 Huang Di Nei Jing Su Wen 黄帝内经素问[The Yellow Emperor's Classic of Internal Medicine – Simple Questions]. People's Health Publishing House, Beijing. First published *c.*100 BC.
3. 1981 Ling Shu Jing 灵枢经 [Spiritual Axis]. People's Health Publishing House, Beijing. First published *c.*100 BC.
4. Tian Dai Hua 2005 Ling Shu Jing 灵枢经 [Spiritual Axis]. People's Health Publishing House, Beijing. First published *c.*100 BC.
5. Nanjing College of Traditional Chinese Medicine 1979 Nan Jing Jiao Shi 难经校释 [A Revised Explanation of the Classic of Difficulties]. People's Health Publishing House, Beijing. First published *c.*AD 100.
6. Qin Yue Ren 2004 Nan Jing Jiao Shi 难经校释[Classic of Difficulties]. Scientific and Technical Documents Publishing House, Beijing. First published *c.*AD 100.
7. Wu Chang Guo 1985 Zhong Zang Jing 中藏经[The Classic of the Central Organ]. Jiangsu Scientific Publishing House, Nanjing. The *Classic of the Central Organ* was written by Hua Tuo *c.*AD 198.
8. Nanjing College of Traditional Chinese Medicine, Shang Han Lun Research Group 1980 Shang Han Lun 伤寒论 [Discussion on Cold-induced Diseases]. Shanghai Scientific Publishing House, Shanghai. The *Discussion on Cold-induced Diseases* was written by Zhang Zhong Jing and first published *c.*AD 220.
9. Duan Guang Zhou et al 1986 Jin Gui Yao Lue Shou Ce 金匮要略手册 [A Manual of the Essential Prescriptions of the Golden Chest]. Science Publishing House. The *Essential Prescriptions of the Golden Chest* was written by Zhang Zhong Jing and first published *c.*AD 220.
10. Traditional Chinese Medicine Research Institute 1959 Jin Gui Yao Lue Yu Yi 金匮要略喻译[An Explanation of the Essential Prescriptions of the Golden Chest]. People's Health Publishing House, Beijing, p. 61. The *Essential Prescriptions of the Golden Chest* was written by Zhang Zhong Jing and first published *c.*AD 220.
11. He Ren 1979 Jin Gui Yao Lue Tong Su Jiang Hua 金匮要略通俗讲话 [A Popular Guide to the Essential Prescriptions of the Golden Chest]. Shanghai Science Publishing House, Shanghai. The *Essential Prescriptions of the Golden Chest* was written by Zhang Zhong Jing and first published *c.*AD 220.
12. 1981 Jin Gui Yao Lue Fang Xin Jie 金匮要略方新解[A New Explanation of the Essential Prescriptions of the Golden Chest]. Zhejiang Scientific Publishing House, Zhejiang. The *Essential Prescriptions of the Golden Chest* was written by Zhang Zhong Jing and first published *c.*AD 220.
13. He Ren 2005 Jin Gui Yao Lue 金匮要略通俗讲话[Essential Prescriptions of the Golden Chest]. People's Health Publishing House, Beijing. The *Essential Prescriptions of the Golden Chest* was written by Zhang Zhong Jing and first published *c.*AD 220.
14. Fuzhou City People's Hospital 1984 Mai Jing 脉经 [The Pulse Classic]. People's Health Publishing House, Beijing. The *Pulse Classic* was written by Wang Shu He and first published *c.*AD 280.
15. Shandong College of Traditional Chinese Medicine 1984 Mai Jing Jiao Shi 脉经校释 [An Explanation of the Pulse Classic]. People's Health Publishing House, Beijing. The *Pulse Classic* was written by Wang Shu He and first published *c.*AD 280.
16. Shandong College of Traditional Chinese Medicine 1979 Zhen Jiu Jia Yi Jing 针灸甲乙经 [The ABC of Acupuncture]. People's Health Publishing House, Beijing. The *ABC of Acupuncture* was written by Huang Fu Mi and first published AD 282.
17. 1981 Huang Di Nei Jing Tai Su 黄帝内经太素[An Elucidation of the Yellow Emperor's Classic of Internal Medicine]. People's Health Publishing House, Beijing. An *Elucidation of the Yellow Emperor's Classic of Internal Medicine* was written by Yang Shang Shan and first published AD 581–618.
18. Ding Guang Di 1991 Zhu Bing Yuan Hou Lun 诸病源候论 [Discussion of the Origin of Symptoms in Diseases]. People's Health Publishing House, Beijing. The *Discussion of the Origin of Symptoms in Diseases* was written by Chao Yuan Fang in AD 610.
19. 1982 Qian Jin Yao Fang 千金要方[Thousand Golden Ducats Prescriptions]. People's Health Publishing House, Beijing. The *Thousand Golden Ducats Prescriptions* was written by Sun Si Miao in AD 652.
20. 1976 Pi Wei Lun 脾胃论 [Discussion on Stomach and Spleen]. People's Publishing House, Beijing. The *Discussion on Stomach and Spleen* was written by Li Dong Yuan and first published in 1249.
21. Jia Cheng Wen 2002 Pi Wei Lun Bai Hua Jie 脾胃论白话解[A Vernacular Explanation of the Discussion on Stomach and Spleen]. San Qin Publishing House, Xian. The *Discussion on Stomach and Spleen* was written by Li Dong Yuan and first published in 1249.
22. Kang Suo Bin 2002 Quan Xin Zhen Jing Zhi Nan 诠新针经指南 [A New Explanation of the Guide to Acupuncture Channels]. Hebei Science and Technology Publishing House, Hebei, Shijiazhuang. The *Guide to Acupuncture Channels* was written by Han Dou in 1295.
23. 1988 Li Xu Yuan Jian 理虚元鉴[Original Mirror on Regulating Exhaustion]. People's Health Publishing House, Beijing. The *Original Mirror on Regulating Exhaustion* was written by Zhu Qi Shi and first published *c.*1520.
24. 1991 Zhen Jiu Ju Ying 针灸聚英[Gatherings from Eminent Acupuncturists]. Shanghai Science and Technology Publishing House, Shanghai. The *Gatherings from Eminent Acupuncturists* was written by Gao Wu and first published in 1529.
25. Wang Luo Zhen 1985 Qi Jing Ba Mai Kao Jiao Zhu 奇经八脉考校注 [A Compilation of the Study of the Eight Extraordinary Vessels]. Shanghai Science Publishing House, Shanghai. The *Study of the Eight Extraordinary Vessels* was written by Li Shi Zhen and first published in 1578.
26. Heilongjiang Province National Medical Research Group 1984 Zhen Jiu Da Cheng Jiao Shi 针灸大成校释 [An Explanation of the Great Compendium of Acupuncture]. People's Health Publishing House, Beijing. The *Great Compendium of Acupuncture* was written by Yang Ji Zhou and first published in 1601.

27. 1980 Zhen Jiu Da Cheng 针灸大成 [The Great Compendium of Acupuncture]. People's Health Publishing House, Beijing. The *Great Compendium of Acupuncture* was written by Yang Ji Zhou and first published in 1601.
28. Wu Zhan Ren, Yu Zhi Gao 1987 Yi Lin Zheng Yin 医林正印[Correct Seal of Medical Circles]. Jiangsu Science Publishing House, Nanjing. The *Correct Seal of Medical Circles* was written by Ma Zhao Sheng and first published in 1605.
29. 1982 Lei Jing 类经 [Classic of Categories]. People's Health Publishing House, Beijing. The *Classic of Categories* was written by Zhang Jie Bin (also called Zhang Jing Yue) and first published in 1624.
30. 1986 Jing Yue Quan Shu 京岳全书[Complete Book of Jing Yue]. Shangai Scientific Publishing House, Shanghai. The *Complete Book of Jing Yue* was written by Zhang Jing Yue and first published in 1624.
31. Chinese Medicine Research Group of the Zhejiang Province 1985 Wen Yi Lun Ping Zhu 温疫论评注[A Discussion of Epidemic Warm Diseases with Notes and Commentary]. People's Health Publishing House, Beijing. The *Discussion of Epidemic Warm Diseases* was written by Wu You Ke in 1642.
32. Shan Chang Hua 1990 Jing Xue Jie 经穴解 [An Explanation of the Acupuncture Points]. People's Health Publishing House, Beijing. An *Explanation of the Acupuncture Points* was written by Yue Han Zhen and first published in 1654.
33. 1977 Yi Zong Jin Jian 医宗金鉴[Golden Mirror of Medicine]. People's Health Publishing House, Beijing. The *Golden Mirror of Medicine* was written by Wu Qian and first published in 1742.
34. Nanjing College of Traditional Chinese Medicine 1978 Wen Bing Xue 温病学 [A Study of Warm Diseases]. Shanghai Science Publishing House, Shanghai. The *Study of Warm Diseases* was written by Ye Tian Shi in 1746.
35. Wang Zhen Kun 1995 Wen Bing Tiao Bian Xin Jie 温病条辨新解[A New Explanation of the Systematic Differentiation of Warm Diseases]. Xue Yuan Publishing House, Beijing. The *Systematic Differentiation of Warm Diseases* was written by Wu Ju Tong in 1798.
36. 1973 Fu Qing Zhu Fu Qing Zhu Nu Ke 傅青主女科 [Fu Qing Zhu's Gynaecology]. Shanghai People's Publishing House, Shanghai. Fu Qing Zhu was born in 1607 and died in 1684. *Fu Qing Zhu's Gynaecology* was first published in 1827.
37. 1979 Xue Zheng Lun 血证论 [Discussion on Blood Patterns]. People's Health Publishing House, Beijing. The *Discussion on Blood Patterns* was written by Tang Zong Hai and first published in 1884.
38. Pei Zheng Xue 1979 Xue Zheng Lun Ping Shi 血证论评释 [A Commentary on the Discussion on Blood Patterns]. People's Health Publishing House, Beijing. The *Discussion on Blood Patterns* was written by Tang Zong Hai and first published in 1884.
39. 1988 Bing Yuan Ci Dian 病源辞典[Origin of Diseases Dictionary]. Tianjin Ancient Texts Publishing House, Tianjin. The *Origin of Diseases Dictionary* was written by Wu Ke Qian.

MODERN TEXTS

(Publications without an author are listed in chronological order. Those with an author are listed in alphabetical order)

Texts in chronological order

1. Nanjing College of Traditional Chinese Medicine – Warm Diseases Research Group 1959 Wen Bing Xue Jiao Xue Can Kao Zi Liao 温病学教学参考资料 [Teaching Reference Material on the School of Warm Diseases]. Jiangsu People's Publishing House, Nanjing.
2. Guangdong College of Traditional Chinese Medicine 1964 Zhong Yi Zhen Duan Xue 中医诊断学 [A Study of Diagnosis in Chinese Medicine]. Shanghai Scientific Publishing House, Shanghai.
3. Guangzhou Army Health Department 1974 Xin Bian Zhong Yi Xue Gai Yao 新编中医学概要[A New General Outline of Chinese Medicine]. People's Health Publishing House, Beijing.
4. Shanghai College of Traditional Chinese Medicine 1974 Zhen Jiu Xue 针灸学 [A Study of Acupuncture]. People's Health Publishing House, Beijing.
5. 1978 Zhong Yi Ji Chu Xue 中医基础学[Fundamentals of Chinese Medicine]. Shandong Scientific Publishing House, Jinan.
6. 1979 Shen Yu Shen Bing de Zheng Zhi 肾与肾病的证治[Patterns and Treatment of Kidney Diseases]. Hebei People's Publishing House, Hebei.
7. Anwei College of Traditional Chinese Medicine 1979 Zhong Yi Lin Chuang Shou Ce 中医临床手册[Clinical Manual of Chinese Medicine]. Anwei Scientific Publishing House, Anwei.
8. Acupuncture Research Group 1980 Zhen Jiu Xue Jian Bian 针灸学简编 [A Simple Compilation of Acupuncture]. People's Health Publishing House, Beijing.
9. Beijing College of Traditional Chinese Medicine 1980 Shi Yong Zhong Yi Xue 实用中医学[Practical Chinese Medicine]. Beijing Publishing House, Beijing.
10. 1980 Jian Ming Zhong Yi Ci Dian 简明中医辞典[Concise Dictionary of Chinese Medicine]. People's Health Publishing House, Beijing.
11. 1981 Nei Ke Bian Bing Yu Bian Zheng 内科辨病与辨证 [Differentiation of Diseases and Patterns in Internal Medicine]. Heilongjiang People's Publishing House, Harbin.
12. 1981 Zang Fu Zheng Zhi 脏腑证治 [Syndromes and Treatment of the Internal Organs]. Tianjin Scientific Publishing House, Tianjin.
13. Anwei College of Traditional Chinese Medicine and Shanghai College of Traditional Chinese Medicine 1987 Zhen Jiu Xue Ci Dian 针灸学辞典 [Dictionary of Acupuncture]. Shanghai Scientific Publishing House, Shanghai.
14. Cheng Bao Shu 1988 Zhen Jiu Da Ci Dian 针灸大辞典 [Great Dictionary of Chinese Acupuncture]. Beijing Science and Technology Press, Beijing.
15. All-China Research Group in Chinese Medicine 1995 Zhong Yi Da Ci Dian 中医大辞典 [Great Dictionary of Chinese Medicine]. People's Health Publishing House, Beijing.

Texts by author

16. Chen Jin Guang 1992 Xian Dai Zhong Yi Lin Zheng Quan Shu 现代中医临证全书 [Complete Textbook of Chinese Patterns in Contemporary Chinese Medicine]. Beijing Publishing House, Beijing.
17. Chen You Bang 1990 Zhong Guo Zhen Jiu Zhi Liao Xue 中国针灸治疗学 [Chinese Acupuncture Therapy]. China Science Publishing House, Shanghai.
18. Cheng Bao Shu 1988 Zhen Jiu Da Ci Dian 针灸大辞典 [Great Dictionary of Acupuncture]. Beijing Science Publishing House, Beijing.
19. Fang Wen Xian 1989 Zhong Yi Nei Ke Zheng Zhuang Xin Zhi Shou Ce 中医内科证状新治手册 [A Manual of New Treatment of Internal Medicine Diseases in Chinese Medicine]. China Standard Publishing House, Beijing.
20. Fang Wen Xian 1989 Zhong Yi Nei Ke Zheng Zhuang Zhi Shou Ce 中医内科证状治手册 [Manual of Differentiation and Treatment of Symptoms in Internal Chinese Medicine]. China Standard Publishing House, Beijing.
21. Gu He Dao 1979 Zhong Guo Yi Xue Shi Lue 中国医学史略 [History of Chinese Medicine]. Shanxi People's Publishing House, Taiyuan.
22. Gu Yu Qi 2005 Zhong Yi Xin Li Xue 中医心理学[Chinese Medicine Psychology]. China Medicine Science and Technology Publishing House, Beijing.
23. Guo Zhen Qiu 1985 Zhong Yi Zhen Duan Xue 中医诊断学[Diagnosis in Chinese Medicine]. Hunan Science Publishing House, Changsha.
24. Guo Zi Guang 1985 Zhong Yi Qi Zheng Xin Bian 中医奇证新编[A New Compilation of Difficult Syndromes in Chinese Medicine]. Hunan Science Publishing House, Changsha.
25. Hu Xi Ming 1989 Zhong Guo Zhong Yi Mi Fang Da Quan 中国中医秘方大全 [Great Treatise of Secret Formulae in Chinese Medicine]. Literary Publishing House, Shanghai.
26. Huang Long Xiang 1997 Zhen Jiu Ming Zhu Ji Cheng 针灸名著集成 [Collected Works of Famous Outstanding Acupuncturists]. Hua Xia Publishing House, Beijing.

27. Huang Tai Tang 2001 Nei Ke Yi Nan Bing Zhong Yi Zhi Liao Xue 内科医难病中医治疗学 [The Treatment of Difficult Diseases in Chinese Internal Medicine]. Chinese Herbal Medicine Science Publishing House, Beijing.
28. Ji Jie Yin 1984 Tai Yi Shen Zhen Jiu Lin Zheng Lu 太乙神针灸临证录 [Clinical Records of Tai Yi Shen Acupuncture]. Shanxi Province Scientific Publishing House, Shanxi.
29. Jiao Shun Fa 1987 Zhong Guo Zhen Jiu Xue Qiu Zhen 中国针灸学求真 [An Enquiry into Chinese Acupuncture]. Shanxi Science Publishing House, Shanxi.
30. Li Shi Zhen 1985 Chang Yong Shu Xue Lin Chuang Fa Hui 常用输穴临床发挥 [Clinical Application of Frequently Used Acupuncture Points]. People's Health Publishing House, Beijing.
31. Li Wen Chuan, He Bao Yi 1987 Shi Yong Zhen Jiu Xue 实用针灸学 [Practical Acupuncture]. People's Health Publishing House, Beijing.
32. Li Zheng Quan 1992 Shi Yong Zhong Yi Pi Wei Xue 实用中医脾胃学 [A Practical Study of the Stomach and Spleen in Chinese Medicine]. Chongqing Publishing House, Chongqing.
33. Liu Guan Jun 1990 Zhen Jiu Ming Li Yu Lin Zheng 针灸明理与临证 [Acupuncture Theory and Clinical Patterns]. People's Health Publishing House, Beijing.
34. Liu Han Yin 1988 Shi Yong Zhen Jiu Da Quan 实用针灸大全[Practical Treatise of Acupuncture]. Beijing Publishing House, Beijing.
35. Lu Fang 1981 Nei Ke Bian Bing Yu Bian Zheng 内科辨病与辨证 [Identification of Diseases and Patterns in Internal Medicine]. Heilongjiang People's Publishing House, Harbin.
36. Luo Yuan Kai 1986 Zhong Yi Fu Ke Xue 中医妇科学[Gynaecology in Chinese Medicine]. Shanghai Science and Technology Press, Shanghai.
37. Qin Bo Wei 1991 Qing Dai Ming Yi Yi An Jing Hua 清代名医医案精华 [The Essence of Medical Records of Famous Doctors of the Qing Dynasty]. Shanghai Science and Technology Press, Shanghai.
38. Shan Yu Dang 1984 Shang Han Lun Zhen Jiu Pei Xue Xuan Zhu 伤寒论针灸配穴选注 [Selection of Acupuncture Point Combinations from the Discussion on Cold-induced Diseases]. People's Health Publishing House, Beijing.
39. Shen Quan Yu, Wu Yu Hua, Shen Li Ling 1989 Dian Kuang Dian Zheng Zhi 癫狂痫证治 [The Treatment of Manic-Depression and Epilepsy]. Ancient Chinese Medicine Texts Publishing House, Beijing.
40. Shi Yu Guang 1988 Dang Dai Ming Yi Lin Zheng Jing Hua 当代名医临证精华 [Essential Clinical Experience of Famous Modern Doctors]. Ancient Chinese Medicine Texts Publishing House, Beijing.
41. Shi Yu Guang 1992 Dang Dai Ming Yi Lin Zheng Jing Hua 当代名医临证精华 [Essential Clinical Experience of Famous Modern Doctors – Manic-Depression and Epilepsy]. Ancient Chinese Medicine Texts Publishing House, Beijing.
42. Wang Jin Quan 1987 Nei Jing Lei Zheng Lun Zhi 内经类证论指 [Discussion on Categories of Syndromes from the Yellow Emperor's Classic of Internal Medicine]. Shanxi Science Publishing House, Xian.
43. Wang Ke Qin 1988 Zhong Yi Shen Zhu Xue Shuo 中医神主学说 [Theory of the Mind in Chinese Medicine]. Ancient Chinese Medical Texts Publishing House, Beijing.
44. Wang Li Cao 1997 Zhong Guo Zhen Jiu Chu Fang Da Cheng 中国针灸处方大成 [A Collection of Chinese Acupuncture Prescriptions]. Shanxi Science Publishing House, Taiyuan.
45. Wang Xin Hua 1983 Zhong Yi Li Dai Yi Lun Xuan 中国历代医论选 [Selected Historical Theories of Chinese Medicine]. Jiangsu Scientific Publishing House, Nanjing.
46. Wang Xue Tai 1988 Zhong Guo Zhen Jiu Da Quan 中国针灸大全 [Great Treatise of Chinese Acupuncture]. Henan Science Publishing House, Zhengzhou.
47. Wang Yong Yan 2004 Zhong Yi Nei Ke Xue 中医内科学[Chinese Internal Medicine]. People's Health Publishing House, Beijing.
48. Wang Zhi Xian 1987 San Shi Zhong Bing Zhi Yan Lu 三十种病治研绿 [A Record of the Treatment of 30 Types of Diseases]. Shanxi Science Publishing House, Taiyuan.
49. Wang Zhong Heng 1995 Nei Ke Za Bing Zheng Zhi Ji Jin 内科杂病证治集锦 [Collection of Patterns and Treatment of Difficult Diseases in Internal Medicine]. Chinese Medicine Ancient Texts Publishing House, Beijing.
50. Xia De Xin 1989 Zhong Yi Nei Ke Lin Chuang Shou Ce 中医内科临床手册 [Clinical Manual of Internal Medicine]. Shanghai Science Publishing House, Shanghai.
51. Xu Ben Ren 1986 Lin Chuang Zhen Jiu Xue 临床针灸学 [Clinical Acupuncture]. Liaoning Scientific Publishing House, Liaoning.
52. Xu Rong Juan 2004 Nei Ke Xue 内科学 [Internal Medicine]. Chinese Herbal Medicine Publishing House, Beijing.
53. Yang Jia San 1988 Zhong Guo Zhen Jiu Da Ci Dian 中国针灸大辞典 [Great Dictionary of Chinese Acupuncture]. Beijing Sports College Publishing House, Beijing.
54. Yang Jia San 1989 Zhen Jiu Xue 针灸学 [A Study of Acupuncture]. Beijing Science Publishing House, Beijing.
55. Ye Ren Gao 2003 Zhong Yi Nei Ke Zheng Hou 中医内科证候 [Patterns of Internal Chinese Medicine]. People's Health Publishing House, Beijing.
56. Yu Zhong Quan 1988 Jing Xue Bian Zheng Yun Yong Xue 经穴辨证运用学 [A Practical Study of the Differentiation of Acupuncture Points]. Sichuan Science Publishing House, Chengdu.
57. Zeng Shi Zu 1992 Zhi Liao Dian Xian, Yi Bing, Xiao Fang, An Mo Shi Liao 治疗癫痫癔病效方按摩食疗 [Dietary Treatment, Massage and Herbal Treatment for Epilepsy and Hysteria]. Shanxi Science and Technology Publishing House, Xian.
58. Zhai Ming Yi 1979 Zhong Yi Lin Chuang Ji Chu 中医临床集础 [Clinical Chinese Medicine]. Henan Publishing House, Henan.
59. Zhang Bo Yu 1986 Zhong Yi Nei Ke Xue 中医内科学[Chinese Internal Medicine]. Shanghai Science Publishing House, Shanghai.
60. Zhang Fa Rong 1989 Zhong Yi Nei Ke Xue 中医内科学[Chinese Internal Medicine]. Sichuan Science Publishing House, Chengdu.
61. Zhang Qi Wen 1995 Yue Jing Bing Zheng 月经病证[Menstrual Diseases]. People's Hygiene Publishing House, Beijing.
62. Zhang Shan Chen 1982 Zhen Jiu Jia Yi Jing Shu Xue Zhong Ji 针灸甲乙经腧穴重集 [Essential Collection of Acupuncture Points from the ABC of Acupuncture]. Shandong Scientific Publishing House, Shandong. First published AD 282.
63. Zhang Shan You 1980 Nei Jing Zhen Jiu Lei Fang Yu Shi 内经针灸类方语释 [An Explanation of Passages Concerning Acupuncture from the Yellow Emperor's Classic of Internal Medicine]. Shandong Scientific Publishing House, Shandong.
64. Zhang Sheng Xing 1984 Jing Xue Shi Yi Hui Jie 经穴释义汇解 [A Compilation of Explanations of the Meaning of the Acupuncture Points Names]. Shanghai Science Publishing House, Shanghai.
65. Zhang Yuan Kai 1985 Meng He Si Jia Yi Ji 孟河四家医集[Medical Collection of Four Doctors from the Meng He Tradition]. Jiangsu Province Scientific Publishing House, Nanjing.
66. Zhou Chao Fan 2000 Li Dai Zhong Yi Zhi Ze Jing Hua 历代中医治则精华 [Essential Chinese Medicine Treatment Principles in Successive Dynasties]. Chinese Herbal Medicine Publishing House, Beijing.

JOURNALS

1. Liao Ning Zhong Yi 了宁中医 [Liao Ning Journal of Chinese Medicine]. Liao Ning, Shenyang.
2. Zhong Yi Za Zhi 中医杂志 [Journal of Chinese Medicine]. China Association of Traditional Chinese Medicine and China Academy of Traditional Chinese Medicine, Beijing.
3. Nanjing Zhong Yi Yao Da Xue Xue Bao 南京中医药大学学报[Journal of Nanjing University of Traditional Chinese Medicine]. Nanjing University of Traditional Chinese Medicine, Nanjing.

ENGLISH LANGUAGE TEXTS

(Listed in alphabetical order)

1. Ames RT (ed) 1994 Self as Person in Asian Theory and Practice. State University of New York Press, New York.

2. Ames RT, Hall D 2001 Focusing the Familiar – A Translation and Philosophical Interpretation of the Zhongyong. University of Hawai'i Press, Honolulu.
3. Ames RT, Rosemont H 1999 The Analects of Confucius – A Philosophical Translation. Ballantine Books, New York.
4. Ames RT, Kasulis TP, Dissanayake W 1998 Self as Image in Asian Theory and Practice. State University of New York Press, New York.
5. Ames RT, Hall DL 2003 Daodejing – "Making This Life Significant": A Philosophical Translation. Ballantine Books, New York.
6. Beaven DW, Brooks SE 1988 Colour Atlas of the Tongue in Clinical Diagnosis. Wolfe Medical Publications, London.
7. Beijing, Shanghai and Nanjing College of Traditional Chinese Medicine 1980 Essentials of Chinese Acupuncture. Foreign Languages Press, Beijing.
8. Bensky D, O'Connor J 1981 Acupuncture, a Comprehensive Text. Eastland Press, Seattle.
9. Bensky D, Clavey S, Stöger E 2004 Materia Medica, 3rd edition. Eastland Press, Seattle.
10. Bockover M (ed) 1991 Rules, Ritual and Responsibility – Essays Dedicated to Herbert Fingarette. Open Court, La Salle, Illinois.
11. Chang C 1977 The Development of Neo-Confucian Thought. Greenwood Press, Westport, Connecticut.
12. Chang LS, Feng Y 1998 The Four Political Treatises of the Yellow Emperor. University of Hawai'i Press, Honolulu.
13. Chen Xin Nong 1987 Chinese Acupuncture and Moxibustion. Foreign Languages Press, Beijing.
14. Claremont de Castillejo I 1997 Knowing Woman – A Feminine Psychology. Shambhala, Boston.
15. Clavey S 2003 Fluid Physiology and Pathology in Traditional Chinese Medicine. Churchil Livingstone, Edinburgh.
16. Crabbe J (ed) 1999 From Soul to Self. Routledge, London.
17. Damasio A 1994 Descartes' Error – Emotion, Reason and the Human Brain. Penguin Books, London.
18. Damasio A 1999 The Feeling of What Happens – Body and Emotion in the Making of Consciousness. Harcourt, San Diego.
19. Damasio A 2003 Looking for Spinoza – Joy, Sorrow and the Feeling Brain. Harcourt, San Diego.
20. Davidson R, Harrington A 2002 Visions of Compassion – Western Scientists and Tibetan Buddhists Examine Human Nature. Oxford University Press, Oxford.
21. Deadman P, Al-Khafaji M 1998 A Manual of Acupuncture. Journal of Chinese Medicine Publications, Hove, England.
22. Edelman GM, Tononi G 2000 A Universe of Consciousness – How Matter Becomes Imagination. Basic Books, New York.
23. Edelman GM 2005 Wider than the Sky – The Phenomenal Gift of Consciousness. Yale University Press, New Haven.
24. Farquhar J 1994 Knowing Practice – The Clinical Encounter of Chinese Medicine. Westview Press, Boulder, Colorado.
25. Fingarette H 1972 Confucius – The Secular as Sacred. Waveland Press, Prospect Heights, Illinois.
26. Fung Yu Lan 1966 A Short History of Chinese Philosophy. Free Press, New York.
27. Gardner DK 2003 Zhu Xi's Reading of the Analects. Columbia University Press, New York.
28. Gernet J 1983 China and the Christian Impact: a Conflict of Cultures. Cambridge University Press, Cambridge.
29. Giles H 1912 Chinese–English Dictionary. Kelly & Walsh, Shanghai.
30. Gluck A 2007 Damasio's Error and Descartes' Truth. University of Scranton Press, London.
31. Graham AC 1986 Yin-Yang and the Nature of Correlative Thinking. Institute of East Asian Philosophies, Singapore.
32. Graham AC 1999 The Book of Lieh-Tzu – A Classic of Tao. Columbia University Press, New York.
33. Greene B 2000 The Elegant Universe. Vintage, London.
34. Greenfield S 2000 The Private Life of the Brain. Penguin Books, London.
35. Hall DL, Ames RT 1998 Thinking from the Han – Self, Truth and Transcendence in Chinese and Western Culture. State University of New York Press, New York.
36. Helms JM 1995 Acupuncture Energetics – A Clinical Approach for Physicians. Medical Acupuncture Publishers, California.
37. Holcombe C 1994 In the Shadow of the Han. University of Hawai'i, Honolulu.
38. Huang Siu-chi 1999 Essentials of Neo-Confucianism. Greenwood Press, Westport, Connecticut.
39. James S 2003 Passion and Action – The Emotions in Seventeenth-Century Philosophy. Clarendon Press, Oxford.
40. Jones D (ed) 2008 Confucius Now. Open Court, Chicago
41. Jung CG 1961 Modern Man in Search of a Soul. Routledge & Kegan Paul, London.
42. Kaptchuk T 2000 The Web that has no Weaver – Understanding Chinese Medicine. Contemporary Books, Chicago.
43. Kasulis TP, Ames RT, Dissanayke W 1993 Self as Body in Asian Theory and Practice. State University of New York Press, New York.
44. Kim Yung Sik 2000 The Natural Philosophy of Chu Hsi. American Philosophical Society, Philadelphia.
45. Kovacs J, Unschuld P 1998 Essential Subtleties on the Silver Sea – The Yin Hai Jing Wei: a Chinese Classic of Ophthalmology. University of California Press, Berkeley.
46. Lange CG, James W 1922 The Emotions, Vol. 1. Williams & Wilkins, Baltimore.
47. Lau DC, Ames RT 1998 Yuan Dao – Tracing Dao to its Source. Ballantine Books, New York.
48. LeDoux J 1996 The Emotional Brain. Simon & Shuster, New York.
49. Lewis T, Amini F, Lannon R 2000 A General Theory of Love. Random House, New York.
50. Lewis M, Haviland-Jones JM (eds) 2004 Handbook of Emotions. Guilford Press, New York.
51. Liu Bing Quan 1988 Optimum Time for Acupuncture – A Collection of Traditional Chinese Chronotherapeutics. Shandong Science and Technology Press, Jinan.
52. Maciocia G 2004 The Diagnosis of Chinese Medicine. Churchill Livingstone, Edinburgh
53. Maciocia G 2005 The Foundations of Chinese Medicine, 2nd edition. Churchill Livingstone, Edinburgh.
54. Maciocia G 2007 The Practice of Chinese Medicine, 2nd edition. Churchill Livingstone, Edinburgh.
55. Marks J, Ames RT 1995 Emotions in Asian Thought. State University of New York Press, New York.
56. Matsumoto K, Birch S 1988 Hara Diagnosis: Reflections on the Sea. Paradigm Publications, Brookline.
57. Needham J 1977 Science and Civilization in China, Vol. 2. Cambridge University Press, Cambridge.
58. Needham J, Lu GD 1980 Celestial Lancets. Cambridge University Press, Cambridge.
59. Ng On-cho 2001 Cheng-Zhu Confucianism in the Early Qing. State University of New York Press, New York.
60. Ni Yitian 1996 Navigating the Channels of Traditional Chinese Medicine. Complementary Medicine Press, San Diego.
61. Nisbett RE 2003 The Geography of Thought – How Asians and Westerners Think Differently and Why. Free Press, New York.
62. Pert C 1997 Molecules of Emotion – The Science of Mind-Body Medicine. Scribner, New York.
63. Qiu Mao Liang 1993 Chinese Acupuncture and Moxibustion. Churchill Livingstone, Edinburgh.
64. Redfield Jamison K 1993 Touched with Fire – Manic-depressive Illness and the Artistic Temperament. Free Press, New York.
65. Redfield Jamison K 1995 An Unquiet Mind. Picador, London.
66. Russell B 2002 History of Western Philosophy. Routledge, London.
67. Sartre JP 2004 Sketch for a Theory of the Emotions. Routledge, London.
68. Searle JR 2004 Mind. Oxford University Press, Oxford.
69. Solomon RC 1993 The Passions – Emotions and the Meaning of Life. Hackett Publishing, Indianapolis.
70. Sorabji R 2002 Emotion and Peace of Mind – From Stoic Agitation to Christian Temptation. Oxford University Press, Oxford.
71. Tallis F 2004 Love Sick. Century, London.
72. Taylor C 2003 Sources of the Self – The Making of the Modern Identity. Cambridge University Press, Cambridge.

73. Trimble MR 2007 The Soul in the Brain. Johns Hopkins University Press, Baltimore.
74. Unschuld P 1985 Medicine in China – A History of Ideas. University of California Press, Berkeley.
75. Unschuld P 1986 Nan-ching – The Classic of Difficult Issues. University of California Press, Berkeley.
76. Unschuld P 2000 Medicine in China – Historical Artefacts and Images. Prestel, Munich.
77. Unschuld P 2003 Huang Di Nei Jing Su Wen: Nature, Knowledge, Imagery in an Ancient Chinese Medical Text. University of California Press, Berkeley.
78. Wang Ai He 1999 Cosmology and Political Culture in Early China. Cambridge University Press, Cambridge.
79. Wilhelm R (translator) 1962 The Secret of the Golden Flower. Harcourt, Brace & World, New York.
80. Wollheim R 1999 On the Emotions. Yale University Press, New Haven.
81. Scalp-Needling Therapy 1975 Medicine and Health Publishing, Hong Kong.

TEXTBOOKS OF WESTERN MEDICINE

1. American Psychiatric Association 1994 Diagnostic and Statistical Manual for Mental Disorders, 4th edition (DSM-IV). American Psychiatric Press, Washington, DC.
2. Baldry PE 1994 Acupuncture, Trigger Points and Musculoskeletal Pain. Churchill Livingstone, Edinburgh.
3. Baldry PE 2001 Myofascial Pain and Fibromyalgia Syndromes. Churchill Livingstone, Edinburgh.
4. Bowlby J 1980 Loss, Sadness and Depression. Hogarth Press, London.
5. Burkitt D 1980 Don't Forget Fibre in Your Diet. Martin Dunitz, London.
6. Everard ML 1998 Respiratory syncytial virus bronchiolitis and pneumonia. In: Taussig L, Landau L (eds) Textbook of Paediatric Respiratory Medicine. Mosby, St Louis.
7. Graf P, Birt A 1996 Explicit and implicit memory retrieval: intentions and strategies. In: Reder L (ed) Implicit Memory and Metacognition. Lawrence Erlbaum Associates, Mahwah, NJ, Chapter 2.
8. Grahame-Smith D, Aronson J 1995 Clinical Pharmacology and Drug Therapy. Oxford University Press, Oxford.
9. Haslett C, Chilvers E, Hunter J, Boon N 1999 Davidson's Principles and Practice of Medicine. Churchill Livingstone, Edinburgh.
10. Hickling P, Golding J 1984 An Outline of Rheumatology. Wright, Bristol.
11. Kay AB 1989 Allergy and Asthma. Blackwell Scientific Publications, Oxford.
12. Kumar PJ, Clark ML 1987 Clinical Medicine. Baillière Tindall, London.
13. Kumar PJ, Clark ML 2005 Clinical Medicine, 6th edition. Saunders, Edinburgh.
14. Lane DJ 1996 Asthma: the Facts, 3rd edition. Oxford University Press, Oxford.
15. Laurence DR 1973 Clinical Pharmacology. Churchill Livingstone, Edinburgh.
16. Mygind N et al 1990 Rhinitis and Asthma. Munksgaard, Lund, Sweden.
17. Robins LN, Regier DA (eds) 1991 Psychiatric Disorders in America: the Epidemiologic Catchment Area Study. Free Press, New York.
18. Seligman MEP 1975 Helplessness. W.H. Freeman, San Francisco.
19. Shepherd C 1989 Living with ME. Cedar, London.
20. Smith DG 1989 Understanding ME. Robinson Publishing, London.
21. Souhami R, Moxham J 1994 Textbook of Medicine. Churchill Livingstone, Edinburgh.
22. Wallace D, Wallace J 2002 All About Fibromyalgia. Oxford University Press, Oxford.

FOREIGN LANGUAGE TEXTS

1. Battaglia F et al 1957 Enciclopedia Filosofica. Casa Editrice Sansoni, Firenze.
2. Eyssalet J-M 1990 Le Secret de la Maison des Ancêtres. Guy Trédaniel Editeur, Paris.
3. Granet M 1973 La Religione dei Cinesi. Adelphi, Milano.
4. Lamanna EP 1967 Storia della Filosofia [History of Philosophy], Vol 1. Le Monnier, Florence.
5. Middleton E et al 1991 Treatise of Allergology, Italian Edition. Momento Medico.

INDEX

Please note that page references relating to non-textual content such as Figures or Tables are in *italic* print, while page numbers with major mentions of topics, acupuncture points or herbal prescriptions are in **bold**. Names of specific acupuncture points will be found under the heading "acupuncture points, by channel"; names of individual herbal prescriptions will be located under "herbal prescriptions/main herbs".

A

ABC of Acupuncture, 253
Absolute, Hegel on, 2
acupuncture points, by channel, 244–281
  see also acupuncture treatment, indications for
  Bladder Channel
    BL-1 Jingming, 453, 456, 457
    BL-8 Luoque, 232, 233, 281
    BL-10 Tianzhu, 232, 233, **255–256**, **260**, 514, **554**, 555
    BL-13 Feishu, 60, 74, 93, 94, 133, 214, 228, 229, **256**, **258**, **260**, **354**, 383, 434, 436, 519
    BL-14 Jueyinshu, 205, 206
    BL-15 Xinshu, 24, 74, 201, 205, 208, 209, 212, 213, 214, 230, 232, **256–257**, **260**, 372, 373, 374, **380–381**, **385**, 430, 431, 433, 434, 458, 466, 467, 468, 469, 488, 489, 494, 495, 514, 515, **551**, 554, 557, 558, 559
    BL-17 Geshu, 205, 206, 207, 366, 367, 370, 461, 462, 463, 527
    BL-18 Ganshu, 34, 74, 201, 206, 207, 208, 214, 215, 219, 220, 224, 225, 258, 456, 457, 514
    BL-21 Weishu, 65, 226, 227, 230, 232, 372, 373, 519
    BL-22 Sanjiaoshu, 65, 490, 491, 492
    BL-23 Shenshu, 69, 74, 132, 154, 216, 232, 233, 234, 235, 239, 240, **257**, **259**, **260**, **346**, **353**, 377, **381**, 469, 489, 492, 494, 495, **554**, 555
    BL-42 Pohu, 93, 214, 228, 229, 235, **257–258**, **260**, **354**, **381**, 383, **385**
    BL-44 Shentang, 205, 206, 208, 209, 212, 213, 214, 228, 229, 230, 232, **258**, **260**, **381**, **385**, 458, 461, 462, 469, 489, 495, 520
    BL-47 Hunmen, 40, 44, 45, 95, 132, 206, 207, 214, 215, 219, 220, 237, 239, **258–259**, **260**, 280, **353**, 358, 359, 360, 363, 364, 371, 372, 377, 378, **381**, **385**, 457, 465, 466, 471, 472, 486, 487, 537, 538, 539, 540, **552**, 555
    BL-49 Yishe, 65, 97, 226, 227, **259**, **260**, **354**, 494, 557, 558, 559
    BL-52 Zhishi, 45, 69, 100, 132, 216, 232, 233, 234, 235, 237, 239, 240, **259**, **260**, **346**, **353**, 377–378, **381**, 381–382, **385**, 469, 489, 492, 494, 495
    BL-62 Shenmai, 69, 92, **259**, **260**, **453**, 456, 457, 515
  Directing Vessel (*Ren Mai*)
    Ren-4 Guanyuan Gate to the Original Qi, 45, 99, 148, 152, 195, 212, 213, 214, 215, 216, 217, 218, 219, 220, 221, 230, 232, 233, 234, 235, 237, 239, 240, **272**, **275**, 281, 377, **384**, 386, 432, 433, 436, 468, 469, 471, 472, 474, 489, 494, 495, 525, 526, 527, 528, 539, 540, 556, 557
    Ren-6 Qihai, 152, 195, 207, 208, 228, 229, 371, 372, 433, 434, 495
    Ren-7 Yinjiao, 239, 240
    Ren-8 Shenque, **249**, **272–273**, **275**, 281
    Ren-9 Shuifen, 45, 65, 226, 227, 459, 460, 486, 490, 491, 516, 517, 518, 519, 521, 523, 524, 525, 526, 527, 528, 538, 558, 559
    Ren-10 Xiawan, 464, 465
    Ren-12 Zhongwan, 45, 65, 96, 97, 131, 152, 195, 208, 209, 226, 227, **273**, **276**, 365, 368, 369, 434, 436, 437, 438, 459, 460, 464, 465, 490, 491, 492, 516, 517, 518, 519, 521, 523, 525, 526, 527, 555, 556, 557, 558, 559
    Ren-13 Shangwan, 464, 465
    Ren-14 Juque, 205, 206, 212, 213, **273–274**, **276**, 366, 367, 430, 431, 432, 433, 434, 436, 437, 466, 467, 468, 514
    Ren-15 Jiuwei, 24, 45, 91, 93, 133, 135, 136, 137, 152, 204, 205, 213, 214, 216, 217, 218, 221, 222, 230, 232, 239, **275**, **276**, 281, **353**, 362, 368, 369, 370, 372, 373, 375, 376, **384**, 386, 435, 436, 437, 438, 458, 460, 461, 462, 463, 464, 465, 466, 469, 486, 488, 489, 520, 527, 528, 537, 539, 540, 541, 555, 556, 557, 558, 559
    Ren-17 Shanzhong, 146, 204, 205, 206, 362, 368, 369, 435, 436, 460, 461, 462
  Gall-Bladder Channel
    G.B.-6 Xuanli, 281
    G.B.-9 Tianchong, **268**, **270**
    G.B.-12 Wangu, 74, **268**, **270**, 456, 457, 459, 460

acupuncture points, by channel—*cont'd*
G.B.-13 Benshen, 45, 93, 125, 140, 200, 201, 202, 206, 207, 214, 215, 219, 220, 221, 224, 225, 226, 227, 239, 240, **268–270**, **271**, 358, 360, 363, 364, 365, 379, **383**, **385**, **428–429**, 429, 437, 438, 456, 457, 465, 466, 471, 472, 474, 514, 537, 538, **553**, 555, 556, 557, 558
G.B.-15 Toulinqi, 221, 222, 224, 226, 227, **270**, **271**, 281, **354**, 366, 367, 456, 457
G.B.-17 Zhengying, 45, 200, 226, 227, **270**, **271**, 281, 365, 514, 521, 523, 527, 538, **553–554**, 555
G.B.-18 Chengling, 45, 200, 205, 206, 207, 226, 227, **270**, **271**, 281, 365, 514, 521, 523, **554**, 555
G.B.-19 Naokong, **270**, **271**, **554**, 555
G.B.-20 Fengchi, 125, 456, 457
G.B.-34 Yanglingquan, 225, 239, 281, 358, 360, 363, 364, 465, 466
G.B.-37 Guangming, 34
G.B.-38 Yangfu, **429**
G.B.-39 Xuanzhong, 281
G.B.-40 Qiuxu, 44, 45, 74, 95, 106, 107, 266, **270**, **271**, 281, **352**, **353**, 430, 431, 470, 471, 487
G.B.-43 Xiaxi, 281, 363, 364
G.B.-44 Zuqiaoyin, **270**, **271**, 456, 457, 486, 487, 524, 525
Governing Vessel
Du-4 Mingmen, 148, 154, 232, 233, **276–277**, **280**, 377, **383**, **385**
Du-9 Zhiyang, 370
Du-10 Lingtai, **277**, **280**
Du-11 Shendao, **277**, **280**, **383**, **385**
Du-12 Shenzhu, 60, 133, **277–278**, **280**, 371, 372, **383**, **385**, 434, 515
Du-14 Dazhau, 208, 209, 232, 233, **278**, **280**, 281, 372, 373, 374, **383–384**, **386**, 433, 494, 495, 515
Du-15 Yamen, 515
Du-16 Fengfu, 69, **278**, **280**, **384**, **386**, 514, 515, **552**, 555
Du-17 Naohu, **278**, **280**, **552**, 555
Du-18 Qiangjian, 207, 219, 220, 224, 225, **278**, **280**, 281
Du-19 Houding, 60, 125, 136, 137, 152, 195, 200, 218, **278**, **280**, 281, 375, 376, 384, **386**, 429, 458, 514, 521, 523, 525, 526, 527, **552–553**, 555
Du-20 Baihui, 44, 45, 65, 69, 100, 135, 152, 195, 200, 208, 209, 226, 227, 228, 229, 230, 232, 233, 234, 239, 240, 266, **278**, **280**, 281, 358, 359, 360, 363, 364, 365, 366, 367, 368, 369, 371, 372, 374, 377, 378, **384**, **386**, 490, 491, 492, 494, 495, 514, 515, 516, 517, 518, 519, 521, **553**, 555, 556, 557
Du-21 Qianding, 368, 369
Du-23 Shangxing, 515
Du-24 Shenting, 24, 91, 93, 129, 131, 133, 140, 152, 195, 200, 201, 202, 206, 207, 214, 215, 219, 220, 221, 224, 225, **278–279**, **280**, 281, **353**, **354**, 365, 375, 376, 379, **384**, 386, **428–429**, 437, 438, 456, 457, 464, 465, 466, 471, 472, 474, 486, 488, 490, 491, 492, 518, 519, 520, 521, 525, 526, 527, 538, 539, 540, 541, **553**, 553, 555, 556, 557, 558, 559
Du-26 Renzhong, 200, 266, 514, 515, 519
Heart Channel
HE-3 Shaohai, **252**, **254**
HE-4 Lingdao, **252**, **254**, 515
HE-5 Tongli, 24, 93, 146, 148, 152, **252–253**, **254**, 281, 362, 366, 367, 371, 372, 374, **380**, **385**, **429**, 430, 431, 433, 434, 435, 437, 460, 461, 462, 487, 488, 495, 518, 519, **551**, 554, 557, 558, 559
HE-6 Yinxi, 213, 216, 217, 218, 375, 376, 432, 433, 469, 489, 525, 527, 528
HE-7 Shenmen, 23–24, 91, 92, 93, 125, 129, 133, 134, 135, 136, 137, 140, 146, 204, 205, 206, 212, 214, 217, 218, 221, 222, 224, 225, 228, 229, 230, 232, **253**, **254**, 281, **353**, 362, 372, 373, **380**, **385**, **427–428**, 430, 431, 432, 433, 434, 435, 436, 458, 460, 461, 462, 466, 467, 468, 469, 470, 471, **480–481**, 486, 487, 488, 489, 514, 515, 518, 519, 520, 524, 525, 527, 528, 539, 540, 541, **551**, 554, 555, 556, 557
HE-8 Shaofu, 45, 91, 93, 221, 222, **253**, **254**, **428**, 437, 458, 463, 515, 520, 521, 523, 524, 537, 538
HE-9 Shaochong, **253**, **254**
Knotted Heat in, 520
Kidney Channel
KI-1 Yongquan, **260–261**, **263**, 281
KI-2 Rangu, 219, 220, 221, 375, 376
KI-3 Taixi, 45, 100, 134, 214, 215, 216, 217, 218, 219, 220, 221, 232, 233, 234, 235, 237, **261**, **263**, 281, **353**, 375, 376, 377, **382**, **385**, 432, 433, 469, 474, 489, 492, 494, 495, 525, 526, 527, 556, 557
KI-4 Dazhong, 92, 100, 134, 135, 140, **261**, **263**, 281, **428**
KI-6 Zhaohai, 216, 217, 218, 234, 235, 237, **261**, **263**, 375, 376, **453**, 456, 457, 469, 489
KI-7 Fuliu, 232, 233, 377, 432, 433
KI-9 Zhubin, 217, 218, **261–262**, **263**, 375, 376, **382**, **385**, **428**
KI-10 Yingu, 217
KI-13 Qixue, 201
KI-14 Siman, 201, 207, 208
KI-16 Huangshu, **249**, **262**, **263**
KI-21 Youmen, 464, 465
Large Intestine Channel
L.I.-1 Shangyang, 514
L.I.-4 Hegu, 60, 65, 74, 104, 146, 201, 202, 204, 205, 208, 209, 224, 225, **247**, **248**, 281, **379**, **383**, **385**, **428**
L.I.-5 Yangxi, **247**, **248**, 514
L.I.-6 Pianli, 103, 104
L.I.-7 Wenliu, 208, 209, **247–248**, 514
L.I.-11 Quchi, 60, 281, 370, 458, 459, 460, 463, 486, 487, 514, 524, 525, 537, 538
Liver Channel
LIV-2 Xingjian, 34, 224, 225, **271**, **272**, 456, 457, 486, 487, 515, 521, 523, 524, 525, 537, 538, 558
LIV-3 Taichong, 45, 93, 95, 102, 125, 140, 201, 202, 206, 207, 219, 220, 221, 224, 225, 239, 266, **271**, **272**, 281, 358, 360, 363, 364, 366, 367, 368, 369, 379, **383**, **385**, **428**, 437, 456, 457, 465, 466, 514, 515, 516, 517, 527, **552**, 555, 556, 557, 558
LIV-8 Ququan, 45, 214, 215, 219, 220, 221, 237, 239, 471, 472, 474, 527, 528, 539, 540, 556, 557

LIV-14 Qimen, 201, 202, 206, 207, 225
Lung Channel
LU-1 Zhongfu, 60, 225
LU-3 Tianfu, 94, 224, 225, 228, 229, **245–246**, **247**, 248, 371, 372, **378–379**, 384, 488, 514
LU-5 Chize, 60, 235, 370, 486
LU-7 Lieque, 53, 60, 65, 89, 93, 94, 128, 129, 131, 133, 146, 204, 205, 208, 209, 225, 235, **246**, **247**, 281, 362, **379**, **385**, **428**, 435, 460, 461, 490, 491
LU-9 Taiyuan, 94, 214, 235, 371, 372, 434, 436, 488, 519
LU-10 Yugi, **246**, **247**, 463
Pericardium Channel, **263–268**
P-3 Quze, **264**, **267**, 267
P-4 Ximen, **264**, **267**
P-5 Jianshi, 45, 154, 200, 205, 206, 208, 209, **264**, **267**, 281, 365, 368, 369, 437, 438, 486, 514, 516, 517, 518, 519, 520, 521, 523, 524, 525, 526, 527, 528
P-6 Neiguan, 44, 60, 102, 110, 113, 132, 146, 154, **155**, 201, 202, 204, 205, 206, 207, 208, 209, 212, 225, **264–266**, **267**, 281, **354**, 358, **359**, 360, 362, 363, 364, 366, 367, 368, 369, 370, 372, 373, **382**, **385**, **428**, 435, 437, 460, 461, 462, 464, 465, 466, 467, **480–481**, 514, 515, 516, 517, 519, 527
P-7 Daling, 45, 60, 102, 113, 137, 140, 148, 152, 154, 195, 206, 207, 208, 209, 217, 218, 221, 222, 224, 225, 226, 227, **266**, **267**, 281, **354**, 365, 375, 376, **428**, 469, 471, 472, 474, 489, 514, 521, 523, 525, 527, 528
P-8 Laogong, 152, 195, **267**, **268**, 486, 487, 515, 520, 521, 523, 524, 537, 538
Small Intestine Channel
S.I.-3 Houxi, 69, 92, 281
S.I.-5 Yanggu, 103, 104, **254–255**
S.I.-7 Zhizheng Branch to *Heart Channel*, 103, 104, **255**
S.I.-16 Tianchuang, **255**, 514
Spleen Channel
BL-20 Pishu, 45, 65, 74, 96, 97, 152, 195, 208, 209, 226, 227, 228, 229, 230, 232, 365, 368, 369, 371, 372, 373, 459, 460, 466, 467, 490, 491, 492, 494, 514, 518, 519, **552**, 555, 556, 557, 558, 559
SP-1 Yinbai, 207, **250**, **251–252**, 459, 460, 514
SP-3 Taibai, 65, 97, 131, 226, 227, 228, 229, **250**, **252**, 491, 492, 494, **551–552**, 555
SP-4 Gongsun, 132, 207, 208, 212, **251**, **252**, 266, 464, 465, 466, 467
SP-5 Shangqiu, **251**, **252**
SP-6 Sanyinjiao, 45, 65, 110, 201, 205, 206, 207, 208, 212, 213, 214, 215, 217, 219, 220, 221, 222, 224, 225, 230, 232, 233, 234, 237, 239, 240, **251**, **252**, 366, 367, 368, 369, 372, 373, 374, 375, 376, **380**, **385**, **428**, 431, 432, 433, 436, 437, 456, 457, 458, 459, 460, 463, 466, 467, 468, 469, 471, 472, 474, 486, 487, 488, 489, 490, 491, 492, 514, 515, 516, 517, 518, 519, 521, 523, 524, 525, 526, 527, 528, 538, 539, 540, **552**, 555, 556, 557, 558, 559
SP-9 Yinlingquan, 65, 365, 368, 369, 459, 460
SP-10 Xuehai, 207, 208, 281, 366, 367, 527
SP-15 Daheng, 524
Stomach Channel
ST-8 Touwei, 65, 226, 227, 365, 459, 460, 490, 491, 492, **554**, 555
ST-21 Liangmen, 464, 465
ST-25 Tianshu, 200, 208, 209, 226, 227, **248–249**, **250**, 514, 524
ST-29 Quilai, 207, 208
ST-30 Qichong, 201
ST-36 Zusanli, 45, 65, 96, 97, 109, 110, 152, 195, 208, 209, 212, 213, 228, 229, 230, 232, 233, 239, 371, 372, 373, 374, **379**, **385**, 430, 431, 432, 433, 434, 466, 467, 468, 487, 488, 490, 491, 492, 494, 515, 518, 519, 539, 540, 551, 557, 558, 559
ST-40 Fenglong, 44–45, 65, 102, 109, 110, 146, 204, 208, 209, 225, 226, 227, **249**, 266, 281, 362, 365, 368, 369, **379**, *380*, **385**, **428**, 435, 437, 438, 459, 460, 461, 463, 464, 465, 486, 491, 514, 515, 516, 517, 519, 521, 523, 524, 525, 527, 528, 538, 558, 559
ST-41 Jiexi, **249**, **250**
ST-42 Chongyang, 74, **249**, **250**, 514
ST-44 Neiting, 464, 465, 524
ST-45 Lidui, **249–250**, 459, 460, 464, 465, 514
Triple Burner Channel
T.B.-3 Zhongzhu, 113, **268**, 281, 358, 360, 363, 364, **382–383**, **385**
T.B.-4 Yangchi, 74
T.B.-5 Waiguan, 113, 152, **354**, 370
T.B.-6 Zhigou, 60, 152, 195, 201, 368, 369, 465, 466, 516, 517
T.B.-10 Tianjing, **268**
acupuncture points, mental and emotional problems
classified by channel *see* acupuncture points, by channel
with *gui* in their name, 84
Hunshe *House of the Ethereal Soul*, 280
from Nanjing Affiliated hospital, **281**
point combinations, examples, 92, 259, 261, 266, 267, **281**
Sun Si Miao's 13 Ghost points, 84, *85*, 259, 515
Yingtang *Seal Hall*, 280–281
acupuncture treatment, indications for
see also herbal treatment, indications for
in ADD, 551–555
clinical trials, 561–562
deficiency of Heart- and Spleen-Blood, 556
Heart- and Kidney-Yin deficiency, 556
Heart and Spleen deficiency, 557
with Phlegm, 558, 559
Kidney- and Liver- Yin deficiency with Liver-Yang rising, 556–557
Liver- and Heart-Fire, 558
in anxiety, 427–430
Heart- and Gall-Bladder deficiency, 430, 431
Heart-Blood deficiency, 431–432
Heart-Blood stasis, 437
Heart-Yang deficiency, 433
Kidney- and Heart-Yin deficiency, with Empty Heat, 432, 433
Lung- and Heart-Qi deficiency or stagnation, 434, 435
Lung- and Heart-Yin deficiency, 436
Phlegm-Heat harassing the Heart, 437, 438
in bipolar disorder/*Dian Kuang*, 515–516
Fire in Bright Yang, 524
Fire injuring Yin with Phlegm, 525–526

acupuncture treatment, indications for—*cont'd*
Gall-Bladder- and Liver-Fire, 524–525
Heart and Spleen deficiency with Phlegm, 518, 519
Knotted Heat in Heart Channel, 520
Phlegm-Fire harassing upwards, 521, 523
Phlegm obstructing Heart orifices, 521
Qi deficiency or stagnation with Phlegm, 516, 517, 519
Qi stagnation, Blood stasis and Phlegm, 527
Yin deficiency with Empty Heat, 527–528
Corporeal Soul, contraction or expansion of, 60
in depression
Blood stasis obstructing the Mind, 366, 367
clinical trials, 392–399
Diaphragm Heat, 370
Heart- and Lung-Qi stagnation, 362
Heart and Spleen deficiency, 372, 373
Heart-Yang deficiency, 374
Kidney- and Heart-Yin deficiency, Empty Heat blazing, 375, 376
Kidney-Yang deficiency, 377–378
Liver-Qi stagnation, 358–359
Phlegm-Heat harassing the Mind, 365
Qi stagnation with Phlegm, 368, 369
stagnant Liver-Qi turning into Heat, 363, 364
Worry injuring the Mind, 371, 372
effect of emotions, 146
Ethereal Soul, stimulation or restraint of movement, 44–45, 95
Lower Burner, Blood stasis in, 207
in Mind Obstructed, 200
Heart- and Lung-Qi stagnation, 204
Heart-Blood stasis, 205
Liver-Blood stasis, 206
Liver-Qi stagnation, 201
Phlegm-Heat harassing the Mind, 208
in Mind Unsettled
Heart- and Kidney-Yin deficiency with Heart Empty Heat, 217
Heart-Blood deficiency, 212
Heart-Fire, 221–222
Heart-Yin deficiency, 213
Kidney-Yin deficiency, 216
Liver-Fire, 224
Liver-Yin deficiency, 214, 219
Phlegm-Fire, 226
in Mind Weakened
Kidney- and Liver- Yin deficiency, 237
Kidney-Essence deficiency, 239
Kidney-Yang deficiency, 232
Kidney-Yin deficiency, 234
Lung- and Kidney-Yin deficiency, 235
Qi deficiency, 228
in night terrors
Liver- and Heart-Blood deficiency, 539
Liver- and Heart-Fire, 537
Liver- and Heart-Yin deficiency, 540
Phlegm-Heat harassing the Mind and Ethereal Soul, 538
shock displacing the Mind, 541
in sleep disorders, 452–453
clinical trials, 478–482
Dampness obstructing the brain, 490
deficiency of Heart and Spleen, 488
deficiency of Qi of Heart and Gall-Bladder, 487
Heart- and Gall-Bladder deficiency, 470, 471
Heart and Kidneys not harmonized, 469, 489
Heart- and Lung-Qi deficiency, 488
Heart- and Spleen-Blood deficiency, 466, 467
Heart-Blood stasis, 461–462
Heart deficiency, 495
Heart-Fire blazing, 458
Heart-Qi stagnation, 460–461
Heart-Yin deficiency, 468
Kidney-Essence deficiency, 494
Kidney-Yang deficiency, 492
Liver- and Kidney-Yin deficiency, 474
Liver-Fire blazing, 456–457, 486–487
Liver-Qi stagnation, 465, 466
Liver-Yin deficiency, 471–472
Phlegm-Heat harassing the Mind, 459, 486
Phlegm misting the brain, 491
residual Heat in diaphragm, 463
retention of food, 464, 465
Spleen deficiency, 491–492, 494
ADD *see* attention deficit disorder (ADD)
ADHD *see* attention deficit hyperactivity disorder (ADHD)
adjustment disorders, and depression, 343
afterlife, and soul, 3
Agitation (*Zang Zao*), 11–12
and anxiety, 419
and depression, 348–349
Alexander of Tralles, 502
altruism, 318
Ames, RT, 5
amygdala, brain, 303
Analects, Confucius's teachings in, 315
ancient Greece, soul in, 3
anger
and depression, 354–355
and emotions, 122–125
and insomnia, 450
and Liver, 117
modern theories, 294
sensation of, 306
anger diaphragm, 360
animal spirits, 2, 290
animus and anima, Jungian psychology, 2, 301
anterior cingulate cortex (ACC), 304
anticonvulsants, 501
antidepressants
in ADD/ADHD, 547
combined reuptake inhibitors and receptor blockers, 414
mechanism of action, 408
monoamine oxidase inhibitors, 414–415
noradrenaline and dopamine reuptake inhibitors, 411–412
selective serotonin reuptake inhibitors, 410–411
serotonin and noradrenaline reuptake inhibitors, 412
side-effects, 410–411
tetracyclics, 408, 413–414
tricyclics, 408, 409, 412–413
antipsychotics, 502
anus, and Corporeal Soul, 55
anxiety
acupuncture treatment, indications for, 265, 272, 427–430
head points, 428–429
Chinese disease entities corresponding to, 419
in Chinese medicine, 418–422
disease entities corresponding to anxiety, 419
Rebellious Qi of Penetrating Vessel, 249, 251, 419–422
and constitutional types, 423
with depression, 379
and emotional stress, 422–423
etiology, 422–423
Fire type prone to, 164
identification of patterns and treatment, 430–438
Heart- and Gall-Bladder deficiency, 430–431
Heart-Blood deficiency, 431–432
Heart-Blood stasis, 436–437
Heart-Yang deficiency, 433–434

Kidney- and Heart-Yin deficiency, Empty Heat blazing, 432–433
Lung- and Heart-Qi deficiency or stagnation, 434–435
Lung- and Heart-Yin deficiency, 435–436
Phlegm-Heat harassing the Heart, 437–438
internal urgency, 420
and irregular diet, 423
and overwork, 423
with palpitations, in ancient Chinese medicine, 12, 350–351, 420
pathology and treatment principles, 423–427
rebellious Qi causing, 249, 251, 419–422
in Western medicine, 417–418
appetites, 288
Aquinas, Thomas, 288, 290
archetypes, 300
Aretaeus of Cappadocia, 502
Aristotle, 3, 286–287
artistic inspiration, and Ethereal Soul, 39
Asberg Rating Scale, depression, 397
asthma, and Corporeal Soul, 49, 50
attention deficit disorder (ADD)
acupuncture points indicated for, by channel
Bladder, 554, 555
Gall-Bladder, 553, 554, 555
Governing Vessel, 552–553, 555
Heart, 551
Liver, 552, 555
Spleen, 551–552, 555
Stomach, 554, 555
and caffeine, 560, 561
case history, 89–90
in Chinese medicine, 548–559
acupuncture points indicated for *see* acupuncture points indicated for, by channel
clinical trials, 561–563
etiology, 550–551
identification of patterns and treatment, 555–559
pathology, 548–549
etiology, 550–551
high-resolution brain SPECT imaging, 559
identification of patterns and treatment, 555–559
deficiency of Heart- and Spleen-Blood, 555–556
Heart- and Kidney-Yin deficiency, 556
Heart and Spleen deficiency, 557, 558–559
Kidney- and Liver-Yin deficiency with Liver-Yang rising, 556–557
Liver and Heart-Fire, 558
Nanjing University of TCM, experience of teachers from, 554
organ pathology, 549, 550
possible causes, 545–546
symptoms, 544–545
treatment of, 546–547
in Western medicine, 544–548
clinical trials, 559–561
attention deficit hyperactivity disorder (ADHD)
see also attention deficit disorder (ADD)
in adults, 547–548
and children, 544
and Ethereal Soul, dysfunction of movement, 40, 89
possible causes, 545–546
treatment of, 546–547
Augustine, St, 288, 328
autism, 40, 89, 561–562

B

Baillarger, Jules, 502
Bard, Philip, 292
basal ganglia, 305
behaviorism, 302
Berkeley, George, 2
bipolar disorder
see also Dian, identification of patterns and treatment; *Dian Kuang*; *Kuang*, identification of patterns and treatment
in ancient Chinese medicine (*Zian Kuang*), 12
course of condition, 501
cyclothymia, 500
depressive phase (*Dian*), 193
diagnosis, 500–501
Dian Kuang compared, 504–506
history, 502
in Chinese medicine, 503–508
mania, symptoms, 498–499
manic phase (*Kuang*), 193
symptoms, 498–500
treatment, 501–502
and *Dian Kuang*, 513–514
in Western medicine, 498–502
Bladder, 110
Bladder Channel *see under* acupuncture points, by channel
Blood deficiency
in childbirth, 423
see also childbirth
and Heart-Blood deficiency, 186, 212–213
and Liver-Blood deficiency, 186
in Mind Weakened, 234
in night terrors, 536
in sleep disorders, 454, 466
blood, effects of mental-emotional problems on, 185–188
Blood-Heat, 187–188
blood loss, 423, 451, 493, 536
Blood stasis
emotions
effect on Qi, 146
effects of mental-emotional problems, 186–187
Heart-Blood stasis, 186–187, 205–206
Liver-Blood stasis, 187, 206–207
in Lower Burner, 207–208
Mind Obstructed, 205–208
Mind Unsettled, 221
obstructing the Mind, 365–367
and Qi stagnation, 356, 506
and Phlegm, 526–527
Bockover, M, 297
"body", concept of in Chinese medicine, 6
Bowlby, J., 302–303, 343
brain
cortex, 158, 292, **308–309**
Dampness obstructing, 489–490
hypothalamus, 292
injury to, in ADD/ADHD, 545
limbic system, 156
Mind and Ethereal Soul, 157–158
minimal function, 563
neocortex, 156, 306
and neurophysiology of emotions, 303–304
paleomammalian, 307–308
quantitative electroencephalographic measurements of activity in, 544, 559
reptilian, 157, 158, **307**
thalamus, 292
as transformation of Marrow, 65
triune, 155–158, 306–309
breathing, 2, 54
Buddhism, 40–41, 323
bupropion (NDRI), 411, 547

C

caffeine, in ADD, 560, 561
calming the Mind
see also anxiety; attention deficit disorder (ADD); bipolar disorder; depression
defined, 605
herbs indicated for *see* herbal prescriptions/main herbs; herbal treatment, indications for
points indicated for, by channel
see also specific acupuncture points and herbs
Bladder Channel, 256, 257, 258

calming the Mind—*cont'd*
Directing Vessel, 272
Gall-Bladder Channel, 268, 270, 553, 554
Governing Vessel, 552–553
Heart Channel, 252, **428**
Kidney Channel, 261, 262
Large Intestine Channel, 247
Liver Channel, 271, **428**, 552
Lung Channel, 245, 246
Pericardium Channel, 264
Small Intestine Channel, 255
Spleen Channel, 250, 552
Stomach Channel, 249, 250, 379
cannabis, 168
Cannon, Walter B., 292
carbamazepine, 501
case histories
anger, 125
anxiety, 443–445
depression, 399–406
Internal Organs, 89–90
Kuang, 523–524, 526
Liver, role in psyche, 95
Mind Obstructed, 198, 202–203
and Phlegm-Heat harassing the Mind, 209–212
Mind Unsettled
Heart- and Kidney-Yin deficiency with Empty Heat, 218–219
Heart-Fire, 222–224
Heart-Yin deficiency, 214
Liver-Fire, 225–226
Liver-Yin deficiency with Empty Heat, 220–221
Phlegm-Fire, 227
Mind Weakened, 229–230, 236, 238–239
sleep disorders, 467–468, 470, 472–473
Stomach, role in psyche, 108–109
Cheng Hao (Neo-Confucian philosopher), 124, 336
childbirth
and anxiety, 423
and night terrors, 536
and sleep disorders, 451, 493
children
and ADHD, 544–545
autism, 40, 89, 561–562
and Ethereal Soul, 38–39
hyperkinesia in, 562–563
Chinese Acupuncture and Moxibustion, 478
Chinese Acupuncture Therapy, 348
Chinese Internal Medicine, 505
Chinese literature
on anxiety, 438–439
on bipolar disorder/*Dian Kuang*, 528–532
classics *see specific works, such as* Yellow Emperor's Classic of Internal Medicine
on depression, 389–392
on sleep disorders, 475–478
Chinese Medical Psychology, 25, 28
Chinese medicine
see also acupuncture points, by channel; acupuncture treatment, indications for; herbal prescriptions/main herbs; herbal treatment, indications for
ancient, mental illness in, 10–12
concept of "body" in, 6
mind-body integration in, 7, 331
Mind in, 8–9
Neo-Confucianism, influence on, 336–338
polarism of philosophy, 5, 81
role in disorders of psyche, 565–569
self, concept of, 327–332
soul in, 6–8
spirit in, 3, 4–6
Choppy pulse, 174, 176
Christchurch Health and Development Study, on cannabis use, 168
Christianity, 2, 288, 328
Chrysippus, 287
Classic of Categories (Lei Jing), **602**
on Corporeal Soul/Ethereal Soul, 55, 56
on emotions, 118, 145
on sleep and dreaming, 30, 31, 485
Classic of Difficulties (Nan Jing), **600–601**
on bipolar disorder/*Dian Kuang*, 503, 506
Gate of Life in, 98
clearing Heat
defined, 605
points indicated for *see specific points under* acupuncture points, by channel
clinical trials
for ADD, 561–563
for anxiety, 439–443
for bipolar disorder/*Dian Kuang*, 532–533
for depression, 392–399
for sleep disorders, 478–484
cocaine, 168–169
cognition, 20
cognitive behavioral therapy, 502
cold diaphragm, 360
coma, and Ethereal Soul, 40
Compendium of Acupuncture see Great Compendium of Acupuncture (Zhen Jiu Da Cheng)
Complete Book of Jing Yue (Jing Yue Quan Shu), 344, 350, 602
Complete Textbook of Chinese Patterns in Contemporary Chinese Medicine, 528–529
complexion, and diagnosis of mental-emotional problems, 171–173
Confucian ethics, 317–320
and Internal Organs, 87
qualities of human being
Li see Li concept, in Neo-Confucianism/Confucianism
Ren, 317–319
Shu, 320
Yi, 319
Zhong, 320
and social relationships, 142, *316*
and society/state, 320–323
Confucianism, 23, 313–323
see also Neo-Confucianism
and anger, 124
and body, 88
and craving, 137
and Daoism, 315, 323
ethics *see* Confucian ethics
Legalist School, 313, 314, 335
and status of women, 338
Confucius, 72, 315–316
consciousness, 15, 19
see also unconscious
core and extended, 52, 328
Ethereal Soul as layer of, 36
focussed, 92
in Jungian psychology, 41
and self, concept of, 328
constitutional types
and anxiety, 423
and *Dian Kuang*, 508–509
Earth, 164
Fire, 163–164
Metal, 164–165
Water, 165–166
Wood, 162, *163*
Corporeal Soul (*Po*), 47–61
and anus, 55
and breathing, 54
clinical application of, 60–61
contraction of, 60
and death, 381
and emotions, 53–54
and Essence, 7, 48–50, 76
and Ethereal Soul, 55–60, *57*
and *gui*, 54–55, 77–79
as movement of Corporeal Soul, 75–76
and individual life, 54
and infancy, 51
and Lungs, 93, 246
and mother-baby bonding, 302–303
movement of, 48
and physiological activity, 52–53

and senses, 51–52
types, 48
and verticality, 59, *60*
cortex, 158, 292, **308–309**
anterior cingulate, 304
insular, 304–305
and limbic system, 305
prefrontal, 303–304
courage, and Ethereal Soul, 34–35
craving, 136–138
restraining, 170
cyclothymia, 500

D

Dai Dong Yuan (of Qing dynasty), 327
Damasio, A
on Corporeal Soul, 52, 53
on emotions, 116, 290, 297–299
on Ethereal Soul, 40
Dampness
obstructing the brain, in somnolence, 489–490
or Phlegm, 147, 167
Dao, meaning, 324
Daoism
and Confucianism, 315, 323
influence on Chinese medicine, 22–23
on tranquil Mind, 169, 170
Darwin, Charles, 291–292
daydreams, guided, 40
death
see also soul; spirit
and Corporeal Soul/Ethereal Soul, 26, 48, 58, 256, 381
and *gui see gui*
Shen as spirit of dead person, 10
deficiency conditions *see specific disorders, such as* Qi deficiency
dementia, 270
demonic medicine, 72, 73, 74, 75
Depakote (valproate), 501
depression
acupuncture points indicated for, by channel
Bladder, 258, 380–382, 385
Directing Vessel, 273, 384
Gall-Bladder, 270, 383, 385
Governing Vessel, 383–384, 385, 386
Heart, 380, 385
Kidney, 382, 385
Large Intestine, 379
Liver, 383, 385
Lung, 378–379
Pericardium, 265, 382, 385
Spleen, 380, 385
Stomach, 379, *380*, 385
Triple Burner, 382–383, 385
Agitation, 348–349
in ancient Chinese medicine (*Yu Zheng*), 11
with anxiety, 379
and bipolar disorder, 500
constitutional types, 355–356
and Ethereal Soul *see under* Ethereal Soul (*Hun*)
etiology, 354–356
Fire type prone to, 164
and Gall-Bladder, 354
identification of patterns and treatment, 357–378
Blood stasis obstructing the Mind, 365–367
Diaphragm Heat, 369–370
Heart- and Lung-Qi stagnation, 361–362
Heart and Spleen deficiency, 372–373
Heart-Yang deficiency, 373–374
Kidney- and Heart-Yin deficiency, Empty Heat blazing, 375–376
Kidney-Yang deficiency, 376–378
Liver-Qi stagnation, 358–361
Phlegm-Heat harassing the Mind, 364–365
Qi stagnation with Phlegm, 367–369
stagnant Liver-Qi turning into Heat, 362–364
Worry injuring the Mind, 370–372
and Intellect, 354
and irregular diet, 356
Lilium Syndrome, 347–348
Liver-Qi deficiency or stagnation in, 351–352, 362–364
major depressive syndrome, 343–344, 398
minor, 397, 442
and neurasthenia, 353
and overwork, 356
pathology of, 356–357
in Chinese medicine, 344–354
patient statistics, 407
Pericardium and Triple Burner, 354
Plum-Stone Syndrome, 349–350
post-stroke, 394–395
in pregnancy, 396
randomized controlled trials, literature on, 395
relapse rates, acupuncture treatment, 397–398
relationship between Mind and Ethereal Soul, 345–346
severe, 346
and stagnation, 345
symptoms, 342, 343
in bipolar disorder/*Dian Kuang*, 499
tiaoshenshugan acupuncture versus routine acupuncture, 395
Western medicine on, 342–344
combined with Chinese, 415
drug treatment, 407–415
and Will-Power, 353
in *Yu/Yu* syndrome, 344–345, 346–347
Descartes, René, 2, 290, 291
desire, 306, 335
diagnosis
in bipolar disorder, 500–501
and complexion, 171–173
and eyes, 173–174
in mania, 499–500
in panic attacks, 418
and pulse *see* pulse
in sleep disorders, 454–456
and tongue *see* tongue diagnosis
Diagnostic and Statistical Manual for Mental Disorders (DSM-IV), 500
Dian, identification of patterns and treatment
see also Kuang, identification of patterns and treatment
Heart- and Spleen deficiency with Phlegm, 518–519
Knotted Heat in Heart Channel, 520
Phlegm obstructing Heart orifices, 520–521
points that open the Mind's orifices, 514, 515
Qi deficiency or stagnation with Phlegm, 516–517, 519–520
Dian Kuang
see also Dian, identification of patterns and treatment; *Kuang*, identification of patterns and treatment
bipolar disorder compared, 504–506
see also bipolar disorder
depressive phase (*Dian*), 193
differentiation between *Dian* and *Kuang*, 512
etiology, 508–509
historical development, 503–504
manic phase (*Kuang*), 193
mental-emotional indications of points, 244, 270
pathology of, 509–511
disharmony of Yin and Yang, 506
Ethereal Soul, disharmony of "coming and going", 507
Fire harassing upwards, 506
Phlegm, 506
Qi stagnation and Blood stasis, 506
symptoms, 12

Dian Kuang—*cont'd*
treatment of, 511–513
adaptation to bipolar disorder treatment, 513–514
Dian syndrome, in depression, 346–347
Diaphragm Heat, in depression, 369–370
dietary factors, in mental-emotional problems
excessive consumption of cold-energy foods, 167
excessive consumption of Damp-producing foods, 166–167
excessive consumption of hot-energy foods, 166
insufficient eating, 167
irregular eating habits, 167
in anxiety, 423
in bipolar disorder/*Dian Kuang*, 508
in depression, 356
in insomnia, 450–451
in night terrors, 536
retention of food, in sleep problems, 450, 452, 464, 465
diffuse awareness, 92
Dionysus, 32
Directing Vessel (*Ren Mai*) *see under* acupuncture points, by channel
Discussion of Blood Patterns, 55
Discussion of the Origin of Symptoms in Diseases (Zhu Bing Yuan Hou Lun), 601
Discussion on Blood Patterns (Xue Zheng Lun), 602
Discussion on Stomach and Spleen (Pi Wei Lun), 601
disharmony
of "coming and going" of Ethereal Soul, 507
of Heart and Kidneys, in sleep problems, 468–470, 488
of Yin and Yang, in *Dian Kuang*, 506
Dong Zhong Shu (Confucian scholar), 324
draining Fire, 512, 605
dreams
"chaotic", 30
and Ethereal Soul, 29–31, 39–40
examples, 454–455
excessive dreaming, 29, 484–489
Blood or Yin deficiency, 454
Heart and Kidneys not harmonized, 488
Heart- and Lung-Qi deficiency, 487–488
Liver-Fire, 486–487
Phlegm-Heat, 486
Qi deficiency of Heart and Gall-Bladder, 487
Freudian theory, 299
insomnia diagnosis, 454–455
"normal", 30
rapid eye movement (REM), 39
drug treatment
anticonvulsants, 501
antipsychotics, 502
for bipolar disorder, 501–502
for depression *see* antidepressants
dualism, of Western philosophy, 5, 331
dullness, 245
Duloxetine (SNRI), 412
dysthymia, and depression, 343, 500

E

Earth, and Spleen, 96
Earth type, 164
eating habits, irregular, 167
in anxiety, 423
in bipolar disorder/*Dian Kuang*, 508
in depression, 356
in insomnia, 450–451
in night terrors, 536
ecstasy (drug), 169
eczema, and Corporeal Soul, 49
ego, Freudian theory, 300
An Elucidation of the Yellow Emperor's Classic of Internal Medicine, 322
emotional life, 19, 60–61
see also emotions
emotional stress *see also* mental-emotional problems, patterns in
in ADD/ADHD, 550–551
and anxiety, 422–423
consequences, *185*
and depression, 354–355
and *Dian Kuang*, 508
and insomnia, 450
and night terrors, 536
emotions, 115–158
see also emotional life
anger, 122–125
balance of, and Ethereal Soul, 32–34
control of emotions by Reason, *289*
and Corporeal Soul, 53, 53–54
craving, 136–138
Damasio on, 116, 297–299
definitions, 2
as disharmonies of Qi, 333
effect on blood, 146
effect on Qi, 143–147
Dampness or Phlegm, 147
derangement of Qi in emotional problems, 143–144
Heat or Fire, 146–147
stagnation, 145–147
fear *see* fear
and feeling, 8, 53, 116
guilt *see* guilt
and human nature, 78
Internal Organs, effect on, 144–145
James-Lange theory of, 7–8, 292–294
joy, 126–127
love, 135–136
mental-emotional problems *see* mental-emotional problems, patterns in
Minister Fire, pathology of, 148–155
Empty Heat, 149–150
Full Heat, 149
Pericardium in mental-emotional problems, 152–155
Yin Fire, 150–152
Neo-Confucianism, 332–336
neurophysiology of, 303–306
pensiveness, 129–131
and pulse qualities, 176–177
sadness and grief, 131–133
shame *see* shame
shock, 134–135
terminology, 115, 116
triune brain and Chinese medicine, 155–158
in Western philosophy, 283–309
ancient theories, 285–291
early modern theories, 291–292
modern theories, 294–299
worry, 127–129
Empty Heat
with Heart-Yin deficiency, 189
with Kidney- and Heart-Yin deficiency, 375–376
with Kidney-Yin deficiency, 190
with Liver-Yin deficiency, 189–190, 219–221
with Lung-Yin deficiency, 190
Minister Fire, pathology of, 149–150
as pathogenic factor in mental-emotional problems, 193–194
with Spleen-Yin deficiency, 190
with Yin deficiency, 189, 190, 217–221, 527–528
An Enquiry into Chinese Acupuncture, 270
enteric nervous system, 102
environmental agents, in ADD/ADHD, 545
Epicurus, 3
epilepsy, 12, 503
Erasistratus, 2
Essence (*Jing*), and Corporeal Soul, 7, 48–50, 76
The Essence of Medical Classics on the Convergence of Chinese and Western Medicine, 20
Essential Method of Dan Xi, 344
Essential Prescriptions of the Golden Chest (Jin Gui Yao Lue), 601
and depression, 348, 349
and *Dian Kuang*, 503
and Lilium Syndrome, 10, 347
and Plum-Stone Syndrome, 349

Ethereal Soul (*Hun*), 25–46
acupuncture points indicated for, 44–45
Bladder Channel, 257, 259, 381
Heart Channel, 253
Spleen Channel, 251
in ADD, 548, 550
balance of emotions, 32–34
and Buddhist psychology, 40–41
clinical application, 44–46
clinical patterns of pathologies, 43
"coming and going" of, 7, 31
and artistic inspiration, 39
in bipolar disorder/*Dian Kuang*, 510
choice of acupuncture points, 258, 259, 265, 266, 270, 271, 367
clinical patterns of pathologies, 43
disharmony of in *Dian Kuang*, 507
giving "horizontality" to life, 59
Liver-Qi, free flow of, 34
and Corporeal Soul, 55–60, *57*
courage, 34–35
and depression, deficient movement in, 345–346, 347, 353, 354, 355, 358, 367, 380, 383, 386, 387, 388
Ethereal Soul, relationship with Mind, *37*, 44–45
examples of the nature of, 38–40
excessive movement of, *37*
restraining, 45, 46
eyes/vision, 34, *35*
gui as movement of, 75–76
and horizontality, 59, *60*
imparted by father after birth, 28, 54
and Jungian psychology, 41–42
and limbic system/Mind, 157–158
and Liver, 427
metaphysical nature of concept, 23
Mind, relationship with, 36–44, 345–346
and modern diseases, 40
movement of, 29
acupuncture points indicated for, 264
deficient in depression *see and depression, deficient movement in*
dysfunction in autism and ADHD, 40
excessive, *37*, 45, 46, 89, 94, 549
and expansion/contraction, 42
and mental activities, 31–32
and Phlegm-Heat harassing the Mind, in night terrors, 537–538
planning, 35, 36
role of, 27
and sleep, 29–31, 449
and soul, 4
stimulation of movement, 44–45, 95
three types, 26
wandering at night, in dreams, 454
Willis on, 290–291
ethics, Confucian *see* Confucian ethics
etiology of mental emotional problems, 161–170
and anxiety, 422–423
attention deficit disorder, 550–551
constitutional types, 162–166
and depression, 354–356
Dian Kuang, 508–509
diet *see* dietary factors, in mental-emotional problems
night terrors, 536
overwork *see* overwork
prevention, 169–170
recreational drugs, 167–169, 493
sexual activity, excessive *see* sexual activity, excessive
sleep disorders, 450–451
expansion/contraction, and Ethereal Soul, movement of, 42
An Explanation of the Acupuncture Points (Jing Xue Jie)
for ADD, 552
for depression, 378, 381
description of points, 245, 246, 248, 249, 250, 252, 253, 254, 255, 258, 261, 266, 275, 278, 279, 602
extroversion/introversion, 301–302
eyes, diagnosis of mental-emotional problems, 173–174
eyesight, 20–21, 34, *35*

F

Falret, Jean Pierre, 502
family therapy, 502
Fan Chen (Daoist philosopher), 4–5
fear
anxiety distinguished, 419
and emotions, 133–134
sensation of, 306
feeling, and emotions, 8, 53, 116
Fire
in bipolar disorder/*Dian Kuang*, 530–531
harassing upwards, in bipolar disorder/*Dian Kuang*, 506
Heart-Fire *see* Heart-Fire
Liver-Fire *see* Liver-Fire blazing
in night terrors, 536
or Heat *see* Heat or Fire
in treatment of mental-emotional problems, 221–226
Fire in Bright Yang, 524
Fire type, 163–164
Five-Element perspective
and Confucianism, 325
constitutional types, 165
and emotions, 118, 123
and Pericardium, 264
focussing, 65, 66
focussed consciousness, 92
food additives and sugar, in ADD/ADHD, 545
Food and Drug Administration, US (FDA), 546
foods, excessive consumption of, 166–167
Forbidden City, and Directing Vessel points, *274*
forgetfulness, 245
Four Political Treatises of the Yellow Emperor, 336
Free and Easy Wanderer Plus (FEWP), herbal medicine, 533
Freud, Sigmund, 299–300
Fright Cry, 533
Fu Qing Zhu (from Qing dynasty), 512
Full Heat, Minister Fire, pathology of, 149
functional magnetic resonance imaging (fMRI), 305

G

gabapentin, 501
GAD (generalized anxiety disorder), 418, 438–439
Gall-Bladder
"courage" of, 354
decision-making capacity, 88, 94
and depression, 354
Gall-Bladder Channel *see under* acupuncture points, by channel
role in psyche, 104–107
Gall-Bladder- and Liver-Fire, in *Kuang*, 524–525
Gate of Life, 98, 99, 273
Du-4 Mingmen *Gate of Life see under* acupuncture points
Gatherings from Eminent Acupuncturists, 245, 246, 247, 248, 251, 255, 256, 258, 261, 266, 277, 278
generalized anxiety disorder (GAD), 418, 438–439
genetic factors
in ADD/ADHD, 545, 550
in bipolar disorder/*Dian Kuang*, 509
nervous system, 162
Governing Vessel *see under* acupuncture points, by channel
Great Compendium of Acupuncture (Zhen Jiu Da Cheng), 245, 248, 253, 254, 255, 258, 261, 267, 270, 274, 277, 602
Great Dictionary of Acupuncture, 269, 272

gui
acupuncture points with *gui* in their name, 84
as centripetal, separating, fragmenting force, 50, 76–77, 78
Chinese character for, *26*, 48
and Corporeal Soul, 54–55, 77–79
as counterpole to *Shen*, 79–83, *80*, 81, 82, 83
as dark force of psyche, 83–84
and Jungian psychology, 301
as movement of the Ethereal Soul and Corporeal Soul, 75–76
as spirit, ghost, 23, 71–75
as symbol of contraction, 79–83, *80*, 81
guilt
and depression, 355
and Earth type, 164
and emotions, 138–140
and insomnia, 450
and Kidneys, 426
gut/gut brain, 102

H

Hamilton Depression Rating Scale (HAMD), 397
Han dynasty, 4, 315, 321
happiness, 306
hearing, and Mind, 21
Heart
and anxiety, 424–425
correspondence to a hall, 258
deficiency, 495, 549
Empty conditions of, 425
Full conditions of, 256, 425
Heart Channel *see under* acupuncture points, by channel
and memory, 64, 493
Mind of, 18, 21–22, 253
as Monarch, 88, 90
pathology in ADD, 549, 550
Phlegm-Heat harassing, in anxiety, 437–438
Phlegm obstructing orifices, 521
and physiological activity, 52
pulse, 175–176
role in psyche, 90–93
Heart- and Gall-Bladder deficiency
in anxiety, 430–431
in sleep disorders, 454, 470–471, 477
excessive dreaming, 487
Heart- and Kidney-Yin deficiency, 217–219, 556
Heart and Kidneys not harmonized, 261
sleep disorders, 468–470, 488, 489
Heart- and Lung-Qi deficiency or stagnation
and depression, 361–362
effects of mental-emotional problems/ emotional stress, 184–185, 355
in Mind Obstructed, 203–205
in sleep disorders, 487–488
Heart- and Spleen-Blood deficiency, in sleep disorders, 466–468, 467
Heart and Spleen deficiency
in ADD, 557, 558–559
in bipolar disorder/*Dian Kuang*, 518
in depression, 372–373
with Phlegm, in ADD, 558–559
in sleep disorders, 476–477, 488
Heart-Blood deficiency
in anxiety, 425, 428, 431–432
in depression, 372
in Mind Unsettled, 212–213
in night terrors, 536
points indicated for, 253
in sleep disorders, 451
Heart-Blood Heat, 187
Heart-Blood stasis
in anxiety, 436–437
in sleep disorders, 451–452, 461–462, 476
Heart crack, tongue, 162, 178–179
combined with Stomach crack, *178*, 180–181
constitutional traits, 355
Heart Empty Heat
acupuncture points for clearing of, 252, 256
and craving, 137
with Heart- and Kidney-Yin deficiency, in Mind Unsettled, 217–218
with Kidney-Yin deficiency, 452
Heart-Fire
acupuncture points for clearing of, 252, 256
in ADD, 554
in anxiety, 428
and craving, 137
in sleep disorders, 457–458
in treatment of mental-emotional problems, 221–224
Heart-Qi stagnation
emotions, effect of, 146
in sleep disorders, 451, 460–461
Heart-Yang deficiency
in anxiety, 433–434
in depression, 373–374
Heart-Yin deficiency
with Empty Heat, 189
in Mind Unsettled, 213–214
in night terrors, 536
in sleep disorders, 468
Heat
blazing upwards, 384
Diaphragm, 369–370
Empty *see* Empty Heat
Full *see* Full Heat
Heart Empty *see* Heart Empty Heat
or Fire *see* Heat or Fire
in sleeping positions, 455
stagnant Liver-Qi turning into, 362–364
Heat- and Spleen Blood, deficiency in ADD, 555–556
heat diaphragm, 360
Heat or Fire
dietary factors, 166
effects of mental-emotional problems, 191–192
emotions, effect on Qi, 146–147
restraining of movement of Ethereal Soul, 45, 46
Heaven, 317
Hegel, G.W.F., 2
helplessness, in depression, 343–344
Heraclitus, 285–286
herbal prescriptions/main herbs
Bai He Di Huang Tang, **571**
Bai He Gu Jin Tang (and variation), 436, **571**
Bai He Zhi Mu Tang, 348, **571**
Bai Zi Yang Xin Wan, 213, 214, **571–572**
Ban Xia Hou Po Tang, 45, 60, 146, 204, 205, 349, 362, 368, 369, 435, 461, **572**
Ban Xia Shu Mi Tang, 464, 465, **572**
plus Wen Dan Tang, 491
Bao Nao Ning Jiao Nang, **572**
Bu Fei Tang (and variations), 61, 434, 488, **572**
Bu Sui Rong Nao Tang, **572**
Bu Xin Dan (and variation), 373, **572–573**
Bu Zhong Yi Qi Tang (and variation), 492, **573**
Cang Bai Er Chen Tang, **573**
Chai Hu Long Gu Mu Li Tang, **573**
Chai Hu Shu Gan Tang (and variation), 359, 361, **573–574**
Da Bu Yin Jian, 237
Da Bu Yin Wan, **574**
Da Bu Yuan Jian, **574**
Da Cheng Qi Tang (and variation), 524, **574**
Dan Zhi Xiao Yao San, 363, 364, **574**
Dang Gui Long Hui Wan, 522, 523, **574**
Dao Chi San (and variation), 46, 222, 458, 520, **574–575**
Dao Tan Tang, **575**
Di Po Tang, 235, 236, **575**
Di Tan Tang, 519, 520, 521, **575**

Dian Kuang Meng Xing Tang, 527, **575**
Ding Kuang Zhu Yu Tang, 527, **575**
Ding Zhi Wan (and variation), 228, 229, 471, **575–576**
Er Chen Tang (and variation), **576**
Er Huang San, **576**
Er Yin Jian (and variations), 525, 526, 528, **576**
Er Zhi Wan (and variation), 474, **576–577**
Fo Shou, 386, 388
Free and Easy Wanderer Plus (FEWP), 533
Fu Shen Tang, **577**
Gan Mai Da Zao Tang (and variation), 12, 231, 232, 349, 371, 372, 518, 519, 541, **577**
plus Gui Pi Tang, 557, 559
Gui Pi Tang (and variations), 230, 232, 372, 373, 380, 432, 466, 467, 488, 494, 539, 555, 556, **577–578**
plus Gan Mai Da Zao Tang, 557, 559
Gui Shen Tang, 209, 438, **578**
Gui Zhi Gan Cao Long Gu Mu Li Tang (and variation), 216, 374, 433, 434, **578–579**
Gui Zhi Jia Long Gu Mu Li Tang, **579**
He Che Da Zao Wan, 239, 240, **579**
He Huan Hua, 387, 388
He Huan Pi, 202, 387, 388
plus Gan Mai Da Zao Tang, 371
Huang Lian E Jiao Tang (and variation), 489, **579**
Huang Lian Wen Dan Tang (and variation), 459, 460, 486, **579**
Ji Sheng Shen Qi Tang (and variation), 518, 519, **579–580**
Jiao Tai Wan, 469, **580**
Jie Fan Yi Xin Tang, 376, **580**
Jie Yu Qing Xin Tang, 363, 364, **580**
Jin Gui Shen Qi Wan, 377, 378, **580**
Jin Suo Gu Jing Wan, **580**
Jing Gong Sha Xiang San, **580**
Kai Yu Yue Shen Tang, **580–581**
Kong Sheng Zhen Zhong Dan, 556, **581**
Liang Ge San, **581**
Ling Jiao Gou Teng Tang, 46, **581**
Liu Jun Zi Tang (and variation), 492, **581**
Liu Wei Di Huang Wan (and variations), 218, 234, 495, **581–582**
Long Dan Xie Gan Tang (and variations), 46, 457, 487, 525, 537, 558, **582–583**
Mai Wei Di Huang Wan (Ba Xian Chang Shou Wan), 235, 236, **583**
Mei Gui Hua, 386–387, 388
Meng Shi Gun Tan Wan, 522, 523, **583**
Mu Xiang Liu Qi Yin, 146, 202, 362, 461, **583**
Nan Geng Tang, 377, 378, **583**
Niu Huang Qing Xin Wan, **583**
Ping Bu Zhen Xin Dan (and variation), 431, **583–584**
Ping Wei San (and variation), 490, **584**
Ping Xin Wang You Tang, **584**
Qi Ju Di Huang Wan (and variation), 557, **584–585**
Qing Pi, 386, 388
Qing Xin Tang, **585**
Rou Fu Bao Yuan Tang, 374, **585**
San Cai Feng Sui Dan, **585**
Sang Dan Xie Bai San (and variation), 60, **585**
Sang Piao Xiao San, **585**
An Shen Ding Zhi Wan (and variation), 228, 430, 431, 471, **571**
Shen Zhong Dan, **585**
Sheng Mai San, **585**
Sheng Tie Luo Yin, 521, 523, **585–586**
Shi Bu Wan, 492, **586**
Shi Chang Pu, 202, 388, 389
plus Xue Fu Zhu Yu Tang, 367
Shi Wei Wen Dan Tang (and variations), 231, 232, 368, 369, 459, 460, 487, 519, 520, **586**
Shi Yu Tang (and variation), **587**
Shun Qi Dao Tan Tang (and variations), 368, 369, 516, 517, **587**
Si Ni San, **587**
plus Yue Ju Wan, 461, 465, 466, **593**
Si Qi Tang (and variation), 205, 517, **587–588**
plus Su He Xiang Wan, 517
Su He Xiang Wan, **588**
plus Si Qi Tang, 517
Suan Zao Ren Tang (and variation), 42, 214, 216, 219, 220, 221, 472, 540, **588**
clinical trials, 482, 483
plus Wen Dan Tang, 365
Tan Yu Tang, **588–589**
Tao He Cheng Qi Tang, 207, 208, **589**
Tao Ren Hong Hua Jian, 437, **589**
Tian Wang Bu Xin Dan, 217–218, 376, 432, 433, 469, 489, **589**
Tiao Wei Cheng Qi Tang, **589**
Tiaoshen Liquor, 562
Tong Qiao Huo Xue Tang, 462, **589**
Wen Dan Tang (and variations), 46, 208, 209, 226, 227, 365, 438, 516, 517, 521, 522, 523, 538, **589–590**
plus Ban Xia Shu Mi Tang, 491
plus Zhu Sha An Shen Wan, 522, 523
Wu Ge Kuan Zhong San, 360, 361, **590**
Wu Wei Zi Tang (and variation), 431, **590**
Xiang Yuan, 386, 388
Xiao Chai Hu Tang, **590**
Xiao Feng San, 60, **590**
Xiao Yao San, 359–360, 361, **590**
plus Zuo Jin Wan, 363, 364
Xie Gan An Shen Wan, 224, 225, **590–591**
Xie Qing Wan (and variation), 457, **591**
Xie Xin Tang (and variation), 458, 522, 523, **591**
Xu Fu Zhu Yu Tang (and variation), **591**
Xuan Fu Dai Zhe Tang, **591**
Xue Fu Zhu Yu Tang, 205, 206, 366, 367, 462
Xue Yu Tang, **592**
Yang Xin Jian Pi Tang, **592**
Yang Xin Tang (I), 212, 373, 433, 434, 518, 519, **592**
Yang Xin Tang (II), 433, 434, 468, 518, 519, **592**
Yi Lu Kang Jiao Nang, **592**
Yi Shen Ning, 369, **592**
Yin Mei Tang (and variation), 215, 216, 472, 540, **592–593**
You Gui Wan, 46, 232, 233, 377, 378, **593**
You Gui Yin, **593**
Yu Jin, 388, 389
plus Xue Fu Zhu Yu Tang, 367
Yuan Zhi, 42, 387, 388
plus Gan Mai Da Zao Tang, 371
plus Wen Dan Tang, 365
Yuan Zhi Wan, **593**
Yue Ju Wan, 45, 201, 202, 206, 207, 344, 359, **593**
plus Si Ni San, 461, 465, 466, **593**
plus Xiao Yao San, *360*
Zhen Zhong Dan, 216, 495, **593**
Zhen Zhu Mu Wan, 215, 216, **593–594**
Zhi Shi Dao Zhi Wan, 464, 465, **594**
Zhi Zi Chi Tang, 370, 463, **594**
Zhu Sha An Shen Wan, **594**
plus Wen Dan Tang, 522, 523
Zhu Ye Shi Gao Tang, 463, **594**

herbal prescriptions/main herbs—*cont'd*
Zi Shui Qing Gan Yin, 375, 376, **594**
Zuo Gui Wan (and variation), 237, 474, **594**
Zuo Gui Yin, **594–595**
Zuo Jin Wan, **595**
plus Xiao Yao San, 363, 364
empirical, **595**
herbal treatment, indications for
see also acupuncture treatment, indications for; herbal prescriptions/main herbs
in ADD
clinical trials, 562–563
deficiency of Heart- and Spleen-Blood, 556
Heart- and Kidney-Yin deficiency, 556
Heart and Spleen deficiency, 557, 559
Kidney- and Liver- Yin deficiency with Liver-Yang rising, 557
Liver- and Heart-Fire, 558
in anxiety
Heart and Gall-Bladder deficiency, 430–431
Heart-Blood deficiency, 432
Heart-Blood stasis, 437
Heart-Yang deficiency, 433, 434
Kidney- and Heart-Yin deficiency, with Empty Heat, 432, 433
Lung- and Heart-Qi deficiency or stagnation, 434, 435, 436
Phlegm-Heat harassing the Heart, 438
in bipolar disorder/*Dian Kuang*
clinical trials, 532–533
Fire in Bright Yang, 524
Fire injuring Yin with Phlegm, 525, 526
Gall-Bladder- and Liver-Fire, 525
Heart and Spleen deficiency with Phlegm, 518, 519
Knotted Heat in Heart Channel, 520
Phlegm-Fire harassing upwards, 521–522, 523
Phlegm obstructing Heart orifices, 521
Qi deficiency or stagnation with Phlegm, 516–517, 519, 520
Qi stagnation, Blood stasis and Phlegm, 527
Yin deficiency with Empty Heat, 528
Corporeal Soul, contraction or expansion of, 60, 61
in depression
Blood stasis obstructing the Mind, 366–367
clinical trials, 399
Diaphragm Heat, 370
Heart- and Lung-Qi stagnation, 362
Heart and Spleen deficiency, 372–373
Heart-Yang deficiency, 374
Kidney- and Heart-Yin deficiency, Empty Heat blazing, 375–376
Kidney-Yang deficiency, 377
Liver-Qi stagnation, 359–360
Phlegm-Heat harassing the Mind, 365
prescriptions, main herbs, 386–389
Qi stagnation with Phlegm, 368–369
stagnant Liver-Qi turning into Heat, 363–364
Worry injuring the Mind, 371–372
effect of emotions, 146
Ethereal Soul, stimulation or restraint of movement, 42, 45–46
in Mind Obstructed, 198–199
Heart- and Lung-Qi stagnation, 204
Heart-Blood stasis, 205–206
Liver-Blood stasis, 206–207
Liver-Qi stagnation, 201–202
Lower Burner, stasis in, 207–208
Phlegm-Heat harassing the Mind, 208–209
in Mind Unsettled, 198–199
Heart- and Kidney-Yin deficiency with Heart Empty Heat, 217–218
Heart-Blood deficiency, 212–213
Heart-Fire, 222–224
Heart-Yin deficiency, 213–214
Kidney-Yin deficiency, 216–217
Liver-Fire, 224–225
Liver-Yin deficiency, 214–216, 219–220
Phlegm-Fire, 226–227
in Mind Weakened, 198–199
Blood deficiency, 234
Kidney- and Liver- Yin deficiency, 237
Kidney-Essence deficiency, 239–240
Kidney-Yang deficiency, 233–234
Kidney-Yin deficiency, 234
Lung- and Kidney-Yin deficiency, 235
Qi and Blood deficiency, 230–231
Qi deficiency, 228–229
in Neo-Confucianism, 337
in night terrors
Liver- and Heart-Blood deficiency, 539
Liver- and Heart-Fire, 537
Liver- and Heart-Yin deficiency, 540
Phlegm-Heat harassing the Mind and Ethereal Soul, 538
shock displacing the Mind, 541
in sleep disorders
clinical trials, 482–484
Dampness obstructing the brain, 490
deficiency of Heart and Spleen, 488
deficiency of Qi of Heart and Gall-Bladder, 487
Heart- and Gall-Bladder deficiency, 471
Heart and Kidneys not harmonized, 469, 489
Heart- and Lung-Qi deficiency, 488
Heart- and Spleen-Blood deficiency, 466, 467
Heart-Blood stasis, 462
Heart deficiency, 495
Heart-Fire blazing, 458
Heart-Qi stagnation, 461
Heart-Yin deficiency, 468
Kidney-Essence deficiency, 495
Kidney-Yang deficiency, 492
Liver- and Kidney-Yin deficiency, 474
Liver-Fire blazing, 457, 487
Liver-Qi stagnation, 465, 466
Liver-Yin deficiency, 472
Phlegm-Heat harassing the Mind, 459–460, 486
Phlegm misting the brain, 491
residual Heat in diaphragm, 463
retention of food, 464, 465
Spleen deficiency, 492, 494
suggested substitutions for Chinese, 597, 598
horizontality, and Ethereal Soul, 59, *60*
Huangshu, meaning, 262
human nature (*Xing*), in Neo-Confucianism, 78, 325–326, 332
humanism, 72
Hume, David, 291
hyper self-consciousness, 328
hyperactivity-impulsiveness, in ADD, 544–545
hyperkinesia, 562–563
hyperventilation syndrome, 441–442
hypomania, 499, 500–501
hypothalamus, 292
hysteria, 270

I

id, Freudian theory, 300
Idealism school of philosophy, 2–3
ideas, generation of, 20, 64, 66
immune function impairment, in anxiety, 442
inattention, in ADD, 545
individualism, 328
infancy, and Corporeal Soul, 51
insight, 19

insomnia/sleep problems *see* sleep disorders
insular cortex, 304–305
Intellect (*Yi*)
in ADD, 548–549, 550
clinical application, 65, 66
and cortex, 158
and depression, 354
focussing, 65, 66
and functions of Mind, 20
and ideas, 64, 66
and memory, 63–64, 65
and Mind, 65, 66
and Postnatal Qi, 7, 63
resident in Spleen, 7
studying/concentrating, 64–65, 66
Internal Organs *see also specific organs, such as* Heart
case history, 89–90
emotions, effect on, 116, 144–145
as "officials", 321
and psyche, 87–112
Internal Wind, effects of mental-emotional problems, 195–196
interpersonal therapy, 502
invigorating Blood, defined, 605
inwardness, and Western notion of self, 328

J

James-Lange theory of emotions, 7–8, 292–294
James, William, 8, 292–294
Journal of Chinese Medicine
on anxiety, 438–439
on bipolar disorder/*Dian Kuang*, 528
on depression, 389–392
on sleep disorders, 475–477
joy, and emotions, 126–127
Jungian psychology
animus and anima, 2, 301
collective unconscious, 300
and Ethereal Soul, 41–42
and *gui*, 301
guided daydreams, 40
psychological types, 301–302
Shadow concept, 83–84, 300–301

K

Kant, Immanuel, 2, 291
Kidney- and Heart-Yin deficiency, Empty Heat blazing
in anxiety, 432–433
in depression, 375–376
Kidney- and Liver- Yin deficiency
with Liver-Yang rising, in ADD, 556–557
in Mind Weakened, 236–239
Kidney-Essence
and brain, 65
deficiency
in anxiety, 429
in memory problems, 494–495
in Mind Weakened, 239–240
and sexual activity, 167
and Pre-Heaven Qi, 553
as source of Marrow, 269, 429, 493
Kidney-Qi stagnation, in anxiety, 426
Kidney-Yang deficiency
in depression, 376–378, 383
and diet, 167
in Mind Weakened, 232–234
in somnolence, 492–493
Kidney-Yin deficiency
acupuncture points indicated for, 262
and ADD/ADHD, 554
and anxiety, 423
with Empty Heat, 190
Heart Empty Heat, 452
Mind Unsettled, 216–217
and overwork, 167, 450
Kidneys
and anxiety, 426
and guilt, 426
importance of, 90
Kidney Channel *see under* acupuncture points, by channel
and memory, 64
role in psyche, 97–100
Zhi of, in depression, 346
Kuang, identification of patterns and treatment
see also Dian, identification of patterns and treatment
Fire in Bright Yang, 524
Fire injuring Yin with Phlegm, 525–526
Gall-Bladder- and Liver-Fire, 524–525
Phlegm-Fire harassing upwards, 521–524
points that open the Mind's orifices, 514–515
Qi stagnation, Blood stasis and Phlegm, 526–527
Yin deficiency with Empty Heat, 527–528

L

Lamictal (lamotrigine), 501
lamotrigine, 501
Lange, Carl, 8, 292–294
language, 306
Large Intestine
Large Intestine Channel *see under* acupuncture points, by channel
role in psyche, 104
Legalist School, Confucianism, 313, 314, 335
Li concept, in Neo-Confucianism/Confucianism, 320, 326–327
and nature of Mind, 9, 23
lifting mood, defined, 605
Lilium Syndrome (*Bai He Bing*), 10–11, 347–348
limbic system, 156, 157–158, 305, 306
lithium, 501, 513
Liver
and anger, 117
and anxiety, 427
and Ethereal Soul, 427
and Gall-Bladder, 94
importance of, 89
Liver Channel *see under* acupuncture points, by channel
pathology in ADD, 549, 550
role in psyche, 94–95
Liver- and Heart-Blood deficiency, 538–539
Liver- and Heart-Fire, 536, 537, 558
Liver- and Heart-Yin deficiency, 539–540
Liver- and Kidney-Yin deficiency, 473–474, 477
Liver-Blood and Liver-Qi balance, 33
Liver-Blood and/or Liver-Qi deficiency
in ADD/ADHD, 549
in depression, 359
and Ethereal Soul, 35, 45, 46
Liver-Blood and/or Liver-Yin deficiency, 30, 45, 46
Liver-Blood Heat, 187–188
Liver-Blood stasis, 187, 206–207
Liver-Fire blazing
in anxiety, 428
in sleep disorders, 270, 456–457
excessive dreaming, 486–487
Liver-Qi deficiency
see also Liver-Blood and/or Liver-Qi deficiency
in depression, 351–352
Ethereal Soul pathologies, 43
Liver-Qi stagnation
in anger, 123
in depression, 265, 355, 358–361, 380
Chinese literature, 390
effects of mental-emotional problems, 184
in Mind Obstructed, 200–203
in Plum-Stone Syndrome, 11, 349
in sleep disorders, 465–466
turning into Heat, 362–364
in Wood type, 162
in worry, 355
Liver-Yang rising
and anger, 123

Liver-Yang rising—*cont'd*
with Kidney- and Liver-Yin deficiency, 556–557
in sleep disorders, 452
in Wood type, 162
Liver-Yin deficiency
with Empty Heat, 189–190, 219–221
Mind Unsettled, 214–216, 219–221
in sleep disorders, 30, 471–473
Locke, John, 2
loss, sadness and grief, 93
love, and emotions, 135–136
Lower Burner, Blood stasis in, 207–208
Lung- and Heart-Qi deficiency or stagnation, in anxiety, 434–435
Lung- and Heart-Yin deficiency, in anxiety, 435–436
Lung- and Kidney-Yin deficiency, Mind Weakened, 235–236
Lung-Qi stagnation, 146, 355, 379
Lung-Yin deficiency, with Empty Heat, 190
Lungs
and anxiety, 425
Lung Channel *see under* acupuncture points, by channel
and physiological activity, 52
as residence of Corporeal Soul, 246
role in psyche, 93–94
and sadness/grief, 89, 93, 94, 246, 425
Lunyu, Confucius's teachings in, 315
lustre condition in diagnosis, *Shen* as, 10

M

major depressive syndrome, 343–344, 398
Malebranche, 284
mania
degrees of, 507–508
diagnosis, 501
manic behavior, 252
mild, 38
signs and symptoms, 38, 498–499
manic-depression *see* bipolar disorder
MAOIs (monoamine oxidase inhibitors), 408–409, 414–415
maprotiline, 397
Mayo Clinic, on depression, 343
MBD (minimal brain function), 563
Mead, Richard, 502
meditation, 54
memory
and cortex, 158
explicit and implicit, 18–19, 63
and Heart, 64, 493
and Intellect, 63–64, 65
problems, 493–495
Zhi as, 67–68, 493
men, importance of treatment of Heart in, 91
mental activities, and movement of Ethereal Soul, 31–32
mental-emotional problems, patterns in
see also emotional stress
effects on blood, 185–188
Blood-Heat, 187–188
Blood stasis, 186–187
effects on Qi, 184–185
effects on yin, 188–190
Heart-Yin deficiency with Empty Heat, 189
Kidney-Yin deficiency with Empty Heat, 190
Liver-Yin deficiency with Empty Heat, 189–190
Lung-Yin deficiency with Empty Heat, 190
Spleen-Yin deficiency with Empty Heat, 190
emotional stress *see* emotional stress
Heart, treatment of, 90
Mind Obstructed *see* Mind Obstructed
Mind Unsettled *see* Mind Unsettled
Mind Weakened *see* Mind Weakened
pathogenic factors, 190–196
Empty Heat, 193–194
Heat or Fire, 191–192
Internal Wind, 195–196
Phlegm, 191
Yin Fire, 194–195
Pericardium, 152–155
mental illness, 10–12, 38, 504
see also specific conditions
Metal type, 164–165
methylphenidate, in ADD, 560–561
metripatheia, 287
Middle Ages and Christianity, 288
Middle Burner, Dampness in, 151
Mind
in ADD, 548, 550
calming *see* calming the Mind
in Chinese medicine, 8–9
clinical application of, 23–24
coordinating and integrating function of, 21–22
and cortex, 158
and depression, 345–346, 353
and Ethereal Soul, 36–44, 345–346
functions, 18–22
of Heart, 18, 21–22, 253
and human nature, 325
and Intellect, 65, 66
nature of in Chinese medicine, 15–22
and Three Treasures, 7, 17–18
Obstructed pattern *see* Mind Obstructed
Phlegm misting, 208–212
and senses, 20–21
shock displacing, in night terrors, 540–541
versus Spirit as a translation of *Shen*, 4, 22–23
terminology, 15–16
Unsettled pattern *see* Mind Unsettled
wandering at night, in dreams, 454
Weakened pattern *see* Mind Weakened
worry injuring, in depression, 370–372
Mind Obstructed
acupuncture points for, 246
anxiety, 422
Blood stasis, 205–208
effects of, 196
herbal treatment for, 198–199
Qi stagnation, 200–205
Heart- and Lung-Qi, 203–205
Liver-Qi, 200–203
Mind Unsettled, 212–227
anxiety, 422
Blood deficiency, 212–213
Blood stasis, 221
effects of, 196–197
Fire
Heart-Fire, 221–224
Liver-Fire, 224–226
herbal treatment for, 198–199
Phlegm-Fire, 226–227
Qi stagnation, 221
Yin deficiency, 213–217
with Empty Heat, 217–221
Mind Weakened
Blood deficiency, 234
effects of, 197–198
herbal treatment for, 198–199
Kidney- and Liver-Yin deficiency, 236–239
Kidney-Essence deficiency, 239–240
Lung- and Kidney-Yin deficiency, 235–236
Qi and Blood deficiency, 230–232
Qi deficiency, 228–230
Yang deficiency, 232–234
Yin deficiency, 234–240
Ming Di, 273
Ming dynasty, 78, 98
Ming Men (Gate of Life), 98, 99, 273
minimal brain function (MBD), 563
Minister Fire
and Kidneys, 97–98
pathology of in emotional problems, 148–155
and Pericardium, 152–155, *265*
as Yang aspect of Essence, 99
and Yin Fire, 150–152
mirtazapine (tetracyclic antidepressant), 413
modern diseases, and Ethereal Soul, 40

monoamine oxidase inhibitors (MAOIs), 408–409, 414–415
mood stabilizers, in bipolar disorder, 501, 502
moon, and Corporeal Soul, 47
More, Henry, 2
mother-baby bonding, and Corporeal Soul, 302–303
moving Qi, 511, 605
Multimodal Treatment Study of Children with Attention Deficit Hyperactivity Disorder (MTA), 546
Myth of the Passions, 295

N

National Institute of Mental Health, 423, 546
natural phenomena (unfathomable), *Shen* as, 9
NDRIs (noradrenaline and dopamine reuptake inhibitors), 411–412
Needham, J, 22, 321
needling sensation, *Shen* as, 10
Neo-Confucianism, 323–327
  see also Confucianism
  emotions in, 332–336
  human nature in, 78, 325–326
  influence on Chinese medicine, 336–338
  Li (principle) in, 326–327
  and Mind in Chinese Medicine, 8
Neo-Platonic school, 2
neocortex, 156, 306
neurasthenia, and depression, 353
neurons, communication of, 408
Neurontin (gabapentin), 501
neurophysiology of emotions, 303–306
neurotransmitters, 408, 409, 546
Nietzsche, Friedrich, 292
night terrors, 535–541
  etiology, 536
  identification of patterns and treatment, 537–541
    Liver- and Heart-Blood deficiency, 538–539
    Liver- and Heart-Fire, 537
    Liver- and Heart-Yin deficiency, 539–540
    Phlegm-Heat harassing the Ethereal Soul and Mind, 537–538
    shock displacing the Mind, 540–541
  pathology of, 536
noradrenaline and dopamine reuptake inhibitors (NDRIs), 411–412
nourishing Blood
  defined, 605
  herbs indicated for, 373
  points indicated for, 251, 380, 382
    see also specific points
nourishing the brain, 493, 552
nourishing the Heart
  in bipolar disorder/*Dian Kuang*, 511
  defined, 606
  points indicated for, 257, 383
    see also specific points

O

obsessive thinking, 259, 270, 278, 554
Oedipus complex, 300
opening the chest, defined, 606
opening the orifices
  in bipolar disorder/*Dian Kuang*, 514–515
  defined, 606
  points indicated for
    see also specific points under acupuncture points, by channel
    Gall-Bladder Channel, 270, 553
    Governing Vessel, 552
    Kidney Channel, 261
    Large Intestine Channel, 247
    Lung Channel, 379
    Pericardium Channel, 264
    Small Intestine Channel, 255
    Stomach Channel, 249
Origin of Medicine, on complexion, 171
Original Sin, and guilt, 139
overwork
  and anxiety, 423
  and depression, 356
  etiology of mental emotional problems, 167
  and insomnia, 450
  and memory problems, 493
  and night terrors, 536

P

paleomammalian brain, 307–308
palpitations
  and anxiety (*Xin Ji Zheng Chong*), 12, 350–351, 420
  in Chinese diagnosis, 422
panic attacks/panic disorder, 249, 418, 423
"Panic Throbbing", in anxiety, 350, 351, 419
passions, 290
Passions of the Soul (Descartes), 2
patient statistics, 407, 484
Paul, St, 2
pensiveness
  choice of acupuncture points, 273
  and emotions, 129–131
  and insomnia, 450
  and memory problems, 493
  and Spleen, 427
Pericardium
  in mental emotional problems, 152–155, 354
  pathology of, 101
  Pericardium Channel *see under* acupuncture points, by channel
  role in psyche, 100–102
Phlegm
  in bipolar disorder/*Dian Kuang*, 506, 509, 518–519, 530–531
  choice of acupuncture points, 264, 269
  in depression, 356
  and diet, 423
  eliminating, 270, 553–554
  with Heart and Spleen deficiency, 518–519
  and mental-emotional problems, pathogenic factors, 191
  obstructing the Heart, 264
  obstructing the Mind's orifices, 347
  or Dampness, 147, 167
  pathology in ADD, 549
  with Qi deficiency or stagnation, 367–369
    and Blood stasis, 526–527
    in *Dian*, 516–517, 519–520
Phlegm-Fire
  effects of mental-emotional problems, 192–193
  harassing upwards, in *Kuang*, 521–524
  Mind Unsettled, 226–227
  restraining of movement of Ethereal Soul, 45, 46
Phlegm-Heat harassing the Heart, in anxiety, 437–438
Phlegm-Heat harassing the Mind
  in depression, 364–365
  and Ethereal Soul, 537–538
  in mental emotional problems, 208–212
  in night terrors, 536
  in sleep disorders, 452, 459–460, 476
    excessive dreaming, 486
Phlegm misting the brain
  acupuncture points indicated for, 264
  in Mind Obstructed, 208–212
  in somnolence, 490–491
physiological activities, 9, 52–53
planning, 35, 36, 94
Plato, 3, 286, 328
Plum-Stone Syndrome (*Mei He Qi*), 11, 349–350
polarism, in Chinese medicine, 5
Posidonius, 287
positron emission tomography (PET), 305

post-traumatic stress disorder (PTSD), 440
Postnatal Essence, 17, 65
Postnatal Qi, and Intellect, 7, 63
Pratensis, Jason, 502
prefrontal cortex, brain, 303–304
pregnancy
  and ADD/ADHD, 551
  Corporeal Soul during, 50
  depression in, 396
  insomnia in, 480
  shock to mother during, 162
Prenatal Essences, 17, 90
prescriptions, herbal *see* herbal prescriptions/main herbs
Principles of Medical Practice, 119, 145, 171
psyche
  conscious, in Jung, 302
  and Internal Organs *see under* Internal Organs
  masculine and feminine aspects of, 92
  soul as, 3
psychiatric problems, in Ecstasy use, 169
psychic spirit, 2
psychoeducation, 502
psychological types, Jungian psychology, 301–302
psychosocial treatments, bipolar disorder, 502
pulse
  in anger, 125
  Choppy, 174, 176
  in craving, 137
  diagnosis of mental-emotional problems, 174–177
  in Empty Heat, 150
  in fear, 134
  in Full Heat, 150
  general qualities and emotions, 176–177
  in guilt, 139
  Heart, 175–176
  in joy, 126
  in obsessive love, 136
  in pensiveness, 130
  Sad, 176
  in sadness, 132
  in shame, 143
  Short, 174, 176
  Weak, 355
  Wiry, 176, 177, 355
The Pulse Classic (Mai Jing), 601
  and *Ming Men*, 98
Pythagoras, 285

Q

Qi
  deficiency of *see* Qi and Blood deficiency; Qi deficiency
  disharmonies of, in Chinese medicine, 333
  effect of emotions or mental-emotional problems on, 143–147, 184–185
    derangement of, 143–144
  and spirit, 5
  stagnation of *see* Qi stagnation
Qi and Blood deficiency
  in depression, 390
  Mind Weakened, 230–232
  points indicated for, 379
Qi deficiency
  see also Qi stagnation
  and anxiety, 420, 425
  and diet, 167
  of Gall-Bladder, 253
  of Heart and Gall-Bladder, 487
  Heart- and Lung-Qi, 487–488
  Liver-Blood and Liver-Qi, 45, 46
  Liver-Qi, 351–352
  Mind Weakened, 228–230
  with Phlegm, 519–520
Qi diaphragm, 360
Qi Jing Ba Mai Kao (Study of the Eight Extraordinary Vessels), 601–602
Qi-Phlegm, in Plum-Stone Syndrome, 11
Qi stagnation
  see also Qi deficiency
  and anger, 124
  and anxiety, 423, 428
  in bipolar disorder/*Dian Kuang*, 510
  and Blood stasis, 356, 506
    and Phlegm, 526–527
  emotions, effect on Qi, 145–147
  in guilt, 450
  Heart- and Lung-Qi
    in depression, 356, 361–362
    effects of mental-emotional problems, 184–185
    Mind Obstructed, 203–205
  Heart-Qi, 146, 460–461
  and Heat, 356
  Liver-Qi
    in depression, 358–364
    effects of mental-emotional problems, 184
    Mind Obstructed, 200–203
    in Plum-Stone Syndrome, 11
    in sleep disorders, 465–466
  Lung- and Heart-Qi, 435
  Lung-Qi, 146
  Mind Obstructed, 200–205
  Mind Unsettled, 221
  with Phlegm
    in bipolar disorder/*Dian Kuang*, 509
    and Blood stasis, 526–527
    in depression, 367–369
    in *Dian*, 516–517
    and stimulation of Ethereal Soul, 44–45
Qin dynasty, 314
qing, as translation of "emotion", 115
Qing dynasty, 424
quantitative electroencephalographic measurements, brain wave activity, 544, 559
que, meaning, 273, 274

R

rapid eye movement (REM), 39
Reason, control of emotions by, *289*
Rebellious Qi of Penetrating Vessel (*Chong Mai*)
  in anxiety, 249, 419–422
  points indicated for, 251
Record of Rites, on Ethereal Soul, 27
"recreational" drugs, 167–169
  cannabis, 168
  cocaine, 168–169
  ecstasy, 169
  and memory problems, 493
red tip, tongue, 177–178
Ren, Confucian ethics, 317–319
reptilian brain, 157, 306, **307**
resentment, 129
resolving Phlegm, in bipolar disorder/ *Dian Kuang*, 511, 512
rituals, 320

S

Sad pulse, 176
SAD (seasonal affective disorder), 343
sadness and grief
  and Corporeal Soul, 53
  and depression, 355
  and emotions, 131–133
  loss, 93, 355
  and Lungs, 89, 93, 94, 246, 425
  and memory problems, 493
  and Metal type, 165
  modern theories, 294
  points indicated for, 246
  Qi stagnation, 349
  sensation of, 306
Sartre, Jean-Paul, 295
Schachter, Stanley, 294
schizophrenia, 270, 505
School of Mind, 8, 15
Sea of Marrow, and Kidneys, 97
sea, unconscious symbolized by, 42
seasonal affective disorder (SAD), 343
Secret of the Golden Flower, 29–30, 34
selective serotonin reuptake inhibitors (SSRIs), 392–394, 408, 409, 410–411
self, concept of in Western and Chinese philosophy, 318, 327–332

Seligman, MEP, 343–344
Seneca, 287, 288
senile dyssomnia, 482–483
senses
  and Corporeal Soul, 51–52
  and Ethereal Soul, 34, 35
  and Mind, 20–21
serotonin and noradrenaline reuptake inhibitors (SNRIs), 412
serotonin syndrome, 410
settling the Corporeal Soul
  defined, 606
  points indicated for
    see also specific points under acupuncture points, by channel
    Gall-Bladder Channel, 383
    Large Intestine Channel, 247
    Lung Channel, 246
settling the Ethereal Soul
  defined, 606
  herbs indicated for, 461
  points indicated for
    see also specific points under acupuncture points, by channel
    Bladder Channel, 381
    Large Intestine Channel, 247
    Liver Channel, 271, **428**, 552
sexual activity, excessive
  effects of mental-emotional problems, 167
  and insomnia, 451
  and memory problems, 493
Shadow concept, Jungian, 300–301
  and *gui*, 83–84
shaman, 72
shame
  and Dampness, 167
  and Earth type, 164
  and emotions, 140–143
  modern theories, 294–295
  sensation of, 306
Shang dynasty, 71–72, 75
Shen
  and body, 331–332
  Chinese characters for, 16
  on complexion, 172
  as consciousness, 15
  Five Shen, 6, 23
  and *gui*, 79–83, *80*, 81, 82, 83
  as lustre condition in diagnosis, 10
  as Mind, 4, 8–9
  Mind versus Spirit as translation of, 22–23
  as needling sensation, 10
  as physiological activities, 9
  as skill of acupuncturist, 10
  as spirit, 4–6, 10
  as term for vital substances, 10
  as unfathomable natural phenomena, 9
shock
  displacing the Mind, in night terrors, 540–541
  and emotions, 134–135
Short pulse, 174, 176
Shu, Confucian ethics, 320
side-effects
  antidepressants, 410–411, 414–415
  stimulants, 546
sight, and Mind, 20–21
Simple Questions
  on anxiety, 423
  on bipolar disorder/*Dian Kuang*, 506
  on complexion, 171
  on depression, 11, 344
  on emotions, 118
    anger, 123
    and Confucianism, 333
    fear, 133
    joy, 126
    pensiveness, 129
    sadness and grief, 131
    shock, 135
  on Ethereal Soul, 27, 33
  on eyesight, 20–21
  on functions of Mind, 18
  on hearing, 21
  on Intellect, 65
  on Internal Organs, 88
    Bladder, 110
    Gall-Bladder, 104, 105
    Heart, 90
    Large Intestine, 104
    Liver, 89, 94
    Lungs, 93
    Pericardium, 100, 152
    Small Intestine, 102
    Spleen, 96
    Stomach, 107
    Triple Burner, 110, 112
  on Lungs, 52
  on patterns in mental-emotional problems, 185
  on *Shen*, 9
  on sleep disorders, 455
  on smell, sense of, 21
  on soul, 6
  on spirit, 4, 72
Singer, Jerome E., 294
Sketch for a Theory of the Emotions (Sartre), 295
skin, and Corporeal Soul, 60
sleep
  and Ethereal Soul, 29–31, 449
  and functions of Mind, 20
  problems *see* sleep disorders
sleep disorders, 448–495
  acupuncture treatment, indications for, 245, 256, 270, 380, 452–453
    auricular, 479–480
  anger, 450
  causes of insomnia, 245
  and childbirth, 451, 493
  diagnosis, 454–456
  difficulty falling asleep, 454
  emotional stress, 450
  excessive dreaming, 29, 484–489
  guilt, 450
  in HIV disease, 481
  identification of patterns and treatment
    Heart and Kidneys not harmonized, 468–470
    Heart- and Spleen-Blood deficiency, 466–468, 467
    Heart-Blood stasis, 461–462
    Heart-Fire blazing, 457–458
    Heart-Qi stagnation, 460–461
    Heart-Yin deficiency, 468
    Liver-Fire blazing, 456–457
    Liver-Qi stagnation, 465–466
    Phlegm-Heat harassing the Mind, 459–460
    residual Heat in diaphragm, 462–463
    retention of food, 464, 465
  insomnia, defined, 448
  irregular eating habits, 450–451
  memory, 493–495
  overwork, 450
  pathology, 451–454
  patient statistics, 484
  in pregnancy, 480
  randomized controlled trials, literature on, 478
  residual Heat, 451
    in diaphragm, 462–463
  sexual activity, excessive, 451
  sleeping positions, 455, 456
  snoring, 456
  somnolence, 489–492
  timid character/constitutional weakness, 450
  waking up early, 454
  worry and pensiveness, 450
sleeping positions, insomnia diagnosis, 455, 456
sleepwalking, and Ethereal Soul, 40
Small Intestine
  role in psyche, 102–104
  Small Intestine Channel *see under* acupuncture points, by channel
smell, sense of, 21
snoring, insomnia diagnosis, 455, 456
SNRIs (serotonin and noradrenaline reuptake inhibitors), 412
social rhythm therapy, 502
Socrates, 286
Solomon, RC, 140, 295–297
somatoform disorder, tinnitus with, 483

somnolence, 489–492
Dampness obstructing the brain, 489–490
Phlegm misting the brain, 490–491
Song dynasty, Neo-Confucian philosophers of, 8, 78, 322, 337
soothing the Liver, moving Qi, defined, 606
soul
see also Corporeal Soul (*Po*); Ethereal Soul (*Hun*)
in Chinese medicine, 6–8
in Western philosophy, 3
Spinoza, Baruch, 291
spirit
in Chinese medicine, 3, 4–6, 10
of dead person, 10, 71
see also gui
defined, 22
five Yin organs as physiological basis of, 7
versus Mind as a translation of *Shen*, 22–23
talking to ghosts, 245, 246
in Western philosophy, 1–3
Spiritual Axis
on bipolar disorder/*Dian Kuang*, 503
on emotions, 118, 119–120
anger, 122
fear, 134
sadness and grief, 132
worry, 128
on Essence, 17, 48
on Ethereal Soul, 27
on functions of Mind, 18
on nature of Mind, 15
on *Shen*, 9
on sleep disorders, 452, 490
on soul, 6
Spleen
and anxiety, 427
and ideas, generation of, 64
pathology in ADD, 549, 550
role in psyche, 96–97
Spleen Channel *see under* acupuncture points, by channel
Spleen- and Heart-Blood deficiency, 251, 552
Spleen- and Kidney-Yang deficiency, 45, 46
Spleen deficiency
in ADD/ADHD, 549
in depression, 359
and Phlegm, 509
in somnolence, 491–492
Spleen-Yin deficiency, with Empty Heat, 190
SSRIs (selective serotonin reuptake inhibitors), 392–394, 408, 409, 410–411
St Augustine, 288, 328
St Paul, 2
stagnation
in bipolar disorder/*Dian Kuang*, 530–531
and depression, 345
eliminated, defined, 605
Liver-Qi, turning into Heat, 362–364
Qi *see* Qi stagnation
Yu as, 344–345
stimulants, in ADD, 546, 560
Stoics, 2, 3, 287–288
Stomach
role in psyche, 107–110
Stomach Channel *see under* acupuncture points, by channel
Stomach crack on tongue, combined with Heart crack, *178*, 180–181
Stomach-Qi deficiency, and diet, 167
Stomach-Yin deficiency, and diet, 167
streams of thinking, 292
strengthening Will-Power *see under* Will-Power
A Study of the Pulse by the Pin Hu Lake Master (Pin Hu Mai Xue), 602
studying/concentrating, 64–65, 66
suicide, desire to commit, 256, 258
Sun Si Miao's 13 Ghost points, 84, *85*, 259
in *Dian Kuang*, 515
super-ego, Freudian theory, 300
supernatural influences on diseases, 338

T

taste, sense of, 21
TCAs (tricyclic antidepressants), 408, 409, 412–413
Tegretol (carbamazepine), 501
tetracyclic antidepressants, 408, 413–414
thalamus, 292
thinking/thought, 18
obsessive, 259, 270, 278, 554
rationality, 302
streams of thinking, 292
Thousand Golden Ducats Prescriptions (Qian Jin Yao Fang), 253, 601
Three Treasures, and Mind, nature of, *7*, 17–18
Tian (Heaven), 316–317
tinnitus, 21
with somatoform disorder, 483
tongue diagnosis
body shape, 179–180, 181
combined Stomach and Heart crack, *178*, 180–181
in Empty Heat, 150
in Full Heat, 149
Heart crack, 162, 178–179, 355
in heat conditions, 152
red tip, 177–178
sides of tongue, 179, 181
Topamax (topiramate), 501
topiramate, 501
touch, sense of, 21
Treatise of Human Nature (Hume), 291
tricyclic antidepressants (TCAs), 408, 409, 412–413
Triple Burner
in depression, 354
role in psyche, 110–113
Triple Burner Channel *see under* acupuncture points, by channel
triune brain, 306–309
and Chinese medicine, 155–158
cortex and Mind, Intellect and Memory, 158
limbic system, 156
Mind and Ethereal Soul, 157–158
reptilian brain, 157, **307**

U

unconscious
see also consciousness
collective, 300
Freudian theory, 299–300
in Jungian psychology, 41, 42
Upper Burner, blocking, 134

V

valproate, 501
venlafaxine (SNRI), 412, 547
ventral striatum, brain, 304
verticality, and Corporeal Soul, 59, *60*
vision, 20–21, 34, *35*
vital spirit, 2
vital substances, *Shen* as, 10

W

Wang Chong (Confucian philosopher), 79, *80*
Wang Ming Sheng (No-Confucianist), 324
Warring-States period
and belief in soul, 26–27
Confucianism, 313
and spirits/ghosts, 72
Water type, 165–166
Watson, John B., 292, 302
weeping, 246
Western medicine
on anxiety, 417–418
on bipolar disorder, 498–502

on depression, 342–344
combined with Chinese, 415
drug treatment, 407–415
Western philosophy
dualism of, 5, 331
emotions in
ancient theories, 285–291
early modern theories, 291–292
modern theories, 294–299
Idealism school, 2–3
mind-body integration, 7, 331
self, concept of, 327–332
soul in, 3
spirit in, 1–3
Will-Power
and depression, 353
and Kidney-Yang deficiency, 376
strengthening of, 257, 259
acupuncture points indicated for, 259
defined, 606
Zhi as, 68–69, 346
Willis, Thomas, 290–291, 502
Wind-Heat
in depression, 369
in sleep disorders, 463
Wiry pulse, 176, 177
wisdom, 20
Wood type, 162, *163*, 427
worry
and depression, 355
and emotions, 127–129
injuring the Mind, in depression, 370–372
and insomnia, 450
and memory problems, 493
and Metal type, 165
worry diaphragm, 360

X

Xi Kang (Daoist philosopher), 4
Xu Chun Fu, 73
xue (acupuncture point), 72

Y

Yang deficiency, 232–234
Yang Quan (Daoist philosopher), 4
Yellow Emperor's Classic of Internal Medicine (Huang Di Nei Jing), 599–600
on bipolar disorder/*Dian Kuang*, 509
Confucianism in, 322
on emotions, 118
on epilepsy, 12
and Neo-Confucianism, 332
on *Shen*, 16
Yi, Confucian ethics, 319, 320
Yi Zong Jin Jian (Golden Mirror of Medicine), 602
Yin deficiency
with Empty Heat, 217–221, 261, 357, 527–528
and Ethereal Soul, 259
Heart- and Kidney-Yin
in ADD, 556
in Mind Unsettled, 217–218
Heart-Yin, 213–214
effects of mental-emotional problems, 189
in mental-emotional problems, 213–214
in sleep disorders, 468
and Heat, 356–357
Kidney- and Heart-Yin, with Empty Heat blazing
in anxiety, 432–433
in depression, 375–376
Kidney- and Liver-Yin
with Liver-Yang rising, in ADD, 556–557
in mental-emotional problems, 236–239
Kidney-Yin, 216–217, 234–235, 262
effects of mental-emotional problems, 190
in mental-emotional problems, 216–217
in Mind Weakened, 234–235
Liver- and Heart-Yin
in night terrors, 539–540
Liver- and Kidney-Yin
in sleep disorders, 473–474
Liver-Yin, 214–216
effects of mental-emotional problems, 189–190
in mental-emotional problems, 214–216
in sleep disorders, 471–473
Lung- and Kidney-Yin, 235–236
Lung-Yin, effects of mental-emotional problems, 190
Mind Unsettled, 213–217
Mind Weakened, 234–240
in night terrors, 536
with Phlegm, 356–357
in sleep disorders, 454
Spleen-Yin
mental-emotional problems, 190
Yin, effects of mental-emotional problems on
Heart-Yin deficiency with Empty Heat, 189
Kidney-Yin deficiency with Empty Heat, 190
Liver-Yin deficiency with Empty Heat, 189–190
Lung-Yin deficiency with Empty Heat, 190
Spleen-Yin deficiency with Empty Heat, 190
Yin Fire, 150–152, 194–195
Yin-Yang, 325
disharmony of in *Dian Kuang*, 506
Yu
as mental depression, 345, 356
as stagnation, 344–345, 356
syndrome of, in depression, 346–347

Z

Zhang Jie Bin
on demonic medicine, 74
on emotions, 118, 119
on *gui*, 73, 75
on Internal Organs, 98
on senses, 51
Zhang Jing Yue, 424, 535
Zhang Zai (Neo-Confucian philosopher), 5, 8, 325
Zhi
clinical application, 69
of Kidneys, in depression, 346
as memory, 67–68, 493
multiple meanings of, 67
as Will-Power, 68–69
Zhong Feng (Wind-Stroke), 73
Zhou Dun Yi (cosmological philosopher), 323
Zhou dynasty, and spirits/ghosts, 72, 75
Zhu Dan Xi, on anxiety, 424
Zhu Xi (Neo-Confucian philosopher), 8, 9, 48, 57, 58, 59, 326